Medical Devices and Human Engineering

THE BIOMEDICAL ENGINEERING HANDBOOK

FOURTH EDITION

Medical Devices and Human Engineering

GEORGE GREEN LIBRARY OF
SCIENCE AND ENGINEERING

Edited by

Joseph D. Bronzino

Founder and President
Biomedical Engineering Alliance and Consortium (BEACON)
Hartford, Connecticut, U.S.A.

Donald R. Peterson

Professor of Engineering
Dean of the College of Science, Technology, Engineering, Mathematics, and Nursing
Texas A&M University – Texarkana
Texarkana, Texas, U.S.A.

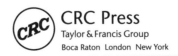

CRC Press
Taylor & Francis Group
Boca Raton London New York

CRC Press is an imprint of the
Taylor & Francis Group, an **informa** business

100345553

CRC Press
Taylor & Francis Group
6000 Broken Sound Parkway NW, Suite 300
Boca Raton, FL 33487-2742

© 2015 by Taylor & Francis Group, LLC
CRC Press is an imprint of Taylor & Francis Group, an Informa business

No claim to original U.S. Government works

Printed on acid-free paper
Version Date: 20141017

International Standard Book Number-13: 978-1-4398-2525-9 (Hardback)

Library of Congress Cataloging-in-Publication Data

Medical devices and human engineering / edited by Joseph D. Bronzino and Donald R. Peterson.
    p. ; cm.
    Preceded by The biomedical engineering handbook / edited by Joseph D. Bronzino. 3rd. 2006.
    Includes bibliographical references and index.
    ISBN 978-1-4398-2525-9 (hardcover : alk. paper)
    I. Bronzino, Joseph D., 1937- , editor. II. Peterson, Donald R., editor.
    [DNLM: 1. Biomedical Engineering--instrumentation. 2. Biosensing Techniques--instrumentation.
3. Electrical Equipment and Supplies. 4. Human Engineering. QT 36]

    R856
    610.28--dc23
                                       2014035624

Visit the Taylor & Francis Web site at
http://www.taylorandfrancis.com

and the CRC Press Web site at
http://www.crcpress.com

Contents

SECTION I   Biomedical Sensors

Michael R. Neuman

SECTION II   Medical Instruments and Devices

Steven Schreiner

SECTION III Human Performance Engineering

Donald R. Peterson

SECTION IV Rehabilitation Engineering

Charles Robinson

SECTION V   Clinical Engineering

Yadin David

Preface

During the past eight years since the publication of the third edition—a three-volume set—of *The Biomedical Engineering Handbook*, the field of biomedical engineering has continued to evolve and expand. As a result, the fourth edition has been significantly modified to reflect state-of-the-field knowledge and applications in this important discipline and has been enlarged to a four-volume set:

- Volume I: *Biomedical Engineering Fundamentals*
- Volume II: *Medical Devices and Human Engineering*
- Volume III: *Biomedical Signals, Imaging, and Informatics*
- Volume IV: *Molecular, Cellular, and Tissue Engineering*

More specifically, this fourth edition has been considerably updated and contains completely new sections, including

- Stem Cell Engineering
- Drug Design, Delivery Systems, and Devices
- Personalized Medicine

as well as a number of substantially updated sections, including

- Tissue Engineering (which has been completely restructured)
- Transport Phenomena and Biomimetic Systems
- Artificial Organs
- Medical Imaging
- Infrared Imaging
- Medical Informatics

In addition, Volume IV contains a chapter on ethics because of its ever-increasing role in the biomedical engineering arts.

Nearly all the sections that have appeared in the first three editions have been significantly revised. Therefore, this fourth edition presents an excellent summary of the status of knowledge and activities of biomedical engineers in the first decades of the twenty-first century. As such, it can serve as an excellent reference for individuals interested not only in a review of fundamental physiology but also in quickly being brought up to speed in certain areas of biomedical engineering research. It can serve as an excellent textbook for students in areas where traditional textbooks have not yet been developed and as an excellent review of the major areas of activity in each biomedical engineering sub-discipline, such as biomechanics, biomaterials, bioinstrumentation, medical imaging, and so on. Finally, it can serve as the "bible" for practicing biomedical engineering professionals by covering such topics as historical perspective of medical technology, the role of professional societies, the ethical issues associated with medical technology, and the FDA process.

Biomedical engineering is now an important and vital interdisciplinary field. Biomedical engineers are involved in virtually all aspects of developing new medical technology. They are involved in the design, development, and utilization of materials, devices (such as pacemakers, lithotripsy, etc.), and techniques (such as signal processing, artificial intelligence, etc.) for clinical research and use, and they serve as members of the healthcare delivery team (clinical engineering, medical informatics, rehabilitation engineering, etc.) seeking new solutions for the difficult healthcare problems confronting our society. To meet the needs of this diverse body of biomedical engineers, this handbook provides a central core of knowledge in those fields encompassed by the discipline. However, before presenting this detailed information, it is important to provide a sense of the evolution of the modern healthcare system and identify the diverse activities biomedical engineers perform to assist in the diagnosis and treatment of patients.

Evolution of the Modern Healthcare System

Before 1900, medicine had little to offer average citizens, since its resources consisted mainly of physicians, their education, and their "little black bag." In general, physicians seemed to be in short supply, but the shortage had rather different causes than the current crisis in the availability of healthcare professionals. Although the costs of obtaining medical training were relatively low, the demand for doctors' services also was very small, since many of the services provided by physicians also could be obtained from experienced amateurs in the community. The home was typically the site for treatment and recuperation, and relatives and neighbors constituted an able and willing nursing staff. Babies were delivered by midwives, and those illnesses not cured by home remedies were left to run their natural, albeit frequently fatal, course. The contrast with contemporary healthcare practices in which specialized physicians and nurses located within hospitals provide critical diagnostic and treatment services is dramatic.

The changes that have occurred within medical science originated in the rapid developments that took place in the applied sciences (i.e., chemistry, physics, engineering, microbiology, physiology, pharmacology, etc.) at the turn of the twentieth century. This process of development was characterized by intense interdisciplinary cross-fertilization, which provided an environment in which medical research was able to take giant strides in developing techniques for the diagnosis and treatment of diseases. For example, in 1903, Willem Einthoven, a Dutch physiologist, devised the first electrocardiograph to measure the electrical activity of the heart. In applying discoveries in the physical sciences to the analysis of the biological process, he initiated a new age in both cardiovascular medicine and electrical measurement techniques.

New discoveries in medical sciences followed one another like intermediates in a chain reaction. However, the most significant innovation for clinical medicine was the development of x-rays. These "new kinds of rays," as W. K. Roentgen described them in 1895, opened the "inner man" to medical inspection. Initially, x-rays were used to diagnose bone fractures and dislocations, and in the process, x-ray machines became commonplace in most urban hospitals. Separate departments of radiology were established, and their influence spread to other departments throughout the hospital. By the 1930s, x-ray visualization of practically all organ systems of the body had been made possible through the use of barium salts and a wide variety of radiopaque materials.

X-ray technology gave physicians a powerful tool that, for the first time, permitted accurate diagnosis of a wide variety of diseases and injuries. Moreover, since x-ray machines were too cumbersome and expensive for local doctors and clinics, they had to be placed in healthcare centers or hospitals. Once there, x-ray technology essentially triggered the transformation of the hospital from a passive receptacle for the sick to an active curative institution for all members of society.

For economic reasons, the centralization of healthcare services became essential because of many other important technological innovations appearing on the medical scene. However, hospitals remained institutions to dread, and it was not until the introduction of sulfanilamide in the mid-1930s and penicillin in the early 1940s that the main danger of hospitalization, that is, cross-infection among patients, was significantly reduced. With these new drugs in their arsenals, surgeons were able to perform their operations without prohibitive morbidity and mortality due to infection. Furthermore, even though the different blood groups and their incompatibility were discovered in 1900 and sodium citrate was used in 1913 to prevent clotting, full development of blood banks was not practical until the 1930s, when technology provided adequate refrigeration. Until that time, "fresh" donors were bled and the blood transfused while it was still warm.

Once these surgical suites were established, the employment of specifically designed pieces of medical technology assisted in further advancing the development of complex surgical procedures. For example, the Drinker respirator was introduced in 1927 and the first heart–lung bypass in 1939. By the 1940s, medical procedures heavily dependent on medical technology, such as cardiac catheterization and angiography (the use of a cannula threaded through an arm vein and into the heart with the injection of radiopaque dye) for the x-ray visualization of congenital and acquired heart disease (mainly valve disorders due to rheumatic fever) became possible, and a new era of cardiac and vascular surgery was established.

In the decades following World War II, technological advances were spurred on by efforts to develop superior weapon systems and to establish habitats in space and on the ocean floor. As a by-product of these efforts, the development of medical devices accelerated and the medical profession benefited greatly from this rapid surge of technological finds. Consider the following examples:

1. Advances in solid-state electronics made it possible to map the subtle behavior of the fundamental unit of the central nervous system—the neuron—as well as to monitor the various physiological parameters, such as the electrocardiogram, of patients in intensive care units.
2. New prosthetic devices became a goal of engineers involved in providing the disabled with tools to improve their quality of life.
3. Nuclear medicine—an outgrowth of the atomic age—emerged as a powerful and effective approach in detecting and treating specific physiological abnormalities.
4. Diagnostic ultrasound based on sonar technology became so widely accepted that ultrasonic studies are now part of the routine diagnostic workup in many medical specialties.
5. "Spare parts" surgery also became commonplace. Technologists were encouraged to provide cardiac assist devices, such as artificial heart valves and artificial blood vessels, and the artificial heart program was launched to develop a replacement for a defective or diseased human heart.
6. Advances in materials have made the development of disposable medical devices, such as needles and thermometers, a reality.
7. Advancements in molecular engineering have allowed for the discovery of countless pharmacological agents and to the design of their delivery, including implantable delivery systems.
8. Computers similar to those developed to control the flight plans of the Apollo capsule were used to store, process, and cross-check medical records, to monitor patient status in intensive care units, and to provide sophisticated statistical diagnoses of potential diseases correlated with specific sets of patient symptoms.
9. Development of the first computer-based medical instrument, the computerized axial tomography scanner, revolutionized clinical approaches to noninvasive diagnostic imaging procedures, which now include magnetic resonance imaging and positron emission tomography as well.
10. A wide variety of new cardiovascular technologies including implantable defibrillators and chemically treated stents were developed.
11. Neuronal pacing systems were used to detect and prevent epileptic seizures.
12. Artificial organs and tissue have been created.
13. The completion of the genome project has stimulated the search for new biological markers and personalized medicine.
14. The further understanding of cellular and biomolecular processes has led to the engineering of stem cells into therapeutically valuable lineages and to the regeneration of organs and tissue structures.

15. Developments in nanotechnology have yielded nanomaterials for use in tissue engineering and facilitated the creation and study of nanoparticles and molecular machine systems that will assist in the detection and treatment of disease and injury.

The impact of these discoveries and many others has been profound. The healthcare system of today consists of technologically sophisticated clinical staff operating primarily in modern hospitals designed to accommodate the new medical technology. This evolutionary process continues, with advances in the physical sciences such as materials and nanotechnology and in the life sciences such as molecular biology, genomics, stem cell biology, and artificial and regenerated tissue and organs. These advances have altered and will continue to alter the very nature of the healthcare delivery system itself.

Biomedical Engineering: A Definition

Bioengineering is usually defined as a basic research-oriented activity closely related to biotechnology and genetic engineering, that is, the modification of animal or plant cells or parts of cells to improve plants or animals or to develop new microorganisms for beneficial ends. In the food industry, for example, this has meant the improvement of strains of yeast for fermentation. In agriculture, bioengineers may be concerned with the improvement of crop yields by treatment of plants with organisms to reduce frost damage. It is clear that future bioengineers will have a tremendous impact on the quality of human life. The potential of this specialty is difficult to imagine. Consider the following activities of bioengineers:

- Development of improved species of plants and animals for food production
- Invention of new medical diagnostic tests for diseases
- Production of synthetic vaccines from clone cells
- Bioenvironmental engineering to protect human, animal, and plant life from toxicants and pollutants
- Study of protein–surface interactions
- Modeling of the growth kinetics of yeast and hybridoma cells
- Research in immobilized enzyme technology
- Development of therapeutic proteins and monoclonal antibodies

Biomedical engineers, on the other hand, apply electrical, mechanical, chemical, optical, and other engineering principles to understand, modify, or control biological (i.e., human and animal) systems as well as design and manufacture products that can monitor physiological functions and assist in the diagnosis and treatment of patients. When biomedical engineers work in a hospital or clinic, they are more aptly called clinical engineers.

Activities of Biomedical Engineers

The breadth of activity of biomedical engineers is now significant. The field has moved from being concerned primarily with the development of medical instruments in the 1950s and 1960s to include a more wide-ranging set of activities. As illustrated below, the field of biomedical engineering now includes many new career areas (see Figure P.1), each of which is presented in this handbook. These areas include

- Application of engineering system analysis (physiological modeling, simulation, and control) to biological problems
- Detection, measurement, and monitoring of physiological signals (i.e., biosensors and biomedical instrumentation)
- Diagnostic interpretation via signal-processing techniques of bioelectric data
- Therapeutic and rehabilitation procedures and devices (rehabilitation engineering)
- Devices for replacement or augmentation of bodily functions (artificial organs)

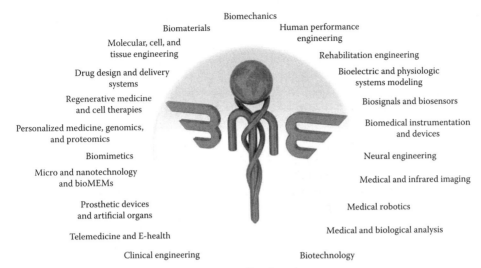

FIGURE P.1 The world of biomedical engineering.

- Computer analysis of patient-related data and clinical decision making (i.e., medical informatics and artificial intelligence)
- Medical imaging, that is, the graphic display of anatomic detail or physiological function
- The creation of new biological products (e.g., biotechnology and tissue engineering)
- The development of new materials to be used within the body (biomaterials)

Typical pursuits of biomedical engineers, therefore, include

- Research in new materials for implanted artificial organs
- Development of new diagnostic instruments for blood analysis
- Computer modeling of the function of the human heart
- Writing software for analysis of medical research data
- Analysis of medical device hazards for safety and efficacy
- Development of new diagnostic imaging systems
- Design of telemetry systems for patient monitoring
- Design of biomedical sensors for measurement of human physiological systems variables
- Development of expert systems for diagnosis of disease
- Design of closed-loop control systems for drug administration
- Modeling of the physiological systems of the human body
- Design of instrumentation for sports medicine
- Development of new dental materials
- Design of communication aids for the handicapped
- Study of pulmonary fluid dynamics
- Study of the biomechanics of the human body
- Development of material to be used as a replacement for human skin

Biomedical engineering, then, is an interdisciplinary branch of engineering that ranges from theoretical, nonexperimental undertakings to state-of-the-art applications. It can encompass research, development, implementation, and operation. Accordingly, like medical practice itself, it is unlikely that any single person can acquire expertise that encompasses the entire field. Yet, because of the interdisciplinary nature of this activity, there is considerable interplay and overlapping of interest and effort between them. For example, biomedical engineers engaged in the development of biosensors may interact with those interested in prosthetic devices to develop a means to detect and use the same bio-electric signal to power a prosthetic device. Those engaged in automating clinical chemistry laboratories may collaborate with those developing expert systems to assist clinicians in making decisions based on specific laboratory data. The possibilities are endless.

Perhaps, a greater potential benefit occurring from the use of biomedical engineering is identification of the problems and needs of our present healthcare system that can be solved using existing engineering technology and systems methodology. Consequently, the field of biomedical engineering offers hope in the continuing battle to provide high-quality care at a reasonable cost. If properly directed toward solving problems related to preventive medical approaches, ambulatory care services, and the like, biomedical engineers can provide the tools and techniques to make our healthcare system more effective and efficient and, in the process, improve the quality of life for all.

Joseph D. Bronzino
Donald R. Peterson
Editors-in-Chief

Editors

Joseph D. Bronzino is currently the president of the Biomedical Engineering Alliance and Consortium (BEACON; www.beaconalliance.org), which is a nonprofit organization dedicated to the promotion of collaborative research, translation, and partnership among academic, medical, and industry people in the field of biomedical engineering to develop new medical technologies and devices. To accomplish this goal, Dr. Bronzino and BEACON facilitate collaborative research, industrial partnering, and the development of emerging companies. Dr. Bronzino earned a BSEE from Worcester Polytechnic Institute, Worcester, Massachusetts, in 1959, an MSEE from the Naval Postgraduate School, Monterey, California, in 1961, and a PhD in electrical engineering from Worcester Polytechnic Institute in 1968. He was recently the Vernon Roosa Professor of Applied Science and endowed chair at Trinity College, Hartford, Connecticut.

Dr. Bronzino is the author of over 200 journal articles and 15 books, including *Technology for Patient Care* (C.V. Mosby, 1977), *Computer Applications for Patient Care* (Addison-Wesley, 1982), *Biomedical Engineering: Basic Concepts and Instrumentation* (PWS Publishing Co., 1986), *Expert Systems: Basic Concepts* (Research Foundation of State University of New York, 1989), *Medical Technology and Society: An Interdisciplinary Perspective* (MIT Press and McGraw-Hill, 1990), *Management of Medical Technology* (Butterworth/Heinemann, 1992), *The Biomedical Engineering Handbook* (CRC Press, 1st Edition, 1995; 2nd Edition, 2000; 3rd Edition, 2006), *Introduction to Biomedical Engineering* (Academic Press, 1st Edition, 1999; 2nd Edition, 2005; 3rd Edition, 2011), *Biomechanics: Principles and Applications* (CRC Press, 2002), *Biomaterials: Principles and Applications* (CRC Press, 2002), *Tissue Engineering* (CRC Press, 2002), and *Biomedical Imaging* (CRC Press, 2002).

Dr. Bronzino is a fellow of IEEE and the American Institute of Medical and Biological Engineering (AIMBE), an honorary member of the Italian Society of Experimental Biology, past chairman of the Biomedical Engineering Division of the American Society for Engineering Education (ASEE), a charter member of the Connecticut Academy of Science and Engineering (CASE), a charter member of the American College of Clinical Engineering (ACCE), a member of the Association for the Advancement of Medical Instrumentation (AAMI), past president of the IEEE-Engineering in Medicine and Biology Society (EMBS), past chairman of the IEEE Health Care Engineering Policy Committee (HCEPC), and past chairman of the IEEE Technical Policy Council in Washington, DC. He is a member of Eta Kappa Nu, Sigma Xi, and Tau Beta Pi. He is also a recipient of the IEEE Millennium Medal for "his contributions to biomedical engineering research and education" and the Goddard Award from WPI for Outstanding Professional Achievement in 2005. He is presently editor-in-chief of the Academic Press/Elsevier BME Book Series.

Donald R. Peterson is a professor of engineering and the dean of the College of Science, Technology, Engineering, Mathematics, and Nursing at Texas A&M University in Texarkana, Texas, and holds a joint appointment in the Department of Biomedical Engineering (BME) at Texas A&M University in College Station, Texas. He was recently an associate professor of medicine and the director of the

Biodynamics Laboratory in the School of Medicine at the University of Connecticut (UConn) and served as chair of the BME Program in the School of Engineering at UConn as well as the director of the BME Graduate and Undergraduate Programs. Dr. Peterson earned a BS in aerospace engineering and a BS in biomechanical engineering from Worcester Polytechnic Institute, in Worcester, Massachusetts, in 1992, an MS in mechanical engineering from the UConn, in Storrs, Connecticut, in 1995, and a PhD in biomedical engineering from UConn in 1999. He has 17 years of experience in BME education and has offered graduate-level and undergraduate-level courses in the areas of biomechanics, biodynamics, biofluid mechanics, BME communication, BME senior design, and ergonomics, and has taught subjects such as gross anatomy, occupational biomechanics, and occupational exposure and response in the School of Medicine. Dr. Peterson was also recently the co-executive director of the Biomedical Engineering Alliance and Consortium (BEACON), which is a nonprofit organization dedicated to the promotion of collaborative research, translation, and partnership among academic, medical, and industry people in the field of biomedical engineering to develop new medical technologies and devices.

Dr. Peterson has over 21 years of experience in devices and systems and in engineering and medical research, and his work on human–device interaction has led to applications on the design and development of several medical devices and tools. Other recent translations of his research include the development of devices such as robotic assist devices and prosthetics, long-duration biosensor monitoring systems, surgical and dental instruments, patient care medical devices, spacesuits and space tools for NASA, powered and non-powered hand tools, musical instruments, sports equipment, computer input devices, and so on. Other overlapping research initiatives focus on the development of computational models and simulations of biofluid dynamics and biomechanical performance, cell mechanics and cellular responses to fluid shear stress, human exposure and response to vibration, and the acoustics of hearing protection and communication. He has also been involved clinically with the Occupational and Environmental Medicine group at the UConn Health Center, where his work has been directed toward the objective engineering analysis of the anatomic and physiological processes involved in the onset of musculoskeletal and neuromuscular diseases, including strategies of disease mitigation.

Dr. Peterson's scholarly activities include over 50 published journal articles, 2 textbook chapters, 2 textbook sections, and 12 textbooks, including his new appointment as co-editor-in-chief for *The Biomedical Engineering Handbook* by CRC Press.

Contributors

Joseph Adam
Premise Development Corporation
Hartford, Connecticut

Dennis D. Autio
Dybonics, Inc.
Portland, Oregon

Pamela J. Hoyes Beehler
University of Texas
Arlington, Texas

Khosrow Behbehani
Department of Biomedical Engineering
University of Texas
Arlington, Texas

and

Southwestern Medical Center
University of Texas
Dallas, Texas

Paul A. Belk
St. Jude Medical
St. Paul, Minnesota

Joseph D. Bronzino
Trinity College
Hartford, Connecticut

Mark E. Bruley
ECRI Institute
Plymouth Meeting, Pennsylvania

Richard P. Buck (deceased)
University of North Carolina
Chapel Hill, North Carolina

Robert D. Butterfield
IVAC Corporation
San Diego, California

Christopher S. Chen
Department of Bioengineering
University of Pennsylvania
Philadelphia, Pennsylvania

Vivian H. Coates
ECRI Institute
Plymouth Meeting, Pennsylvania

David D. Cunningham
Eastern Kentucky University
Richmond, Kentucky

Yadin David
Biomedical Engineering Consultants
Houston, Texas

Gary Drzewiecki
Department of Biomedical Engineering
Rutgers University
Piscataway, New Jersey

Jeffrey L. Eggleston
Covidien Energy-Based Devices
Valleylab Inc.
Boulder, Colorado

Larry Fennigkoh
Milwaukee School of Engineering
Milwaukee, Wisconsin

Kevin Fite
Clarkson University
Potsdam, New York

Ross Flewelling
Nellcor Inc.
Pleasant, California

Leslie A. Geddes (deceased)
Purdue University
West Lafayette, Indiana

John Gill
John Gill Technology Ltd
Buckinghamshire, UK

Sverre Grimnes
Department of Physics
University of Oslo
and
Department of Clinical and Biomedical
Engineering
Oslo University Hospital
Oslo, Norway

Katya Hill
University of Pittsburgh
and
AAC Institute
Pittsburgh, Pennsylvania

Douglas Hobson
University of Pittsburgh
Pittsburgh, Pennsylvania

Sheik N. Imrhan
University of Texas
Arlington, Texas

Richard D. Jones
New Zealand Brain Research Institute
and
Canterbury District Health Board
Ashburton, New Zealand

and

University of Canterbury
Christchurch, New Zealand

and

University of Otago
Dunedin, New Zealand

Thomas M. Judd
Kaiser Permanente
Atlanta, Georgia

Millard M. Judy
Baylor Research Institute
Dallas, Texas

Kurt A. Kaczmarek
University of Wisconsin
Madison, Wisconsin

George V. Kondraske
University of Texas
Arlington, Texas

Chung-Chiun Liu
Case Western Reserve University
Cleveland, Ohio

Marilyn Lord
King's College Hospital
London, United Kingdom

Ørjan G. Martinsen
Department of Physics
University of Oslo
and
Department of Clinical and Biomedical
Engineering
Oslo University Hospital
Oslo, Norway

Ken Maxwell
IBM
and
MaxwellX
Fort Worth, Texas

Joseph P. McClain
Walter Reed Army Medical Center
Washington, DC

Yitzhak Mendelson
Worcester Polytechnic Institute
Worcester, Massachusetts

Gary C.H. Mo
Departments of Chemical Engineering and
    Applied Chemistry and Biochemistry
and
Institute of Biomaterials and Biomedical
    Engineering
University of Toronto
Toronto, Ontario, Canada

Robert L. Morris
Dybonics, Inc.
Portland, Oregon

Thomas J. Mullen
Medtronic
Minneapolis, Minnesota

Joachim H. Nagel
Institute of Biomedical Engineering
University of Stuttgart
Stuttgart, Germany

Michael R. Neuman
Department of Biomedical Engineering
Michigan Technological University
Houghton, Michigan

Keat Ghee Ong
Department of Biomedical Engineering
Michigan Technological University
Houghton, Michigan

Mohamad Parnianpour
Department of Mechanical Engineering
Sharif University of Technology
Tehran, Iran

A. William Paulsen
Quinnipiac University
Hamden, Connecticut

P. Hunter Peckham
Case Western Reserve University
Cleveland, Ohio

Brandon D. Pereles
Department of Biomedical Engineering
Michigan Technological University
Houghton, Michigan

Dejan B. Popović
University of Belgrade
Belgrade, Serbia

and

Aalborg University
Aalbrog, Denmark

Jeremiah J. Remus
Clarkson University
Potsdam, New York

Pat Ridgely
Medtronic, Inc.
Minneapolis, Minnesota

Richard L. Roa
Baylor University Medical Center
Dallas, Texas

Charles J. Robinson
Clarkson University
Potsdam, New York

and

VA Medical Center
Syracuse, New York

Barry Romich
Prentke Romich Company
and
AAC Institute
Pittsburgh, Pennsylvania

Eric Rosow
Hartford Hospital
and
Premise Development Corporation
Hartford, Connecticut

Steven Schreiner
School of Engineering
The College of New Jersey
Ewing, New Jersey

Susan S. Smith
Texas Women's University
Denton, Texas

Nathan J. Sniadecki
Department of Mechanical Engineering and
    Department of Bioengineering
University of Washington
Seattle, Washington

Orhan Soykan
Medtronic, Inc.
and
Michigan Technological University
Houghton, Michigan

Primoz Strojnik
Case Western Reserve University
Cleveland, Ohio

Karl Syndulko
UCLA School of Medicine
Los Angeles, California

Willis A. Tacker Jr.
Purdue University
West Lafayette, Indiana

Elaine Trefler
University of Pittsburgh
Pittsburgh, Pennsylvania

Alan Turner-Smith
King's College Hospital
London, United Kingdom

Gregg Vanderheiden
Trace R&D Center
Biomedical Engineering
University of Wisconsin, Madison
Madison, Wisconsin

Paul J. Vasta
University of Texas
Arlington, Texas

Wolf W. von Maltzahn
Rensselaer Polytechnic Institute
Troy, New York

Gregory I. Voss
IVAC Corporation
San Diego, California

Alvin Wald
Columbia University
New York, New York

Christopher M. Yip
Departments of Chemical Engineering and
    Applied Chemistry and Biochemistry
University of Toronto
Toronto, Ontario, Canada

MATLAB Statement

MATLAB® and Simulink® are registered trademarks of The MathWorks, Inc. For product information, please contact:

The MathWorks, Inc.
3 Apple Hill Drive
Natick, MA 01760-2098 USA
Tel: 508 647 7000
Fax: 508-647-7001
E-mail: info@mathworks.com
Web: www.mathworks.com

I

Biomedical Sensors

Michael R. Neuman
Michigan Technological University

1

Michael R. Neuman
Michigan Technological
University

Introduction

Any instrumentation system has three fundamental components: a sensor, a signal processor, and a display and/or storage device as illustrated in Figure 1.1. Although all these components of the instrumentation system are important, the sensor serves a special function in that it interfaces the instrument with the system being measured. In the case of biomedical instrumentation, a biomedical sensor (that in some cases may be referred to as a biosensor) is the interface between the electronic instrument and the biological system. There are some general concerns that are very important for any sensor in an instrumentation system regarding its ability to effectively carry out the interface function. These concerns are especially important for biomedical sensors because the sensor can affect the system being measured as well as the system can affect the sensor. Sensors must be designed in such a way that they minimize their interaction with the biological host. It is important that the presence of the sensor does not affect the variable being measured as a result of the interaction between the sensor and the biological system. If the sensor is placed in a living organism, that organism will probably recognize the sensor as a foreign body and react to it. This may result in a local change in the quantity being sensed in the vicinity of the sensor so that the measurement reflects the foreign body reaction rather than a central characteristic of the host. When a sensor is implanted, proteins and cells are likely to be deposited on its surface, and eventually a fibrous capsule is formed around it. These aspects of the foreign body reaction will change the way the sensor appears to the remaining surrounding tissue and the microenvironment encompassing the sensor is likely to be different from the environment in the rest of the body. Thus, the sensor's response to the physiological quantity being measured may yield a different result from the systemic value of the variable. For example, chronically implanted sensors often appear to drift over time during the implant duration although the variable being measured remains constant. When these sensors are removed from the tissue, their calibration and baseline appear to be the same as they were immediately before being implanted. One can conclude from this that the sensors' interactions with their surrounding tissue were the causes of the drift, not the sensor itself. Therefore, it is important to consider the materials from which a sensor is made and their physical configuration as well as the functional properties of the sensor itself. The former issues can have a significant effect on how the body perceives the sensor and the resulting interaction that can lead to measurement errors.

Similarly, the biological system can affect the performance of the sensor. The foreign body reaction might cause the host to attempt to break down the materials of the sensor in an attempt to remove it. This may, in fact, degrade the sensor package so that the sensor can no longer perform in an adequate manner. Even if the foreign body reaction is not sufficiently strong to affect the measurement, the fact that the sensor is placed in a warm, aqueous, and often caustic environment may cause water and ions to eventually invade the package and degrade the function of the sensor.

Finally, as will be described in the following chapters, sensors that are implanted in the body are usually not accessible for calibration. Thus, such sensors must have extremely stable characteristics, so that frequent calibrations are not necessary.

Biomedical sensors can be classified according to how they are used with respect to the biological system. Table 1.1 shows that sensors can range from noninvasive to invasive as far as the biological host is

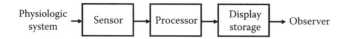

FIGURE 1.1   Block diagram of a general biomedical instrument.

concerned. The most noninvasive of biomedical sensors do not even contact the biological system being measured. Sensors of radiant heat or sound energy coming from an organism are examples of noncontacting sensors. Noninvasive sensors can also be placed on the body surface. Skin-surface thermometers, biopotential electrodes, pulse oximeter probes, and strain gauges placed on the skin are examples of noninvasive sensors. Indwelling sensors are those that can be placed into a natural body cavity that communicates with the outside. Sensors placed orally, rectally, or in the auditory canal (ear) are examples of this class of sensor. These are sometimes referred to as minimally invasive sensors and include familiar sensors such as oral–rectal thermometers, intrauterine pressure transducers, and stomach pH sensors. The most invasive sensors are those that need to be surgically placed and that results in some tissue damage associated with their placement. For example, a needle electrode for picking up electromyographic signals directly from muscles; a blood pressure sensor placed in an artery, vein, or the heart itself; or a blood flow transducer positioned on a major artery are all examples of invasive sensors.

We can also classify sensors in terms of the quantities that they measure. Physical sensors are used in measuring physical quantities, such as displacement, pressure, and flow, whereas chemical sensors are used to determine the concentration of chemical substances within the host. A subgroup of the chemical sensors that are concerned with sensing the presence and the concentration of biochemical materials

TABLE 1.1   Classification of Biomedical Sensors

Physical Sensors	Chemical Sensors
• Displacement	• Gas
• Linear	• Electrochemical
• Angular	• Electrical conductivity
• Volume	• Thermal
• Mechanical	• Electrochemical
• Force	• Conductimetric
• Mass	• Amperometric
• Torque	• Potentiometric
• Hydraulic	• Bioanalytic
• Pressure	• Enzyme mediated
• Flow	• Antigen–antibody
• Thermal	• Ligand–receptor
• Temperature	• Photometric
• Heat flux	• Colorimetric
• Convection	• Intensity
• Electrical	• Fluorescence
• Voltage	
• Current	
• Impedance	
• Frequency	
• Optical	
• Intensity	
• Wavelength (color)	

in the host are known as bioanalytical sensors, or sometimes, they are referred to as biosensors. These sensors use biological reactions in the measurement process.

In the following chapters, we will discuss each type of sensor and present some examples as well as describe some of the important issues surrounding such sensors. We will analyze physical and chemical sensors and consider their applications in diagnosis and patient monitoring.

2

Physical Sensors

Michael R. Neuman
Michigan Technological
University

2.1 Introduction

Physical variables associated with biomedical systems are measured by a group of sensors called physical sensors. A list of typical variables that are frequently measured by these devices and examples of sensors of these variables used in biomedical measurements are given in Table 2.1. These quantities are similar to physical quantities measured by sensors for nonbiomedical applications, and the devices used for biomedical and nonbiomedical sensing are, therefore, quite similar. Thus, sensors of linear displacement can frequently be used equally well for measuring the displacement of the heart muscle during the cardiac cycle or the movement of a robot arm. There is, however one notable exception regarding the similarity of these sensors: the packaging of the sensor and attachment to the system being measured. Although physical sensors used in nonbiomedical applications need to be packaged so as to be protected from their environment, few of these sensors have to deal with the harsh environment of biological tissue, especially with the mechanisms inherent to biological tissue having the sole purpose of trying to eliminate foreign objects such as a sensor from the body. Other notable exceptions to this similarity of sensors for measuring physical quantities in biological and nonbiological systems are the sensors used for fluidic measurements such as pressure and flow. Special needs for these measurements in biological systems have resulted in special sensors and instrumentation systems for these measurements that can be quite different from systems for measuring pressure and flow in nonbiological environments.

In this chapter, we will attempt to review various examples of sensors used for physical measurement in biological systems. Although it would be beyond the scope of this chapter to cover all of these in detail, the principal sensors applied for biological measurement will be described. Each section will include a brief description of the principle of operation of the sensor and the underlying physical principles, examples of some of the more common forms of these sensors for application in living systems, methods of signal processing for these sensors where appropriate, and important considerations for when the sensor is applied.

TABLE 2.1   Physical Variables and Sensors

Physical Quantity	Sensor	Variable Sensed
Geometric	Strain gauge	Strain
	LVDT	Displacement
	Ultrasonic transit time	Displacement
Kinematic	Velocimeter	Velocity
	Accelerometer	Acceleration
Force–torque	Load cell	Applied force or torque
Fluidic	Pressure transducer	Pressure
	Flow meter	Flow
Thermal	Thermometer	Temperature
	Thermal flux sensor	Heat flux

2.2 Description of Sensors

2.2.1 Linear and Angular Displacement Sensors

A comparison of various characteristics of displacement sensors described in detail here is outlined in Table 2.2.

2.2.1.1 Variable Resistance Sensor

One of the simplest sensors for measuring linear or angular displacement is a variable resistor similar to the volume control on an audio electronic device [1]. The resistance between two terminals, one end of a resistance and a movable contact on this resistance, of this device is related to the linear or angular displacement of the movable sliding contact along the resistance element. Precision devices are available that have highly reproducible, linear relationships between resistance and displacement. These devices can be connected in circuits that measure resistance such as an ohm meter or Wheatstone bridge, or they can be used as a part of a circuit that provides a voltage that is proportional to the displacement. Such circuits include the voltage divider (as illustrated in Figure 2.1a) or driving a known constant current through the resistance and measuring the resulting voltage across it. This sensor is simple and inexpensive and can be used for measuring relatively large displacements. Variable resistances for measuring

TABLE 2.2   Comparison of Displacement Sensors

Sensor	Electrical Variable	Measurement Circuit	Sensitivity	Precision	Range
Variable resistor	Resistance	Voltage divider, ohmmeter, bridge, current source	High	Moderate	Large
Foil strain gauge	Resistance	Bridge	Low	Moderate	Small
Liquid metal strain gauge	Resistance	Ohmmeter, bridge	Moderate	Moderate	Large
Silicon strain gauge	Resistance	Bridge	High	Moderate	Small
Mutual inductance coils	Inductance	Impedance bridge, inductance meter	Moderate to high	Moderate to low	Moderate to large
Variable reluctance	Inductance	Impedance bridge, inductance meter	High	Moderate	Large
LVDT	Inductance	Voltmeter	High	High	High
Parallel plate capacitor	Capacitance	Impedance bridge, capacitance meter	Moderate to high	Moderate	Moderate to large
Sonic/ultrasonic	Time	Timer circuit	High	High	Large

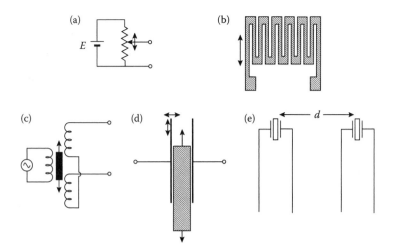

FIGURE 2.1 Examples of displacement sensors: (a) variable resistance sensor, (b) foil strain gauge, (c) linear variable differential transformer (LVDT), (d) parallel plate capacitive sensor, and (e) ultrasonic transit time–displacement sensor.

linear displacements can be several centimeters in length, and precision 10- or 15-turn angular displacement sensors are commercially available.

There are certain things to keep in mind when applying this type of displacement sensor. When the circuit is a simple voltage divider, it is important that the electrical load on the output is very small such that there is very little current in the slider circuit. Significant current will introduce nonlinearities in the voltage versus displacement characteristics. To avoid this from happening, an operational amplifier voltage follower circuit can be used to keep the slider circuit current at a very low level. The sensor requires mechanical attachment to the structure being displaced and to some reference point. This can present difficulties in certain biological situations. Furthermore, because the slider must move along the resistance element, this can introduce some friction that may alter the actual displacement. Because the slider is moving across the resistance element and must contact it, there can be mechanical wear involved that may eventually cause a change in the resistance element that can lead to introducing nonlinearities and noise in the measurement and ultimately to failure of the resistance element.

There are also digital devices that can measure linear and angular displacements, the latter often being called digital shaft encoders. These devices produce an electrical pulse or digital word when they are displaced by a small amount, their resolution. Linear digital displacement sensors can measure displacements as great as several meters with resolutions as small as 1 μm, and digital angular displacement sensors can measure very small angular changes. These devices are particularly useful when signal processing is done by digital means, such as a computer, microprocessor, or microcontroller. In these cases there is no need for an analog-to-digital converter because the sensor's output is already in digital form.

2.2.1.2 Strain Gauge

A different type of displacement sensor based on an electrical resistance change is the strain gauge [2]. If a long narrow electrical conductor, such as a piece of metal foil or a fine gauge wire, is stretched within its elastic limit it will increase in length and decrease in cross-sectional area. The electrical resistance between both ends of the foil or wire can be given by

$$R = \rho \frac{L}{A}$$

(2.1)

where ρ is the electrical resistivity of the foil or wire material, L its length, and A its cross-sectional area. From Equation 2.1 it can be seen that this stretching will result in an increase in resistance. When the tension on the wire or foil is released, their elastic properties will restore their original shape, and the electrical resistance will return to the baseline values. The change in length can only be very small for the foil or wire to remain within their elastic limits, so the change in electrical resistance will also be very small. The relative sensitivity of this device is given by its gauge factor, γ, which is defined as

$$\gamma = \frac{\Delta R/R}{\Delta L/L}$$

(2.2)

where ΔR is the change in resistance when the structure is stretched by an amount ΔL. Foil strain gauges are the most frequently applied sensors of small displacements or strain and are available commercially in different sizes, materials, and shapes. They consist of a structure as shown in Figure 2.1b. A piece of metal foil that is bonded to an insulating polymeric film, such as polyimide that is more compliant than the metal foil itself, is chemically etched into a pattern similar to that shown in Figure 2.1b. When a strain is applied in the sensitive direction, the long direction of the individual elements of the strain gauge, the length of the gauge will be slightly increased, and this will result in an increase in the electrical resistance seen between the terminals. Because the displacement or strain that this sensor can measure is quite small for it to remain within its elastic limit, it can only be used to measure small displacements that occur as loads are applied to structural beams. If one wants to increase the range of a foil strain gauge, one has to attach it to some sort of mechanical impedance converter such as a cantilever beam. If the strain gauges are attached to one surface of this beam as shown in Figure 2.2a, a fairly large displacement at the unsupported end of the beam can be translated to a relatively small displacement on the beam's surface. It is, therefore, possible for the structure to be used to measure larger displacements at the cantilever beam tip using a strain gauge bonded on the beam surface near its point of support.

Because the electrical resistance changes for a strain gauge are quite small, the measurement of resistance change can be challenging. Generally, Wheatstone bridge circuits are used. It is important to note,

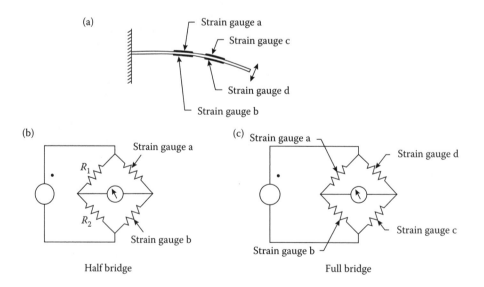

FIGURE 2.2 Strain gauges on a cantilever structure to provide temperature compensation: (a) cross-sectional view of the cantilever and placement of the strain gauges in a (b) half bridge or (c) full bridge for temperature compensation and enhanced sensitivity.

however, that changes in temperature can also result in electrical resistance changes that are of the same order of magnitude or even larger than the resistance changes due to the strain. Thus, it is important to temperature compensate strain gauges in most applications. A simple method of temperature compensation is to use a double or quadruple strain gauge and a bridge circuit for measuring the resistance change. This is illustrated in Figures 2.2b and 2.2c. If one can use the strain gauge in an application, such as the cantilever beam application described earlier, one can place one or two of the strain gauge structures on the concave side of the beam and the other one or two on the convex side. Thus, as the beam deflects, the strain gauge on the convex side will experience tension, and that on the concave side will experience compression. By putting these gauges in adjacent arms of the Wheatstone bridge, this can double the sensitivity of the circuit in the case of using two strain gauges and quadruple it in the case where the entire bridge is made up of strain gauges on the cantilever beam.

In addition to increased sensitivity, the bridge circuit minimizes temperature effects on the strain gauge measurements. Placing strain gauges that are on opposite sides of the beam in adjacent arms of the bridge results in a change in bridge output voltage when the beam is deflected; this occurs because the strain gauges on one side of the beam will increase in resistance, whereas those on the other side will decrease in resistance when the beam is deflected. However, when the temperature of the beam changes all of the strain gauges will have the same change in resistance, and this change will not affect the bridge output voltage.

In some applications it is not possible to place strain gauges so that one gauge is undergoing tension while the other is undergoing compression. In this case, a second strain gauge can still be used for temperature compensation if it can be oriented such that its sensitive axis is in a direction where the strain is minimal. Thus, it is still possible to have temperature compensation by having two identical strain gauges at the same temperature in adjacent arms of the bridge circuit, but the sensitivity improvement described in the previous paragraph is not seen in this case.

Another constraint imposed by temperature is that the material to which the strain gauge is attached and the strain gauge itself both have temperature coefficients of expansion. Thus, even if a gauge is attached to a structure under conditions of no strain, if the temperature is changed, the strain gauge could experience some strain due to the different expansion that it will have compared to the structure to which it is attached. To avoid this problem, strain gauges have been developed using materials that have identical temperature coefficients of expansion to various common materials to which they might be attached. In selecting a strain gauge, one should choose a device with thermal expansion characteristics as close as possible to those of the object on which the strain gauge is to be attached for measurement.

A more compliant structure that has found applications in biomedical instrumentation is the liquid metal strain gauge [3]. Instead of using a solid electrical conductor such as the wire or metal foil that make up the strain gauges mentioned earlier, mercury confined to within a compliant, thin-wall, narrow bore elastomeric tube is used. The compliance of this strain gauge is determined by the elastic properties of the tube. Because only the elastic limit of the tube is of concern, this sensor can be used to detect much larger displacements than conventional strain gauges. Its sensitivity is roughly the same as that of a foil or wire strain gauge, but it is not as reliable. Mercury can easily become oxidized or small gaps can occur in the mercury column thereby interrupting the electrical circuit. These effects make the sensor's characteristics noisy and sometimes results in failure of the structure. Liquid metal strain gauges have been used to measure breathing movements by placing them around the chest or abdomen, venous return from the leg by placing them circumferentially around the leg, and as a means of measuring nocturnal penile tumescence.

Another variation on the strain gauge is the semiconductor strain gauge. These devices are generally made of pieces of silicon with strain gauge patterns formed using semiconductor microelectronic technology. The principal advantage of these devices is that their gauge factors can be more than 50 times greater than that of the solid and liquid metal devices. They are available commercially, but they are a bit more difficult to handle and attach to structures being measured due to their small size, brittleness, and fine gauge lead wires.

2.2.1.3 Inductance Sensors

2.2.1.3.1 *Mutual Inductance*

The mutual inductance between two coils is related to many geometric factors, one of which is the separation of the coils. Thus, one can create a very simple displacement sensor by having two coils that are coaxial but have variable separation. By driving one coil with an ac signal and measuring the voltage signal induced in the second coil, this voltage will be related to how far apart the coils are from one another. When the coils are close together, the mutual inductance will be relatively high, and so a higher voltage will be induced in the second coil; when the coils are more widely separated, the mutual inductance will be lower as will be the induced voltage. The relationship between voltage and separation will be determined by the specific geometry of the coils and in general will not have a linear relationship with separation unless the change of displacement is relatively small. Nevertheless, this is a simple method for measuring displacement that works reasonably well provided the coils remain coaxial. If there is movement of the coils transverse to their axes, it is difficult to separate the effects of transverse displacement from those of displacement along the axis.

2.2.1.3.2 *Variable Reluctance*

A variation on this sensor is the variable reluctance sensor wherein a single coil or two coaxial coils remain fixed on a form which allows a high reluctance material such as piece of iron to move into or out of the center of the coil or coils along their axis. Since the position of this core material determines the number of flux linkages through the coil or coils, this can affect the self-inductance of a single coil or mutual inductance between two coils. In the case of mutual inductance, this can be measured using the technique described in the previous section, whereas self-inductance changes can be measured by various instrumentation circuits used for measuring inductance. This method is also a simple method for measuring displacements, but the characteristics are generally nonlinear, and the sensor often has only moderate precision.

2.2.1.3.3 *Linear Variable Differential Transformer*

By far the most frequently applied displacement transducer based on inductance is the linear variable differential transformer (LVDT) [4,5]. This device is illustrated in Figure 2.1c and is essentially a three-coil variable reluctance transducer. The two secondary coils are situated symmetrically about and coaxial with the primary coil and connected such that the induced voltages in each secondary oppose each other. When a high-reluctance core is located in the center of the structure equidistant from each secondary coil, the voltage induced in each secondary will be the same. Because these voltages oppose one another, the output voltage from the device will be zero. As the core is moved closer to one or the other secondary coils, the voltages in each coil will no longer be equal, and there will be an output voltage proportional to the displacement of the core from the central, zero-voltage position. Because of the symmetry of the structure, this voltage is linearly related to the core displacement over a range of displacements determined by the geometric arrangements of the coils. When the core passes through the central, zero point, the phase of the output voltage from the sensor changes by 180°. Thus, by measuring the phase angle as well as the voltage, one can determine the position of the core. The circuit associated with the LVDT not only measures the voltage but also often measures the phase angle as well. Linear variable differential transformers are available commercially in many sizes and shapes. Depending on the configuration of the coils, they can measure displacements ranging from tens of micrometers through several centimeters.

More details on inductance and other magnetically based sensors can be found in Chapter 3, Magnetic Biosensors.

2.2.1.4 Capacitive Sensors

Displacement sensors can be based on measurements of capacitance as well as inductance. The fundamental principle of operation is the capacitance of a parallel plate capacitor as given by

$$C = \varepsilon \frac{A}{d}$$

$$(2.3)$$

where ε is the dielectric constant of the medium between the plates, d the separation between the plates, and A the overlapping surface area of the plates. Each of the quantities in Equation 2.3 can be varied as a displacement, thereby changing the capacitance. By moving one of the plates with respect to the other, Equation 2.3 shows us that the capacitance will vary inversely with respect to the plate separation. This will give a hyperbolic capacitance–displacement characteristic. However, if the plate separation is maintained at a constant value and the plates are displaced laterally with respect to one another so that the area of overlap changes, this can produce a capacitance–displacement characteristic that can be linear, depending on the shape of the actual plates.

The third way that a variable capacitance transducer can measure displacement is by having a fixed parallel plate capacitor with a slab of dielectric material having a dielectric constant different from that of air that can slide between the plates (Figure 2.1d). The effective dielectric constant for the capacitor will depend on how much of the slab is between the plates and how much of the region between the plates is occupied only by air. This, also, can yield a transducer with linear capacitance as a function of displacement characteristics.

The electronic circuits used with variable capacitance transducers, are essentially the same as any other circuit used to measure capacitance. As with the inductance transducers, these circuits can take the form of a bridge circuit or specific circuits that measure capacitive reactance. One concern with capacitive sensors is that the sensor should be electrically shielded if there are electrically conductive objects in the vicinity of the sensor. Otherwise stray capacitances may affect the measurement.

2.2.1.5 Sonic and Ultrasonic Sensors

If the velocity of sound in a medium is constant, the time it takes a short burst of that sound energy to propagate from a source to a receiver will be proportional to the displacement between the two transducers. This is given by

$$d = cT$$

$$(2.4)$$

where c is the velocity of sound in the medium, T the transit time, and d the displacement. A simple system for making such a measurement is shown in Figure 2.1e [6]. A brief sonic or ultrasonic pulse is generated at the transmitting transducer and propagates through the medium. It is detected by the receiving transducer at time T after the burst was initiated. The displacement can then be determined by applying Equation 2.4.

In practice, this method is best used with ultrasound because the wavelength is shorter, and the device will neither produce annoying sounds nor respond to extraneous sounds in the environment. Small piezoelectric transducers to generate and receive ultrasonic pulses are readily available. The electronic circuit used with this instrument carries out three functions (1) generation of the sonic or ultrasonic burst, (2) detection of the received burst, and (3) measurement of the time of propagation of the ultrasound. A signal processing or a computing device can then calculate the displacement from the measured propagation time. An advantage of this system is that the two transducers are coupled to one another only sonically. There is no physical connection between them as was the case for the other sensors described in this section.

2.2.2 Velocity Measurement

Velocity is the time derivative of displacement, and therefore all the displacement transducers mentioned earlier can be used to measure velocity if their signals are processed by passing them through a differentiator circuit or computing their time derivative. There are, however, two additional methods, magnetic induction and Doppler ultrasound, that can be applied to measure velocity directly. They are described in the following two sections.

2.2.2.1 Magnetic Induction

If a magnetic field that passes through a conducting coil varies with time, a voltage is induced in that coil that is proportional to the time-varying magnetic field. This relationship is given by

$$\upsilon = N \frac{d\phi}{dt}$$

(2.5)

where υ is the voltage induced in the coil, N the number of turns in the coil, and ϕ the total magnetic flux passing through the coil (the product of the flux density and area within the coil). Thus, a simple way to apply this principle is to attach a small permanent magnet to an object whose velocity is to be determined, and attach a coil to a nearby structure that will serve as the reference against which the velocity is to be measured. A voltage will be induced in the coil whenever the structure containing the permanent magnet moves, and this voltage will be related to the velocity of that movement. The exact relationship will be determined by the field distribution for the particular magnet and the orientation of the magnet with respect to the coil.

2.2.2.2 Doppler Ultrasound

When the receiver of a signal in the form of a wave such as electromagnetic radiation or sound is moving at a nonzero velocity with respect to the emitter of that wave, the frequency of the wave perceived by the receiver will be different from the frequency of the transmitter. This frequency difference, known as the Doppler shift is determined by the relative velocity of the receiver with respect to the emitter and is given by

$$f_d = \frac{f_o u}{c}$$

(2.6)

where f_d is the Doppler frequency shift, f_o the frequency of the transmitted wave, u the relative velocity between the transmitter and receiver, and c the velocity of sound in the medium. This principle can be applied in biomedical applications as a Doppler velocimeter. A piezoelectric transducer can be used as the ultrasound source with a similar transducer as the receiver. When there is no relative movement between the two transducers, the frequency of the signal at the receiver will be the same as that at the emitter, but when there is relative motion, the frequency at the receiver will be shifted according to Equation 2.6. The ultrasonic velocimeter can be applied in the same way that the ultrasonic displacement sensor is used. In this case the electronic circuit at the emitter generates a continuous ultrasonic wave; and, instead of detecting the transit time of the signal, it now detects the frequency difference between the transmitted and received signals. This frequency difference can then be converted to a signal proportional to the relative velocity between the two transducers.

2.2.3 Accelerometers

Acceleration is the time derivative of velocity and the second derivative with respect to time of displacement. Thus, sensors of displacement and velocity can be used to determine acceleration when their signals are appropriately processed. In addition, there are direct sensors of acceleration based on Newton's second law and Hooke's law. The fundamental structure of an accelerometer is shown in Figure 2.3. A known seismic mass is attached to the housing by an elastic element. As the structure is accelerated in the sensitive direction of the elastic element, a force is applied to that element according to Newton's

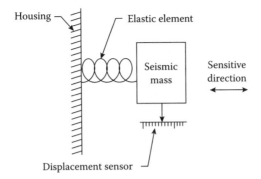

FIGURE 2.3 Fundamental structure of an accelerometer.

second law. This force causes the elastic element to be distorted according to Hooke's law, which results in a displacement of the mass with respect to the accelerometer housing. This displacement is measured by a displacement sensor. The relationship between the displacement and the acceleration is found by combining Newton's second law and Hooke's law

$$a = \frac{k}{m}x$$

(2.7)

where x is the measured displacement, m the known mass, k the spring constant of the elastic element, and a the acceleration. Any of the displacement sensors described earlier can be used in an accelerometer. The most frequently used displacement sensors are strain gauges or the LVDT. One type of accelerometer uses a piezoelectric sensor as both the displacement sensor and the elastic element. A piezoelectric sensor generates an electric signal that is related to the dynamic change in shape of the piezoelectric material as a force is applied. Thus, piezoelectric materials can only directly measure time-varying forces. A piezoelectric accelerometer is, therefore, better for measuring changes in acceleration than for measuring constant accelerations. A principal advantage of piezoelectric accelerometers is that they can be made very small, which is useful in many biomedical applications.

Very small and relatively inexpensive accelerometers are currently made on a single silicon chip using microelectromechanical systems (MEMS) technology. An example is shown in Figure 2.4. A small piece of silicon is etched to give the paddle-like structure that is attached to the silicon frame at one end and is free to move with respect to the frame by flexing the "handle" of the paddle. This movement results in strains being induced on the surfaces of the "handle," and a strain gauge integrated into this handle structure detects the strain and converts it into an electrical signal. The paddle serves as the seismic mass, and the "handle" is the elastic element. Inexpensive three-dimensional semiconductor chip accelerometers are commercially available. They utilize variable capacitance sensors integrated into their structure for sensing displacement in each of the Cartesian directions. Miniature silicon chip accelerometers are included in "smart" mobile telephones and tablet computers and are used to determine the orientation of the device to appropriately orient the display. They also can be used in applications that measure quantities that are associated with acceleration such as detecting accelerations associated with individual steps in a pedometer.

2.2.4 Force Measurement

Force is measured by converting the force into a displacement and measuring the displacement with a displacement sensor. The conversion takes place as a result of the elastic properties of a material on which the force is applied. This force distorts the material's shape, and this distortion can be measured

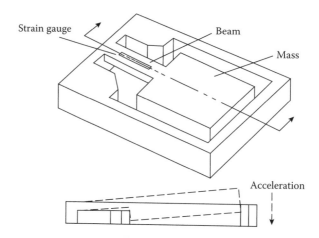

FIGURE 2.4   Example of a silicon chip accelerometer fabricated using MEMS technology. The lower figure shows the upward deflection of the seismic mass with a downward acceleration. Typical dimensions of the silicon chip are 1 and 2 mm length and width, respectively and less than a mm thick. This means that the packaged chip can be very small.

by a displacement sensor. For example, the cantilever structure shown in Figure 2.2a could be a force sensor. Applying a vertical force at the tip of the beam will cause the beam to deflect according to its elastic properties. Beam theory such as used on a macro scale in civil engineering can be applied here to relate displacement of the beam to applied forces. This deflection can be detected using a displacement sensor such as a strain gauge on the beam surface as described previously.

A common form of force sensor is the load cell. This consists of a block of material with known elastic properties that has strain gauges attached to it. Applying a force to the load cell stresses the material, resulting in a strain that can be measured by the strain gauges. Applying Hooke's law, one finds that the strain is proportional to the applied force. The strain gauges on a load cell are usually in a half- or full-bridge configuration to minimize the temperature sensitivity of the device. Load cells come in various sizes and configurations, and they can measure a wide range of forces.

2.2.5 Measurement of Fluid Dynamic Variables

The measurement of the fluid pressure and flow in both liquids and gases is important in many biomedical applications. These two variables, however, often are the most difficult variables to measure in biological applications because of interactions with the biological system and stability problems. Some of the most frequently applied sensors for these measurements are described in the following sections.

2.2.5.1 Pressure Measurement

Sensors of pressure for biomedical measurements such as blood pressure [7] consist of a structure such as shown in Figure 2.5. In this case a fluid coupled to the fluid whose pressure is to be measured is housed in a chamber with a flexible diaphragm making up a portion of the wall, with the other side of the diaphragm at atmospheric pressure. When a pressure difference exists across the diaphragm, it causes the diaphragm to deflect. This deflection is then measured by a displacement sensor. In the example in Figure 2.5, the displacement sensor consists of four fine-gauge wires drawn between a structure attached to the diaphragm and the housing of the pressure sensor so that these wires serve as strain gauges. When pressure causes the diaphragm to deflect, two of the fine-wire strain gauges will be extended by a small amount causing their resistance to slightly increase, and the other two will contract by the same amount causing their resistances to decrease by a small amount. By connecting these wires into a bridge circuit, a voltage proportional to the deflection of the diaphragm and hence the pressure can be obtained.

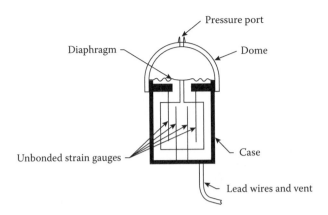

FIGURE 2.5 Structure of an unbonded strain gauge pressure sensor. (Reproduced from Neuman M.R. 1993. In R.C. Dorf (Ed.), *The Electrical Engineering Handbook,* Boca Raton, FL, CRC Press. With permission.)

Semiconductor technology has been applied to the design of pressure transducers such that the entire structure can be fabricated from silicon. A portion of a silicon chip can be formed into a diaphragm and semiconductor strain gauges incorporated directly into that diaphragm to produce a small, inexpensive, and sensitive pressure sensor. Such sensors can be used as disposable, single-use devices for measuring blood pressure without the need for additional sterilization before being used on the next patient. This minimizes the risk of transmitting blood-borne infections in the cases where the transducer is coupled directly to the patient's blood for direct blood pressure measurement. These types of sensors work essentially the same as the unbonded strain gauge sensor shown in Fgure 2.5, but they can be made much smaller than the unbonded strain gauge sensor which gives them significantly improved characteristics. They also can be manufactured and sold at much lower cost. Figure 2.6 shows an example of this type of sensor and a cross sectional view of its components.

In using this type of sensor to measure blood pressure, it is necessary to couple the chamber containing the diaphragm to the blood or other fluids being measured. This is usually done using a small, flexible plastic tube known as a catheter that can have one end placed in an artery of the subject while the other is connected to the pressure sensor. This catheter is filled with a physiological saline solution so that the arterial blood pressure is coupled to the sensor diaphragm. This external blood pressure-measurement

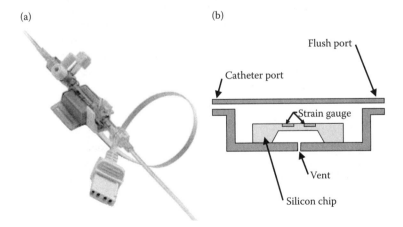

FIGURE 2.6 Silicon chip pressure sensors for biomedical applications: (a) a typical clinical pressure sensor and (b) a cross sectional view of a silicon chip-based biomedical pressure sensor.

method is used quite frequently in the clinic and research laboratory, but it has the limitation that the properties of the fluid in the catheter and the catheter itself can affect the measurement. For example, both ends of the catheter must be at the same vertical level to avoid a pressure offset due to hydrostatic effects. Also, the compliance of the tube will affect the frequency response of the pressure measurement. Air bubbles in the catheter or obstructions due to clotted blood or other materials can introduce distortion of the waveform due to resonance and damping. These problems can be minimized by using a miniature semiconductor pressure transducer that is located at the tip of a catheter and can be placed in the blood vessel rather than being positioned external to the body. Such internal pressure sensors are available commercially and have the advantages of a much broader frequency response, no hydrostatic pressure error, and generally clearer signals than the external system.

Although it is possible to measure blood pressure using the techniques described, this remains one of the major problems in biomedical sensor technology. Long-term stability of pressure transducers can be a significant problem. This is especially true for pressure measurements of venous blood, cerebrospinal fluid, or fluids in the gastrointestinal tract, where pressures are usually relatively low. Long-term changes in baseline pressure for most pressure sensors require that they be frequently adjusted to be certain of the zero pressure level. Although this can be done relatively easily when the pressure transducer is located external to the body, this can be a major problem for indwelling or implanted pressure sensors. Thus, these transducers must be extremely stable and have low baseline drift to be useful in long-term applications.

The packaging of the pressure transducer is also a problem that needs to be addressed, especially when the transducer is in contact with blood for long periods of time. Not only must the package be biocompatible, but it also must allow the appropriate pressure to be transmitted from the biological fluid to the diaphragm. Thus, a material that is mechanically stable under corrosive and aqueous environments in the body is needed. Chronically implanted objects are usually coated with a fibrous capsule by the body as a part of the foreign body response, and this capsule can exert a force on the pressure sensor that will affect its baseline pressure. Thus, it is important to package pressure sensors with materials that will minimize this encapsulation.

2.2.5.2 Flow Measurement

The measurement of true volumetric flow in the body represents one of the most difficult problems in biomedical sensing [8]. The sensors that have been developed measure velocity rather than volume flow, and they can only be used to measure flow if the velocity is measured for a tube of known cross section. Thus, most flow sensors constrain the vessel to have a specific cross-sectional area.

The most frequently used flow sensor in biomedical systems is the electromagnetic flow meter illustrated in Figure 2.7. This device consists of a means of generating a magnetic field transverse to the flow vector in a vessel. A pair of very small biopotential electrodes is attached to the wall of the vessel such that the vessel diameter between them is at right angles to the direction of the magnetic field. As the blood flows in this structure, ions in the blood deflect in the direction of one or the other electrodes due to the magnetic field and their velocity. This results in a voltage across the electrodes that is given by

$$v = Blu$$

(2.8)

where B is the magnetic field strength, l the distance between the electrodes, and u the average instantaneous velocity of the fluid within the vessel. If the sensor constrains the blood vessel to have a circular cross section of known diameter, then its cross-sectional area will be known, and multiplying this area by the measured velocity will give the volume flow. Although dc flow sensors have been developed and are available commercially, the preferred method is to use ac excitation of the magnetic field so that offset potential effects from the biopotential electrodes do not generate errors in this measurement.

Small ultrasonic transducers can also be attached to a blood vessel to measure flow as illustrated in Figure 2.8. In this case the transducers are oriented such that one transmits a continuous ultrasound

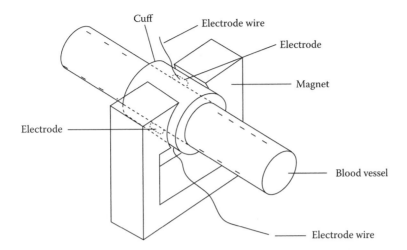

FIGURE 2.7 Fundamental structure of an electromagnetic flowmeter. (Reproduced from Neuman M.R. 1986. In J.D. Bronzino (Ed.), *Biomedical Engineering and Instrumentation: Basic Concepts and Applications*, Boston, PWS Publishers. With permission.)

signal that illuminates the blood. Cells within the blood diffusely reflect this signal in the direction of the second sensor so that the received signal undergoes a Doppler shift in frequency that is proportional to the velocity of the reflecting cells and, hence, the blood. By measuring the frequency shift and knowing the cross-sectional area of the vessel, it is possible to determine the flow.

Another method of measuring flow that has had biomedical application is the measurement of cooling of a heated object by convection. The object is usually a thermistor (see Section 2.2.6.2) placed either in a blood vessel or in tissue, and the thermistor serves as both the heating element and the temperature sensor. In one mode of operation, the amount of power required to maintain the thermistor at a temperature slightly above that of the blood upstream is measured. As the flow around the thermistor increases more heat is removed from the thermistor by convection, and so more power is required to keep it at a constant temperature. Relative flow is then measured by determining the amount of power supplied to the thermistor.

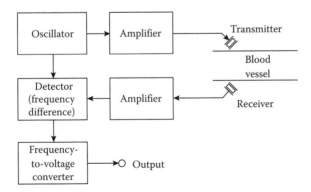

FIGURE 2.8 Structure of an ultrasonic Doppler flowmeter with the major blocks of the electronic signal processing system. The oscillator generates a signal that, after amplification, drives the transmitting transducer. The oscillator frequency is usually in the range of 1–10 MHz. The reflected ultrasound from the blood is sensed by the receiving transducer and amplified before being processed by a detector circuit. This block generates the frequency difference between the transmitted and received ultrasonic signals. This difference frequency can be converted into a voltage proportional to frequency, and hence flow velocity, by the frequency to voltage converter circuit.

TABLE 2.3   Properties of Temperature Sensors

Sensor	Form	Sensitivity	Stability	Range (°C)
Metal resistance thermometer	Coil of fine platinum wire	Low	High	−100 to 700
Thermistor	Bead, disk, chip, or rod	High	Moderate	−50 to 150
Thermocouple	Pair of wires	Low	High	−100 to >1500
Mercury in glass thermometer	Column of Hg in glass capillary	Moderate	High	−50 to 400
Silicon *p–n* diode	Electronic component	Moderate	High	−50 to 150

In a second approach, the thermistor is heated by applying a short duration current pulse and subsequently measuring the cooling curve of the thermistor as the blood flows across it. The thermistor will cool more quickly as the blood flow increases. Both these methods are relatively simple to achieve electronically, but both also have severe limitations. They are essentially qualitative measures and strongly depend on how the thermistor probe is positioned in the vessel being measured and the characteristics of the local flow around it. If the probe is closer to the periphery or even in contact with the vessel wall, the measured flow will be different than if the sensor is in the center of the vessel.

2.2.6 Temperature Measurement

There are different sensors of temperature [9,19,20], but three find particularly wide application to biomedical problems. Table 2.3 summarizes the properties of various temperature sensors, and these three, including metallic resistance thermometers, thermistors, and thermocouples, are described in the following sections.

2.2.6.1 Metallic Resistance Thermometers

The electrical resistance of a piece of metal or wire generally increases as the temperature of that electrical conductor increases. A linear approximation of this relationship is given by

$$R = R_0[1 + \alpha(T - T_0)]$$

(2.9)

where R_0 is the resistance at temperature T_0, α the temperature coefficient of resistance, and T the temperature at which the resistance is being measured. This principle serves as the basis of metallic resistance thermometers, sometimes referred to as resistance temperature devices (RTD). Most metals have temperature coefficients of resistance of the order of 0.1–0.4%/°C, as indicated in Table 2.4. The noble metals are preferred for resistance thermometers because they do not corrode easily and, when drawn into fine wires, their cross section will remain constant. This will help to minimize drift in the resistance over time which could result in an unstable sensor. It is also seen from Table 2.4 that the noble metals, gold and platinum, have some of the highest temperature coefficients of resistance of the common metals.

TABLE 2.4   Temperature Coefficient of Resistance for Common Metals and Alloys

Metal or Alloy	Resistivity at 20°C (μΩ cm)	Temperature Coefficient of Resistance (%/°C)
Platinum	9.83	0.3
Gold	2.22	0.368
Silver	1.629	0.38
Copper	1.724	0.393
Constantan (60% Cu, 40% Ni)	49.0	0.0002
Nichrome (80% Ni, 20% Cr)	108.0	0.013

Source: Pender H. and McIlwain K. 1957. *Electrical Engineers' Handbook*, 4th ed., New York, John Wiley & Sons.

Metal resistance thermometers are often fabricated from fine-gauge insulated wire that is wound into a small coil. It is important in doing so to make certain that there are not other sources of resistance change that could affect the sensor. For example, the structure should be used in such a way that no external strains are applied to the wire because the wire could also behave as a strain gauge. Metallic films and foils can also be used as temperature sensors, and commercial products are available in the wire, foil, or film forms. The electrical circuits used to measure resistance, and hence the temperature, are similar to those used with the wire or foil strain gauges. A bridge circuit is the most desirable, although ohmmeter circuits can also be used. It is important to make sure that the electronic circuit does not pass a large current through the resistance thermometer for that would cause self-heating due to the Joule conversion of electric energy into heat.

2.2.6.2 Thermistors

Unlike metals, semiconductor materials have an inverse relationship between resistance and temperature. This characteristic is nonlinear and cannot be characterized by a linear equation such as Equation 2.9. The thermistor is a semiconductor temperature sensor. Its resistance as a function of temperature is given by

$$R = R_0 e^{\beta\left[\frac{1}{T}-\frac{1}{T_0}\right]}$$

(2.10)

where β is a constant determined by the materials that make up the thermistor. Thermistors can take a variety of forms and cover a wide range of resistances. The most common forms used in biomedical applications are the bead, disk, rod, or chip forms of the sensor as illustrated in Figure 2.9. These structures can be formed from a variety of semiconductors ranging from elements such as silicon and germanium to mixtures of various semiconducting metallic oxides. Most commercially available thermistors are manufactured from the latter materials, and the specific materials as well as the process for fabricating them are closely held industrial secrets. These materials are chosen not only to have high sensitivity but also to have the greatest stability because thermistors are generally not as stable as the metallic resistance thermometers. However, thermistors can be close to an order of magnitude more sensitive.

2.2.6.3 Thermocouples

When different regions of an electric conductor or semiconductor are at different temperatures, there is an electric potential between these regions that is directly related to the temperature differences. This phenomenon, known as the Seebeck effect, can be used to produce a temperature sensor, a thermocouple, by taking a wire of metal or alloy A and another wire of metal or alloy B and connecting

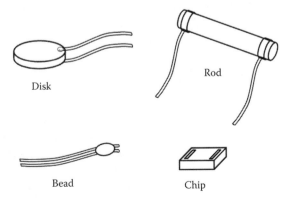

FIGURE 2.9 Common commercially available forms for thermistors.

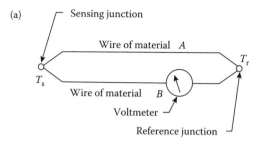

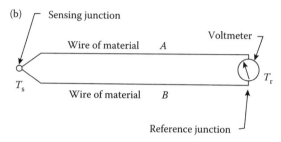

FIGURE 2.10 Circuit arrangement for a thermocouple showing the voltage-measuring device, the voltmeter, interrupting one of the thermocouple wires (a) and at the cold junction (b).

them as shown in Figure 2.10. One of the junctions is known as the sensing junction, and the other is the reference junction. When these junctions are at different temperatures, a voltage proportional to the temperature difference will be seen at the voltmeter when metals or alloys A and B have different Seebeck coefficients. This voltage can be represented over the relatively small temperature differences encountered in biomedical applications by the linear equation

$$V = S_{AB}(T_s - T_r)$$

(2.11)

where S_{AB} is the Seebeck coefficient for the thermocouple made up of metals or alloys A and B, T_s the measured temperature at the sensing junction, and T_r the known temperature at the reference junction. Although this equation is a reasonable approximation, more accurate data are usually found in tables of actual voltages as a function of temperature difference. In some applications the voltmeter is located at the reference junction, and one uses some independent means such as mercury in a glass thermometer to measure the reference junction temperature. Where precision measurements are made, the reference junction is often placed in an environment of known temperature such as an ice bath. Electronic measurement of reference junction temperature can also be carried out and used to compensate for the reference junction temperature so that the voltmeter reads a signal equivalent to what would be seen if the reference junction had been at 0°C. This electronic reference junction compensation is usually carried out using a metal resistance temperature sensor to determine reference junction temperature.

The voltages generated by thermocouples used for temperature measurement are generally quite small being on the order of tens of microvolts per °C. Thus, for most biomedical measurements where there is only a small difference in temperature between the sensing and reference junction, very sensitive voltmeters or amplifiers must be used to measure these potentials. Thermocouples have been used in industry for temperature measurement for many years. Several standard alloys to provide optimal sensitivity and stability of these sensors have evolved. Table 2.5 lists these common alloys, the Seebeck coefficient for thermocouples of these materials at room temperature, and the full range of temperatures over which these thermocouples can be used.

TABLE 2.5 Common Thermocouples

Type	Materials	Seebeck Coefficient (μV/°C)[a]	Temperature Range (°C)
S	Platinum/platinum 10% rhodium	6	0 to 1700
T	Copper/constantan	50	−190 to 400
K	Chromel/alumel	41	−200 to 1370
J	Iron/constantan	53	−200 to 760
E	Chromel/constantan	78	−200 to 970

[a] Seebeck coefficient value is at a temperature of 25°C.

Thermocouples can be fabricated in different ways depending on their applications. They are especially suitable for measuring temperature differences between two objects because the sensing junction can be placed on one while the other has the reference junction. Higher output thermocouples or thermopiles can be produced by connecting several thermocouples in series. Thermocouples can be made from very fine wires that can be implanted in biological tissues for temperature measurements, and it is also possible to place these fine-wire thermocouples within the lumen of a hypodermic needle to make short-term temperature measurements in tissue. Microfabrication technology has made it possible to make thermocouples sufficiently small so as to fit within a living cell.

2.3 Biomedical Applications of Physical Sensors

Just as it is not possible to cover the full range of physical sensors in this chapter, it is also impossible to consider the many biomedical applications that have been reported for these sensors. Instead, some representative examples will be given. These are summarized in Table 2.6 and will be briefly described in the following paragraphs.

Liquid metal strain gauges are especially useful in biomedical applications because they are mechanically compliant and provide a better mechanical impedance match to most biomedical tissues than other types of strain gauges. By wrapping one of these strain gauges around a circumference of the abdomen it will stretch and contract with the abdominal breathing movements. The signal from the strain gauge can then be used to monitor breathing in patients or experimental animals. The advantage of this sensor is its compliance so that it does not interfere with the breathing movements or substantially increase the required breathing effort. Foil strain gauges can be used in

TABLE 2.6 Examples of Biomedical Applications of Physical Sensors

Sensor	Application	Signal Range	Reference
Liquid metal strain gauge	Breathing movement	0–0.05 (strain)	
	Limb plethysmography	0–0.02 (strain)	3
Magnetic displacement sensor	Breathing movement	0–10 mm	10
LVDT	Muscle contraction	0–20 mm	
	Uterine contraction sensor	0–5 mm	11
Load cell	Electronic scale	0–440 lbs (0–200 kg)	12
Accelerometer	Subject activity	0–20 m/s^2	13
Miniature silicon pressure sensor	Intraarterial blood pressure	0–50 Pa (0–350 mmHg)	
	Urinary bladder pressure	0–10 Pa (0–70 mmHg)	
	Intrauterine pressure	0–15 Pa (0–100 mmHg)	14
Electromagnetic flow sensor	Cardiac output (with integrator)	0–500 mL/min	
	Organ blood flow	0–100 mL/min	15

a similar way, but their limited displacement range and low compliance requires that they be used with some sort of a spring structure that will be more compliant and not interfere with breathing movement or effort.

One of the original applications of the liquid metal strain gauge was in limb plethysmography [3]. One or more of these sensors are wrapped around an arm or leg at various points and can be used to measure changes in circumference that are related to the cross-sectional area and hence the volume of the limb at those points. If the venous drainage from the limb is occluded, the limb volume will increase as it fills with blood. Releasing the occlusion allows the volume to return to normal. The rate of this decrease in volume can be monitored using the liquid metal strain gauges, and this can be used to identify venous blockage when the return to baseline volume is too slow.

Breathing movements, although not volume, can be seen using a simple magnetic velocity detector. By placing a small permanent magnet on the anterior side of the chest or abdomen and a flat, large-area coil on the posterior side opposite from the magnet, voltages are induced in the coil as the chest of abdomen moves during breathing. The voltage itself can be used to detect the presence of breathing movements, or it can be electronically integrated to give a signal related to displacement.

The LVDT is a displacement sensor that can be used for applications that require more precise measurements. For example, it can be used in studies of muscle physiology where one wants to measure the displacement of a muscle or where one is measuring the isometric force generated by the muscle (using a load cell) and must ensure that there is no muscle movement. It can also be incorporated into other physical sensors, such as a pressure sensor or a tocodynamometer, a sensor used to electronically "feel" uterine contractions of patients in labor or those at risk of premature labor and delivery.

In addition to studying muscle forces, load cells can be used in various types of electronic scales for weighing patients or studying animals. The simplest electronic scale consists of a platform placed on top of a load cell. The weight of any object placed on the platform will produce a force that can be sensed by the load cell. In some critical care situations in the hospital, it is important to carefully monitor the weight of a patient. For example, this is important in watching water balance in patients receiving fluid therapy or peritoneal dialysis. The electronic scale concept can be extended by placing a load cell under each leg of the patient's bed and summing the forces seen by each load cell to get the total weight of the patient and the bed. Because the bed weight remains fixed, weight changes seen will reflect changes in patient weight which are often associated with fluid retention or loss.

Accelerometers can be used to measure patient or research subject activity. By attaching a small accelerometer to the individual being studied, any movements can be detected. This can be useful in sleep studies where movement can help to determine the sleep state. Miniature accelerometers and recording devices can also be worn by patients to study activity patterns and determine effects of disease or treatments on patient activity [15].

Miniature silicon pressure sensors are used for the indwelling measurement of fluid pressure in most body cavities. The measurement of intraarterial blood pressure is the most frequent application, but pressures in other cavities such as the urinary bladder and the uterus are also measured. The small size of these sensors and the resulting ease of introduction of the sensor into the cavity make these sensors important for these applications.

The electromagnetic flow sensor has been a standard method in use in the physiology laboratory for many years [16]. Its primary application has been for measurement of cardiac output and blood flow to specific organs in research animals. Miniature inverted electromagnetic flow sensors make it possible to temporarily introduce a flow probe into an artery through its lumen to make clinical measurements.

The measurement of body temperature using instruments employing thermistors as the sensor has greatly increased in recent years. Rapid response times of these low-mass sensors make it possible to quickly assess patients' body temperatures so that more patients can be evaluated in a given period. This can then help to reduce healthcare costs. Inexpensive versions of electronic thermometers have replaced mercury in glass thermometers because the latter have the risk of mercury exposure if broken. The rapid response time of low-mass thermistors makes them a simple sensor to be used for sensing breathing. By placing small thermistors near the nose and mouth, the elevated temperature of exhaled air can be sensed to document a breath [10].

The potential applications of physical sensors in medicine and biology are almost limitless. To be able to use these devices, however, scientists must first be familiar with the underlying sensing principles [17,18,21–23]. It is then possible to apply these in a form that addresses the problems at hand.

References

1. Doebelin E.G. 2003. *Measurement Systems: Applications and Design,* New York, McGraw-Hill.
2. Dechow P.E. and Wang, Q. 2006. Strain gauges. In J. Webster (Ed.), *Encyclopedia of Medical Devices and Instrumentation,* Vol. 6: pp. 282–290, New York, John Wiley & Sons.
3. Whitney R.J. 1949. The measurement of changes in human limb-volume by means of a mercury in-rubber strain gauge. *F. Physiol.* 109: 5.
4. Schaevitz H. 1947. The linear variable differential transformer. *Proc. Soc. Stress Anal.* 4: 79.
5. Reddy N.P. and Kesavan S.K. 2006. Linear variable differential transformers. In J. Webster (Ed.), *Encyclopedia of Medical Devices and Instrumentation,* Vol. 4: pp. 252–257, New York, John Wiley & Sons.
6. Stegall H.F., Kardon M.B., Stone H.L. et al. 1967. A portable simple sonomicrometer. *J. Appl. Physiol.* 23: 289.
7. Geddes L.A. 1991. *Handbook of Blood Pressure Measurement,* Totowa, NJ, Humana.
8. Roberts V.E. 1972. *Blood Flow Measurements,* Baltimore, Williams & Wilkins.
9. Herzfeld E.M. (Ed.). 1962. *Temperature: Its Measurement and Control in Science and Industry,* New York, Reinhold.
10. Sekey A. and Seagrave E. 1981. Biomedical subminiature thermistor sensor for analog control by breath flow, *Biomater. Med. Dev. Artif Organs* 9: 73–90
11. Angelsen B.A. and Brubakk A.O. 1976. Transcutaneous measurement of blood flow velocity in the human aorta. *Cardiovasc. Res.* 10: 368.
12. Rolfe P. 1971. A magnetometer respiration monitor for use with premature babies. *Biomed. Eng.* 6: 402.
13. Roe P.C. 1966. New equipment for metabolic studies. *Nurs. Clin. N. Am.* 1: 621.
14. Fleming D.G., Ko W.H., and Neuman M.R. (Eds.) 1977. *Indwelling and Implantable Pressure Transducers,* Cleveland, CRC Press.
15. Patterson S.M., Krantz D.S., Montgomery L.E. et al. 1993. Automated physical activity monitoring: Validation and comparison with physiological and self-report measures. *Psychophysiology* 30: 296.
16. Wyatt D.G. 1971. Electromagnetic blood flow measurements. In B.W. Watson (Ed.), *IEE Medical Electronics Monographs,* London, Peregrinus.
17. Bently J.P. 2005. *Principles of Measurement Systems* 4th ed., Englewood Cliffs, NJ, Pearson Prentice-Hall.
18. Webster J.G. 1999. *Mechanical Variables Measurement—Solid, Fluid, and Thermal,* Boca Raton, FL, CRC Press.
19. Michalski L., Eckersdorf K., Kucharski J., and McGhee J. 2001. *Temperature Measurement,* 2nd ed., New York, John Wiley & Sons.
20. Childs P.R.N. 2001. *Practical Temperature Measurement,* Oxford, Butterworth-Heinemann.
21. Webster J.G. (Ed.) 2004. *Bioinstrumentation,* New York, John Wiley & Sons.
22. Ratha N.K. and Govindaraju V. (Eds.) 2008. *Advances in Biometrics: Sensors, Algorithms and Systems,* London, Springer.
23. Harsányi G. 2000. Sensors in *Biomedical Applications: Fundamentals, Technology & Applications,* Boca Raton, FL, CRC Press.

Further Information

Good overviews of physical sensors are available in the following books: Doebelin E.O. 2003. *Measurement Systems: Application and Design,* 4th ed., New York, McGraw-Hill; Harvey, G.P. (Ed.). 1969. *Transducer Compendium,* 2nd ed., New York, Plenum. One can also find good descriptions of physical sensors in chapters of two works edited by John Webster. Chapters 2, 7, and 8 of his textbook (2010) *Medical Instrumentation: Application and Design,* 4th ed., New York, John Wiley & Sons, and several articles in his *Encyclopedia on Medical Devices and Instrumentation,* published by Wiley in 1988, cover topics on physical sensors. Although a bit old, the text *Transducers for Biomedical Measurements* (New York, John Wiley & Sons, 1974) by Richard S.C. Cobbold, remains one of the best descriptions of biomedical sensors available. By supplementing the material in this book with recent manufacturers' literature, the reader can obtain a wealth of information on physical (and for that matter chemical) sensors for biomedical application. The journals *IEEE Transactions on Biomedical Engineering and Medical and Biological Engineering and Computing* are good sources of recent research on biomedical applications of physical sensors. The journal *Physiological Measurement and Sensors and Actuators* is also a good source for this material as well as papers on the sensors themselves. The *IEEE Sensors Journal* covers different types of sensors, but biomedical devices are included in its scope.

The international journal *Medical and Biological Engineering and Computing* is published bimonthly by the International Federation for Medical and Biological Engineering. This journal also contains frequent reports on biomedical sensors and related topics. Subscription information can be obtained from Peter Peregrinus Ltd., P.O. Box 96, Stevenage, Herts SG12SD, United Kingdom.

The journal *Biomedical Instrumentation and Technology* is published by the Association for the Advancement of Medical Instrumentation. This bimonthly journal has reports on biomedical instrumentation for clinical applications, and these include papers on biomedical sensors.

There are also several scientific meetings that include biomedical sensors. The major meetings in the area include the international conference of the IEEE Engineering in Medicine and Biology Society and the Annual Meeting of the Biomedical Engineering Society. Extended abstracts for these meetings are published on CD-ROM each year.

3

Magnetic and Radio Frequency Induction Sensors

Brandon D. Pereles
Michigan Technological University

Keat Ghee Ong
Michigan Technological University

Magnetic materials and principles form the basis for many sensors and sensing transduction mechanisms. For example, the linear variable differential transformer (LVDT) is a widely used displacement sensors made of simple ferromagnetic materials and electromagnetic coils that operate on the principle of magnetic induction. Despite their simplicity, LVDTs have seen long-term use in many areas, including biomedical applications because of their cost-effectiveness and robustness in harsh environments. Another good example of a sensor comprised of unique magnetic materials is the magnetoelastic resonant sensor, which converts mass variations into remotely detectable magnetic field changes. Similarly, electromagnetic induction provides the foundation for sensor platforms as a signal carrier to wirelessly and passively transmit sensor information to the user. An illustrative example is the radio frequency identification (RFID) sensor, which uses electromagnetic waves at the radio frequency range to remotely power and receive information wirelessly from miniature sensors.

This chapter describes the operating principle, fabrication, and application of a variety of sensors made of magnetic materials and based on the principle of electromagnetic induction. To well describe these systems, fundamental magnetic principles, such as magnetic induction theory and material properties, are also briefly described along with representative examples of these sensors and their applications, with a focus on the area of biomedical engineering.

3.1 Magnetic Induction-Based Sensors

Faraday's induction law, as a fundamental magnetic principle, states that a voltage across a closed electrically conducting loop is proportional to the time rate of change of the magnetic flux that passes through it. By coupling this phenomenon with different types of magnetic materials, several unique sensors, mostly applied to tracking displacement, dimension changes, or stress/pressure, have been designed and successfully deployed in biomedical applications. This section introduces Faraday's induction law and the basic properties of magnetic materials, followed by descriptions of some related sensors and their biomedical applications.

3.1.1 Magnetic Induction and Magnetic Materials

According to Faraday's induction law, an electromotive force (emf) or voltage will be induced in a closed-path electrical circuit if there is a change of magnetic flux linking to the circuit. In equation form, Faraday's law is expressed as

$$\text{emf} = -A\frac{dB}{dt} \tag{3.1}$$

where A is the surface area and B is the magnetic flux. Faraday's induction law is the fundamental operating principle for devices such as variable differential transformers (VDT), where changes in voltage are measured as a result of variations in the induced magnetic fields from changes in the position of a ferromagnetic material.

Most magnetic-based sensors rely on materials with strong magnetic properties to function. Additionally, although all materials exhibit unique magnetization behavior, the most useful materials for magnetic induction sensors are ferromagnetic or ferrimagnetic. These materials are self-saturating, or "spontaneously magnetized," in the absence of an external field, resulting in the generation of a magnetic field. However, to minimize their energy potential, these materials contain many small regions called "domains," which spontaneously magnetize but orient themselves in different directions resulting in a net zero macroscopic magnetization. When an external field is applied, these domains align with the field, and a large magnetization is observed. If the sample is free from structural defects and stress, the magnetization will return to zero when the applied field is removed; this type of material is classified as "magnetically soft." Conversely, materials with structural defects that prevent the magnetization from returning to zero are "magnetically hard," making them excellent permanent magnets.

The magnetization process of a magnetic material causes the generation of additional magnetic flux B by an applied field H characterized by the magnetic permeability μ, where

$$B = \mu H \tag{3.2}$$

For ferromagnetic and ferrimagnetic materials, μ is a nonlinear function depending on the previous state of magnetization (hysteresis). Figure 3.1 plots B versus H, known as the BH loop, where μ is the tangent of the curve at different operating values of H. The BH loop begins with an initial curve obtained by applying a field to a demagnetized sample. As the field increases, the sample magnetizes until reaching the saturation magnetization B_s. When the H field is reduced to zero, the magnetization does not completely decrease, but instead remains at the magnetic remanence B_r. The magnetization becomes zero only when H reaches the coercive field, $H = -H_c$. As the H field continues to decrease, the sample saturates at $-B_s$. When the H field increases again, the BH curve reaches B_r, H_c, and B_s sequentially, although by taking a different path from that of the original curve. One may notice important features of a typical BH curve such as shown in Figure 3.1. Specifically, the BH curve is nonlinear with a characteristic that saturates in the positive and negative directions. Additionally, the curve seen with increasing applied magnetic field differs from the curve seen with a decreasing applied magnetic field. This hysteresis is characterized by the area within the BH loop.

Magnetically soft materials have a low coercivity ($H_c < 1000$ A/m) and high permeability because of their reversible magnetization and correspondingly low hysteresis loss. They are largely used in field

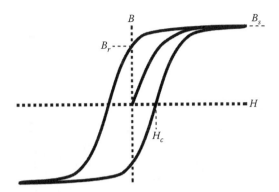

FIGURE 3.1 A *BH* loop of a magnetic sample showing the saturation magnetization B_s, remenance B_r, and coercive force H_c.

sensors, power transformers, induction motors, and so on. Soft magnetic materials include various crystalline alloys, such as iron–nickel (FeNi) alloys (Permalloy, Supermalloy, Mumetal), cobalt–iron (CoFe) alloys, and silicon steels (SiFe). Another class of magnetically soft material consists of amorphous alloys, specifically those containing iron, nickel, and cobalt with stabilizing elements, such as silicon, boron, and molybdenum. Magnetically soft amorphous alloys are also made with transition metals (Zr, Nb, Hf) or rare earth metals (Tb, Dy, Er, Gd).

Magnetically hard materials, however, are categorized by their large coercive force (10^4–10^6 A/m), making them hard to magnetize and giving them large magnetic remanence. This allows them to have a significant spontaneous magnetization under zero applied field. Early magnets, such as magnetite (Fe_3O_4) and iron carbon magnets (Fe_3C), were iron based and later replaced by tungsten, Co–Mo, Co–Cr, and Alnico (Fe_2NiAl) magnets. Today, most magnetically hard materials are rare earth–transition metal magnets, such as $SmCo_5$, R_2Co_7, and $Sm_2(CoFe)_{17}$. These materials are generally applied as permanent magnets and in magnetic data storage devices and sensors.

3.1.2 Variable Differential Transformer (VDT) Sensors

VDTs, based on mutual inductance coupling between two or more magnetic coils, have been in use since the early 20th century and provide precise force and displacement sensing. The basic structure of a VDT device, as illustrated in Figure 3.2, consists of a primary coil and two secondary coils. An ac signal is sent through the primary coil, resulting in an induced voltage in the secondary coils (Nyce 2004). By introducing a magnetic permeable core, the inductance of the secondary coils alters as a function of their proximity to the core. Position measurements are achieved by observing the difference in the ac output from the secondary coils (Nyce 2004). VDT sensors are widely used for their linear output, high resolution and sensitivity, ruggedness, low hysteresis and power consumption, and resistance to high temperatures and pressures (Wolf 1979). There are two main types of VDT devices: linear (LVDTs) and rotatory-variable differential transformers (RVDTs). The difference between the systems is how the magnetic core moves: in an LVDT, the core moves between the coils in a straight line (i.e., linearly), whereas the RVDT rotates for angular displacement measurements (Silva 2005).

LVDTs find numerous applications in the medical field. In hospitals, LVDT sensors were used to monitor the displacement of a CPR manikin during chest compression on pliable surfaces, such as mattresses (Noordergraaf et al. 2009). In medical research, LVDT sensors were used to measure the thermal expansion of a blood vessel under low cryogenic conditions (Rios and Rabin 2006). LVDTs have also been incorporated into implants. For example, a sensor for monitoring micromotion and migration in total knee and total hip arthroplasty implants was realized with a modified LVDT consisting of two coaxial cylindrical coils and two pairs of resistors forming a Wheatstone bridge. The hip model

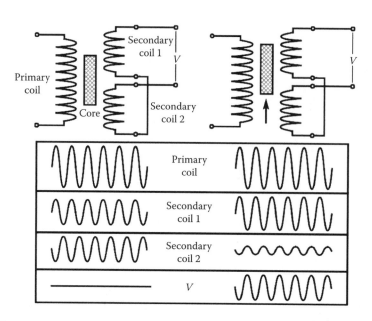

FIGURE 3.2 Illustration of the basic operating principle of linear variable differential transformer displacement sensors. When the core is positioned at the exact center between secondary coils 1 and 2, the differential voltage between the two secondary coils, *V*, is zero. Movement of the core creates an imbalance, increasing *V*. The signals at the primary coil, secondary coils 1 and 2, and the differential voltage *V* are also shown.

positioned the LVDT in the bone cavity with the coils attaching to the bone and a ferrite rod (the core) connecting to the implant. The movement of the implant caused the ferrite rod to move and thus altered the mutual inductance of the coils (Hao et al. 2008).

LVDTs were used as pressure sensors by connecting the coils to a reference pressure point and the core to a pressure responsive flexible membrane. Just like a diaphragm pressure sensor, the membrane of the capsule deflected under pressure, moving the core and changing the mutual inductance of the secondary coils (Wheeler and Ganji 2009). The same principle was applied to physiological monitoring systems, such as a catheter-tip blood pressure measurement device (Rao and Guha 2001).

Not surprisingly, LVDTs have also been deployed for monitoring vibrations, which are essentially time-varying displacements. An LVDT was connected to the sensor structure such that movement in the sensor caused the core of the LVDT to displace, allowing real-time tracking of vibration amplitude and frequency (Wheeler and Ganji 2009). For medical sensing, this technique has been applied to monitor the effects of vibrations on the human body (Rao and Guha 2001).

3.1.3 Magnetic Markers for Biosensing

Magnetic particles have been used as markers for chemical or microbial detection as they are easily detected through magnetic fields. Compared to other chemical or microbial detection techniques, such as polymerase chain reaction (PCR), ELISA, lateral flow assay, and flow cytometry, magnetic markers are simpler and cheaper to operate and easier to incorporate in portable measuring instruments. This allows the development of point-of-care diagnostic systems that have a high degree of mobility. Magnetic particles are often functionalized to specifically bind to target antigens or analytes. Highly specific antibodies, proteins, phages, and other microbial affinity materials are generally used as the functionalization agents, thus playing a direct role in determining the reliability and sensitivity of the sensor. Magnetic particles are made of iron oxide (magnetite) and are commonly available in different sizes, ranging from nanometers to micrometers, for a variety of applications. To achieve a high degree of reactivity and improve the sensing quality, they are often fabricated to have a high surface area to volume ratio. In addition, magnetic particle cores are frequently coated with a layer of organic polymer, such as polyvinyl alcohol (PVA) (Meyer et al. 2007a, Oster et al. 2001), to provide a different surface for functionalization and improve biocompatibility.

Traditionally, magnetic particles were primarily used for preparing samples before measurements with other techniques. For instance, magnetic particles were used to enhance the sensitivity of a fluorescent method for antigen detection (Alefantis et al. 2004). As shown in Figure 3.3, functionalized magnetic particles were used to extract targeted antigens from a sample solution followed by the addition of fluorophore substances that bound to the targets. The intensity of light emission was measured to give the concentration of the targeted antigens. Because only magnetic particles coated with the correct antibodies bind to the extracted antigens, this technique provides a better sensitivity and selectivity compared to standard fluorescent methods.

In recent years, magnetic particles have been increasingly exploited as markers for direct quantification of bacteria by measuring their magnetic signals. When magnetic particles are exposed to a magnetic field generated by an inductive coil, they alter the magnetic field, the degree of which is monitored in terms of measured voltage. Quantification of analytes with magnetic markers is more favorable than conventional techniques mainly because they are less expensive, easy to handle, consume less time, and exhibit remote control and query nature. Furthermore, the specificity of magnetic markers can be enhanced by controlling the applied magnetic field, a process known as "magnetic washing" (Baselt et al. 1998). As a result, specific and nonspecific analytes are easily differentiated by simply varying the applied magnetic field.

In clinical and research studies, nanosized magnetic particles are often interrogated with superconducting quantum interference devices (SQUIDs) because of their high sensitivity (Flynn et al. 2007). Another technique to monitor magnetic particles is the ABICAP column. As illustrated in Figure 3.4, the ABICAP column consists of an ABICAP filter commonly made of polyethylene capable of experiencing further modification to bind with specific antibodies. When the sample solution is added into the column, target analytes bind to the antibody coated on the ABICAP filter. Following this, secondary antibody-coated magnetic beads are added into the column, with subsequent binding of secondary antibodies to bound antigens immobilizing the magnetic particles. Changes in magnetic flux because of incoming magnetic particles can then be measured with a detection coil, which indirectly quantifies the concentration of targeted antigens. This technique has been used for detecting microbial species including *Yersinia pestis* (Meyer et al. 2007a) and *Francisella tularensis* (Meyer et al. 2007b).

For certain applications, magnetic particles are not directly used in bacterial quantification but simply act as a means to assist other techniques for bacterial detection. Magnetic particles are used as components to enhance the sensitivity of detection techniques by specifically selecting target analytes. In

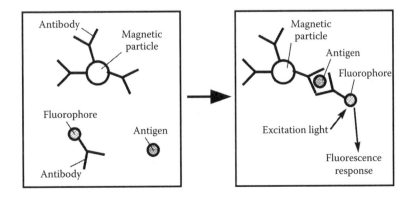

FIGURE 3.3 Diagram illustrating binding of functionalized magnetic particles to target analytes and subsequent binding of fluorophore to target analytes.

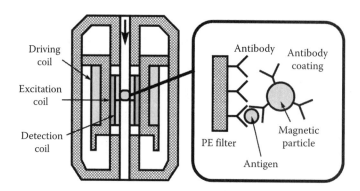

FIGURE 3.4 Schematic diagram of an ABICAP column and binding of target analytes to primary (capturing) antibody and secondary-antibody-coated magnetic beads.

some assays that require multiple washing steps, the utilization of magnetic particles reduces or shortens the washing step thereby decreasing damage and degradation to and of the analytes, respectively. Functionalized magnetic particles also enhance the sensitivity of ELISA while maintaining accuracy by specifically selecting targeted antigens before proceeding to the following steps (Nagasaki et al. 2007, Chou et al. 2001). For example, to detect the HLA-B27 antigen, Chou and coworkers used anti-B27-coated magnetic particles to first extract B27-positive cells, isolating them from peripheral blood mononuclear cells before identification with ELISA (Chou et al. 2001).

3.1.4 Sensors Based on Magnetic Harmonic Field Tuning

A sensing mechanism was realized by tracking the response of a magnetically soft material placed adjacent to a position-varying permanent magnet. While under the excitation of an ac magnetic field, the magnetically soft material generated higher order harmonic fields because of its magnetic softness (low energy loss with large and nonlinear magnetization). Because the amplitudes of the higher order harmonic fields were also dependent on the magnitude of a constant (dc) magnetic field, the magnetically soft material generated a harmonic field pattern when exposed to a varying dc field along with the ac field (see Figure 3.5a). The dc field dependency of the harmonic fields can be explained with the *BH* loop. In the absence of a dc field, the ac excitation field forces the magnetic material to exhibit an odd symmetry magnetization (see Figure 3.6a), resulting in the generation of maximum odd harmonic fields and zero even harmonic fields (see Point A in Figure 3.5a). When a dc field is applied, the odd symmetry of the *BH* curve is destroyed (see Figure 3.6b), resulting in the increase in even harmonic fields and decrease in the odd harmonic fields (see Point B in Figure 3.6a).

Placing a permanent magnet adjacent to the magnetically soft material shifted the pattern of the higher order harmonic field depending on the separation distance. The effect of the permanent magnet is similar to exerting a secondary dc field along with the excitation ac and dc fields, thus shifting the harmonic field pattern as shown in Figure 3.5b (the shift is quantified by H_z). By designing the sensor such that the separation distance varied with a parameter of interest, wireless sensors, known as magnetic harmonic sensors, have been developed to measure pressure, stress, liquid flow rate, and even chemicals by tracking the shift in the harmonic pattern.

Magnetic harmonic sensors allowed for monitoring of stress/strain by relating shifts in the magnetic higher order harmonic fields (H_z) to applied stress/strain. For this sensor to function, a deformable material was situated between the magnetically soft material and the permanent magnet as shown in Figure 3.7a. As the material deformed under a compressive stress, the separation between the sensing and biasing elements decreased, resulting in an observable shift in the higher order harmonic field pattern allowing for the monitoring of stress/strain in a structure (Tan et al. 2008).

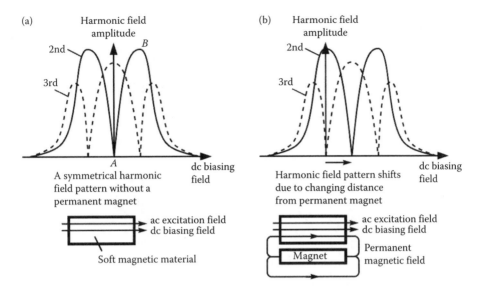

FIGURE 3.5 The higher order harmonic fields, generated by a soft magnetic material under a constant ac magnetic field, change their amplitudes when a dc magnetic (biasing) field is also applied. The higher order harmonic field versus dc biasing field plots have a distinct pattern as shown in (a). When a magnet is placed adjacent to the soft magnetic material, it generates an additional field that shifts the harmonic field pattern shown in (b).

For pressure monitoring, the magnetically soft material was adhered to the bottom of an airtight chamber and the permanent magnet was attached to a flexible rubber membrane (see Figure 3.7b). Deflection of the membrane because of pressure variations altered the separation distance between these two magnetic elements, shifting the observed magnetic harmonic field (Pereles et al. 2008). A flow sensor was also realized by attaching the magnetically soft material to the side of a flow channel at an angle to the permanent magnet across the channel (see Figure 3.7c, top cover not shown). Increasing the flow rate deflected the magnetically soft material away from the permanent magnet, resulting in a shift of the magnetic higher order harmonic field for tracking the flow rate (Pereles et al. 2009).

In addition to physical parameters, chemical sensing was also accomplished by applying a chemically sensitive hydrogel made of (poly)vinyl alcohol and (poly)acrylic acid (PVA/PAA) hydrogel between the magnetically soft material and a permanent magnet (see Figure 3.7d) (Horton et al. 2009). The pH in the test solution caused the hydrogel's dimensions to change, thus varying the separating distance between the two magnetic elements. This in turn altered the shift in the magnetic higher order harmonic field allowing for remote tracking of pH variations (Horton et al. 2009).

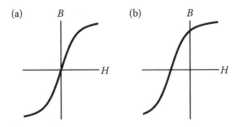

FIGURE 3.6 The *BH* curve of a soft magnetic material while (a) under zero dc magnetic field and (b) biased by a dc magnetic field.

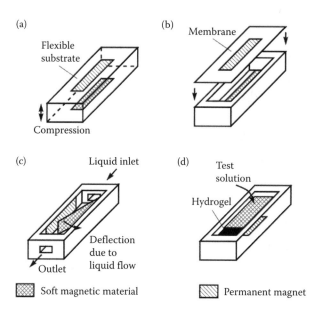

FIGURE 3.7   Various designs of magneto-harmonic sensors for measuring (a) stress/strain, (b) pressure, (c) liquid flow, and (d) pH.

3.2 Magnetoelasticity for Biosensing

Magnetostriction is a phenomenon where the dimensions of a magnetic object change when subjected to the influence of an external magnetic field. The magnetostriction of a material is generally quantified by the saturation magnetostriction λ_s, defined as the ratio of the change in length, Δl, from the original length, l, expressed as a strain at magnetic saturation. In contrast, the magnetoelastic effect describes the coupling between elastic energy and magnetic energy and is usually quantified with the magnetoelastic coupling coefficient k, defined as the ratio of the coupled elastic–magnetic energy to the pure elastic and magnetic energies. Magnetoelastic and magnetostriction effects are related but not necessarily proportional to one another because of the influence of other parameters, such as applied stress and annealing conditions. For example, rare-earth-based alloys have a very high λ_s, but their magnetoelastic coupling is lower than the Fe-rich alloys having a lower λ_s.

The most common magnetoelastic materials are rare-earth intermetallic compounds and amorphous magnetically soft ferromagnetic glasses. Crystalline rare-earth intermetallic compounds, such as Terfenol-D ($Tb_{0.3}Dy_{0.7}Fe_{5.95}$), have a magnetostriction on the order of 10^{-3}, a magnetoelastic coupling of $k = 0.7$, and a low compliance. As a result, such materials are useful actuators for a range of applications, including sonar transducers. Amorphous ferromagnetic alloys, with high iron content, exhibit magnetostrictions on the order of 10^{-5}, and a magnetoelastic coupling close to 1 after annealing. Amorphous ferromagnetic alloys are widely used as stress/strain sensors, field sensors, and as cores of power transformers.

Different types of sensors have been realized based on the principle of magnetoelasticity. A magnetoelastic material can be directly used to quantify parameters such as stress and pressure by measuring the changes in magnetization behavior. Conversely, a class of mass and elasticity sensors, known as magnetoelastic resonant sensors, monitor stress/pressure in addition to performing chemical and biological detection, with proper functionalization. In this case, there is a shift in frequency related to their elasticity change secondary to a mass change because of the analyte.

3.2.1 Magnetoelastic Resonant Sensors

Made of amorphous ferromagnetic ribbons, magnetoelastic resonant sensors are highly attractive for physical, chemical, and biological monitoring not only because of their small size and low cost but also because of their passive and wireless nature. Magnetoelastic resonant sensors are commonly used to measure physical parameters, such as stress, pressure, and strain. By applying a mass and/or an elasticity-changing biological-responsive layer, magnetoelastic sensors become ideal for measuring biological targets such as *Escherichia coli* O157:H7 (Ruan et al. 2003a) and chemical markers such as ricin by detecting changes in the resonant behavior because of the analyte of interest. The sensors mechanically vibrate at the frequency of an applied magnetic field, with the greatest vibration amplitude occurring at the mechanical resonant frequency of the sensor. As illustrated in Figure 3.8, the mechanical vibrations of the sensor produce a time-varying magnetic flux that can be observed remotely by a detection coil. The sensor can be interrogated by performing a frequency sweep to obtain the resonant spectrum (Zeng et al. 2002). Alternatively, the sensor can also be interrogated using a transient frequency-counting operation (Zeng et al. 2002), which first excites the sensor at a frequency near the resonant frequency of the sensor, and then captures the transient response of the sensor to determine the resonant frequency. The resonant frequency, f_0, of an unmodified sensor is related to its mechanical properties and physical length as (Grimes et al. 2002)

$$f_0 = \frac{1}{2L} \sqrt{\frac{E}{\rho}} \tag{3.3}$$

where L is the sensor length, ρ is the density of the sensor, and E is the elasticity of the sensor. Applying a mass changing coating to the sensor alters the resonant frequency in response to an analyte of interest. For small mass loads, the change in resonant frequency Δf is given by (Grimes et al. 2002)

$$\Delta f = -f_0 \frac{\Delta m}{2M} \tag{3.4}$$

where M is the mass of the sensor and Δm is the mass load. Based on Equation 3.4, magnetoelastic sensors can be used to directly measure mass loading (or stress and strain). Additionally, by applying chemical and/or biological affinity coatings, which specifically increase mass loading in response to a target chemical or biological agent, the sensor platform can be used for biological and chemical sensing.

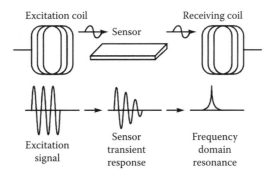

FIGURE 3.8 Schematic drawing illustrating the remote query nature of the passive, wireless magnetoelastic sensor. Magnetic field pulses, at a frequency near the resonant frequency of the sensor, are generated to vibrate the sensor. The excitation field is then turned off allowing the sensor to continue vibration at its resonant frequency. The transient sensor response is then converted to the frequency domain to extract the resonant information.

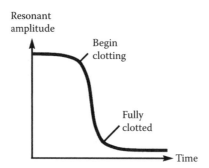

FIGURE 3.9   The response of a magnetoelastic sensor, while immersed in a clotting blood sample, allowed for the determination of blood coagulation time and the clotting profile.

3.2.1.1 Physical Monitoring

In medical research, magnetoelastic sensors have been used to measure viscosity change during blood clotting to precisely determine blood coagulation time, which is critical for therapeutic anticoagulants. As shown in Figure 3.9, soft fibrin clot formation on the surface changes the damping, shifting the characteristic resonant frequency and resonant amplitude, thereby enabling real-time continuous monitoring of the biological event. Benefits of the magnetoelastic sensor system for this application include requiring only a very small volume of blood samples and the noncontact nature of the electronic detection system, rendering it a viable option for portable blood coagulation monitoring (Puckett et al. 2003). In addition to coagulation time, magnetoelastic sensors can also monitor the coagulation and/or dissolution profile of blood, allowing for the observation of hemostasis (Puckett et al. 2005).

3.2.1.2 Chemical Detection

Magnetoelastic sensing technology has also been developed for pH monitoring in various biomedical applications, such as remote gastric/esophageal pH monitoring for the diagnosis of gastroesophageal reflux disease (GERD). GERD is a digestive disorder related to the retrograde movement of gastric acid into the esophagus from the stomach. The continuous monitoring of pH at the lower esophagus or in the stomach itself is useful in establishing a good GERD diagnosis. The magnetoelastic pH sensor consisted of a magnetoelastic sensor coated with a mass-changing pH-responsive polymer made of acrylic acid *iso*-octyl acrylate (Bouropoulos et al. 2005). While the sensor showed good response toward the pH by measuring the change in the resonant frequency, the polymer was sensitive to salt concentrations and altered the sensor response (Cai and Grimes 2000). A similar pH sensor was fabricated by spin coating poly (vinylbenzylchloride-*co*-2,4,5-trichlorophenyl acrylate) (VBC-TCPA) polymer spheres onto the surface of a magnetoelastic sensor (Ruan et al. 2003b). For the polymer spheres to attach to the metallic sensor surface, polyurethane resin was first dip coated as an adhesion promoting layer. Unlike the previous system, this device's response was mostly independent of the interfering potassium chloride concentration (Ruan et al. 2003b).

A glucose sensor was also developed by coimmobilizing glucose oxidase (GOD) and catalase onto a pH-sensitive-polymer-coated magnetoelastic sensor. The GOD catalyzes the hydrolyzation of glucose, producing gluconic acid and shrinking the pH-responsive polymer. The change in pH-sensitive-polymer dimension alters the resonant frequency of the sensor when tested with urine samples. Although the presence of acetaminophen, lactose, saccharose, and galactose does not significantly interfere with detection of glucose, interference from ascorbic acid was observed. The ascorbic acid effect can be eliminated through cross-correlation with a pH-responsive magnetoelastic reference sensor or by preadjusting the sample to pH 7 (Gao et al. 2007).

Magnetoelastic sensors have been used to detect chemicals for disease diagnosis. For example, a sensor was used to detect lithogenetic salts, such as calcium oxalate and brushite (Bouropoulos et al. 2005), major causes of kidney and bladder stones and the deposition of salts on urinary catheters and stents. The sensor was immobilized with a layer of starch gel for α-amylase detection (Wu et al. 2007a) for the diagnosis of acute pancreatitis. Magnetoelastic sensors have also been used to detect acid phosphatase (ACP) (Wu et al. 2007b), which has a great clinical significance in the diagnosis of hypophosphatasia, human prostatic disease, and prostate cancer. The sensor was coated with bovine serum albumin (BSA), followed by 5-bromo-4-chloro-3-indolyl phosphate (BCIP). ACP causes dephosphorylation of BCIP producing an insoluble blue BCIP dimer. This blue dimer strongly adsorbed on the sensor surface changes the mass loading of the sensor and decreases the resonant frequency (Wu 2008).

Magnetoelastic sensors have also been used to monitor environmental contaminants, such as organophosphate (OP) pesticide (Zourob et al. 2007). The sensor was immobilized by applying a pH-sensitive polymer coating and the enzyme OP hydrolase (OPH) onto the sensor surface. OPH catalyzes the hydrolysis of OP compounds, changing the pH in the hydrogel and causing the pH-responsive polymer to either swell or shrink. The sensor is capable of detecting paraoxane and parathion, a subclass of the highly toxic OP compound family, down to a detection limit of $10^{-6} \sim 10^{-7}$ M (Zourob et al. 2007).

3.2.1.3 Bacteria/Virus and Biotoxin Detection

Owing to their high sensitivity toward mass changes, magnetoelastic sensors have been used for the detection of bacteria/viruses and biotoxins. In most cases, biological responsive coatings are applied on the sensors to convert biological information to mass or elasticity variations.

The magnetoelastic sensor has been used to detect *Mycobacterium tuberculosis* (*M. TB*), the cause of tuberculosis (TB) and the world's second most common cause of morbidity and mortality from infectious disease. The sensor was immersed in a culture medium of *M. TB*. The growth and reproduction process produced changes in viscosity and density of the culture medium and, consequently, altered the resonant frequency of the sensor. The device showed logarithmic response proportional to the *M. TB* concentration in the range 10^4–10^9 cells/mL (Pang et al. 2008).

Magnetoelastic sensors have also been used for the detection of food pathogens, such as *Salmonella typhimurium*, *Escherichia coli* 0157:H7, and staphylococcal enterotoxin B (SEB). For the detection of *S. typhimurium*, a polyclonal antibody was immobilized onto the sensor surface. The binding of *S. typhimurium* bacteria to the antibody resulted in mass loading of the sensor, which in turn shifted the sensor's resonant frequency. Although the sensitivity of this sensor was size dependent, a detection limit of 5×10^3 cfu/mL was obtained for the smaller sensors (Guntupalli et al. 2007). The *E. coli* sensor was immobilized using affinity-purified antibodies attached to the surface. As illustrated in Figure 3.10, alkaline phosphatase (AP) was used as a labeled enzyme to the anti-*E. coli* O157:H7 antibody, which helped amplify the mass change by biocatalytic precipitation of BCIP to produce an insoluble dimer that was strongly bound to the surface. This increased the sensor mass loading, thus lowering the sensor's resonant frequency. The detection limit of the biosensor was 10^2 cells/mL with a linear response of up to 10^6 cells/mL (Ruan et al. 2003a). An SEB sensor was developed by immobilizing affinity-purified rabbit anti-SEB antibody on a magnetoelastic sensor surface. The affinity reaction of biotin–avidin and biocatalytic precipitation was used to amplify antigen–antibody binding events on the sensor surface. Horseradish peroxidase and AP were used as the labeled enzymes to induce biocatalytic precipitation with BCIP. The biosensor demonstrates a linear shift in resonant frequency with SEB concentration and a detection limit of 0.5 ng/mL (Ruan et al. 2004).

Magnetoelastic sensors have also been used for the detection of biological agents, such as *Bacillus anthracis* spores (anthrax) and ricin. *B. anthracis* are biological warfare agents that can cause death in humans. To detect *B. anthracis* spores in liquids, micro-sized, freestanding, magnetoelastic particles (MEPs) of iron–boron have been fabricated as sensors using microelectronic fabrication techniques. Affinity-selected filamentous bacteriophage for *B. anthracis* spores were used as the biomolecular recognition agents and were immobilized onto MEPs by physical adsorption. When exposed to dilute spore

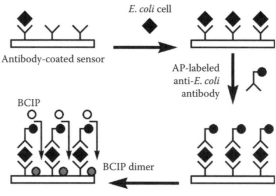

FIGURE 3.10   Schematic representation of the sandwich enzyme-linked immunosorbent assay procedure used with the magnetoelastic *E. coli* O157:H7 sensor.

solutions, the mass on the MEPs changed because of binding of bacteria, reducing the resonant frequency of the resonating particles. During in-liquid testing, a detection limit of 10^3 cfu/mL was reported (Wan et al. 2007).

Ricin, a highly toxic glycoprotein that can pose a serious health hazard resulting in death due to respiratory distress and hypoxemia, was also detected with magnetoelastic sensors by sandwiching a complex of antiricinus antibody-ricin AP and conjugated rabbit antiricinus antibody on the sensor surface. Detection was realized by biocatalytic precipitation of AP through specific binding of AP-antiricinus antibody to ricin in the sample. The sensor demonstrated linear resonant frequency shifts in the range of 10 ng/mL–100 μg/mL.

Magnetoelastic sensors have also been used for the detection of endotoxin, which can cause sepsis in immunocompromised patients. The system was based on the use of magnetoelastic sensors to monitor gel formation (clot formation), which changes the viscosity of the limulus amoebocyte lysate (LAL) assay in response to endotoxin. By correlating different endotoxin concentration and the LAL assay clot rate, it was found that the maximum clot rate was directly proportional to the endotoxin concentration. Endotoxin concentrations as low as 0.0105 EU/mL have been detected in approximately 20 min (Ong et al. 2006).

3.2.2 Magnetoelastic Stress/Strain Sensors

The magnetic properties of magnetoelastic materials change when exposed to an external loading force. By detecting this change via external coils, magnetoelastic stress/strain sensors have been realized (Arms and Townsend 2002), many of which have been used for biomedical applications such as monitoring of various joints, such as shoulder and knee, and lung ventilation (Klinger et al. 1992). In addition, magnetoelastic materials have been used to monitor healing of bone fractures by determining the stress/strain applied to sensors attached to the bone or to prostheses. The sensor detects changes in the axial stress seen on a prosthetic bone plate as the fracture heals by monitoring variations in the magnetic field, which are in turn affected by stress variations as the healing bone is able to support more of the stress (Oess et al. 2009).

Magnetoelastic materials were also used for noninvasive assessment of cardiovascular oscillations of the carotid artery as a skin curvature sensor (SC-sensor) (Kaniusas et al. 2008). The SC-sensor was fabricated with a bending-sensitive magnetoelastic bilayer partly enclosed by a coil. The bilayer consists of a magnetoelastic layer attached to a nonmagnetic counter layer such that when the bilayer is mechanically bent, its permeability changes and this variation transfers into a measurable signal. The sensor records alterations in artery radius through mechanical oscillations of the skin and thus provides relevant physiological data, such as cardiac and respiratory activities and blood pressure changes (Kaniusas et al. 2008).

Another biomedical application for magnetoelastic materials involves monitoring the laryngeal muscles for investigation of unilateral laryngeal paralysis. The sensor consisted of a ring-shaped magnetic circuit with a core made of a high susceptibility magnetostrictive amorphous ribbon surrounded by an excitation and pick-up coil. The sensor configuration was designed to respond to stresses along any direction of the insertion plane and the ring shape provided sensitivity to mechanical deformations along the ring plane. *In vivo* implantation in larynxes of dogs allowed for the detection of physiological functions in the larynx, such as phonation and deglutition. The simple sensor design and working principle make it a potential tool for measuring stresses inside any kind of muscle in the body (Pina et al. 2001).

3.3 Radio Frequency Identification Devices

A RFID system consists of a transceiver and one or more RFID tags communicating through high-frequency electromagnetic signals. The transceiver sends out a signal detected by the RFID tag whose response is acquired and interpreted by the transceiver (Domdouzis et al. 2007). Two main categories of RFID tags exist: read/write or read only and active or passive. A read/write tag allows for storing data and later "writing" over the information, whereas a read-only tag contains an unchangeable piece of unique data. Active tags are powered by an onboard supply, allowing for a longer detection range with detection of more tags and larger data storage. Passive tags are powered by an electromagnetic signal and have a shorter detection range. While they read fewer tags at a time and have more limited data storage capacity, passive tags require no power source and, as a result, are not limited by the size of a battery or the need to eventually replace the tag/battery over time (Domdouzis et al. 2007).

As a whole, RFID technology is robust, versatile, and easy to miniaturize, and can have a low cost per unit. Although the system is more complex compared to magnetic-based wireless sensor technologies, the capacity for coupling with other devices, data storage and transmission, and the versatility of the sensor platform as a wireless communication device make it a highly attractive technology for wireless sensing applications.

3.3.1 RFID for Biomedical Applications

The most common use of RFID technology in biomedical applications involves the tracking and location of objects and people. In hospitals, tags can take advantage of preexisting wireless networks to send and receive information allowing for hospital-wide tracking of patients, charts, doctors, and so on (Sangwan et al. 2005). This becomes especially useful for monitoring infants, who may be taken or accidentally swapped for someone else's baby, and patients who are likely to try and leave a designated area, such as those with dementia (Smith 2008). Another application in hospitals couples the RFID tag to a central database allowing for quick access to patient information, such as allergies, current medications being taken, and so on (Smith 2008), from multiple locations in the hospital (Dalton et al. 2005). RFID tags also have been employed to ensure proper matching and labeling of donated and transfused blood to improve safety during blood donation and transfusion (Dalton et al. 2005). Pharmaceutical companies use RFID tags to prevent counterfeit drug purchases (Dianmin et al. 2008) and hospitals can take advantage of this to track drugs from the factory all the way to the hospital and the patients taking them (Wu et al. 2005). RFID tags have even been used in dentures to allow for simple identification of bodies (Nuzzolese et al. 2010). Another application for hospitals embeds RFID tags into surgical equipment, such as sponges, allowing for localized tracking and identification of surgical objects and equipment before, during, and after a surgery (Gibbs et al. 2007). The system tracks tags with a wand containing an antenna attached to necessary equipment and sends and receives data via electromagnetic signals (Gibbs et al. 2007). Such technology can be useful in avoiding the problem of retained objects in surgical sites.

Most RFID sensors deployed as physical or chemical/biological sensors couple to other devices. For example, an RFID-based sensor system known as wireless identification and sensing platform (WISP) can utilize a variety of physical sensors for applications such as analysis of foot pronation while running. This particular sensor application allows for the analysis of running efficiency by using a 3D accelerometer from a WISP device powered by an RFID tag (Erickson et al. 2009). Similarly, a humidity-sensitive material was incorporated into an RFID tag for moisture monitoring. The tag demonstrates a change in power properties as increased absorption of moisture leads to an increase in the detuning of the sensor (Floerkemeier et al. 2010). An optical chemical sensor was coupled to an RFID chip by incorporating a thin sol–gel film with a pH-sensitive dye for wireless passive pH monitoring (Steinberg and Steinberg 2009). The sensor uses LEDs and a silicon photodiode to monitor changes in the optical absorption of the indicator dye. Collected data were then transmitted externally by the RFID tag (Steinberg and Steinberg 2009).

Several RFID sensors directly monitor physiological events. For instance, a system to monitor and utilize the electroencephalogram (brain waves) to restore body functions was developed for immobilized patients to interact with external devices such as computers and robotic arms. In this system, RFID tags were used for noninvasive collection of the EEG signal for controlling neurobotic prostheses and other devices (Eleni 2008). A similar system applies the RFID technology to power WISP for recording neural data. This device, referred to as NeuralWisp, was tested for feasibility by recording activity in the brains of macaque monkeys (Otis et al. 2009). RFID tags were also incorporated into a retinal prosthetic along with 1000 MEMS electrodes. The RFID tag acted as a wireless data transmitter and power source for the electrodes with the aim of restoring vision to the blind (Weiland et al. 2008). Another reported technology used a small coupled microphone or electrocardiogram to measure the heartbeat spike-pulse in laboratory rats and took advantage of the RFID technology to power the device and send data (Yamakawa et al. 2007).

Chemical and gas sensors for monitoring medically relevant analytes also make use of RFID technology. An RFID glucose sensor was developed for long-term wireless monitoring of insulin levels in diabetic patients without frequent blood drawing. The system consisted of RFID tags, typically embedded in animals for identification purposes, and a coupled glucose sensor. Sensor implantation occurs without surgery using a veterinary needle in an area such as the upper arm. The device could then be scanned with a low-frequency interrogator in a mobile phone, PDA, or a variety of other commonly used mobile devices (Moore 2009). In terms of gas sensing, a commercial metal-oxide CO_2 monitor with an RFID tag system for monitoring the carbon dioxide release of an infant was developed. The RFID sensors installed on the bars of a crib monitor the baby's breathing as an early warning system for sudden infant death syndrome (Cao et al. 2007).

In addition to medically relevant chemicals and gases, liquid monitoring for medical applications also makes use of RFID sensors. A radio frequency integrated circuit (RFIC) was combined with a wetness sensor for monitoring diapers in elderly patients and babies. The sensor could assist in notifying nurses and other staff when a patient incapable of changing themselves is in need of assistance, thus avoiding unnecessary rashes, discomfort, and other problems (Yang et al. 2008).

Not all RFID sensors are coupled to other technologies. Displacement tracking in a variety of structures was accomplished by observing the change in tag backscatter power and minimum reader transmitted power of a sensor tag attached to a metal plate (Bhattacharyya et al. 2009). The sensor functioned by monitoring the degradation of the tag signal due to an attached metal plate that interferes with signal transduction and affects the backscatter signal strength and the minimum power required to turn on the tag. As the distance between the RFID tag and the metal plate varied due to displacement in the structure the plate is adhered to, these parameters change as well and are interpreted as material deformation of the structure (Bhattacharyya et al. 2009).

3.4 Inductive–Capacitive Resonant Circuit Sensors

Generally, an inductive–capacitive resonant circuit (inductance and capacitance (LC) tank circuit) consists of an inductor and capacitor, with the inductor coupled to a nearby coil (see Figure 3.11). Changes in capacitance/inductance of the LC tank circuit are measured indirectly by observing changes in the resonant frequency by sensing circuit impedance through coupling with the coil, allowing for short range wireless sensing. If the inductance or capacitance of the circuit varies with a physiological variable of interest, for example, pressure, then a physical or biological/chemical sensor is realized by measuring the variations in resonant frequency, f_0, given by

$$ f_0 = \frac{1}{2\pi\sqrt{LC}} \tag{3.5} $$

where L and C are the inductance and capacitance, respectively.

As shown in Figure 3.12, LC sensors, as technology platforms, are small, easy to manufacture, reliable, and capable of not only being read through biologic tissue but can also provide a source of wireless passive power for a variety of implantable devices. In comparison to the RFID sensor technologies, the LC sensor is a simpler version of an inductively coupled sensor with no data storage or processing capacity.

LC tank circuits designed for *in vivo* pressure monitoring were originally developed by Stuart Mackay and Bob Merkevitch in the 1950s. The sensor consisted of a coil connected in parallel to a

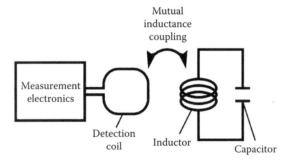

FIGURE 3.11 Illustration of the coupling between the inductive–capacitive resonant circuit and a detection coil.

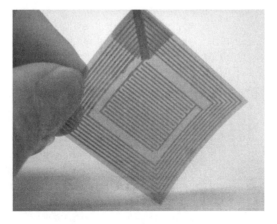

FIGURE 3.12 The inductive–capacitive sensor could be easily fabricated on a flexible substrate.

capacitor placed near a pressure-sensitive diaphragm with an attached magnetic material. As pressure deflects the diaphragm, the external magnetic field experienced by the sensor changes, resulting in measurable variations in sensor resonant frequency, which can be interpreted as pressure changes (Mackay 1983). Thirty-five years later, this device has been modified and refined and now finds use in a wide variety of medical applications. For instance, following an endovascular repair procedure, LC tank sensors, incorporated into stent devices, allow for the detection of an impending aortic aneurysm before the actual event occurs. The sensor consists of an LC circuit with a variable capacitance, which changes in relation to the pressure of the environment, allowing clinical personnel to wirelessly monitor patients postoperatively (Ohki et al. 2004). An intraocular pressure sensor was developed in both a variable capacitance form, by placing a capacitor plate on a deformable diaphragm, and a capacitive/inductive form, through placing the upper layer of the capacitor and inductor in a deformable diaphragm. As the pressure increases within the chamber, the separation distance between the capacitor and/or inductor components increases, resulting in a rise in the resonant frequency of the LC circuit, which can be interpreted as a change in pressure. The device was successfully tested in a 6-month animal study and is expected for use in clinical testing (Chen et al. 2008). Based on the same design, an LC pressure sensor was employed for continuous monitoring of pressure inside the bladder (Coosemans and Puers 2005).

For applications requiring a large sensing surface area, such as those measuring permittivity and conductivity of tissue, an interdigital capacitor was introduced as the capacitive element in an LC circuit. The change in capacitance resulted in a variation of the impedance and resonant frequency of the LC sensor, which can be interpreted as alterations in the permittivity and conductivity of tissue. The sensor was implanted into the phantom tissue and a saturation depth was achieved such that data were only collected from the tissue layer of interest (Yvanoff and Venkataraman 2009).

An LC circuit was also coupled with a varactor for *in vivo* biopotential monitoring. Electrodes sense the variation in biopotential, which was used to alter the bias voltage of the varactor, thus causing its capacitance to change. The alteration in capacitance caused a variation in the LC resonant frequency, which was reflected in the impedance of the detection coil (Riistama 2007).

Glucose-sensitive hydrogels coupled to LC circuits allow for wireless glucose monitoring. A two-plate capacitor, with one fixed and one mobile plate, incorporated into an LC circuit was designed such that the mobile plate attached to a glass membrane on one side and a hydrogel on the other. When exposed to a flowing media with changing glucose concentration, the hydrogel swelled/shrank causing a variation in the deflection of the glass membrane. This altered the separation distance between the capacitor plates, thereby changing the resonant frequency (Ziaie 2007).

A microdosimeter for monitoring radiation uses an LC variable capacitance circuit and an electret material. The sensor measured radiation as a function of the change in surface charge density resulting from attraction to the electret (Son and Ziaie 2006). The variable capacitor consisted of a fixed plate and a mobile plate. This structure changed as the mobile plate was attracted to the fixed plate due to the electric field between them. When exposed to ionizing radiation, the electret inside the capacitor collected the surface charge in the air gap between the capacitor plates, thus reducing the strength of the electric field and, as a result, the attractive force on the mobile plate. This change in plate separation distance altered the capacitance and, as a result, the resonant frequency of the LC circuit (Son and Ziaie 2006).

The LC tank circuit is also used as an energy scavenging unit and communication channel for implantable devices. For instance, an implantable drug delivery system was coupled with an LC tank circuit as an onboard battery for *in vivo* drug delivery. The device controlled drug release by selectively sending an electrical pulse stream between an anode and a cathode on either side of a drug reservoir sealed with a gold membrane. The pulse caused the gold membrane to oxidize and dissolve and thus release the contained drug. Two inductively coupled LC circuits provided power and communication to the device, improving upon a previous system requiring onboard power (Tang et al. 2008).

3.5 Conclusion

Magnetic and electromagnetic principles play an important role in biomedical sensing. From a common concept such as Faraday's induction law to magnetostriction, physical and chemical sensors have improved our ability to diagnosis many diseases and provide better long-term care for patients. Although this chapter describes various magnetic and electromagnetic-based sensor technologies and their biomedical application, these are just a sample of the many available technologies.

References

Alefantis T., Grewal P., Ashton J., Khan A.S., Valdes J.J., and Vecchio V.G.D. 2004. A rapid and sensitive magnetic bead-based immunoassay for the detection of staphylococcal enterotoxin B for high-throughput screening. *Molecular and Cellular Probes* 18:379–382.

Arms S.W. and Townsend C.P. 2002. Microminiature, temperature compensated, magnetoelastic strain gauge. *Smart Structures and Material: Smart Electronics, MEMS, and Nanotechnology* 4700:304–314.

Baselt D., Lee G.U., Natesan M., Metzger S.W., Sheehan P.E., and Colton R.J. 1998. A biosensor based on magnetoresistance technology. *Biosensors and Bioelectronics* 13:731.

Bhattacharyya R., Floerkemeier C., and Sarma S. 2009. Towards tag antenna based sensing: An RFID displacement sensor. *2009 IEEE International Conference on RFID*:95–102, Orlando, FL.

Bouropoulos N., Kouzoudis D., and Grimes C. 2005. The real-time, *in situ* monitoring of calcium oxalate and brushite precipitation using magnetoelastic sensors. *Sensors and Actuators B* 109:227–232.

Cai Q.Y. and Grimes C.A. 2000. A remote query magnetoelastic pH sensor. *Sensors and Actuators B* 71:112–117.

Cao H., Hsu L, Ativanichayaphong T., Sin J., Stephanou H.E., and Chiao J. 2007. An infant monitoring system using CO_2 sensors. *2007 IEEE International Conference on RFID*:134–140, Grapevine, TX.

Chen P., Rodger D.C., Saati S., Humayun M.S., and Tai Y. 2008. Implantable parylene-based wireless intraocular pressure sensor. *2008 21st IEEE International Conference on Micro Electro Mechanical Systems—MEMS '08*:58–61, Tucson, AZ.

Chou C., Tsai Y., Liu J., Wei J.C.C., Liao T., Chen M., and Liu L. 2001. The detection of the HLA-B27 antigen by immunomagnetic separation and enzyme-linked immunosorbent assay—Comparison with a flow cytometric procedure. *Journal of Immunological Methods* 255:15–22.

Coosemans J. and Puers, R. 2005. An autonomous bladder pressure monitoring system. *Sensors and Actuators A* 123–24:155–161.

Dalton J., Ippolito C., Poncet I., and Raffaele S.R. 2005. Using RFID technologies to reduce blood transfusion errors. *White Paper by Intel Corporation*, Autentica, Cisco Systems, and San Raffaele Hospital:8.

Dianmin Y., Xiaodan W., and Junbo B. 2008. RFID application framework for pharmaceutical supply chain. *2008 IEEE International Conference on Service Operations and Logistics, and Informatics (SOLI)*:1125–1130, Beijing, China.

Domdouzis, K., Kumar B., and Anumba C. 2007. Radio-frequency identification (RFID) applications: A brief introduction. *Advanced Engineering Informatics* 21:350–355.

Eleni A. 2008. Control of medical robotics and neurorobotic prosthetics by noninvasive brain-robot interfaces via EEG and RFID technology. *2008 8th IEEE International Conference on Bioinformatics and BioEngineering*:1–4, Athens, Greece.

Erickson V., Kamthe A.U., and Cerpa A.E. 2009. Measuring foot pronation using RFID sensor networks. *Proceedings of the 7th ACM Conference on Embedded Networked Sensor Systems*. Berkeley, California, ACM:325–326.

Floerkemeier C., Bhattacharyya R., and Sarma S. 2010. Beyond the ID in RFID. In *The Internet of Things*. Giusto D., Iera A., Morabito G., and Atzori L. (Eds.), Springer, New York:219–227.

Flynn E.R., Bryant H.C., Bergemann C., Larson R.S., Lovato D., and Sergatskov D.A. 2007. Use of a SQUID array to detect T-cells with magnetic nanoparticles in determining transplant rejection. *Journal of Magnetism and Magnetic Materials* 311:429–435.

Gao X., Yang W., Pang P., Liao S., Cai Q., Zeng K., and Grimes C.A. 2007. A wireless magnetoelastic biosensor for rapid detection of glucose concentrations in urine samples. *Sensors and Actuators B* 128:161–167.

Gibbs V.C., Coakley F.D., and Reines H.D. 2007. Preventable errors in the operating room: Retained foreign bodies after surgery—Part I. *Current Problems in Surgery* 44(5):281–337.

Grimes C.A., Mungle C.S., Zeng K., Jain M.K., Dreschel W.R., Paulose M., and Ong K.G. 2002. Wireless magnetoelastic resonance sensors: A critical review. *Sensors* 2:294–313.

Guntupalli R., Hu J., Lakshmanan R.S., Huang T.S., Barbaree J.M., and Chin B.A. 2007. A magnetoelastic resonance biosensor immobilized with polyclonal antibody for the detection of *Salmonella typhimurium*. *Biosensors and Bioelectronics* 22:1474–1479.

Hao S., Taylor J., Miles A.W., and Bowen C.R. 2008. An implantable system for the *in vivo* measurement of hip and knee migration and micromotion. *2008 International Conference on Signals and Electronic Systems (ICSES)*:445–448, Krakow, Poland.

Horton B. E., Pereles B. D., Tan E. L., and Ong K. G. 2009. A wireless, passive pH sensor based on magnetic higher-order harmonic fields. *Sensor Letters* 7:599–604.

Kaniusas E., Pfützner H., Mehnen L., Kosel J., Varoneckas G., Alonderis A., and Zakarevicius L. 2008. Cardiovascular oscillations of the carotid artery assessed by magnetoelastic skin curvature sensor. *IEEE Transactions on Biomedical Engineering* 55:369–372.

Klinger T., Pfutzner H., Schonhuber P., Hoffmann K., and Bachl N. 1992. Magnetostrictive amorphous sensor for biomedical monitoring. *IEEE Transactions on Magnetics* 28(5):2400–2402.

Mackay S. 1983. Biomedical relemetry: The formative years. *Engineering in Medicine and Biology Magazine*:11–17.

Meyer M.H.F., Krause H.J., Hartmann M., Miethe P., Oster J., and Keusgen M. 2007a. *Francisella tularensis* detection using magnetic labels and a magnetic biosensor based on frequency mixing. *Journal of Magnetism and Magnetic Materials* 311:259–263.

Meyer M.H.F., Stehr M., Bhuju S., Krause H.J., Hartmann M., Miethe P., Singh M., and Keusgen M. 2007b. Magnetic biosensor for the detection of *Yersinia pestis*. *Journal of Microbiological Methods* 68:218–224.

Moore B. 2009. The potential use of radio frequency identification devices for active monitoring of blood glucose levels. *Journal of Diabetes Science and Technology* 3(1):180–183.

Nagasaki Y., Kobayashi H., Katsuyama Y., Jomura T., and Sakura T. 2007. Enhanced immunoresponse of antibody/mixed-PEG co-immobilized surface construction of high-performance immunomagnetic ELISA system. *Journal of Colloid and Interface Science* 309:524–530.

Noordergraaf G.J., Paulussen I.W.F., Venema A., Berkom P.F.J, Woerlee P.H., Scheffer G.J., and Noordergraaf A. 2009. The impact of compliant surfaces on in-hospital chest compressions: Effects of common mattresses and a backboard. *Resuscitation* 80(5):546–552.

Nuzzolese E., Marcario V., and Di Vella G. 2010. Incorporation of radio frequency identification tag in dentures to facilitate recognition and forensic human identification. *Open Dentistry Journal* 4:33–36.

Nyce D.S. 2004. *Linear Position Sensors: Theory and Application*. Hoboken, NJ, Wiley-IEEE.

Oess N.P., Weisse B., and Nelson B.J. 2009. Magnetoelastic strain sensor for optimized assessment of bone fracture fixation. *IEEE Sensors Journal* 9(8):961–968.

Ohki T., Stern D., Allen M., and Yadav J. 2004. Wireless pressure sensing of aneurysms: Will the use of this technology after EVAR make CT scanning obsolete? *Endovascular Today*:47.

Ong K. G. and Grimes C.A. 2006. Nano-structural magnetoelastic materials for sensor applications. In *Handbook of Advanced Magnetic Materials*. Liu Y., Shindo D., Sellmyer D. J. (Eds.), New York and Berlin, Springer 1:1802.

Ong K.G., Leland J.M., Zeng K., Barrett G., Zourob M., and Grimes C.A. 2006. A rapid highly-sensitive endotoxin detection system. *Biosensors and Bioelectronics* 21:2270–2274.

Oster J., Parker J., and Brassard L. 2001. Polyvinyl-alcohol-based magnetic beads for rapid and efficient separation of specific or unspecific nuclei acid sequences. *Journal of Magnetism and Magnetic Materials* 225:145–150.

Otis B., Moritz C., Holleman J., Mishra A., Pandey J., Rai S., Yeager D., and Zhang F. 2009. Circuit techniques for wireless brain interfaces. *2009 31st Annual International Conference of the IEEE Engineering in Medicine and Biology Society.* EMBC:3213–3216, Minneapolis, MN.

Pang P., Cai Q., and Yao S. 2008. The detection of *Mycobacterium tuberculosis* in sputum sample based on a wireless magnetoelastic sensing device. *Talanta* 76(2):360–364.

Pereles B.D., Shao R., Tan E.L., and Ong K.G. 2008. A remote query pressure sensor based on magnetic higher order harmonic fields. *IEEE Sensors Journal* 8(11–12):1824–1829.

Pereles B.D., Shao R., Tan E.L., and Ong K.G. 2009. A wireless flow sensor based on magnetic higher-order harmonic fields. *Smart Materials & Structures* 18(9):095002.

Pina E., Burgos E., Prados C., González J.M., Hernando A., Iglesias M.C., Poch J, and Franco C. 2001. Magnetoelastic sensor as a probe for muscular activity: An in-vivo experiment. *Sensors and Actuators A* 91(1–2):99–102.

Puckett L.G., Barrett G., Kouzoudis D., Grimes C., and Bachas L.G. 2003. Monitoring blood coagulation with magnetoelastic sensors. *Biosensors and Bioelectronics* 18:675–681.

Puckett L.G., Lewis J.K., Urbas A., Cui X., Gao D., and Bachas L.G. 2005. Magnetoelastic transducers for monitoring coagulation, clot inhibition, and fibrinolysis. *Biosensors and Bioelectronics* 20:1737–1743.

Rao C.R. and Guha S.K. 2001. *Principles of Medical Electronics and Biomedical Instrumentation*. Hyderabad, India, Universities Press.

Riistama J. 2007. Characterisation of wearable and implantable physiological measurement devices. *Automation, Mechanical and Materials Engineering*. Tampere, Tampere University of Technology:76.

Rios J.L.J. and Rabin Y. 2006. Thermal expansion of blood vessels in low cryogenic temperatures Part I: A new experimental device. *Cryobiology* 52(2):269–283.

Ruan C., Ong K.G., Mungle C., Paulose M., Nickl N.J., and Grimes C.A. 2003b. A wireless pH sensor based on the use of salt-independent micro-scale polymer spheres. *Sensors and Actuators B* 96:61–69.

Ruan C., Zeng K., Varghese O.K., and Grimes C.A. 2003a. Magnetoelastic immunosensors: Amplified mass immunosorbent assay for detection of *Escherichia coli* O157:H7. *Analytical Chemistry* 75:6494–6498.

Ruan C., Zeng K., Varghese O.K., and Grimes C.A. 2004. A staphylococcal enterotoxin B magnetoelastic immunosensor. *Biosensors and Bioelectronics* 20:585–591.

Sangwan R. S., Qiu R. G., and Jessen D. 2005. Using RFID tags for tracking patients, charts and medical equipment within an integrated health delivery network. *2005 IEEE Networking, Sensing and Control Proceedings*:1070–1074.

Silva C.W.D. 2005. *Mechatronics: An Integrated Approach*. Boca Raton, FL, CRC Press.

Smith C.E. 2008. Human microchip implantation. *Journal of Technology Management & Innovation* 3(3):151–160.

Son, C. and Ziaie B. 2006. A micromachined electret-based transponder for *in situ* radiation measurement. *IEEE Electron Device Letters* 27(11):884–886.

Steinberg I.M. and Steinberg M.D. 2009. Radio-frequency tag with optoelectronic interface for distributed wireless chemical and biological sensor applications. *Sensors and Actuators B* 138(1):120–125.

Tan E.L., Pereles B.D., Ong J., and Ong K.G. 2008. A wireless, passive strain sensor based on the harmonic response of magnetically soft materials. *Smart Materials and Structures* 17(2):025015–025011–025016.

Tang T. B., Smith S., Flynn B.W., Stevenson J.T.M., Gundlach A.M., Reekie H.M., Murray A.F. et al. 2008. Implementation of wireless power transfer and communications for an implantable ocular drug delivery system. *IET Nanobiotechnology* 2(3):72–79.

Wan J., Johnson M.L., Guntupalli R., Petrenko V.A., and Chin B.A. 2007. Detection of *Bacillus anthracis* spores in liquid using phage-based magnetoelastic micro-resonators. *Sensors and Actuators B* 127:559–566.

Weiland J. D., Fink W., Humayun M. S., Wentai L., Wen L., Sivaprakasam M., Yu-Chong T., and Tarbell M. 2008. Systems design of a high resolution retinal prosthesis. IEDM 2008. *IEEE International Electron Devices Meeting. Technical Digest*:1–4, San Francisco, CA.

Wheeler A.J. and Ganji A.R. 2009. *Introduction to Engineering Experimentation.* Prentice Hall.

Wolf J. R. 1979. Linear variable differential transformer and its uses for in-core fuel rod behavior measurements. *International Colloquium on Irradiation for Reactor Safety Programmes.* Petten, Netherlands:23.

Wu F., Kuo F., and Liu L.W. 2005. The application of RFID on drug safety of inpatient nursing healthcare. *Proceedings of the 7th International Conference on Electronic Commerce.* Xi'an, China, ACM:85–92.

Wu S., Gao X., Cai Q., and Grimes C.A. 2007b. A wireless magnetoelastic biosensor for convenient and sensitive detection of acid phosphatase. *Sensors and Actuators B* 123:856–859.

Wu S., Zhu Y., Cai Q., Zeng K., and Grimes C.A. 2007a. A wireless magnetoelastic α-amylase sensor. *Sensors and Actuators B* 121:476–481.

Yamakawa T., Inoue T., Harada M., and Tsuneda A. 2007. Design of a CMOS heartbeat spike-pulse detection circuit integrable in an RFID tag tor heart rate signal sensing. *IEICE Transactions on Electronics* E90C (6):1336–1343.

Yang C., Chien J., Wang B., Chen P., and Lee D. 2008. A flexible surface wetness sensor using a RFID technique. *Biomedical Microdevices* 10(1):47–54.

Yvanoff M. and Venkataraman J.A. 2009. A feasibility study of tissue characterization using LC sensors. *IEEE Transactions on Antennas and Propagation* 57(4):885–893.

Zeng K, Ong K.G., Mungle C.S., and Grimes C.A. 2002. Time domain characterization of oscillating sensors: Application of frequency counting for resonance frequency determination. *Review of Scientific Instruments* 73:4375–4380.

Ziaie B. 2007. Implantable wireless microsystems. In *BioMEMS and Biomedical Nanotechnology.* Ferrari M., Bashir R., and Wereley S. (Eds.), US, Springer:205–221.

Zourob M., Ong K.G., Zeng K., Mouffouk F., and Grimes C.A. 2007. A wireless magnetoelastic biosensor for direct detection of organophosphorus pesticides. *Analyst* 132(4):338–343.

4

Biopotential Electrodes

Michael R. Neuman
Michigan Technological University

Biologic systems frequently have electrical activity associated with them. This activity can be a constant dc electric field, a constant flux of charge-carrying particles or current, or a time-varying electric field or current, which are associated with some time-dependent biologic or biochemical phenomenon. Bioelectric phenomena are associated with the distribution of ions or charged molecules in a biologic structure and also the changes in this distribution resulting from specific processes. These changes can occur as a result of biochemical reactions, or they can emanate from phenomena that alter local anatomy.

One can find bioelectric phenomena associated with just about every organ system in the body. Nevertheless, a large proportion of these signals are associated with phenomena that currently has not generated a lot of interest and are not especially useful in clinical medicine. These signals usually represent time-invariant, low-level signals that are not easily measured in practice. There are, however, several signals that are of diagnostic significance or that provide a means of electronic assessment to aid in understanding biologic systems. These signals, their usual abbreviations, and the systems they measure are listed in Table 4.1. Of these, the most familiar is the electrocardiogram, a signal derived from the electrical activity of the heart. This signal is widely used in diagnosing disturbances in cardiac rhythm, signal conduction through the heart, and damage to the heart muscle because of cardiac ischemia and infarction. The electromyogram is used for diagnosing neuromuscular diseases, and the electroencephalogram is important in identifying brain dysfunction and evaluating sleep. The other signals listed in Table 4.1 are currently of lesser diagnostic significance but are, nevertheless, used for studies of the associated organ systems. Although Table 4.1 and the above discussion are concerned with bioelectric phenomena in animals, bioelectric signals also arise from plants. These signals are generally steady-state or slowly changing, as opposed to the time-varying signals listed in Table 4.1. An extensive literature exists on the origins of bioelectric signals, and the interested reader is referred to the text by Plonsey and Barr for a general overview of this area [1].

TABLE 4.1 Bioelectric Signals Sensed by Biopotential Electrodes and Their Sources

Bioelectric Signal	Abbreviation	Biologic Source
Electrocardiogram	ECG	Heart—as seen from body surface
Cardiac electrogram	—	Heart—as seen from within
Electromyogram	EMG	Muscle
Electroencephalogram	EEG	Brain
Electrooptigram	EOG	Eye dipole field
Electroretinogram	ERG	Eye retina
Action potential	—	Nerve or muscle
Electrogastrogram	EGG	Stomach
Galvanic skin reflex	GSR	Skin

4.1 Sensing Bioelectric Signals

The mechanism of electrical conductivity in the body involves ions as charge carriers. Thus, detecting bioelectric signals involves interacting with these ionic charge carriers and transducing ionic currents into electronic currents required by wires and electronic instrumentation. This transducing function is carried out by electrodes that consist of electrical conductors in contact with the aqueous ionic solutions of the body. The interaction between electrons in the electrodes and ions in the body can greatly affect the performance of these sensors and requires that specific considerations be made in their application. At the interface between an electrode and an ionic solution redox (oxidation–reduction), reactions need to occur for a charge to be transferred between the electrode and the solution. These reactions can be represented, in general, by the following equations:

$$C \rightleftharpoons C^{n+} + ne^-$$
(4.1)

$$A^{m-} \rightleftharpoons A + me^-$$
(4.2)

n is the valence of cation material C, and m the valence of anion material, A. For most electrode systems, the cations in solution and the metal of the electrodes are the same, hence the atoms C are oxidized when they give up electrons and go into solution as positively charged ions. These ions are reduced when the process occurs in the reverse direction. In the case of the anion reaction, Equation 4.2, the directions for oxidation and reduction are reversed. For best operation of the electrodes, these two reactions should be reversible, that is, it should be just as easy for them to occur in one direction as the other.

The interaction between a metal in contact with a solution of its ions produces a local change in the concentration of the ions in solution near the metal surface. This causes charge neutrality not to be maintained in this region, which can result in causing the electrolyte surrounding the metal to be at a different electrical potential from the rest of the solution. Thus, a potential difference known as the half-cell potential is established between the metal and the bulk of the electrolyte. It is found that different characteristic potentials occur for different materials and different redox reactions of these materials. Some of these potentials are summarized in Table 4.2. These half-cell potentials can be important when using electrodes for low-frequency or dc measurements.

The relationship between electrical potential and ionic concentrations or, more precisely, ionic activities is frequently considered in electrochemistry. Most commonly, two ionic solutions of different activity are separated by an ion-selective semipermeable membrane that allows one type of ion to pass freely through the membrane. It can be shown that an electric potential E exist between the solutions on either

TABLE 4.2 Half-Cell Potentials for Materials and Reactions Encountered in Biopotential Measurement

Metal and Reaction	Half-Cell Potential (V)
$Al \rightarrow Al^{3+} + 3e^-$	-1.706
$Ni \rightarrow Ni^{2+} + 2e^-$	-0.230
$H_2 \rightarrow 2H^+ + 2e^-$	0.000 (by definition)
$Ag^+Cl^- \rightarrow AgCl + e^-$	+0.223
$Ag \rightarrow Ag^+ + e^-$	+0.799
$Au \rightarrow Au^+ + e^-$	+1.680

side of the membrane, based on the relative activity of the permeable ions in each of these solutions. This relationship is known as the Nernst equation

$$E = -\frac{RT}{nF} \ln\left(\frac{a_1}{a_2}\right) \tag{4.3}$$

where a_1 and a_2 are the activities of the ions on either side of the membrane, R is the universal gas constant, T the absolute temperature, n the valence of the ions, and F the Faraday's constant. More details on this relationship can be found in Chapter 5.

The Nernst equation also applies to a metal electrode in contact with a solution containing ions of that metal. In this case, its form is slightly different:

$$E = E^0 - \frac{RT}{nF} \ln(a) \tag{4.4}$$

where E^0 is the half-cell potential for the redox reaction of the electrode metal and its ions in solution (Equation 4.1) and a the activity of the electrode metal ions in solution. The activity of the solid electrode metal is considered to be 1 in this case. When no electric current flows between an electrode and the solution of its ions or across an ion-permeable membrane, the potential observed should be the half-cell potential or the Nernst potential, respectively. If, however, there is a current, these potentials can be altered. The difference between the potential at zero current and the measured potentials while the current is passing is known as the overvoltage and is the result of an alteration in the charge distribution in the solution in contact with the electrodes or the ion-selective membrane. This effect is known as polarization and can result in diminished electrode performance, especially under conditions where there is motion of the electrode with respect to the object to which it is attached. There are three basic components to the polarization overpotential: the ohmic, the concentration, and the activation overpotentials. More details of these overpotentials can be found in electrochemistry or biomedical instrumentation texts [2].

Perfectly polarizable electrodes pass a current between the electrode and the electrolytic solution by changing the charge distribution within the solution near the electrode. Thus, no actual current crosses the electrode–electrolyte interface. Nonpolarized electrodes, however, allow the current to pass freely across the electrode–electrolyte interface without changing the charge distribution in the electrolytic solution adjacent to the electrode. Although these types of electrodes can be described theoretically, neither can be realized in practice. It is possible, however, to come up with electrode structures that approximate their characteristics.

Electrodes made from noble metals, such as platinum, are often highly polarizable. A charge distribution different from that of the bulk electrolytic solution is found in the solution close to the electrode surface. Such a distribution can create serious limitations when movement is present and the measurement involves low-frequency or even dc signals. If the electrode moves with respect to the electrolytic

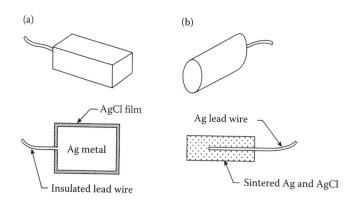

FIGURE 4.1 Silver–silver electrodes for biopotential measurements: (a) metallic silver with a silver chloride surface layer and (b) sintered electrode structure. The lower views show the electrodes in cross section.

solution, the charge distribution in the solution adjacent to the electrode surface will change, and this will induce a voltage change at the electrode that will appear as noise or motion artifact in the measurement. Thus, for most biomedical measurements, nonpolarizable electrodes are preferred to those that are polarizable to minimize this interference.

The silver–silver chloride electrode has characteristics similar to a perfectly nonpolarizable electrode and is practical for use in many biomedical applications. The electrode (Figure 4.1a) consists of a silver base structure that is coated with a layer of the ionic compound silver chloride. Some of the silver chloride when exposed to light is reduced to metallic silver; hence, a typical silver–silver chloride electrode has finely divided metallic silver within a matrix of silver chloride on its surface. Because silver chloride is relatively insoluble in aqueous solutions, this surface remains stable. Moreover, because there is minimal polarization associated with this electrode, motion artifact is reduced compared to polarizable electrodes such as the platinum electrode. Furthermore, owing to the reduction in polarization, there is also a smaller effect of frequency on electrode impedance, especially at low frequencies.

Silver–silver chloride electrodes of this type can be fabricated by starting with a silver base and electrolytically growing the silver chloride layer on its surface [2]. Although an electrode produced in this manner can be used for most biomedical measurements, it is not a robust structure, and pieces of the silver chloride film can be chipped away after repeated use of the electrode. A structure with greater mechanical stability is the sintered silver–silver chloride electrode in Figure 4.1b. This electrode consists of a silver lead wire surrounded by a cylinder made up of finely divided silver and silver chloride powder sintered together.

In addition to its nonpolarizable behavior, the silver–silver chloride electrode exhibits less electrical noise than the equivalent polarizable electrodes. This is especially true at low frequencies, and so silver–silver chloride electrodes are recommended for measurements involving very low voltages for signals that are made up primarily of low frequencies. A more detailed description of silver–silver chloride electrodes and methods to fabricate these devices can be found in Reference 3 and biomedical instrumentation textbooks [4].

4.2 Electrical Characteristics

The electrical characteristics of biopotential electrodes are generally nonlinear and are a function of the current density at their surface. Thus, having the devices represented by linear models requires that they be operated at low potentials and currents.* Under these idealized conditions, electrodes can be represented by an equivalent circuit of the form shown in Figure 4.2. In this circuit, R_d and C_d are components

---

* Or at least at an operating point where the voltage and the current are relatively fixed.

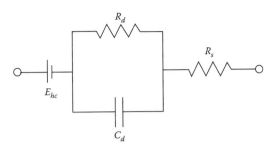

FIGURE 4.2 The equivalent circuit for a biopotential electrode.

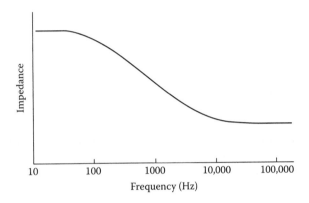

FIGURE 4.3 An example of biopotential electrode impedance as a function of frequency. Characteristic frequencies will be somewhat different for different electrode geometries and materials.

that represent the impedance associated with the electrode–electrolyte interface and polarization at this interface. R_s is the series resistance associated with interfacial effects and the resistance of the electrode materials themselves. The battery E_{hc} represents the half-cell potential described earlier. It is seen that the impedance of this electrode will be frequency dependent, as illustrated in Figure 4.3. At low frequencies, the impedance is dominated by the series combination of R_s and R_d, whereas at higher frequencies, C_d bypasses the effect of R_d so that the impedance is now close to R_s. Thus, by measuring the impedance of an electrode at high and low frequencies, it is possible to determine the component values for the equivalent circuit for that electrode.

The electrical characteristics of electrodes are affected by many physical properties of these electrodes. Table 4.3 lists some of the more common physical properties of electrodes and qualitatively indicates how these can affect electrode impedance.

TABLE 4.3 Effect of Electrode Properties on Electrode Impedance

Property	Change in Property	Changes in Electrode Impedance
Surface area	↑	↓
Polarization	↑	↑ At low frequencies
Surface roughness	↑	↓
Radius of curvature	↑	↓
Surface contamination	↑	↑

Note: ↑—Increase in quantity; ↓—decrease in property.

4.3 Practical Electrodes for Biomedical Measurements

Different forms of electrodes have been developed for different types of biomedical measurements. To describe each of these would go beyond the constraints of this chapter, but some of the more commonly used electrodes are presented in this section. The reader is referred to the monograph by Geddes for more details and a wider selection of practical electrodes [5].

4.3.1 Body-Surface Biopotential Electrodes

This category includes electrodes that can be placed on the body surface for recording bioelectric signals. The integrity of the skin is not compromised when these electrodes are applied, and they can be used for short-term diagnostic recording, such as taking a clinical electrocardiogram or long-term chronic recording as that which occurs in cardiac monitoring or exercise studies.

4.3.2 Metal Electrodes

The basic metal electrode consists of a metallic conductor usually in the form of a sheet, plate, or foil in contact with the skin with a thin layer of an electrolyte gel between the metal and the skin to establish this contact. Examples of metal plate electrodes are presented in Figure 4.4a. Metals commonly used for this type of electrode include German silver (a nickel–silver alloy), silver, gold, and platinum. Sometimes, these electrodes are made of a foil of the metal so as to be flexible, and sometimes they are produced in the form of a suction electrode (Figure 4.4b) to make it easier to attach the electrode to the skin to make a measurement and then move it to another point to repeat the measurement. These types of electrodes are used primarily for diagnostic recordings of biopotentials such as the electrocardiogram or the electroencephalogram. Metal disk electrodes with a gold surface in a conical shape such as shown in Figure 4.4c are frequently used for EEG recordings. The apex of the cone is open so that the electrolyte gel or paste can be introduced to both make good contact between the electrode and the head and to allow this contact medium to be replaced should it dry out during the electrode's use. For many years these types of electrodes were the primary types used for obtaining diagnostic electrocardiograms. Today, disposable electrodes such as described in the following section are frequently used. These do not require as much preparation or strapping to the limbs as the older electrodes did, and because they are disposable they do not need to be cleaned between applications to patients. Also because they are usually silver–silver chloride electrodes, they have less noise and motion artifact than the electrodes made only of metal.

4.3.3 Electrodes for Chronic Patient Monitoring

Long-term monitoring of biopotentials such as the electrocardiogram as performed by cardiac monitors places special constraints on the electrodes used to detect the signals. These electrodes must have a stable interface between them and the body, and frequently nonpolarizable electrodes are, therefore, the best for this application. Mechanical stability of the interface between the electrode and the skin can help to reduce motion artifact, and so there are various approaches to reduce interfacial motion between the electrode and the coupling electrolyte or the skin. Figure 4.4d is an example of one approach to reduce motion artifact by recessing the electrode in a cup of electrolytic fluid or gel. The cup is then securely fastened to the skin surface using a double-sided adhesive ring. Movement of the skin with respect to the electrode may affect the electrolyte near the skin–electrolyte interface, but the electrode–electrolyte interface can be several millimeters away from this location and protected because it is recessed in the cup. The fluid movement is unlikely to affect the recessed electrode–electrolyte interface as compared to what would happen if the electrode was separated from the skin by just a thin layer of electrolyte.

    The advantages of the recessed electrode can be realized in a simpler design that lends itself to mass production through automation. This results in low per-unit cost so that these electrodes can be considered

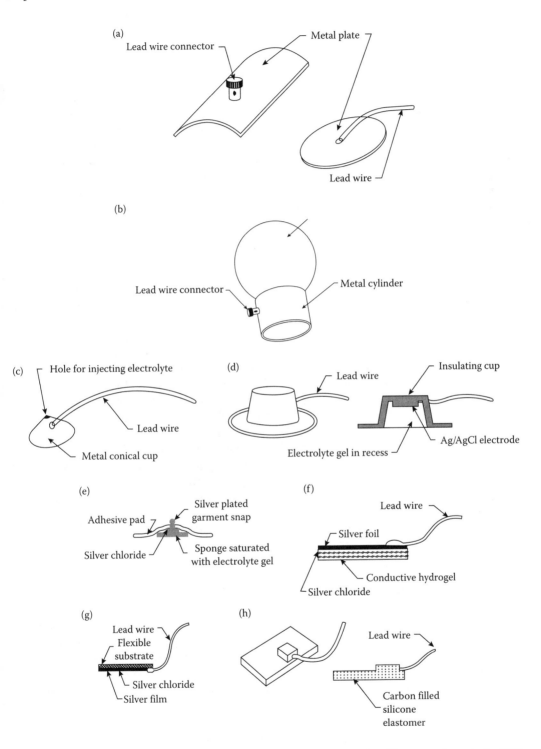

FIGURE 4.4 Examples of different skin electrodes: (a) metal plate electrodes, (b) suction electrode for ECG, (c) metal cup EEG electrode, (d) recessed electrode, (e) disposable electrode with electrolyte-impregnated sponge (shown in cross section), (f) disposable hydrogel electrode (shown in cross section), (g) thin-film electrode for use with neonates (shown in cross section), and (h) carbon-filled elastomer dry electrode.

disposable. Figure 4.4e illustrates such an electrode in cross section. The electrolyte layer now consists of an open-celled sponge saturated with a thickened (high-viscosity) electrolytic solution. The sponge serves the same function as the recess in the cup electrodes and is coupled directly to a silver–silver chloride electrode. Frequently, the electrode itself is attached to a clothing snap through an insulating adhesive disk that holds the structure against the skin. This snap serves as the point of connection to a lead wire. Many commercial versions of these electrodes are available in various sizes, including electrodes with a silver–silver chloride interface or ones that use metallic silver as the electrode material.

A modification of this basic monitoring electrode structure is shown in Figure 4.4f. In this case, the metal electrode is a silver foil with a surface coating of silver chloride. The foil gives the electrode increased flexibility to fit more closely over body contours. Instead of using the sponge, a hydrogel film (really a sponge on a microscopic level) saturated with an electrolytic solution and formed from materials that are very sticky is placed over the electrode surface. The opposite surface of the hydrogel layer can be attached directly to the skin, and because it is very sticky, no additional adhesive or tape is needed. The mobility and concentration of ions in the hydrogel layer is generally lower than for the electrolytic solution used in the sponge or the cup. This results in an electrode that has higher source impedance as compared with electrodes that use the standard gel electrolytic solution. An important advantage of the hydrogel electrode structure is its ability to have the electrolyte stick directly on the skin. This greatly reduces interfacial motion between the skin surface and the electrolyte, and hence the electrode itself, so there is a smaller amount of motion artifact in the signal from these electrodes. This type of hydrogel electrode is, therefore, especially valuable in monitoring patients who move a great deal or during exercise.

Thin-film flexible electrodes such as shown in Figure 4.4g have been used for monitoring neonates. They are basically the same as the metal plate electrodes; only the thickness of the metal in this case is less than a micrometer. These metal films need to be supported on a flexible plastic substrate, such as polyester or polyimide. The advantage of using only a thin metal layer for the electrode lies in the fact that these electrodes are x-ray transparent. This is especially important in infants, in whom repeated placement and removal of electrodes, so that x-rays may be taken, can cause substantial skin irritation.

Electrodes that do not use artificially applied electrolyte solutions or gels and, therefore, are often referred to as dry electrodes have been used in some monitoring applications. These sensors as illustrated in Figure 4.4h can be placed on the skin and held in position by an elastic band or tape. They are made up of graphite or metal-filled polymer, such as silicone. The conducting particles are ground into a fine powder, and this is added to the silicone elastomer before it cures so as to produce a conductive material with physical properties similar to that of the elastomer. When held against the skin surface, these electrodes establish contact with the skin without the need for an electrolytic fluid or gel. In actuality, such a layer is formed by sweat under the electrode surface. For this reason, these electrodes tend to perform better after they have been left in place for an hour or two so that this layer forms. Some investigators have found that placing a drop of physiologic saline solution on the skin before applying the electrode can quickly establish a good connection. This type of electrode has found wide application in home infant cardiorespiratory monitoring because of the ease with which it can be applied by untrained caregivers.

Dry electrodes are also used on certain consumer products, such as stationary exercise bicycles and treadmills, to detect an electrocardiographic signal to determine the heart rate. When a subject grabs the metal contacts, there is generally enough sweat to establish good electrical contact so that a Lead I electrocardiogram can be obtained and used to determine the heart rate. The signals, however, are much noisier than those obtained from other electrodes described in this section.

4.4 Intracavitary and Intratissue Electrodes

Electrodes can be placed within the body for biopotential measurements. These electrodes are generally smaller than skin surface electrodes and do not require special electrolytic coupling fluid because natural body fluids serve this function. There are different designs for these internal electrodes, and only a few examples are given in the following paragraphs. Basically, these electrodes can be classified as needle electrodes, which can be used to penetrate the skin and tissue to reach the point where the measurement is to be made, or they are electrodes that can be placed in a natural cavity or surgically produced cavity in tissue. Figure 4.5 illustrates some of these internal electrodes.

A catheter tip or probe electrode is placed in a naturally occurring cavity in the body, such as in the gastrointestinal system. A metal tip or segment on a catheter makes up the electrode. In the case where there is no hollow lumen, the catheter or probe is inserted into the cavity so that the metal electrode makes contact with the tissue. A lead wire down the lumen of the catheter or down the center of the probe connects the electrode to the external circuitry. Multiple electrodes can be placed along the probe as illustrated in Figure 4.5a.

The basic needle electrode, shown in Figure 4.5b, consists of a solid needle, usually made of stainless steel, with a sharp point. An insulating material coats the shank of the needle up to a millimeter or two from the tip so that the very tip of the needle remains exposed. When this structure is placed in tissue such as skeletal muscle, electrical signals can be detected by the exposed tip. One can also make needle

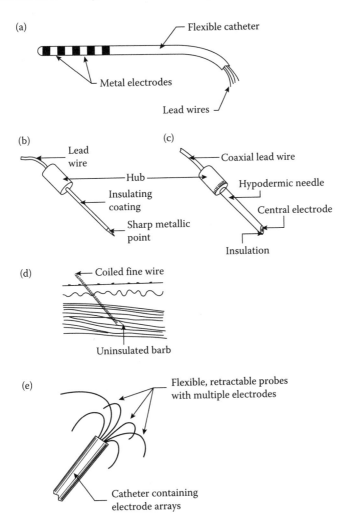

FIGURE 4.5 Examples of different internal electrodes: (a) catheter or probe electrode, (b) needle electrode, (c) coaxial needle electrode, (d) coiled wire electrode, and (e) catheter with electrode arrays. (Webster J.G. (Ed.). *Medical Instrumentation: Application and Design,* 1992. New York, Copyright Wiley-VCH Verlag GmbH & co. KGaA. Reproduced with permission.)

electrodes by running one or more insulated wires down the lumen of a standard hypodermic needle. The electrode as shown in Figure 4.5c is shielded by the metal of the needle and can be used to detect very localized signals in tissue.

Fine wires can also be introduced into tissue using a hypodermic needle, which is then withdrawn. This wire can remain in tissue for acute or chronic measurements. Caldwell and Reswick [6] and Knutson et al. [7] have used fine coiled wire electrodes that were placed through the skin into the skeletal muscle for several years without adverse effects. The advantage of the coil is that it makes the electrode very flexible and compliant. This helps it and the lead wire to endure the frequent flexing and stretching that occurs in the body without breaking.

The relatively new clinical field of cardiac electrophysiology makes use of electrodes that can be advanced into the heart to identify aberrant regions of myocardium that cause life-threatening arrhythmias. These electrodes may be similar to the multiple electrode probe or catheter shown in Figure 4.5a, or they might be much more elaborate such as the "umbrella" electrode array shown in Figure 4.5e. In this case, the electrode array with multiple electrodes on each umbrella rib is advanced into the heart in collapsed form through a blood vessel in the same way as a catheter is passed into the heart. The umbrella is then opened inside the heart such that the electrodes on the ribs contact the endocardium and are used to record and map intracardiac electrograms. Once the procedure is completed, the umbrella is collapsed and withdrawn through the blood vessel. A similar approach can be taken with an electrode array on the surface of a balloon. The collapsed lumen is advanced into one of the chambers of the heart and then distended. Simultaneous recordings are quickly made from each electrode of the array, and then the balloon is collapsed and withdrawn [8,9].

4.5 Transparent Electrodes

Transparent electrodes have also been developed for sensing biopotentials. Their structure is similar to the thin-film electrodes illustrated in Figure 4.4g. A thin film of indium tin oxide 200–500 nm thick is deposited on a transparent substrate, such as a glass microscope slide. This film is electrically conductive and transparent, although it does absorb some light. Because the conductor is a thin film, it can be etched into a geometric pattern consisting of multiple electrodes by using conventional microelectronic photolithographic techniques. Either lead wires can be a part of the indium tin oxide film or thin-film metallic conductors can be used. A transparent insulating material can cover the lead wires and only expose that part of the indium tin oxide film that is the actual electrode. These electrodes have been used for research purposes on contact lenses and as an electrode array for looking at cardiac tissue [10].

4.6 Microelectrodes

The electrodes described in the previous paragraphs have been applied to study bioelectric signals at the organism, organ, or tissue level but not at the cellular level. To study the electrical behavior of cells, electrodes that are themselves smaller than the cells being studied need to be used. Three types of electrodes have been described for this purpose: etched metal electrodes, micropipette electrodes, and metal-film-coated micropipette electrodes. The metal microelectrode is essentially a subminiature version of the needle electrode described in the previous section (Figure 4.5b). This electrode is essentially a stiff wire that has been chemically etched at one end to a very narrow tip. In this case, a strong metal, such as tungsten, is used. The end of this wire is etched electrolytically to give tip diameters on the order of a few micrometers. The structure is insulated up to its tip, and it can be passed through the membrane of a cell to contact the cytosol. The advantage of these electrodes is that they are both small and robust and can be used for neurophysiologic studies. Their principal disadvantage is the difficulty encountered in their fabrication and their high source impedance. A variation on this structure is illustrated in Figure 4.6a. Here, a metal such as gold is placed in the lumen of a thin-wall, small-diameter glass tube that has a softening temperature close to the melting point of the internal

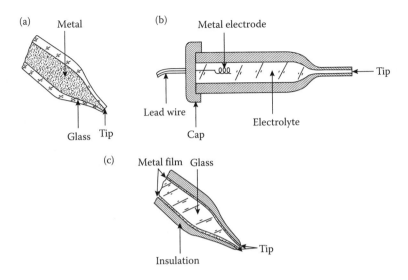

FIGURE 4.6 Microelectrodes: (a) metal, (b) micropipette, and (c) thin metal film on micropipette. (Reprinted with permission from Webster J.C. (Ed.). 1992. *Medical Instrumentation: Application and Design*, Boston, Houghton Mifflin.)

metal. The tube is heated in a flame or an electric coil and drawn to a very fine tip at one end, and the metal being ductile is also drawn to a fine tip. The end of the glass tube can then be cut and polished, yielding a very small-diameter metal disk surrounded by glass insulation. Tip diameters of the order of 1 μm are possible with this technique.

The most frequently used type of microelectrode is the glass micropipette. This structure, as illustrated in Figure 4.6b, consists of a fine glass capillary drawn to a very narrow point and filled with an electrolytic solution. The point can be as narrow as a fraction of a micrometer, and the dimensions of this electrode are strongly dependent on the skill of the individual drawing the tip. The electrolytic solution in the lumen serves as the contact between the interior of the cell through which the tip has been impaled and a larger conventional electrode located in the shank of the pipette. These electrodes also suffer from high source impedances and fabrication difficulty.

A combined form of these two types of electrodes can be achieved by depositing a metal film over the outside surface of a glass micropipette as shown in Figure 4.6c. In this case, the strength and smaller dimensions of the micropipette can be used to support films of various metals that are insulated by an additional film up to a point very close to the actual tip of the electrode structure. These electrodes have been manufactured in quantity and made available as commercial products. Because they combine the features of both the metal and the micropipette electrodes, they also suffer from many of the same limitations. They do, however, have the advantage of being able to be made of a wide selection of metals because of the ability to deposit films of different metals on the micropipette surface without having to worry about the strength of the metal, as would be the case if the metal were used alone.

4.7 Electrodes Fabricated Using Microelectronic Technology

Modern microelectronic technology can be used to fabricate different types of electrodes for specific biomedical applications. For example, dry electrodes used in applications with high source resistances because of the absence of electrolytic gel or microelectrodes with similar high resistance characteristics can be improved by incorporating a microelectronic amplifier for impedance conversion right on the electrode itself. In the case of the conventional-sized electrodes, a metal disk 5–10 mm in diameter can have a high input impedance microelectronic amplifier configured as a follower integrated into the back of the electrode so that localized processing of the high source impedance signal can produce one of lower, more practical impedance for signal transmission [11]. Single- and multiple-element electrodes can be made from thin-film or silicon technology. Mastrototaro and colleagues have demonstrated probes for measuring intramyocardial potentials using thin, patterned gold films on polyimide or oxidized molybdenum substrates [12]. When electrodes are made from pieces of micromachined silicon, it is possible to integrate an amplifier directly into the electrode [13]. Multichannel amplifiers or multiplexers can be used with multiple electrodes on the same probe. Electrodes for contact with individual nerve fibers can be fabricated using micromachined holes in a silicon chip that are just big enough to pass a single growing axon. Electrical contacts on the sides of these holes can then be used to detect electrical activity from these nerves [14]. Arrays of individual miniature electrodes that are microfabricated using silicon micromachining techniques have been described and applied by Normann [15]. This dense array of needle electrodes has been used for making multiple contacts to the brain cortex. These examples are just a few of the many possibilities that can be realized using microelectronics and three-dimensional micromachining technology to fabricate specialized electrodes.

4.8 Biomedical Applications

Electrodes can be used to perform a wide variety of measurements of bioelectric signals. An extensive review of this would be beyond the scope of this chapter, but some typical examples of applications are highlighted in Table 4.4. Biopotential electrodes are most widely used in obtaining the electrocardiogram for diagnostic and patient-monitoring applications. A substantial commercial market exists for various types of electrocardiographic electrodes, and many of the forms described in the previous section are available commercially. Other electrodes for measuring bioelectric potentials for application in diagnostic medicine are indicated in Table 4.4. Research applications of biopotential electrodes are highly varied and specific for individual studies. Although a few examples are given in this chapter and Table 4.4, the field is far too broad to be completely covered here.

Biopotential electrodes are one of the most common biomedical sensors used in clinical medicine. Although their basic principle of operation is the same for most applications, they take on many forms and are used in the measurement of many types of bioelectric phenomena. They will continue to play an important role in biomedical instrumentation systems.

TABLE 4.4 Examples of Applications of Biopotential Electrodes

Application	Biopotential	Type of Electrode
Cardiac monitoring	ECG	Ag/AgCl with sponge
		Ag/AgCl with hydrogel
Infant cardiopulmonary monitoring	ECG impedance	Ag/AgCl with sponge
		Ag/AgCl with hydrogel
		Thin film
		Filled elastomer dry
Sleep encephalography	EEG	Gold cups
		Ag/AgCl cups
		Active electrodes
Diagnostic muscle activity	EMG	Needle
Cardiac electrograms	Electrogram	Intracardiac probe
Implanted telemetry of biopotentials	ECG	Stainless-steel wire loops
	EMG	Platinum disks
Eye movement	EOG	Ag/AgCl with hydrogel

References

1. Plonsey R. and Barr R.E. 2007. *Bioelectricity: A Quantitative Approach,* New York, Springer.
2. Lide D.R. (Ed.) 2004. *Handbook of Chemistry and Physics,* 85th ed., Boca Raton, FL, CRC Press.
3. Janz G.L and Ives D.J.G. 1968. Silver-silver chloride electrodes. *Ann. NY Acad. Sci.* 148: 210.
4. Webster J.G. (Ed.) 2010. *Medical Instrumentation: Application and Design,* 4th ed., New York, J. Wiley.
5. Geddes L.A. 1972. *Electrodes and the Measurement of Bioelectric Events,* New York, John Wiley & Sons.
6. Caldwell C.W. and Reswick J.B. 1975. A percutaneous wire electrode for chronic research use. *IEEE Trans. Biomed. Eng.* 22: 429.
7. Knutson J.S., Naples G.G., Peckham P.H., and Keith M.W. 2002. Fracture rates and occurrences of infection and granuloma associated with percutaneous intramuscular electrodes in upper extremity functional electrical simulation applications. *Rehab. Res. Dev.* 39: 671–684.
8. Rao L., He R., Ding E. et al. 2004. Novel noncontact catheter system for endocardial electrical and anatomical imaging. *Ann. Biomed. Eng.* 32: 573–584.
9. Chen T.E., Parson L.D., and Downar E. 1991. The construction of endocardial balloon arrays for cardiac mapping. *Pacing Clin. Electrophysiol.* 14: 470–479.
10. Knisley S.B. and Neuman M.R. 2003. Simultaneous electrical and optical mapping in rabbit hearts. *Ann. Biomed. Eng.* 31: 32–41.
11. Ko W.H. and Hynecek I. 1974. Dry electrodes and electrode amplifiers. In H.A. Miller and D.C. Harrison (Eds.), *Biomedical Electrode Technology,* pp. 169–181, New York, Academic Press.
12. Mastrototaro J,J., Massoud H.Z., Pilkington T.E. et al. 1992. Rigid and flexible thin-film microelectrode arrays for transmural cardiac recording. *IEEE Trans. Biomed. Eng.* 39: 271.
13. Wise K.D., Najafi K., Ii J. et al. 1990. Micromachined silicon microprobes for CNS recording and stimulation. *Proc. Ann. Conf. IEEE Eng. Med. Biol. Soc.* 12: 2334.
14. Edell D.J. 1986. A peripheral nerve information transducer for amputees: Long-term multichannel recordings from rabbit peripheral nerves. *IEEE Trans. Biomed. Eng.* 33: 203.
15. Normann R.A., Greger B., House P., Romero S.F., Pelayo F., and Fernandez E. 2009. Toward the development of a cortically based visual neuroprosthesis. *J. Neural Eng.* 6: 1741–2560.
16. Yoshida T., Hayashi K., and Toko K. 1988. The effect of anoxia on the spatial pattern of electric potential formed along the root. *Ann. Bot.* 62: 497.
17. Ives J.R. 2005. New chronic EEG electrode for critical/intensive care unit monitoring. *Clin. Neurophysiol.* 22: 119–123.
18. Griss P., Tolvanen-Laakso H.K., Merilainen P. et al. 2002. Characterization of micromachined spiked biopotential electrodes. *IEEE Trans. Biomed. Eng.* 49: 597–604.
19. Konings K.T., Kirchhof E.L, Smeets J.R. et al. 1994. High-density mapping of electrically induced atrial fibrillation in humans. *Circulation* 89: 1665–1680.
20. Kang T.H., Merritt C.R., Grant E., Pourdeyhimi B., and Nagle H.T. 2008. Nonwoven fabric active electrodes for biopotential measurement during normal daily activity. *IEEE Trans. Biomed. Eng.* 55(1): 188–195.

Further Information

Good overviews of biopotential electrodes are found in Geddes L.A. 1972. *Electrodes and the Measurement of Bioelectric Events,* New York, John Wiley & Sons; and Ferris C.D. 1974. *Introduction to Bioelectrodes,* New York, Plenum. Even though these references are more than 20 years old, they clearly cover the field, and little has changed since these books were written. Overviews of biopotential electrodes are found in chapters of two works edited by John Webster. Chapter 5 of his textbook, *Medical Instrumentation: Application and Design,* covers the material of this chapter in more detail, and there is a section on "bioelectrodes" in the *Encyclopedia of Medical Devices and Instrumentation* that he edited and was published by Wiley in 2006. The journals *IEEE Transactions on Biomedical Engineering*, *Medical Engineering & Physics*, *Physiological Measurements*, and *Medical and Biological Engineering & Computing* are also good sources of recent research on biopotential electrodes. A good source of information on bioelectric phenomena is the book *Bioelectricity: A Quantitative Approach* by Robert Plonsey and Roger Barr published by Springer in 2007.

5

Electrochemical Sensors

Chung-Chiun Liu
Case Western Reserve
University

Electrochemical sensors have been used extensively either as a whole or an integral part of a chemical and biomedical sensing element. For instance, blood gas (PO_2, PCO_2, and pH) sensing can be accomplished entirely by electrochemical means. Many important biomedical enzymatic sensors, including glucose sensors, incorporate an enzymatic catalyst and an electrochemical sensing element. The Clark type of oxygen sensor (Clark, 1956) is a well-known practical biomedical sensor based on electrochemical principles, an amperometric device. Electrochemical sensors generally can be categorized as conductivity/capacitance, potentiometric, amperometric, and voltammetric sensors. The amperometric and voltammetric sensors are characterized by their current–potential relationship with the electrochemical system and are less well-defined. Amperometric sensors can also be viewed as a subclass of voltammetric sensors.

Electrochemical sensors are essentially an electrochemical cell which employs a two- or three-electrode arrangement. Electrochemical sensor measurement can be made at steady-state or transient. The applied current or potential for electrochemical sensors may vary according to the mode of operation, and the selection of the mode is often intended to enhance the sensitivity and selectivity of a particular sensor. The general principles of electrochemical sensors have been extensively discussed in many electroanalytic references. However, many electroanalytic methods are not practical in biomedical sensing applications. For instance, dropping mercury electrode polarography is a well-established electroanalytic method, yet its usefulness in biomedical sensor development, particularly for potential *in vivo* sensing, is rather limited. In this chapter, we shall focus on the electrochemical methodologies which are useful in biomedical sensor development.

5.1 Conductivity/Capacitance Electrochemical Sensors

Measurement of the electric conductivity of an electrochemical cell can be the basis for an electrochemical sensor. This differs from an electrical (physical) measurement, for the electrochemical sensor measures the conductivity change of the system in the presence of a given solute concentration. This solute is often the sensing species of interest. Electrochemical sensors may also involve measuring capacitive impedance resulting from the polarization of the electrodes and/or the faradaic or charge transfer processes.

It has been established that the conductance of a homogeneous solution is directly proportional to the cross-sectional area perpendicular to the electrical field and inversely proportional to the segment of solution along the electrical field. Thus, the conductance of this solution (electrolyte), G (S), can be expressed as

$$G = \sigma A/L \qquad (5.1)$$

where A is the cross-sectional area (in cm²), L is the segment of the solution along the electrical field (in cm), and σ (in S/cm) is the specific conductivity of the electrolyte and is related quantitatively to the concentration and the magnitude of the charges of the ionic species. For a practical conductivity sensor, A is the surface of the electrode, and L is the distance between the two electrodes.

Equivalent and molar conductivities are commonly used to express the conductivity of the electrolyte. Equivalent conductance depends on the concentration of the solution. If the solution is a strong electrolyte, it will completely dissociate the components in the solution to ionic forms. Kohlrauch (MacInnes, 1939) found that the equivalent conductance of a strong electrolyte was proportional to the square root of its concentration. However, if the solution is a weak electrolyte which does not completely dissociate the components in the solution to respective ions, the above observation by Kohlrauch is not applicable.

The formation of ions leads to consideration of their contribution to the overall conductance of the electrolyte. The equivalent conductance of a strong electrolyte approaches a constant limiting value at infinite dilution, namely,

$$\Lambda_o = \Lambda_{\lim \to 0} = \lambda_0^+ + \lambda_0^- \qquad (5.2)$$

where Λ_o is the equivalent conductance of the electrolyte at infinite dilution and λ_0^+ and λ_0^- are the ionic equivalent conductance of cations and anions at infinite dilution, respectively.

Kohlrauch also established the law of independent mobilities of ions at infinite dilution. This implies that Lo at infinite dilution is a constant at a given temperature and will not be affected by the presence of other ions in the electrolytes. This provides a practical estimation of the value of Λ_0 from the values of λ_0^+ and λ_0^-. As mentioned, the conductance of an electrolyte is influenced by its concentration. Kohlrausch stated that the equivalent conductance of the electrolyte at any concentration C in mol/L or any other convenient units can be expressed as

$$\Lambda = \Lambda_0 - \beta C^{0.5} \qquad (5.3)$$

where β is a constant depending on the electrolyte.

In general, electrolytes can be classified as weak electrolytes, strong electrolytes, and ion-pair electrolytes. Weak electrolytes only dissociate to their component ions to a limited extent, and the degree of the dissociation is temperature dependent. However, strong electrolytes dissociate completely, and Equation 5.3 is applicable to evaluate its equivalent conductance. Ion-pair electrolytes can by characterized by their tendency to form ion pairs. The dissociation of ion pairs is similar to that of a weak electrolyte and is affected by ionic activities. The conductivity of ion-pair electrolytes is often nonlinear related to its concentration.

The electrolyte conductance measurement technique, in principle, is relatively straightforward. However, the conductivity measurement of an electrolyte is often complicated by the polarization of the electrodes at the operating potential. Faradaic or charge transfer processes occur at the electrode surface, complicating the conductance measurement of the system. Thus, if possible, the conductivity electrochemical sensor should operate at a potential where no faradaic processes occur. Also, another important consideration is the formation of the double layer adjacent to each electrode surface when a potential is imposed on the electrochemical sensor. The effect of the double layer complicates the interpretation of the conductivity measurement and is usually described by the Warburg impedance. Thus, even in the absence of faradaic processes, the potential effect of the double layer on the conductance of the electrolyte must be carefully assessed. The influence of a faradaic process can be minimized by maintaining a high center constant, L/A, of the electrochemical conductivity sensor, so that the cell resistance lies in the region of 1 to 50 kΩ. This implies the desirable feature of a small electrode surface area and a relatively large distance between the two electrodes. Yet, a large electrode surface area enhances the accuracy of the measurement, since a large deviation from the null point facilitates the balance of the Wheatstone bridge, resulting in improvement of sensor sensitivity. These opposing features can be resolved by using a multiple-sensing electrode configuration in which the surface area of each electrode element is small compared to the distance between the electrodes. The multiple electrodes are connected in parallel, and the output of the sensor represents the total sum of the current through each pair of electrodes. In this mode of measurement, the effect of the double layer is included in the conductance measurement. The effects of both the double layers and the faradaic processes can be minimized by using a high-frequency, low-amplitude alternating current. The higher the frequency and the lower the amplitude of the imposed alternating current, the closer the measured value is to the true conductance of the electrolyte.

5.2 Potentiometric Sensors

When a redox reaction, Ox + Ze = Red, takes place at an electrode surface in an electrochemical cell, a potential may develop at the electrode–electrolyte interface. This potential may then be used to quantify the activity (or concentration) of the species involved in the reaction forming the fundamental of potentiometric sensors.

The above reduction reaction occurs at the surface of the cathode and is defined as a half-cell reaction. At thermodynamic equilibrium, the Nernst equation is applicable and can be expressed as:

$$E = E^\circ + \frac{RT}{ZF} \ln\left(\frac{a_{ox}}{a_{red}}\right), \tag{5.4}$$

where E and E° are the measured electrode potential and the electrode potential at standard state, respectively, a_{ox} and a_{red} are the activities of Ox (reactant in this case) and Red (product in this case), respectively; Z is the number of electrons transferred, F the Faraday constant, R the gas constant, and T the operating temperature in the absolute scale. In the electrochemical cell, two half-cell reactions will take place simultaneously. However, for sensing purposes, only one of the two half-cell reactions should involve the species of interest, and the other half-cell reaction is preferably reversible and noninterfering. As indicated in Equation 5.4, a linear relation exists between the measured potential E and the natural logarithm of the ratio of the activities of the reactant and product. If the number of electrons transferred, Z, is one, at ambient temperature (25°C or 298°K) the slope is approximately 60 mV/decade. This slope value governs the sensitivity of the potentiometric sensor.

Potentiometric sensors can be classified based on whether the electrode is inert or active. An inert electrode does not participate in the half-cell reaction and merely provides the surface for the electron transfer or provides a catalytic surface for the reaction. However, an active electrode is either an ion donor or acceptor in the reaction. In general, there are three types of active electrodes: the metal/metal ion, the metal/insoluble salt or oxide, and metal/metal chelate electrodes.

Noble metals such as platinum and gold, graphite, and glassy carbon are commonly used as inert electrodes on which the half-cell reaction of interest takes place. To complete the circuitry for the potentiometric sensor, the other electrode is usually a reference electrode on which a noninterference half-cell reaction occurs. Silver/silver chloride and calomel electrodes are the most commonly used reference electrodes. Calomel consists of $Hg/HgCl_2$ and is less desirable for biomedical systems in terms of the toxicity of mercury.

An active electrode may incorporate chemical or biocatalysts and is involved as either an ion donor or acceptor in the half-cell reaction. The other half-cell reaction takes place on the reference electrode and should also be noninterfering.

If more than a single type of ion contributes to the measured potential in Equation 5.4, the potential can no longer be used to quantify the ions of interest. This is the interference in a potentiometric sensor. Thus, in many cases, the surface of the active electrode often incorporates a specific functional membrane which may be ion-selective, ion-permeable, or have ion-exchange properties. These membranes tend to selectivity permit the ions of interest to diffuse or migrate through. This minimizes the ionic interference.

Potentiometric sensors operate at thermodynamic equilibrium conditions. Thus, in practical potentiometric sensing, the potential measurement needs to be made under zero-current conditions. Consequently, a high-input impedance electrometer is often used for measurements. Also, the response time for a potentiometric sensor to reach equilibrium conditions in order to obtain a meaningful reading can be quite long. These considerations are essential in the design and selection of potentiometric sensors for biomedical applications.

5.3 Voltammetric Sensors

The current-potential relationship of an electrochemical cell provides the basis for voltammetric sensors. Amperometric sensors, that are also based on the current–potential relationship of the electrochemical cell, can be considered a subclass of voltammetric sensors. In amperometric sensors, a fixed potential is applied to the electrochemical cell, and a corresponding current, due to a reduction or oxidation reaction, is then obtained. This current can be used to quantify the species involved in the reaction. The key consideration of an amperometric sensor is that it operates at a fixed potential. However, a voltammetric sensor can operate in other modes such as linear cyclic voltammetric modes. Consequently, the respective current potential response for each mode will be different.

In general, voltammetric sensors examine the concentration effect of the detecting species on the current–potential characteristics of the reduction or oxidation reaction involved.

The mass transfer rate of the detecting species in the reaction onto the electrode surface and the kinetics of the faradaic or charge transfer reaction at the electrode surface directly affect the current–potential characteristics. This mass transfer can be accomplished through (a) an ionic migration as a result of an electric potential gradient, (b) a diffusion under a chemical potential difference or concentration gradient, and (c) a bulk transfer by natural or forced convection. The electrode reaction kinetics and the mass transfer processes contribute to the rate of the faradaic process in an electrochemical cell. This provides the basis for the operation of the voltammetric sensor. However, assessment of the simultaneous mass transfer and kinetic mechanism is rather complicated. Thus, the system is usually operated under definitive hydrodynamic conditions. Various techniques to control either the potential or current are used to simplify the analysis of the voltammetric measurement. A description of these techniques and their corresponding mathematical analyses are well documented in many texts on electrochemistry or electroanalysis (Adams, 1969; Bard and Faulkner, 1980; Lingane, 1958; Macdonald, 1977; Murray and Reilley, 1966).

A preferred mass transfer condition is total diffusion, which can be described by Fick's law of diffusion. Under this condition, the cell current, a measure of the rate of the faradaic process at an electrode, usually increases with increases in the electrode potential. This current approaches a limiting value when the rate of the faradaic process at the electrode surface reaches its maximum mass transfer rate. Under this condition, the concentration of the detecting species at the electrode surface is considered as zero and the flux is governed by diffusional mass transfer. Consequently, the limiting current and the bulk concentration of the detecting species can be related by

$$i = ZFkmC^*$$

(5.5)

where km is the mass transfer coefficient and C^* is the bulk concentration of the detecting species. At the other extreme, when the electrode kinetics are slow compared with the mass transfer rate, the electrochemical system is operated in the reaction kinetic control regime. This usually corresponds to a small overpotential. The limiting current and the bulk concentration of the detecting species can be related as

$$i = ZFkcC^* \tag{5.6}$$

where kc is the kinetic rate constant for the electrode process. Both Equations 5.5 and 5.6 show the linear relationship between the limiting current and the bulk concentration of the detecting species. In many cases, the current does not tend to a limiting value with an increase in the electrode potential. This is because other faradaic or nonfaradaic processes become active, and the cell current represents the cumulative rates of all active electrode processes. The relative rates of these processes, expressing current efficiency, depend on the current density of the electrode. Assessment of such a system is rather complicated, and the limiting current technique may become ineffective.

When a voltammetric sensor operates with a small overpotential, the faradaic reaction rate is also small; consequently, a high-precision instrument for the measurement is needed. An amperometric sensor is usually operated under limiting current or relatively small overpotential conditions. Amperometric sensors operate under an imposed fixed electrode potential. Under this condition, the cell current can be correlated with the bulk concentration of the detecting species (the solute). This operating mode is commonly classified as amperometric in most sensor work, but it is also referred to as the chronosuperometric method, since time is involved.

Voltammetric sensors can be operated in a linear or cyclic sweep mode. Linear sweep voltammetry involves an increase in the imposed potential linearly at a constant scanning rate from an initial potential to a defined upper potential limit. This is the so-called potential window. The current–potential curve usually shows a peak at a potential where the oxidation or reduction reaction occurs. The height of the peak current can be used for the quantification of the concentration of the oxidation or reduction species. Cyclic voltammetry is similar to the linear sweep voltammetry except that the electrode potential returns to its initial value at a fixed scanning rate. The cyclic sweep normally generates the current peaks corresponding to the oxidation and reduction reactions. Under these circumstances, the peak current value can relate to the corresponding oxidation or reduction reaction. However, the voltammogram can be very complicated for a system involving adsorption (nonfaradaic processes) and charge processes (faradaic processes). The potential scanning rate, diffusivity of the reactant, and operating temperature are essential parameters for sensor operation, similar to the effects of these parameters for linear sweep voltammograms. The peak current may be used to quantify the concentration of the reactant of interest, provided that the effect of concentration on the diffusivity is negligible. The potential at which the peak current occurs can be used in some cases to identify the reaction, or the reactant. This identification is based on the half-cell potential of the electrochemical reactions, either oxidation or reduction. The values of these half-cell reactions are listed extensively in handbooks and references.

The described voltammetric and amperometric sensors can be used very effectively to carry out qualitative and quantitative analyses of chemical and biochemical species. The fundamentals of this sensing technique are well established, and the critical issue is the applicability of the technique to a complex, practical environment, such as in whole blood or other biologic fluids. This is also the exciting challenge of designing a biosensor using voltammetric and amperometric principles.

5.4 Reference Electrodes

Potentiometric, voltammetric, and amperometric sensors employ a reference electrode. The reference electrode in the case of potentiometric and amperometric sensors serves as a counter electrode to complete the circuitry. In either case, the reaction of interest takes place at the surface of the working electrode, and this reaction is either an oxidation or reduction reaction. Consequently, the reaction at the counter electrode, that is, the reference electrode, is a separate reduction or oxidation reaction, respectively. It is necessary that the reaction occurring at the reference electrode does not interfere with the reaction at the working electrode. For practical applications, the reaction occurring at the reference electrode should be highly reversible and, as stated, does not contribute to the reaction at the working electrode. In electrochemistry, the hydrogen electrode is universally accepted as the primary standard with which other electrodes are compared. Consequently, the hydrogen electrode serves extensively as a standard reference. A hydrogen reference electrode is relatively simple to prepare. However, for practical applications hydrogen reference electrodes are too cumbersome to be useful.

A class of electrode called the electrode of the second kind, which forms from a metal and its sparingly soluble metal salt, finds use as the reference electrode. The most common electrode of this type includes the calomel electrode, $Hg/HgCl_2$ and the silver–silver chloride electrode, $Ag/AgCl$. In biomedical applications, particularly in *in vivo* applications, $Ag/AgCl$ is more suitable as a reference electrode.

An $Ag/AgCl$ electrode can be small, compact, and relatively simple to fabricate. As a reference electrode, the stability and reproducibility of an $Ag/AgCl$ electrode is very important. Contributing factors to instability and poor reproducibility of $Ag/AgCl$ electrodes include the purity of the materials used, the aging effect of the electrode, the light effect, and so on. When in use, the electrode and the electrolyte interface contribute to the stability of the reference electrode. It is necessary that a sufficient quantity of Cl^- ions exists in the electrolyte when the $Ag/AgCl$ electrode serves as a reference. Therefore, other silver–silver halides such as $Ag/AgBr$ or Ag/AgI electrodes are used in cases where these other halide ions are present in the electrolyte.

In a voltammetric sensor, the reference electrode serves as a true reference for the working electrode, and no current flows between the working and reference electrodes. Nevertheless, the stability of the reference electrode remains essential for a voltammetric sensor.

5.5 Summary

Electrochemical sensors are used extensively in many biomedical applications including blood chemistry sensors, PO_2, PCO_2, and pH electrodes. Many practical enzymatic sensors, including glucose and lactate sensors, also employ electrochemical sensors as sensing elements. Electrochemically based biomedical sensors are found to have *in vivo* and *in vitro* applications. We believe that electrochemical sensors will continue to be an important aspect of biomedical sensor development.

References

Adams, R. N. 1969. *Electrochemistry at Solid Electrodes*, New York, Marcel Dekker.

Bard, A. J. and Faulkner, L. R. 2000. *Electrochemical Methods: Fundamentals and Applications*, 2nd Ed., New York, John Wiley & Sons.

Clark, L. C. Jr. 1956. Monitor and control of blood and tissue oxygen tension, *Trans. Am. Soc. Artif. Organs*, 2:41.

Lingane, J. J. 1966. *Electroanalytical Chemistry*, 2nd Ed. New York, Interscience.

Macdonald, D. D. 1977. *Transient Techniques in Electrochemistry*, New York, Plenum.

MacInnes, D. A. 1939. *The Principles of Electrochemistry*, New York, Reinhold.

Monk, P. M. S. 2001. *Fundamentals of Electro-Analytical Chemistry*, New York, John Wiley & Sons.

Murray, R. W. and Reilley, C. N. 1996. *Electroanalytical Principles*, New York-London, Interscience.

6

Optical Sensors

Yitzhak Mendelson
Worcester Polytechnic
Institute

Optical methods are among the oldest and best-established techniques for sensing biochemical analytes. Instrumentation for optical measurements generally consists of a light source, a number of optical components to generate a light beam with specific characteristics and to direct this light to some modulating agent, and a photodetector for processing the optical signal. The central part of an optical sensor is the modulating component, and a major part of this chapter will focus on how to exploit the interaction of an analyte with optical radiation in order to obtain essential biochemical information.

The number of publications in the field of optical sensors for biomedical applications has grown significantly during the past two decades. Numerous scientific reviews and historical perspectives have been published, and the reader interested in this rapidly growing field is advised to consult these sources for additional details. This chapter will emphasize the basic concept of typical optical sensors intended for continuous *in vivo* monitoring of biochemical variables, concentrating on those sensors which have generally progressed beyond the initial feasibility stage and reached the promising stage of practical development or commercialization.

Optical sensors are usually based on optical fibers or on planar waveguides. Generally, there are three distinctive methods for quantitative optical sensing at surfaces:

1. The analyte directly affects the optical properties of a waveguide, such as evanescent waves (electromagnetic waves generated in the medium outside the optical waveguide when light is reflected from within) or surface plasmons (resonances induced by an evanescent wave in a thin film deposited on a waveguide surface).
2. An optical fiber is used as a plain transducer to guide light to a remote sample and return light from the sample to the detection system. Changes in the intrinsic optical properties of the medium itself are sensed by an external spectrophotometer.
3. An indicator or chemical reagent placed inside, or on, a polymeric support near the tip of the optical fiber is used as a mediator to produce an observable optical signal. Typically, conventional techniques, such as absorption spectroscopy and fluorimetry, are employed to measure changes in the optical signal.

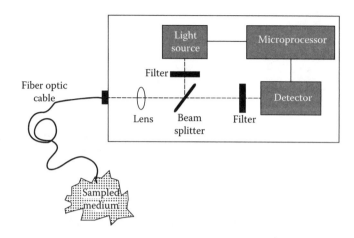

FIGURE 6.1   General diagram representing the basic building blocks of an optical instrument for optical sensor applications.

6.1 Instrumentation

The actual implementation of instrumentation designed to interface with optical sensors will vary greatly depending on the type of optical sensor used and its intended application. A block diagram of a generic instrument is illustrated in Figure 6.1. The basic building blocks of such an instrument are the light source, various optical elements, and photodetectors.

6.1.1 Light Source

A wide selection of light sources are available for optical sensor applications. These include highly coherent gas and semiconductor diode lasers, broad spectral band incandescent lamps, and narrow-band, solid-state, light-emitting diodes (LEDs). The important requirement of a light source is obviously good stability. In certain applications, for example in portable instrumentation, LEDs have significant advantages over other light sources because they are small and inexpensive, consume lower power, produce selective wavelengths, and are easy to work with. In contrast, tungsten lamps provide a broader range of wavelengths, higher intensity, and better stability but require a sizable power supply and can cause heating problems inside the apparatus.

6.1.2 Optical Elements

Various optical elements are used routinely to manipulate light in optical instrumentation. These include lenses, mirrors, light choppers, beam splitters, and couplers for directing the light from the light source into the small aperture of a fiber optic sensor or a specific area on a waveguide surface and collecting the light from the sensor before it is processed by the photodetector. For wavelength selection, optical filters, prisms, and diffraction gratings are the most common components used to provide a narrow bandwidth of excitation when a broadwidth light source is utilized.

6.1.3 Photodetectors

In choosing photodetectors for optical sensors, a number of factors must be considered. These include sensitivity, detectivity, noise, spectral response, and response time. Photomultipliers and semiconductor quantum photodetectors, such as photoconductors and photodiodes, are all suitable. The choice, however, is somewhat dependent on the wavelength region of interest. Generally, both types give adequate performance. Photodiodes are usually more attractive because of the compactness and simplicity of the circuitry involved.

Typically, two photodetectors are used in optical instrumentation because it is often necessary to include a separate reference detector to track fluctuations in source intensity and temperature. By taking a ratio between the two detector readings, whereby a part of the light that is not affected by the measurement variable is used for correcting any optical variations in the measurement system, a more accurate and stable measurement can be obtained.

6.1.4 Signal Processing

Typically, the signal obtained from a photodetector provides a voltage or a current proportional to the measured light intensity. Therefore, either simple analog computing circuitry (e.g., a current-to-voltage converter) or direct connection to a programmable gain voltage stage is appropriate. Usually, the output from a photodetector is connected directly to a preamplifier before it is applied to sampling and analog-to-digital conversion circuitry residing inside a computer.

Quite often two different wavelengths of light are utilized to perform a specific measurement. One wavelength is usually sensitive to changes in the species being measured, and the other wavelength is unaffected by changes in the analyte concentration. In this manner, the unaffected wavelength is used as a reference to compensate for fluctuation in instrumentation over time. In other applications, additional discriminations, such as pulse excitation or electronic background subtraction utilizing synchronized lock-in amplifier detection, are useful, allowing improved selectivity and enhanced signal-to-noise ratio.

6.2 Optical Fibers

Several types of biomedical measurements can be made by using either plain optical fibers as a remote device for detecting changes in the spectral properties of tissue and blood or optical fibers tightly coupled to various indicator-mediated transducers. The measurement relies either on direct illumination of a sample through the endface of the fiber or by excitation of a coating on the side wall surface through evanescent wave coupling. In both cases, sensing takes place in a region outside the optical fiber itself. Light emanating from the fiber end is scattered or fluoresced back into the fiber, allowing measurement of the returning light as an indication of the optical absorption or fluorescence of the sample at the fiber optic tip.

Optical fibers are based on the principle of total internal reflection. Incident light is transmitted through the fiber if it strikes the cladding at an angle greater than the so-called critical angle, so that it is totally internally reflected at the core/cladding interface. A typical instrument for performing fiber optic sensing consists of a light source, an optical coupling arrangement, the fiber optic light guide with or without the necessary sensing medium incorporated at the distal tip, and a light detector.

A variety of high-quality optical fibers are available commercially for biomedical sensor applications, depending on the analytic wavelength desired. These include plastic, glass, and quartz fibers which cover the optical spectrum from the UV through the visible to the near IR region. On one hand, plastic optical fibers have a larger aperture and are strong, inexpensive, flexible, and easy to work with but have poor UV transmission below 400 nm. On the other hand, glass and quartz fibers have low attenuation and better transmission in the UV but have small apertures, are fragile, and present a potential risk in *in vivo* applications.

6.2.1 Probe Configurations

There are many different ways to implement fiber optic sensors. Most fiber optic chemical sensors employ either a single-fiber configuration, where light travels to and from the sensing tip in one fiber, or a double-fiber configuration, where separate optical fibers are used for illumination and detection.

A single fiber optic configuration offers the most compact and potentially least expensive implementation. However, additional challenges in instrumentation are involved in separating the illuminating signal from the composite signal returning for processing.

The design of intravascular catheters requires special considerations related to the sterility and biocompatibility of the sensor. For example, intravascular fiberoptic sensors must be sterilizable and their material nonthrombogenic and resistant to platelet and protein deposition. Therefore, these catheters are typically made of materials covalently bound with heparin or antiplatelet agents. The catheter is normally introduced into a peripheral artery or vein via a cut-down and a slow heparin flush is maintained until the device is removed from the blood.

6.2.2 Optical Fiber Sensors

Advantages cited for fiber sensors include their small size and low cost. In contrast to electrical measurements, where the difference of two absolute potentials must be measured, fiber optics are self-contained and do not require an external reference signal. Because the signal is optical, there is no electrical risk to the patient, and there is no direct interference from surrounding electric or magnetic fields. Chemical analysis can be performed in real-time with almost an instantaneous response. Furthermore, versatile sensors can be developed that respond to multiple analytes by utilizing multiwavelength measurements.

Despite these advantages, optical fiber sensors exhibit several shortcomings. Sensors with immobilized dyes and other indicators have limited long-term stability, and their shelf life degrades over time. Moreover, ambient light can interfere with the optical measurement unless optical shielding or special time-synchronous gating is performed. As with other implanted or indwelling sensors, organic materials or cells can deposit on the sensor surface due to the biologic response to the presence of the foreign material. All of these problems can result in measurement errors.

6.2.3 Indicator-Mediated Transducers

Only a limited number of biochemical analytes have an intrinsic optical absorption that can be measured with sufficient selectivity directly by spectroscopic methods. Other species, particularly hydrogen, oxygen, carbon dioxide, and glucose, which are of primary interest in diagnostic applications, are not susceptible to direct photometry. Therefore, indicator-mediated sensors have been developed using specific reagents that are properly immobilized on the surface of an optical sensor.

The most difficult aspect of developing an optical biosensor is the coupling of light to the specific recognition element so that the sensor can respond selectively and reversibly to a change in the concentration of a particular analyte. In fiber-optic-based sensors, light travels efficiently to the end of the fiber where it exists and interacts with a specific chemical or biologic recognition element that is immobilized at the tip of the fiber optic. These transducers may include indicators and ionophores (i.e., ion-binding compounds) as well as a wide variety of selective polymeric materials. After the light interacts with the sample, the light returns through the same or a different optical fiber to a detector which correlates the degree of change with the analyte concentration.

Typical indicator-mediated fiber-optic-sensor configurations are shown schematically in Figure 6.2. In (a) the indicator is immobilized directly on a membrane positioned at the end of a fiber. An indicator in the form of a powder can be either glued directly onto a membrane, as shown in (b), or physically retained in position at the end of the fiber by a special permeable membrane (c), a tubular capillary/ membrane (d), or a hollow capillary tube (e).

6.3 General Principles of Optical Sensing

Two major optical techniques are commonly available to sense optical changes at sensor interfaces. These are usually based on evanescent wave and surface plasmon resonance principles.

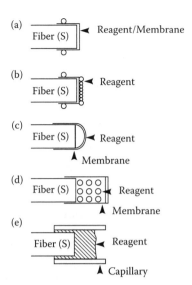

FIGURE 6.2 Typical configuration of different indicator-mediated fiber optic sensor tips. (a) Indicator is immobilized on the fiber surface, (b) indicator is immobilized on the surface of a membrane attached to the fiber, (c) indicator contained within a chamber created between a membrane and the fiber, (d) indicator contained in a chamber created by a tubular capillary at the end of the fiber, (e) indicator retained in a hollow open capillary at the end of the fiber. (Taken from Otto S. Wolfbeis, *Fiber Optic Chemical Sensors and Biosensors*, Vol. 1, CRC Press, Boca Raton, FL, 1990.)

6.3.1 Evanescent Wave Spectroscopy

When light propagates along an optical fiber, it is not confined to the core region but penetrates to some extent into the surrounding cladding region. In this case, an electromagnetic component of the light penetrates a characteristic distance (on the order of one wavelength) beyond the reflecting surface into the less optically dense medium where it is attenuated exponentially according to Beer–Lambert's law (Figure 6.3).

The evanescent wave depends on the angle of incidence and the incident wavelength. This phenomenon has been widely exploited to construct different types of optical sensors for biomedical applications. Because of the short penetration depth and the exponential decay of the intensity, the evanescent wave is absorbed mainly by absorbing compounds very close to the surface. In the case of particularly weak absorbing analytes, sensitivity can be enhanced by combining the evanescent wave principle with multiple internal reflections along the sides of an unclad portion of a fiber optic tip.

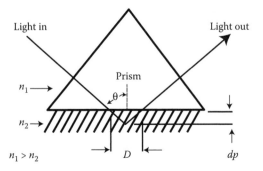

FIGURE 6.3 Schematic diagram of the path of a light ray at the interface of two different optical materials with index of refraction n_1 and n_2. The ray penetrates a fraction of a wavelength (*dp*) beyond the interface into the medium with the smaller refractive index.

Instead of an absorbing species, a fluorophore can also be used. Light is absorbed by the fluorophore emitting detectable fluorescent light at a higher wavelength, thus providing improved sensitivity. Evanescent wave sensors have been applied successfully to measure the fluorescence of indicators in solution, for pH measurement, and in immunodiagnostics.

6.3.2 Surface Plasmon Resonance

Instead of the dielectric/dielectric interface used in evanescent wave sensors, it is possible to arrange a dielectric/metal/dielectric sandwich layer such that when monochromatic polarized light (e.g., from a laser source) impinges on a transparent medium having a metallized (e.g., Ag or Au) surface, light is absorbed within the plasma formed by the conduction electrons of the metal. This results in a phenomenon known as surface plasmon resonance (SPR). When SPR is induced, the effect is observed as a minimum in the intensity of the light reflected off the metal surface.

As is the case with the evanescent wave, an SPR is exponentially decaying into solution with a penetration depth of about 20 nm. The resonance between the incident light and the plasma wave depends on the angle, wavelength, and polarization state of the incident light and the refractive indices of the metal film and the materials on either side of the metal film. A change in the dielectric constant or the refractive index at the surface causes the resonance angle to shift, thus providing a highly sensitive means of monitoring surface reactions.

The method of SPR is generally used for sensitive measurement of variations in the refractive index of the medium immediately surrounding the metal film. For example, if an antibody is bound to or absorbed into the metal surface, a noticeable change in the resonance angle can be readily observed because of the change of the refraction index at the surface, assuming all other parameters are kept

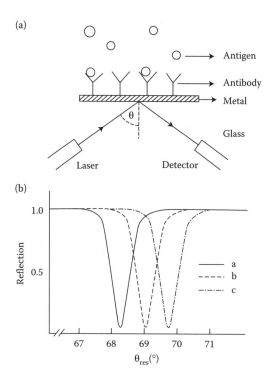

FIGURE 6.4 Surface plasmon resonance at the interface between a thin metallic surface and a liquid (a). A sharp decrease in the reflected light intensity can be observed in (b). The location of the resonance angle is dependent on the refractive index of the material present at the interface.

constant (Figure 6.4). The advantage of this concept is the improved ability to detect the direct interaction between antibody and antigen as an interfacial measurement.

SPR has been used to analyze immunochemicals and to detect gases. The main limitation of SPR, however, is that the sensitivity depends on the optical thickness of the adsorbed layer, and, therefore, small molecules cannot be measured in very low concentrations.

6.4 Applications

6.4.1 Oximetry

Oximetry refers to the colorimetric measurement of the degree of oxygen saturation of blood, that is, the relative amount of oxygen carried by the hemoglobin in the erythrocytes, by recording the variation in the color of deoxyhemoglobin (Hb) and oxyhemoglobin (HbO_2). A quantitative method for measuring blood oxygenation is of great importance in assessing the circulatory and respiratory status of a patient.

Various optical methods for measuring the oxygen saturation of arterial (SaO_2) and mixed venous (SvO_2) blood have been developed, all based on light transmission through, or reflecting from, tissue and blood. The measurement is performed at two specific wavelengths: λ_1, where there is a large difference in light absorbance between Hb and HbO_2 (e.g., 660 nm red light), and λ_2, which can be an isobestic wavelength (e.g., 805 nm infrared light), where the absorbance of light is independent of blood oxygenation, or a different wavelength in the infrared region (>805 nm), where the absorbance of Hb is slightly smaller than that of HbO_2.

Assuming for simplicity that a hemolyzed blood sample consists of a two-component homogeneous mixture of Hb and HbO_2, and that light absorbance by the mixture of these two components is additive, a simple quantitative relationship can be derived for computing the oxygen saturation of blood:

$$\text{Oxygen saturation} = A - B\left[\frac{OD(\lambda_1)}{OD(\lambda_2)}\right] \tag{6.1}$$

where A and B are coefficients which are functions of the specific absorptivities of Hb and HbO_2, and OD is the corresponding absorbance (optical density) of the blood [4].

Since the original discovery of this phenomenon over 50 years ago, there has been progressive development in instrumentation to measure oxygen saturation along three different paths: bench-top oximeters for clinical laboratories, fiber optic catheters for invasive intravascular monitoring, and transcutaneous sensors, which are noninvasive devices placed against the skin.

6.4.1.1 Intravascular Fiber Optic SvO_2 Catheters

In vivo fiberoptic oximeters were first described in the early 1960s by Polanyi and Heir [1]. They demonstrated that in a highly scattering medium such as blood, where a very short path length is required for a transmittance measurement, a reflectance measurement was practical. Accordingly, they showed that a linear relationship exists between oxygen saturation and the ratio of the infrared-to-red (IR/R) light backscattered from the blood

$$\text{oxygen saturation} = a - b(IR/R) \tag{6.2}$$

where a and b are catheter-specific calibration coefficients.

Fiber optic SvO_2 catheters consist of two separate optical fibers. One fiber is used for transmitting the light to the flowing blood, and a second fiber directs the backscattered light to a photodetector. In some commercial instruments (e.g., Oximetrix), automatic compensation for hematocrit is employed utilizing three, rather than two, infrared reference wavelengths. Bornzin et al. [2] and Mendelson et al. [3] described a 5-lumen, 7.5F thermodilution catheter that is comprised of three unequally spaced optical

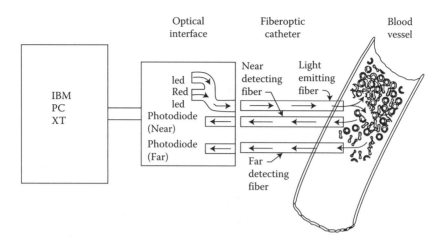

FIGURE 6.5   Principle of a three-fiber optical catheter for SvO$_2$/HCT measurement. (Taken from Bornzin G.A., Mendelson Y., Moran B.L. et al. 1987. *Proc. 9th Ann. Conf. Eng. Med. Bio. Soc.* pp. 807–809. With permission.)

fibers, each fiber 250 μm in diameter, and provides continuous SvO$_2$ reading with automatic corrections for hematocrit variations (Figure 6.5).

Intravenous fiberoptic catheters are utilized in monitoring SvO$_2$ in the pulmonary artery and can be used to indicate the effectiveness of the cardiopulmonary system during cardiac surgery and in the ICU. Several problems limit the wide clinical application of intravascular fiberoptic oximeters. These include the dependence of the individual red and infrared backscattered light intensities and their ratio on hematocrit (especially for SvO$_2$ below 80%), blood flow, motion artifacts due to catheter tip "whipping" against the blood vessel wall, blood temperature, and pH.

6.4.1.2 Noninvasive Pulse Oximetry

Noninvasive monitoring of SaO$_2$ by pulse oximetry is a well-established practice in many fields of clinical medicine [4]. The most important advantage of this technique is the capability to provide continuous, safe, and effective monitoring of blood oxygenation at the patient's bedside without the need to calibrate the instrument before each use.

Pulse oximetry, which was first suggested by Aoyagi and colleagues [5] and Yoshiya and colleagues [6], relies on the detection of the time-variant photoplethysmographic signal, caused by changes in arterial blood volume associated with cardiac contraction. SaO$_2$ is derived by analyzing only the time-variant changes in absorbance caused by the pulsating arterial blood at the same red and infrared wavelengths used in conventional invasive type oximeters. A normalization process is commonly performed by which the pulsatile (ac) component at each wavelength, which results from the expansion and relaxation of the arterial and capillary bed, is divided by the corresponding nonpulsatile (dc) component of the photoplethysmogram, which is composed of the light absorbed by the blood-less tissue and the nonpulsatile portion of the blood compartment. This effective scaling process results in a normalized red/infrared ratio which is dependent on SaO$_2$ but is largely independent of the incident light intensity, skin pigmentation, skin thickness, and tissue vasculature.

Pulse oximeter sensors consist of a pair of small and inexpensive red and infrared LEDs and a single, highly sensitive, silicon photodetector. These components are mounted inside a reusable rigid spring-loaded clip, a flexible probe, or a disposable adhesive wrap (Figure 6.6). The majority of the commercially available sensors are of the transmittance type in which the pulsatile arterial bed, for example, ear lobe, fingertip, or toe, is positioned between the LEDs and the photodetector. Other probes are available for reflectance (backscatter) measurement where both the LEDs and photodetectors are mounted side-by-side facing the skin [7,8].

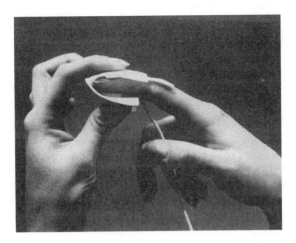

FIGURE 6.6 Disposable finger probe of a noninvasive pulse oximeter.

6.4.1.3 Noninvasive Cerebral Oximetry

Another substance whose optical absorption in the near infrared changes corresponding to its reduced and oxidized state is cytochrome aa3, the terminal member of the respiratory chain. Although the concentration of cytochrome aa3 is considerably lower than that of hemoglobin, advanced instrumentation including time-resolved spectroscopy and differential measurements is being used successfully to obtain noninvasive measurements of hemoglobin saturation and cytochrome aa3 by transilluminating areas of the neonatal brain [9–11].

6.4.2 Blood Gases

Frequent measurement of blood gases, that is, oxygen partial pressure (PO_2), carbon dioxide partial pressure (PCO_2), and pH, is essential to clinical diagnosis and management of respiratory and metabolic problems in the operating room and the ICU. Considerable effort has been devoted over the last two decades to developing disposable extracorporeal and in particular intravascular fiber optic sensors that can be used to provide continuous information on the acid-base status of a patient.

In the early 1970s, Lübbers and Opitz [12] originated what they called optodes (from the Greek, optical path) for measurements of important physiologic gases in fluids and in gases. The principle upon which these sensors was designed was a closed cell containing a fluorescent indicator in solution, with a membrane permeable to the analyte of interest (either ions or gases) constituting one of the cell walls. The cell was coupled by optical fibers to a system that measured the fluorescence in the cell. The cell solution would equilibrate with the PO_2 or PCO_2 of the medium placed against it, and the fluorescence of an indicator reagent in the solution would correspond to the partial pressure of the measured gas.

6.4.2.1 Extracorporeal Measurement

Following the initial feasibility studies of Lübbers and Opitz, Cardiovascular Devices (CDI, USA) developed a GasStat™ extracorporeal system suitable for continuous online monitoring of blood gases ex vivo during cardiopulmonary bypass operations. The system consists of a disposable plastic sensor connected inline with a blood loop through a fiber optic cable. Permeable membranes separate the flowing blood from the system chemistry. The CO_2-sensitive indicator consists of a fine emulsion of a bicarbonate buffer in a two-component silicone. The pH-sensitive indicator is a cellulose material to which hydroxypyrene trisulfonate (HPTS) is bonded covalently. The O_2-sensitive chemistry is composed of a solution of oxygen-quenching decacyclene in a one-component silicone covered with a thin layer of black PTFE for optical isolation and to render the measurement insensitive to the halothane anesthetic.

The extracorporeal device has two channels, one for arterial blood and the other for venous blood, and is capable of recording the temperature of the blood for correcting the measurements to 37°C. Several studies have been conducted comparing the specifications of the GasStat™ with that of intermittent blood samples analyzed on bench-top blood gas analyzers [13–15].

6.4.2.2 Intravascular Catheters

In recent years, numerous efforts have been made to develop integrated fiber optic sensors for intravascular monitoring of blood gases. Recent literature reports of sensor performance show considerable progress has been made mainly in improving the accuracy and reliability of these intravascular blood gas sensors [16–19], yet their performance has not yet reached a level suitable for widespread clinical application.

Most fiber optic intravascular blood gas sensors employ either a single- or a double-fiber configuration. Typically, the matrix containing the indicator is attached to the end of the optical fiber as illustrated in Figure 6.7. Since the solubility of O_2 and CO_2 gases, as well as the optical properties of the sensing chemistry itself, are affected by temperature variations, fiber optic intravascular sensors include a thermocouple or thermistor wire running alongside the fiber optic cable to monitor and correct for temperature fluctuations near the sensor tip. A nonlinear response is characteristic of most chemical indicator sensors, so they are designed to match the concentration region of the intended application. Also, the response time of the optode is somewhat slower compared to electrochemical sensors.

Intravascular fiber optic blood gas sensors are normally placed inside a standard 20-gauge catheter, which is sufficiently small to allow adequate spacing between the sensor and the catheter wall. The resulting lumen is large enough to permit the withdrawal of blood samples, introduction of a continuous heparin flush, and the recording of a blood pressure waveform. In addition, the optical fibers are encased in a protective tubing to contain any fiber fragments in case they break off.

6.4.2.3 pH Sensors

In 1976, Peterson et al. [20] originated the development of the first fiber optic chemical sensor for physiological pH measurement. The basic idea was to contain a reversible color-changing indicator at the end of a pair of optical fibers. The indicator, phenol red, was covalently bound to a hydrophilic polymer in the form of water-permeable microbeads. This technique stabilized the indicator concentration. The indicator beads were contained in a sealed hydrogen-ion-permeable envelope made out of a hollow cellulose tubing. In effect, this formed a miniature spectrophotometric cell at the end of the fibers and represented an early prototype of a fiber optic chemical sensor.

The phenol red dye indicator is a weak organic acid, and the acid form (un-ionized) and base form (ionized) are present in a concentration ratio determined by the ionization constant of the acid and the

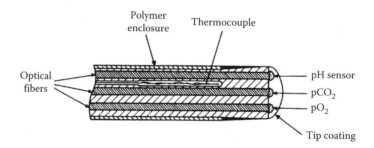

FIGURE 6.7 Structural diagram of an integrated fiber optic blood gas catheter. (Taken from Otto S. Wolfbeis, *Fiber Optic Chemical Sensors and Biosensors*, Vol. 2, CRC Press, Boca Raton, FL, 1990.)

pH of the medium according to the familiar Henderson–Hasselbalch equation. The two forms of the dye have different optical absorption spectra, so the relative concentration of one of the forms, which varies as a function of pH, can be measured optically and related to variations in pH. In the pH sensor, green (560 nm) and red (longer than 600 nm) light emerging from the end of one fiber passes through the dye and is reflected back into the other fiber by light-scattering particles. The green light is absorbed by the base form of the indicator. The red light is not absorbed by the indicator and is used as an optical reference. The ratio of green to red light is measured and is related to pH by an S-shaped curve with an approximate high-sensitivity linear region where the equilibrium constant (pK) of the indicator matches the pH of the solution.

The same principle can also be used with a reversible fluorescent indicator, in which case the concentration of one of the indicator forms is measured by its fluorescence rather than absorbance intensity. Light in the blue or UV wavelength region excites the fluorescent dye to emit longer wavelength light, and the two forms of the dye may have different excitation or emission spectra to allow their distinction.

The original instrument design for a pH measurement was very simple and consisted of a tungsten lamp for fiber illumination, a rotating filter wheel to select the green and red light returning from the fiber optic sensor, and signal processing instrumentation to give a pH output based on the green-to-red ratio. This system was capable of measuring pH in the physiologic range between 7.0 and 7.4 with an accuracy and precision of 0.01 pH units. The sensor was susceptible to ionic strength variation in the order of 0.01 pH unit per 11% change in ionic strength.

Further development of the pH probe for practical use was continued by Markle and colleagues [21]. They designed the fiber optic probe in the form of a 25-gauge (0.5 mm OD) hypodermic needle, with an ion-permeable side window, using 75-μm-diameter plastic optical fibers. The sensor had a 90% response time of 30 s. With improved instrumentation and computerized signal processing and with a three-point calibration, the range was extended to $\pm$3 pH units, and a precision of 0.001 pH units was achieved.

Several reports have appeared suggesting other dye indicator systems that can be used for fiber optic pH sensing [22]. A classic problem with dye indicators is the sensitivity of their equilibrium constant to ionic strength. To circumvent this problem, Wolfbeis and Offenbacher [23] and Opitz and Lübbers [24] demonstrated a system in which a dual sensor arrangement can measure ionic strength and pH and simultaneously can correct the pH measurement for variations in ionic strength.

6.4.2.4 PCO_2 Sensors

The PCO_2 of a sample is typically determined by measuring changes in the pH of a bicarbonate solution that is isolated from the sample by a CO_2-permeable membrane but remains in equilibrium with the CO_2. The bicarbonate and CO_2, as carbonic acid, form a pH buffer system, and, by the Henderson–Hasselbalch equation, hydrogen ion concentration is proportional to the pCO_2 in the sample. This measurement is done with either a pH electrode or a dye indicator in solution.

Vurek [25] demonstrated that the same techniques can also be used with a fiber optic sensor. In his design, one plastic fiber carries light to the transducer, which is made of a silicone rubber tubing about 0.6 mm in diameter and 1.0 mm long, filled with a phenol red solution in a 35-mM bicarbonate. Ambient PCO_2 controls the pH of the solution which changes the optical absorption of the phenol red dye. The CO_2 permeates through the rubber to equilibrate with the indicator solution. A second optical fiber carries the transmitted signal to a photodetector for analysis. The design by Zhujun and Seitz [26] uses a PCO $_2$ sensor based on a pair of membranes separated from a bifurcated optical fiber by a cavity filled with bicarbonate buffer. The external membrane is made of silicone, and the internal membrane is HPTS immobilized on an ion-exchange membrane.

6.4.2.5 PO_2 Sensors

The development of an indicator system for fiber optic PO_2 sensing is challenging because there are very few known ways to measure PO_2 optically. Although a color-changing indicator would have been desirable, the development of a sufficiently stable indicator has been difficult. The only principle applicable to fiber optics appears to be the quenching effect of oxygen on fluorescence.

Fluorescence quenching is a general property of aromatic molecules, dyes containing them, and some other substances. In brief, when light is absorbed by a molecule, the absorbed energy is held as an excited electronic state of the molecule. It is then lost by coupling to the mechanical movement of the molecule (heat), reradiated from the molecule in a mean time of about 10 ns (fluorescence), or converted into another excited state with much longer mean lifetime and then reradiated (phosphorescence). Quenching reduces the intensity of fluorescence and is related to the concentration of the quenching molecules, such as O_2.

A fiber optic sensor for measuring PO_2 using the principle of fluorescence quenching was developed by Peterson and colleagues [27]. The dye is excited at around 470 nm (blue) and fluoresces at about 515 nm (green) with an intensity that depends on the PO_2. The optical information is derived from the ratio of green fluorescence to the blue excitation light, which serves as an internal reference signal. The system was chosen for visible light excitation, because plastic optical fibers block light transmission at wavelengths shorter than 450 nm, and glass fibers were not considered acceptable for biomedical use.

The sensor was similar in design to the pH probe continuing the basic idea of an indicator packing in a permeable container at the end of a pair of optical fibers. A dye perylene dibutyrate, absorbed on a macroreticular polystyrene adsorbent, is contained in an oxygen-permeable porous polystyrene envelope. The ratio of green to blue intensity was processed according to the Stren–Volmer equation:

$$\frac{I_0}{I} = 1 + KPO_2 \tag{6.3}$$

where I and I_0 are the fluorescence emission intensities in the presence and absence of a quencher, respectively, and I is the Stern–Volmer quenching coefficient. This provides a nearly linear readout of PO_2 over the range of 0–150 mmHg (0–20 kPa), with a precision of 1 mmHg (0.13 kPa). The original sensor was 0.5 mm in diameter, but it can be made much smaller. Although its response time in a gas mixture is a fraction of a second, it is slower in an aqueous system, about 1.5 min for 90% response.

Wolfbeis et al. [28] designed a system for measuring the widely used halothane anesthetic which interferes with the measurement of oxygen. This dual-sensor combination had two semipermeable membranes (one of which blocked halothane) so that the probe could measure both oxygen and halothane simultaneously. The response time of their sensor, 15–20 s for halothane and 10–15 s for oxygen, is considered short enough to allow gas analysis in the breathing circuit. Potential applications of this device include the continuous monitoring of halothane in breathing circuits and in the blood.

6.4.3 Glucose Sensors

Another important principle that can be used in fiber optic sensors for measurements of high sensitivity and specificity is the concept of competitive binding. This was first described by Schultz et al. [29] to construct a glucose sensor. In their unique sensor, the analyte (glucose) competes for binding sites on a substrate (the lectin concanavalin A) with a fluorescent indicator-tagged polymer [fluorescein isothiocyanate (FITC)-dextran]. The sensor, which is illustrated in Figure 6.8, is arranged so that the substrate is fixed in a position out of the optical path of the fiber end. The substrate is bound to the inner wall of a glucose-permeable hollow fiber tubing (300 m O.D. × 200 m ID) and fastened to the end of an optical fiber. The hollow fiber acts as the container and is impermeable to the large molecules of the fluorescent indicator. The light beam that extends from the fiber "sees" only the unbound indicator in solution inside the hollow fiber but not the indicator bound on the container wall. Excitation light passes through the fiber and into the solution, fluorescing the unbound indicator, and the fluorescent light passes back along the same fiber to a measuring system. The fluorescent indicator and the glucose are in competitive

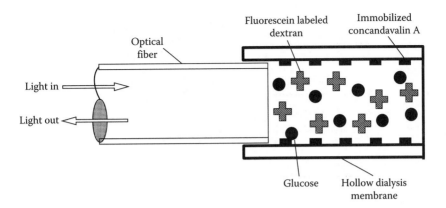

FIGURE 6.8 Schematic diagram of a competitive binding fluorescence affinity sensor for glucose measurement. (Taken from Schultz J.S., Mansouri S., and Goldstein I.J. 1982. *Diabetes Care* 5: 245. With permission.)

binding equilibrium with the substrate. The interior glucose concentration equilibrates with its concentration exterior to the probe. If the glucose concentration increases, the indicator is driven off the substrate to increase the concentration of the indicator. Thus, fluorescence intensity as seen by the optical fiber follows the glucose concentration.

The response time of the sensor was found to be about 5 min. *In vivo* studies demonstrated fairly close correspondence between the sensor output and actual blood glucose levels. A time lag of about 5 min was found and is believed to be due to the diffusion of glucose across the hollow fiber membrane and the diffusion of FTIC-dextran within the tubing.

In principle, the concept of competitive binding can be applied to any analysis for which a specific reaction can be devised. However, long-term stability of these sensors remains the major limiting factor that needs to be solved.

6.4.4 Immunosensors

Immunologic techniques offer outstanding selectivity and sensitivity through the process of antibody–antigen interaction. This is the primary recognition mechanism by which the immune system detects and fights foreign matter and has therefore allowed the measurement of many important compounds at trace levels in complex biologic samples.

In principle, it is possible to design competitive binding optical sensors utilizing immobilized antibodies as selective reagents and detecting the displacement of a labeled antigen by the analyte. Therefore, antibody-based immunologic optical systems have been the subject of considerable research [30–34]. In practice, however, the strong binding of antigens to antibodies and vice versa causes difficulties in constructing reversible sensors with fast dynamic responses.

Several immunologic sensors based on fiber optic waveguides have been demonstrated for monitoring antibody–antigen reactions. Typically, several centimeters of cladding are removed along the fiber's distal end, and the recognition antibodies are immobilized on the exposed core surface. These antibodies bind fluorophore–antigen complexes within the evanescent wave as illustrated in Figure 6.9. The fluorescent signal excited within the evanescent wave is then transmitted through the cladded fiber to a fluorimeter for processing.

Experimental studies have indicated that immunologic optical sensors can generally detect micromolar and even picomolar concentrations. However, the major obstacle that must be overcome to achieve high sensitivity in immunologic optical sensors is the nonspecific binding of immobilized antibodies.

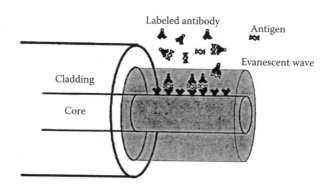

FIGURE 6.9 Basic principle of a fiber optic antigen–antibody sensor. (Taken from Anderson G.P., Golden J.P., and Ligler F.S. 1993. *IEEE Trans. Biomed. Eng.* 41: 578.)

6.5 Summary

Optical sensors have been used in many ways to detect physiological variables both *in vitro* and *in vivo*. The most frequent biomedical application involves the use of fiber optics within an interluminal catheter or tissue probe with some sort of optical indicator at or near its distal tip. This indicator communicates with body fluids or tissues through a membrane permeable to the analyte but not the indicator so the latter remains in the sensor. The intensity of the light produced or modulated by the indicator is determined by optoelectronic systems back at the proximal end of the catheter or probe. Such devices have many applications in clinical medicine but are particularly important in critical care medicine.

References

1. Polanyi M.L. and Heir R.M. 1962. *In vivo* oximeter with fast dynamic response. *Rev. Sci. Instrum.* 33: 1050.
2. Bornzin G.A., Mendelson Y., Moran B.L. et al. 1987. Measuring oxygen saturation and hematocrit using a fiberoptic catheter. *Proc. 9th Ann. Conf. Eng. Med. Bio. Soc,* Boston, pp. 807–809.
3. Mendelson Y., Galvin J.J., and Wang Y. 1990. *In vitro* evaluation of a dual oxygen saturation/hematocrit intravascular fiberoptic catheter. *Biomed. Instrum. Tech.* 24: 199.
4. Mendelson Y. 1992. Pulse oximetry: Theory and application for noninvasive monitoring. *Clin. Chem.* 28: 1601.
5. Aoyagi T., Kishi M., Yamaguchi K. et al. 1974. Improvement of the earpiece oximeter. *Jpn. Soc. Med. Electron. Biomed. Eng.* 90–91.
6. Yoshiya I., Shimada Y., and Tanaka K. 1980. Spectrophotometric monitoring of arterial oxygen saturation in the fingertip. *Med. Biol. Eng. Comput.* 18: 27.
7. Mendelson Y. and Solomita M.V. 1992. The feasibility of spectrophotometric measurements of arterial oxygen saturation from the scalp utilizing noninvasive skin reflectance pulse oximetry. *Biomed. Instrum. Technol.* 26: 215.
8. Mendelson Y. and McGinn M.J. 1991. Skin reflectance pulse oximetry: *In vivo* measurements from the forearm and calf. *J. Clin. Monit.* 7: 7.
9. Chance B., Leigh H., Miyake H. et al. 1988. Comparison of time resolved and un-resolved measurements of deoxyhemoglobin in brain. *Proc. Natl Acad. Sci. USA* 85: 4971.
10. Jobsis F.F., Keizer J.H., LaManna J.C. et al. 1977. Reflection spectrophotometry of cytochrome aa3 *in vivo. Appl. Physiol: Respirat. Environ. Excerc. Physiol.* 43: 858.
11. Kurth C.D., Steven I.M., Benaron D. et al. 1993. Near-infrared monitoring of the cerebral circulation. *J. Clin. Monit.* 9: 163.

12. Lübbers D.W. and Opitz N. 1975. The pCO$_2$/pO$_2$-optode: A new probe for measurement of pCO$_2$ or pO$_2$ in fluids and gases. *Z. Naturforsch. C: Biosci.* 30C: 532.
13. Clark C.L., O'Brien J., McCulloch J. et al. 1986. Early clinical experience with GasStat. *J. Extra Corporeal. Technol.* 18: 185.
14. Hill A.G., Groom R.C., Vinansky R.P. et al. 1985. On-line or off-line blood gas analysis: Cost vs. time vs. accuracy. *Proc. Am. Acad. Cardiovasc. Perfusion* 6: 148.
15. Siggaard-Andersen O., Gothgen I.H., Wimberley et al. 1988. Evaluation of the GasStat fluorescence sensors for continuous measurement of pH, pCO$_2$ and pO$_3$ during CPB and hypothermia. *Scand. J. Clin. Lab. Invest.* 48: 77.
16. Zimmerman J.L. and Dellinger R.P. 1993. Initial evaluation of a new intra-arterial blood gas system in humans. *Crit. Care Med.* 21: 495.
17. Gottlieb A. 1992. The optical measurement of blood gases—Approaches, problems and trends: Fiber optic medical and fluorescent sensors and applications. *Proc. SPIE* 1648: 4.
18. Barker S.L. and Hyatt J. 1991. Continuous measurement of intraarterial pHa, PaCO$_2$, and PaO$_2$ in the operation room. *Anesth. Analg.* 73: 43.
19. Larson C.P., Divers G.A., and Riccitelli S.D. 1991. Continuous monitoring of PaO$_2$ and PaCO$_2$ in surgical patients. *Abstr. Crit. Care Med.* 19: 525.
20. Peterson J.I., Goldstein S.R., and Fitzgerald R.V. 1980. Fiber optic pH probe for physiological use. *Anal. Chem.* 52: 864.
21. Markle D.R., McGuire D.A., Goldstein S.R. et al. 1981. A pH measurement system for use in tissue and blood, employing miniature fiber optic probes. In D.C. Viano (Ed.), *Advances in Bioengineering*, p. 123, New York, American Society of Mechanical Engineers.
22. Wolfbeis O.S., Furlinger E., Kroneis H. et al. 1983. Fluorimeter analysis: 1. A study on fluorescent indicators for measuring near neutral (physiological) pH values. *Fresenius' Z. Anal. Chem.* 314: 119.
23. Wolfbeis O.S. and Offenbacher H. 1986. Fluorescence sensor for monitoring ionic strength and physiological pH values. *Sens. Actuat.* 9: 85.
24. Opitz N. and Lübbers D.W. 1983. New fluorescence photomatrical techniques for simultaneous and continuous measurements of ionic strength and hydrogen ion activities. *Sens. Actuat.* 4: 473.
25. Vurek G.G., Feustel P.J., and Severinghaus J.W. 1983. A fiber optic pCO$_2$ sensor. *Ann. Biomed. Eng.* 11: 499.
26. Zhujun Z. and Seitz W.R. 1984. A carbon dioxide sensor based on fluorescence. *Anal. Chim. Acta* 160: 305.
27. Peterson J.I., Fitzgerald R.V., and Buckhold D.K. 1984. Fiber-optic probe for *in vivo* measurements of oxygen partial pressure. *Anal. Chem.* 56: 62.
28. Wolfbeis O.S., Posch H.E., and Kroneis H.W. 1985. Fiber optical fluorosensor for determination of halothane and/or oxygen. *Anal. Chem.* 57: 2556.
29. Schultz J.S., Mansouri S., and Goldstein I.J. 1982. Affinity sensor: A new technique for developing implantable sensors for glucose and other metabolites. *Diabetes Care* 5: 245.
30. Andrade J.D., Vanwagenen R.A., Gregonis D.E. et al. 1985. Remote fiber optic biosensors based on evanescent-excited fluoro-immunoassay: Concept and progress. *IEEE Trans. Elect. Devices* ED-32: 1175.
31. Sutherland R.M., Daehne C., Place J.F. et al. 1984. Optical detection of antibody–antigen reactions at a glass–liquid interface. *Clin. Chem.* 30: 1533.
32. Hirschfeld T.E. and Block M.J. 1984. Fluorescent immunoassay employing optical fiber in a capillary tube. US Patent No. 4,447,546.
33. Anderson G.P., Golden J.P., and Ligler F.S. 1993. An evanescent wave biosensor: Part I. Fluorescent signal acquisition from step-etched fiber optic probes. *IEEE Trans. Biomed. Eng.* 41: 578.
34. Golden J.P., Anderson G.P., Rabbany S.Y. et al. 1994. An evanescent wave biosensor: Part II. Fluorescent signal acquisition from tapered fiber optic probes. *IEEE Trans. Biomed. Eng.* 41: 585.

7

Bioanalytic Sensors

Richard P. Buck
University of North Carolina

7.1 Classification of Biochemical Reactions in the Context of Sensor Design and Development

7.1.1 Introduction and Definitions

Since sensors generate a measurable material property, they belong in some grouping of transducer devices. Sensors specifically contain a recognition process that is characteristic of a material sample at the molecular–chemical level, and a sensor incorporates a transduction process (step) to create a useful signal. Biomedical sensors include a whole range of devices that may be chemical sensors, physical sensors, or some kind of mixed sensor.

Chemical sensors use chemical processes in the recognition and transduction steps. Biosensors are also chemical sensors, but they use particular classes of biological recognition/transduction processes. A pure physical sensor generates and transduces a parameter that does not depend on the chemistry per se, but is a result of the sensor responding as an aggregate of point masses or charges. All these when used in a biologic system (biomatrix) may be considered bioanalytic sensors without regard to the chemical, biochemical, or physical distinctions. They provide an "analytic signal of the biologic system" for some further use.

The chemical recognition process focuses on some molecular-level chemical entity, usually a kind of chemical structure. In classical analysis this structure may be a simple functional group: SiO—in a glass electrode surface, a chromophore in an indicator dye, or a metallic surface structure, such as silver metal that recognizes Ag+ in solution. In recent times, the biologic recognition processes have been better understood, and the general concept of recognition by receptor or chemoreceptor has come into fashion. Although these are often large molecules bound to cell membranes, they contain specific structures that permit a wide variety of different molecular recognition steps including recognition of large and small species and of charged and uncharged species. Thus, chemoreceptor appears in the sensor literature as a generic term for the principal entity doing the recognition. For a history and examples, see References 1–6.

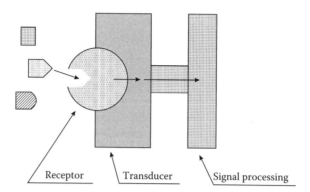

FIGURE 7.1   Generic bioanalytic sensor.

Biorecognition in biosensors has especially stressed "receptors" and their categories. Historically, application of receptors has not necessarily meant measurement directly of the receptor. Usually there are coupled chemical reactions, and the transduction has used measurement of the subsidiary products: change of pH, change of dissolved O_2, generation of H_2O_2, changes of conductivity, changes of optical adsorption, and changes of temperature. Principal receptors are enzymes because of their extraordinary selectivity. Other receptors can be the more subtle species of biochemistry: antibodies, organelles, microbes, and tissue slices, not to mention the trace level "receptors" that guide ants, such as pheromones, and other unusual species. A sketch of a generic bioanalytic sensor is shown in Figure 7.1.

7.1.2 Classification of Recognition Reactions and Receptor Processes

The concept of recognition in chemistry is universal. It almost goes without saying that all chemical reactions involved recognition and selection on the basis of size, shape, and charge. For the purpose of constructing sensors, general recognition based on these factors is not usually enough. Frequently in inorganic chemistry a given ion will react indiscriminantly with similar ions of the same size and charge. Changes in charge from unity to two, for example, do change the driving forces of some ionic reactions. By control of dielectric constant of phases, heterogeneous reactions can often be "tailored" to select divalent ions over monovalent ions and to select small versus large ions or vice versa.

Shape, however, has more special possibilities, and natural synthetic methods permit product control. Nature manages to use shape together with charge to build organic molecules, called enzymes, that have acquired remarkable selectivity. It is in the realm of biochemistry that these natural constructions are investigated and catalogued. Biochemistry books list large numbers of enzymes and other selective materials that direct chemical reactions. Many of these have been tried as the basis of selective sensors for bioanalytic and biomedical purposes. The list in Table 7.1 shows how some of the materials can be grouped into lists according to function and to analytic substrate, both organic and inorganic. The principles seem general, so there is no reason to discriminate against the inorganic substrates in favor or the organic substrates. All can be used in biomedical analysis.

7.2 Classification of Transduction Processes: Detection Methods

Some years ago, the engineering community addressed the topic of sensor classification—Richard M. White in *IEEE Trans. Ultra., Ferro., Freq. Control* (UFFC), UFFC-34 (1987) 124, and Wen H. Ko in IEEE/EMBS Symposium Abstract T.1.1 84CH2068-5 (1984). It is interesting because the physical and chemical properties are given equal weight. There are many ideas given here that remain without embodiment.

TABLE 7.1   Recognition Reactions and Receptor Processes

1. Insoluble salt-based sensors
   a. $S^+ + R^-$ 1 (insoluble salt)

   Ion exchange with crystalline SR (homogeneous or heterogeneous crystals)

Chemical signal S^{+n}	Receptor R^{-n}
Inorganic cations	Inorganic anions
Examples: Ag^+, Hg_2^{2+}, Pb^{2+}, Cd^{2+}, Cu^{2+}	$S^=$, $Se^{2=}$, SCN^-, I^-, Br^-, Cl^-

   b. $S^{-n} + R^{+n}$ 1SR (insoluble salt)

   Ion exchange with crystalline SR (homogeneous or heterogeneous crystals)

Chemical signal S^{-n}	Receptor R^{+n}
Inorganic anions	Inorganic cations
Examples: F^-, $S^=$, $Se^{2=}$, SCN^-, I^-, Br^-, Cl^-	LaF_2^+, Ag^+, Hg_2^{2+}, Pb^{2+}, Cd^{2+}, Cu^{2+}

2. Solid ion exchanges
   a. $S^{+n} + R^{-n}$ (sites) $lS^{+n} R^{-n} = SR$ (in ion exchanger phase)

   Ion exchange with synthetic ion exchangers containing negative fixed sites (homogeneous or heterogeneous, inorganic or organic materials)

Chemical signal S^{+n}	Receptor R^{-n}
Inorganic and organic ions	Inorganic and organic ion sites
Examples: H^+, Na^+, K^+	Silicate glass $Si\text{-}0^-$
H^+, Na^+, K^+, other M^{+n}	Synthetic sulfonated, phosphorylated, EDTA-substituted polystyrenes

   b. $S^{-n} + R^{+n}$ (sites) $1S^{-n} R^{+n} = SR$ (in ion exchanger phase)

   Ion exchange with synthetic ion exchangers containing positive fixed sites (homogeneous or heterogeneous, inorganic or organic materials)

Chemical signal S^{-n}	Receptor R^{+n}
Organic and inorganic ions	Organic and inorganic ion sites
Examples: hydrophobic anions	Quaternized polystyrene

3. Liquid ion exchanger sensors with electrostatic selection
   a. $S^{-n} + R^{-n}$ (sites) $lS^{+n} R^{-n} = SR$ (in ion exchanger phase)

   Plasticized, passive membranes containing mobile trapped negative fixed sites (homogeneous or heterogeneous, inorganic or organic materials)

Chemical signal S^{+n}	Receptor R^{-n}
Inorganic and organic ions	Inorganic and organic ion sites
Examples: Ca^{2+}	Diester of phosphoric acid or monoester of a phosphonic acid
M^{+n}	Dinonylnaphthalene sulfonate and other organic, Hydrophobic anions
R_1, R_2, R_3 R_4 N^+ and bis-Quaternary cations cationic drugs tetrasubstituted arsonium$^-$	Tetraphenylborate anion or substituted derivatives

   b. $S^{-n} + R^{+n}$ (sites) $1S^{-n} R^{+n} = SR$ (in ion exchanger phase)

   Plasticized, passive membranes containing mobile, trapped negative fixed sites (homogeneous or heterogeneous, inorganic or organic materials)

Chemical signal S^{-n}	Receptor R^{+n}
Inorganic and organic ions	Inorganic and organic sites
Examples: anions, simple Cl^-, Br^-, ClO_4^-	Quaternary ammonium cations: for example, tridodecylmethyl-ammonium
Anions, complex, drugs	Quaternary ammonium cations: for example, tridodecylmethyl-ammonium

4. Liquid ion exchanger sensors with neutral (or charged) carrier selection
   a. $S^{+n} + X$ and R^{-n} (sites) $lS^{+n} X R^{-n} = SXR$ (in ion exchanger phase)

continued

TABLE 7.1 (continued) Recognition Reactions and Receptor Processes

Plasticized, passive membranes containing mobile, trapped negative fixed sites (homogeneous or heterogeneous, inorganic or organic materials)

Chemical signal S^{+n}	Receptor R^{-n}
Inorganic and organic ions	Inorganic and organic ion sites
Examples: Ca^{2+}	X = synthetic ionophore complexing agent selective to Ca^{2+}
	R^{-n} usually a substituted tetra phenylborate salt
Na^+, K^+, H^+	X = selective ionophore complexing agent

b. $S^{-n} + X$ and R^{+n} (sites) $1S^{-n}\, X\, R^{+n} = SXR$ (in ion exchanger phase)

Plasticized, passive membranes containing mobile, trapped negative fixed sites (homogeneous or heterogeneous, inorganic or organic materials)

Chemical signal S^{-n}	Receptor R^{+n}
Inorganic and organic ions	Inorganic and organic ion sites
Examples: $HPO_4^{2=}$	R^{+n} = quaternary ammonium salt
	X = synthetic ionophore complexing agent; aryl organotin compound or suggested cyclic polyamido-polyamines
HCO_3^-	X = synthetic ionophore: trifluoro acetophenone
Cl^-	X = aliphatic organotin compound

5. Bioaffinity sensors based on change of local electron densitites

$S + R\ 1SR$

Chemical signal S	Receptor R
Protein	Dyes
Saccharide	Lectin
Glycoprotein	
Substrate	Enzyme
Inhibitor	Transferases
	Hydrolases (peptidases, esterases, etc.)
	Lyases
	Isomerases
	Ligases
Prosthetic group	Apoenzyme
Antigen	Antibody
Hormone	"Receptor
Substrate analogue	Transport system

6. Metabolism sensors based on substrate consumption and product formation

$S + R\ 1SR \rightarrow P + R$

Chemical signal S	Receptor R
Substrate	Enzyme
Examples: lactate (SH_2)	Hydrogenases catalyze hydrogen transfer from S to acceptor A (not molecular oxygen!) reversibly pyruvate + NADH +
$SH_2 + A\ 1S + AH_2$ lactate+ NAD^+	H^+ using lactate dehydrogenase
Glucose (SH_2)	
$SH_2 + \frac{1}{2}O_2\,1S + H_2O$ or	Oxidases catalyze hydrogen transfer to molecular oxygen
$SH_2 + O_2\ 1S + H_2O_2$	Using glucose oxidase
Glucose $+ O_2$ 1gluconolactone $+ H_2O_2$	

continued

TABLE 7.1 (continued) Recognition Reactions and Receptor Processes

Reducing agents (S)	Peroxidases catalyze oxidation of a substrate by H_2O_2 using horseradish peroxidase
$2S + 2H^+ + H_2O_2$ $12S^+ + 2H_2O$	
$Fe^{2+} + H_2O_2 + 2H^+$ $1Fe^{3+} + 2H_2O$	
Reducing agents	Oxygenates catalyze substrate oxidations by molecular O_2
L-lactate + O_2 lactate + CO_2 + H_2O	
Cofactor	Organelle
Inhibitor	Microbe
Activator	Tissue slice
Enzyme activity	
7. Coupled and hybrid systems using sequences, competition, anti-interference, and amplification concepts and reactions.	
8. Biomimetic sensors	
Chemical signal S	Receptor R
Sound	Carrier enzyme
Stress	
Light	

Source: Adapted from Scheller F. and Schubert F. 1989. Biosensors, #18 in *Advances in Research Technologies (Beitrage zur Forschungstec technologies)*, Berlin, Akademie-Verlag, Amsterdam, Elsevier; Cosofret V.V. and Buck R.P. 1992. *Pharmaceutical Applications of Membrane Sensors*, Boca Raton, FL, CRC Press.

This list is reproduced as Table 7.2. Of particular interest in this section are "detection means used in sensors" and "sensor conversion phenomena." At present the principle transduction schemes use electrochemical, optical, and thermal detection effects and principles.

7.2.1 Calorimetric, Thermometric, and Pyroelectric Transducers

Especially useful for enzymatic reactions, the generation of heat (enthalpy change) can be used easily and generally. The enzyme provides the selectivity and the reaction enthalpy cannot be confused with other reactions from species in a typical biologic mixture. The ideal aim is to measure total evolved heat, that is, to perform a calorimetric measurement. In real systems there is always heat loss, that is, heat is conducted away by the sample and sample container so that the process cannot be adiabatic as required for a total heat evolution measurement. As a result, temperature difference before and after evolution is measured most often. It has to be assumed that the heat capacity of the specimen and container is constant over the small temperature range usually measured.

The simplest transducer is a thermometer coated with the enzyme that permits the selected reaction to proceed. Thermistors are used rather than thermometers or thermocouples. The change of resistance of certain oxides is much greater than the change of length of a mercury column or the microvolt changes of thermocouple junctions.

Pyroelectric heat flow transducers are relatively new. Heat flows from a heated region to a lower temperature region, controlled to occur in one dimension. The lower temperature side can be coated with an enzyme. When the substrate is converted, the lower temperature side is warmed. The pyroelectric material is from a category of materials that develops a spontaneous voltage difference in a thermal gradient. If the gradient is disturbed by evolution or adsorption of heat, the voltage temporarily changes.

In biomedical sensing, some of the solid-state devices based on thermal sensing cannot be used effectively. The reason is that the sensor itself has to be heated or is heated quite hot by catalytic surface reactions. Thus pellistors (oxides with catalytic surfaces and embedded platinum wire thermometer), chemiresistors, and "Figaro" sensor "smoke" detectors have not found many biologic applications.

TABLE 7.2   Detection Means and Conversion Phenomena Used in Sensors

Detection means
Biologic
Chemical
Electric, magnetic, or electromagnetic wave
Heat, temperature
Mechanical displacement of wave
Radioactivity, radiation
Other
Conversion phenomena
Biologic
Biochemical transformation
Physical transformation
Effect on test organism
Spectroscopy
Other
Chemical
Chemical transformation
Physical transformation
Electrochemical process
Spectroscopy
Other
Physical
Thermoelectric
Photoelectric
Photomagnetic
Magnetoelectric
Elastomagnetic
Thermoelastic
Elastoelectric
Thermomagnetic
Thermooptic
Photoelastic
Others

7.2.2 Optical, Optoelectronic Transducers

Most optical detection systems for sensors are small, that is, they occupy a small region of space because the sample size and volume are themselves small. This means that common absorption spectrophotometers and photofluorometers are not used with their conventional sample-containing cells, or with their conventional beam-handling systems. Instead light-conducting optical fibers are used to connect the sample with the more remote monochromator and optical readout system. The techniques still remain absorption spectrophotometry, fluorimetry including fluorescence quenching, and reflectometry.

The most widely published optical sensors use a miniature reagent contained or immobilized at the tip of an optical fiber. In most systems a permselective membrane coating allows the detected species to penetrate the dye region. The corresponding absorption change, usually at a sensitive externally preset wavelength, is changed and correlated with the sample concentration. Similarly, fluorescence can be stimulated by the higher-frequency external light source and the lower-frequency emission detected. Some configurations are illustrated in References 1 and 2. Fluorimetric detection of coenzyme

A, NAD+/NADH, is involved in many so-called pyridine-linked enzyme systems. The fluorescence of NADH contained or immobilized can be a convenient way to follow these reactions. Optodes, miniature encapsulated dyes, can be placed *in vivo*. Their fluorescence can be enhanced or quenched and used to detect acidity, oxygen, and other species.

A subtle form of optical transduction uses the "peeled" optical fiber as a multiple reflectance cell. The normal fiber core glass has a refractive index greater than that of the exterior coating; there is a range of angles of entry to the fiber so that all the light beam remains inside the core. If the coating is removed and materials of lower index of refraction are coated on the exterior surface, there can be absorption by multiple reflections, since the evanescent wave can penetrate the coating. Chemical reagent can be added externally to create selective layers on the optical fiber.

Ellipsometry is a reflectance technique that depends on the optical constants and thickness of surface layer. For colorless layers, a polarized light beam will change its plane of polarization upon reflection by the surface film. The thickness can sometimes be determined when optical constants are known or approximated by constants of the bulk material. Antibody–antigen surface reaction can be detected this way.

7.2.3 Piezoelectric Transducers

Cut quartz crystals have characteristic modes of vibration that can be induced by painting electrodes on the opposite surfaces and applying a megaHertz ac voltage. The frequency is searched until the crystal goes into a resonance. The resonant frequency is very stable. It is a property of the material and maintains a value to a few parts per hundred million. When the surface is coated with a stiff mass, the frequency is altered. The shift in frequency is directly related to the surface mass for thin, stiff layers. The reaction of a substrate with this layer changes the constants of the film and further shifts the resonant frequency. These devices can be used in air, in vacuum, or in electrolyte solutions.

7.2.4 Electrochemical Transducers

Electrochemical transducers are commonly used in the sensor field. The main forms of electrochemistry used are potentiometry (zero-current cell voltage [potential difference measurements]), amperometry (current measurement at constant applied voltage at the working electrode), and ac conductivity of a cell.

7.2.4.1 Potentiometric Transduction

The classical generation of an activity-sensitive voltage is spontaneous in a solution containing both nonredox ions and redox ions. Classical electrodes of types 1, 2, and 3 respond by ion exchange directly or indirectly to ions of the same material as the electrode. Inert metal electrodes (sometimes called type 0)—Pt, Ir, Rh, and occasionally carbon C—respond by electrons exchange from redox pairs in solution. Potential differences are interfacial and reflect ratios of activities of oxidized to reduced forms.

7.2.4.2 Amperometric Transduction

For dissolved species that can exchange electrons with an inert electrode, it is possible to force the transfer in one direction by applying a voltage very oxidizing (anodic) or reducing (cathodic). When the voltage is fixed, the species will be, by definition, out of equilibrium with the electrode at its present applied voltage. Locally, the species (regardless of charge) will oxidize or reduce by moving from bulk solution to the electrode surface where they react. Ions do not move like electrons. Rather they diffuse from high to low concentration and do not usually move by drift or migration. The reason is that the electrolytes in solutions are at high concentrations, and the electric field is virtually eliminated from the bulk. The field drops through the first 1000 A at the electrode surface. The concentration of the moving species is from high concentration in bulk to zero at the electrode surface where it reacts. This process is called concentration polarization. The current flowing is limited by mass transport and so is proportional to the bulk concentration.

7.2.4.3 Conductometric Transducers

Ac conductivity (impedance) can be purely resistive when the frequency is picked to be about 1000–10,000 Hz. In this range the transport of ions is sufficiently slow that they never lose their uniform concentration. They simply quiver in space and carry current forward and backward each half cycle. In the lower and higher frequencies, the cell capacitance can become involved, but this effect is to be avoided.

7.3 Tables of Sensors from the Literature

The longest and most consistently complete references to the chemical sensor field is the review issue of *Analytical Chemistry Journal*. In the 1970s and 1980s these appeared in the April issue, but more recently they appear in the June issue. The editors are Jiri Janata and various colleagues [7–10]. Note all possible or imaginable sensors have been made according to the list in Table 7.2. A more realistic table can be constructed from the existing literature that describes actual devices. This list is Table 7.3. Book references are listed in Table 7.4 in reverse time order to about 1986. This list covers most of the major source books and many of the symposium proceedings volumes. The reviews [7–10] are a principal source of references to the published research literature.

TABLE 7.3 Chemical Sensors and Properties Documented in the Literature

I. General topics including items II–V; selectivity, fabrication, data processing
II. Thermal sensors
III. Mass sensors
  Gas sensors
  Liquid sensors
IV. Electrochemical sensors
  Potentiometric sensors
   Reference electrodes
   Biomedical electrodes
   Applications to cations, anions
   Coated wire/hybrids
   ISFETs and related
   Biosensors
   Gas sensors
  Amperometric sensors
   Modified electrodes
   Gas sensors
   Biosensors
    Direct electron transfer
    Mediated electron transfer
    Biomedical
  Conductimetric sensors
   Semiconducting oxide sensors
   Zinc oxide based
   Chemiresistors
   Dielectrometers
V. Optical sensors
   Liquid sensors
   Biosensors
   Gas sensors

TABLE 7.4 Books and Long Reviews Keyed to Items in Table 7.3 (Reviewed Since 1988 in Reverse Time Sequence)

I. *General Topics*

Yamauchi S. (ed). 1992. *Chemical Sensor Technology*, Vol 4, Tokyo, Kodansha Ltd.

Flores J.R. and Lorenzo E. 1992. Amperometric biosensors, In M.R. Smyth, J.G. Vos (eds), *Comprehensive Analytical Chemistry*, Amsterdam, Elsevier

Vaihinger S. and Goepel W. 1991. Multicomponent analysis in chemical sensing. In W. Goepel, J. Hesse, J. Zemel (eds), *Sensors*, Vol. 2, Part 1, pp. 191–237, Weinheim, Germany, VCH Publishers

Wise D.L. (ed). 1991. *Bioinstrumentation and Biosensors*, New York, Marcel Dekker; Scheller F., Schubert F. 1989. *Biosensors*, Basel, Switzerland, Birkhauser Verlag, see also [2].

Madou M. and Morrison S.R. 1989. *Chemical Sensing with Solid State Devices*, New York, Academic Press.

Janata J. 1989. *Principles of Chemical Sensors*, New York, Plenum Press.

Edmonds T.E. (ed). 1988. *Chemical Sensors*, Glasgow, Blackie.

Yoda K. 1988. Immobilized enzyme cells. *Methods Enzymology*, 137:61.

Turner A.P.F., Karube I., Wilson G.S. (eds). 1987. *Biosensors: Fundamentals and Applications*, Oxford, Oxford University Press.

Seiyama T. (ed). 1986. *Chemical Sensor Technology*, Tokyo, Kodansha Ltd.

II. *Thermal Sensors*

There are extensive research and application papers and these are mentioned in books listed under I. However, the up-to-date lists of papers are given in References 7–10.

III. *Mass Sensors*

There are extensive research and application papers and these are mentioned in books listed under I. However, the up-to-date lists of papers are given in References 7–10. Fundamentals of this rapidly expanding field are recently reviewed:

Buttry D.A. and Ward M.D. 1992. Measurement of interfacial processes at electrode surfaces with the electrochemical quartz crystal microbalance, *Chemical Reviews* 92:1355.

Grate J.W., Martin S.J., and White R.M. 1993. Acoustic wave microsensors, Part 1, *Analyt Chem* 65:940A; part 2, *Analyt. Chem.* 65:987A.

Ricco A.T. 1994. SAW Chemical sensors, *The Electrochemical Society Interface Winter*: 38–44.

IVA. *Electrochemical Sensors—Liquid Samples*

Scheller F., Schmid R.D. (eds). 1992. *Biosensors: Fundamentals, Technologies and Applications*, GBF Monograph Series, New York, VCH Publishers.

Erbach R., Vogel A., and Hoffmann B. 1992. Ion-sensitive field-effect structures with Langmuir–Blodgett membranes. In F. Scheller, R.D. Schmid (eds). *Biosensors: Fundamentals, Technologies, and Applications*, GBF Monograph 17, pp. 353–357, New York, VCH Publishers.

Ho May Y.K. and Rechnitz G.A. 1992. An introduction to biosensors, In R.M. Nakamura, Y. Kasahara, G.A. Rechnitz (eds), *Immunochemical Assays and Biosensors Technology*, pp. 275–291, Washington, DC, American Society Microbiology.

Mattiasson B. and Haakanson H. Immunochemically-based assays for process control, 1992. *Advances in Biochemical Engineering and Biotechnology* 46:81.

Maas A.H. and Sprokholt R. 1990. Proposed IFCC Recommendations for electrolyte measurements with ISEs in clinical chemistry, In A. Ivaska, A. Lewenstam, R. Sara (eds), *Contemporary Electroanalytical Chemistry, Proceedings of the ElectroFinnAnalysis International Conference on Electroanalytical Chemistry*, pp. 311–315, New York, Plenum.

Vanrolleghem P., Dries D., and Verstreate W. RODTOX: Biosensor for rapid determination of the biochemical oxygen demand, 1990. In C. Christiansen, L. Munck, J. Villadsen (eds), *Proceedings of the 5th European Congress Biotechnology*, Vol 1, pp. 161–164, Copenhagen, Denmark, Munksgaard.

Cronenberg C., Van den Heuvel H., Van den Hauw M., and Van Groen B. Development of glucose microelectrodes for measurements in biofilms, 1990. In C. Christiansen, L. Munck, J. Villadsen (eds), *Proceedings of the 5th European Congress Biotechnology*, Vol. 1, pp. 548–551, Copenhagen, Denmark, Munksgaard.

Wise D.L. (ed). 1989. *Bioinstrumentation Research, Development and Applications*, Boston, MA, Butterworth-Heinemann.

Pungor E. (ed). 1989. *Ion-Selective Electrodes—Proceedings of the 5th Symposium* [Matrafured, Hungary 1988], Oxford, Pergamon.

continued

TABLE 7.4 (continued)   Books and Long Reviews Keyed to Items in Table 7.3 (Reviewed Since 1988 in Reverse Time Sequence)

Wang J. (ed). 1988. *Electrochemical Techniques in Clinical Chemistry and Laboratory Medicine*, New York, VCH Publishers.

Evans A. 1987. *Potentiometry and Ion-Selective Electrodes*, New York, Wiley.

Ngo T.T. (ed). 1987. *Electrochemical Sensors in Immunological Analysis*, New York, Plenum.

IVB. *Electrochemical Sensors—Gas Samples*

Sberveglieri G. (ed). 1992. *Gas Sensors*, Dordrecht, The Netherlands, Kluwer.

Moseley P.T., Norris J.O.W., and Williams D.E. 1991. *Technology and Mechanisms of Gas Sensors*, Bristol, UK, Hilger.

Moseley P.T., Tofield B.D. (eds). 1989. *Solid State Gas Sensors*, Philadelphia, Taylor & Francis, Publishers.

V. *Optical Sensors*

Coulet P.R. and Blum L.J. Luminescence in biosensor design, 1991. In D.L. Wise, L.B. Wingard, Jr (eds). *Biosensors with Fiberoptics*, pp. 293–324, Clifton, NJ, Humana.

Wolfbeis OS. 1991. Spectroscopic techniques, In O.S. Wolfbeis (ed). *Fiber Optic Chemical Sensors and Biosensors*, Vol. 1, pp. 25–60. Boca Raton, FL, CRC Press.

Wolfbeis O.S. 1987. Fibre-optic sensors for chemical parameters of interest in biotechnology, In R.D. Schmidt (ed). GBF (Gesellschaft fur Biotechnologische Forschung) *Monogr. Series*, Vol. 10, pp. 197–206, New York, VCH Publishers

7.4 Applications of Microelectronics in Sensor Fabrication

The reviews of sensors since 1988 cover fabrication papers and microfabrication methods and examples [7–10]. A recent review by two of the few chemical sensor scientists (chemical engineers) who also operate a microfabrication laboratory is C. C. Liu, Z.-R. Zhang. 1992. Research and development of chemical sensors using microfabrication techniques. *Selective Electrode* 14:147.

References

1. Janata J. 1989. *Principles of Chemical Sensors*, New York, Plenum.
2. Scheller F. and Schubert F. 1989. *Biosensors, #18 in Advances in Research Technologies (Beitrage zur Forschungstechnologie)*, Berlin, Akademie-Verlag, Amsterdam, Elsevier (English translation).
3. Turner A.P.F., Karube I., and Wilson G.S. 1987. *Biosensors: Fundamentals and Applications*, Oxford, Oxford University Press.
4. Hall E.A.H. 1990. *Biosensors*, Milton Keynes, England, Open University Press.
5. Eddoes M.J. 1990. Theoretical methods for analyzing biosensor performance. In A.E.G. Cass (ed), *Biosensor—A Practical Approach*, Oxford, IRL Press at Oxford University, Ch. 9, pp. 211–262.
6. Cosofret V.V. and Buck R.P. 1992. *Pharmaceutical Applications of Membrane Sensors*, Boca Raton, FL, CRC Press.
7. Janata J. and Bezegh A. 1988. Chemical sensors, *Analyt. Chem.* 60: 62R.
8. Janata J. 1990. Chemical sensors, *Analyt. Chem.* 62: 33R.
9. Janata J. 1992. Chemical sensors, *Analyt. Chem.* 66: 196R.
10. Janata J., Josowicz M., and DeVaney M. 1994. Chemical sensors, *Analyt. Chem.* 66: 207R.

8

Biological Sensors for Diagnostics

Orhan Soykan
Michigan Technological University

8.1 Diagnostics Industry

Many biologically relevant molecules can be measured from the samples taken from the body, which constitutes the foundation of the medical diagnostics industry. In 2003, the global clinical diagnostic market was more than U.S. $2 billion. Of that, sales of the laboratory instruments constituted slightly less than half, while the point of care systems and the diagnostic kits made up the rest. Even though this amount accounts for only a few percent of the total spending on healthcare, it continues to grow, and not surprisingly, a significant number of biomedical engineers are employed in the research, design, and manufacturing of these products.

Utilization of these devices for various functions is shown in Table 8.1.

In this chapter, we will discuss some examples to illustrate the principles and the technologies used for these measurements. They will be categorized in three groups (a) sensors for proteins and enzymes, (b) sensors for nucleic acids, and (c) sensors for cellular processes.

8.2 Diagnostic Sensors for Measuring Proteins and Enzymes

We are all born with the genes that we will carry throughout our lives, and our genetic makeup remains relatively constant except in parts of the immune and reproductive systems. Expression patterns of genes on the other hand are noting but constant. These changes can be due to aging, environmental and physiological conditions we experience, or due to diseases. Hence, many of the diseases can be detected by sensing the presence, or measuring the level of activity of proteins and enzymes in the tissue and blood for diagnostic purposes. In this section, we will review some of these techniques.

TABLE 8.1 Diagnostics Industry by Discipline

Discipline	Percentage
Clinical chemistry tests	42.0
Immunodiagnostics	30.6
Hematology/flow cytometry	7.7
Microbiology	6.9
Molecular diagnostics	5.8
Coagulation	3.4
Other	3.5

Source: Simonsen M., *BBI Newsletter*, 27, 221–228, 2004.

8.2.1 Spectrophotometry

Spectrophotometry utilizes the principle of atomic absorption to determine the concentration of a substance in a volume of solution. Transmission of light through a clear fluid containing an analyte has a reciprocal relationship to the concentration of the analyte, as shown in Figure 8.1b [2]. Percent transmission can be calculated as

$$\%T = \frac{I_T}{I_O}100$$

where, I_T and I_O are intensities of transmitted and incident light respectively.

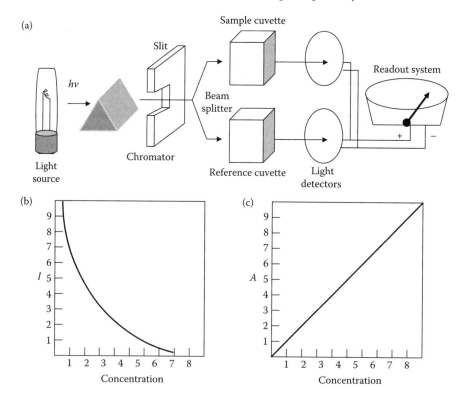

FIGURE 8.1 Principle of spectrophotometry: monochromated light is split into two beams and passed through a sample cuvette as well as a reference solution. Intensities of the transmitted light beams are compared to determine the concentration of the analyte in the sample. Lower two graphs show the percent transmission of light and absorption as a function of the concentration of the analyte of interest in a given solution.

Absorption (*A*) can be defined as $A = -\log(\%T)$, which yields a linear relationship between absorption and the concentration (*C*) of the solute, as shown in Figure 8.1c.

A schematic diagram of a spectrophotometer is shown in Figure 8.1a. Light from an optical source is first passed through a monochromator, such as a prism or a diffraction grating. Then, a beam splitter produces two light beams where one passes through a cuvette containing the patient sample, and the other through a cuvette containing a reference solution. Intensities of the transmitted light beams are detected and compared to each other to determine the concentration of the analyte in the sample [3].

The exponential form of the Beer–Lambert law can be used to calculate the absorption of light passing through a solution.

$$\frac{I_T}{I_O} = e^{-A}$$

where I_T is the transmitted light intensity, I_O is the incident light intensity, and *A* is the absorption occurring in the light amplitude as it travels through the media.

Absorption in a cuvette can be calculated as follows:

$$A = abC$$

where *a* is the absorptivity coefficient, *b* is the optical path length in the solution, and *C* is the concentration of the colored analyte of interest.

If A_S and A_R are the absorption in the sample and the reference cuvettes, and the C_S and C_R are the analyte concentrations in the sample and reference cuvettes, then the concentration in the sample cuvette can be calculated as follows:

$$\frac{A_S}{A_R} = \frac{C_S}{C_R} \Rightarrow C_S = \frac{A_S}{A_R}C_R = \frac{\log(I_R)}{\log(I_S)}C_R$$

where I_S and I_R are the intensity of the light transmitted through the cuvettes and detected by the photo-sensors.

A common use of spectrophotometry in clinical medicine is for the measurement of hemoglobin. Hemoglobin is made of heme, an iron compound, and globin, a protein. The iron gives blood its red color and the hemoglobin tests make use of this red color. A chemical is added to a sample of blood to make the red blood cells burst and to release the hemoglobin into the surrounding fluid, coloring it clear red. By measuring this color change using a spectrophotometer, and using the above equations, the concentration of hemoglobin in the blood can be determined [4,5].

For substances that are not colored, one can monitor the absorption at wavelengths that are outside of the visible spectrum, such as infrared and ultraviolet. Additionally, fluorescence spectroscopy can also be utilized.

8.2.2 Immunoassays

When the concentration of the analyte in the biological solution is too low for detection using spectrophotometry, more sensitive methods such as immunoassays are used for the measurement. Immunoassays utilize antibodies developed against the analyte of interest. Since the antigen and the antibody have a very specific interaction and has very high affinity toward each other, the resulting detection system also has a very high sensitivity. A specific example, the enzyme linked immunosorbent assay (ELISA), will be described here.

First, antibodies against the protein to be measured are developed in a host animal. For example, protein can be the human cardiac troponin-T (h-cT), which is a marker of myocardial infarction. Purified h-cT is injected into a rabbit to raise IgG molecules against h-cT, and these antibodies can either be recovered from the blood or produced recombinantly in a bioprocessor. A secondary antibody is also needed, which reacts with the first antibody and provides a colored solution. For example, this secondary antibody can be the goat antirabbit IgG antibody, which is tagged with a coloring compound or a fluorescent molecule. This second antibody can be used for any ELISA test that utilizes rabbit IgGs, regardless of the analyte, and such secondary antibodies are usually available commercially [6].

In the first step, a solution containing the protein of interest is placed on a substrate forming the sensor, such as a polystyrene dish. Then, the first antibody is added to the solution and allowed to react with the analyte. Unbound antibody is washed away and the second antibody is added. After a sufficient time is allowed for the second antibody to react with the first one, a second wash is performed to remove the unbound second antibody. Now the remaining solution contains the complexes formed by the protein of interest as well as the first and the second antibodies. Therefore, the color or the fluorescence produced is a function of the protein concentration. Figure 8.2 shows the steps used in an ELISA process. ELISAs are used for many clinical tests such as determining pregnancy or infectious disease tests such as detecting HIV. Its high sensitivity is due to the extremely high specificity of the antigen–antibody interaction [7,8].

8.2.3 Mass Spectrometry

Sometimes a test for more than one protein is needed and mass spectrometry is the method of choice for that purpose. A good example for this would be the use of tandem mass spectrometry to screen neonates for metabolic disorders such as amino acidemias (e.g., phenylketonuria—PKU), organic acidemias (e.g., propionic acidemia—PPA), and fatty acid oxidation disorders (e.g., Medium-chain acyl-CoA Dehydrogenase deficiency—MCAD) [9]. Although the price of this capital equipment could be high, costs of using it as a sensor is quite low (usually < U.S. $50.00 to screen for more than 20 metabolic disorders), and many states in the United States provide the service to newborns during the first week of life.

A mass spectrometer can be considered as a giant sensor, which measures the mass/charge (m/z) ratio as well as the relative abundance of multiple molecules in a given sample. Mass spectrometers consist of three main components: an ionization source, a physical separation environment, and a detector. Ionization of the molecules in the sample can be done by the deposition of energy from a laser source to remove an electron, a technique known as laser desorption ionization, which is depicted on the left side of Figure 8.3. Alternatively, it is possible to ionize molecules in a fluid flow by applying an electrical voltage to cause them to charge and subsequently spray, a technique known as electrospray ionization.

Following the ionization step, the molecules are sent into a physical separation chamber, where they are separated based on their m/z ratio. This can be achieved by first accelerating them in an electric field to give them a speed of

$$v = \sqrt{\frac{2Uz}{m}}$$

where U is the accelerating potential, z and m are the charge and the mass of the molecule respectively.

Since the velocity is a function of the mass, a determination of the mass of the molecules becomes possible in the physical separation environment. One option is to measure the time of flight in a flight tube, as shown in the middle section of Figure 8.3. This technique is known as the time-of-flight measurement, and makes use of the fact that larger molecules will fly slowly and require more time to cross the flight tube. Molecular mass can be calculated as

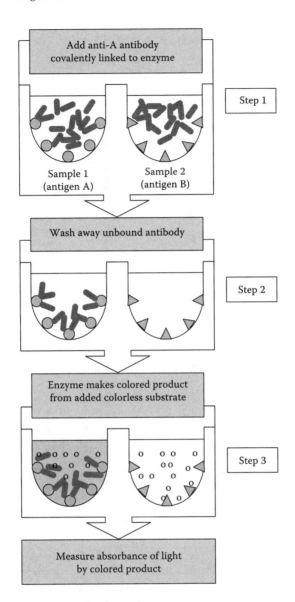

FIGURE 8.2 Steps of ELISA process. (1) Specimen containing the target molecule antigen A, shown as round circles, is exposed to the primary antibody, shown as rectangular shapes. (2) Unbound antibody is washed, leaving the plate on the right-hand side with no primary antibodies. (3) Secondary antibody depicted with oval shapes is added to the wells. (4) Unbound secondary antibody is also washed away, leaving the primary–secondary antibody complex along with the target molecule in the wells (step not shown). Test on the left plate would give a positive response to this test.

$$m = 2\frac{T^2}{L^2}Uz$$

where T is the flight time and L is the length of the flight tube.

Alternatively, one can apply a fixed magnetic field, perpendicular to the flight path of the ions, and cause a deviation in the flight path of the moving ions to separate them.

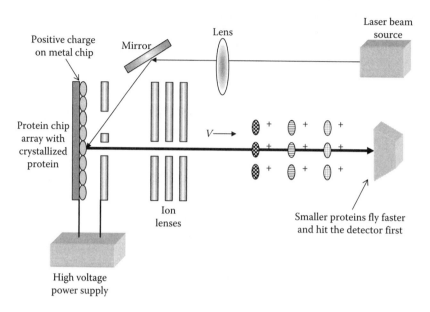

FIGURE 8.3 Mass spectrophotometry: proteins are released from the chip surface by the application of the laser pulse. A secondary pulse is used to charge the proteins, which are later accelerated in an electric field. A time-of-flight measurement can be used to determine the mass of the protein.

Although the mass spectrometer can separate the molecules based on their molecular weight, additional analysis is needed to separate molecules with identical or similar masses. This can be achieved by tandem mass spectrometry, where the ions coming from the first spectrometer enter into an argon collision chamber, and the resulting molecular fragments are catalogued by a secondary mass spectrometer. By studying the fragments, composition of the original mixture and the relative amount of the ions in the solution can be calculated [10–12].

8.2.4 Electrophoresis

Electrophoresis can be used to obtain a rapid separation of the proteins. A typical apparatus used for this purpose is shown in Figure 8.4. Proteins are first exposed to negatively charged sodium dodecyl sulfate, or SDS, which binds to the hydrophobic regions of the proteins, and causes them to unfold. The mixtures are placed into the wells on top of vertically placed gel slabs, as shown in Figure 8.4. Application of the electric potential, usually on the order of hundreds of volts, across the gel creates a force to move the protein molecules downward. Mobility of the proteins in the gel is given by

$$\mu = \frac{Q}{6\pi r \eta}$$

where μ is the electrophoretic mobility (cm/s), Q, the ionic charge (due to SDS), r, the radius of the protein, and η is the viscosity of the cellulose acetate or polyacrylamide gel.

Therefore, the movement of the ions within the gel is directly proportional to the applied voltage, and inversely proportional to the size of the protein. Gel electrophoresis is run for a fixed amount of time, allowing the small proteins to migrate further than the larger ones, resulting in their separation based on their size. Coomassie blue or silver staining can be used to detect the bands across the gel to confirm the presence of proteins with known molecular masses.

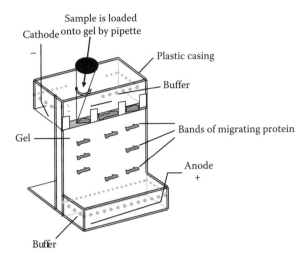

Sample is loaded
Cathode onto gel by pipette

Plastic casing

Buffer

Gel

Bands of migrating protein

Anode
+

Buffer

FIGURE 8.4 Gel electrophoresis: proteins loaded on the slab of gel are separated based on their size as they migrate under a constant electric field. Smaller proteins move faster and travel further than the larger ones.

Unlike mass spectroscopy, gel electrophoresis does not provide a quantitative value for the amount of given protein. However, it provides a low cost and relatively rapid method for the analysis of multiple proteins in a specimen, especially when implemented as a capillary electrophoresis system. Therefore, it has been used for the separation of enzymes (e.g., creatinine phosphokinase), mucopolysaccharides, plasma, serum, cerebrospinal fluid, urine, and other bodily fluids [13]. It is also used for quality control applications for the manufacturing of biological compounds to verify the purity or to examine the manufacturing yield [14].

8.2.5 Chromatography

Chromatography is also a simple technique that has applications in the toxicology and serum drug level measurements. In paper chromatography, a solution containing the analytes wicks up an absorbent paper for a period of time, and separation is achieved by the relative position of the analytes while the analyte and the solvent move up in the paper. A more precise technique known as column chromatography uses affinity columns, where the sample is applied to the top of the column and the fractionated molecules are eluted and collected at the bottom of the column (Figure 8.5). Since the smaller molecules with lower affinity to the column material will come out sooner than the larger molecules and ones with the higher affinity to the column, separation is achieved as a function of time. Further analysis can be done in the fractionated samples if desired.

8.3 Sensors for Measuring Nucleic Acids

Nucleic acids present in the body exist in the form of DNA and RNA. Determination of DNA sequences would allow the clinicians to determine the presence to congenital or genetically inherited diseases. On the other hand, measurement of RNA levels would indicate if gene is turned on or off. Discussions in this section focus on the basics of few of the tools used in practice beginning with some enabling technologies.

8.3.1 Enabling Technologies: DNA Extraction and Amplification

Cells in the human body contain the genetic material, DNA, which consists of a very long series of nucleic acids. Three nucleic acids in a row in the genome is called a codon, which determines the amino

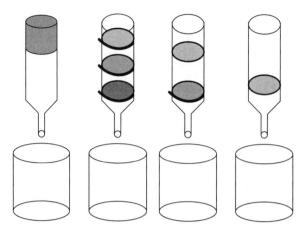

FIGURE 8.5 Affinity chromatography: a chemical column with relatively high affinity to proteins is loaded with a mixture of proteins, and allowed to run downward with the aid of gravity. Eluted fractions are collected in different tubes, each of which would contain different group of proteins.

acid to be used when synthesizing a protein. This genetic code is shown in Table 8.2. Table 8.2 has $4^3 = 64$ entries, but since there are only 20 amino acids, many of the codons do code the same amino acid, a fact known as the redundancy of the genetic code. Therefore, a change in the genetic sequence may or may not cause a change in the protein synthesis. If the variation in the genetic sequence causes a change in the amino acid sequence altering the function of the protein, then an altered phenotype may emerge. Although the results of some of these changes are benign, such as different hair and eye colors, others are not, such as increased susceptibility to various diseases. This genetic information can be read from the genes of interest. However, before that can be done, the DNA must be extracted and amplified.

TABLE 8.2 Genetic Code

1st Base in Codon	2nd Base in Codon					3rd Base in Codon
	U	C	A	G		
U	Phe	Ser	Tyr	Cys	U	
	Phe	Ser	Tyr	Cys	C	
	Leu	Ser	**STOP**	**STOP**	A	
	Leu	Ser	**STOP**	Trp	G	
C	Leu	Pro	His	Arg	U	
	Leu	Pro	His	Arg	C	
	Leu	Pro	Gln	Arg	A	
	Leu	Pro	Gln	Arg	G	
A	Ile	Thr	Asn	Ser	U	
	Ile	Thr	Asn	Ser	C	
	Ile	Thr	Lys	Arg	A	
	Met	Thr	Lys	Arg	G	
G	Val	Ala	Asp	Gly	U	
	Val	Ala	Asp	Gly	C	
	Val	Ala	Glu	Gly	A	
	Val	Ala	Glu	Gly	G	

Note: Amino acids coded by three nucleic acid bases are shown as the entries of the table.

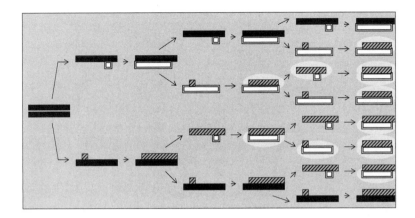

FIGURE 8.6 Polymerase chain reaction: double-stranded DNA is first heated to denature the bonds between the two strands. In the second step, primers are allowed to attach to their complementary strands. In the third step, double stranded DNA is formed by the enzyme DNA polymerase. Process is repeated many times, doubling the amount of DNA at each step.

Extraction of DNA from biological samples can be accomplished by precipitation or affinity methods [15]. Amplification of the amount of DNA is also needed before any sequence detection can be done. This can be done by a method known as polymerase chain reaction or PCR in short. This process is depicted in Figure 8.6. Briefly, original double stranded DNA molecules, shown as black rectangles, are heated to more than 90°C for separation. Afterward, DNA primers, shown as squares, as well as nucleic acids are added to the solution to initiate the DNA synthesis, forming two pairs of double stranded DNA at the end of the first cycle. The process is repeated for more than 30 times, doubling the amount of DNA at each step [16]. RNA can also be amplified using a similar process known as reverse transcription-polymerase chain reaction (RT-PCR) [17].

8.3.2 DNA/RNA Probes

Gene chip arrays are being utilized as sensors to measure the level of gene expression to discover the genetic causes or to validate the presence of various disorders such as cancer. The most common form of these sensors is the RNA chips that consist of an array of probes. Each spot on the array contains multiple copies of a single genetic sequence immobilized to the sensor surface. These probe sequences are complementary to the RNA sequences being studied. Amplified RNA from the patient is labeled with a fluorescent dye, for example one that fluoresces red in this case. A second set of RNA, the reference RNA, with known concentration is labeled with another fluorescent dye, for example, green in this case. The RNA solutions are mixed and exposed to the sensor. Since sections of RNA from the patient and the reference are complementary to individual probe sequence, there would be a competitive binding during the exposure period (Figure 8.7). Following the incubation period, unbound RNA is removed, and the sensor array is exposed to a light source for the measurement of the fluorescence from each spot on the array. If a spot fluoresces red, the indication would be that the most of the RNA bound to this spot came from the patient, meaning that the patient is expressing this gene at high levels. On the other hand, a green fluorescence would indicate that the binding is from the reference RNA, and the patient is not expressing high levels of the gene. A yellow color would indicate a moderate gene expression, since some of each type of RNA molecule must bind to the probe to produce the mixed response. The advantage of these sensors is the same as any other sensor array, which is the ability to probe a large number of genes simultaneously [18].

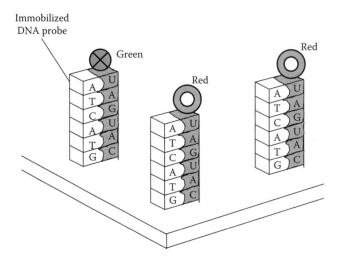

FIGURE 8.7 Gene array: reference RNA labeled with green fluorescence molecules compete with the RNA from the patient labeled with red fluorescent molecules to bind to the immobilized probes on the gene array.

8.3.3 SNP Detection

Single nucleotide polymorphism, or SNP, occurs when only one nucleotide in the genetic sequence is altered. It could be a mutation, and it could be inherited from a parent. Reading a single nucleotide from the genome that had been substituted for another one might stop the reading process of that gene or cause a different protein to be synthesized. Thus detecting a SNP could be important in diagnosing genetically related diseases or a patient's tendency toward being more susceptible to this type of disease.

There are many methods developed for the detection of a SNP, and one of them will be described later, which is illustrated in Figure 8.8. In the first step, a primer consisting of 20–50 nucleic acids having a sequence complementary to the gene sequence adjacent to the SNP is synthesized and allowed to anneal

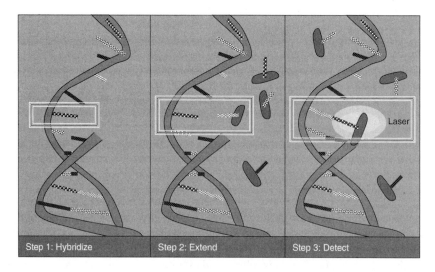

FIGURE 8.8 SNP detection by primer extension method: first the amplified DNA is hybridized to the primers that are specific to the genetic region of interest. Second, a labeled terminating base at the target SNP site extends the primer. Finally, the extended primer is read by fluorescence.

to a single strand of the DNA from the patient. In the second step, terminal nucleic acids (A, T, C, and G) with different fluorescent tags are added allowing the double stand to grow by only one base pair. As the third step, the solution is exposed to a laser light for detecting the fluorescence to read the nucleic acid at the SNP location. Since the patient sample will contain two copies for each gene, one from each parent, the sensor might detect one or two nucleic acids for each SNP site [19].

Detection of SNPs can be used as a clinical test to diagnose various diseases. Some examples of these are SNPs for BRAC-1 gene to detect patients with high susceptibility to a type of breast cancer, and long-quantitative trait (QT) genes, which make patients prone to fatal cardiac arrhythmias [20,21].

8.4 Sensors for Cellular Processes

Flow cytometry is used to separate populations of cells in a mixture from one another by means of fluorescently labeled antibodies and DNA-specific dyes. Antibodies used are usually against the molecules expressed on the cell surface, such as cell-surface receptors. The labeled cells are diluted in a solution and passed through a nozzle in a single-cell stream while being illuminated by a laser beam. Fluorescence is detected by photomultiplier tubes (PMTs) with optical filters to determine the emission wavelength, which in turn helps to identify the surface receptors (Figure 8.9). Fluorescence data are used to measure the relative proportions of various cell types in the mixture, and to derive the diagnostic information [22].

Flow cytometry is commonly used in the clinical diagnostics, for immunophenotyping leukemia, counting stem cells for optimizing autologous transplants for the treatment of leukemia, counting CD4+/CD8+ lymphocytes in HIV-infected patients to determine the progression of the disease, and the analysis of stained DNA from solid tumors [23].

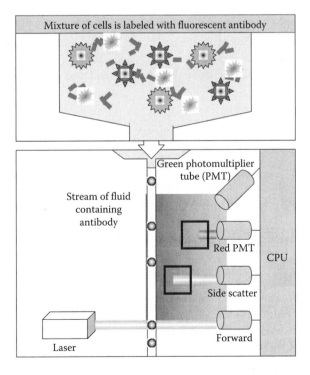

FIGURE 8.9 Flow cytometry: fluorescently labeled cells are passed in front of light detectors (labeled as PMTs in the figure) to detect their labeling color, which indicates the phenotype of the cell.

8.5 Personalized Medicine

Today the personalization of the treatment for the needs of individual patients is done by healthcare providers. In some cases, clinicians can neither predict reliably the best treatment pathway for a patient, nor anticipate the optimal drug regimen. However, it would be possible to improve the treatment and tailor the therapy to the specific needs of the patients if their genetic information is known. For example, some drugs are known to cause cardiac arrhythmias in patients with certain genotypes and should be avoided. It might be possible that in the future, patients coming to hospitals might be asked to bring their genome cards along with their insurance cards. Knowledge of the genome of individual patients would not only predict their medical vulnerabilities, but also help with the selection of their treatment [24].

Some of these studies have already begun. For example, in the United States, the Food and Drug Administration is already encouraging the pharmaceutical industry to submit the results of genomic tests when seeking approval for new drugs [25]. This new field of research is now being recognized as pharmacogenetics.

Another early application of personalized medicine is the use of microphysiometry, a device that measures the extracellular acidification rate of cells, to establish their sensitivity to chemotherapy [26]. This sensor measures the chemosensitivity by comparing the acidification rate of cells treated with cytostatic agents, such as anticancer drugs, to that of nontreated cells, before a drug is prescribed to the patient.

8.6 Final Comments

As the aging of the population in the Western world, and the increase in the population of the World in general continues, the need for diagnostic procedures will also increase. Due to the need for cost containment, the emphasis will continue to shift from therapeutics to early diagnosis for prevention. Both of these factors will increase the need for diagnostic procedures and additional diagnostic technologies. While the basic methodology for the traditional diagnostics is becoming well established, the techniques needed for personalized medicine are still being developed, and the biomedical engineers will be able to participate in both the research and implementation aspects of these very important areas.

References

1. Simonsen, M., Nucleic acid testing, proteomics to drive future of diagnostics, *BBI Newsletter*, 27, 221–228, 2004.
2. Skoog, D.A. and Leary, J.J., *Principles of Instrumental Analysis*, 4th ed., Saunders, Orlando, FL, 1992.
3. Kellner, R., Mermet, J.-M., Otto, M., and Widmer, H.M., *Analytical Chemistry*, Wiley, Weinheim, GR, 1998.
4. Kaplan, A., Jack, R., Opheim, K.E., Toivola, B., and Lyon, A.W., *Clinical Chemistry*, 4th ed., Williams & Wilkins, Malvern, PA, 1995.
5. Burtis, C.A. and Ashwood, E.R., *Tietz Fundamentals of Clinical Chemistry*, 5th ed., W.B. Saunders, Philadelphia, PA, 2001.
6. Alberts, B., Bray, D., Lewis, J., Raff, M., Roberts, K., and Watson, J.D., *Molecular Biology of the Cell*, 3rd ed., Garland, New York, NY, 1994,
7. Liu, S., Boyer-Chatenet, L., Lu, H., and Jiang, S., Rapid and automated fluorescence-linked immunosorbent assay for high-throughput screening of HIV-1 fusion inhibitors targeting gp41. *J. Biomol. Screen.* 8, 685–693, 2003.
8. Bandi, Z.L., Schoen, I., and DeLara, M., Enzyme-linked immunosorbent urine pregnancy tests, *Am. J. Clin. Pathol.*, 87, 236–242, 1987.

9. Schulze, A., Lindner, M., Kohlmuller, D., Olgemoller, K., Mayatepek, E., and Hoffmann, G.F., Expanded newborn screening for inborn errors of metabolism by electrospray ionization-tandem mass spectrometry: Results, outcome, and implications, *Pediatrics*, 111, 1399–1406, 2003.

10. Liebler, D.C., *Introduction to Proteomics*, Humana Press, Totowa, NJ, 2002.

11. Pennington, S.R. and Dunn, M.J., *Proteomics*, Springer-Verlag, New York, NY, 2001.

12. Kambhampati, D., *Protein Microarray Technology*, Wiley, Heppenheim, GR, 2004.

13. Chen, F.T., Liu, C.M., Hsieh, Y.Z., and Sternberg, J.C., Capillary electrophoresis—A new clinical tool, *Clin. Chem.*, 37, 14–19, 1991.

14. Reilly, R.M., Scollard, D.A., Wang, J., Monda, H., Chen, P., Henderson, L.A., Bowen, B.M., and Vallis, K.A., A kit formulated under good manufacturing practices for labeling human epidermal growth factor with 111In for radiotherapeutic applications, *J. Nucl. Med.*, 45, 701–708, 2004.

15. Bowtell, D. and Sambrook, J., *DNA Microarrays: A Molecular Cloning Manual*, Cold Spring Harbor Press, Cold Spring Harbor, NY, 2003.

16. Malacinski, G.M., *Essentials of Molecular Biology*, 4th ed., Jones and Bartlett, Sudbury, MA, 2003.

17. Stahlberg, A., Hakansson, J., Xian, X., Semb, H., and Kubista, M., Properties of the reverse transcription reaction in mRNA quantification, *Clin. Chem.*, 50, 509–515, 2004.

18. Blalock, E., *A Beginner's Guide to Microarrays*, Kluwer, Dordrecht, NL, 2003.

19. Kwok, P.-Y., *Single Nucleotide Polymorphisms: Methods and Protocols*, Humana, Totowa, NJ, 2003.

20. Burke, W., Genomic medicine: Genetic testing, *N. Engl. J. Med.*, 347, 1867–1875, 2002.

21. Haack, B., Kupka, S., Ebauer, M., Siemiatkowska, A., Pfister, M., Kwiatkowska, J., Erecinski, J., Limon, J., Ochman, K., and Blin, N., Analysis of candidate genes for genotypic diagnosis in the long QT syndrome, *J. Appl. Genet.*, 45, 375–381, 2004.

22. Lodish, H., Berk, A., Zipursky, S.L., Matsudaira, P., Baltimore, D., and Barnell, J., *Molecular Cell Biology*, 4th ed., W.H. Freeman, New York, NY, 2000.

23. Rose, N.R., Friedman, H., and Fahey, J.L., *Manual of Clinical Laboratory Immunology*, 3rd ed., American Society for Microbiology, Washington, D.C., 1986.

24. Brown, S.M., *Essentials of Medical Genomics*, Wiley, Hoboken, NJ, 2003.

25. Guidance for Industry: Pharmacogenomic Data Submissions, U.S. Department of Health and Human Services, Food and Drug Administration, November 2003.

26. Waldenmaier, D.S., Babarina, A., and Kischkel, F.C., Rapid *in vitro* chemosensitivity analysis of human colon tumor cell lines, *Toxicol. Appl. Pharmacol.*, 192, 237–245, 2003.

II

Medical Instruments and Devices

Steven Schreiner
The College of New Jersey

Preface

This section of the *Biomedical Engineering Handbook* covers the broad topic of medical instruments and devices. Given the breadth of this topic, it is an impossible task to include all aspects within the confines of this medium. This section has been created to provide information on a range of instruments and devices that span not only a range of physiological systems, but also span the physiological scale: from molecule to cell to organ to organ system. Each chapter provides the reader a solid foundation on the topic and offers resources for deeper investigation. I would like to acknowledge the work of the previous editor, Dr. Wolf W. von Maltzahn of Rensselaer Polytechnic Institute whose editorial prowess is still clearly visible in the design of this section.

Sadly, during the writing of this edition, Dr. Leslie A. Geddes passed away at the age of 88. With BS and MS in electrical engineering from McGill University and a PhD in physiology from Baylor University College of Medicine, Dr. Geddes was a pioneer in biomedical engineering and spent his life teaching and conducting biomedical engineering research. At the time of his death, he was the Showalter Distinguished Professor Emeritus of Bioengineering and the former director of the Hillenbrand Biomedical Engineering Center at Purdue University. Internationally renowned, he was the recipient of numerous awards and prizes, as well as the inventor for many patents. I send my condolences to Dr. Geddes' family; he will be missed by the entire biomedical engineering community. I am pleased to offer you his two foundational chapters in this section on cardiac output and respiration.

9

Biopotential Amplifiers

Joachim H. Nagel
University of Stuttgart

9.1 Introduction

Biosignals are recorded as potentials, voltages, and electrical field strengths generated by nerves and muscles. The measurements involve voltages at very low levels, typically ranging between 1 μV and 100 mV, with high source impedances and superimposed high-level interference signals and noise. The signals need to be amplified to make them compatible with devices such as displays, recorders, or analog/digital (A/D) converters for computerized equipments. Amplifiers suitable to measure these signals have to satisfy very specific requirements. They have to provide amplification selective to the physiological signal, reject superimposed noise and interference signals, and guarantee protection from damages through voltage and current surges for both patient and electronic equipment. Amplifiers featuring these specifications are known as biopotential amplifiers. The basic requirements and features as well as some specialized systems will be presented.

9.2 Basic Amplifier Requirements

The basic requirements that a biopotential amplifier has to satisfy are

- The physiological process to be monitored should not be influenced in any way by the amplifier
- The measured signal should not be distorted
- The amplifier should provide the best possible separation of signal and interferences
- The amplifier has to offer protection of the patient from any hazard of electrical shock
- The amplifier itself has to be protected against damages that might result from high input voltages as they occur during the application of defibrillators or electrosurgical instrumentation

A typical configuration for the measurement of biopotentials is shown in Figure 9.1. Three electrodes, two of them detecting the biological signal and the third providing the reference potential, connect the

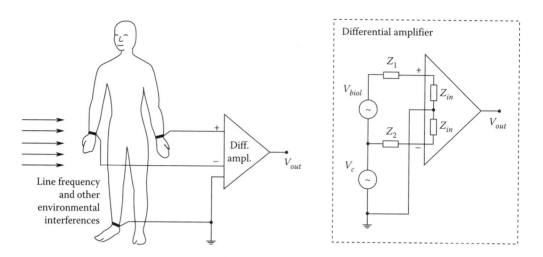

FIGURE 9.1 Typical configuration for the measurement of biopotentials. The biological signal V_{biol} appears between the two measuring electrodes at the right and left arm of the patient, and is fed to the inverting and the noninverting inputs of the differential amplifier. The right leg electrode provides the reference potential for the amplifier with a common mode voltage V_c as indicated.

subject to the amplifier. The input signal to the amplifier consists of five components: the desired biopotential, undesired biopotentials, a power line interference signal of 60 Hz (50 Hz in some countries) and its harmonics, interference signals generated by the tissue/electrode interface, and noise. Accurate design of the amplifier provides rejection of a large portion of the signal interferences. The main task of the differential amplifier as shown in Figure 9.1 is to reject the line frequency interference that is electrostatically or magnetically coupled to the subject. The desired biopotential appears as a voltage between the two input terminals of the differential amplifier and is referred to as the *differential signal*. The line frequency interference signal shows only very small differences in amplitude and phase between the two measuring electrodes, causing approximately the same potential at both inputs, and thus appears only between the inputs and ground and is called the *common mode signal*. Strong rejection of the common mode signal is one of the most important characteristics of a good biopotential amplifier.

The *common mode rejection ratio* or CMRR of an amplifier is defined as the ratio of the differential mode gain over the common mode gain. As seen in Figure 9.1, the rejection of the common mode signal in a biopotential amplifier is both a function of the amplifier CMRR and the source impedances Z_1 and Z_2. For the ideal biopotential amplifier with $Z_1 = Z_2$ and infinite CMRR of the differential amplifier, the output voltage is the pure biological signal amplified by G_D, the differential mode gain: $V_{out} = G_D \cdot V_{biol}$. With finite CMRR, the common mode signal is not completely rejected, adding the interference term $G_D \cdot V_c/CMRR$ to the output signal. Even in the case of an ideal differential amplifier with infinite CMRR, the common mode signal will not completely disappear unless the source impedances are equal. The common mode signal V_c causes currents to flow through Z_1 and Z_2. The related voltage drops show a difference if the source impedances are unequal, thus generating a differential signal at the amplifier input, which, of course, is not rejected by the differential amplifier. With amplifier gain G_D and input impedance Z_{in}, the output voltage of the amplifier is

$$V_{out} = G_D V_{biol} + \frac{G_D V_c}{CMRR} + G_D V_c \left(1 - \frac{Z_{in}}{Z_{in} + Z_1 - Z_2}\right) \qquad (9.1)$$

The output of a real biopotential amplifier will always consist of the desired output component owing to a differential biosignal, an undesired component because of incomplete rejection of common mode interference signals as a function of CMRR and an undesired component because of source impedance unbalance allowing a small proportion of a common mode signal to appear as a differential signal to the amplifier. Because source impedance unbalances of 5000–10,000 Ω, mainly caused by electrodes, are not uncommon and sufficient rejection of line frequency interferences requires a minimum CMRR of 100 dB, the input impedance of the amplifier should be at least 10^9 Ω at 60 Hz to prevent source impedance unbalances from deteriorating the overall CMRR of the amplifier. State-of-the-art biopotential amplifiers provide a CMRR of 120–140 dB.

To provide optimum signal quality and adequate voltage level for further signal processing, the amplifier has to provide a gain of 100–50,000 and needs to maintain the best possible signal-to-noise ratio. The presence of high-level interference signals not only deteriorates the quality of the physiological signals, but also restricts the design of the biopotential amplifier. Electrode half-cell potentials, for example, limit the gain factor of the first amplifier stage because their amplitude can be several orders of magnitude larger than the amplitude of the physiological signal. To prevent the amplifier to go into saturation, this component has to be eliminated before the required gain can be provided for the physiological signal.

A typical design of the various stages of a biopotential amplifier is shown in Figure 9.2. The electrodes that provide the transition between the ionic flow of currents in biological tissue and the electronic flow of current in the amplifier represent a complex electrochemical system that is described elsewhere in this handbook. The electrodes determine to a large extent the composition of the measured signal. The preamplifier represents the most critical part of the amplifier itself as it sets the stage for the quality of the biosignal. With appropriate design, the preamplifier can eliminate, or at least minimize most of the signals interfering with the measurement of biopotentials.

In addition to electrode potentials and electromagnetic interferences, noise—generated by the amplifier and the connection between biological source and amplifier—has to be taken into account when designing the preamplifier. The total source resistance R_s, including the resistance of the biological source and all transition resistances between signal source and amplifier input, causes thermal voltage noise with a root mean square (rms) value of

$$E_{rms} = \sqrt{4kTR_sB} \cdot (V)$$

(9.2)

where k = Boltzmann constant, T = absolute temperature, R_s = resistance in ohms, and B = bandwidth in Hertz.

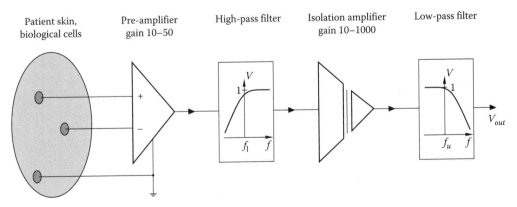

FIGURE 9.2 Schematic design of the main stages of a biopotential amplifier. Three electrodes connect the patient to a preamplifier stage. After removing DC and low-frequency interferences, the signal is connected to an output low-pass filter through an isolation stage that provides electrical safety to the patient, prevents ground loops, and reduces the influence of interference signals.

Additionally, there is the inherent amplifier noise. It consists of two frequency-dependent components, the internal voltage noise source e_n and the voltage drop across the source resistance R_s caused by an internal current noise generator i_n. The total input noise for the amplifier with a bandwidth of $B = f_2 - f_1$ is calculated as the sum of its three independent components:

$$E_{rms}^2 = \int_{f_1}^{f_2} e_n^2 df + R_s^2 \int_{f_1}^{f_2} i_n^2 df + 4kTR_s B \qquad (9.3)$$

High signal-to-noise ratios thus require the use of very low noise amplifiers and the limitation of bandwidth. The current technology offers differential amplifiers with voltage noise of less than 10 nV/√Hz and current noise less than 1 pA/√Hz. Both parameters are frequency dependent and decrease approximately with the square root of frequency. The exact relationship depends on the technology of the amplifier input stage. Field effect transistor (FET) preamplifiers exhibit about 5 times the voltage noise density compared to bipolar transistors but a current noise density that is about 100 times smaller.

The purpose of the high- and low-pass filters, shown in Figure 9.2, is to eliminate interference signals such as electrode half-cell potentials and preamplifier offset potentials and to reduce the noise amplitude by the limitation of the amplifier bandwidth. Because the biosignal should not be distorted or attenuated, higher order sharp-cutting linear-phase filters have to be used. Active Bessel filters are preferred filter types because of their smooth transfer function. Separation of biosignal and interference is in most cases incomplete because of the overlap of their spectra.

The isolation stage serves the galvanic decoupling of the patient from the measuring equipment and provides safety from electrical hazards. This stage also prevents galvanic currents from deteriorating the signal to noise ratio, especially by preventing ground loops. Various principles can be used to realize the isolation stage. Analog isolation amplifiers use either transformer, optical, or capacitive couplers to transmit the signal through the isolation barrier. Digital isolation amplifiers use a voltage/frequency converter to digitize the signal before it is transmitted easily by optical or inductive couplers to the output frequency/voltage converter. The most important characteristics of an isolation amplifier are low leakage current, isolation impedance, isolation voltage (or mode) rejection (IMR), and maximum safe isolation voltage.

9.2.1 Interferences

The most critical point in the measurement of biopotentials is the contact between electrodes and biological tissue. Both the electrode offset potential and the electrode/tissue impedance are subject to changes because of relative movements of electrode and tissue. Thus, two interference signals are generated as motion artifacts: the changes of the electrode potential and motion-induced changes of the voltage drop caused by the input current of the preamplifier. These motion artifacts can be minimized by providing high input impedances for the preamplifier, usage of nonpolarized electrodes with low half-cell potentials such as Ag/AgCl electrodes, and by reducing the source impedance by use of electrode gel. Motion artifacts, interferences from external electromagnetic fields, and noise can also be generated in the wires connecting electrodes and amplifier. Reduction of these interferences is achieved by using twisted pair cables, shielded wires, and input guarding.

Recording of biopotentials is often done in an environment that is equipped with many electrical systems that produce strong electrical and magnetic fields. In addition to 60 Hz (or 50 Hz) power line frequency and some strong harmonics, high-frequency electromagnetic fields are encountered. At power line frequency, the electric and magnetic components of the interfering fields can be considered separately. Electrical fields are caused by all conductors that are connected to power, even with no flow

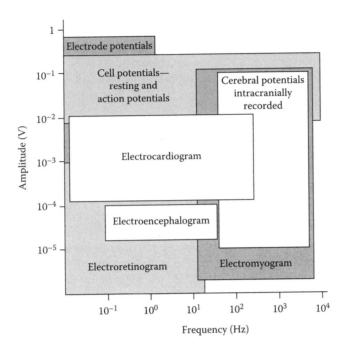

FIGURE 9.3 Amplitudes and spectral ranges of some important biosignals. The various biopotentials completely cover the area from 10^{-6} to almost 1 V and from DC to 10 kHz.

of current. A current is capacitively coupled into the body where it flows to the ground electrode. If an isolation amplifier is used without patient ground, the current is capacitively coupled to the ground. In this case, the body potential floats with a voltage of up to 100 V toward the ground. Minimizing interferences requires increasing the distance between power lines and the body, use of isolation amplifiers, separate grounding of the body at a location as far away from the measuring electrodes as possible, and use of shielded electrode cables.

The magnetic field components produce eddy currents in the body. Amplifier, electrode cable, and the body form an induction loop that is subject to the generation of an interference signal. Minimizing this interference signal requires increasing the distance between interference source and patient, twisting the connecting cables, shielding of the magnetic fields, and relocating the patient to a place and orientation that offers minimum interference signals. In many cases, an additional narrow-band-rejection filter (notch filter) is implemented as an additional stage in the biopotential amplifier to provide sufficient suppression of line frequency interferences.

To achieve optimum signal quality, the biopotential amplifier has to be adapted to the specific application. On the basis of signal parameters, both appropriate bandwidth and gain factor are chosen. Figure 9.3 shows an overview of the most commonly measured biopotentials and specifies the normal ranges for amplitude and bandwidth.

A final requirement for biopotential amplifiers is the need for calibration. Because the amplitude of the biopotential often has to be determined very accurately, there must be provisions to easily determine the gain or the amplitude range referenced to the input of the amplifier. For this purpose, the gain of the amplifier must be well calibrated. To prevent difficulties with calibrations, some amplifiers that need to have adjustable gain use various fixed gain settings rather than providing a continuous gain control. Some amplifiers have a standard signal source of known amplitude built in that can be momentarily connected to the input by the push of a button to check the calibration at the output of the biopotential amplifier. Table 9.1 gives an example for the specifications of a typical electrocardiogram (ECG) amplifier.

TABLE 9.1 Typical Specifications for an ECG Amplifier

Gain	500, 1000, 2000, and 5000
Frequency response	Maximum bandwidth (0.05 Hz–10 kHz)
Low-pass filter	20 Hz, 35 Hz, 50 Hz, 150 Hz, 1 kHz, and 10 kHz
High-pass filter	0.05 Hz, 0.1 Hz, 0.5 Hz, 1.0 Hz, and 10 Hz
Filter type	Slope Butterworth, flattest response, and −12 dB/octave
Notch interference filter	50 dB rejection at 50 or 60 Hz
Noise voltage (0.05–35 Hz)	0.1 μV (rms)
Z_{in}	2 MΩ (differential), 1000 MΩ (common mode)
CMRR	110 dB min (50/60 Hz)
Common mode input voltage range	±10 V
Output range	±10 V (analog)
Input voltage range	
Gain	V_{in} (mV)
500:	±20
1000:	±10
2000:	±5
5000:	±2
AC calibrator	1 mV P–P square wave, 10 Hz
Subject isolation	>4 kV

9.2.2 Special Circuits

9.2.2.1 Instrumentation Amplifier

An important stage of all biopotential amplifiers is the input preamplifier that substantially contributes to the overall quality of the system. The main tasks of the preamplifier are to sense the voltage between two measuring electrodes while rejecting the common mode signal and minimizing the effect of electrode polarization overpotentials. Crucial to the performance of the preamplifier is the input impedance that should be as high as possible. Such a differential amplifier cannot be realized using a standard single *operational amplifier* (op-amp) design because this does not provide the necessary high input impedance. The general solution to the problem involves voltage followers or noninverting amplifiers, to attain high input impedances. A possible realization is shown in Figure 9.4a. The main disadvantage

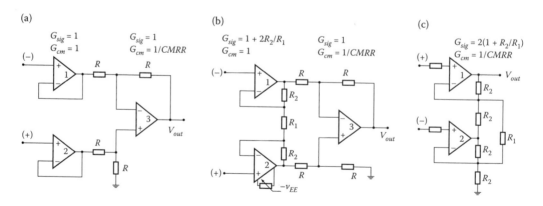

FIGURE 9.4 Circuit drawings for three different realizations of instrumentation amplifiers for biomedical applications. (a) Voltage follower input stage, (b) improved, amplifying input stage, and (c) 2-op-amp version.

of this circuit is that it requires high CMRR both in the followers and in the final op-amp. With the input buffers working at unity gain, all the common mode rejection must be accomplished in the output amplifier, requiring very precise resistor matching. Additionally, the noise of the final op-amp is added at a low signal level, decreasing the signal-to-noise ratio unnecessarily. The circuit in Figure 9.4b eliminates this disadvantage. It represents the standard instrumentation amplifier configuration. The two input op-amps provide high differential gain and unity common mode gain without the requirement of close resistor matching. The differential output from the first stage represents a signal with substantial relative reduction of the common mode signal and is used to drive a standard differential amplifier that further reduces the common mode signal. CMRR of the output op-amp as well as resistor matching in its circuit are less critical than in the follower-type instrumentation amplifier. Offset trimming for the whole circuit can be done at one of the input op-amps. Complete instrumentation amplifier integrated circuits based on this standard instrumentation amplifier configuration are available from several manufacturers. All components except R_1, which determines the gain of the amplifier, and the potentiometer for offset trimming are contained on the integrated circuit chip. Figure 9.4c shows another configuration that offers high input impedance with only two op-amps. For good CMRR, however, it requires precise resistor matching.

In applications where direct current (DC) and very-low-frequency biopotentials are not to be measured, it would be desirable to block those signal components at the preamplifier inputs by simply adding a capacitor working as a passive high-pass filter. This would eliminate the electrode offset potentials and permit a higher gain factor for the preamplifier *and thus a higher CMRR*. A capacitor between electrodes and amplifier input would, however, result in charging effects from the input bias current. Owing to the difficulty of precisely matching capacitors for the two input leads, they would also contribute to an increased source impedance unbalance and thus reduce CMRR. Avoiding the problem of charging effects by adding a resistor between the preamplifier inputs and ground, as shown in Figure 9.5a, also results in a decrease of CMRR because of the diminished and mismatched input impedance. A 1% mismatch for two 1 MΩ resistors can already create a −60 dB loss in CMRR. The loss in CMRR is much greater if the capacitors are mismatched, which cannot be prevented in real systems. Nevertheless, such realizations are used where the specific situation permits. In some applications, a further reduction of the amplifier to a two-electrode amplifier configuration would be convenient, even at the expense of some loss in the CMRR. Figure 9.6 shows a preamplifier design working with two electrodes and providing alternating current (AC) coupling as proposed by Pallás-Areny and Webster (1990).

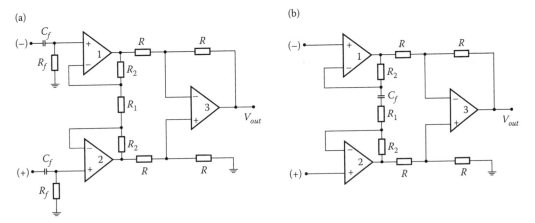

FIGURE 9.5   AC-coupled instrumentation amplifier designs. The classical design using an RC high-pass filter at the inputs (a) and a high CMRR "quasi-high-pass" amplifier as proposed by C.C. Lu (b).

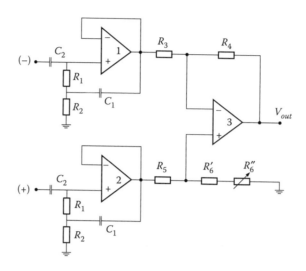

FIGURE 9.6 Composite instrumentation amplifier based on an AC-coupled first stage. The second stage is based on a one op-amp differential amplifier that can be replaced by an instrumentation amplifier.

A third alternative of eliminating DC and low frequencies in the first amplifier stage, a directly coupled quasi-high-pass amplifier design can be used that maintains the high CMRR of DC-coupled high input impedance instrumentation amplifiers (Song et al. 1998). In this design, the gain determining resistor R_1 (Figure 9.5a) is replaced by a first-order high-pass filter consisting of R_1 and a series capacitor C_f. The signal gain of the amplifier is

$$G = 1 + \frac{2R_2}{R_1 + (1/j\omega C)} \tag{9.4}$$

Thus, DC gain is 1, whereas the high-frequency gain remains at $G = 1 + 2R_2/R_1$. A realization using an off-the-shelf instrumentation amplifier (Burr-Brown INA 118) operates at low power (0.35 mA) with low offset voltage (11 µV typical) and low input bias current (1 nA typical), and offers a high CMRR of 118 dB at a gain of $G = 50$. The very high input impedance (10 GΩ) of the instrumentation amplifier renders it insensitive to fluctuations of the electrode impedance. Therefore, it is suitable for bioelectric measurements using pasteless electrodes applied to unprepared, that is, high impedance skin.

The preamplifier, often implemented as a separate device that is placed adjacent to the electrodes or even directly attached to the electrodes, also acts as an impedance converter that allows the transmission of even weak signals to the remote monitoring unit. Owing to the low output impedance of the preamplifier, the input impedance of the following amplifier stage can be low, and still the influence of interference signals coupled into the transmission lines is reduced.

9.3 Isolation Amplifier and Patient Safety

Isolation amplifiers can be used to break ground loops, eliminate source ground connections, and provide isolation protection to the patient and electronic equipment. In a biopotential amplifier, the main purpose of the isolation amplifier is the protection of the patient by eliminating the hazard of electric shock resulting from the interaction among patient, amplifier, and other electric devices in the patient's environment, specifically defibrillators and electrosurgical equipment. It also adds to the prevention of line frequency interferences.

Isolation amplifiers are realized in three different technologies: transformer isolation, capacitor isolation, and optoisolation. An isolation barrier provides a complete galvanic separation of the input side, that is, patient and preamplifier, from all equipment on the output side. Ideally, there will be no flow of electric current across the barrier. The isolation mode voltage is the voltage that appears across the isolation barrier, that is, between the input common and the output common (Figure 9.7). The amplifier has to withstand the largest expected isolation voltages without damage. Two isolation voltages are specified for commercial isolation amplifiers: the continuous rating and the test voltage. To eliminate the need for longtime testing, the device is tested at about 2 times the rated continuous voltage. Thus, for a continuous rating of 2000 V, the device has to be tested at 4000–5000 V for a reasonable period of time.

Because there is always some leakage across the isolation barrier, the isolation mode rejection ratio (IMRR) is not infinite. For a circuit as shown in Figure 9.7, the output voltage is

$$V_{out} = \frac{G}{R_{G1} + R_{G2} + R_{IN}}\left[V_D + \frac{V_{CM}}{CMRR}\right] + \frac{V_{ISO}}{IMRR} \tag{9.5}$$

where G is the amplifier gain, V_D, V_{CM}, and V_{ISO} are differential, common mode, and isolation voltages, respectively, and CMRR is the common mode rejection ratio for the amplifier (Burr-Brown, 1994).

Typical values of IMRR for a gain of 10 are 140 dB at DC, and 120 dB at 60 Hz with a source unbalance of 5000 Ω. The isolation impedance is approximately 1.8 pF $\|$ 10^{12} Ω.

Transformer-coupled isolation amplifiers perform on the basis of inductive transmission of a carrier signal that is amplitude modulated by the biosignal. A synchronous demodulator on the output port reconstructs the signal before it is fed through a Bessel response low-pass filter to an output buffer. A power transformer, generally driven by a 400–900 kHz square wave, supplies isolated power to the amplifier.

Optically coupled isolation amplifiers can principally be realized using only a single light-emitting diode (LED) and photodiode combination. Although useful for a wide range of digital applications, this design has fundamental limitations as to its linearity and stability as a function of time and temperature. A matched photodiode design, as used in the Burr-Brown 3650/3652 isolation amplifier, overcomes these difficulties (Burr-Brown, 1994). Operation of the amplifier requires an isolated power supply to drive the input stages. Transformer-coupled low-leakage current-isolated DC/DC converters

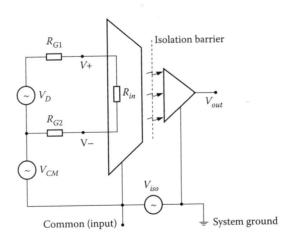

FIGURE 9.7 Equivalent circuit of an isolation amplifier. The differential amplifier on the left transmits the signal through the isolation barrier by a transformer, capacitor, or an optocoupler.

are commonly used for this purpose. In some particular applications, especially in cases where the signal is transmitted over a longer distance by fiber optics, for example, ECG amplifiers used for gated magnetic resonance imaging, batteries are used to power the amplifier. Fiber optic coupling in isolation amplifiers is another option that offers the advantage of higher flexibility in the placement of parts on the amplifier board.

Biopotential amplifiers have to provide sufficient protection from electrical shock to both user and patient. Electrical-safety codes and standards specify the minimum safety requirements for the equipment, especially the maximum leakage currents for chassis and patient leads, and the power distribution system (Webster, 1992; AAMI, 1993).

Special attention to patient safety is required in situations where biopotential amplifiers are connected to personal computers (PCs) that are increasingly used to process and store physiological signals and data. Owing to the design of the power supplies used in standard PCs permitting high leakage currents—an inadequate situation for a medical environment—there is a potential risk involved even when the patient is isolated from the PC through an isolation amplifier stage or optical signal transmission from the amplifier to the computer. This holds especially in those cases where because of the proximity of the PC to the patient, an operator might touch the patient and computer at the same time, or the patient might touch the computer. It is required that a special power supply with sufficient limitation of leakage currents is used in the computer, or that an additional, medical grade isolation transformer is used to provide the necessary isolation between power outlet and PC.

9.4 Surge Protection

The isolation amplifiers described in the preceding section are primarily used for the protection of the patient from electric shock. Voltage surges between electrodes as they occur during the application of a defibrillator or electrosurgical instrumentation also present a risk to the biopotential amplifier. Biopotential amplifiers should be protected against serious damage to the electronic circuits. This is also part of the patient safety because defective input stages could otherwise apply dangerous current levels to the patient. To achieve this protection, voltage-limiting devices are connected between each measuring electrode and electric ground. Ideally, these devices do not represent a shunt impedance and thus do not lower the input impedance of the preamplifier as long as the input voltage remains in a range considered safe for the equipment. They appear as an open circuit. As soon as the voltage drop across the device reaches a critical value V_b, the impedance of the device changes sharply and current passes through it to such an extent that the voltage cannot exceed V_b because of the voltage drop across the series resistor R as indicated in Figure 9.8.

The devices used for amplifier protection are diodes, Zener diodes, and gas-discharge tubes. Parallel silicon diodes limit the voltage to approximately 600 mV. The transition from nonconducting to conducting state is not very sharp and signal distortion begins at about 300 mV that can be within the range of input voltages depending on the electrodes used. The breakdown voltage can be increased by connecting several diodes in series. Higher breakdown voltages are achieved by Zener diodes connected back to back. One of the diodes will be biased in the forward direction and the other in the reverse direction. The breakdown voltage in the forward direction is approximately 600 mV but the breakdown voltage in the reverse direction is higher, generally in the range of 3–20 V, with a sharper voltage–current characteristic than the diode circuit.

A preferred voltage-limiting device for biopotential amplifiers is the gas-discharge tube. Owing to its extremely high impedance in the nonconducting state, this device appears as an open circuit until it reaches its breakdown voltage. At the breakdown voltage that is in the range of 50–90 V, the tube switches to the conducting state and maintains a voltage that is usually several volts less than the breakdown voltage. Although the voltage maintained by the gas-discharge tube is still too high for some amplifiers, it is sufficiently low to allow the input current to be easily limited to a safe value by simple

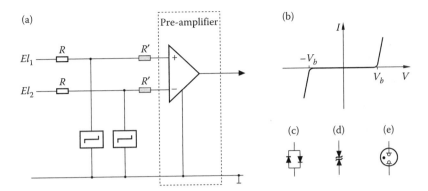

FIGURE 9.8 Protection of the amplifier input against high-voltage transients. The connection diagram for voltage-limiting elements is shown in panel (a) with two optional resistors R' at the input. A typical current–voltage characteristic is shown in panel (b). Voltage-limiting elements shown are the antiparallel connection of diodes (c), antiparallel connection of Zener diodes (d), and gas-discharge tubes (e).

circuit elements such as resistors like the resistor R' indicated in Figure 9.8a. Preferred gas-discharge tubes for biomedical applications are miniature neon lamps that are very inexpensive and have a symmetric characteristic.

9.5 Input Guarding

The common mode input impedance and thus the CMRR of an amplifier can be greatly increased by guarding the input circuit (Strong 1970). The common mode signal can be obtained by two averaging resistors connected between the outputs of the two input op-amps of an instrumentation amplifier as shown in Figure 9.9. The buffered common mode signal at the output of op-amp 4 can be used as guard voltage to reduce the effects of cable capacitance and leakage.

In many modern biopotential amplifiers, the reference electrode is not grounded. Instead, it is connected to the output of an amplifier for the common mode voltage, op-amp 3 in Figure 9.10, which works as an inverting amplifier. The inverted common mode voltage is fed back to the reference electrode. This

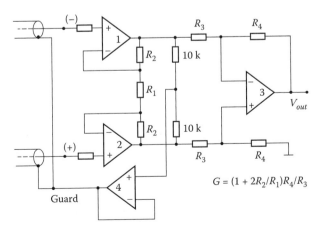

$$G = (1 + 2R_2/R_1)R_4/R_3$$

FIGURE 9.9 Instrumentation amplifier providing input guarding.

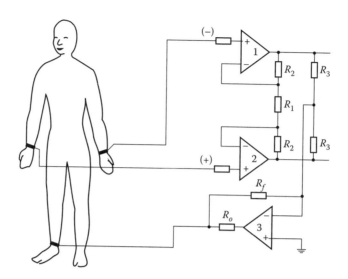

FIGURE 9.10   Driven-right-leg circuit reducing common mode interference.

negative feedback reduces the common mode voltage to a low value (Webster, 1992). Electrocardiographs based on this principle are called driven-right-leg systems replacing the right-leg ground electrode of ordinary electrocardiographs by an actively driven electrode.

9.6 Dynamic Range and Recovery

With an increase of either the common mode or differential input voltage, there will be a point where the amplifier will overload and the output voltage will no longer be representative for the input voltage. Similarly, with a decrease of the input voltage, there will be a point where the noise components of the output voltage cover the output signal to a degree that a measurement of the desired biopotential is no longer possible. The dynamic range of the amplifier, that is, the range between the smallest and largest possible input signal to be measured, has to cover the whole amplitude range of the physiological signal of interest. The required dynamic range of biopotential amplifiers can be quite large. In an application such as fetal monitoring, for example, two signals are recorded simultaneously from the electrodes that are quite different in their amplitudes: the fetal and the maternal ECG. Although the maternal ECG shows an amplitude of up to 10 mV, the fetal ECG often does not reach more than 1 µV. Assuming that the fetal ECG is separated from the composite signal and fed to an A/D converter for digital signal processing with a resolution of 10 bit (signed integer), the smallest voltage to be safely measured with the biopotential amplifier is 1/512 µV or about 2 nV versus 10 mV for the largest signal, or even up to 300 mV in the presence of an electrode offset potential. This translates to a dynamic range of 134 dB for the signals alone and 164 dB if the electrode potential is included into the consideration. Although most applications are less demanding, even such extreme requirements can be realized through careful design of the biopotential amplifier and the use of adequate components. The penalty for using less-expensive amplifiers with diminished performance would be a potentially severe loss of information.

Transients appearing at the input of the biopotential amplifier, such as voltage peaks from a cardiac pacemaker or a defibrillator, can drive the amplifier into saturation. An important characteristic of the amplifier is the time it takes to recover from such overloads. The recovery time depends on the characteristics of the transient, such as amplitude and duration, the specific design of the amplifier, such as bandwidth, and the components used. Typical biopotential amplifiers may take several seconds to recover from severe overload. The recovery time can be reduced by disconnecting the amplifier inputs at the discovery of a transient using an electronic switch.

9.6.1 Passive Isolation Amplifiers

Increasingly, biopotentials have to be measured within implanted devices and need to be transmitted to an external monitor or controller. Such applications include cardiac pacemakers transmitting the intra-cardiac ECG and functional electrical stimulation where, for example, action potentials measured at one eyelid serve to stimulate the other lid to restore the physiological function of a damaged lid at least to some degree. In these applications, the power consumption of the implanted biopotential amplifier limits the life span of the implanted device. The usual solution to this problem is an inductive transmission of power into the implanted device that serves to recharge an implanted battery. In applications where the size of the implant is of concern, it is desirable to eliminate the need for the battery and the related circuitry by using a quasi-passive biopotential amplifier, that is, an amplifier that does not need a power supply.

The function of passive telemetric amplifiers for biopotentials is based on the ability of the biological source to drive a low-power device such as an FET and the sensing of the biopotentials through inductive or acoustic coupling of the implanted and external devices (Nagel et al. 1982). In an inductive system, an FET serves as a load to an implanted secondary resonator, that is, an LC circuit containing a secondary coil with the inductance L and a capacitor with the capacitance C that is stimulated inductively by an extracorporeal oscillator (Figure 9.11). Depending on the special realization of the system, the biopotential is available in the external circuit from either an amplitude or frequency-modulated carrier signal. The input impedance of the inductive transmitter as a function of the secondary load impedance Z_2 is given by

$$Z_1 = j\omega L_1 + \frac{(\omega M)^2}{Z_2 + j\omega L_2}$$
(9.6)

In an amplitude-modulated system, the resistive part of the input impedance Z_1 must change as a linear function of the biopotential. The signal is obtained as the envelope of the carrier signal is measured across a resistor R_m. A frequency-modulated system is realized when the frequency of the signal generator is determined at least in part by the impedance Z_1 of the inductive transmitter. In both cases, the signal-dependent changes of the secondary impedance Z_2 can be achieved by a junction–FET. Using the FET as a variable load resistance changing its resistance in proportion to the source–gate voltage that is determined by the electrodes of this two-electrode amplifier, the power supplied by the biological source is sufficient to drive the amplifier. The input impedance can be in the range of 10^{10} Ω.

Optimal transmission characteristics are achieved with amplitude modulation (AM) systems. Different combinations of external and implanted resonance circuits are possible to realize an AM system, but primary parallel with secondary serial resonance yields the best characteristics. In this case, the input impedance is given by

$$Z_1 = \frac{1}{j\omega C_1} + \left(\frac{L_1}{M}\right)^2 \cdot R_2$$
(9.7)

The transmission factor $(L_1/M)^2$ is optimal because the secondary inductivity, that is, the implanted inductivity L_2 can be small, only the external inductivity determines the transmission factor, and the mutual inductivity M should be small, a fact that favors the loose coupling that is inherent to two coils

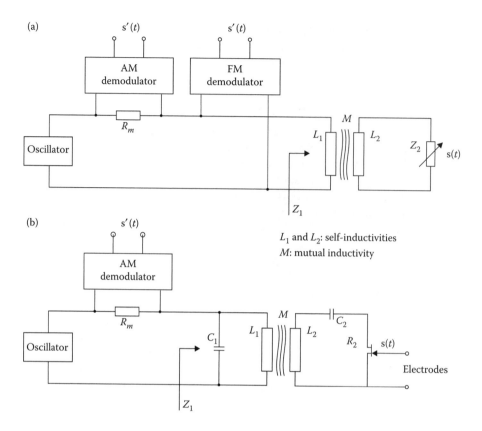

FIGURE 9.11 *Passive* isolation amplifier can be operated without the need for an isolated power supply (a). The biological source provides the power to modulate the load impedance of an inductive transformer. As an easy realization shown in (b), an FET can be directly connected to two electrodes. The source–drain resistance changes as a linear function of the biopotential that is then reflected by the input impedance of the transformer.

separated by skin and tissue. There are, of course, limits to M that cannot be seen from Equation 9.7. In a similar fashion, two piezoelectric crystals can be employed to provide the coupling between input and output.

This two-lead isolation amplifier design is not limited to telemetric applications, it can also be used in all other applications where its main advantage lies in its simplicity and the resulting substantial cost savings as compared to other isolation amplifiers that require additional amplifier stages and an additional isolated power supply.

9.7 Digital Electronics

The ever-increasing density of integrated digital circuits together with their extremely low-power consumption permits digitizing and preprocessing of signals already on the isolated patient side of the amplifiers, thus improving signal quality and eliminating the problems normally related to the isolation barrier, especially those concerning isolation voltage interferences and long-term stability of the isolation amplifiers. Digital signal transmission to a remote monitoring unit, a computer system, or computer network can be achieved without any risk of detecting transmission line interferences, especially when implemented with fiber optical cables.

Digital techniques also offer easy means of controlling the front end of the amplifier. Gain factors can be easily adapted, and changes of the electrode potential resulting from electrode polarization or from interferences that might drive the differential amplifier into saturation can be easily detected and compensated.

9.8 Summary

Biopotential amplifiers are a crucial component in many medical and biological measurements, and largely determine the quality and information content of the measured signals. The extremely wide range of necessary specifications with regard to bandwidth, sensitivity, dynamic range, gain, CMRR, and patient safety leaves only little room for the application of general-purpose biopotential amplifiers and mostly requires the use of special-purpose amplifiers.

Defining Terms

Common mode rejection ratio (CMRR): CMRR of a differential amplifier is defined as the ratio between the amplitude of a common mode signal and the amplitude of a differential signal that would produce the same output amplitude or as the ratio of the differential gain over the common mode gain: CMRR = GD/GCM. Expressed in decibels, the common mode rejection is 20 log 10 CMRR. The common mode rejection is a function of frequency and source impedance unbalance.

Isolation mode rejection ratio (IMRR): IMRR of an isolation amplifier is defined as the ratio between the isolation voltage, V_{ISO}, and the amplitude of the isolation signal appearing at the output of the isolation amplifier or as isolation voltage divided by output voltage V_{OUT} in the absence of differential and common mode signal: IMRR = V_{ISO}/V_{OUT}.

Operational amplifier (op-amp): Op-amp is a very high-gain DC-coupled differential amplifier with single-ended output, high-voltage gain, high input impedance, and low output impedance. Owing to its high open-loop gain, the characteristics of an op-amp circuit only depend on its feedback network. Therefore, the integrated circuit op-amp is an extremely convenient tool for the realization of linear amplifier circuits (Horowitz and Hill, 1980).

References

AAMI. 1993. *AAMI Standards and Recommended Practices, Biomedical Equipment*, Vol. 2, 4th ed. AAMI, Arlington, VA.

Burr-Brown. 1994. *Burr-Brown Integrated Circuits Data Book, Linear Products*, Burr-Brown Corp., Tucson, AZ.

Horowitz, P. and W. Hill. 1980. *The Art of Electronics*, Cambridge University Press, Cambridge, UK.

Nagel, J.H., M. Ostgen, and M. Schaldach. 1982. Telemetriesystem. *German Patent Application*, P3233240. 8–15.

Pallás-Areny, R. and J.G. Webster. 1990. Composite instrumentation amplifier for biopotentials. *Annals of Biomedical Engineering*. 18, 251–262.

Song, Y., O. Ozdamar, and C.C. Lu. 1998. Pasteless electrode/amplifier system for auditory brainstem response (ABR) recording. *Annals of Biomedical Engineering*. 26, S-103.

Strong, P. 1970. *Biophysical Measurements*, Tektronix, Inc., Beaverton, OR.

Webster, J.G. (ed.), 1992. *Medical Instrumentation, Application and Design*, 2nd ed. Houghton Mifflin Company, Boston, MA.

Further Information

Detailed information on the realization of amplifiers for biomedical instrumentation and the availability of commercial products can be found in the references and in the data books and application notes of various manufacturers of integrated circuit amplifiers, such as Burr-Brown, Analog Devices, and Linear Technology Corporation, as well as manufacturers of laboratory equipment, such as Biopac Systemy Inc., Gould, and Grass.

10

Bioimpedance Measurements

Sverre Grimnes
University of Oslo
Oslo University Hospital

Ørjan G. Martinsen
University of Oslo
Oslo University Hospital

10.1 What Is Bioimpedance?

Bioimpedance is an electrical property of a biomaterial: the ability to oppose alternating current (AC) flow. Impedance is a physical variable, which may be of interest as such, but often, it is converted into another variable or parameter of special, for example, clinical interest. Active electrodes are always used in bioimpedance sensors; the method is exogenous with two current-carrying (CC) electrodes sending the measuring current through the tissue volume of interest. This is in contrast to measuring, for example, a biopotential difference caused by living tissue activity (bioelectricity) with passive pickup (PU) electrodes, an endogenous method.

The biomaterial may be living tissue measured *in situ* and *in vivo*, or it may be dead, for example, hair or meat. The biomaterial may also be excised tissue or cell suspensions kept alive outside the body (*ex vivo*) or passively dying or dead tissue in a glass container (*in vitro*). In this chapter, we will focus on living person and patient tissue.

The books that include our field are, for instance: Malmivuo and Plonsey (1995), which also covers magnetic aspects; Schwan (2001), which is a collection of many of the classical papers by Herman P.

Schwan; Plonsey and Barr (2000), which focuses on bioelectricity; and Grimnes and Martinsen (2008) on bioimpedance and bioelectricity.

10.2 Conductors and Dielectrics

A tissue as a biomaterial may be considered as a conductor or a dielectric. Figure 10.1 shows a model of the biomaterial between two metal electrode plates. In principle, a dielectric is dry without direct current (DC) conductance and living tissue is wet with appreciable DC conductance and polarization impedance caused by the double layer at the surface of the wetted metal plates. Charge carriers are electrons in metal, but ions in tissue.

Let us consider the AC case in Figure 10.1. The AC is a sinusoidal signal with voltage u and current i. Admittance Y and impedance Z are found by measuring i and u.

However, as illustrated in Figure 10.2, living tissue has capacitive properties because of, for example, cell membranes. Therefore, the u and i signals are not in-phase, and impedance and admittance are complex quantities. They are written in **bold** characters and can be decomposed in their in-phase and quadrature components

$$\mathbf{Y} = \mathbf{i}/u = G + jB = G + j\omega C_p \qquad \text{[siemens]} \quad (10.1)$$

$$\mathbf{Z} = \mathbf{u}/i = R + jX = R - j/\omega C_s \qquad \text{[ohm]} \quad (10.2)$$

where j is the imaginary unit, G is the conductance, B is the susceptance, ω is the angular frequency, and C_p is the parallel capacitance. R is the resistance, X is the reactance, and C_s is the series capacitance.

Material constants such as conductivity can be used instead of conductance if geometrical dimensions such as A and d are known

$$\mathbf{Y} = (\sigma' + j\sigma'') A/d \qquad (10.3)$$

where σ is the conductivity [siemens/m], σ' the in-phase part, and σ'' the 90° (capacitive) part.

$$\mathbf{Z} = 1/\mathbf{Y} = (\rho' - j\,\rho'')d/A \qquad (10.4)$$

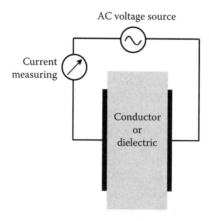

FIGURE 10.1 Basic model of a conductor or a dielectric placed between two metal plates of contact area *A* and distance *d*.

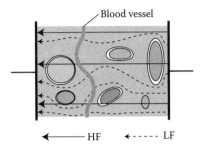

FIGURE 10.2 Tissue, cells, membranes, and a blood vessel. Note the difference between (<1 kHz) and HF (>100 kHz) current flow lines.

where ρ is the resistivity [ohm m], ρ' the in-phase part, and ρ'' the 90° (capacitive) part.

$$\varepsilon = \varepsilon' - j\varepsilon'' = (C' - jC'')d/A \qquad \text{[farad/m]} \quad (10.5)$$

where ε is complex permittivity, ε' capacitive permittivity expressing the capacitor's ability to store electric energy, ε'' dielectric loss permittivity, and **C** complex capacitance.

Equations 10.3 through 10.5 show that if a biomaterial is to be regarded as a conductor, complex resistivity or conductivity parameters are used; if the material is to be regarded as a dielectric, permittivity parameters are used. In linear cases, the information content is the same.

The circuit of Figure 10.1 is an AC circuit. Capacitance and permittivity cannot be measured at frequency 0 Hz; they are instead defined with static values (ε_s) found from capacitor DC voltage U and charge Q (C = Q/U).

Without phase data, the modulus of the quantities is simple and useful. If the biomaterial is considered as an ideal, dry capacitor ($C'' = 0$), the capacitance C is

$$C = \varepsilon \, A/d \qquad \text{[farad]} \quad (10.6)$$

If it is considered as an ideal conductor, the conductance is

$$G = \sigma \, A/d \qquad \text{[siemens]} \quad (10.7)$$

Material constants may be derived from measured values if the biomaterial is measured *in vitro* in simple geometries, such as circular or rectangular tubes. Tissue is a very heterogeneous material and *in vivo* measurements are not sharply limited to a defined volume. It may be very difficult or virtually impossible to go from, for example, measured conductance, resistance, and capacitance to conductivity, resistivity, and permittivity.

Living tissue is neither an ideal capacitor nor an ideal conductor. Many types of membranes with special electrical properties are found—from the dead, horny layer at the human skin surface to cell membranes and the large peritoneum membrane in the abdominal cavity. At a frequency of, for example, 1000 Hz, an imposed current may partly pass the extracellular electrolytes and partly the intracellular electrolytes through the capacitive cell membranes. This is illustrated in Figure 10.2, showing how a high-frequency (HF) current passes right through the intracellular volume, whereas the low-frequency (LF) current must go around the membrane obstacles. The current division leads to a frequency-dependent phase shift between measured voltage and current, and by measuring a frequency spectrum, additional data can be obtained.

10.3 Living Tissue Electrical Models

Electrical circuits with lumped components are often used as models mimicking the electrical properties of tissue. The simplest models are with three components. If all components are ideal (not frequency-dependent values), the model is a Debye model.

10.3.1 Debye Models

The model to the left in Figure 10.3 is often used to model skin impedance. For instance, R may represent the deeper viable parts and the parallel R and C components represent the poorly conducting stratum corneum (SC). The model to the right may be used for tissue as shown in Figure 10.2. Then G models the extracellular electrolyte, C_m the cell membranes, and R the intracellular resistance. Fixed component values in the two models can be found so that they have exactly the same impedance spectrum.

Figure 10.4 shows dielectric models of the same tissue as shown in Figure 10.2. They have no DC conductance and basically have quite different spectra than the models of Figure 10.4. Fixed component values in the two dielectric models can be found so that they have exactly the same impedance spectrum. The same impedance spectrum with 2R-1C and 1R-2C models is not possible.

10.3.2 Dispersions

Take a look again at Figure 10.2. At LF, the membrane impedances are high and AC current through the membranes is very small; the tissue behaves as a frequency-independent AC conductor without contribution from the cell membranes and intracellular electrolytes. At HF, the membranes have low impedance and the current contribution of the intracellular electrolytes is high. The tissue also then behaves as an AC conductor but with a higher conductance than at LF.

Both the models of Figure 10.3 have the same general impedance spectrum as the one shown in Figure 10.5. Such a spectrum represents a *dispersion,* characterized by the following behavior: At LF

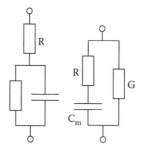

FIGURE 10.3   Two popular *impedance* models (2R-1C).

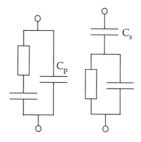

FIGURE 10.4   Two popular *dielectric* models (1R-2C).

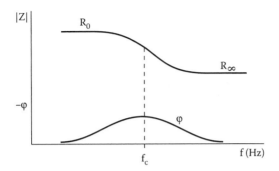

FIGURE 10.5 Frequency spectrum of the tissue electrical model shown in Figure 10.3.

and HF, the impedance is resistive with zero phase shift. The resistance R_∞ at HF is lower than the LF value R_0. At a characteristic frequency, the phase shift is maximum (and negative) and the impedance is complex. Because the capacitor is ideal in a Debye model, all energy dissipation occurs in the two resistors.

10.3.3 Memristive Systems and Constant Phase Elements

Traditionally, special components have been used for making bioimpedance electrical models. A new component that appeared recently is the memristor (memory resistor). It was first described by Chua (1971). It is a passive two-terminal circuit element, which complements the resistor, coil, and capacitor. There is a relationship between charge and magnetic flux in the memristor in such a way that the resistance is dependent on the net amount of charge having passed the device in a given direction. The theory was extended to memristive systems (Chua and Kang 1976), comprising memristors, memcapacitors, and meminductors. All these elements typically show pinched hysteretic loops in the two constitutive variables that define them: current–voltage for the memristor, charge–voltage for the memcapacitor, and current–flux for the meminductor (Di Ventra et al. 2009). Memristor theory has, for example, been used within bioimpedance for the modeling of electro-osmosis in the human epidermis (Johnsen et al. 2011).

Constant phase elements (CPEs) have been used in bioimpedance models since the late 1920s. A CPE can be modeled by a resistor and capacitor, both having frequency-dependent values, in such a way that the phase angle is frequency independent. A CPE is mathematically simple, but not so simple as to realize with discrete, passive components in the real world. A particular type of CPE is the Warburg element, known from electrochemistry and solid state physics. It is diffusion controlled with a constant phase angle of 45° (Warburg 1899).

10.3.4 Cole Models

The similarity between the spectra of a model with just three components and a complex material such as tissue is of course limited. The first step of refinement is often to replace an ideal capacitor found in the Debye models of Figures 10.3 and 10.4 with a CPE. They are then called Cole impedance models (Cole 1940) and Cole–Cole permittivity models (Cole and Cole 1941).

10.3.5 Schwan Multiple α, β, and γ Dispersion Model

Schwan published his dispersion models many times, sometimes only with permittivity ε', sometimes also with ε'', or σ' as shown on Figure 10.6. Schwan (1957) named the LF part α dispersion. It is caused by

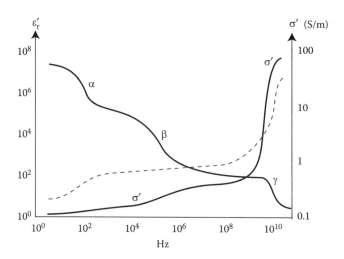

FIGURE 10.6 Schwan general model of α, β, and γ dispersions. Dashed curve is an example of measured muscle longitudinal conductivity.

cell-surface processes. The medium-frequency (MF) part is called β dispersion and is caused by capacitive membranes dividing intracellular and extracellular electrolytes. The HF part is called γ dispersion and is caused by water and protein processes. A clear separation between the dispersions is of course only possible if their characteristic frequencies are sufficiently apart. If this is not the case, dispersions may merge into a more or less straight line. The difference between tissue electrical parameters may be very large, from SC (low conductivity) to blood tissue (high conductivity). In addition to the generic curves shown in Figure 10.6, an example of measured conductivity from longitudinal muscle tissue (Gabriel et al. 1996) is shown.

In the literature, there is abundant data on conductivity/resistivity dispersions of biomaterials (Gabriel et al. 1996), biopolymers and membranes (Takashima 1989), dielectric and electronic properties (Pethig 1979), and physical properties (Duck 1990). Table 10.1 shows a few examples of LF (<1 kHz) data, followed by some comments on different tissues to illustrate the complexity of giving the exact data. As the tissue is so heterogeneous both on the micro- and macro- (organ) scale, the given values must be regarded as some sort of mean values of a given volume. Also, the question of difference between normal and pathological tissue is of great interest.

Tissue anisotropy may be strong, as shown in Table 10.1 for a muscle with 10 times higher longitude than perpendicular conductivity (Epstein and Foster 1983). They found that the anisotropy almost disappeared at 1 MHz; it is an LF phenomenon. The conductivity of muscle tissue is dependent on other factors such as mechanical contraction (Shiffman et al. 2003).

Tissue values change rapidly if the tissue becomes ischemic or dies (Gersing 1998; Schäfer et al. 1998; Casas et al. 1999; Martinsen et al. 2000).

10.3.5.1 Skin

SC resistivity in Table 10.1 is quoted from Yamamoto and Yamamoto (1976). The resistivity is higher the lower the water content of the SC. This is also the case with many (dead) protein powders (Takashima and Schwan 1965; Smith and Foster 1985). The water content of SC is dependent on the relative humidity of the air in contact with the SC surface. Methods for diagnosis of, for example, cancer tissue by information extraction from impedance dispersions in skin and oral mucosa have been found (Ollmar 1998), or correlation of impedance response patterns to histological findings in irritant skin reactions induced by various surfactants (Nicander et al. 1996).

TABLE 10.1 Conductivity and Resistivity Data

Material	Conductivity σ (S/m)	Resistivity ρ (Ω m)
Metals (implants)	5×10^6	2×10^{-7}
Saline (0.9% NaCl 37°C)	2	0.5
Muscle (longit/perpend)	0.6/0.06	1.6/16
Skin (SC)	10^{-5}	10^5
Diamond	10^{-14}	10^{14}

10.3.5.2 Cell Suspensions

Electrical properties of tissue and cell suspensions were reviewed by Schwan (1957). Membrane capacitance and conductance for pancreatic β-cells were measured by an electrokinetic method (Pethig et al. 2005; Grimnes and Martinsen 2008). The conductivity of blood is dependent on blood velocity; this is the Sigman effect (Sigman et al. 1937).

Also, deoxyribonucleic acid (DNA) molecules and their electrical conduction have been examined: the electrical conduction through DNA molecules (Fink and Schönenberger 1999) and resonances in the dielectric absorption of DNA (Foster et al. 1987). Recently, the Pethig group (Chung et al. 2011) has shown that measurement results in a cell suspension up to 10 MHz that is dependent on the cytoplasma membrane capacitance and resistance, the cell diameter, and the suspension conductivity. By using special interdigitated electrodes, the cell membrane capacitive reactance sort out the resistance above 100 MHz so that the electric field penetrates into the cell interior and intracellular dielectric properties can be measured.

10.4 Electrodes and Electrode Polarization

Electrodes are the most important part of an impedance-measuring system (Geddes 1972). They determine the sensitivity field (Section 10.5), which determines the contribution of each small voxel to the overall result. Three- and four-electrode systems are more complicated because, as we shall see, they introduce volumes of negative sensitivity because they measure *transfer* impedance.

10.4.1 Electrode Types

10.4.1.1 Skin Surface Electrodes

Skin electrodes have the largest commercial product volume, most of them are pregelled ready-to-use nonsterile products. Some of them have a snap-action wire contact; others are prewired, for instance, adapted for babies. There is a contact electrolyte between the skin and the electrode metal. Dry SC is a poor conductor and this easily results in poor (high impedance) contact and noise. The contact area with the skin should be as large as practically possible, and reducing the SCs thickness by sandpaper abrasion is useful. Hydrating the skin with contact electrolyte or by the covering effect of the electrode will usually reduce the contact impedance with time (minutes to hours).

Figure 10.7 shows to the left a classical wet gel type with an adhesive foam ring holding a sponge with gel in position and pressed against the skin. The AgCl metal part is recessed to reduce movement artifacts. If the electrolyte has higher salt concentration than, for example, seawater, it may irritate the skin and should be used as a short-time (hours) electrode. Long-term use (days) must have weaker electrolytes to be nonirritating on the skin. Often, the adhesive part of the foam is more irritating to the skin than the electrolyte. The wet electrolyte penetrates the SC and may fill the sweat ducts steadily increasing the electrical contact with the body.

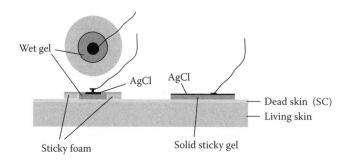

FIGURE 10.7 Two common types of skin surface electrodes.

Figure 10.7 to the right shows a solid gel electrode where the gel is also the sticky part. The gel (solid- or hydrogel) does not penetrate the skin but may to a small extent participate in receiving and storing water from the skin or delivering water to the skin (Tronstad et al. 2010).

10.4.1.1.1 Needle and Catheter Sterile Electrodes

With an invasive needle, it is possible to obtain rapid low impedance contact with the body. In neurology, the needles may be in the form of a tube with thin noble metal wires coming out through perpendicular holes on the shaft or coaxially at the tube end. The catheter version is often with metal rings and a metal tip at the end. They are used as CC or PU electrodes. If the needle shaft is insulated, the contact area can be small and the space resolution high in CC or PU applications. The needle tip position can be guided by measuring impedance spectra with the tip (Kalvøy et al. 2009). The needle may be of massive metal or hollow allowing liquid infusion together with impedance measurements.

10.4.1.1.2 Micro- and Nanotechnology Electrodes

By using interdigitated microelectrodes, it is possible to sort different cells in a suspension (Becker et al. 1994); it is a parallel to the Coulter counter technique described in Section 10.8 Micromachined electrodes for biopotential measurements are described in Griss et al. (2001). Pethig's group (Chung et al. 2011) describes interdigitated nanoelectrodes in a cellular suspension being able to measure intracellular dielectric properties.

10.4.2 Electrode Polarization

Electrode polarization is an important source of error in tissue impedance measurements (Schwan 1968). Current carriers in the electrode metal are electrons and those in living tissue are ions. The electric contact between metal and electrolyte (tissue liquids or applied electrolyte) has special electric nonlinear properties because of the formation of a double layer in the electrolyte. The double layer is very thin (nanometer) and depleted of current carriers. It generates a DC voltage and generates special polarization impedance. Figure 10.8 shows the polarization spectrum of an electrode with wet gel and AgCl metal surface. They have been obtained with two pregelled electrodes face to face and are taking half the impedance value. The Bode plot (Section 10.7) in Figure 10.8 shows a maximum phase shift of about 25° at 20 kHz. The impedance modulus is from about 300 Ω (1 Hz) down to 25 Ω (1 MHz). Above about 500 kHz, the phase goes through zero and the impedance becomes inductive. This is because of the self-inductance of the lead wires. Figure 10.9 shows a Wessel plot (Section 10.7) of the impedance. It reveals that the polarization impedance has two dispersions. The HF dispersion has a characteristic frequency of 46 kHz, determined by a circular arc drawn by regression analysis. Electrode polarization impedance dispersions are dependent on the metal, surface geometrical properties, and contact electrolyte (Mirtaheri et al. 2005) (Figure 10.9).

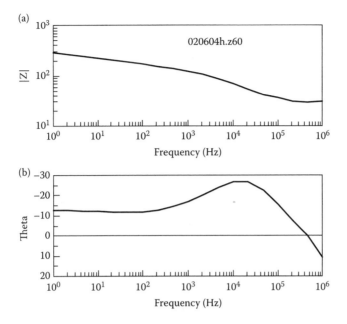

FIGURE 10.8 Polarization impedance by Bode plot. Two electrodes face to face, contribution of one electrode. Commercial ECG skin electrode with wet gel and AgCl metal surface of 0.7 cm².

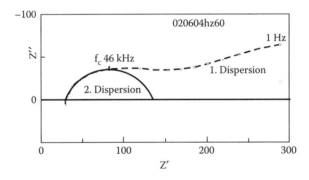

FIGURE 10.9 Polarization impedance Wessel plot showing a part of a first dispersion, and a second dispersion with a complete circular arc regression line. Same data as Figure 10.8a.

10.5 Electrode Systems and Their Sensitivity Fields

Bipolar (Figure 10.10) means that two electrodes contribute equally to the measurement result. Used as DC CC electrodes, they are polarized and become anode and cathode with different electrolytic processes. Measured AC impedance will include the polarization impedance of each electrode and the contribution of the tissue in between each electrode. As signal PU electrodes, they are used with negligible current flow and are then not polarized. They measure the potential difference between the electrodes. The potential difference may be generated as a result of remote organ activity setting up a volume current flow spreading out from the organ (endogenous currents generating, e.g., ECG or EMG). The potential difference may also be neurogenic, for example, originating from a sweat gland being excited by a nerve signal from a remote source.

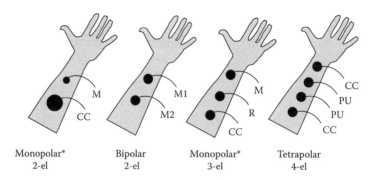

| Monopolar* | Bipolar | Monopolar* | Tetrapolar |
| 2-el | 2-el | 3-el | 4-el |

FIGURE 10.10　Skin surface electrode systems. Monopolar* systems are usually not ideally monopolar, see text below. The three- and four- electrode systems measure transfer immittance. Electrode functions: M, measuring; CC, current carrying; R, reference; PU, pick up.

A bipolar PU electrode system is also a local electric field strength sensor because $\mathbf{E} \cdot \mathbf{d} = U$ where $\mathbf{E}$ is he local electric field strength (V/m) in magnitude and direction (space vector), $\mathbf{d}$ the distance and direction between the electrodes (space vector), and U the potential difference. By using two bipolar electrode systems perpendicular to each other, the direction of the E-field can be determined. And if tissue conductivity σ is known, the local current density $\mathbf{J}$ can be estimated according to $\mathbf{J} = \sigma\,\mathbf{E}$.

Monopolar means that one of the electrodes contributes more to the measurement result than the other.

An *ideal* monopolar two-electrode system means that the large electrode has negligible influence on the result. The monopolar system shown in Figure 10.10 (left) has two very different electrode areas. With DC current flow, they are polarized and will become anode and cathode with different electrolytic processes. However, the large electrode will have much smaller current density and is, therefore, often regarded as an indifferent or neutral electrode. AC impedance will be dominated by the impedance of the small electrode (electrode polarization impedance included). As PU electrodes with negligible current flow, the size of the electrodes is not important but the metal of each electrode is very important. A potential difference will be measured if the large electrode is positioned at an indifferent skin site and the small electrode at a nerve-activated skin site. If both electrodes are placed on an active site, the recorded voltage difference may be very low.

Monopolar three-electrode system (Figure 10.10, number 3 to the right) means that it functions as a monopolar system when used on high-resistivity SC, cf. Figure 10.16. Then the *M* electrode contributes much more to the measurement result than the two other electrodes. However, in direct contact with low resistivity, the living tissue in Figure 10.13 shows that the *R* electrode is surrounded by high-sensitivity zones (and also small negative sensitivity zones) even if the *R* electrode is not CC.

The four-electrode tetrapolar system of Figure 10.10 is very different from the two-electrode mono- and bipolar systems (Grimnes and Martinsen 2007). It measures *transfer* impedance because the potential is recorded at a separate PU port and not at the CC port. If the two ports are far apart, no signal will be transferred from the CC to the PU port and the transfer impedance will be virtually 0 Ω.

10.5.1　Sensitivity Field

When measuring the impedance of a material with, for example, surface electrodes, it is obvious that not all small subvolumes in the material contribute equally to the measured impedance. Volumes between and close to the electrodes contribute more than volumes far away from the electrodes. Hence, a careful choice of electrode size and placement will enable the user to focus the measurements on the desired part of the material.

It is sometimes assumed that if the electrodes are placed in a linear fashion, with the voltage PU electrodes between the CC electrodes, only the volume between the PU electrodes is measured. Not only is this wrong, but there will also be zones of negative sensitivity between the PU electrodes and the CC electrodes (Grimnes and Martinsen 2007). Negative sensitivity means that if the complex resistivity is increased in that specific volume, lower total impedance will be measured.

The sensitivity of a small volume dv (voxel) within a material is a measure of how much this volume contributes to the total measured impedance (Geselowitz 1971), provided that the electrical properties (e.g., resistivity) are uniform throughout the material. If, in this case, the resistivity varies within the material, the local resistivity must be multiplied with the sensitivity to give a measure of the volume's contribution to the total measured resistance.

If we look at a simple example of a DC resistance measurement with a four-electrode system, the sensitivity will be computed in the following manner:

1. Imagine that you inject a current I between the two CC electrodes. Compute the current density J_1 in each small volume element in the material as a result of this current.
2. Imagine that you instead inject the same current between the PU electrodes and again compute the resulting current density J_2 in each small volume element.
3. The vector dot product between J_1 and J_2 in each volume element, divided by the current squared, is now the sensitivity of the volume element and if we multiply with the resistivity ρ in each volume, we will directly obtain this volume's contribution to the total measured resistance R.

Hence, the local (voxel) sensitivity S and the total measured volume resistance R will be

$$S = J_1 \cdot J_2/I^2 \qquad R = \int_V \rho S \, dv \qquad (10.8)$$

Note that sensitivity is not dependent on voxel resistivity. These equations demonstrate the reciprocal nature of tetrapolar systems (or any other electrode system where this theory applies); under linear conditions, the CC electrodes and PU electrodes can be interchanged without any change in measured values.

A positive value for the sensitivity means that if the resistivity of this volume element is increased, a higher total resistance will be measured. The higher the value of sensitivity, the greater the influence on measured resistance. A negative value for the sensitivity, however, means that increased resistivity in that volume gives a lower total resistance. Two-electrode systems will not have volumes with negative sensitivity, but both the three- and four-electrode systems will typically have volumes with negative sensitivity. The commercial software package Comsol Multiphysics has been used for making Figures 10.11 through 10.14. All the finite-element calculations were made with half-cylinders immersed into the surface of the tissue and with the tissue volume extending far outside the figure in side and bottom directions.

Figure 10.11 is with a vertical slice with a resistivity 5 times that of the surrounding medium. It has little influence on the sensitivity field. Multiplying the sensitivity field with the local resistivity yields the volume resistance density field, as shown in Figure 10.12. The result is quite different and illustrates that with respect to the overall transfer resistance of the system, the increased resistivity of the slice is very important. The transfer resistance is not determined by the sensitivity value alone, the sensitivity is to be multiplied by the resistivity to obtain resistance values.

Sensitivity calculations can be utilized equally well for two-, three-, and four-electrode systems. In each case, you must identify the two CC electrodes used for driving an electrical current through the

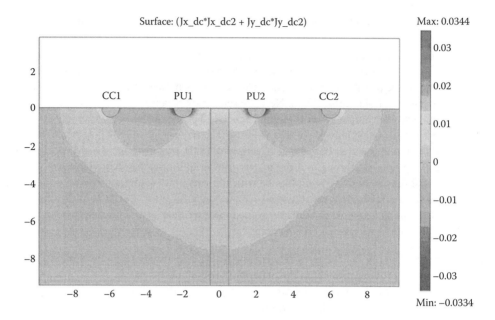

FIGURE 10.11 Volume sensitivity field of a biomaterial with a tetrapolar electrode system with two CC electrodes and two PU electrodes. Two homogeneous biomaterial regions, the vertical slice has 5 times the resistivity of the surrounding medium.

material and the two PU electrodes used for measuring the potential drop in the material. Figure 10.13 shows the sensitivity field for a three-electrode system (Grimnes 1983a).

In the case of a two-electrode system, the driving and PU electrode pairs are the same, and the sensitivity in a given volume will hence be the square of the current density divided by the square of the total injected current. The sensitivity can only have positive values (Figure 10.14).

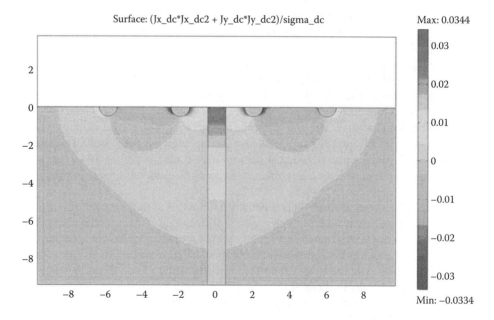

FIGURE 10.12 Volume *resistance density* plot of the model shown in Figure 10.11.

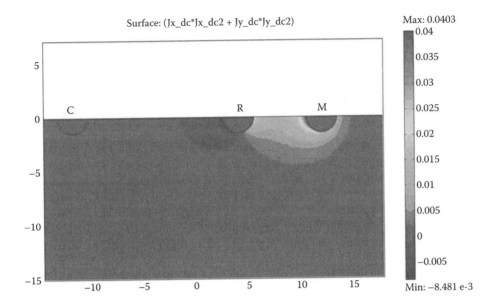

FIGURE 10.13 Volume *sensitivity* field of a quasi-monopolar three-electrode system. Notice zones of negative sensitivity at the left side of the *R* electrode.

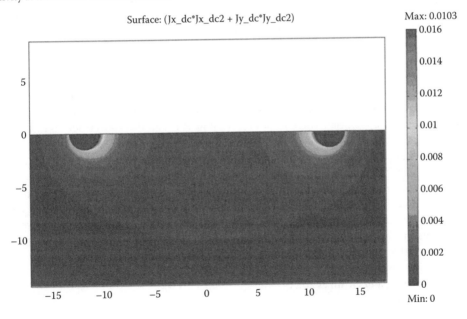

FIGURE 10.14 Volume *sensitivity* field of a bipolar two-electrode system. Notice the lack of negative sensitivity volumes.

10.6 Instrumentation and Quality Controls

With two electrodes, impedance or admittance can be calculated by measuring the voltage u and current i in the electrode wires. The two electrodes function as both CC and PU pairs. It is often practical to monitor *admittance* directly by applying a constant (amplitude) voltage and measuring current because the admittance is then proportional to current according to $Y = i/u$. *Impedance* is measured

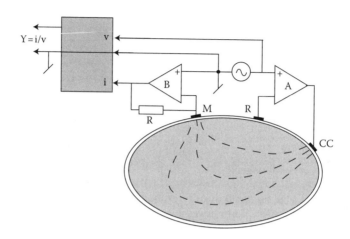

FIGURE 10.15 Monopolar admittance measuring circuit with three skin surface electrodes. SC thickness is exaggerated. Current flow lines are shown as dashed lines.

directly by applying a constant current i and measuring voltage because it is proportional to the voltage, $Z = u/i$.

Figure 10.15 shows an example of a skin surface admittance measuring circuit. It is a quasi-monopolar system with three electrodes: M is the measuring electrode, R a potential recording reference electrode, and CC is a current-carrying control electrode.

Two operational amplifiers are used: amplifier A for setting up a current through the body so that the voltage recorded by R becomes equal to the excitation voltage (30 mV). Amplifier B is an ideal (zero-voltage drop) current-reading amplifier. If the skin has sufficiently high resistivity, the R and CC electrodes are merely control electrodes with negligible influence on the admittance result (this is in contrast to Figure 10.13 because there the skin was not modeled). The well-conducting living body is considered isopotential. There is no current flow through the R electrode so that amplifier A brings the internal body potential to be equal to the excitation voltage. As the M electrode is on reference potential, $Y = i/u$ where i is the measured current and u is the constant AC potential difference across the SC.

Because of the capacitive properties of the skin, the measured current will be phase shifted with respect to the excitation voltage. By using a synchronous rectifier circuit with the excitation voltage as reference, the admittance can be decomposed so that only the in-phase conductance component G is measured. Susceptance B can be measured simultaneously according to $Y = G + jB$ by using a second synchronous rectifier with the reference signal 90° phase shifted.

More detailed descriptions of measuring methods can be found in Schwan (1963), Grimnes (1983a), Yelamos et al. (1999), and Grimnes and Martinsen (2008).

10.6.1 Synchronous Rectifiers

To measure impedance, an external current must be applied; it is an exogenous method. Thus, impedance measurements are ideally suited for synchronous rectification (SR) because the external excitation signal is available. The SR acts as a sort of sharp tracking filter with a bandwidth dependent on the time constant of the output of the low-pass filter. The result is a very noisy robust system.

SR is obtained by multiplying the input signal with the reference signal. Two types of circuit are in common use: the simplest method (Figure 10.16a) is with a reference signal in the form of a square wave. The multiplier circle may contain only on–off switches. The most elaborate method (Figure 10.16b) is with the reference signal as a sinusoidal waveform and the multiplication may be done digitally after

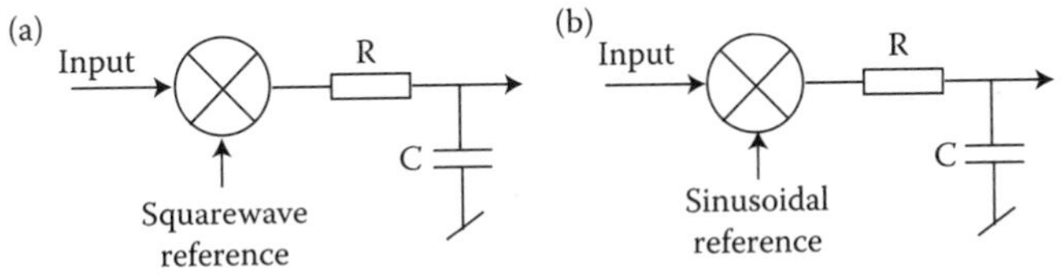

(a) Input — ⊗ — R —→

C

Squarewave
reference

(b) Input — ⊗ — R —→

C

Sinusoidal
reference

FIGURE 10.16 Synchronous rectifier circuits (a) with square wave and (b) with sinusoidal reference signal. Each circle mathematically multiplies the input signal with the reference signal.

both signals have been sampled and *A–D* converted. Such a circuit can be made insensitive to the DC level of the input signal (Grimnes and Martinsen 2008).

10.6.2 Quality Controls

10.6.2.1 Linearity

Bioimpedance is measured with an electric current applied to the CC electrodes. If the current wave-form is sinusoidal, the signal from the PU electrodes should also be a sine. If it is not, the system is nonlinear and the current amplitude should then be reduced until the PU signal is sinusoidal. Signal-to-noise ratio is also reduced; so, a trade-off may be necessary in the choice of the best amplitude.

There are sources of nonlinearity both in electrode polarization and tissue impedance (Schwan 1992). Onaral and Schwan (1982) studied electrode *polarization impedance* and found that the limit voltage of linearity was about 100 mV and frequency independent. The corresponding limit current is of course impedance dependent and therefore frequency dependent, and may be about 5 $\mu A/cm^2$ at a frequency of 1 Hz.

Yamamoto and Yamamoto (1981) studied *human skin tissue* and found the limit current of linearity to be about 10 $\mu A/cm^2$ at a frequency of 10 Hz. Grimnes (1983b) studied electro-osmosis in human skin *in vivo* and found a strong polarity-dependent nonlinearity. The effect was stronger; the lower the frequency, Figure 10.17 shows the dramatic effect with ±20 V and 0.2 Hz, soon leading to skin breakdown. Nonlinearity of cardiac pacemaker CC electrodes made of noble metals and intended for use with pulses has been extensively studied (Jaron et al. 1969).

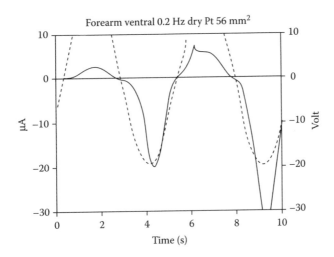

FIGURE 10.17 Electro-osmotic nonlinearity on the skin. Dashed line shows the applied voltage.

10.6.2.2 Kramers–Kronig Control

The Kramers–Kronig theorem in linear systems links, for example, the modulus spectrum of the imped-ance |Z| to the phase spectrum (Grimnes and Martinsen 2008). Take a look at the Bode plot of Figure 10.8a. The steeper the fall of the Z-modulus with frequency, the more negative the phase. Phase zero means that the impedance level is constant. The change to positive phase corresponds to increasing impedance with higher frequency. The results shown in Figure 10.8a are Kramers–Kronig compatible. Noncompatibility may be because of nonlinearity, change of measured volume, or drift in volume prop-erties (e.g., temperature) during spectrum recording.

10.6.2.3 Reciprocity Control of Transfer Impedance

According to the theorem, PU and CC electrodes can be swapped without change in measured transfer impedance. This may sound contraintuitive, but it is so. Reciprocity is destroyed if the system is nonlin-ear, for example, if the CC electrodes have larger contact area than the PU electrodes. After swapping, the small CC electrodes may then be driven into nonlinearity because of the increased current density. Reciprocity may also be destroyed if the properties of the biomaterial have changed.

10.6.3 Electrical Safety

For humans, bioimpedance methods use currents, which are not perceptible and of course not harmful. Only AC sinusoidal currents and DC are considered in this section, not pulse excitation. The biological effects of externally applied electromagnetic fields (through the air) are treated elsewhere (Polk and Postow 1996). For practical reasons, perception and hazard levels are usually quoted as current, energy, or charge in the external circuit (Dalziel 1954, 1972). The current density field in the tissue is usually unknown.

10.6.3.1 Threshold of Perception

10.6.3.1.1 Direct Current

The sensation of AC and DC currents is quite different. DC produces electrolytic products in the tissue near the electrode metal. The sensation may come after minutes, and after the DC has been switched off, the sensation may persist for a long time (minutes and more). Such perception is, therefore, not related to direct electric current nerve excitation. If a DC current is suddenly switched on or off, a transient sensa-tion may be felt on the skin; this is direct nerve excitation. Table 10.2 shows that the maximum 10 μA DC is allowable auxiliary current.

10.6.3.1.2 Sine Waves

The lowest level (<1 μA) of 50/60 Hz perception is caused by *electrovibration* (Grimnes 1983c). It is per-ceived when dry skin slides on a CC conductor; the frictional force is modulated by the electrostatic force and can be felt as a lateral mechanical vibration.

The second level (1 mA) of 50/60 Hz is due to the *direct electric excitation* of nerves. The level increases as frequency is increased above 1 kHz (Figure 10.18). For example, 10 mA at 100 kHz is without percep-tion, but temperature rise caused by the current may then be a limiting factor. Interpersonal variations

TABLE 10.2 Allowable Values of Continuous Leakage and Patient Auxiliary Currents (μA) (IEC-60601 2005)

Currents	Type B		Type BF		Type CF		
	NC	Single fault	NC	Single fault	NC	Single fault	
Patient leakage	100	500	100	500	10	50	
Patient auxiliary	100	500	100	500	10	50	AC
Patient auxiliary	10	50	10	50	10	50	DC

Note: NC = normal conditions.

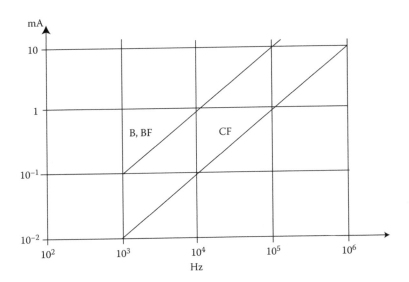

FIGURE 10.18 Allowable excitation (auxiliary) currents, AC (>0.1 Hz) rms values (according to IEC-60601 (2005)).

and the dependence on age and sex are small. The skin condition is not important as long as there are no wounds. The skin site may be important.

10.6.3.2 Electrical Hazards

If the current density is sufficiently high, an electric current triggers nerve and muscle tissue. If the current flow is through the heart or the brain stem, this may be lethal.

10.6.3.2.1 Macroshock

A macroshock situation is when current is applied to tissue far away from the heart or brain stem. The current is spread out more or less uniformly, and rather, large currents are needed in the external circuit (usually quoted >50 mA at 50/60 Hz) to attain dangerous levels in local tissue volumes such as heart and lungs.

10.6.3.2.2 Microshock

Small area contacts occur, for example, with pacemaker electrodes, catheter electrodes, and CC fluid-filled cardiac catheters. Small area contact implies a monopolar system with possible high local current densities but low current levels in the external circuit. This is called a *microshock* situation. The 50/60 Hz safe current limit for a small area contact with the heart is 10 μA in normal modes. The difference between macro- and microshock dangerous current levels is, therefore, more than three orders of magnitude.

10.6.3.3 Electrical Safety of Electromedical Equipment

Special safety precautions are taken for *electromedical equipment* and its use in the patient environment and in physical contact with the patient. Safety is regulated by international standards such as (IEC-60601 2005) used in Table 10.2.

The part of the equipment intended to be in physical contact with the patient is called the *applied part*. The applied part may ground the patient (type B) or keep the patient floating with respect to ground (BF—body floating or CF—cardiac floating) by *galvanic separation* circuitry (magnetic or optical coupling, battery-operated equipment).

Leakage currents are currents at power line frequency (50 or 60 Hz), they may be because of capacitive currents even with perfect insulation, and are thus difficult to avoid completely. *Patient leakage currents* are the leakage currents flowing to the patient via the applied part. Patient *auxiliary currents* are important for bioimpedance measurements. They are functional currents flowing *between* leads of the applied part, for example, as used with impedance plethysmography. They are not leakage currents and therefore usually not at power line frequency. It can be seen that not more than 10 μA DC can be used in an applied part under normal conditions, but 100 μA AC (>0.1 Hz) can be used except in CF (cardiac) applications.

Nerve and muscle tissue is less sensitive at higher frequencies. The allowable currents increase (Figure 10.18), for example, to 10 mA at 100 kHz in B and BF applications.

10.7 Result Presentations

10.7.1 Spectrum Plots

Bode plots are with logarithmic frequency and impedance scales, and with linear phase scale. An example is given in Figure 10.8a. The advantage is that a broad frequency spectrum can be shown combined with frequency-independent resolution.

Wessel (Argand, Nyquist, and Cole) plots are plots in the imaginary plane with real and imaginary axes (Figure 10.8b). The frequency scale is along the curve. The advantage is easily discernible dispersion arcs. The problem is the lack of linear frequency scale and the narrow high-resolution zone around the characteristic frequency.

10.7.2 Time-Series Plots

These plots are with fixed measuring frequency. An important parameter may be the sampling frequency because the recording of an LF spectrum may take a minute or more.

10.7.3 Converting Measured Variables to Clinical Variables or Parameters

Living tissue is a very heterogeneous and complex biomaterial. Impedance as a quantity is valid for a tissue volume and the contribution of the different volume elements (voxels) can be very different according to the electrode system sensitivity field. The results always represent some sort of mean values valid for a body region.

Geddes and Baker (1989) used the expression "Detection of Physiological Events by Impedance." The physiological variable may, for instance, be blood volume or flow and air volume or flow as described in Section 10.8.1. Impedance-based transducers convert the measured variable online into a signal from which the clinical parameter can be continuously calculated. Users are often not aware of which variable is the primary (actually measured) variable.

The measured variable can also be converted into the clinical parameter by a process of combining information from more than one sensor (polygraphy). Such calculation may be based on multivariate analysis. The result may be a numerical value or be placed in a group, for example, "normal" or "pathological." The end result may be variables such as CO_2 level, glucose level, lactic acid level, sweat activity (SA), total body water (TBW), meat quality, fruit freshness, and so on. For an interesting clinical parameter, it is often necessary to define a range of normal values to find a diagnosis or prognosis. To evaluate a proposed measuring method, a protocol is set up describing how measurements on healthy persons or organs are to be performed. The results are compared with a golden standard giving correct answers; for example, the hope is that lactic acid level can be measured with bioimpedance. Healthy persons are selected for impedance measurement, for example, of a large muscle performing mechanical work. Blood samples are taken and examined *in vitro* in a biochemical instrument (golden standard). Correlation coefficients between *in vivo* and *in vitro* results give the answer.

10.8 Application Examples

The application field of bioimpedance is very wide—from single-cell measurements with micro- and nanoelectrodes to whole-body composition analysis; from healthy to ischemic, pathological, and dead tissue. We have selected some typical bioimpedance application examples.

10.8.1 Volume and Flow Measurements

Volume measurements by impedance were proposed early and became one of the first widespread impedance applications in hospital instrumentation. It is a part of the usual bedside patient monitor present in all intensive-care units; impedance adds respiration to the ECG and blood pressure channels. It is embedded in the monitors rather anonymously, uses the ECG electrodes already there, and passes unnoticed as a clinical bioimpedance method by most users.

10.8.1.1 Plethysmographic *One-Compartment Model*

Plethysmography is a volume-measuring method, for example, of blood or air volumes in the lungs. Figure 10.19 illustrates a basic one-compartment model of a blood vessel segment of length L. As a one-compartment model, the electrical contribution of the vessel wall has been neglected. The resistance R of the blood volume is $R = \rho L/A$, where A is the cross-sectional area and ρ is the resistivity of the blood. The volume $v = LA$ and $A = v/L$ is put into the equation so that $v = \rho L^2/R$.

The variable G is preferred to variable R because it is directly proportional to v; so, the equation above is changed to

$$v = G\,\rho L^2 \qquad [\text{m}^3] \text{ or } [\text{L}] \text{ liter}$$
$$\text{Validity: A is constant along the length and } \rho \text{ is uniformly distributed.} \qquad (10.9)$$

10.8.1.2 Volume Sensor

In our simplified model, a choice must now be made: Let us consider that the segment volume is increased by a blood pressure increase. The elastic vessel wall is stretched so that a volume Δv is added to the tube content; does it result in a swelling of length or cross-sectional area? A blood vessel is usually considered to swell in cross-sectional area. Then L is constant and by measuring G, we have a calibrated volume-measuring system if ρ is considered constant with a known value.

Equation 10.9 represents a basic example of an impedance-based sensor in the form of a transducer. The transducer is the vessel segment, which is biological. It converts the volume variable into an electrical signal in a way so that the measured quantity is conductance G [siemens S]. By multiplying the conductance value with the constant ρL^2 [ohm m^3], the measured result can be presented as volume [m^3]. It is a common misunderstanding that the transducer measures volume. The measured variable, however, is electrical conductance. The elasticity of the wall determines the compliance $C = \Delta v/\Delta p$ of the vessel segment volume, with p as blood pressure. $C = 0$ is a stiff wall with no volume increase with increasing blood pressure and so no plethysmography.

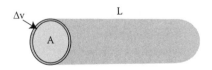

FIGURE 10.19 One-compartment blood vessel plethysmographic model.

10.8.1.3 Flow Sensor

Consider that the vessel segment is closed in one end. From Equation 10.9, $\Delta v = \Delta G \, \rho L^2$ and

$$dv/dt = (dG/dt) \, \rho L^2 \qquad \text{for example, [L/s].} \qquad (10.10)$$

The time derivative of volume is flow, flow into, or out of a closed segment.

10.8.1.4 Plethysmographic Two-Compartment Model

In the two-compartment model, the inner volume is, for example, a blood volume and the outer volume is the surrounding tissue volume.

Figure 10.20 shows the two-compartment model with a volume increase Δv. All tissue is considered incompressible (no air). If the inner volume $vA = A \cdot L$ is supplied with extra volume Δv, it swells to $\Delta v + vA$. The outer tube also swells to an increased outer diameter, but the volume vt remains constant. If all the volumes have the same resistivity, it can be shown that

$$\Delta G/G = \Delta v/(\Delta v + v_A + v_t) \qquad (10.11)$$

where v_A is the volume of the inner cylinder and v_t is the volume of the outer tissue cylinder. It is evident that the surrounding tissue also diminishes the sensitivity of the method because the compliance of the blood vessel is reduced by the support of the tissue surroundings. Further details can be found (Grimnes and Martinsen 2008), also for the case when the resistivities of the compartments are unequal and when the Sigman effect is relevant.

10.8.2 Three Different Variables Measured with Two Electrodes

With only two chest ECG electrodes, it is possible to monitor

- Blood: Mechanical pumping action of the heart
- Electrical activity of the heart
- Air: Mechanical respiration activity

The two electrodes are attached to the skin of the chest. As ECG PU electrodes, they record the signal corresponding to the electrical activity of the heart. It is well known that electrical activity is not necessarily followed by mechanical blood pumping. For the impedance measurement, an AC current of, for example, 50 kHz is applied to the same electrodes. The impedance as a function of time shows two different signals (Figure 10.21). The large-amplitude signal is due to the emptying and filling of the lungs with air. The smaller waves correspond to the mechanical emptying of the heart with well-conducting blood (ICG—impedance cardiography). Figure 10.21 shows a result also comprising an *apnea* period of about eight heartbeats where only the mechanical pumping activity of the heart is visible. The division

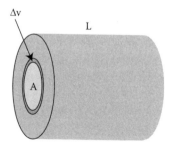

FIGURE 10.20   Two-compartment plethysmographic model.

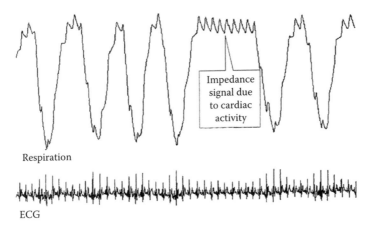

Respiration

ECG

FIGURE 10.21 Simultaneous registration of (1) heart mechanical pumping activity, (2) heart electrical activity, and (3) lung mechanical ventilation, using only two electrodes. (From Patterson R. 1995. *The Biomedical Engineering Handbook*. Boca Raton, FL, CRC Press, 3rd edition, pp. 1223–1230.)

between the air and blood plethysmographies is only possible because the two variables have rather different repetition frequencies.

10.8.3 Bioimpedance in Electrosurgery

Electrosurgery (ES) units are used in all operating rooms throughout the world. HF currents are used for tissue cutting, coagulation, desiccation, and sealing. Several bioimpedance systems are used to increase performance and safety.

10.8.3.1 Monitoring Return Electrode Safety

In monopolar ES, the safe functioning of the return electrode is most important. If the HF current (often around 500 kHz) does not have a safe return path back to the unit, the current spreads uncontrolled into the air (antenna effect) and jump to metal objects of all kinds because of capacitive coupling. Patients being in touch with such objects will also couple current from the patient body to the metal, resulting in tissue burns. One method to reduce the risk of accidents is to split the return electrode plate in two halves and monitor by impedance that both halves have good contact with the skin. The halves are coupled with a HF capacitor and both function as the return electrode for the ES HF current. A small sensing current is sent out to the halves to check the continuity of leads and skin contact. The current is supposed to go through one half-electrode and the skin to the other half. If the contact area is too small or a lead is broken, the impedance becomes too high and a trigger alarm is activated. During alarm, the surgeon cannot activate the ES unit any longer.

Figure 10.22 shows how the impedance is measured at 50 kHz and the impedance value is sampled at the start of the procedure. The sampled value is used as reference for the remaining procedure, and the impedance is continuously monitored and compared with the reference. If the deviation is too large, an alarm is triggered and further activation of the ES unit is inhibited. There are two alarm levels. The low level gives warning of a short-circuit condition, the high level gives warning of poor skin contact or wire break.

10.8.3.2 Bipolar Forceps Activation

Forceps are used for bipolar microsurgery and the unit is activated by a pedal or a microswitch on the forceps. However, some surgeons prefer impedance-based activation so that when both tips have sufficient tissue contact, a low impedance level is reached, which triggers activation.

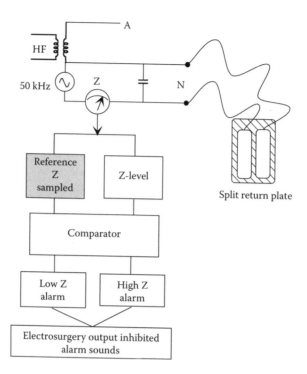

FIGURE 10.22   Impedance-based ES safety monitoring of the return plate system.

10.8.3.3 Vessel Sealing

Safe sealing of blood vessels is very important to prevent postoperative bleeding and reoperations. A special technique for sealing is based on the discovery that under tight control, it is possible to prevent too much tissue destruction and obtain a melting process between connective protein tissue parts of the blood vessel walls. The method is based on a special bipolar jaw with large contact surfaces and a high mechanical pressure to the tissue between the surface blades (Figure 10.23). The electrical contact to the tissue between the upper and lower jaw is very efficient, and it is possible to use much lower voltage and higher current than in ordinary cut and coagulation procedures. The impedance of the tissue is monitored during the clamping and current flow, and within a few seconds, the sealing process starts and this is registered by the impedance system. The impedance system registers when melting is optimum and activation is automatically stopped by the system, not the surgeon. The cutting device is used immediately after activation stops so that both vessel ends can be effectively sealed.

10.8.4 Body Composition

The parameters of interest in body composition analysis (bioelectric impedance analysis, BIA) are (a) TBW, (b) extracellular/intracellular fluid balance, (c) muscle mass, and (d) fat mass. Application areas are as diversified as sports, medicine, nutrition, and fluid balance in renal dialysis and transplantations.

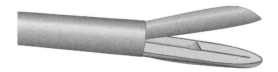

FIGURE 10.23   Vessel-sealing bipolar electrode system with cutting device. (Courtesy: Tormod Martinsen.)

10.8.4.1 Method

The most validated method is prediction of TBW from four-electrode whole-body transfer impedance measurements at 50 kHz. It is not really a whole-body measurement because the results are dominated by the wrist and ankle segments with very little influence from the chest because of the large cross-sectional area. By using more than four electrodes, it is possible to measure more than one body segment. With two electrodes at each hand and foot, the body impedance can, for instance, be modeled in five segments: arms, legs, and chest.

Either the series impedance electrical model (often with the reactance component X neglected) or the parallel equivalent has been used. Several indexes have been introduced to increase the accuracy. Gender, age, and anthropometric results, such as total body weight and height, are parameters used. An often-used index is H^2/R_{segm}, where H is the body height and R_{segm} the resistance of a given segment. Because of the $1/R_{segm}$ term, this is therefore actually a *conductance* index. Calibration, for example, can be done by determining the k-constants in the equation

$$TBW = k_1 \frac{H^2}{R_{segm}} + k_2 \tag{10.12}$$

Such an equation is not directly derived from biophysical laws, but has been empirically selected because it gives the best correlation.

10.8.4.2 Results

The correlation according to Equation 10.12 can be better than 0.95. Hundreds of validation studies with isotope dilution have established a solid relation between whole-body impedance at 50 kHz and body fluid volume (Kyle et al. 2004). Improved prediction of extracellular and TBW has been obtained using impedance loci generated by multiple-frequency BIA (Cornish et al. 1993). Predicting body cell mass with bioimpedance by using more theoretical methods has also been proposed (De Lorenzo et al. 1997). Assessment of hydration change in women during pregnancy and postpartum with bioelectrical impedance vectors has been used (Lukaski et al. 2007).

Complex impedance data can also be given as modulus and phase. Phase has been used as an index of *nutrition*. This is true only in comparison between vectors with the same modulus. For instance, short vectors with a small phase angle are associated with edema, whereas long vectors with an increased phase angle indicate dehydration. The prediction error of fat mass is too high for clinical use (standard error of the estimate in the order of 3–4 L for TBW and 3–4 kg for the fat-free mass) (Sun et al. 2003).

10.8.4.3 Calibration

Calibration can be done with alternative but cumbersome methods using, for example, deuterium, underwater weighing, or dual-energy x-ray absorption. Standardization of the type of electrodes used and their placement is a major concern (Cornish et al. 1999; Kyle et al. 2004).

10.8.5 Electrical Impedance Tomography

There are many examples in medicine where the spatial distribution of a variable is more important than a single value valid for the whole body or just one small volume. For example, in cancer, the spread (metastases) must be mapped; in lungs, it is not just the vital capacity, but how different parts of the lung respond to treatment differently and where in the airway or blood perfusion obstructions occur; with impedance, it is possible to map a tissue layer (EIT, electrical impedance tomography) defined by a skin surface multiple-electrode system; clinical application areas are imaging and imaging of small regions, which can be parameterized and compared (e.g., left and right lung); with thorax imaging,

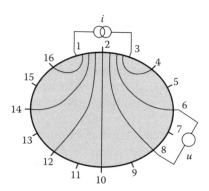

FIGURE 10.24 EIT 16-electrode skin surface system. Current is applied to one bipolar electrode pair; the corresponding equipotential lines are shown. Signals are picked up with all six corresponding bipolar pairs. A homogeneous material model is shown.

determining stroke volume (cardiac output [CO]), pulmonary blood perfusion, and regional lung function; and furthermore, imaging for brain function, breast cancer screening, gastrointestinal function, and hyperthermia (Holder 2005).

Electric current is typically injected in one CC electrode pair and the voltages of all the other PU electrode pairs are recorded. Current injection can then be successively shifted until all electrode pairs have been used as a CC pair. The quantity measured is a group of transfer impedances.

Typical EIT systems involve 16–32 electrodes in any one plane and operate at frequencies between 10 kHz and 1 MHz. The Sheffield Mark III system (Brown et al. 1994a,b) uses 16 electrodes and injects current and measures potential drop between interleaved neighboring electrodes to reduce cross talk (Figure 10.24). Figure 10.24 shows equipotential lines because of a single CC electrode pair. A total of 64 measurements are made at each frequency when driving odd-numbered electrodes and measuring at even-numbered electrodes. Because of reciprocity (see Section 10.5), this gives 32 independent measurements. Voltage differences can be sampled from all PU electrode pairs (not just neighboring) with any combination of single or multiple CC electrode pair combinations.

As explained in Section 10.5, the sensitivity to a given local change in resistivity is given by the dot product of the current vectors resulting from injecting current through the two CC pairs and two PU pairs, respectively. The sensitivity may hence be highest close to the CC or PU electrodes and lowest toward the center of the medium. Figure 10.24 shows the equipotential lines, not the sensitivity field of the CC–PU four-electrode system.

10.8.5.1 Multifrequency EIT

One of the fundamental problems of anatomical imaging based on single-frequency impedance measurements was that the absolute impedance is difficult to determine sufficiently accurately because of the errors in the positioning of the electrodes, boundary shape, and contact impedance density. Impedance imaging was, therefore, concerned with impedance changes because of physiological or pathological processes. With the introduction of multifrequency EIT, the possibility of tissue characterization based on impedance spectroscopy was introduced. If the frequency response varies significantly between different organs and tissues, it will be easier to achieve anatomical images because the images will be based on characteristic impedance changes rather than the absolute value of impedance. Indexes, that is, the relation between measured data at two frequencies may be used, but because of the different characteristic frequencies for different tissues, it has been proved difficult to choose only two frequencies to match all types of tissue. Hence, typically 8–16 frequencies are used (Brown et al. 1994a) computed from the measured data several parameters from a three-component electrical model. They also adapted the measured data to the Cole impedance equation (Cole 1940). Furthermore, indexes were made by using the lowest frequency of 9.6 kHz data as a reference and Brown et al. concluded that it may be possible to identify tissues on the basis of their impedance spectrum and the spectrum of the changes in impedance.

10.8.5.2 Contactless Data-Acquisition Techniques

Contactless data-acquisition techniques can also be used in EIT. Such systems may involve coils for inducing currents but with usual PU electrodes. Totally, contactless circuitry is also possible with magnetic coils or capacitive coupling both for the current excitation and for measuring the tissue current response. Contactless systems have been presented at frequencies up to 20 MHz.

10.8.5.3 Invasive EIT

Classical EIT in medicine is with surface electrodes. However, an array with insulated needles but exposed tips can perform a two-dimensional (2D) recording when measuring during rapid withdrawal of the array. Intended use is in resuscitation outside hospitals (Martinsen et al. 2010).

10.8.5.4 Image Reconstruction

The algorithms for image reconstruction started with the Sheffield group using back-projection methods. On the basis of the equipotential lines shown in Figure 10.24, a conformal transformation could be performed so that the equipotential lines became straight lines. Through many refinement steps, the end result was that uniform resolution across the image was not possible, the spatial accuracy was about 15% of the body diameter; best at the edge (12%) and gradually worse toward the center where the spatial accuracy may be 20% (Holder 2005). The back projection is based on some conditions that are not fulfilled: that the problem can be treated as a 2D problem and that the initial resistivity is uniform. Even if back projection had little theoretical support, it gave the best *in vivo* results. An alternative to back projection was the use of a sensitivity matrix. The sensitivity matrix is the matrix of values by which the conductivity values can be multiplied to give the electrode voltages. The matrix describes how different parts of the measured object influence on the recorded voltages because of the geometrical shape of the object. Iterative methods can be used for static imaging; an intelligent guess of the distribution of, for example, conductivities in the tissue is made initially. The forward problem is then solved to calculate the theoretical boundary potentials that are compared to the actual measured potentials. The initial guess is then modified to reduce the difference between calculated and measured potentials and this process is repeated until the difference is acceptably small. The sensitivity matrix has to be inverted to enable image reconstruction. This operation is not uncomplicated and many techniques have been suggested.

10.8.5.5 Advantages and Problems

EIT is basically not tomographic in the way, for instance, computer tomography (CT) is. Photons reaching a CT detector have followed straight lines after scattered photons have been absorbed in collimators. Electric current lines out from a CC electrode spread out in all directions and do not clearly define a tomographic plane and its thickness. Some important achievements in the pursuit of three-dimensional (3D) EIT were presented in *Nature* (Metherall et al. 1996). This leads to a 3D multilayer aspect as a parallel to the magnetic resonance imaging (MRI) volume-imaging technique. However, the complexity of both the EIT hardware and software increases considerably by introducing this third dimension.

A sufficiently precise positioning of the electrodes is difficult and it is easier to work with dynamic images, which do not depend so much on absolute impedance values. If the tissue shows sufficient dispersion, a multifrequency approach has been found useful. Also, time series from changes in the tissue during recording, for instance, respiration, has proven useful.

EIT is a fast technique because an image uptake can take less than 1/10 s. The sensors are small and low priced, and the instrumentation can also be low priced, small, and light weighted.

A new and very interesting application is the monitoring of the distribution of ventilation in the lungs. Dräger has developed a special EIT application using 15 or 16 electrodes around the chest. It is used in intensive-care and neonatal units. To operate ventilators in a manner that is correct for each patient, doctors need reliable data not only on classical respiration parameters valid for the lung volume, but also on the distribution of the ventilation to assess treatment. The EIT instrumentation is small and well suited for bedside use delivering information directly in real time. This is in contrast to x-ray, CT, and MRI instrumentation where the patient usually must be brought to a special examination room.

New application examples are coming up all the time, such as imaging of gastric function, pulmonary ventilation, perfusion, brain hemorrhage, hyperthermia, swallowing disorders, and breast cancer. A fundamental difficulty is the considerable anisotropy found in the electrical properties of, for example, muscle tissue.

10.8.6 Some Additional Applications

10.8.6.1 Impedance Cardiography and Cardiac Output

ICG has been around for a long time (Kubicek et al. 1970) and appreciable activity has been going on toward clarifying the best method (Hettrick and Zielinski 2006). The electrode systems consist of either four band electrodes, two in the region of the neck and two around the thorax, or the use of spot electrodes (Kauppinen et al. 1998). The origin of the impedance changes during the cardiac cycle is known. Physiologically, it is the filling and emptying of the heart, the opening and closing of the valves, the rapid filling and slow emptying of the aorta, the filling and emptying of the lung vessels, lung tissue, and surrounding tissue. Clinically, the need for a bedside CO monitor has resulted in intensive research and many interventional trials (Bernstein 1986). New ways, for example, with the use of the Sigman effect are still under development (Bernstein 2010).

10.8.6.2 Intrathoracic Impedance and Fluid Status

Active implants, such as pacemakers, cardioverters (ICDs), and neurostimulators, are increasingly using impedance measurements (Yu et al. 2005; Vollmann et al. 2007). The implants are already equipped with advanced electronic circuitry and advanced multielectrode catheter systems together with data storage and communication facilities. Parameters of interest are, for instance, CO, myocardial contractility, ischemia, and thoracic fluid accumulation.

10.8.6.3 Implant Rejection Monitoring

Transplanted organs, such as heart or kidney, can be followed with impedance measurements using skin electrodes or implanted leads or catheters (Ollmar 1997).

10.8.6.4 Cancer Detection

For many years, there has been hope that the impedance difference between normal and cancerous tissue is sufficiently large to clinically obtain useful diagnoses. An impedance method is rapid and practical, but cancer is a serious diagnosis and both sensitivity and specificity must be high. Interesting results have been obtained with the cervix in nonpregnant and pregnant women. Skin cancer in the breast has been examined (Jossinet 1996). Perhaps, the most promising results have been presented by Stig Ollmar's group (Ollmar et al. 1995) on skin cancer, using a special electrode surface with many very small and very short needles as a microinvasive technique (Emtestam et al. 1998; Åberg et al. 2004).

10.8.6.5 Sweat Activity

Human skin conductance is very dependent on SA. The SA instrumentation uses skin surface electrodes for unipolar admittance measurements (Tronstad et al. 2008). Small, portable, and multichannel loggers are now available enabling recording of SA under circumstances such as daily errands, exercise, and sleep. Results show that SA is related to physical exercise, dermatomes, distribution of sweat glands, and sympathetic activity. With the normal sweating patterns of the healthy population better known, measurements on hyperhidrosis patients can yield a distinguishing parameter, which can be used for diagnosis and treatment evaluation.

10.8.6.6 Skin Hydration

SC complex resistivity is very dependent on SC hydration. The hydration is dependent on the SA and also the relative humidity of the surrounding air in contact with the SC surface. They both influence the measured admittance but in different ways. The capacitive part of the skin admittance (susceptance) gives information on SC hydration (Martinsen and Grimnes 2001).

Gravimetric and other methods have been used for *in vitro* calibration of skin hydration measurements (Martinsen et al. 2008).

10.8.6.7 Needle Positioning

The method is based on precise determinations of local impedance values in tissue surrounding the tip of a needle (Kalvøy et al. 2009). Such impedance spectra allow determination of the tissue type and thereby an anatomical positioning of the needle. In some clinical applications, the separation of fat and muscle is, for instance, crucial. For clinical use, sufficient spatial resolution is obtained cause of the small sensitivity zone. A needle may be a solid needle or a cannula for simultaneous infusion or biopsy taking. The method requires a needle with an insulated shaft and a conducting tip in galvanic contact with the tissue. The method may also be applied in further characterization of tissue state, for example, oxygenation, content of substances such as lactic acid, and so on.

10.8.6.8 Electrodermal Response

Palmar skin changes both skin potential level and skin conductance as a response to psychophysiological stimuli (answering questions, doing mathematical calculations, taking a deep breath, being in a stressed situation, etc.). A committee report (Fowles et al. 1981) recommended the use of DC conductance and this has been the most popular method since. 0.5 V DC is applied to two electrodes, the current is measured and the DC conductance calculated. However, a new committee report also recommends using AC conductance for electrodermal response measurements (Boucsein et al. 2012). By using AC conductance, it is possible to measure skin potential simultaneously with the same electrode (Grimnes et al. 2011). The waves are very dependent on the electrode contact and electrolyte used (Tronstad et al. 2010). Potential response waves may be different from AC response waves and the generation mechanism is unknown.

10.8.6.9 Cell- and Bacteria Suspensions, Coulter Counter

Schwan (1957) wrote an introduction to impedance measurement on cell and bacteria suspensions. A Coulter counter is a streaming blood cell counter. Two different electrolyte reservoirs equipped with impedance CC electrodes are connected via a short capillary. The reservoir with the cell suspension is on higher pressure so that the electrolyte with cells stream through the capillary. Measured impedance is dominated by the capillary because of its very small diameter. At passage, the impedance goes through a peak because of the cell membrane. The frequency of the peaks is the number of cells passed per second; the impedance waveforms are characteristic for different cell types. The cell suspension must have a concentration so that the probability of two cells in the capillary at the same time is low. The electrolyte concentration must be adapted to the impedance increase caused by each cell.

10.8.6.10 Rheoencephalography

Although not evident from the title, rheoencephalography is a plethysmographic technique based on bioimpedance and with focus on cerebral blood flow (Bodo et al. 2004; Grimnes and Martinsen 2008; Bodo 2010).

10.8.6.11 Cell Nanometer Motion

Some cells must be in contact with a surface to thrive. When a cell is in contact with a small electrode surface, the cell's covering effect results in an impedance increase. The electrode can be of gold and can have a surface area not very larger than the spread of a single cell. The suspension can contain protein molecules, which first cover the golden surface so that the cell is attracted to the protein surface. The basic polarization impedance is, therefore, modified by the protein layer. The impedance is measured, for example, at 4 kHz. Living cells that are attached to a surface will move around on the electrode surface giving varying impedance. This cell motion corresponds to nanometer movements giving information about cell status and behavior (Giaever and Keese 1993).

10.8.6.12 EMG and Neurology Impedance

The action potential is the endogenous bioelectric signal from an excited nerve cell. The process can be followed by impedance changes as well (Sauter et al. 2009) and in electrical impedance myography (EIM) (Nie et al. 2006).

10.8.6.13 Electroporation

Electroporation is generation of pores in the cell membranes by short voltage pulses (Weaver and Chizmadzhev 1996; Pliquett et al. 2007). The cells may die (a sort of nonthermal ablation) or survive. The generation of pores implies an impedance decrease, which can be detected by an impedance reduction. Bioimpedance can, therefore, monitor the pore-generating process. In the Coulter counter the cells pass rapidly through a capillary connecting two electrolytic chambers and are counted and analyzed. Here, a single cell is mechanically trapped in a hole between two chambers and by pulsing the two chambers the cell can be electroporated even with low voltages pulses, and the process can be followed in the stationary cell.

References

Åberg P, Nicander I, Hansson J, Geladi P, Holmgren U, Ollmar S. 2004. Skin cancer identification using multi-frequency electrical impedance—A potential screening tool. *IEEE Trans Biomed Eng* 51, 2097–2102.

Becker FF, Wang X-B, Huang Y, Pethig R, Vykoukal J, Gascoyne PRC. 1994. The removal of human leukaemia cells from blood using interdigitated microelectrodes. *J Phys D: Appl Phys* 27, 2659–2662.

Bernstein DP. 1986. A new stroke volume equation for thoracic electrical bioimpedance: Theory and rationale. *Crit Care Med* 14 (10), 904–909.

Bernstein, DP. 2010. Impedance cardiography: Pulsatile blood flow and the biophysical and electrodynamic basis for the stroke volume equations. *J Electr Bioimp* 1, 2–17.

Bodo M. 2010. Studies in rheoencephalography (REG). *J Electr Bioimp* 1, 18–40.

Bodo M, Pearce FJ, Armonda RA. 2004. Cerebrovascular reactivity: Rat studies in rheoencephalography. *Physiol Meas* 25, 1371–1384.

Boucsein W, Fowles DC, Grimnes S, Ben-Shakhar G, Roth WT, Dawson ME, Filion DL. 2012. Publication recommendations for electrodermal response. *Psychophysiology*, 49, 1017–1034.

Brown BH, Barber DC, Leathard AD, Lu L, Wang W, Smallwood RH, Wilson AJ. 1994b. High frequency EIT data collection and parametric imaging. *Innov Tech Biol Med* 15(1), 1–8.

Brown BH, Barber DC, Wang W, Lu L, Leathard AD, Smallwood RH, Hampshire AR, Mackay R, Hatzigalanis K. 1994a. Multi-frequency imaging and modeling of respiratory related electrical impedance changes. *Physiol Meas*. 15(suppl.), 1–12.

Casas O, Bragos R, Riu P, Rosell J, Tresanchez M, Warren M, Rodriguez-Sinovas A, Carreño A, Cinca J. 1999. *In-vivo* and *in-situ* ischemic tissue characterisation using electrical impedance spectroscopy. *Ann N Y Acad Sci* 873, 51–59.

Chua LO. 1971. Memristor—The missing circuit element. *IEEE Trans Circuit Theory* CT-18(5), 507–519.

Chua LO, Kang SM. 1976. Memristive devices and systems. *Proc IEEE*, 64, 209–223.

Chung C, Waterfall M, Pells S, Menachery A, Smith S, Pethig R. 2011. Dielectrophoretic characterisation of mammalian cells above 100 MHz. *J Electr Bioimp* 2, 64–71.

Cole KS. 1940. Permeability and impermeability of cell membranes for ions. *Cold Spring Harbor Sympos Quant Biol* 8, 110–122.

Cole KS, Cole RH. 1941. Dispersion and absorption in dielectrics. I. Alternating current characteristics. *J Chem Phys* 9, 341–351.

Cornish BH, Jacobs A, Thomas BJ, Ward LC. 1999. Optimising electrode sites for segmental bioimpedance measurements. *Physiol Meas* 20, 241–250.

Cornish BH, Thomas BJ, Ward LC. 1993. Improved prediction of extracellular and total body water using impedance loci generated by multiple frequency bioelectrical impedance analysis. *Phys Med Biol* 38, 337.

Dalziel CF. 1954. The threshold of perception currents. *AIEE Trans Power App Syst* 73, 990–996.

Dalziel, CF. 1972. Electric shock hazard. *IEEE Spectr*, 9, 41.

De Lorenzo A, Andreoli A, Matthie J, Withers P. 1997. Predicting body cell mass with bioimpedance by using theoretical methods: A technology review. *J Appl Physiol* 82, 1542–1558.

Di Ventra M, Pershin YV, Chua LO. 2009. Circuit elements with memory: Memristors, memcapacitors, and meminductors. *Proc IEEE* 97, 1717–1724.

Duck FA.1990. *Physical Properties of Tissue. A Comprehensive Reference Book*. London, Academic Press.

Emtestam L, Nicander I, Stenström M, Ollmar S. 1998. Electrical impedance of nodular basal cell carcinoma: A pilot study. *Dermatology* 197, 313–316.

Epstein BR, Foster KR. 1983. Anisotropy in the dielectric properties of skeletal muscles. *Med Biol Eng Comp* 21, 51.

Fink H-W, Schönenberger C. 1999. Electrical conduction through DNA molecules. *Nature* 398, 407–410.

Foster KR, Epstein BR, Gealt MA. 1987. "Resonances" in the dielectric absorption of DNA? *Biophys J* 52, 421–425.

Fowles DC, Christie MJ, Edelberg R, Grings WW, Lykken DT, Venables PH. 1981. Publication recommendations for electrodermal measurements. *Psychophysiology* 18, 232–239.

Gabriel S, Lau RW, Gabriel C. 1996. The dielectric properties of biological tissue: II. Measurements in the frequency range 10 Hz to 20 GHz. *Phys Med Biol* 41, 2251–2269.

Geddes LA. 1972. *Electrodes and the Measurement of Bioelectric Events*. New York, Wiley-Interscience.

Geddes LA, Baker LE. 1989. *Applied Biomedical Instrumentation*. New York, Wiley Interscience.

Gersing E. 1998. Impedance spectroscopy on living tissue for determination of the state of organs. *Bioelectrochem Bioenerg* 45(2), 145–149.

Geselowitz DB. 1971. An application of electrocardiographic lead theory to impedance plethysmography. *IEEE Trans Biomed Eng* 18, 38–41.

Giaever I, Keese CR. 1993. A morphological biosensor for mammalian cells. *Nature* 366, 591–592.

Grimnes S. 1983a. Impedance measurement of individual skin surface electrodes. *Med Biol Eng Comput* 21, 750–755.

Grimnes S. 1983b. Skin impedance and electro-osmosis in the human epidermis. *Med Biol Eng Comput* 21, 739–749.

Grimnes S. 1983c. Electrovibration, cutaneous sensation of microampere current. *Acta Physiol Scand* 118, 19–25.

Grimnes S, Jabbari A, Martinsen ØG, Tronstad C. 2011. Electrodermal activity by DC potential and AC conductance measured simultaneously at the same skin site. *Skin Res Technol* 17, 26–34.

Grimnes S, Martinsen ØG. 2007. Sources of error in tetrapolar impedance measurements on biomaterials and other ionic conductors. *J Phys D: Appl Phys* 40, 9–14.

Grimnes S, Martinsen ØG. 2008. *Bioimpedance and Bioelectricity Basics*. Amsterdam, Elsevier-Academic Press.

Griss P, Enoksson P, Tolvanen-Laakso HK, Meriläinen P, Ollmar S, Stemme G. 2001. Micromachined electrodes for biopotential measurements. *IEEE J Microelectro-mechanical Systems* 10, 10–16.

Hettrick DA, Zielinski TM. 2006. *Bioimpedance in Cardiovascular Medicine. Encyclopedia of Medical Devices and Instrumentation*, 2nd edition. New York, John Wiley & Sons, Inc. pp. 197–216.

Holder DS (ed). 2005. *Electrical Impedance Tomography. Method, History and Applications*. Bristol, Institute of Physics Publishing (IoP).

IEC-60601. 2005. Medical electrical equipment. General requirements for basic safety and essential performance. International standard.

Jaron D, Briller A, Schwan HP, Geselowitz DB. 1969. Nonlinearity of cardiac pacemaker electrodes. *IEEE Trans Biomed Eng* 16, 132–138.

Johnsen GK, Lütken CA, Martinsen ØG, Grimnes S. 2011. Memristive model of electro-osmosis in skin. *Phys Rev E* 83, 031916.

Jossinet J. 1996. Variability of impedivity in normal and pathological breast tissue. *Med Biol Eng Comput* 34(5), 346–350.

Kalvøy H, Frich L, Grimnes S, Martinsen ØG, Hol PK, Stubhaug A. 2009. Impedance-based tissue discrimination for needle guidance. *Physiol Meas* 30, 129–140.

Kauppinen PK, Hyttinen JA, Malmivuo JA. 1998. Sensitivity distributions of impedance cardiography using band and spot electrodes analyzed by a three-dimensional computer model. *Ann Biomed Eng* 26(4), 694–702.

Kubicek WG, Patterson RP, Witsoe DA, Mattson RH. 1970. Impedance cardiography as a non-invasive method for monitoring cardiac function and other parameters of the cardiovascular system. *Ann NY Acad Sci* 170, 724–732.

Kyle UG, Bosaeus I, De Lorenzo AD, Deurenberg P, Elia M, Gomez JM, Heitmann BL et al. 2004. Bioelectrical impedance analysis—Part I: Review of principles and methods. *Clin Nutr* 23, 1226–1243.

Lukaski HC, Hall CB, Siders WA. 2007. Assessment of change in hydration in women during pregnancy and postpartum with bioelectrical impedance vectors. *Nutrition* 8, 543–550.

Malmivuo J, Plonsey R. 1995. *Bioelectromagnetism*. New York, Oxford University Press.

Martinsen ØG, Grimnes S. 2001. Facts and myths about electrical measurement of stratum corneum hydration state. *Dermatology*, 202, 87–89.

Martinsen ØG, Grimnes S, Mirtaheri P. 2000. Non-invasive measurements of post mortem changes in dielectric properties of haddock muscle—A pilot study. *J Food Eng* 43, 189–192.

Martinsen ØG, Grimnes S, Nilsen JK, Tronstad C, Jang W, Kim H, Shin K. 2008. Gravimetric method for *in vitro* calibration of skin hydration measurements. *IEEE Trans Biomed Eng* 55(2), 728–732.

Martinsen ØG, Kalvøy H, Grimnes S, Nordbotten B, Hol PK, Fosse E, Myklebust H, Becker LB. 2010. Invasive electrical impedance tomography for blood vessel detection. *Open Biomed Eng J* 4, 135–137.

Metherall P, Barber DC, Smallwood RH, Brown BH. 1996. Three dimensional electrical impedance tomography. *Nature* 380(6574), 509–512.

Mirtaheri P, Grimnes S, Martinsen ØG. 2005. Electrode polarization impedance in weak NaCl aqueous solutions. *IEEE Trans Biomed Eng.* 52(12), 2093–2099.

Nicander I, Ollmar S, Eek A, Lundh Rozell B, Emtestam L. 1996. Correlation of impedance response patterns to histological findings in irritant skin reactions induced by various surfactants. *Br J Dermatol* 134, 221–228.

Nie R, Chin AB, Lee KS, Sunmonu NA, Rutkove SB. 2006. Electrical impedance myography: Transitioning from human to animal studies. *Clin Neurophys* 117, 1844–1849.

Ollmar S. 1997. Noninvasive monitoring of transplanted kidneys by impedance spectroscopy—A pilot study. *Med Biol Eng Comput* 35 (suppl.), Part 1, 336.

Ollmar S. 1998. Methods for information extraction from impedance spectra of biological tissue, in particular skin and oral mucosa—A critical review and suggestions for the future. *Bioelectrochem Bioenerg* 45, 157–160.

Ollmar S, Eek A, Sundstrøm F, Emtestam L. 1995. Electrical impedance for estimation of irritation in oral mucosa and skin. *Med Prog Technol* 21, 29–37.

Onaral B, Schwan HP. 1982. Linear and nonlinear properties of platinum electrode polarisation. Part I: Frequency dependence at very low frequencies. *Med & Biol Eng & Comp* 20, 299–306.

Patterson R. 1995. Bioelectric impedance measurement. In: Bronzino JD (ed.) *The Biomedical Engineering Handbook*. Boca Raton, FL, CRC Press, 3rd edition, pp. 1223–1230.

Pethig R. 1979. *Dielectric and Electronic Properties of Biological Materials*. Chichester, John Wiley.

Pethig R, Jakubek LM, Sanger RH, Heart E, Corson ED, Smith PJS. 2005. Electrokinetic measurements of membrane capacitance and conductance for pancreatic β-cells. *IEE Proc Nanobiotechnol* 152(6), 189–193.

Pliquett U, Joshi RP, Sridhara V, Schoenbach KH. 2007. High electric field effects on cell membranes. *Bioelectrochemistry* 27, 275–282.

Plonsey, R, Barr C. 2007. *Bioelectricity, a Quantitative Approach*. 3rd edition, New York, Springer.

Polk C, Postow E. 1996. *Biological Effects of Electromagnetic Fields*. Boca Raton, FL, CRC Handbook.

Sauter AR, Dodgson MS, Kalvøy H, Grimnes S, Stubhaug A, Klaastad Ø. 2009. Current threshold for nerve stimulation depends on electrical impedance of the tissue: A study of ultrasound-guided electrical nerve stimulation of the median nerve. *Anesth Analog* 108(4), 1338–1343.

Schäfer M, Schlegel C, Kirlum H-J, Gersing E, Gebhard MM. 1998. Monitoring of damage to skeletal muscle tissue caused by ischemia. *Bioelectrochem Bioenerg* 45, 151–155.

Schwan HP. 1957. Electrical properties of tissue and cell suspensions. In: *Advances in Biological and Medical Physics*. Lawrence JH, Tobias CA, eds. Vol. V, pp. 147–209, Academic Press.

Schwan HP. 1963. Determination of biological impedances. In: *Physical Techniques in Biological Research*. Nastuk WL, ed. Vol. 6, pp. 323–406, Academic Press.

Schwan HP. 1968. Electrode polarization impedance and measurements in biological materials. *Ann NY Acad Sci* 148, 191–208.

Schwan HP. 1992. Linear and non-linear electrode polarisation and biological materials. *Ann Biomed Eng* 20, 269–288.

Schwan HP. 2001. In: *Selected Papers by Herman P. Schwan*. Grimnes S, Martinsen ØG, eds. Medisinkteknisk avdelings forlag (Oslo). ogm//www.med-tek.no/t-Bokhandel.aspx

Shiffman CA, Aaron R, Rutkove SB. 2003. Electrical impedance of muscle during isometric contraction. *Physiol Meas* 24, 213–234.

Sigman E, Kolin A, Katz LN, Jochim K. 1937. Effect of motion on the electrical conductivity of the blood. *Am J Physiol* 118, 708–719.

Smith SR, Foster KR. 1985. Dielectric properties of low-water content tissues. *Phys Med Biol* 30, 965.

Sun SS, Chumlea WC, Heimsfield SB et al. 2003. Development of bioelectrical impedance analysis prediction equations for body composition with the use of a multicomponent model for use in epidemiological surveys. *Am J Clin Nutr* 77, 331–340.

Takashima S. 1989. *Electrical Properties of Biopolymers and Membranes*. Bristol, Adam Hilger.

Takashima S, Schwan HP. 1965. Dielectric dispersion of crystalline powders of amino acids, peptides and proteins. *J Phys Chem* 69, 4176–4182.

Tronstad C, Gjein GE, Grimnes S, Martinsen ØG, Krogstad A-L, Fosse E. 2008. Electrical measurement of sweat activity. *Physiol Meas* 29(6), S407–S415.

Tronstad C, Johnsen GK, Grimnes S, Martinsen ØJ. 2010. A study on electrode gels for skin conductance measurements. *Physiol Meas* 31, 1395–1410.

Vollmann D, Nagele H, Schauerte P et al. 2007. Clinical utility of intrathoracic impedance monitoring to alert patients with an implanted device of deteriorating chronic heart failure. *Eur Heart J* 19, 1835–1840.

Warburg E. 1899. Über das Verhalten sogenannte unpolarisierbare Elektroden gegen Wechselstrom. *Ann Phys Chem* 67, 493–499.

Weaver JC, Chizmadzhev YA. 1996. Theory of electroporation: A review. *Bioelectrochem. Bioenerg.* 41, 135–160.

Yamamoto T, Yamamoto Y. 1976. Electrical properties of the epidermal stratum corneum. *Med Biol Eng* 14, 592–594.

Yamamoto T, Yamamoto Y. 1981. Non-linear electrical properties of the skin in the low frequency range. *Med Biol Eng Comp* 19, 302–310.

Yelamos D, Casas O, Bragos R, Rosell J. 1999. Improvement of a front end for bioimpedance spectroscopy. *Ann N Y Acad Sci* 873, 306–312.

Yu C, Wang L, Chau E et al. 2005. Intrathoracic impedance monitoring in patients with heart failure. Correlation with fluid status and feasibility of early warning preceding hospitalization. *Circulation* 112, 841–848.

11

Implantable Cardiac Pacemakers

Pat Ridgely
Medtronic, Inc.

11.1 Introduction

The practical use of an implantable device for delivering a controlled, rhythmic electric stimulus to maintain the heartbeat is now approximately 50 years old and has become a standard cardiac therapy. During this period, circuit density has increased by a factor of more than a million, and devices have become steadily smaller (from 250 g in 1960 to less than a tenth of that today). Early devices provided only single-chamber, asynchronous, nonprogrammable pacing coupled with questionable reliability and short device longevity. Today, advances in a variety of technologies provide dual-chamber multiprogrammability, rate response, data collection, diagnostic functions, and exceptional reliability. Moreover, lithium-iodide power sources have extended device longevity to beyond a decade.

The modern pacing system still comprises three distinct components: pulse generator, lead, and programmer (Figure 11.1). The pulse generator houses the battery; the circuitry, which senses electrical (and in some cases, physical) activity, configures an appropriate response, and generates the stimulus; and a transceiver. The lead is an insulated wire that carries the stimulus from the generator to the heart and relays intrinsic cardiac signals back to the generator. The programmer is a telemetry device used to provide two-way communications between the generator and the clinician. It can alter the therapy delivered by the pacemaker and retrieve diagnostic data that are essential for optimally titrating that therapy over time. Ultimately, the therapeutic success of the pacing prescription rests on the clinician's choice of an appropriate system, the use of sound implant technique, and programming focused on patient outcomes.

This chapter discusses in further detail the components of the modern pacing system and the significant evolution that has occurred since its inception. The emphasis here is on system operation; an in-depth discussion of the fundamental electrophysiology of tissue stimulation can be found in Ellenbogen et al. (2007).

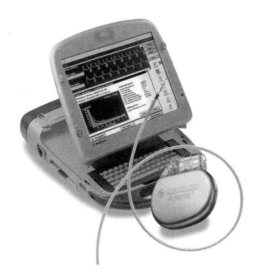

FIGURE 11.1   A pacing system comprises a programmer, pulse generator, and lead.

11.2 Indications

The decision to implant a permanent pacemaker usually is based on the major goals of symptom relief (at rest and with physical activity), restoration of functional capacity and quality of life, and reduced mortality. As with other healthcare technologies, the appropriate use of pacing is the intent of indications guidelines published by professional societies in cardiology. (The most recent version of guidelines for the United States can be found on the website of the Heart Rhythm Society.)

Historically, pacing has been indicated when there is a dramatic slowing of the heart rate or a failure in the connection between the atria and ventricles, resulting in decreased cardiac output manifested by symptoms such as syncope, light-headedness, fatigue, and exercise intolerance. Though this failure of impulse formation and/or conduction resulting in bradycardia has been the overriding theme of pacemaker indications, two additional uses have become important:

- Antitachycardia pacing to terminate inappropriately fast rhythms, typically in the ventricle
- Cardiac resynchronization therapy (CRT) to restore the normal activation sequence of contraction in the hearts of some patients with heart failure

11.3 Pulse Generators

The pulse generator contains a power source, output circuit, sensing circuit, and a timing circuit.

A telemetry coil is used to send and receive information between the generator and the programmer. Rate-adaptive pulse generators include the sensor components, along with the circuit, to process the information measured by the sensor (Figures 11.2 and 11.3).

Modern pacemakers use both read-only memory (ROM) and random-access memory (RAM). Although RAM provides the ability to store diagnostic data and change feature sets after implantation, the need to minimize device size and current drain keeps RAM typically on the order of tens of kilobytes in older devices. (Newer devices may have a megabyte or more.) ROM is less susceptible to data errors; therefore, it is typically used to store essential execution codes. Pacemakers usually have less ROM than RAM.

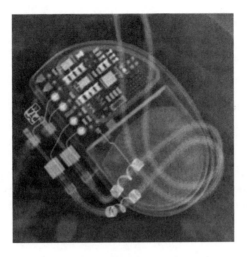

FIGURE 11.2 X-ray view of a pulse generator and two leads.

All components of the pulse generator are housed in a hermetically sealed titanium case with an epoxy header block that accepts the lead(s). Because pacing leads are available with a variety of connector sites and configurations, the pulse generator is available with an equal variety of connectors. The outer casing is laser etched with the manufacturer, model name, type (e.g., single- versus dual-chamber), model number, serial number, and the lead-connection diagram for each identification. Once implanted, it may be necessary to use an x-ray to reveal the identity of the generator. Some manufacturers use radiopaque symbols and ID codes for this purpose, whereas others give their generators characteristic shapes.

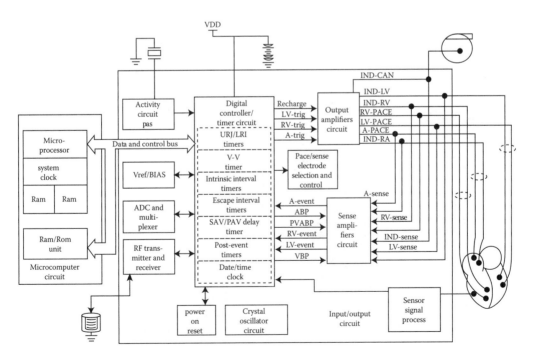

FIGURE 11.3 Sample block diagram of a pacemaker.

11.3.1 Sensing Circuit

Pulse generators have two basic functions, sensing and pacing. Sensing refers to the recognition of intrinsic cardiac depolarization from the chamber or chambers in which the leads are placed. It is imperative for the sensing circuit to discriminate between these intracardiac signals and unwanted electrical interference such as far-field cardiac events, diastolic potentials, skeletal muscle contraction, and pacing stimuli. Because the desired signals are low-amplitude, extensive amplification and filtering are typically required. An intracardiac electrogram shows the waveform as seen by the pacemaker; it is typically quite different from the corresponding event as shown on the surface ECG (Figure 11.4).

Sensing (and pacing) is accomplished with one of two configurations, bipolar and unipolar (Figure 11.5). In bipolar configuration, the anode and cathode are close together, with the anode at the tip of the lead and the cathode a ring electrode about 2 cm proximal to the tip. In unipolar configuration,

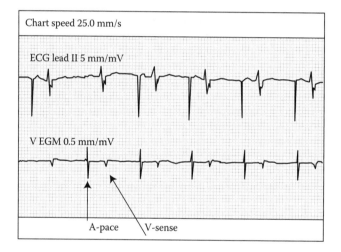

FIGURE 11.4 The surface ECG (ECG LEAD II) represents the sum total of the electrical potentials of all depolarizing tissue. The intracardiac electrogram (V EGM) shows only the potentials measured between the lead electrodes. This allows the evaluation of signals that may be hidden within the surface ECG.

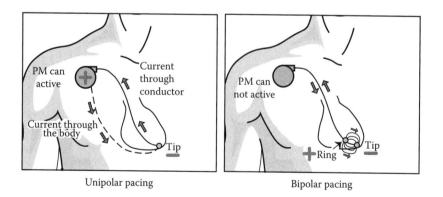

FIGURE 11.5 Unipolar versus bipolar pacing.

the anode and cathode may be 5–10 cm apart. The anode is at the lead tip and the cathode is the pulse generator itself (usually located in the pectoral region).

In general, bipolar and unipolar sensing configurations have equal performance. A drawback of the unipolar approach is the increased possibility of sensing noncardiac signals. The large electrode separation may, for example, sense myopotentials from skeletal muscle movement, leading to inappropriate inhibition of pacing. Many newer pacemakers can be programmed to sense or pace in either configuration.

Once the electrogram enters the sensing circuit, it is scrutinized by a bandpass filter. The frequency of an R-wave is 10–30 Hz. The center frequency of most sensing amplifiers is 30 Hz. T-waves are slower, broad signals that are composed of lower frequencies (approximately 5 Hz or less). Far-field signals are also lower frequency signals, whereas skeletal muscle falls in the range of 10–200 Hz (Figure 11.6).

At implant, the voltage amplitude of the R-wave (and the P-wave, in the case of dual-chamber pacing) is measured to ensure the availability of an adequate signal. R-wave amplitudes are typically 5–25 mV, and P-wave amplitudes are 2–6 mV. The signals passing through the sense amplifier are compared to an adjustable reference voltage called the sensitivity; some pacemakers allow sensitivity settings as low as a tenth of a millivolt. Any signal below the reference voltage is not sensed, and those above it are sensed. Higher sensitivity settings (high reference voltage) may lead to substandard sensing, and a lower reference voltage may result in oversensing. A minimum 2:1 safety margin should be maintained between the sensitivity setting and the amplitude of the intracardiac signal. The circuit is protected from extremely high voltages by a Zener diode.

The slope of the signal is also surveyed by the sensing circuit and is determined by the slew rate (the time rate of change in voltage). A slew rate that is too flat or too steep may be eliminated by the bandpass filter. On average, the slew rate measured at implant should be between 0.75 and 2.50 V/s.

The most drastic way to deal with undesirable signals is to "blind" the circuit at specific times during the cardiac cycle. This is accomplished with blanking and refractory periods. Some of these periods

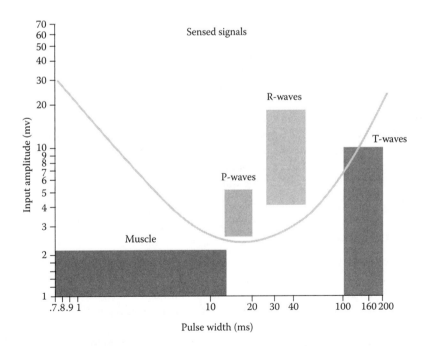

FIGURE 11.6 A conceptual depiction of the bandpass filter, demonstrating the typical filtering of unwanted signals by discriminating between those with slew rates that are too low and/or too high.

are programmable. During the blanking period, the sensing circuit is turned off; during the refractory period, the circuit can see the signal but does not initiate any of the basic timing intervals. Virtually all paced and sensed events begin concurrent blanking and refractory periods, typically ranging from 10 to 400 ms. These are especially helpful in dual-chamber pacemakers in which there exists the potential for the pacing output of the atrial side to inhibit the ventricular pacing output, with dangerous consequences for patients in complete heart block.

Probably, the most common question asked by the general public about pacing systems is the effect of electromagnetic interference (EMI) on their operation. EMI outside of the hospital is an infrequent problem, although patients are advised to avoid sources of strong electromagnetic fields such as arc welders, high-voltage generators, and radar antennae. Some clinicians suggest that patients avoid standing near antitheft devices used in retail stores. Airport screening devices are generally safe. Microwave ovens, ham radio equipment, video games, computers, and office equipment rarely interfere with the operation of modern pacemakers. A common recommendation regarding cell phones is to keep them 15 cm from the pacemaker.

Several medical devices and procedures can affect pacemakers, however: electrocautery, cardioversion and defibrillation, lithotripsy, diathermy, neurostimulation units, RF ablation, radiation therapy, and MRI, among others. MRI can have effects through multiple mechanisms other than EMI: force and torque, current induction, and heating (Al-Ahmad et al. 2010).

Pacemakers affected by interference typically respond with temporary loss of output or temporary reversion to asynchronous pacing (pacing at a fixed rate, with no inhibition from intrinsic cardiac events). The usual consequence for the patient is a return of symptoms that originally led to the pacemaker implant, and pacemaker-dependent patients are placed at clinical risk. Pacemaker manufacturers provide extensive information on interference issues via their websites and technical service phone centers.

11.3.2 Output Circuit

Pacing stimuli are of low energy and short duration: on the order of 10 µJ, delivered in pulses lasting on the order of a millisecond. Modern permanent pulse generators use a constant-voltage approach: the voltage remains at the programmed value while the current varies. Pulse amplitudes are typically on the order of a volt, but in some generators can be as high as 10 V (used for troubleshooting or for pediatric patients).

The output pulse is generated from the discharge of a capacitor charged by the battery. Most modern pulse generators contain a 2.8 V battery. The higher voltages are achieved using voltage multipliers (smaller capacitors used to charge the large capacitor). The voltage can be doubled by charging two smaller capacitors in parallel, with the discharge delivered to the output capacitor in series. Output pulses are emitted at a rate controlled by the timing circuit; output is commonly inhibited by sensed cardiac signals.

11.3.3 Timing Circuit

The timing circuit regulates parameters such as the pacing cycle length, refractory and blanking periods, pulse duration, and specific timing intervals between atrial and ventricular events. A crystal oscillator generating frequencies in the kilohertz range sends a signal to a digital timing and logic control circuit, which in turn operates internally generated clocks at divisions of the oscillatory frequency.

A rate-limiting circuit is incorporated into the timing circuit to prevent the pacing rate from exceeding an upper limit, should a random component failure occur (an extremely rare event). This is also referred to as "runaway" protection and is typically 180–200 pulses per minute.

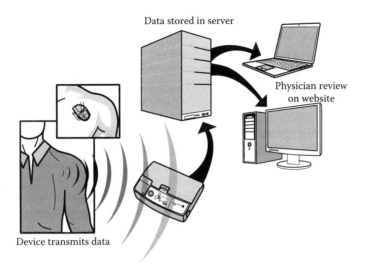

FIGURE 11.7 Remote monitoring systems connect cardiac device patients from home or other location to their clinics via a secure Internet website.

11.3.4 Telemetry Circuit

Pulse generators have long been capable of two-way communication using near-field inductive coupling between the pulse generator and the programmer. This has enabled real-time telemetry in which the pulse generator during clinic visits provides information such as pulse amplitude, pulse duration, lead impedance, battery impedance, lead current, charge, and energy. The programmer, in turn, delivers coded messages to the pulse generator to alter any of the programmable features and to retrieve diagnostic data. Signal fidelity is accomplished by using pulse-strings, typically 16 digital pulses in length; each manufacturer's devices communicate only with programmers from that manufacturer.

Historically, device monitoring away from the clinic was accomplished transtelephonically. In these sessions, the patient dons wristband electrodes attached to a device that transmits a rhythm strip over a landline. More recently, advances in telecommunication technology have enabled the use of cell-phone-based transmission of essential data directly to a clinic, where it can be viewed via the Internet. This remote monitoring can provide valuable alerts when certain clinical criteria are met (Figure 11.7).

Most manufacturers in the United States use the medical implant communications service (MICS) band, established since 1999. This band sets aside the 402–405 MHz frequency range, a range that has reasonable signal-propagation characteristics in the human body. The increase in wireless and network connectivity has led to concerns over data privacy and security, and calls to the FDA to establish a policy in this area (Maisel and Kohno 2010).

11.3.5 Power Source

The longevity of very early pulse generators was measured in hours, but current devices can function for more than a decade before they need to be replaced due to battery depletion. The clinical desire to have a generator that is small and full featured, yet also long-lasting, poses a formidable challenge to battery designers.

Over the years, several different battery technologies have been tried, including mercury-zinc, rechargeable silver-modified-mercuric-oxide-zinc, rechargeable nickel-cadmium, radioactive plutonium or promethium, and lithium with a variety of different cathodes. Lithium-cupric-sulfide and mercury-zinc batteries were associated with corrosion and early failure. Mercury-zinc produced hydrogen gas as a by-product of the battery reaction; the venting required made it impossible to hermetically seal the generator. This led to fluid infiltration followed by the risk of sudden failure.

Lithium-iodide technology has been the workhorse for pacemaker battery applications, with more than 10 million such devices having been implanted. Their high energy density (on the order of 1 W-h/cc) and low rate of self-discharge enable small size and good longevity, and their simplicity contributes to excellent reliability. Typical capacity is in the range of 1–3 A-h. The semisolid layer of lithium-iodide that separates the anode and the cathode gradually thickens over the life of the cell, increasing the internal resistance of the battery. The voltage produced by lithium-iodide batteries is inversely related to this resistance and is linear from 2.8 V to approximately 2.4 V, representing about 90% of the usable battery life. It then declines exponentially to 1.8 V as the internal battery resistance increases dramatically to 10,000 Ω or more.

When the battery reaches between 2.0 and 2.4 V (depending on the manufacturer), certain functions of the pulse generator are altered so as to alert the clinician. These alterations are called the elective replacement indicators (ERI). They vary from one pulse generator to another and include signature decreases in rate, a change to a specific pacing mode, pulse duration stretching, and the telemetered battery voltage. When the battery voltage reaches 1.8 V, the pulse generator may operate erratically or cease to function and is said to have reached "end of life." The time period between appearance of the ERI and end-of-life status averages about 3–4 months (Figure 11.8).

More recently, demands for higher power (e.g., for faster, longer range telemetry) have led to the emergence of newer battery technologies. One example is the lithium/hybrid-cathode battery, which has an energy density similar to that of lithium-iodide batteries but power output that is roughly two orders of magnitude greater. An excellent discussion of battery technology is given in Ellenbogen et al. (2007).

Many factors besides battery capacity affect longevity, for example, pulse amplitude and duration, pacing amount and rate, single- versus dual-chamber pacing, use of specialized algorithms, lead design, and so-called housekeeping functions (those functions other than actual delivery of pacing stimuli). The total current drain is typically on the order of 10 μA, with most of this in the form of housekeeping current rather than stimulus current. The programming choices made by clinicians can have a dramatic effect on longevity: a pacemaker with a projected longevity of 8 years under nominal settings could have an actual longevity several years more or less than that value.

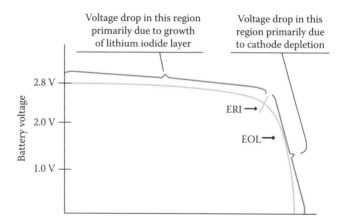

FIGURE 11.8   The initial decline in battery voltage is slow and then more rapid after the battery reaches the ERI voltage. An important aspect of battery design is the predictability of this decline so that timely generator replacement can be anticipated.

11.4 Leads

Standard pacing has traditionally involved the stimulation of one or both chambers (dual-chamber) on the right side of the heart. Cardiac resynchronization therapy (CRT) typically involves pacing at least three chambers (currently the right atrium, right ventricle, and left ventricle), and is thus sometimes called biventricular pacing (Figures 11.9 and 11.10).

Regardless of the specific configuration, implantable pacing leads must be designed not only for consistent performance within the hostile environment of the body but also for easy handling by the implanting physician. Every lead has four major components: electrode, conductor, insulation, and connector pin(s) (Figure 11.11). The electrode is located at the tip of the lead and is in direct contact with the myocardium. Bipolar leads have a tip electrode and a ring electrode (located about 2 cm proximal to the tip); unipolar leads have tip electrodes only. A small-radius electrode provides increased current density, resulting in lower stimulation thresholds; it also increases impedance at the electrode–myocardium interface, thus lowering the current drain further and improving battery longevity. A "high-impedance" lead may have a tip surface area as low as 1.5 mm², whereas standard leads have areas four times as large. A typical value for the impedance "seen" by the pulse generator is 500–1000 Ω; of this, most arises at the electrode–myocardium interface rather than in the lead itself.

Small electrodes, however, historically have been associated with inferior sensing performance. Lead designers were able to achieve both good pacing and good sensing by creating porous-tip electrodes containing thousands of pores in the 20–100 µm range. The pores allow the ingrowth of tissue, resulting in

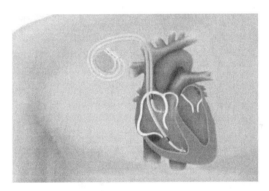

FIGURE 11.9   Illustration of a dual-chamber pacing system.

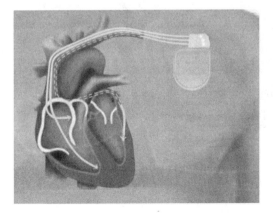

FIGURE 11.10   Illustration of a CRT pacing system.

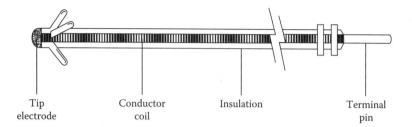

| Tip electrode | Conductor coil | Insulation | Terminal pin |

FIGURE 11.11   The four major lead components.

necessary increase in the effective sensing area while maintaining a small pacing area. Some commonly used electrode materials include platinum-iridium, Elgiloy (an alloy of cobalt, iron, chromium, molybdenum, nickel, and manganese), platinum coated with platinized titanium, and vitreous or pyrolytic carbon coating a titanium or graphite core.

Another major breakthrough in lead design is the steroid-eluting electrode (Figure 11.12). About 1 mg of a corticosteroid (dexamethasone sodium phosphate) is contained in a silicone core that is surrounded by the electrode material. The "leaking" of the steroid into the myocardium occurs slowly over several years and reduces the inflammation that results from the lead placement. It also retards the growth of the fibrous sack that forms around the electrode, which separates it from viable myocardium. As a result, the dramatic rise in acute thresholds that is seen with nonsteroid leads during the 8–16 weeks postimplant is nearly eliminated.

Once a lead has been implanted, it must remain stable (or fixated). The fixation device is either active or passive. Active-fixation leads incorporate corkscrew mechanisms, barbs, or hooks to attach themselves to the myocardium. Passive-fixation leads are held in place with tines that become entangled in the net-like lining (trabeculae) of the heart. Passive-fixation leads generally have better acute pacing and sensing performance but are difficult to remove chronically. Active-fixation leads are easier to remove chronically and have the advantage of unlimited placement sites. Some implanters prefer to use active-fixation leads in the atrium and passive-fixation leads in the ventricle.

The conductor carries electric signals to the pulse generator and delivers the pacing pulses to the heart. It must be strong and flexible to withstand the repeated flexing stress placed on it by the beating

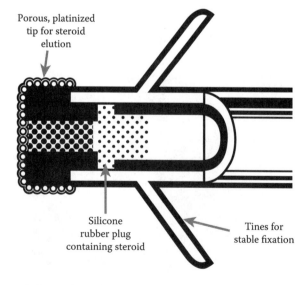

FIGURE 11.12   The steroid-eluting electrode.

heart. The early conductors were a single, straight wire that was vulnerable to fracturing. They have evolved into conductors that are coiled (for increased flexibility) and multifilar (to prevent complete failure with partial fractures). Common conductor materials are Elgiloy and MP35N (an alloy of cobalt, nickel, chromium, and molybdenum). Because of the need for two conductors, bipolar leads are usually larger in diameter than unipolar leads. Current bipolar leads have a coaxial design that has significantly reduced the overall lead diameter.

Insulation materials (typically silicone and polyurethane) are used to isolate the conductor. Silicone has high biostability and a longer history. Because of low tear strength, however, silicone leads historically tended to be thicker than polyurethane leads. Another relative disadvantage of silicone is its high coefficient of friction in blood, which makes it difficult for two leads to pass through the same vein; a coating applied during manufacturing has diminished this problem. Some forms of polyurethane have shown relatively high failure rates.

A variety of generator-lead connector configurations and adapters are available. Because incompatibility can result in disturbed (or even lost) pacing and sensing, an international standard (IS-1) has been developed in an attempt to minimize incompatibility and allow leads from one manufacturer to be used with generators from another.

Leads can be implanted epicardially and endocardially. Epicardial leads are placed on the outer surface of the heart and require the surgical exposure of a small portion of the heart. They are used when venous occlusion makes it impossible to pass a lead transvenously, when abdominal placement of the pulse generator is needed (as in the case of radiation therapy to the pectoral area), or in children (to allow for growth). Endocardial leads are far more common and perform better in the long term. These leads are passed through the venous system and into the right side of the heart. The subclavian or cephalic veins in the pectoral region are common entry sites. Positioning is facilitated by a thin, firm wire stylet that passes through the central lumen of the lead, stiffening it. Fluoroscopy is used to visualize lead positioning and to confirm the desired location.

Improvements in lead design are often overlooked, as compared to improvements in generator design, but the leads used in 1960 required a pulse generator output of 675 μJ for effective stimulation. The evolution in lead technology since then has reduced that figure by two orders of magnitude.

11.5 Programmers and Ongoing Follow-Up

Noninvasive, reversible alteration of the functional parameters of the pacemaker is critical to ongoing clinical management. For a pacing system to remain effective throughout its lifetime, it must be able to adjust to the patient's changing clinical status. The programmer is the primary clinical tool for changing settings, retrieving diagnostic data, and conducting noninvasive tests.

The pacing rate for programmable pacemakers of the early 1960s was adjusted via a Keith needle manipulated percutaneously into a knob on the side of the pacemaker; rotating the needle changed the pacing rate. Through the late 1960s and early 1970s, magnetically attuned reed switches in the pulse generator made it possible to noninvasively change certain parameters, such as rate, output, sensitivity, and polarity. The application of a magnet could alter the parameters, which were usually limited to only one of two choices. It was not until the late 1970s that RF-technology-enabled programmability began realizing its full potential.

Manufacturers have moved away from dedicated special-use programmers toward a PC-based design. The newer designs are more flexible, intuitive to use, and easily updated when new devices are released. They also enable the use of diagnostic and programming options of increasing complexity (Figure 11.13).

Manufacturers and clinicians alike are becoming more sensitive to the role that time-efficient programming and follow-up can play in the productivity of pacing clinics, which may provide follow-up for thousands of patients a year. The management of the resulting mountains of data is a major challenge, and sophisticated systems are appearing to help with this task.

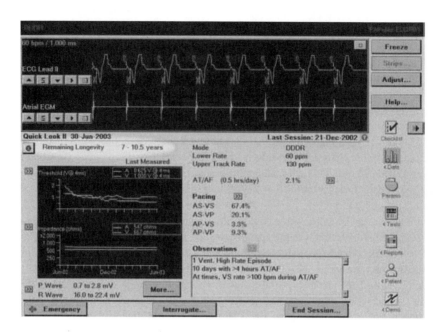

FIGURE 11.13   Typical programmer screen seen during a pacemaker check.

11.6 System Operation

Much of the apparent complexity of the timing rules that determine pacemaker operation is because of a design goal of mimicking normal cardiac function without interfering with it. One example is the dual-chamber feature that provides a sequential stimulation of the atrium before the ventricle. Another example is rate response, designed for patients who lack the normal ability to increase their heart rate in response to a variety of physical conditions (e.g., exercise). Introduced in the mid-1980s, rate-responsive systems use some sort of a sensor to measure the change in a physical variable correlated to heart rate. The sensor output is signal-processed and then used by the output circuit to specify a target pacing rate. The clinician controls the aggressiveness of the rate increase through a variety of parameters (including a choice of transfer function). Pacemaker-resident diagnostics provide data helpful in titrating the rate-response therapy, but most systems operate in "open-loop" fashion: that is, the induced rate changes do not provide negative feedback to the sensor parameter.

The most common sensor is the activity sensor, which uses any of a variety of technologies (e.g., piezo-electric crystals and accelerometers) to detect body movement. Systems using a transthoracic-impedance sensor to estimate pulmonary minute ventilation or cardiac contractility are also commercially available. Numerous other sensors (e.g., stroke volume, blood temperature or pH, oxygen saturation, and right ventricular pressure) have been researched or market-released at various times. Some systems are dual-sensor, combining the best features of each sensor in a single pacing system.

To make it easier to understand the gross-level system operation of modern pacemakers, a five-letter code was developed in 1987 by the North American Society of Pacing and Electrophysiology (NASPE) and the British Pacing and Electrophysiology Group (BPEG), and was subsequently revised (Bernstein et al. 2002). In this "Revised NBG Code," the first letter indicates the chamber (or chambers) that are paced (Table 11.1). The second letter reveals those chambers in which sensing takes place, and the third letter describes how the pacemaker will respond to a sensed event. The pacemaker will "inhibit" the pacing output when intrinsic activity is sensed or will "trigger" a pacing output based on a specific previously sensed event. For example, in the DDD mode:

TABLE 11.1 The NASPE/BPEG Generic (NBG) Pacemaker Code

Position	I	II	III	IV	V
Category	Chamber(s) paced	Chamber(s) sensed	Response to sensing	Rate modulation	Multisite pacing
	O = None	O = None	O = None	O = None	O = None
	A = Atrium	A = Atrium	T = Triggered	R = Rate modulation	A = Atrium
	V = Ventricle	V = Ventricle	I = Inhibited		V = Ventricle
	D = Dual (A+V)	D = Dual (A+V)	D = Dual (T+I)		D = Dual (A+V)
Mfr designation only	S = Single	S = Single			
	(A or V)	(A or V)			

Source: Bernstein, A., Daubert J., Fletcher R. et al. 2002. The revised NASPE/BPEG generic code for antibradycardia, adaptive-rate, and multisite pacing. *PACE* 23:260–64.

D: Pacing takes place in the atrium and the ventricle.

D: Sensing takes place in the atrium and the ventricle.

D: Both inhibition and triggering are the response to a sensed event. An atrial output is inhibited with an atrial-sensed event, whereas a ventricular output is inhibited with a ventricular-sensed event; a ventricular pacing output is triggered by an atrial-sensed event (assuming no ventricular event occurs during the A–V interval).

The fourth letter in the code reflects the ability of the device to provide a rate response. For example, a DDDR device is one that is programmed to pace and sense in both chambers and is capable of sensor-driven rate variability. The fifth letter is used to indicate the device's ability to do multisite pacing.

Pacing in the right ventricle can have deleterious effects in terms of the development of heart failure and atrial fibrillation. This has led to the development of algorithms that minimize ventricular pacing in patients whose bradycardia is because of the dysfunction of their sinus node (which functions as the heart's natural pacemaker), rather than the dysfunction of their heart's intrinsic conduction system. Excellent discussions of this issue and other sophisticated pacemaker algorithms can be found in Al-Ahmad et al. (2010).

11.7 Performance and Reliability

Standard pacing is remarkably effective in treating bradycardia, a condition for which there is no acceptable pharmacological therapy for chronic use. Biventricular pacing is effective in the majority of patients for which it is indicated, but as many as a third of patients who receive the device are the so-called nonresponders; major efforts at better defining patient selection criteria are ongoing.

Pacemakers are among the most reliable electronic devices ever built: device survival probabilities of 99.9% (excluding normal battery depletion) at 10 years are not unheard of. But despite intensive quality assurance efforts by manufacturers, the devices do remain subject to occasional failures: the annual pacemaker replacement rate due to generator malfunction has been estimated at roughly one per 1000 devices implanted, a marked improvement in reliability since the early 1980s (Maisel et al. 2006; Maisel 2006). There have been multiple major advisories and recalls issued by the FDA regarding pacing leads, with more of these because of problems with the lead insulation than with the lead conductor.

Manufacturers maintain product performance reports on their websites; reports from the largest manufacturer (Medtronic) date back to the early 1980s. Manufacturers have also established processes by which a product can be returned to them for failure analysis.

11.8 Future of Pacing Technology

Permanent cardiac pacing is the beneficiary of four decades of advances in a variety of key technologies: biomaterials, electrical stimulation, sensing of bioelectrical events, power sources, microelectronics, transducers, signal analysis, telecommunications, and software development. These advances, informed and guided by a wealth of clinical experience acquired during that time, have made pacing a cost-effective cornerstone of cardiac arrhythmia management.

The development of biological pacemakers through the use of, for example, gene therapy, is an active area of cutting-edge pacing research. Other areas of likely evolution include the following:

- Increased automaticity and optimization of arrhythmia monitoring and therapy delivery, with greater provision of feedback to clinicians on their programming choices
- More efficient integration of device-generated data into electronic medical record (EMR) systems
- Increased sophistication of resynchronization therapy, with broader ranges of multisite pacing
- Integration of sensors for monitoring a broader range of patients' clinical status in areas such as cardiac hemodynamics and ischemia status. (At least one manufacturer already provides a feature that uses monitoring of transthoracic impedance as a way to assess pulmonary congestion in heart failure patients with a CRT device)
- Improved battery technology and circuit density, enabling higher power features without increasing device size
- Greater attention to obtaining cost-effectiveness data for new and existing features

References

Al-Ahmad, A., Ellenbogen, K.A., Natale, A., and Wang, P.J. (eds). 2010. *Pacemakers and Implantable Cardioverter Defibrillators: An Expert's Manual.* Minneapolis: Cardiotext.

Bernstein, A., Daubert J., Fletcher R. et al. 2002. The revised NASPE/BPEG generic code for antibradycardia, adaptive-rate, and multisite pacing. *PACE* 23:260–64.

Ellenbogen, K.A., Kay, G.N., Lau, C.P., and Wilkoff B.J. (eds). 2007. *Clinical Cardiac Pacing, Defibrillation, and Resynchronization Therapy.* Philadelphia: Saunders Elsevier.

Heart Rhythm Society website (www.hrsonline.org).

Maisel, W.H. 2006. Pacemaker and ICD generator reliability: Meta-analysis of device registries. *JAMA* 295:1929–34.

Maisel, W.H. and Kohno, T. 2010. Improving the security and privacy of implantable medical devices. *NEJM* 362:1164–66.

Maisel, W.H., Moynahan M., Zuckerman B.D. et al. 2006. Pacemaker and ICD generator malfunctions: Analysis of Food and Drug Administration annual reports. *JAMA* 295:1901–06.

12

Model Investigation of Pseudo-Hypertension in Oscillometry

Gary Drzewiecki
Rutgers University

12.1 Pseudo-Hypertension

Pentz (1999) and Osler (1892) defined pseudo-hypertension as a condition in which the cuff pressure is higher than the intra-arterial pressure resulting from the presence of an atheromatosis. He hypothesized that a higher cuff pressure was needed to compress a calcified and sclerotic artery than a normal vessel. Osler suggested a method for diagnosis of pseudo-hypertension, which was named as Osler's Maneuver by Messerli et al. in 1985. The method is as follows: by palpating the pulse less radial or brachial artery distal to the point of occlusion of the artery with a sphygmomanometer cuff, one can perform the Osler's maneuver. The patient is Osler positive if either of these arteries remains palpable despite being pulse less. However, the patient is Osler negative if the artery collapses and becomes impalpable. In 1985, Messerli et al. assessed "the palpability of the pulse less radial, or brachial artery distal to a point of occlusion of the artery manually or by cuff pressure." They then measured the intra-arterial pressure, arterial compliance, and systemic hemodynamics of the Osler-positive and Osler-negative patients. The degree of pseudo-hypertension in the Osler-positive patients, those with pseudo-hypertension, ranged from 10 to 54 mmHg, which was the difference between cuff and intra-arterial pressure. Osler-positive subjects had lower arterial compliance, which related to the difference between the cuff and intra-arterial pressures. This explained the fact that the stiffer the artery, the higher the degree of pseudo-hypertension. Pseudo-hypertension is thought to occur mostly in the elderly. It advances as arterial compliance decreases and the sclerosis of the arteries increases with age.

Messerli et al. believed that Osler's maneuver was the simplest and best test to discriminate patients with true hypertension from those with a false elevation in blood pressure. However, automatic blood pressure monitors are currently not capable of discriminating the presence of pseudo-hypertension. The frequency of pseudo-hypertension is not certain, but the prevalence of pseudo-hypertension among the adult population has been estimated to be 7% of the adult population (Oparil et al. 1988). Because the total healthcare costs of treating hypertension and its complications range from $15.0 billion to $60.0 billion (Balu and Thomas 2006), the cost of pseudo-hypertension therapy in the United States is estimated to be $4 billion. Other clinical features of pseudo-hypertension are postural hypotension in spite of antihypertensive therapy, drug-resistant hypertension, and the absence of end-organ damage. Pseudo-hypertension may also result in dangerous outcome of unnecessary treatments if it is not recognized (Campbell et al. 1994). The main theory of pseudo-hypertension is the artery disease and stiffening theory.

There has not been any prior analytical investigation of the arterial stiffening theory of pseudo-hypertension. The low arterial compliance theory is tested in this chapter via a mathematical model of oscillometric blood pressure measurement. The computational model will be used to evaluate measurement error introduced by arterial disease or alterations in arterial mechanics in general. Once these errors are established, the model will then be used to investigate the means by which automated blood pressure monitor may detect the occurrence of pseudo-hypertension or provide a correction method by which blood pressure accuracy is improved even in the presence of arterial disease.

12.2 Automatic Oscillometry

Current automatic oscillometric blood pressure monitors use an occlusive arm cuff wrapped around the subject's upper arm. The air tubing of the cuff is connected to a pump, a pressure transducer, and an air-release valve all under computer control. Drzewiecki et al. (1994) proposed a mathematical model of the oscillometric method in addition to the systolic and diastolic ratios. The oscillometric model included the mechanics of the occlusive arm cuff, the arterial pressure pulse waveform, and the mechanics of the brachial artery. The buckling of an artery under a cuff occurred near −2 to 0 mmHg transmural pressure. This effect resulted in a maximum arterial compliance and maximum cuff pressure oscillations when the cuff pressure was nearly equal to mean arterial pressure. The model indicated the basic features of experimental oscillometry: the increasing and decreasing amplitude in oscillations as cuff pressure decreases, the oscillations corresponding to cuff pressure above systolic pressure, maximum oscillation amplitudes in the range of 1–4 mmHg, and an oscillatory maximum at cuff pressure equal to mean arterial pressure, or MAP. This model computed values for the systolic and diastolic detection ratios of 0.593 and 0.717, respectively, that compared well to the experimental values determined by other researchers (Geddes 1983). This model is applied to study pseudo-hypertension in this chapter.

12.3 Modeling Methods

The mathematical model of the oscillometry was implemented in MATLAB® according to the details provided by Drzewiecki et al. (1994). The main elements of the model are brachial artery mechanics, arterial pressure pulse, and automatic blood pressure detection. A brief review of these elements is now provided (Pedley 1980, Shapiro 1977).

12.3.1 Artery Mechanics Model

An empirical relation describing nonlinear geometric collapse and nonlinear elastic distension of an artery is given by

$$A = (d \log ((a^* p) + b))/(1 + \exp (-cp)) \tag{12.1}$$

where A is the area of the lumen, p transmural pressure, and a, b, c, d are empirical constants calibrated for the normal human brachial artery (Drzewiecki et al. 1994, Brower and Noordergraaf 1978).

12.3.2 Arterial Pulse Pressure Model

The arterial pulse pressure Fourier series of the first two terms of the Fourier series of the human arterial blood pressure pulse is given by

$$Pa(t) = MAP + A0 \sin (2\Pi\ Fhr/60) + A1\ (\sin (4\Pi\ Fhr)/60 + \emptyset 1) \tag{12.2}$$

where Pa(t) is the Fourier synthesized arterial pressure as a function of time, Fhr the heart rate, Ø1 the phase angle, A0 and A1 are the Fourier constants that approximate the waveform of a human brachial artery pulse.

It is assumed that arterial blood pressure is independent of any other quantity. This results in systolic and diastolic pressures that are constant at this location.

Transmural pressure is given by

$$P = Pa - Pc \tag{12.3}$$

where P is the transmural pressure, Pa arterial pressure, and Pc cuff pressure. Cuff pressure simulates a blood pressure recording such that the cuff is inflated to 150 mmHg and then allowed to decrease at a linear rate according to

$$Pc = -13/3\ t + 150 \tag{12.4}$$

12.4 Model Parameters

Table 12.1 provides the control values of the model constants that we have applied in the MATLAB model. Parameters *a* and *b* are related to the arterial wall stiffness and parameters *c* and *d* are related to the arterial closure due to disease and external pressure.

12.5 Computer Modeling

On the basis of the above Drzewiecki et al. mathematical model, a MATLAB program was generated to model oscillometry for normal and diseased arteries. Pressure was input to Equation 12.1 to generate the pulsatile lumen area at each value of cuff pressure. The lumen area pulse is then computed continuously while cuff pressure falls.

The local minimum and maximum of the area pulse were found, and their difference provided the area pulse amplitudes. It was assumed that cuff pressure oscillations are proportionate to the area pulse so that cuff pressure was not computed directly. This is a good approach because it was shown that the

TABLE 12.1 Control Parameters for Oscillometric Model for Typical Normal Human

Quantity	Value	Units	Function
a	0.03	mmHg	Arterial stiffness
b	3.30		Arterial stiffness
c	0.10		Closure stiffness
d	0.08		Closure stiffness
MAP	95.0	mmHg	Mean arterial pressure
A0	10.0		First Fourier pulse magnitude
A1	9.0		Second Fourier pulse magnitude
Ø1	1.2	rad	First Fourier pulse phase
Fhr	75.0	beats/min	Heart rate frequency

cuff pressure is simply responding as an arterial volume transducer. The pulse amplitudes were normalized by maximum pulse amplitude to provide the pressure detection ratios. Spline interpolation was used to accurately calculate the detection ratios: 0.55 and 0.85 that correspond to a diastolic pressure of 68.4 mmHg and a systolic pressure of 107.3 mmHg, respectively. These values are equal to those found experimentally by Geddes et al. (1983). The arterial pressure input values were a diastolic reading of 82.5 mmHg and a systolic reading of 114 mmHg that corresponded to 0.88 and 0.67, respectively. Hence, for normal control conditions the oscillometric simulation resulted in 100% accuracy in arterial pressure measurement.

12.5.1 Control Condition Model (Normal Artery)

The control model of the oscillometric blood pressure measurement was represented by the normal parameters of Table 12.1.

12.5.2 Experimental Condition Model (Pseudo-Hypertension)

To develop the experimental model (stiff artery theory), the arterial mechanics was completely modeled by Equation 12.1. The parameters of this equation represent the artery stiffness over varied ranges of pressure. Because it was not fully understood how the arterial mechanics and its pressure area function change with disease, the approach taken here was to perform an evaluation of parametric sensitivity. The mechanical parameters *a*, *b*, *c*, and *d* were varied to detect their influence on blood pressure accuracy. The results of the model for control and experimental conditions are provided below.

12.6 Results

The arterial pressure pulse as a function of time is illustrated in Figure 12.1. It has fixed waveform that sets systolic pressure at 112 mmHg and diastolic pressure at 73 mmHg.

Hence, this pulse is the input to the model and is only dependent on time. For any model condition, the systolic and diastolic pressure would remain fixed at these values. The modeled computer subject will always have a constant known blood pressure of 112/73 mmHg so that accuracy of blood pressure measurement can be easily assessed.

Cuff pressure and arterial pressure are input to the arterial mechanics model to yield the arterial lumen area pulse which is also related to the cuff pressure oscillations as shown in Figure 12.2. In this example, the cuff pressure was allowed to linearly decrease in pressure according to Equation 12.4.

The control and experimental models each generate lumen area data similar to that of Figure 12.2 because oscillometry is only concerned with the lumen pulse magnitude and lumen area is further analyzed to find blood pressure.

1. *Normal conditions.* The maximum and minimum values of each area pulse was computed and then subtracted from each other to obtain the pulse amplitude at all values of cuff pressure. The amplitude curve is then normalized by the maximum overall amplitude. This analysis yields the oscillation amplitude curve shown in Figure 12.3. The amplitudes of the oscillations may be further analyzed to determine the arterial blood pressure provided the systolic and diastolic detection ratios are known. Hence, the oscillation amplitude curve is all that is required to determine blood pressure by means of oscillometry. If the oscillation amplitude curve is altered by any parameter, it will result in blood pressure determination error.

2. *Experimental conditions.* To identify sources of blood pressure error, the model parameters were varied to discover their effect on the oscillation amplitude curve. The model parameters that are related to arterial mechanics are the parameters *a*, *b*, *c*, *d* of Equation 12.1. The variation in

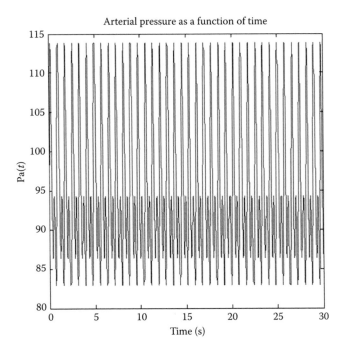

FIGURE 12.1 Arterial pressure pulse versus time. Pressure is in mmHg.

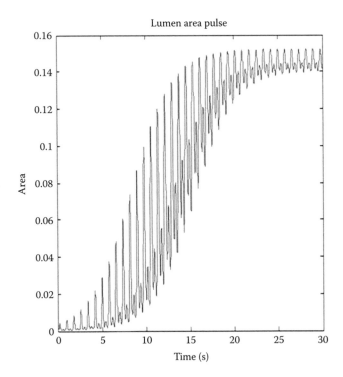

FIGURE 12.2 Lumen area pulse as a function of time and transmural pressure.

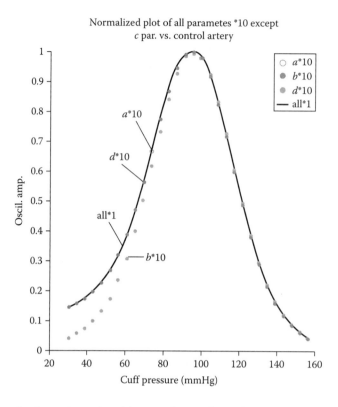

FIGURE 12.3 Control and experimental models: control artery diseased.

parameters a, b, and d by any number did not change their resulting oscillation amplitude curves. They are shown to be superimposed with the control curve and after normalization. This can be seen in Figure 12.3 for the results of both the control model shown and variation parameters a, b, and d. In summary, it is clear that the oscillation amplitude curve is independent of the arterial mechanics following the normalization process. Because actual experimental oscillometry always applies normalization before blood pressure determination, it is clear that this aspect of arterial mechanics does not result in blood pressure errors and is not responsible for pseudo-hypertension. However, the variation of parameter c resulted in a very different oscillation amplitude curve as compared to control. Because parameter c alters the closure mechanics of an artery it is most closely reflecting arterial disease.

Figure 12.4 shows the control of an experimental oscillation amplitude curve for parameter c. The blood pressure determination errors resulting from c parameter included pseudo-systolic hypotension and pseudo-diastolic hypertension. These errors are evident from Figure 12.4 as a shift of the parameter curve c toward higher cuff pressure in both the systolic and diastolic ranges.

To illustrate the change in arterial mechanics, the cuff pressure area curve was graphed for the model of the control and diseased arteries in Figures 12.5 and 12.6.

In Figures 12.5 and 12.6, positive and negative values of the pressure are because of dilation and constriction of the brachial artery, respectively. In comparison with the normal artery shown in Figure 12.5, the lumen area of the diseased artery is less at all pressures and especially for negative pressures.

The pulse error is the problem of every blood pressure monitor, therefore, by varying the pulse error in the first derivative of the control and experimental models, we observe that for the small and large pulses, the derivative goes below 0.1 only for the diseased artery. Hence, one can conclude that if

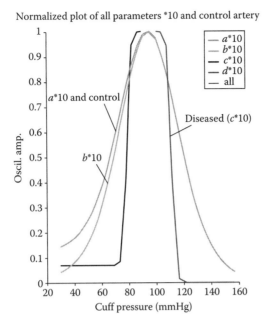

FIGURE 12.4 Control and experimental models: Control and arteries.

oscillations and maximum derivatives are less than 0.1, the artery is diseased, and it collapses easily and we also know that artery collapses in pseudo-hypertension (Figures 12.7 through 12.10).

Because the arterial pressure pulse sets the systolic and diastolic pressure at 112 and 73 mmHg, respectively, the effect of any artery parameter may be easily observed. To discover the effect of each arterial parameter on blood pressure determination accuracy, each artery parameter was varied separately by a

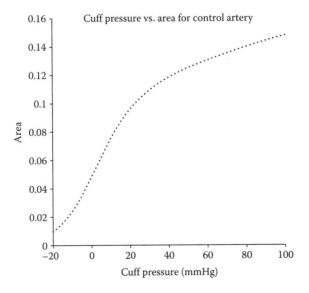

FIGURE 12.5 Cuff pressure versus area for control artery.

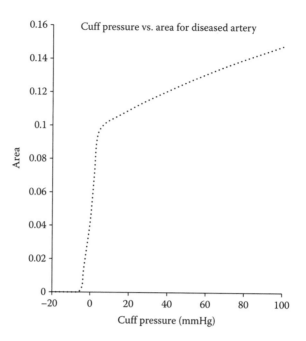

FIGURE 12.6 Cuff pressure versus area for diseased artery.

factor of 10. Therefore, variations in *a*, *b*, *c*, and *d* parameters will not affect the above values for systolic and diastolic pressure. The results are shown in Table 12.2.

Table 12.2 includes the values of systolic and diastolic pressure, % error for the derivative of the oscillometric model for control and the cases when each parameter is multiplied by 10. The negative% errors correspond to a decrease in pressure, whereas the positive ones correlate with an increase in pressure. The *c* parameter causes the largest positive error in blood pressure for diastolic pressure.

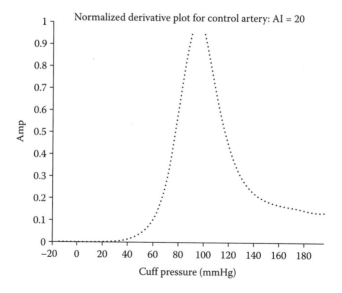

FIGURE 12.7 Normalized arterial oscillations of the control model for control artery: AI = 20.

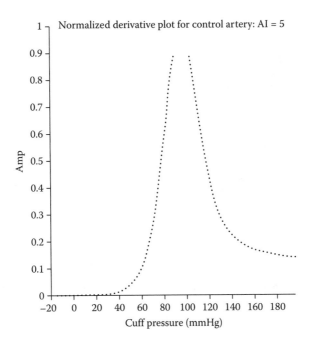

FIGURE 12.8 Normalized oscillations of the control model for control artery: AI = 5.

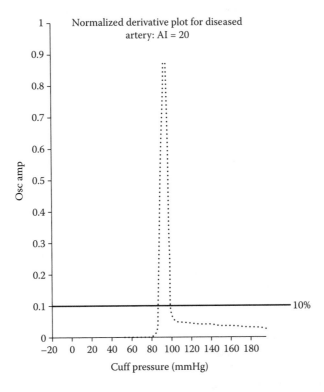

FIGURE 12.9 Normalized arterial oscillations of the experimental model for the diseased artery: AI = 20.

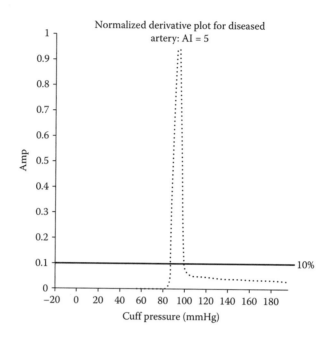

FIGURE 12.10 Normalized arterial oscillations of the model of the DISEASED artery AI = 5.

TABLE 12.2 Derivative of the Oscillometric Model for Control and Diseased Arteries

Multiplier	Parameter	Ps	Pd	% error (Ps)	% error (Pd)
*1 (control)	a, b, c, and d	105.2	74.9	−6.07	2.71
*10	d	107.3	68.3	−4.2	−6.44
*10	c	108.9	78.7	−2.77	7.8
*10	b	107.6	70.8	−3.85	−4.1
*10	a	107.3	68.3	−4.2	−6.8

12.7 Discussion and Analysis

The alteration of parameters *a*, *b*, *c*, or *d* represent some alteration in the arterial mechanics of the subject under study. The analysis here reveals that the parameters *a*, *b*, and *d* caused very little error in blood pressure measurement and no pseudo-hypertension. This result was also evident from Figure 12.3, in which the oscillometric oscillation curves for *a*, *b*, and *d* superimposed on the control curve and expect no change in error. Conversely, the oscillometric oscillations for the *c* parameter (Figure 12.4) looked very different from the control oscillations. Parameter *c* resulted in pseudo-hypertension for diastolic pressure as seen in Table 12.2. Referring to Figure 12.5 and the arterial model, parameters *a*, *b*, and *d* affect the positive pressure region, whereas only parameter *c* affects the negative pressure portion of the lumen area curve. Negative transmural pressure corresponds with high cuff pressure and the mechanics of arterial closure and collapse. The presence of arterial disease is most likely to affect the arterial closure because it would enable the artery to close at higher transmural pressure. Hence, the *c* parameter is most closely related to artery disease and the model thereby confirms that artery disease causes pseudo-hypertension in oscillometry as suggested earlier in this section.

In the cuff pressure VS area model, the *c* parameter was still the source of error, especially for diastolic pressure. It caused pseudo-systolic hypotension and pseudo-diastolic hypertension. By comparing a large pulse to a small one, we noticed that the derivative went low in the high-pressure zone for the diseased artery and this did not happen for the normal artery; therefore, we came up with a new rule that we call the oscillometry of false hypertension. At high blood pressure zone with the derivative less than 0.1, the artery is diseased and stiff, and it collapses easily. As mentioned earlier, the true measurement of the blood pressure should be independent of the arterial mechanics. However, in every modeling experiment, it was found that *c* was the source of error and its related plot was very different from the rest. Other parameters like *a*, *b*, and *d* did not change the accuracy of blood pressure measurement before and after normalization. Normalization did not even correct the inaccuracy caused by the *c* parameter. In the case of the diseased artery, the arterial stiffness did increase diastolic pressure by almost 8% (Table 12.2) and this was consistent with the theory of pseudo-hypertension.

Acknowledgment

The author would like to thank the Rutgers' graduate student Farah Rahimy for her work in completing the oscillometric blood pressure model computations related to pseudo-hypertension for this chapter that also resulted in the completion of her MS in biomedical engineering.

References

Balu, S., Thomas, J. Incremental expenditures of treating hypertension in U.S. Al. *Am. J. Hypertens.* 19:810–816, 2006.

Brower, R.W., Noordergraaf, A. Theory of steady flow in collapsible tubes and veins. In: Baan, J., Noordergraaf, A., Raines, J. eds, *Cardiovascular System Dynamics.* Cambridge, MA: Cambridge, pp. 256–265, 1978.

Campbell N.R., Hogan D.B., McKay D.W. Pitfalls to avoid in the measurement of blood pressure in the elderly. *Can. J. Public Health* 85(Suppl 2):S26–28, 1994.

Drzewiecki G., Hood R., Apple H. Theory of the oscillometric maximum and the systolic and diastolic detection ratios. *Ann. Biomed. Eng.* 22(1):88–96, 1994.

Geddes, L.A., Voelz, M., Combs, C., Reiner, D. Characterization of the oscillometric method for measuring indirect blood pressure. *Ann. Biomed. Eng.* 10:271–280, 1983.

High Blood Pressure: Heart & Blood Vessel Disorders. 2007. www.merck.com/mmhe/sec022/ch022a.html

Messerli F.H., Ventura H.O., Amodeo C. Osler's maneuver and Pseudohypertension. *New Eng. J. of Med.* 312:1548–1551, 1985.

Oparil S., Calhoun D.A. Managing the patient with hard-to-control hypertension. *Am. Fam. Physician.* 57(5):1007–1014, 1988.

Osler, W. *The Principles and Practice of Medicine: Designed for the Use of Practitioners and Students of Medicine.* New York: D Appleton and Company, pp. 656, 668, 1892.

Pedley, T.J. Flow in collapsible tubes. In: *The Fluid Mechanics of Large Blood Vessels.* Oxford: Cambridge University Press; Chap. 6, pp. 301–368, 1980.

Pentz, W.H. Controlling isolated systolic hypertension. *Post Graduate Medicine, Osler's Maneuver & Pseudo hypertension,* 105(5), May, 1999.

Shapiro, A.H. Steady flow in collapsible tubes. Trans. ASME (ser. K.) *J. Biomech. Eng.* 99:126–147, 1977.

Skalak R., Chien S. *Handbook of Bioengineering.* New York, NY: McGraw-Hill, 1987.

Zuschke, C.A. Pseudo hypertension. *South Medical Journal.* 88(12):1185–1190, 1995.

Cardiac Output Measurement

Leslie A. Geddes
Purdue University

13.1 Introduction

Cardiac output is the amount of blood pumped by the right or left ventricle per unit of time. It is expressed in liters per minute (L/min) and normalized by division by body surface area in square meters (m²). The resulting quantity is called the cardiac index. Cardiac output is sometimes normalized to body weight, being expressed as mL/min per kilogram. A typical resting value for a wide variety of mammals is 70 mL/min per kg.

With exercise, cardiac output increases. In well-trained athletes, cardiac output can increase fivefold with maximum exercise. During exercise, heart rate increases, venous return increases, and the ejection fraction increases. Parenthetically, physically fit subjects have a low resting heart rate, and the time for the heart rate to return to the resting value after exercise is less than that for subjects who are not physically fit.

There are many direct and indirect (noninvasive) methods of measuring cardiac output. Of equal importance to the number that represents cardiac output is the left-ventricular ejection fraction (stroke volume divided by diastolic volume), which indicates the ability of the left ventricle to pump blood.

13.2 Indicator–Dilution Method

The principle underlying the indicator–dilution method is based on the upstream injection of a detectable indicator and on measuring the downstream concentration–time curve, which is called a *dilution curve*. The essential requirement is that the indicator mixes with all the blood flowing through the central mixing pool. Although the dilution curves in the outlet branches may be slightly different in shape, they all have the same area.

Figure 13.1a illustrates the injection of m g of indicator into an idealized flowing stream having the same velocity across the diameter of the tube. Figure 13.1b shows the dilution curve recorded downstream. Because of the flow–velocity profile, the cylinder of indicator and fluid becomes teardrop in shape, as shown in Figure 13.1c. The resulting dilution curve has a rapid rise and an exponential fall, as shown in Figure 13.1d. However, the area of the dilution curve is the same as that shown in Figure 13.1a. Derivation of the flow equation is shown in Figure 13.1, and the flow is simply the amount of indicator (m g) divided by the area of the dilution curve (g/mL × s), which provides the flow in mL/s.

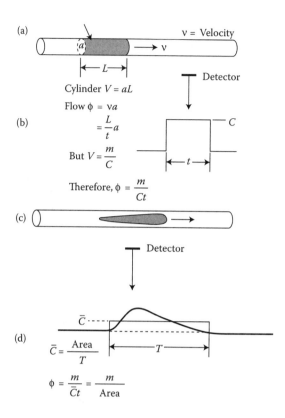

FIGURE 13.1 Genesis of the indicator–dilution curve.

13.2.1 Indicators

Before describing the various indicator–dilution methods, it is useful to recognize that there are two types of indicators, diffusible and nondiffusible. A diffusible indicator will leak out of the capillaries. A nondiffusible indicator is retained in the vascular system for a time that depends on the type of indicator. Whether cardiac output is overestimated with a diffusible indicator depends on the location of the injection and measuring sites. Table 13.1 lists many of the indicators that have been used for measuring cardiac output and the types of detectors used to obtain the dilution curve. It is obvious that the indicator selected must be detectable and not alter the flow being measured. Importantly, the indicator must be nontoxic and sterile.

When a diffusible indicator is injected into the right heart, the dilution curve can be detected in the pulmonary artery, and there is no loss of indicator because there is no capillary bed between these sites; therefore, the cardiac output value will be accurate.

13.2.2 Thermal Dilution Method

Chilled 5% dextrose in water (D5W) or 0.9% NaCl can be used as indicators. The dilution curve represents a transient reduction in pulmonary artery blood temperature following injection of the indicator into the right atrium. Figure 13.2 illustrates the method and a typical thermodilution curve. Note that the indicator is really negative calories. The thermodilution method is based on heat exchange measured in calories, and the flow equation contains terms for the specific heat (C) and the specific gravity (S) of the indicator (i) and blood (b). The expression employed when a #7F thermistor-tipped catheter is used and chilled D5W is injected into the right atrium is as follows:

TABLE 13.1   Indicators

Material	Detector	Retention Data
Evans blue (T1824)	Photoelectric 640 μ	50% loss in 5 days
Indocyanine green	Photoelectric 800 μ	50% loss in 10 min
Coomassie blue	Photoelectric 585–600 μ	50% loss in 15–20 min
Saline (5%)	Conductivity cell	Diffusible[a]
Albumin 1[131]	Radioactive	50% loss in 8 days
Na[24], K[42], D$_2$O, DHO	Radioactive	Diffusible[a]
Hot-cold solutions	Thermodetector	Diffusible[a]

^{a} It is estimated that there is about 15% loss of diffusible indicators during the first pass through the lungs.

$$CO = \left[\frac{V(T_b - T_i)60}{A} \right]\left[\frac{S_iC_i}{S_bC_b} \right]F \qquad (13.1)$$

where
- V = Volume of indicator injected in mL
- T_b = Temperature (average of pulmonary artery blood in °C)
- T_i = Temperature of the indicator (°C)
- 60 = Multiplier required to convert mL/s into mL/min
- A = Area under the dilution curve in (s × °C)
- S = Specific gravity of indicator (i) and blood (b)
- C = Specific heat of indicator (i) and blood (b)
- (S_iC_i/S_bC_b = 1.08 for 5% dextrose and blood of 40% packed-cell volume)
- F = Empiric factor employed to correct for heat transfer through the injection catheter (for a #7F catheter, $F = 0.825$ [2]).

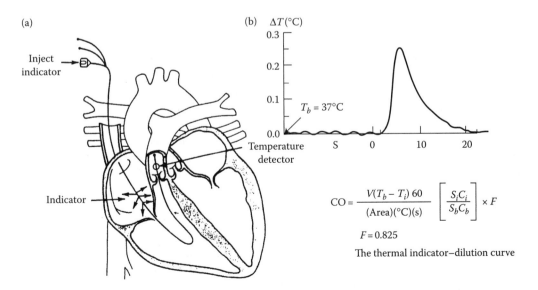

(a)

Inject indicator

Indicator

(b) ΔT(°C)

$T_b = 37°C$

Temperature detector

$$CO = \frac{V(T_b - T_i)\,60}{(\text{Area})(°C)(s)}\left[\frac{S_iC_i}{S_bC_b} \right] \times F$$

$F = 0.825$

The thermal indicator–dilution curve

FIGURE 13.2   The thermodilution method (a) and a typical dilution curve (b).

Entering these factors into the expression gives

$$CO = \frac{V(T_b - T_i)53.46}{A} \qquad (13.2)$$

where CO = cardiac output in mL/min

$$53.46 = 60 \times 1.08 \times 0.825$$

To illustrate how a thermodilution curve is processed, cardiac output is calculated below using the dilution curve shown in Figure 13.2.

$$
\begin{aligned}
V &= \text{5 mL of 5\% dextrose in water} \\
T_b &= 37°C \\
T_i &= 0°C \\
A &= 1.59°C\ \text{s}
\end{aligned}
$$

$$CO = \frac{5(37 - 0)53.46}{1.59} = 6220\,\text{mL/min}$$

Although the thermodilution method is *the standard in clinical medicine*, it has a few disadvantages. Because of the heat loss through the catheter wall, several series 5-mL injections of indicator are needed to obtain a consistent value for cardiac output. If cardiac output is low, that is, the dilution curve is very broad, it is difficult to obtain an accurate value for cardiac output. There are respiratory-induced variations in PA blood temperature that confound the dilution curve when it is of low amplitude. Although room-temperature D5W can be used, chilled D5W provides a better dilution curve and a more reliable cardiac output value. Furthermore, it should be obvious that if the temperature of the indicator is the same as that of blood, there will be no dilution curve.

13.2.3 Indicator Recirculation

An ideal dilution curve shown in Figure 13.2 consists of a steep rise and an exponential decrease in indicator concentration. Algorithms that measure the dilution-curve area have no difficulty with such a curve. However, when cardiac output is low, the dilution curve is typically low in amplitude and very broad. Often the descending limb of the curve is obscured by recirculation of the indicator or by low-amplitude artifacts. Figure 13.3a is a dilution curve in which the descending limb is obscured by recirculation of the indicator. Obviously it is difficult to determine the practical end of the curve, which is often specified as the time when the indicator concentration has fallen to a chosen percentage (e.g., 1%) of the maximum amplitude (C_{max}). Because the descending limb represents a good approximation of a decaying exponential curve (e^{-kt}), fitting the descending limb to an exponential allows reconstruction of the curve without a recirculation error, thereby providing a means for identifying the end for what is called the *first pass of the indicator*.

In Figure 13.3b, the amplitude of the descending limb of the curve in Figure 13.3a has been plotted on semilogarithmic paper, and the exponential part represents a straight line. When recirculation appears, the data points deviate from the straight line and therefore can be ignored, and the linear part (representing the exponential) can be extrapolated to the desired percentage of the maximum concentration, say 1% of C_{max}. The data points representing the extrapolated part were replotted in Figure 13.3a to reveal the dilution curve undistorted by recirculation.

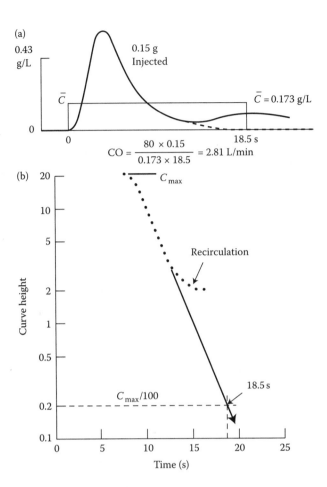

FIGURE 13.3 Dilution curve obscured by recirculation (a) and a semilogarithmic plot of the descending limb (b).

Commercially available indicator–dilution instruments employ digitization of the dilution curve. Often the data beyond about 30% of C_{max} are ignored, and the exponential is computed on digitally extrapolated data.

13.3 Fick Method

The Fick method *employs oxygen as the indicator* and the increase in oxygen content of venous blood as it passes through the lungs, along with the respiratory oxygen uptake, as the quantities that are needed to determine cardiac output (CO = O_2 uptake/$A - V\, O_2$ difference). Oxygen uptake (mL/min) is measured at the airway, usually with an oxygen-filled spirometer containing a CO_2 absorber. The $A - V\, O_2$ difference is determined from the oxygen content (mL/100 mL blood) from any arterial sample and the oxygen content (mL/100 mL) of pulmonary arterial blood. The oxygen content of blood used to be difficult to measure. However, the new blood–gas analyzers that measure, pH, pO_2, pCO_2, hematocrit, and hemoglobin provide a value for O_2 content by computation using the oxygen-dissociation curve.

There is a slight technicality involved in determining the oxygen uptake because oxygen is consumed at body temperature but measured at room temperature in the spirometer. Consequently, the volume of

O_2 consumed per minute displayed by the spirometer must be multiplied by a factor, F. Therefore, the Fick equation is

$$CO = \frac{O_2 \text{ uptake/min}(F)}{A - V \, O_2 \text{ difference}} \qquad (13.3)$$

Figure 13.4 is a spirogram showing a tidal volume riding on a sloping baseline that represents the resting expirating level (REL). The slope identifies the oxygen uptake at room temperature. In this subject, the uncorrected oxygen consumption was 400 mL/min at 26°C in the spirometer. With a barometric pressure of 750 mmHg, the conversion factor F to correct this volume to body temperature (37°C) and saturated with water vapor is

$$F = \frac{273 + 37}{273 + T_s} \times \frac{P_b - PH_2O}{P_b - 47} \qquad (13.4)$$

where T_s is the spirometer temperature, P_b is the barometric pressure, and PH_2O at T_s is obtained from the water-vapor table (Table 13.2).

A sample calculation for the correction factor F is given in Figure 13.4, which reveals a value for F of 1.069. However, it is easier to use Table 13.3 to obtain the correction factor. For example, for a spirometer temperature of 26°C and a barometric pressure of 750 mmHg, $F = 1.0691$.

Note that the correction factor F in this case is only 6.9%. The error encountered by not including it may be less than the experimental error in making all other measurements.

(a)

Subject: 36-Year-old male
Height: 59' 10½"
Weight: 175 lb
Body surface area: $A = W^{0.425} \times H^{0.725} \times 71.84$

where W = weight in kg
H = height in cm
A = area in cm^2
A = 1.98m^2

O_2 Uptake at 26°C: 400 mL/min
Barometer: 750 mmHg P_{H_2O} at 26°C: 25.2 mmHg
O_2 Uptake correction factor: F

$$F = \frac{273 + 37}{273 + 26} \times \frac{750 - 25.2}{750 - 47}$$

$F = 1.069$

F from table 4.5 = 1.069

O_2 Uptake BTPS: 400 × 1.069 = 427.6
Blood O_2:

Arterial = 20 V%
Mixed venous = 15 V%

Cardiac output:

$$CO = \frac{427.6}{(20 - 15)/100} = 8552 \text{ mL/min}$$

Cardiac index:

$$CI = \frac{8.552}{1.98} = 4.32 \text{ L/min/m}^2$$

(b)

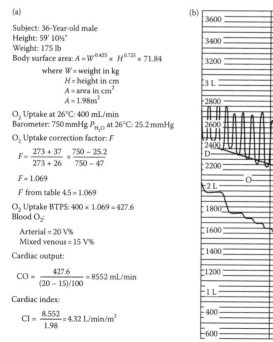
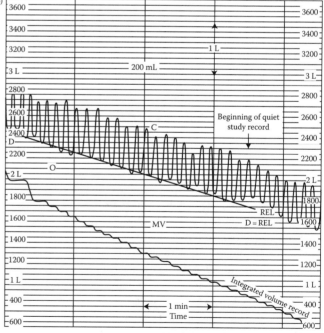

FIGURE 13.4 Measurement of oxygen uptake with a spirometer (b) and the method used to correct the measured volume (a).

TABLE 13.2 Vapor Pressure of Water

Temp. (°C)	0.0	0.2	0.4	0.6	0.8
15	12.788	12.953	13.121	13.290	13.461
16	13.634	13.809	13.987	14.166	14.347
17	14.530	14.715	14.903	15.092	15.284
18	15.477	15.673	15.871	16.071	16.272
19	16.477	16.685	16.894	17.105	17.319
20	17.535	17.753	17.974	18.197	18.422
21	18.650	18.880	19.113	19.349	19.587
22	19.827	20.070	20.316	20.565	20.815
23	21.068	21.324	21.583	21.845	22.110
24	22.377	22.648	22.922	23.198	23.476
25	23.756	24.039	24.326	24.617	24.912
26	25.209	25.509	25.812	26.117	26.426
27	26.739	27.055	27.374	27.696	28.021
28	28.349	28.680	29.015	29.354	29.697
29	30.043	30.392	30.745	31.102	31.461
30	31.825	32.191	32.561	32.934	33.312
31	33.695	34.082	34.471	34.864	35.261
32	35.663	36.068	36.477	36.891	37.308
33	37.729	38.155	38.584	39.018	39.457
34	39.898	40.344	40.796	41.251	41.710
35	42.175	42.644	43.117	43.595	44.078
36	44.563	45.054	45.549	46.050	46.556
37	47.067	47.582	48.102	48.627	49.157
38	49.692	50.231	50.774	51.323	51.879
39	42.442	53.009	53.580	54.156	54.737
40	55.324	55.910	56.510	57.110	57.720
41	58.340	58.960	59.580	60.220	60.860

The example selected shows that the A–V O_2 difference is $20 - 15$ mL/100 mL blood and that the corrected O_2 uptake is 400×1.069; therefore the cardiac output is

$$CO = \frac{400 \times 1.069}{(20 - 15)/100} = 8552 \text{ mL/min} \tag{13.5}$$

The Fick method does not require the addition of a fluid to the circulation and may have value in such a circumstance. However, its use requires stable conditions because an average oxygen uptake takes many minutes to obtain.

13.4 Ejection Fraction

The ejection fraction (EF) is one of the most convenient indicators of the ability of the left (or right) ventricle to pump the blood that is presented to it. Let v be the stroke volume (SV) and V be the end-diastolic volume (EDV); the ejection fraction is v/V or SV/EDV.

Measurement of ventricular diastolic and systolic volumes can be achieved radiographically, ultrasonically, and by the use of an indicator that is injected into the left ventricle where the indicator concentration is measured in the aorta on a beat-by-beat basis.

TABLE 13.3   Correction Factor F for Standardization of Collected Volume

°C/P_B	640	650	660	670	680	690	700	710	720	730	740	750	760	770	780
15	1.1388	1.1377	1.1367	1.1358	1.1348	1.1339	1.1330	1.1322	1.1314	1.1306	1.1298	1.1290	1.1283	1.1276	1.1269
16	1.1333	1.1323	1.1313	1.1304	1.1295	1.1286	1.1277	1.1269	1.1260	1.1253	1.1245	1.1238	1.1231	1.1224	1.1217
17	1.1277	1.1268	1.1266	1.1249	1.1240	1.1232	1.1224	1.1216	1.1208	1.1200	1.1193	1.1186	1.1179	1.1172	1.1165
18	1.1222	1.1212	1.1203	1.1194	1.1186	1.1178	1.1170	1.1162	1.1154	1.1147	1.1140	1.1133	1.1126	1.1120	1.1113
19	1.1165	1.1156	1.1147	1.1139	1.1131	1.1123	1.1115	1.1107	1.1100	1.1093	1.1086	1.1080	1.1073	1.1067	1.1061
20	1.1108	1.1099	1.1091	1.1083	1.1075	1.1067	1.1060	1.1052	1.1045	1.1039	1.1032	1.1026	1.1019	1.1014	1.1008
21	1.1056	1.1042	1.1034	1.1027	1.1019	1.1011	1.1004	1.0997	1.0990	1.0984	1.0978	1.0971	1.0965	1.0960	1.0954
22	1.0992	1.0984	1.0976	1.0969	1.0962	1.0964	1.0948	1.0941	1.0935	1.0929	1.0923	1.0917	1.0911	1.0905	1.0900
23	1.0932	1.0925	1.0918	1.0911	1.0904	1.0897	1.0891	1.0884	1.0878	1.0872	1.0867	1.0861	1.0856	1.0850	1.0845
24	1.0873	1.0866	1.0859	1.0852	1.0846	1.0839	1.0833	1.0827	1.0822	1.0816	1.0810	1.0805	1.0800	1.0795	1.0790
25	1.0812	1.0806	1.0799	1.0793	1.0787	1.0781	1.0775	1.0769	1.0764	1.0758	1.0753	1.0748	1.0744	1.0739	1.0734
26	1.0751	1.0710	1.0738	1.0732	1.0727	1.0721	1.0716	1.0710	1.0705	1.0700	1.0696	1.0691	1.0686	1.0682	1.0678
27	1.0688	1.0682	1.0677	1.0671	1.0666	1.0661	1.0656	1.0651	1.0640	1.0641	1.0637	1.0633	1.0629	1.0624	1.0621
28	1.0625	1.0619	1.0614	1.0609	1.0604	1.0599	1.0595	1.0591	1.0586	1.0582	1.0578	1.0574	1.0570	1.0566	1.0563
29	1.0560	1.0555	1.0550	1.0546	1.0548	1.0537	1.0533	1.0529	1.0525	1.0521	1.0518	1.0514	1.0519	1.0507	1.0504
30	1.0494	1.0496	1.0486	1.0482	1.0478	1.0474	1.0470	1.0467	1.0463	1.0460	1.0450	1.0453	1.0450	1.0447	1.0444

Source: From Kovach J.C., Paulos P., and Arabadjis C. 1955. *J. Thorac. Surg.* **29**: 552.

Note: $V_s = FV_c$, where V_s is the standardized condition and V_c is the collected condition: $V = \dfrac{1+37/273}{1+t^\circ C/273} \times \dfrac{P_B - PH_2O}{P_B - 47}$ $V_c = FV_c$

13.4.1 Indicator–Dilution Method for Ejection Fraction

Holt [1] described the method of injecting an indicator into the left ventricular during diastole and measuring the stepwise decrease in aortic concentration with successive beats (Figure 13.5). From this concentration–time record, end-diastolic volume, stroke volume, and ejection fraction can be calculated. No assumption need be made about the geometric shape of the ventricle. The following describes the theory of this fundamental method.

Let V be the end-diastolic ventricular volume. Inject m g of indicator into this volume during diastole. The concentration (C_1) of indicator in the aorta for the first beat is m/V. By knowing the amount of indicator (m) injected and the calibration for the aortic detector, C_1 is established, and ventricular end-diastolic volume $V = m/C_1$.

After the first beat, the ventricle fills, and the amount of indicator left in the left ventricle is $m - mv/V$. The aortic concentration (C_2) for the second beat is therefore $m - mV/V = m(1 - v/V)$. Therefore, the aortic concentration (C_2) for the second beat is

$$C_2 = \frac{m}{V}\left[1 - \frac{v}{V}\right]\tag{13.6}$$

By continuing the process, it is easily shown that the aortic concentration (C_n) for the nth beat is

$$C_n = \frac{m}{V}\left[1 - \frac{v}{V}\right]^{n-1}\tag{13.7}$$

Figure 13.6 illustrates the stepwise decrease in aortic concentration for ejection fractions (v/V) of 0.2 and 0.5, that is, 20% and 50%.

It is possible to determine the ejection fraction from the concentration ratio for two successive beats. For example,

$$C_n = \frac{m}{V}\left[1 - \frac{v}{V}\right]^{n-1}\tag{13.8}$$

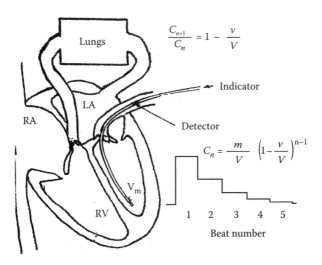

$$\frac{C_{n+1}}{C_n} = 1 - \frac{v}{V}$$

$$C_n = \frac{m}{V}\left(1 - \frac{v}{V}\right)^{n-1}$$

FIGURE 13.5   The saline method of measuring ejection fraction, involving injection of m g of NaCl into the left ventricle and detecting the aortic concentration (C) on a beat-by-beat basis.

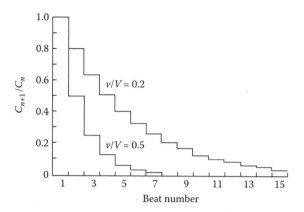

FIGURE 13.6 Stepwise decrease in indicator concentration (C) vs. beat number for ejection fraction (v/V) of 0.5 and 0.2.

$$C_{n+1} = \frac{m}{V}\left[1 - \frac{v}{V}\right]^n \tag{13.9}$$

$$\frac{C_{n+1}}{C_n} = 1 - \frac{v}{V} \tag{13.10}$$

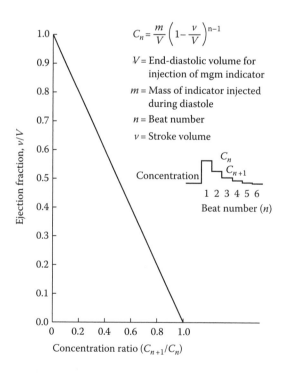

FIGURE 13.7 Ejection fraction (v/V) vs. the ratio of concentrations for successive beats (C_{n+1}/C_n).

from which

$$\frac{v}{V} = 1 - \frac{C_{n+1}}{C_n} \tag{13.11}$$

where v/V is the ejection fraction and C_{n+1}/C_n is the concentration ratio for two successive beats, for example, C_2/C_1 or C_3/C_2. Figure 13.7 illustrates the relationship between the ejection fraction v/V and the ratio of C_{n+1}/C_n. Observe that the detector need not be calibrated as long as there is a linear relationship between detector output and indicator concentration in the operating range.

References

1. Holt, J.P. 1956. Estimation of the residual volume of the ventricle of the dog heart by two indicator–dilution techniques. *Circ. Res.* 4: 181.
2. Weissel, R.D., Berger, R.L., and Hechtman, H.B. 1975. Measurement of cardiac output by thermodilution. *N. Engl. J. Med.* 292: 682.

14

External Defibrillators

Willis A. Tacker Jr.
Purdue University

14.1 Introduction

Cardiac defibrillators are electronic devices that have been used for decades to provide a strong electrical shock to a patient in an attempt to convert a *very* rapid (and often chaotic), ineffective heart rhythm to a slower, coordinated, and more effective rhythm. When used to treat ventricular fibrillation (VF) or very rapid ventricular tachycardia the shock may be lifesaving because the heart output is nil or is too low to sustain life. Occurrence of VF is a medical emergency and rapid treatment (within seconds to minutes) is essential for survival.

In the case of a *moderately* accelerated ventricular tachycardia (and impaired heart function), the electrical shock may be useful for slowing the heart rate so that the heart will beat with a more effective rhythm and force. The problem in this other category of patients is that the shortened filling time between contractions does not allow adequate cardiac filling and so blood flow is impaired, but not eliminated. The circuitous pathway that creates the fast heart rate is interrupted by the shock and slowing of the heart rate after the shock corrects this problem. Usually, this non-VF impairment is compatible with life and, therefore, the urgency for treatment is less, because there is less risk of sudden death.

Another use for defibrillators is to shock either atrial flutter or fibrillation, which are abnormally rapid atrial rhythms. These atrial rhythms are much less likely to spontaneously proceed rapidly to death than ventricular arrhythmias. Using electrical shock to treat rapid heart arrhythmias other than VF is usually referred to as "cardioversion" and hence some users refer to the tachycardia treatment devices as cardiovertor—defibrillators. Cardiovertor and defibrillator treatment is different from pacemaker treatment (discussed elsewhere in this book) because a pacemaker stimulates a *slowly* beating heart and uses much weaker shocks. Pacemaking increases the rate of the relatively healthy heart, which increases blood flow.

14.2 Mechanism of Fibrillation

Fibrillation is chaotic electric excitation of the myocardium and results in loss of coordinated mechanical contraction characteristic of normal heart beats. Description of the mechanisms leading to, and maintaining, fibrillation and other rhythm disorders are reviewed elsewhere [1–3] and are beyond the scope of this chapter. In summary, however, these rhythm disorders are commonly held to be a result of reentrant excitation pathways within the heart. The underlying abnormality that leads to the mechanism is the combination of an area of conduction block of cardiac excitation, plus rapidly recurring depolarization of the membranes of the cardiac cells. This leads to rapid repetitive propagation of a single excitation wave or multiple excitatory waves throughout the heart. If the waves are multiple, the rhythm may degrade into total loss of synchronization of cardiac fiber contraction. Without synchronized contraction, the chamber affected will not contract, and this is fatal in the situation of VF. The most common cause of these conditions, and therefore of these rhythm disorders, is cardiac ischemia or infarction as a complication of atherosclerosis. Additional relatively common causes include other cardiac disorders, drug toxicity, electrolyte imbalances in the blood, hypothermia, and electric shocks (especially from alternating current).

14.3 Mechanism of Defibrillation

The corrective measure is to extinguish the rapidly occurring waves of excitation by simultaneously depolarizing all or most of the cardiac cells with a strong electric shock. The cells can then simultaneously repolarize themselves, and this will put them back in phase with each other.

Despite years of intensive research there is still no single theory for the mechanism of defibrillation that explains all the phenomena observed. However, it is generally held that the defibrillating shock must be adequately strong and have adequate duration to affect most of the heart cells. In general, longer duration shocks require less current than shorter duration shocks. This relationship is called the strength–duration relationship and is demonstrated by the curve shown in Figure 14.1. Shocks of strength and duration above and to the right of the current curve (or above the energy curve) have adequate strength to defibrillate, whereas shocks below and to the left do not. From the exponentially decaying current curve an energy curve can also be determined (also shown in Figure 14.1), which is high at very short durations because of high current requirements at short durations, but which is also high at longer durations owing to additional energy being delivered as the pulse duration is lengthened at nearly constant current. Thus, for most electrical waveforms there is a minimum energy for

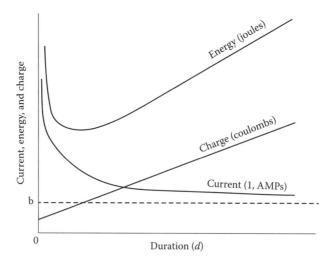

FIGURE 14.1 Strength–duration curves for current, energy, and charge. Adequate current shocks are above and to the right of the current curve. (Modified from Tacker WA, Geddes LA. 1980. *Electrical Defibrillation*, Boca Raton, FL, CRC Press. With permission.)

defibrillation at approximate pulse durations of 3–10 ms. A strength–duration charge curve can also be determined as shown in Figure 14.1, which demonstrates that the minimum charge for defibrillation occurs at the shortest pulse duration tested. Very short duration pulses are not used, however, because the high current and voltage required is damaging to the myocardium. It is also important to note that excessively strong or long shocks may cause damage that leads to immediate refibrillation, thus failing to restore the heart function.

In practice, for a shock applied to the electrodes on the skin surface of the patient's chest, durations are on the order of 3–10 ms and deliver 10s of amperes. The energy delivered to the subject by these shocks is selectable by the operator and for adults is on the order of 50–360 J. The exact shock intensity required at a given duration of electric pulse depends on several variables, including the intrinsic characteristics of the patient (such as body size, the underlying disease problem or the presence of certain drugs, and the length of time the arrhythmia has been present), the techniques for electrode application, and the particular rhythm disorder being treated (highly organized rhythms usually require less energy than extremely disorganized rhythms).

14.4 Clinical Defibrillators

Defibrillator design has evolved through the years, based on technologic improvements in waveform shaping, combined with studies of the effectiveness of different waveforms to defibrillate or cardiovert the various rhythm disorders. Also, decreased time to diagnose the exact rhythm problem is paramount for success under emergency VF conditions and automated signal processing is important to speed up rhythm identification and treatment using the best shock strength. Most defibrillators have automated diagnosis and treatment operating modes and many have manual, nonautomated controls available for specific uses. The optimal amount of automation depends on how the unit will be used. For example, highly automatic external defibrillators (AEDs) are optimal for use by lay persons who may have no training, such as in an airport. The important goal is to prevent sudden death from VF and quick response to simple instructions on the defibrillator is desirable. Another use is for home defibrillation if a defibrillator is kept in the home of a patient who is at high risk for VF. Depending on how, where, and by whom they will be operated, AEDs may be considered automatic or semiautomatic. Figure 14.2 shows an AED and Figure 14.3 shows a wearable defibrillator.

However, a defibrillator intended for use in a hospital electrophysiology laboratory, or perhaps in an ambulance, or a hospital crash cart would have multiple, controllable variables for use by the physician

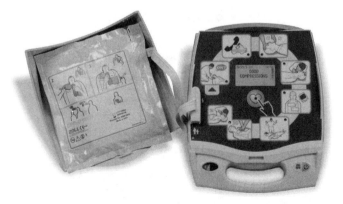

FIGURE 14.2 AED, showing packaged electrodes in the pouch on the left and the electrical shock generator on the right. Drawings and text provide visual instructions and audible voice instructions are provided by speakers in the defibrillator case.

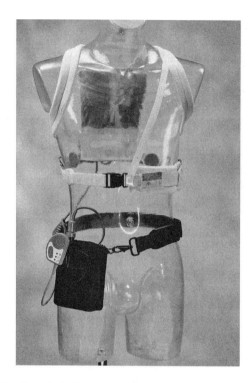

FIGURE 14.3   Wearable defibrillator for high risk patients.

or EMT who is testing or monitoring for arrhythmias and who may have to diagnose and treat the full spectrum of cardiac rhythm disorders, sometimes with great urgency. Hence, most defibrillators routinely used by medical personnel have a built-in control panel, monitor, and synchronizer. Figure 14.4 shows a hospital defibrillator.

Improved defibrillator waveforms have been developed and been advocated during the years from [1] multiple pulse sine waveform to [2] simple capacitor discharge waveform to [3] damped sine (RLC) waveform, to [4] monophasic truncated exponential decay waveform, to [5] a pair of truncated exponential waveforms, to [6] paired, biphasic truncated exponential decay waveforms. It is evident that the

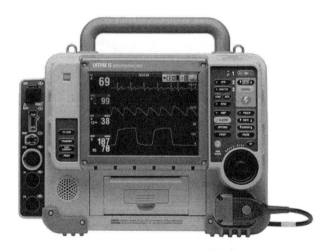

FIGURE 14.4   Defibrillator with monitor and control panel for us by trained medical personnel.

sine waveform and capacitor discharge are less effective and more damaging to the heart than the other waveforms, but there is still controversy about the benefits and limitations of the other waveforms. All of them defibrillate reliably but long-term patient survival with low morbidity is often low. (Of course, many variables other than waveform affect the final outcome.) At present, the biphasic truncated exponential decay waveform is the most widely used.

Optimal *shock intensity* for defibrillation is also controversial because in adult patients stronger shocks have a modestly higher success rate, but probably are more likely to damage the myocardium. Accordingly, experts and users take the position that a weaker first shock should be used for cardioversion, with gradual increase until success occurs. However, for the emergency situation of ventricular defibrillation, the best sequence (strength of first shock and extent of increases with subsequent shocks) has not yet been determined.

14.5 Electrodes

Electrodes for external defibrillation are connected to the defibrillator and are of two types; hand held and self-adhesive. The hand-held ones, shown in Figure 14.5, are most often used by medical personnel and have a metal surface area between 70 and 100 cm^{2}in. They must be coupled to the skin with an electrically conductive gel material that is specifically formulated for defibrillation to achieve low impedance across the electrode–patient interface. Hand-held electrodes are reusable.

The self-adhesive electrodes are patches wired to the patient through conductive flexible adhesive which holds the electrode in place, tightly against the skin. Adhesive electrodes are shown in Figure 14.6. They are disposable and are applied to the chest before the delivery of shock. Adhesive electrodes are left in place for reuse in case subsequent shocks are needed. Electrodes are usually applied with both electrodes on the anterior chest as shown in Figure 14.7, or in an anterior-to-posterior position, as shown in Figure 14.8.

14.6 Synchronization

Most defibrillators for use by medical personnel have the feature of synchronization, which is an electronic sensing and triggering mechanism for application of shock during the QRS complex of the ECG. This is required when treating arrhythmias other than VF (i.e., cardioverting), because when a patient does not have VF, inadvertent application of a shock during the T wave of the ECG often produces VF. Selection by the operator of the synchronized mode of defibrillator operation will cause the defibrillator to automatically sense the QRS complex and apply the shock during the QRS complex. Furthermore, on the ECG display, the timing of the shock on the QRS is graphically displayed so that the operator can be certain that the shock will not fall during the T wave (see Figure 14.9). This prevents production of VF by the defibrillator.

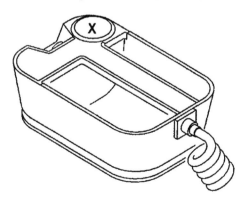

FIGURE 14.5 Hand held electrodes for external use.

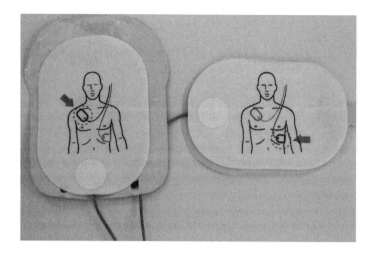

FIGURE 14.6   Disposable adhesive electrodes for external defibrillation.

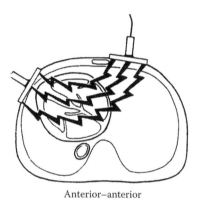

Anterior–anterior

FIGURE 14.7   Cross-sectional view of the chest showing position for standard anterior wall (precordial) electrode placement. Lines of presumed current flow are shown between the electrodes on the skin surface. (Modified from Tacker WA (ed). 1994. *Defibrillation of the Heart: ICDs, AEDs and Manual*, St. Louis, Mosby-Year Book. With permission.)

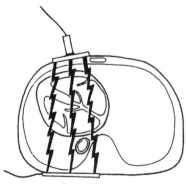

L-anterior–posterior

FIGURE 14.8   Cross-sectional view of the chest showing position for front-to-back electrode placement. Lines of presumed current flow are shown between the electrodes on the skin surface. (Modified from Tacker WA (ed). 1994. *Defibrillation of the Heart: ICDs, AEDs and Manual*, St. Louis, Mosby-Year Book. With permission.)

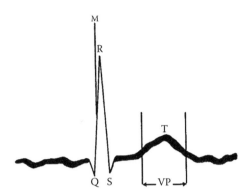

FIGURE 14.9 Timing mark (M) as shown on a synchronized defibrillator monitor. The M designates when in the cardiac cycle a shock will be applied. The T wave must be avoided, since a shock during the vulnerable period (VP) may fibrillate the ventricles. This tracing shows atrial fibrillation as identified by the irregular wavy baseline of the ECG. (Modified from Fein berg B. 1980. *Handbook Series in Clinical Laboratory Science*, vol. 2, Boca Raton, FL, CRC Press. With permission.)

14.7 Defibrillator Safety

Defibrillators are potentially dangerous devices because of their high electrical output. The danger to the patient is that of delivering unsynchronized shocks to a beating heart, a situation which can cause VF. Other problems include inadvertent shocking of the operator or others in the vicinity of use. Proper training and careful use are required for safety. Another risk is injuring the patient by applying excessively strong and/or excessive number of shocks. Failure of a defibrillator to operate correctly is a safety issue because a patient may die of his/her VF.

References

1. Tacker, W. A. Jr. (ed), 1994. *Defibrillation of the Heart: ICDs, AEDs, and Manual.* St. Louis, Mosby-Year Book.
2. Tacker, W. A. Jr. and Geddes, L. A. 1980. *Electrical Defibrillation.* Boca Raton, FL, CRC Press.
3. Paradis, N. A. (ed), 2007. *Cardiac Arrest: The Science and Practice of Resuscitation Medicine.* Cambridge CB2 8RU, United Kingdom, Cambridge University Press.
4. American National Standard ANSI/AAMI DF2, 1989. (second edition, revision of ANSI/AAMI DF2-1981) Safety and performance standard: Cardiac defibrillator devices.
5. Canadian National Standard CAN/CSA C22.2 No. 601.2.4-M90, 1990. Medical electrical equipment, part 2: Particular requirements for the safety of cardiac defibrillators and cardiac defibrillator/monitors.
6. International Standard IEC 601-2-4, 1983. Medical electrical equipment, part 2: Particular requirements for the safety of cardiac defibrillators and cardiac defibrillator/monitors.

Further Information

Detailed presentation of material on defibrillator waveforms, algorithms for ECG analysis, and automatic defibrillation using AEDs, electrodes, design, clinical use, effects of drugs on shock strength required to defibrillate, damage because of defibrillator shocks, and use of defibrillators during open-thorax surgical procedures or trans-esophageal defibrillation are beyond the scope of this chapter. Also, the historical aspects of defibrillation are not presented here. For more information, the reader is referred to the publications at the end of the chapter [1–3]. For American, Canadian, and European defibrillator standards, the reader is referred to the published standards [3–6].

15

Implantable Defibrillators

Paul A. Belk
St. Jude Medical

Thomas J. Mullen
Medtronic

15.1 Introduction

The heart is an electromechanical system, in which mechanical pumping function is initiated and coordinated by automatic rhythmic cardiac electrical activity. Transient electrical disturbances in this activity (cardiac arrhythmias) can immediately cause death. The implantable cardioverter defibrillator (ICD) is a medical device that can be implanted in a human body and will automatically detect and treat cardiac arrhythmias. Mirowski et al. [1] first reported on a demonstration of a functioning ICD in 1970. In his demonstration, he induced a fatal ventricular tachyarrhythmia in a dog. The dog was then successfully and dramatically rescued by the automatic operation of a previously implanted ICD. The first report of successful ICD implantation in humans soon followed [2]. In subsequent decades, advances in ICD technology have reduced ICD size from more than 200 cm³, originally, to as little as 25 cm³, while markedly improving functionality, reliability, and longevity. ICDs are now considered as standard of care for patients at risk for ventricular arrhythmia and are implanted in more than 150,000 patients per year in the United States alone [3].

Sudden cardiac death (SCD) is defined as abrupt loss of consciousness caused by failure of cardiac pumping function, generally because of an electrical problem. In certain cases, cardiac activity ceases completely because cardiac electrical impulse generation fails (bradycardic sudden death). Most commonly, however, cardiac electrical activity is present, but is either too rapid for effective mechanical response or too disorganized for coordinated mechanical response (tachycardic sudden death). Despite the term, resuscitation from SCD is possible, but lack of prompt treatment is almost invariably fatal. SCD is responsible for at least 160,000 deaths each year in the United States alone [4].

For most patients, treatment of SCD requires using an external defibrillator, but given the typical delay between identification of SCD and application of an external device, the chance of surviving SCD is less than 7% [4]. In contrast to external defibrillators, ICDs virtually guarantee prompt electrical therapy and one study showed that patients who receive ICD therapy for a lethal ventricular arrhythmia have greater than 75% chance of surviving for at least a year following the episode [5].

However, the expense of the device and associated complications and side effects limit ICD therapy to identifiable high-risk groups. Large numbers of patients in lower-risk groups, in fact, make up the majority of SCD victims and are currently not indicated or eligible to receive a device. As devices become less expensive and as therapy improves, more people become eligible. Improvement of device function would, therefore, potentially save lives of patients not currently indicated and reduce unpleasant side effects in patients who are.

15.2 Hardware

An ICD system consists of the "generator," which contains all the circuitry and energy storage and the "leads" that provide electrical connection to the heart (Figure 15.1).

15.2.1 Generator

To understand the construction of the ICD generator, it would be useful to review its required functions. The generator is implanted subcutaneously, usually in the left upper chest (Figure 15.1), but sometimes in other locations (abdominally or right chest). It normally remains implanted for between 4 and 10 years, until it reaches end of service life (through battery depletion). During this time, it must operate without fail and therefore must be built to the highest standards of quality and reliability. To survive for years implanted within the human body, the generator must be encased in a hermetically sealed casing that can withstand the harsh conditions of the human body. The casing is normally constructed of titanium because of its durability and biocompatibility. Attached to the casing is a "header" that provides ports into which the leads are inserted. The header provides externalization of the electrical connections without compromising the hermetic seal of the casing. Figure 15.2 shows typical components of a generator.

15.2.1.1 Low-Voltage Requirements

The ICD continuously monitors electrical activity in the heart. It may monitor one or more locations usually by analyzing the voltage across a bipolar electrode which is in intimate contact with cardiac tissue. Potentials across this electrode are generally between 1 and 20 mV. They are low-pass filtered with cutoff frequency between 30 and 100 Hz. Electrode impedances vary between 200 and 3000 Ω. In addition to providing therapy for tachyarrhythmias, almost all modern ICDs are capable of providing constant

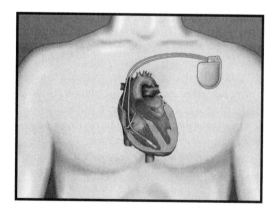

FIGURE 15.1 Schematic representation of a dual-chamber ICD. The generator is implanted in the pectoral region. The defibrillation lead (lower) is in the right ventricle, where it is fixed by a helix at the distal (far) end of the lead. The atrial lead (upper) is secured by flexible tines in the right atrial appendage. (Reproduced with permission of Medtronic, Inc.)

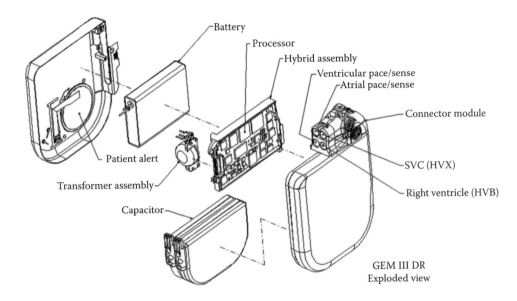

Battery

Processor

Hybrid assembly

Ventricular pace/sense

Atrial pace/sense

Connector module

Patient alert

Transformer assembly

Capacitor

SVC (HVX)

Right ventricle (HVB)

GEM III DR
Exploded view

FIGURE 15.2 Exploded view of ICD generator components. (Reproduced with permission of Medtronic, Inc.)

low-voltage pacing (at rates of 40–80 beats per minute) in the event of unacceptably slow heart rates (bradycardia). Pacing outputs are on the order of 1–5 V into an impedance of roughly 1 kΩ.

15.2.1.2 High-Voltage Requirements

Cardioversion or defibrillation is the electrical termination of arrhythmias using field stimulation. Unlike pacing, in which cardiac excitation is initiated in and propagates from a small region of tissue near the electrode, cardioversion must arrest electrical activity by simultaneous stimulation of most of the heart. In practice, this means establishing a "critical field" across a "critical mass" of cardiac tissue. This requires a compromise between the electrical response of the tissue and the electrical capabilities of the device. The electrical response of cardiac cells is complex, but stimulation mostly depends on the first-order properties of the membrane [6]. Theoretical and experimental studies have shown that the optimum voltage waveform for stimulation of cardiac tissue is a waveform with a characteristic rise time comparable to the cell membrane time constant [7,8].

The easiest waveform to deliver from an implantable device, however, is an exponentially decaying, capacitive discharge waveform because the capacitor is the natural high-voltage storage device. Optimum energy transfer occurs when the time constant of the waveform is similar to the first-order time constant of the cardiac tissue [6], and the polarity of the pulse is reversed at a prespecified voltage and then truncated [9,10]. The resulting pulse rises to as much as 750 V, with a duration of several milliseconds, into an impedance of 30–80 Ω. The need for phase reversal and truncation requires multiple high-voltage switches, usually arranged as an "H-bridge." Typical cardioversion energies are approximately 30 J, although completely subcutaneous systems (in which the leads are outside the chest cavity) may require twice that. Modern ICDs are designed for longevities of 4–9 years under the assumption that they will deliver up to four cardioversion shocks per year or about 500 J of high-voltage output.

15.2.1.3 Battery

Most of the volume of an ICD is required for the long- and short-term energy-storage devices: the battery and high-voltage capacitor. There is a minimum power, the quiescent energy drain, required for continuous function of the device; generally about 1 μW, which the battery must deliver continuously for many years, but it must also be able to deliver more than 4 W for 10 s necessary to charge the high-voltage capacitors for a 30–40 J cardioversion. The voltage characteristics of the battery must also be predictable, so that monitoring battery voltage gives adequate warning of end of battery life.

In modern ICDs, the battery chemistry is based on a lithium anode and a silver vanadium oxide cathode, giving relatively high-energy density and a predictable discharge curve. There are many ways of using this chemistry, and there are trade-offs between energy density and internal resistance. Internal battery resistance limits instantaneous power; therefore, it is often useful to sacrifice available energy density to control internal resistance. Some battery designers choose to make one of the battery electrodes larger than necessary, which limits the increase in internal resistance as the battery depletes, although at the cost of energy storage.

15.2.1.4 High-Voltage Capacitor

A cardioversion shock is usually a pulse of duration approximately 5 ms, delivered into a resistive load of approximately 50 Ω (3.2 kW). Because no miniature battery is even nearly capable of that voltage or that power, ICD generators require high-voltage capacitors. Originally, the capacitors were commodity electronic parts, such as those used for camera flashes, but modern ICD capacitors are designed specifically for that purpose and are optimized for volume, shape, and resistance. Because energy density at high voltage is the key design criterion, high-density technologies such as wet electrolytics are chosen despite their tendency to be leaky and to require periodic recharges to maintain their performance. Typical high-voltage capacitors have a capacitance of approximately 75 μF and a rating of at least 750 V.

15.2.1.5 High-Voltage Hybrid Circuitry

The high-voltage circuitry in an ICD controls high-voltage pulse duration and polarity, as well as charging the capacitors. The need to reverse the polarity of the pulse during delivery necessitates an H-bridge of high-voltage switching components. The need to charge the capacitors from a miniature battery requires high-voltage DC-to-DC conversion using, for example, a fly-back transformer. In addition to miniaturization and very high reliability, efficiency is a critical consideration, not only because of device longevity but also because all components are sealed inside the body, and excessive heat dissipation would result in tissue damage near the device.

15.2.1.6 Low-Voltage Analog Circuitry

Analog ICD circuitry continuously processes the voltage across the bipolar sensing electrode in contact with the cardiac tissue. This circuitry filters and rectifies the voltage waveform and provides a time series of cardiac depolarizations by comparing the amplitude of the processed voltage signal to a continuously adapting threshold. When the resulting time series is sufficiently fast, the signal is sampled for digital processing and storage. Depending on the configuration of the signal processing path, some of these operations are now performed by digital signal processing (DSP) hardware, in which case the analog components provide anti-alias filtering and sampling.

Most ICDs also monitor other analog signals. Taking regular measurements of the impedance of the lead systems can give early warning of lead failure. Also, there are signals that can augment ICD function. ICD patients often have diseases that limit the response of their heart rate to physical activity. Because virtually all transvenous ICDs are capable of pacing the heart, many ICDs are capable of modulating the pacing rate in response to external cues of activity, such as signals from an accelerometer or changes in impedance associated with respiration.

15.2.1.7 Digital Circuitry

A modern ICD contains a complete digital computing system, including a microprocessor, random-access memory (RAM), read-only memory (ROM), programmable nonvolatile memory (such as flash), and often low-power DSP chips. The most important requirements of this system are ultrahigh reliability and very low-power consumption; therefore, microprocessor bandwidth is usually very small compared to other systems, but the microprocessor generally handles all high-level tasks, including the analysis of the rhythm (determining whether therapy is needed) and sequencing of therapy. It also handles processing and storage of data records capturing device function and detected arrhythmic episodes and communication with external devices by telemetry. Critical functions of the ICD often use code from ROM, but it is increasingly possible to specify device functions in nonvolatile memory or even RAM, allowing sophisticated modification of ICD behavior and even the temporary implementation of research functionality.

Because of the susceptibility of writable memory to corruption, memory that contains critical instructions always has automatic integrity checks. Any evidence of data or code corruption initiates a "power-on reset (POR)" operation, in which the device returns to a "safe" set of parameters and trusted programs. POR operation is designed to ensure safety while providing only minimal sophistication.

15.2.2 Leads

Although intimate electrical contact with heart tissue is not necessary for defibrillator operation [11], direct electrical contact with cardiac tissue facilitates sensing of cardiac activity, especially by avoiding noise associated with skeletal muscle activity, and also reduces the voltage and energy that must be delivered to achieve therapeutic effects. Currently, all approved ICDs require direct electrical contact with heart muscle. This contact is accomplished with "leads," or insulated conducting systems that connect from a header on the ICD generator to electrodes in contact with the heart or vascular blood pool (Figure 15.3).

Cardiac lead systems are either epicardial or transvenous. Transvenous lead systems are introduced through the peripheral veins and routed to the endocardial surface through the superior vena cava and the atrium, which significantly constrains the geometry of the electrodes and the efficiency of energy delivery. Epicardial systems, in which the electrodes are in contact with the outer surface of the heart, historically required thoracic surgery and were therefore largely replaced by less-invasive transvenous electrodes. Modern epicardial systems can be implanted minimally invasively, but are still not commonly used. Epicardial systems generally provide more surface area than transvenous systems and, therefore, require less energy, and so were used in early ICD systems. They are also often used in pediatric patients because the lead system tends to be less distorted as the patient grows.

High-voltage lead systems consist of several components [12,13]. The proximal end has the connectors that make electrical contact to the header block on the ICD. The lead body is composed of insulators and conductors that link the poles of the connector to the pace-sensing electrodes and the one or two high-voltage coil electrodes near the distal end of the lead (Figure 15.4). Lead connectors and ICD headers are standardized so that leads from one manufacturer are fully compatible with ICDs from any manufacturer. The contemporary low-voltage standard (IS-1) uses a single port for the low-voltage bipolar electrode and the contemporary high-voltage standard (DF-1) uses one port for each high-voltage electrode, necessitating a bulky set of connectors and header ports for a single ICD lead. A new, lower profile standard (DF-4) has been developed by an industry task force, based on a quadrapolar lead connector that incorporates two high-voltage circuits and a pace-sense circuit within one connector.

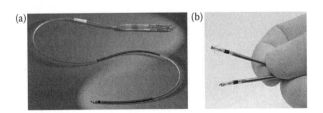

FIGURE 15.3 (a) A dual-coil, true bipolar ICD lead system. (b) Tips of two leads: one active fixation (helix at tip) and one passive fixation (tines at tip). (Reproduced with permission of Medtronic, Inc.)

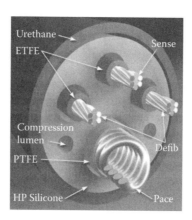

FIGURE 15.4 Transverse section of high-voltage lead body. (Reproduced with permission of Medtronic, Inc.)

The distal end of the lead has electrodes for delivery of defibrillation therapies, delivery of pacing therapies, and sensing of cardiac electrograms (EGMs). The pace-sense electrodes are similar to those in leads for standard implantable pacemakers. "True bipolar" leads have one electrode on the lead tip and a full ring electrode around the circumference of the lead body approximately 1 cm from the tip. "Integrated bipolar" leads have a tip electrode and use the distal high-voltage electrode as the other low-voltage pole. Sensing and pacing can be achieved between the tip and ring electrodes (termed bipolar) or between one of the lead electrodes and the ICD casing (termed unipolar).

Electrodes are constructed of platinum, iridium, titanium, or alloys of these metals. Delivery of high-voltage, high-current defibrillation shocks requires significantly larger surface area; hence, transvenous high-voltage electrodes are designed as exposed coils that spiral along the circumference of the lead and for multiple centimeters of the lead length. The external casing of the ICD itself usually serves as the return electrode in the high-voltage therapy current path, but the return path may also include a second coil electrode on the same lead (dual coil lead), a transvenous coil electrode on an independent lead, or even a nontransvenous, subcutaneous electrode on an independent lead. Although epicardial leads share similar electrode and lead body designs, the electrodes are unconstrained by the requirements for transvenous delivery and typically consist of coil electrodes organized across the surface of a broad patch that can be affixed to the epicardium.

Some older ICD lead bodies were designed with conductors organized as coaxial coils, but in modern ICD leads conductors pass through multiple, parallel lumens enclosed in layers of specialized insulating materials. The conductors are fabricated as cables or multifilar coils or a combination of each, using materials capable of withstanding the continual mechanical stresses without fracture and having low resistance to minimize heating and voltage drops. An alloy of nickel, cobalt, chromium and molybdenum, and MP-35N® is commonly used because of its resistance to fatigue damage, although usually combined with silver to minimize electrical resistance. Modern ICD leads also incorporate materials that slowly release steroid so as to limit the electrical degradation of the lead tissue interface due to inflammatory encapsulation.

Transvenous ICD leads are anchored in the right ventricle by small flexible tines at the lead tip that intertwine in small structures in the chamber ("passive fixation") or by a helix at the lead tip that can be screwed into the myocardial tissue ("active fixation"). The distal defibrillation coil rests within the right ventricle. Dual coil leads are designed such that the proximal coil is positioned in the superior vena cava.

In many ICD systems, pacing and sensing are limited to the right ventricle (single-chamber ICDs), and usually, only a single lead is required. More often, a pace-sense lead is also inserted via the same transvenous route and is fixed in the right atrium (dual-chamber ICD). The right atrial lead provides atrial pacing and sensing and permits the use of more complex dual-chamber tachyarrhythmia sensing, detection, and discrimination algorithms. In triple-chamber or cardiac resynchronization ICDs, a pace-sense lead is also placed in a coronary vein of the left ventricle, to allow independent (though limited) control of left- and right-ventricular depolarization timing.

Although it is tempting to regard them simply as wires, ICD leads are complex medical devices in their own right. The ICD lead must be capable of sensing millivolt-level cardiac electrical activity, delivering low-voltage pacing pulses (occasionally in short-cycle length bursts) and delivering high-voltage, high-current rescue shocks while withstanding the associated thermal and electrical stresses. It must also withstand the significant biochemical stresses to which any implanted medical device is subjected as well as large mechanical stresses imposed by the movement of the arm and upper body and the repetitive mechanical (torsional and bending) stresses associated with implant in or on a beating heart.

15.2.3 Programmer

The automatic behavior of ICDs is controlled by a large number (often more than 100) of adjustable parameters. These parameters allow clinicians to tune arrhythmia detection behaviors, determine the sequences and types of arrhythmia therapies to be delivered, and set the characteristics of bradycardia pacing. In addition, ICDs often store large amounts of diagnostic data about the device function as well as physiologic parameters such as time-dependent electrical response of the heart and a history of selected arrhythmia episodes. Transfer, modification, and interpretation of this information are traditionally controlled by an external device (a "programmer"), which communicates with the ICD via radio frequency (RF) telemetry (Figure 15.5). Historically, communication between the implanted device and the programmer required placement of a transmitter/receiver unit on the skin in close (a few centimeters) proximity to the location of the implanted device. More recently, with the definition of a dedicated medical devices frequency band, long distance (multiple meters) or "non-contact" telemetry is becoming more widely available. In this way, a clinician can program the function of the device or retrieve diagnostic information from a programmer located in the same room with the patient.

Telemetry communication to and from the implanted device can also be used in the home. In fact, home monitors are available for most ICDs. The home monitor can interrogate a device and provide valuable diagnostic data to clinicians via telephone or Internet uplinks. Although the technology already

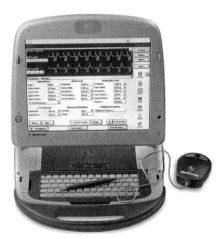

FIGURE 15.5 Programmer with transmitter/receiver unit that is placed in the vicinity of the implanted ICD. Long-range telemetry now eliminates the need for the transmitter/receiver in many ICD systems. (Reproduced with permission of Medtronic, Inc.)

exists to allow it, at this time, due in part to safety concerns, there is limited remote programmability of device parameters permitted.

15.3 Arrhythmia Detection

Arrhythmia detection is and has been a critical area of development for modern ICDs. All ICDs are designed with a bias for overtreatment because the consequence of undertreatment may be death. This was initially relatively unimportant because patients indicated for ICD therapy had already survived multiple episodes of SCD. As indications expand to lower risk groups, however, the risk of overtreatment increases substantially and overtreatment is often unacceptable to otherwise healthy patients at risk for SCD. More sophisticated detection is the primary means for addressing this problem.

The steps that lead from analysis of cardiac rhythm to delivery of ICD therapy can be considered as three distinct subprocesses: sensing, detection, and discrimination. Although the technology is evolving, it is useful to think of *sensing* as primarily a problem in analog signal processing and *detection* as the digital processing of the sensed information. Given that a potentially dangerous tachyarrhythmia is *detected*, the *discrimination* subsystem analyzes aspects of the rhythm to determine whether it can be reliably classified as benign, usually meaning that the arrhythmia is the result of rapid atrial depolarization, and therefore does not significantly degrade cardiac pumping function. The discrimination subsystem can then *withhold* therapy for as long as the rhythm can be classified as benign, although many ICDs include a "high-rate timeout" feature that guarantees therapy delivery (i.e., overrides the discrimination subsystem), after a fixed period of time. Yet, despite advances in detection, the basis of ICD therapy delivery is ventricular rate and duration, just as was the case for the first commercial ICD systems.

15.3.1 Sensing

ICDs continuously monitor the voltage across a bipolar electrode (the near-field EGM). The signal is affected by any nearby electrical activity, including local and distant cardiac activity, activity of skeletal muscles, and external fields such as household power and alternating current motors. In practice, the only aspect of the EGM that is of interest for initial detection of ventricular arrhythmia is associated with local tissue depolarization. This part of the EGM is called the *R-wave*, in analogy to a similar signal on the surface of the electrocardiogram. (Note that dual-chamber ICDs perform similar operations on the atrial EGM.) The purpose of sensing is to reliably identify the timing of the *R*-wave, without being affected by other deflections in the EGM. This has generally been an analog operation, although the incorporation of low-power DSP components has steadily grown and digital operation will soon become the dominant implementation.

Sensing is accomplished through filtering, rectifying, and then thresholding. Filtering effectively isolates the *R*-waves from the other components in the EGM signals. The other cardiac signals, including Ventricular repolarization (*T*-wave), are lower in frequency than the *R*-wave; therefore, most devices use high-pass filtering with cutoff between 10 and 20 Hz. External signals, including skeletal muscle depolarizations and electrical interference are largely common-mode signals, although they are diminished by low-pass filtering. Many ICDs, therefore, use low-pass cutoffs of less than 50 Hz, and most filter below 100 Hz.

After filtering, *R*-waves may be identified by rectification and comparison to a threshold, although a static threshold would be inadequate because the amplitude of filtered *R*-waves is unpredictable. In particular, pathological *R*-waves, which the device must detect to deliver therapy, can change substantially as a result of the pathology. In ventricular fibrillation (VF), the most lethal of ventricular arrhythmias, the *R*-waves can become much smaller than normal and often exhibit high variability.

In practice, this problem is solved by continuous adaptation of either the threshold or the signal gain. The detection sensitivity is lowest (highest threshold) immediately after identification of an *R*-wave, and generally set to a level that would only identify features of similar magnitude. In the absence of further identified activity, the sensitivity increases continuously toward a predefined maximum, ensuring that the largest features in a time-varying signal will be identified.

15.3.2 Detection

ICD detection algorithms primarily rely on the time sequence of *R*-waves determined by the sensing subsystem. It is fundamentally rate based. When the rate of identified *R*-waves is higher than a prespecified threshold, and for a prespecified duration, therapy is presumed to be required unless secondary considerations classify the tachycardia as benign.

15.3.3 Discrimination

Tachycardias are generally classified as ventricular or supraventricular. Ventricular tachycardia (VT) is due to primary ventricular dysfunction and is often acutely dangerous. Supraventricular tachycardia (SVT) is almost never immediately dangerous and does not necessarily respond to ICD therapy; hence, the treatment of SVT by an ICD is generally considered undesirable. The discrimination subsystem identifies rhythms that are sufficiently fast to treat (tachycardia), but are not ventricular in origin (SVT). Again, the bias of the device is to overtreat because the erroneous treatment of SVT is considered preferable to failure to treat a potentially lethal Ventricular.

Discrimination can be pattern based, morphology based, or a combination of the two approaches. In pattern-based discrimination, specific features of the time sequence of events are used to classify the rhythm as SVT. The patterns indicative of SVT include timing irregularity (unless all R-R intervals are shorter than a fixed cutoff), gradual acceleration of the R-R intervals, or, in dual-chamber ICDs, certain specific relationships between the timing of atrial and ventricular events.

Morphology-based discrimination uses the shape of the *R*-wave to identify SVT. SVT, like normal cardiac rhythm, uses the specialized cardiac conduction system to depolarize the ventricle. Therefore, there is a characteristic *R*-wave morphology that is preserved in SVT but not in Ventricular. Morphology analysis is most informative when it samples large regions of the heart; therefore, it usually makes use of the vector between the high-voltage electrodes, unlike sensing, which uses the low-voltage electrodes. It also requires a method for storing the characteristics of the normal morphology. The storage system can be as simple as a characteristic *R*-wave width or may include many components of the morphology using a system such as wavelet decomposition.

15.4 Arrhythmia Therapy

Modern ICDs provide low- and high-voltage therapy that can support the cardiac rhythm when the heart is beating too slowly (bradycardia) or when the electrical rhythm becomes uncontrolled and too fast (tachycardia).

15.4.1 Bradycardia Therapy

Bradycardia therapy in a modern ICD is virtually indistinguishable from that in a modern pacemaker. All ICDs are capable of ventricular demand pacing at adjustable rates and many are capable of rate-responsive pacing, in which the rate of pacing is modulated by external activity cues such as accelerometer signals or measured respiration rate. Dual-chamber ICDs have the same pacing capabilities as dual-chamber pacemakers, providing rate-responsive pacing in the atrium and ventricle, as well as coordinated AV pacing. Triple-chamber or cardiac resynchronization therapy ICDs can stimulate the ventricles independently to improve pumping function when the specialized ventricular conduction system is damaged.

15.4.2 High-Voltage Antitachycardia Therapy

Ventricular tachycardia (VT) is the result of uncontrolled electrical activity in the ventricle. This activity may be coordinated or uncoordinated. The definitive therapy for Ventricular is external stimulation by an electric field sufficiently large to reset the electrical activity of most ventricular cells. This ends the previous (uncontrolled) electrical activity and allows the reestablishment of normal cardiac activity. As explained earlier, this requires depolarization of a "critical mass" of tissue by a high-voltage discharge. When high-voltage therapy is delivered, an attempt is made to synchronize the delivery with a detected *R*-wave. A synchronized shock is termed "cardioversion," whereas an unsynchronized shock is termed "defibrillation" because VF has no coherent electrical activity, and therefore no basis for synchronization (Figure 15.6).

15.4.3 Low-Voltage Antitachycardia Therapy

Although high-voltage therapy is highly effective, it can be an unpleasant experience to the patient and also requires significant energy from the battery. Studies have shown that most Ventricular occurring in patients with ICDs is monomorphic, meaning that ventricular electrical activity, although uncontrolled, is still coordinated [14,15]. The same studies have shown that as many as 75% of these episodes can be terminated by overdrive pacing, termed "antitachycardia pacing (ATP)" (Figure 15.7). The exact timing of the ATP pulses seems to be a significant factor in ATP efficacy and many timing algorithms are available in ICDs. The most commonly used algorithms are "burst" ATP, in which a fixed number of pacing pulses are delivered at a constant fraction of the Ventricular cycle length, and "ramp," or "scan" ATP, in which the interval between pulses is decreased by a specified amount for each pulse. More complex algorithms for ATP have been studied, including combinations of burst and ramp, and methods for choosing the ideal ATP parameters automatically. As yet, nothing has proven to be superior to the delivery of eight pulses at 88% of the Ventricular cycle length [16].

15.5 Diagnostics and Monitoring

Due to memory and energy limitations, early ICDs had limited capability for recording diagnostic data. Today, all ICDs provide some capability for recording of cardiac EGMs and of counters that provide a history of ventricular arrhythmic events and therapies delivered. These data are clinically valuable for determining the appropriateness of device detection and therapy settings. The devices typically supplement the EGM data with simultaneous information about beat-to-beat device function in a "marker channel" (Figures 15.6 and 15.7). Devices also report on battery status to provide early warning for elective device replacement and continuously monitor lead integrity.

An implanted device also offers a unique opportunity for continuous ambulatory collection and trending of physiologic information. Today's devices can provide a history of the incidence and duration of atrial arrhythmias, track heart rate 24 hours/day, and provide estimates of heart rate variability on a daily basis (Figure 15.8). In addition, many devices are equipped with accelerometers that can be used to estimate and track patient activity [17,18]. Other devices track the impedance between electrodes and the ICD housing as a measure of fluid volume in the chest that can be useful in the management of patients with heart failure [19,20]. The addition of implanted sensors to ICDs promises to offer new opportunities for providing important clinical information.

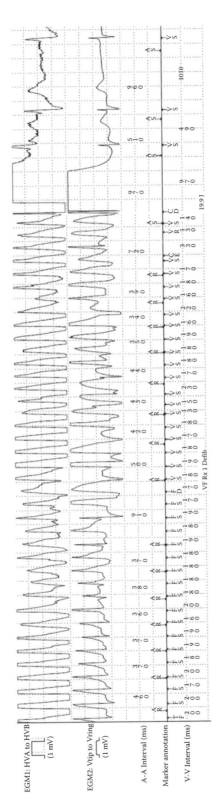

FIGURE 15.6 Record stored by an ICD of successful delivery of a defibrillation. An atrial EGM, (top tracing), ventricular electrogram (middle tracing), and ICD marker channel are shown. Markers include ventricular sense (VS), atrial sense (AS), ventricular pace (VP), atrial pace (AP), end of ICD capacitor charge (CE), and delivery of shock (CD). (Reproduced with permission of Medtronic, Inc.)

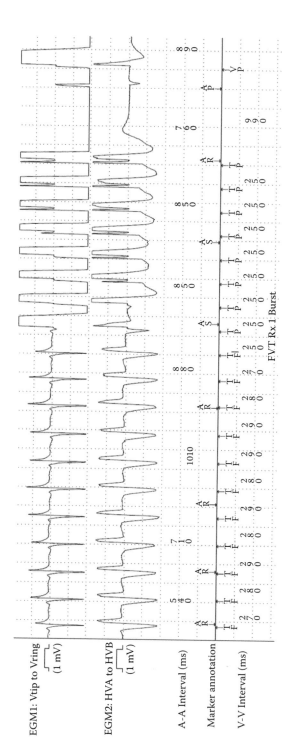

FIGURE 15.7 Stored record of successful delivery of ATP. An atrial EGM (top tracing), ventricular electrogram (middle tracing), and ICD marker channel are shown. TS markers indicate sensing of tachyarrhythmia beats, TP markers indicate delivery of ATP, and VS marker indicates sensing of a normally timed ventricular beat. (Reproduced with permission of Medtronic, Inc.)

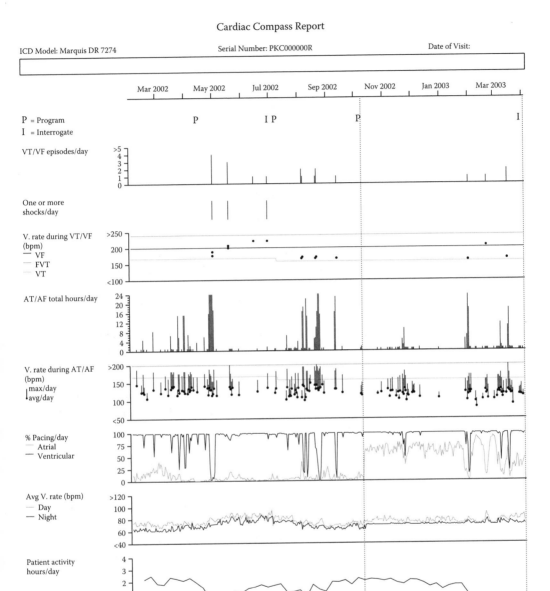

FIGURE 15.8   A diagnostics report issued from an ICD based on stored data. (Reproduced with permission of Medtronic, Inc.)

15.6 Conclusion

The ICD is an established therapy for patients at risk of life-threatening ventricular arrhythmias. It is a complex medical device that incorporates many advances in low-energy electronics and biomaterials.

To date, it is one of the few therapies proven to extend life in patients at risk of SCD and is the only effective therapy for patients who experience an episode of SCD. Beyond this fundamental therapy, the modern ICD is also a fully functional pacemaker and cardiac resynchronization device and provides diagnostic capabilities. The future use of the ICD, particularly in the large fraction of patients who currently do not survive their first episode of SCD will depend on reducing the cost of manufacture and implantation, increasing reliability and longevity, reducing undesirable device side effects such as painful or inappropriate high-voltage therapy, and extending diagnostic capabilities to increase the usefulness of the ICD in the management of patients.

References

1. M. Mirowski, M. M. Mower, W. S. Staewen, B. Tabatznik, and A. I. Mendeloff. Standby automatic defibrillator. An approach to prevention of sudden coronary death. *Arch Intern Med*, 126(1):158–161, July 1970.
2. M. Mirowski, P. R. Reid, M. M. Mower, L. Watkins, E. V. Platia, L. S. Griffith, E. P. Veltri, T. Guarnieri, and J. M. Juanteguy. Clinical experience with the automatic implantable defibrillator. *Arch Mal Coeur Vaiss*, 78:39–42, October 1985.
3. A. J. Camm and S. Nisam. European utilization of the implantable defibrillator: Has 10 years changed the enigma? *Europace*, 12(8):1063–1069, August 2010.
4. Writing Group Members, D. Lloyd-Jones, R. J. Adams, T. M. Brown, M. Carnethon, S. Dai, G. D. Simone, T. B. Ferguson et al. American Heart Association Statistics Committee, and Stroke Statistics Subcommittee. Heart disease and stroke statistics—2010 update: A report from the American Heart Association. *Circulation*, 121(7):e46–e215, February 2010.
5. J. E. Poole, G. W. Johnson, A. S. Hellkamp, J. Anderson, D. J. Callans, M. H. Raitt, R. K. Reddy et al. Prognostic importance of defibrillator shocks in patients with heart failure. *N Engl J Med*, 359(10):1009–1017, September 2008.
6. S. R. Shorofsky, E. Rashba, W. Havel, P. Belk, P. Degroot, C. Swerdlow, and M. R. Gold. Improved defibrillation efficacy with an ascending ramp waveform in humans. *Heart Rhythm*, 2(4):388–394, April 2005.
7. R. D. Klafter. An optimally energized cardiac pacemaker. *IEEE Trans Biomed Eng*, 20(5):350–356, September 1973.
8. R. D. Klafter and L. Hrebien. An *in vivo* study of cardiac pacemaker optimization by pulse shape modification. *IEEE Trans Biomed Eng*, 23(3):233–239, May 1976.
9. S. Saksena, H. An, R. Mehra, P. DeGroot, R. B. Krol, E. Burkhardt, D. Mehta, and T. John. Prospective comparison of biphasic and monophasic shocks for implantable cardioverter-defibrillators using endocardial leads. *Am J Cardiol*, 70(3):304–310, August 1992.
10. M. O. Sweeney, A. Natale, K. J. Volosin, C. D. Swerdlow, J. H. Baker, and P. Degroot. Prospective randomized comparison of 50%/50% versus 65%/65% tilt biphasic waveform on defibrillation in humans. *Pacing Clin Electrophysiol*, 24(1):60–65, January 2001.
11. G. H. Bardy, W. M. Smith, M. A. Hood, I. G. Crozier, I. C. Melton, L. Jordaens, D. Theuns et al. An entirely subcutaneous implantable cardioverter-defibrillator. *N Engl J Med*, 363(1):36–44, May 2010.
12. G. Kalahasty and K. A. Ellenbogen. *ICD Lead Design*, pp. 239–263. Cardiotext Publishing, Minneapolis, MN, 2010.
13. H. M. Haqqani and H. G. Mond. The implantable cardioverter-defibrillator lead: Principles, progress, and promises. *Pacing Clin Electrophysiol*, 32(10):1336–1353, October 2009.
14. M. S. Wathen, P. J. DeGroot, M. O. Sweeney, A. J. Stark, M. F. Otterness, W. O. Adkisson, R. C. Canby et al. Rx II investigators. Prospective randomized multicenter trial of empirical antitachycardia pacing versus shocks for spontaneous rapid ventricular tachycardia in patients with implantable cardioverter-defibrillators: Pacing fast ventricular tachycardia reduces shock therapies (pain-free Rx II) trial results. *Circulation*, 110(17):2591–2596, October 2004.

15. M. S. Wathen, M. O. Sweeney, P. J. DeGroot, A. J. Stark, J. L. Koehler, M. B. Chisner, C. Machado, and W. O. Adkisson. Shock reduction using antitachycardia pacing for spontaneous rapid ventricular tachycardia in patients with coronary artery disease. *Circulation*, 104(7):796–801, August 2001.

16. B. L. Wilkoff, K. T. Ousdigian, L. D. Sterns, Z. J. Wang, R. D. Wilson, and J. M. Morgan. A comparison of empiric to physician-tailored programming of implantable cardioverter-defibrillators: Results from the prospective randomized multicenter empiric trial. *J Am Coll Cardiol*, 48(2):330–339, 2006.

17. R. Germany and C. Murray. Use of device diagnostics in the outpatient management of heart failure. *Am J Cardiol*, 99(10A):11G–16G, May 2007.

18. A. Gardini, P. Lupo, E. Zanelli, S. Bisetti, and R. Cappato. Diagnostic capabilities of devices for cardiac resynchronization therapy. *J Cardiovasc Med (Hagerstown)*, 11(3):186–189, March 2010.

19. R. Germany. The use of device-based diagnostics to manage patients with heart failure. *Congest Heart Fail*, 14(5 Suppl 2):19–24, 2008.

20. D. J. Whellan, K. T. Ousdigian, S. M. Al-Khatib, W. Pu, S. Sarkar, C. B. Porter, B. B. Pavri, C. M. O'Connor, and Partners study investigators. Combined heart failure device diagnostics identify patients at higher risk of subsequent heart failure hospitalizations: Results from partners HF (program to access and review trending information and evaluate correlation to symptoms in patients with heart failure) study. *J Am Coll Cardiol*, 55(17):1803–1810, April 2010.

16

Implantable Stimulators for Neuromuscular Control

Primoz Strojnik
Case Western Reserve University

P. Hunter Peckham
Case Western Reserve University

16.1 Functional Electrical Stimulation

Implantable stimulators for neuromuscular control are the technologically most advanced versions of functional electrical stimulators. Their function is to generate contraction of muscles, which cannot be controlled volitionally because of the damage or dysfunction in the neural paths of the central nervous system (CNS). Their operation is based on the electrical nature of conducting information within nerve fibers, from the neuron cell body (soma), along the axon, where a traveling action potential is the carrier of excitation. While the action potential is naturally generated chemically in the head of the axon, it may also be generated artificially by depolarizing the neuron membrane with an electrical pulse. A train of electrical impulses with certain amplitude, width, and repetition rate, applied to a muscle innervating nerve (a motor neuron) will cause the muscle to contract, very much like in natural excitation. Similarly, a train of electrical pulses applied to the muscular tissue close to the motor point will cause muscle contraction by stimulating the muscle through the neural structures at the motor point.

16.2 Technology for Delivering Stimulation Pulses to Excitable Tissue

A practical system used to stimulate a nerve consists of three components (1) a *pulse generator* to generate a train of pulses capable of depolarizing the nerve, (2) a *lead wire*, the function of which is to deliver the pulses to the stimulation site, and (3) an *electrode*, which delivers the stimulation pulses to the excitable tissue in a safe and efficient manner.

In terms of location of the above three components of an electrical stimulator, stimulation technology can be described in the following terms:

Surface or transcutaneous stimulation, where all three components are outside the body and the electrodes are placed on the skin above or near the motor point of the muscle to be stimulated. This method has been used extensively in medical rehabilitation of nerve and muscle. Therapeutically, it has been used to prevent atrophy of paralyzed muscles, to condition paralyzed muscles before the application of functional stimulation, and to generally increase the muscle bulk. As a functional tool, it has been used in rehabilitation of plegic and paretic patients. Surface systems for functional stimulation have been developed to correct drop-foot condition in hemiplegic individuals (Liberson et al., 1961), for hand control (Rebersek and Vodovnik, 1973), and for standing and stepping in individuals with *paralysis* of the lower extremities (Kralj and Bajd, 1989). This fundamental technology was commercialized by Sigmedics, Inc. (Graupe and Kohn, 1998). The inability of surface stimulation to reliably excite the underlying tissue in a repeatable manner and to selectively stimulate deep muscles has limited the clinical applicability of surface stimulation.

Percutaneous stimulation employs electrodes which are positioned inside the body close to the structures to be stimulated. Their lead wires permanently penetrate the skin to be connected to the external pulse generator. State of the art embodiments of percutaneous electrodes utilize a small-diameter insulated stainless steel lead that is passed through the skin. The electrode structure is formed by removal of the insulation from the lead and subsequent modification to ensure stability within the tissue. This modification includes forming barbs or similar anchoring mechanisms. The percutaneous electrode is implanted using a hypodermic needle as a trochar for introduction. As the needle is withdrawn, the anchor at the electrode tip is engaged into the surrounding tissue and remains in the tissue. A connector at the skin surface, next to the skin penetration point, joins the percutaneous electrode lead to the hard-wired external stimulator. The penetration site has to be maintained and care must be taken to avoid physical damage of the lead wires. In the past, this technology has helped develop the existing implantable systems, and it may be used for short and long term, albeit not permanent, stimulation applications (Marsolais and Kobetic, 1986; Memberg et al., 1993).

The term *implantable stimulation* refers to stimulation systems in which all three components, pulse generator, lead wires, and electrodes, are permanently surgically implanted into the body and the skin is solidly closed after the implantation procedure. Any interaction between the implantable part and the outside world is performed using telemetry principles in a contact-less fashion. This chapter is focused on implantable neuromuscular stimulators, which will be discussed in more detail.

16.3 Stimulation Parameters

In functional *electrical stimulation*, the typical stimulation waveform is a train of rectangular pulses. This shape is used because of its effectiveness as well as relative ease of generation. All three parameters of a stimulation train, that is, frequency, amplitude, and pulse-width, have effect on muscle contraction. Generally, the stimulation frequency is kept as low as possible, to prevent muscle fatigue and to conserve stimulation energy. The determining factor is the muscle fusion frequency at which a smooth muscle response is obtained. This frequency varies; however, it can be as low as 12–14 Hz and as high as 50 Hz. In most cases, the stimulation frequency is kept constant for a certain application. This is true both for surface as well as implanted electrodes.

With surface electrodes, the common way of modulating muscle force is by varying the stimulation pulse amplitude at a constant frequency and pulse-width. The stimulation amplitudes may be as low as 25 V at 200 μs for the stimulation of the peroneal nerve and as high as 120 V or more at 300 μs for activation of large muscles such as the gluteus maximus.

In implantable stimulators and electrodes, the stimulation parameters greatly depend on the implantation site. When the electrodes are positioned on or around the target nerve, the stimulation amplitudes are on the order of a few milliamperes or less. Electrodes positioned on the muscle surface (epimysial electrodes) or in the muscle itself (intramuscular electrodes), employ up to ten times higher amplitudes. For muscle force control, implantable stimulators rely either on pulse-width modulation or amplitude modulation. For example, in upper extremity applications, the current amplitude is usually a fixed parameter set to 16 or 20 mA, while the muscle force is modulated with pulse widths within 0–200 μs.

16.4 Implantable Neuromuscular Stimulators

Implantable stimulation systems use an encapsulated pulse generator that is surgically implanted and has subcutaneous leads that terminate at electrodes on or near the desired nerves. In low power consumption applications such as the cardiac pacemaker, a primary battery power source is included in the pulse generator case. When the battery is close to depletion, the pulse generator has to be surgically replaced.

Most implantable systems for neuromuscular application consist of an external and an implanted component. Between the two, an inductive radio-frequency link is established, consisting of two tightly coupled resonant coils. The link allows transmission of power and information, through the skin, from the external device to the implanted pulse generator. In more advanced systems, a back-telemetry link is also established, allowing transmission of data outwards, from the implanted to the external component.

Ideally, implantable stimulators for neuromuscular control would be stand alone, totally implanted devices with an internal power source and integrated sensors detecting desired movements from the motor cortex and delivering stimulation sequences to appropriate muscles, thus bypassing the neural damage. At the present developmental stage, they still need a control source and an external controller to provide power and stimulation information. The control source may be either operator driven, controlled by the user, or triggered by an event such as the heel-strike phase of the gait cycle. Figure 16.1 depicts a neuromuscular prosthesis developed at the Case Western Reserve University (CWRU) and Cleveland Veterans Affairs Medical Center for the restoration of hand functions using an implantable

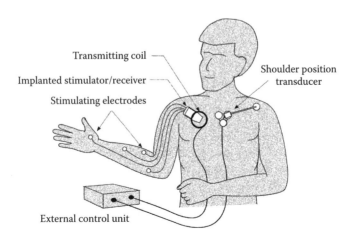

FIGURE 16.1 Implanted FES hand grasp system.

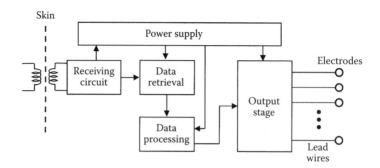

FIGURE 16.2   Block diagram of an implantable neuromuscular stimulator.

neuromuscular stimulator. In this application, the patient uses the shoulder motion to control opening and closing of the hand.

The internal electronic structure of an implantable neuromuscular stimulator is shown in Figure 16.2. It consists of receiving and data retrieval circuits, power supply, data processing circuits, and output stages.

16.4.1 Receiving Circuit

The stimulator's receiving circuit is an LC circuit tuned to the resonating frequency of the external transmitter, followed by a rectifier. Its task is to provide the raw DC power from the received rf signal and at the same time allow extraction of stimulation information embedded in the rf carrier. There are various encoding schemes allowing simultaneous transmission of power and information into an implantable electronic device. They include amplitude and frequency modulation with different modulation indexes as well as different versions of digital encoding such as Manchester encoding where the information is hidden in a logic value transition position rather than the logic value itself. Synchronous and asynchronous clock signals may be extracted from the modulated carrier to drive the implant's logic circuits.

The use of radiofrequency transmission for medical devices is regulated and in most countries limited to certain frequencies and radiation powers. (In the United States, the use of the rf space is regulated by the Federal Communication Commission [FCC].) Limited rf transmission powers as well as conservation of power in battery operated external controllers dictate high coupling efficiencies between the transmitting and receiving antennas. Optimal coupling parameters cannot be uniformly defined; they depend on application particularities and design strategies.

16.4.2 Power Supply

The amount of power delivered into an implanted electronic package depends on the coupling between the transmitting and the receiving coil. The coupling is dependent on the distance as well as the alignment between the coils. The power supply circuits must compensate for the variations in distance for different users as well as for the alignment variations due to skin movements and consequent changes in relative coil-to-coil position during daily usage. The power dissipated on power supply circuits must not raise the overall implant case temperature.

In implantable stimulators that require stimulation voltages in excess of the electronics power supply voltages (20–30 V), the stimulation voltage can be provided directly through the receiving coil. In that case, voltage regulators must be used to provide the electronics supply voltage (usually 5 V), which heavily taxes the external power transmitter and increases the implant internal power dissipation.

16.4.3 Data Retrieval

Data retrieval technique depends on the data-encoding scheme and is closely related to power supply circuits and implant power consumption. Most commonly, amplitude modulation is used to encode the in-going data stream. As the high quality factor of resonant LC circuits increases the efficiency of power transmission, it also effectively reduces the transmission bandwidth and therefore the transmission data rate. Also, high quality circuits are difficult to amplitude modulate since they tend to continue oscillating even with power removed. This has to be taken into account when designing the communication link in particular for the start-up situation when the implanted device does not use the power for stimulation and therefore loads the transmitter side less heavily, resulting in narrower and higher resonant curves. The load on the receiving coil may also affect the low pass filtering of the received rf signal.

Modulation index (m) or depth of modulation affects the overall energy transfer into the implant. At a given rf signal amplitude, less energy is transferred into the implanted device when 100% modulation is used ($m = 1$) as compared to 10% modulation ($m = 0.053$). However, retrieval of 100% modulated signal is much easier than retrieval of a 10% modulated signal.

16.4.4 Data Processing

Once the information signal has been satisfactorily retrieved and reconstructed into logic voltage levels, it is ready for logic processing. For synchronous data processing a clock signal is required. It can be generated locally within the implant device, reconstructed from the incoming data stream, or can be derived from the rf carrier. A crystal has to be used with a local oscillator to assure stable clock frequency. Local oscillator allows for asynchronous data transmission. Synchronous transmission is best achieved using Manchester data encoding. Decoding of Manchester encoded data recovers the original clock signal, which was used during data encoding. Another method is using the downscaled rf carrier signal as the clock source. In this case, the information signal has to be synchronized with the rf carrier. Of course, 100% modulation scheme cannot be used with carrier-based clock signal. Complex command structure used in multichannel stimulators requires intensive data decoding and processing and consequently extensive electronic circuitry. Custom-made, application specific circuits (ASIC) are commonly used to minimize the space requirements and optimize the circuit performance.

16.4.5 Output Stage

The output stage forms stimulation pulses and defines their electrical characteristics. Even though a mere rectangular pulse can depolarize a nervous membrane, such pulses are not used in clinical practice due to their noxious effect on the tissue and *stimulating electrodes*. These effects can be significantly reduced by charge balanced stimulating pulses where the cathodic stimulation pulse is followed by an anodic pulse containing the same electrical charge, which reverses the electrochemical effects of the cathodic pulse. Charge balanced waveforms can be assured by capacitive coupling between the pulse generator and stimulation electrodes. Charge balanced stimulation pulses include symmetrical and asymmetrical waveforms with anodic phase immediately following the cathodic pulse or being delayed by a short, 20–60 µs interval.

The output stages of most implantable neuromuscular stimulators have constant current characteristics, meaning that the output current is independent on the electrode or tissue impedance. Practically, the constant current characteristics ensure that the same current flows through the excitable tissues regardless of the changes that may occur on the electrode–tissue interface, such as the growth of fibrous tissue around the electrodes. Constant current output stage can deliver constant current only within the supply voltage–compliance voltage. In neuromuscular stimulation, with the electrode impedance being on the order of 1 kΩ, and the stimulating currents in the order of 20 mA, the compliance voltage must be above 20 V. Considering the voltage drops and losses across electronic components, the compliance voltage of the output stage may have to be as high as 33 V.

The stimulus may be applied through either monopolar or bipolar electrodes. The monopolar electrode is one in which a single active electrode is placed near the excitable nerve and the return electrode is placed remotely, generally at the implantable unit itself. Bipolar electrodes are placed at the stimulation site, thus limiting the current paths to the area between the electrodes. Generally, in monopolar stimulation the active electrode is much smaller than the return electrode, while bipolar electrodes are the same size.

16.5 Packaging of Implantable Electronics

Electronic circuits must be protected from the harsh environment of the human body. The packaging of implantable electronics uses various materials, including polymers, metals, and ceramics. The encapsulation method depends somewhat on the electronic circuit technology. Older devices may still use discrete components in a classical form, such as leaded transistors and resistors. The newer designs, depending on the sophistication of the implanted device, may employ application-specific integrated circuits (ASICs) and thick film hybrid circuitry for their implementation. Such circuits place considerable requirements for hermeticity and protection on the implanted circuit packaging.

Epoxy encapsulation was the original choice of designers of implantable neuromuscular stimulators. It has been successfully used with relatively simple circuits using discrete, low impedance components. With epoxy encapsulation, the receiving coil is placed around the circuitry to be "potted" in a mold, which gives the implant the final shape. Additionally, the epoxy body is coated with silicone rubber that improves the *biocompatibility* of the package. Polymers do not provide an impermeable barrier and therefore cannot be used for encapsulation of high density, high impedance electronic circuits. The moisture ingress ultimately will reach the electronic components, and surface ions can allow electric shorting and degradation of leakage-sensitive circuitry and subsequent failure.

Hermetic packaging provides the implant electronic circuitry with a long-term protection from the ingress of body fluids. Materials that provide hermetic barriers are metals, ceramics, and glasses. Metallic packaging generally uses a titanium capsule machined from a solid piece of metal or deep-drawn from a piece of sheet metal. Electrical signals, such as power and stimulation, enter and exit the package through hermetic feedthroughs, which are hermetically welded onto the package walls. The *feedthrough* assembly utilizes a ceramic or glass insulator to allow one or more wires to exit the package without contact with the package itself. During the assembly procedures, the electronic circuitry is placed in the package and connected internally to the feedthroughs, and the package is then welded closed. Tungsten Inert Gas (TIG), electron beam, or laser welding equipment is used for the final closure. Assuming integrity of all components, hermeticity with this package is ensured. This integrity can be checked by detecting gas leakage from the capsule. Metallic packaging requires that the receiving coil be placed outside the package to avoid significant loss of rf signal or power, thus requiring additional space within the body to accommodate the volume of the entire implant. Generally, the hermetic package and the receiving antenna are jointly embedded in an epoxy encapsulant, which provides electric isolation for the metallic antenna and stabilizes the entire implant assembly. Figure 16.3 shows such an implantable stimulator designed and made by the CWRU/Veterans Administration Program. The hermetic package is open, displaying the electronic *hybrid circuit*. More recently, alumina-based ceramic packages have been developed that allow hermetic sealing of the electronic circuitry together with enclosure of the receiving coil (Strojnik et al., 1994). This is possible due to the rf transparency of ceramics. The impact of this type of enclosure is still not fully investigated. The advantage of this approach is that the volume of the implant can be reduced, thus minimizing the biologic response, which is a function of volume. Yet, an unexplored issue of this packaging method is the effect of powerful electromagnetic fields on the implant circuits, lacking the protection of the metal enclosure. This is a particular concern with high gain (EMG, ENG, or EKG sensing) amplifiers, which in the future may be included in the implant

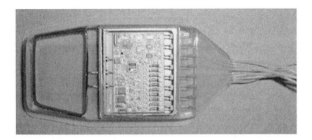

FIGURE 16.3 Photograph of a multichannel implantable stimulator telemeter. Hybrid circuit in titanium package is shown exposed. Receiving coil (left) is embedded in epoxy resin together with titanium case. Double feedthroughs are seen penetrating titanium capsule wall on the right.

package as part of back-telemetry circuits. Physical strength of ceramic packages and their resistance to impact will also require future investigation.

16.6 Leads and Electrodes

Leads connect the pulse generator to the electrodes. They must be sufficiently flexible to move across the joints while at the same time sufficiently sturdy to last for the decades of the intended life of the device. They must also be stretchable to allow change of distance between the pulse generator and the electrodes, associated with body movements. Ability to flex and to stretch is achieved by coiling the lead conductor into a helix and inserting the helix into a small-diameter silicone tubing. This way, both flexing movements and stretching forces exerted on the lead are attenuated, while translated into torsion movements and forces exerted on the coiled conductor. Using multi-strand rather than solid conductors further enhances the longevity. Several individually insulated multi-strand conductors can be coiled together, thus forming a multiple conductor lead wire. Most lead configurations include a connector at some point between the implant and the terminal electrode, allowing for replacement of the implanted receiver or leads in the event of failure. The connectors used have been either single pin in-line connectors located somewhere along the lead length or a multiport/multilead connector at the implant itself. Materials used for lead wires are stainless steels, MP35N (Co, Cr, Ni alloy), and noble metals and their alloys.

Electrodes deliver electrical charge to the stimulated tissues. Those placed on the muscle surface are called epimysial, while those inserted into the muscles are called intramuscular. Nerve stimulating electrodes are called epineural when placed against the nerve, or cuff electrodes when they encircle the nerve. Nerve electrodes may embrace the nerve in a spiral manner individually, or in an array configuration. Some implantable stimulation systems merely use exposed lead-wire conductor sutured to the epineurium as the electrode. Generally, nerve electrodes require approximately one-tenth of the energy for muscle activation as compared to muscle electrodes. However, they require more extensive surgery and may be less selective, but the potential for neural damage is greater than, for example, nerve encircling electrodes.

Electrodes are made of corrosion resistant materials, such as noble metals (platinum or iridium) and their alloys. For example, a platinum–iridium alloy consisting of 10% iridium and 90% platinum is commonly used as an electrode material. Epimysial electrodes developed at CWRU use Ø4 mm Pt90Ir10 discs placed on Dacron reinforced silicone backing. CWRU intramuscular electrodes employ a stainless steel lead-wire with the distal end de-insulated and configured into an electrode tip. A small, umbrella-like anchoring barb is attached to it. With this arrangement, the diameter of the electrode tip does not differ much from the lead wire diameter and this electrode can be introduced into a deep muscle with a trochar-like insertion tool. Figure 16.4 shows enlarged views of these electrodes.

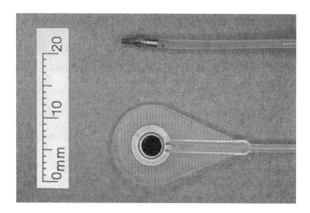

FIGURE 16.4 Implantable electrodes with attached lead wires. Intramuscular electrode (top) has stainless steel tip and anchoring barbs. Epimysial electrode has PtIr disk in the center and is backed by silicone-impregnated Dacron mesh.

16.7 Safety Issues of Implantable Stimulators

The targeted lifetime of implantable stimulators for neuromuscular control is the lifetime of their users, which is measured in tens of years. Resistance to premature failure must be assured by manufacturing processes and testing procedures. Appropriate materials must be selected that will withstand the working environment. Protection against mechanical and electrical hazards that may be encountered during the device lifetime must be incorporated in the design. Various procedures are followed and rigorous tests must be performed during and after its manufacturing to assure the quality and reliability of the device.

- *Manufacturing and testing*—Production of implantable electronic circuits and their encapsulation in many instances falls under the standards governing production and encapsulation of integrated circuits. To minimize the possibility of failure, the implantable electronic devices are manufactured in controlled clean-room environments, using high quality components and strictly defined manufacturing procedures. Finished devices are submitted to rigorous testing before being released for implantation. Also, many tests are carried out during the manufacturing process itself. To assure maximum reliability and product confidence, methods, tests, and procedures defined by military standards, such as MILSTD-883, are followed.
- *Bio-compatibility*—Since the implantable stimulators are surgically implanted in living tissue, an important part of their design has to be dedicated to biocompatibility, that is, their ability to dwell in living tissue without disrupting the tissue in its functions, creating adverse tissue response, or changing its own properties due to the tissue environment. Elements of biocompatibility include tissue reaction to materials, shape, and size, as well as electrochemical reactions on stimulation electrodes. There are known biomaterials used in the making of implantable stimulators. They include stainless steels, titanium and tantalum, noble metals such as platinum and iridium, as well as implantable grades of selected epoxy and silicone-based materials.
- *Susceptibility to electromagnetic interference (EMI) and electrostatic discharge (ESD)*— Electromagnetic fields can disrupt the operation of electronic devices, which may be lethal in situations with life support systems, but they may also impose risk and danger to users of neuromuscular stimulators. Emissions of EMI may come from outside sources; however, the external control unit is also a source of electromagnetic radiation. Electrostatic discharge shocks are not uncommon during the dry winter season. These shocks may reach voltages as high as 15 kV and more. Sensitive electronic components can easily be damaged by these shocks unless protective

design measures are taken. The electronic circuitry in implantable stimulators is generally protected by the metal case. However, the circuitry can be damaged through the feedthroughs either by handling or during the implantation procedure by the electrocautery equipment. ESD damage may happen even after implantation when long lead-wires are utilized. There are no standards directed specifically towards implantable electronic devices. The general standards put in place for electromedical equipment by the International Electrotechnical Commission provide guidance. The specifications require survival after 3 and 8 kV ESD discharges on all conductive and nonconductive accessible parts, respectively.

16.8 Implantable Stimulators in Clinical Use

16.8.1 Peripheral Nerve Stimulators

- *Manipulation*—Control of complex functions for movement, such as hand control, requires the use of many channels of stimulation. At the Case Western Reserve University and Cleveland VAMC, an eight-channel stimulator has been developed for grasp and release (Smith et al., 1987). This system uses eight channels of stimulation and a titanium-packaged, thick-film hybrid circuit as the pulse generator. The implant is distributed by the Neurocontrol Corporation (Cleveland, OH) under the name of Freehand®. It has been implanted in approximately 150 patients in the United States, Europe, Asia, and Australia. The implant is controlled by a dual-microprocessor external unit carried by the patient with an input control signal provided by the user's remaining volitional movement. Activation of the muscles provides two primary grasp patterns and allows the person to achieve functional performance that exceeds his or her capabilities without the use of the implanted system. This system received pre-market approval from the FDA in 1998.
- *Locomotion*—The first implantable stimulators were designed and implanted for the correction of the foot drop condition in hemiplegic patients. Medtronic's Neuromuscular Assist (NMA) device consisted of an rf receiver implanted in the inner thigh and connected to a cuff electrode embracing the peroneal nerve just beneath the head of fibula at the knee (McNeal et al., 1977; Waters et al., 1984). The Ljubljana peroneal implant had two versions (Vavken and Jeglic, 1976; Strojnik et al., 1987) with the common feature that the implant–rf receiver was small enough to be implanted next to the peroneal nerve in the fossa poplitea region. Epineural stimulating electrodes were an integral part of the implant. This feature and the comparatively small size make the Ljubljana implant a precursor of the microstimulators described in Section 16.9. Both NMA and the Ljubljana implants were triggered and synchronized with gait by a heel switch.

The same implant used for hand control and developed by the CWRU has also been implanted in the lower extremity musculature to assist incomplete quadriplegics in standing and transfer operations (Triolo et al., 1996). Since the design of the implant is completely transparent, it can generate any stimulation sequence requested by the external controller. For locomotion and transfer-related tasks, stimulation sequences are preprogrammed for individual users and activated by the user by means of pushbuttons. The implant (two in some applications) is surgically positioned in the lower abdominal region. Locomotion application uses the same electrodes as the manipulation system; however, the lead wires have to be somewhat longer.

- *Respiration*—Respiratory control systems involve a two-channel implantable stimulator with electrodes applied bilaterally to the phrenic nerve. Most of the devices in clinical use were developed by Avery Laboratories (Dobelle Institute) and employed discrete circuitry with epoxy encapsulation of the implant and a nerve cuff electrode. Approximately 1000 of these devices have been implanted in patients with respiratory disorders such as high-level tetraplegia (Glenn et al.,

1986). Activation of the phrenic nerve results in contraction of each hemidiaphragm in response to electrical stimulation. In order to minimize damage to the diaphragms during chronic use, alternation of the diaphragms has been employed, in which one hemidiaphragm will be activated for several hours followed by the second. A review of existing systems was given by Creasy et al. (1996). Astrotech of Finland also recently introduced a phrenic stimulator. More recently, DiMarco et al. (1997) have investigated use of CNS activation of a respiratory center to provide augmented breathing.

- *Urinary control*—Urinary control systems have been developed for persons with spinal cord injury. The most successful of these devices has been developed by Brindley et al. (1982) and is manufactured by Finetech, Ltd. (England). The implanted receiver consists of three separate stimulator devices, each with its own coil and circuitry, encapsulated within a single package. The sacral roots (S2, S3, and S4) are placed within a type of encircling electrode, and stimulation of the proper roots will generate contraction of both the bladder and the external sphincter. Cessation of stimulation results in faster relaxation of the external sphincter than of the bladder wall, which then results in voiding. Repeated trains of pulses applied in this manner will eliminate most urine, with only small residual amounts remaining. Approximately 1500 of these devices have been implanted around the world. This technology also has received FDA pre-market approval and is currently distributed by NeuroControl Corporation.

- *Scoliosis treatment*—Progressive lateral curvature of the adolescent vertebral column with simultaneous rotation is known as idiopathic scoliosis. Electrical stimulation applied to the convex side of the curvature has been used to stop or reduce its progression. Initially rf powered stimulators have been replaced by battery powered totally implanted devices (Bobechko et al., 1979; Herbert and Bobechko, 1989). Stimulation is applied intermittently, stimulation amplitudes are under 10.5 V (510 Ω), and frequency and pulsewidth are within usual FES parameter values.

16.8.2 Stimulators of Central Nervous System

Some stimulation systems have electrodes implanted on the surface of the central nervous system or in its deep areas. They do not produce functional movements; however, they "modulate" a pathological motor brain behavior and by that stop unwanted motor activity or abnormality. Therefore, they can be regarded as stimulators for neuromuscular control.

- *Cerebellar stimulation*—Among the earliest stimulators from this category are cerebellar stimulators for control of reduction of effects of cerebral palsy in children. Electrodes are placed on the cerebellar surface with the leads penetrating cranium and dura. The pulse generator is located subcutaneously in the chest area and produces intermittent stimulation bursts. There are about 600 patients using these devices (Davis, 1997).

- *Vagal stimulation*—Intermittent stimulation of the vagus nerve with 30 s on and 5 min off has been shown to reduce frequency of epileptic seizures. A pacemaker-like device, developed by Cyberonics, is implanted in the chest area with a bipolar helical electrode wrapped around the left vagus nerve in the neck. The stimulation sequence is programmed (most often parameter settings are 30 Hz, 500 µs, 1.75 mA); however, patients have some control over the device using a handheld magnet (Terry et al., 1991). More than 3000 patients have been implanted with this device, which received the pre-marketing approval (PMA) from the FDA in 1997.

- *Deep brain stimulation*—Recently, in 1998, an implantable stimulation device (Activa by Medtronic) was approved by the FDA that can dramatically reduce uncontrollable tremor in patients with Parkinson's disease or essential tremor (Koller et al., 1997). With this device, an electrode array is placed stereotactically into the ventral intermediate nucleus of thalamic region of the brain. Lead wires again connect the electrodes to a programmable pulse generator implanted in the chest area. Application of high frequency stimulation (130 Hz, 60–210 μs, 0.25–2.75 V) can immediately suppress the patient's tremor.

16.9 Future of Implantable Electrical Stimulators

16.9.1 Distributed Stimulators

One of the major concerns with multichannel implantable neuromuscular stimulators is the multitude of leads that exit the pulse generator and their management during surgical implantation. Routing of multiple leads virtually increases the implant size and by that the burden that an implant imposes on the tissue. A solution to that may be distributed stimulation systems with a single outside controller and multiple single-channel implantable devices implanted throughout the structures to be stimulated. This concept has been pursued both by the Alfred E. Mann Foundation (Strojnik et al., 1992; Cameron et al., 1997) and the University of Michigan (Ziaie et al., 1997). Microinjectable stimulator modules have been developed that can be injected into the tissue, into a muscle, or close to a nerve through a lumen of a hypodermic needle. A single external coil can address and activate a number of these devices located within its field, on a pulse-to-pulse basis. A glass-encapsulated microstimulator developed at the AEMF is shown in Figure 16.5.

16.9.2 Sensing of Implantable Transducer-Generated and Physiological Signals

External command sources such as the shoulder-controlled joystick utilized by the Freehand system impose additional constraints on the implantable stimulator users, since they have to be donned by an attendant. Permanently implanted control sources make neuroprosthetic devices much more attractive and easier to use. An implantable joint angle transducer (IJAT) has been developed at the CWRU that consists of a magnet and an array of magnetic sensors implanted in the distal and the proximal end of a joint, respectively (Smith et al., 1998). The sensor is connected to the implantable stimulator package, which provides the power and also transmits the sensor data to the external controller, using a back-telemetry link. Figure 16.6 shows a radiograph of the IJAT implanted in a patient's wrist. Myoelectric signals (MES) from muscles not affected by paralysis are another attractive control source for implantable neuromuscular stimulators. Amplified and bin-integrated EMG signal from uninvolved muscles, such as the sterno-cleido-mastoid muscle, has been shown to contain enough information to control an upper extremity neuroprosthesis (Scott et al., 1996). EMG signal is being utilized by a multichannel stimulator–telemeter developed at the CWRU, containing 12 stimulator channels and 2 MES channels integrated into the same platform (Strojnik et al., 1998).

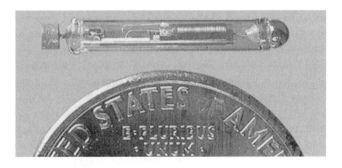

FIGURE 16.5 Microstimulator developed at A.E. Mann Foundation. Dimensions are roughly 2 × 16 mm. Electrodes at the ends are made of tantalum and iridium, respectively.

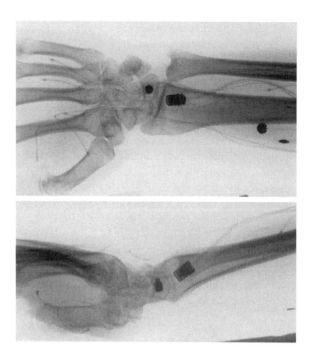

FIGURE 16.6 Radiograph of the joint angle transducer (IJAT) implanted in the wrist. The magnet is implanted in the lunate bone (top) while the magnetic sensor array is implanted in the radius. Leads going to the implant case can be seen as well as intramuscular and epimysial electrodes with their individual lead wires.

16.10 Summary

Implantable stimulators for neuromuscular control are an important tool in rehabilitation of paralyzed individuals with preserved neuromuscular apparatus, as well as in the treatment of some neurological disorders that result in involuntary motor activity. Their impact on rehabilitation is still in its infancy; however, it is expected to increase with further progress in microelectronics technology, development of smaller and better sensors, and with improvements of advanced materials. Advancements in neurophysiological science are also expected to bring forward wider utilization of possibilities offered by implantable neuromuscular stimulators.

Defining Terms

Biocompatibility: Ability of a foreign object to coexist in a living tissue.
Electrical stimulation: Diagnostic, therapeutic, and rehabilitational method used to excite motor
        nerves with the aim of contracting the appropriate muscles and obtain limb movement.
EMG activity: Muscular electrical activity associated with muscle contraction and production of force.
Feedthrough: Device that allows passage of a conductor through a hermetic barrier.
Hybrid circuit: Electronic circuit combining miniature active and passive components on a single
        ceramic substrate.
Implantable stimulator: Biocompatible electronic stimulator designed for surgical implantation and
        operation in a living tissue.
Lead wire: Flexible and strong insulated conductor connecting pulse generator to stimulating electrodes.
Paralysis: Loss of power of voluntary movement in a muscle through injury to or disease to its nerve
        supply.

rf-radiofrequency: Pertaining to electromagnetic propagation of power and signal in frequencies above those used in electrical power distribution.

Stimulating electrode: Conductive device that transfers stimulating current to a living tissue. On its surface, the electric charge carriers change from electrons to ions or vice versa.

References

Bobechko, W.P., Herbert, M.A., and Friedman, H.G. 1979. Electrospinal instrumentation for scoliosis: Current status. *Orthop. Clin. North. Am.* 10: 927.

Brindley, G.S., Polkey, C.E., and Rushton, D.N. 1982. Sacral anterior root stimulators for bladder control in paraplegia. *Paraplegia* 20: 365.

Cameron, T., Loeb, G.E., Peck, R.A., Schulman, J.H., Strojnik, P., and Troyk, P.R. 1997. Micromodular implants to provide electrical stimulation of paralyzed muscles and limbs. *IEEE Trans. Biomed. Eng.* 44: 781.

Creasey, G., Elefteriades, J., DiMarco, A., Talonen, P., Bijak, M., Girsch, W., and Kantor, C. 1996. Electrical stimulation to restore respiration. *J. Rehab. Res. Dev.* 33: 123.

Davis, R. 1997. Cerebellar stimulation for movement disorders. In P.L. Gildenberg and R.R. Tasker (eds.), *Textbook of Stereotactic and Functional Neurosurgery*, McGraw-Hill, New York.

DiMarco, A.F., Romaniuk, J.R., Kowalski, K.E., and Supinski, G.S. 1997. Efficacy of combined inspiratory intercostal and expiratory muscle pacing to maintain artificial ventilation. *Am. J. Respir. Crit. Care Med.* 156: 122.

Glenn, W.W., Phelps, M.L., Elefteriades, J.A., Dentz, B., and Hogan, J.F. 1986. Twenty years of experience in phrenic nerve stimulation to pace the diaphragm pacing. *Clin. Electrophysiol.* 9: 780.

Graupe, D. and Kohn, K.H. 1998. Functional neuromuscular stimulator for short-distance ambulation by certain thoracic-level spinal-cord-injured paraplegics. *Surg. Neurol.* 50: 202.

Herbert, M.A. and Bobechko, W.P. 1989. Scoliosis treatment in children using a programmable, totally implantable muscle stimulator (ESI). *IEEE Trans. Biomed. Eng.* 36: 801.

Koller, W., Pahwa, R., Busenbark, K., Hubble, J., Wilkinson, S., Lang, A., Tuite, P. et al. 1997. High-frequency unilateral thalamic stimulation in the treatment of essential and parkinsonian tremor. *Ann. Neurol.* 42: 292.

Kralj, A. and Bajd, T. 1989. *Functional Electrical Stimulation: Standing and Walking after Spinal Cord Injury*, CRC Press, Inc., Boca Raton, FL.

Liberson, W.T., Holmquest, H.J., Scot, D., and Dow, M. 1961. Functional electrotherapy: Stimulation of the peroneal nerve synchronized with the swing phase of the gait of hemiplegic patients. *Arch. Phys. Med. Rehab.* 42: 101.

Marsolais, E.B. and Kobetic, R. 1986. Implantation techniques and experience with percutaneous intramuscular electrodes in lower extremities. *J. Rehab. Res. Dev.* 23: 1.

McNeal, D.R., Waters, R., and Reswick, J. 1977. Experience with implanted electrodes. *Neurosurgery* 1: 228.

Memberg, W., Peckham, P.H., Thorpe, G.B., Keith, M.W., and Kicher, T.P. 1993. An analysis of the reliability of percutaneous intramuscular electrodes in upper extremity FNS applications. *IEEE Trans. Biomed. Eng.* 1: 126.

Rebersek, S. and Vodovnik, L. 1973. Proportionally controlled functional electrical stimulation of hand. *Arch. Phys. Med. Rehab.* 54: 378.

Scott, T.R.D., Peckham, P.H., and Kilgore, K.L. 1996. Tri-state myoelectric control of bilateral upper extremity neuroprostheses for tetraplegic individuals. *IEEE Trans. Rehab. Eng.* 2: 251.

Smith, B., Peckham, P.H., Keith, M.W., and Roscoe, D.D. 1987. An externally powered, multichannel, implantable stimulator for versatile control of paralyzed muscle. *IEEE Trans. Biomed. Eng.* 34: 499.

Smith, B., Tang, Z., Johnson, M.W., Pourmehdi, S., Gazdik, M.M., Buckett, J.R., and Peckham, P.H. 1998. An externally powered, multichannel, implantable stimulator–telemeter for control of paralyzed muscle. *IEEE Trans. Biomed. Eng.* 45: 463.

Strojnik, P., Acimovic, R., Vavken, E., Simic, V., and Stanic, U. 1987. Treatment of drop foot using an implantable peroneal underknee stimulator. *Scand. J. Rehab. Med.* 19: 37.

Strojnik, P., Meadows, P., Schulman, J.H., and Whitmoyer, D. 1994. Modification of a cochlear stimulation system for FES applications. *Basic Appl. Myol.* BAM 4: 129.

Strojnik, P., Pourmehdi, S., and Peckham, P. 1998. Incorporating FES control sources into implantable stimulators. *Proceedings of the 6th Vienna International Workshop on Functional Electrostimulation*, Vienna, Austria.

Strojnik, P., Schulman, J., Loeb, G., and Troyk, P. 1992. Multichannel FES system with distributed microstimulators. *Proceedings of the 14th Annual International Conference IEEE*, MBS, Paris, p. 1352.

Terry, R.S., Tarver, W.B., and Zabara, J. 1991. The implantable neurocybernetic prosthesis system. *Pacing Clin. Electrophysiol.* 14: 86.

Triolo, R.J., Bieri, C., Uhlir, J., Kobetic, R., Scheiner, A., and Marsolais, E.B. 1996. Implanted functional neuromuscular stimulation systems for individuals with cervical spinal cord injuries: Clinical case reports. *Arch. Phys. Med. Rehabil.* 77: 1119.

Vavken, E. and Jeglic, A. 1976. Application of an implantable stimulator in the rehabilitation of paraplegic patients. *Int. Surg.* 61: 335–339.

Waters, R.L., McNeal, D.R., and Clifford, B. 1984. Correction of footdrop in stroke patients via surgically implanted peroneal nerve stimulator. *Acta Orthop. Belg.* 50: 285.

Ziaie, B., Nardin, M.D., Coghlan, A.R., and Najafi, K. 1997. A single-channel implantable microstimulator for functional neuromuscular stimulation. *IEEE Trans. Biomed. Eng.* 44: 909.

Further Information

Additional references on early work in FES which augment peer review publications can be found in Proceedings from Conferences in Dubrovnik and Vienna. These are the *External Control of Human Extremities* and the *Vienna International Workshop on Electrostimulation*, respectively.

17

Respiration

Leslie A. Geddes

Purdue University

17.1 Lung Volumes

The amount of air flowing into and out of the lungs with each breath is called the tidal volume (TV). In a typical adult this amounts to about 500 mL during quiet breathing. The respiratory system is capable of moving much more air than the tidal volume. Starting at the *resting expiratory level* (REL in Figure 17.1), it is possible to inhale a volume amounting to about seven times the tidal volume; this volume is called the *inspiratory capacity* (IC). A measure of the ability to inspire more than the tidal volume is the *inspiratory reserve volume* (IRV), which is also shown in Figure 17.1. Starting from REL, it is possible to forcibly exhale a volume amounting to about twice the tidal volume; this volume is called the *expiratory reserve volume* (ERV). However, even with the most forcible expiration, it is not possible to exhale all the air from the lungs; a *residual volume* (RV) about equal to the expiratory reserve volume remains. The sum of the expiratory reserve volume and the residual volume is designated the *functional residual capacity* (FRC). The volume of air exhaled from a maximum inspiration to a maximum expiration is called the *vital capacity* (VC). The *total lung capacity* (TLC) is the total air within the lungs, that is, that which can be moved in a vital-capacity maneuver plus the residual volume. All except the residual volume can be determined with a volume-measuring instrument such as a spirometer connected to the airway.

17.2 Pulmonary Function Tests

In addition to the static lung volumes just identified, there are several time-dependent volumes associated with the respiratory act. The *minute volume* (MV) is the volume of air per breath (tidal volume) multiplied by the respiratory rate (R), that is, MV = (TV) R. It is obvious that the same minute volume can be produced by rapid shallow or slow deep breathing. However, the effectiveness is not the same, because not all the respiratory air participates in gas exchange, there being a dead space volume. Therefore the alveolar ventilation is the important quantity which is defined as the tidal volume (TV) minus the dead space (DS) multiplied by the respiratory rate R, that is, alveolar ventilation = (TV–DS) R. In a normal adult subject, the dead space amounts to about 150 mL, or 2 mL/kg.

17.2.1 Dynamic Tests

Several timed respiratory volumes describe the ability of the respiratory system to move air. Among these are *forced vital capacity* (FVC), *forced expiratory volume* in *t* seconds (FEV$_t$), the *maximum ventilatory*

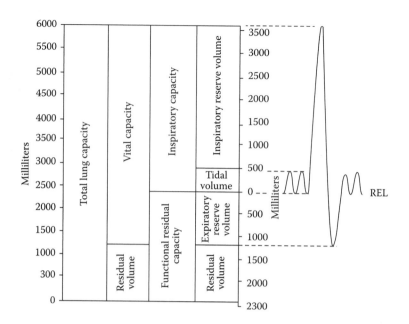

FIGURE 17.1   Lung volumes.

volume (MVV), which was previously designated the *maximum breathing capacity* (MBC), and the *peak flow* (PF). These quantities are measured with a spirometer without valves and CO_2 absorber or with a pneumotachograph coupled to an integrator.

17.2.1.1 Forced Vital Capacity

Forced vital capacity (FVC) is shown in Figure 17.2 and is measured by taking the maximum inspiration and forcing all of the inspired air out as rapidly as possible. Table 17.1 presents normal values for males and females.

17.2.1.2 Forced Expiratory Volume

Forced expiratory volume in t seconds (FEV_t) is shown in Figure 17.2, which identifies $FEV_{0.5}$ and $FEV_{1.0}$, and Table 17.1 presents normal values for $FEV_{1.0}$.

17.2.1.3 Maximum Voluntary Ventilation

Maximum voluntary ventilation (MVV) is the volume of air moved in 1 min when breathing as deeply and rapidly as possible. The test is performed for 20 s and the volume scaled to a 1-min value; Table 17.1 presents normal values.

17.2.1.4 Peak Flow

Peak flow (PF) in L/min is the maximum flow velocity attainable during an FEV maneuver and represents the maximum slope of the expired volume–time curve (Figure 17.2); typical normal values are shown in Table 17.1.

17.2.1.5 The Water-Sealed Spirometer

The water-sealed spirometer was the traditional device used to measure the volume of air moved in respiration. The Latin word *spirare* means to breathe. The most popular type of spirometer consists of a hollow cylinder closed at one end, inverted and suspended in an annular space filled with water to

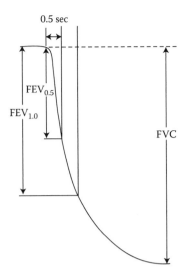

FIGURE 17.2 The measurement of timed forced expiratory volume (FEV_t) and forced vital capacity (FVC).

provide an air-tight seal. Figure 17.3 illustrates the method of suspending the counterbalanced cylinder (bell), which is free to move up and down to accommodate the volume of air under it. Movement of the bell, which is proportional to volume, is usually recorded by an inking pen applied to a graphic record which is caused to move with a constant speed. Below the cylinder, in the space that accommodates the volume of air, are inlet and outlet breathing tubes. At the end of one or both of these tubes is a check valve designed to maintain a unidirectional flow of air through the spirometer. Outside the spirometer the two breathing tubes are brought to a Y tube which is connected to a mouthpiece. With a pinch clamp placed on the nose, inspiration diminishes the volume of air under the bell, which descends, causing the stylus to rise on the graphic record. Expiration produces the reverse effect. Thus, starting with the spirometer half-filled, quiet respiration causes the bell to rise and fall. By knowing the "bell factor," the volume of air moved per centimeter excursion of the bell, the volume change can be quantitated. Although a variety of flowmeters are now used to measure respiratory volumes, the spirometer with a CO_2 absorber is ideally suited to measure oxygen uptake.

TABLE 17.1   Dynamic Volumes

Males

FVC (L) = 0.133H − 0.022A − 3.60(SEE = 0.58)[a]
FEV1 (L) = 0.094H − 0.028A − 1.59(SEE = 0.52)[a]
MVV (L/min) = 3.39H − 1.26A − 21.4(SEE = 29)[a]
PF (L/min) = (10.03 − 0.038A)H[b]

Females

FVC (L) = 0.111H − 0.015A − 3.16(SD = 0.42)[c]
FEV1 (L) = 0.068H − 0.023A − 0.92(SD = 0.37)[c]
MVV (L/min) = 2.05H − 0.57A − 5.5(SD = 10.7)[c]
PF (L/min) = (7.44 − 0.0183A) H[c]

Note: H = height in inches, A = age in years, L = liters, L/min = liters per minute, SEE = standard error of estimate, SD = standard deviation.
[a] Kory et al. 1961. *Am. J. Med.* 30: 243.
[b] Leiner et al. 1963. *Am. Rev. Resp. Dis.* 88: 644.
[c] Lindall, Medina, and Grismer. 1967. *Am. Rev. Resp. Dis.* 95: 1061.

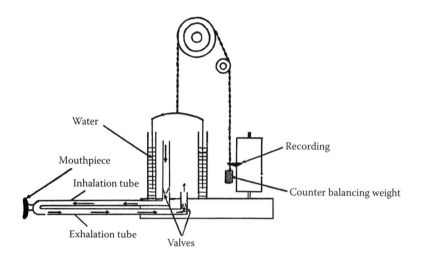

FIGURE 17.3   The simple spirometer.

17.2.1.6 Oxygen Uptake

A second and very important use for the water-filled spirometer is measurement of oxygen used per unit of time, designated the O_2 *uptake*. This measurement is accomplished by incorporating a soda-lime, carbon-dioxide absorber into the spirometer as shown in Figure 17.4. Soda-lime is a mixture of calcium hydroxide, sodium hydroxide, and silicates of sodium and calcium. The exhaled carbon dioxide combines with the soda-lime and becomes solid carbonates. A small amount of heat is liberated by this reaction.

Starting with a spirometer filled with oxygen and connected to a subject, respiration causes the bell to move up and down (indicating tidal volume) as shown in Figure 17.5. With continued respiration the baseline of the recording rises, reflecting disappearance of oxygen from under the bell. By measuring the slope of the baseline on the spirogram, the volume of oxygen consumed per minute can be determined. Figure 17.5 presents a typical example along with calculation.

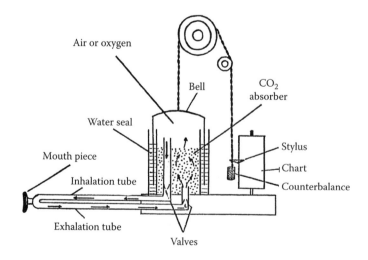

FIGURE 17.4   The spirometer with CO_2 absorber and a record of oxygen uptake.

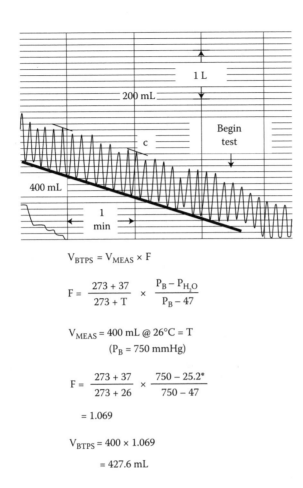

$$V_{BTPS} = V_{MEAS} \times F$$

$$F = \frac{273 + 37}{273 + T} \times \frac{P_B - P_{H_2O}}{P_B - 47}$$

$$V_{MEAS} = 400 \text{ mL @ } 26°C = T$$
$$(P_B = 750 \text{ mmHg})$$

$$F = \frac{273 + 37}{273 + 26} \times \frac{750 - 25.2^*}{750 - 47}$$

$$= 1.069$$

$$V_{BTPS} = 400 \times 1.069$$

$$= 427.6 \text{ mL}$$

FIGURE 17.5 Oxygen consumption.

17.2.1.7 The Dry Spirometer

The water-sealed spirometer was the most popular device for measuring the volumes of respiratory gases; however, it is not without its inconveniences. The presence of water causes corrosion of the metal parts. Maintenance is required to keep the device in good working order over prolonged periods. To eliminate these problems, manufacturers have developed dry spirometers. The most common type employs a collapsible rubber or plastic bellows, the expansion of which is recorded during breathing. The earlier rubber models had a decidedly undesirable characteristic which caused their abandonment. When the bellows were in its mid-position, the resistance to breathing was a minimum; when fully collapsed, it imposed a slight negative resistance; and when fully extended it imposed a slight positive resistance to breathing. Newer units with compliant plastic bellows minimize this defect.

17.2.2 The Pneumotachograph

The pneumotachograph is a device which is placed directly in the airway to measure the velocity of air flow. The volume per breath is therefore the integral of the velocity–time record during inspiration or expiration. Planimetric integration of the record, or electronic integration of the velocity–time signal, yields the tidal volume. Although tidal volume is perhaps more easily recorded with the spirometer, the

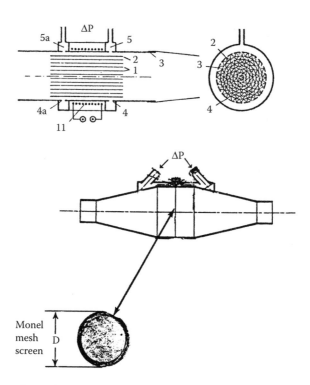

FIGURE 17.6 Pneumotachographs.

dynamics of respiration are better displayed by the pneumotachograph, which offers less resistance to the air stream and exhibits a much shorter response time—so short in most instruments that cardiac impulses are often clearly identifiable in the velocity–time record.

If a specially designed resistor is placed in a tube in which the respiratory gases flow, a pressure drop will appear across it. Below the point of turbulent flow, the pressure drop is linearly related to air-flow velocity. The resistance may consist of a wire screen or a series of capillary tubes; Figure 17.6 illustrates both types. Detection and recording of this pressure differential constitutes a pneumotachogram; Figure 17.7 presents a typical air–velocity record, along with the spirogram, which is the integral of the flow signal. The small-amplitude artifacts in the pneumotachogram are cardiac impulses.

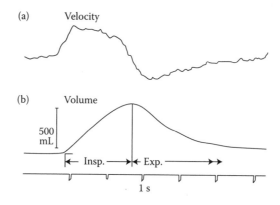

FIGURE 17.7 Velocity (a) and volume changes (b) during normal, quiet breathing; b is the integral of a.

For human application, linear flow rates up to 200 L/min should be recordable with fidelity. The resistance to breathing depends upon the flow rate, and it is difficult to establish an upper limit of tolerable resistance. Silverman and Whittenberger (1950) stated that a resistance of 6 mm H_2O is perceptible to human subjects. Many of the high-fidelity pneumotachographs offer 5–10 mm H_2O resistance at 100 and 200 L/min. It would appear that such resistances are acceptable in practice.

Response times of 15–40 ms seem to be currently in use. Fry et al. (1957) analyzed the dynamic characteristics of three types of commercially available, differential-pressure pneumotachographs which employed concentric cylinders, screen mesh, and parallel plates for the air resistors. Using a high-quality, differential-pressure transducer with each, they measured total flow resistance ranging from 5 to 15 cm H_2O. Frequency response curves taken on one model showed fairly uniform response to 40 Hz; the second model showed a slight increase in response at 50 Hz, and the third exhibited a slight drop in response at this frequency.

17.2.3 The Nitrogen-Washout Method for Measuring FRC

The *functional residual capacity* (FRC) and the *residual volume* (RV) are the only lung compartments that cannot be measured with a volume-measuring device. Measuring these requires use of the nitrogen analyzer and application of the dilution method.

Because nitrogen does not participate in respiration, it can be called a *diluent*. Inspired and expired air contains about 80% nitrogen. Between breaths, the FRC of the lungs contains the same concentration of nitrogen as in environmental air, that is, 80%. By causing a subject to inspire from a spirometer filled with 100% oxygen and to exhale into a second collecting spirometer, all the nitrogen in the FRC is replaced by oxygen, that is, the nitrogen is "washed out" into the second spirometer. Measurement of the concentration of nitrogen in the collecting spirometer, along with a knowledge of its volume, permits calculation of the amount of nitrogen originally in the functional residual capacity and hence allows calculation of the FRC, as now will be shown.

Figure 17.8 illustrates the arrangement of equipment for the nitrogen-washout test. Note that two check valves, (I, EX) are on both sides of the subject's breathing tube, and the nitrogen meter is connected to the mouthpiece. Valve V is used to switch the subject from breathing environmental air to the measuring system. The left-hand spirometer contains 100% oxygen, which is inhaled by the subject via valve I. Of course, a nose clip must be applied so that all the respired gases flow through the breathing tube connected to the mouthpiece. It is in this tube that the sampling inlet for the nitrogen analyzer is located. Starting at the resting expiratory level, inhalation of pure oxygen causes the nitrogen analyzer

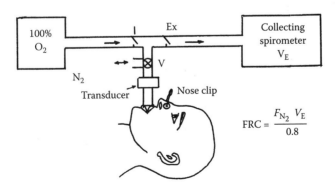

FIGURE 17.8 Arrangement of equipment for the nitrogen-washout technique. Valve V allows the subject to breathe room air until the test is started. The test is started by operating valve V at the end of a normal breath, that is, the subject starts breathing 100% O_2 through the inspiratory valve (I) and exhales the N_2 and O_2 mixture into a collecting spirometer via the expiratory valve EX.

to indicate zero. Expiration closes valve I and opens valve EX. The first expired breath contains nitrogen derived from the FRC (diluted by the oxygen which was inspired); the nitrogen analyzer indicates this percentage. The exhaled gases are collected in the right-hand spirometer. The collecting spirometer and all the interconnecting tubing was first flushed with oxygen to eliminate all nitrogen. This simple procedure eliminates the need for applying corrections and facilitates calculation of the FRC. With continued breathing, the nitrogen analyzer indicates less and less nitrogen because it is being washed out of the FRC and is replaced by oxygen. Figure 17.9 presents a typical record of the diminishing concentration of expired nitrogen throughout the test. In most laboratories, the test is continued until the concentration of nitrogen falls to about 1%. The nitrogen analyzer output permits identification of this concentration. In normal subjects, virtually all the nitrogen can be washed out of the FRC in about 5 min.

If the peaks on the nitrogen-washout record are joined, a smooth exponential decay curve is obtained in normal subjects. A semilog of N_2 vs. time provides a straight line. In subjects with trapped air, or poorly ventilated alveoli, the nitrogen-washout curve consists of several exponentials as the multiple poorly ventilated regions give up their nitrogen. In such subjects, the time taken to wash out all the nitrogen usually exceeds 10 min. Thus, the nitrogen concentration–time curve provides useful diagnostic information on ventilation of the alveoli.

If it is assumed that all the collected (washed-out) nitrogen was uniformly distributed within the lungs, it is easy to calculate the FRC. If the environmental air contains 80% nitrogen, then the volume of nitrogen in the functional residual capacity is 0.8 (FRC). Because the volume of expired gas in the collecting spirometer is known, it is merely necessary to determine the concentration of nitrogen in this volume. To do so requires admitting some of this gas to the inlet valve of the nitrogen analyzer. Note that this concentration of nitrogen (F_{N2}) exists in a volume which includes the volume of air expired (V_E) plus the original volume of oxygen in the collecting spirometer (V_0) at the start of the test and the volume of the tubing (V_t) leading from the expiratory collecting valve. It is therefore advisable to start with an empty collecting spirometer ($V_0 = 0$). Usually the tubing volume (V_t) is negligible with respect to the volume of expired gas collected in a typical washout test. In this situation the volume of nitrogen collected is $V_E F_{N_2}$, where F_{N_2} is the fraction of nitrogen within the collected gas. Thus, 0.80 (FRC) $= F_{N_2}(V_E)$. Therefore,

$$\text{FRC} = \frac{F_{N_2} V_E}{0.80} \tag{17.1}$$

It is important to note that the value for FRC so obtained is at ambient temperature and pressure and is saturated with water vapor (ATPS). In respiratory studies, this value is converted to body temperature and saturated with water vapor (BTPS).

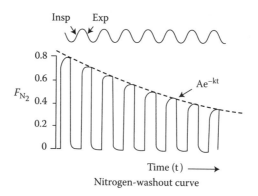

FIGURE 17.9   The nitrogen-washout curve.

In the example shown in Figure 17.9, the washout to 1% took about 44 breaths. With a breathing rate of 12/min, the washout time was 220 s. The volume collected (V_E) was 22 L and the concentration of nitrogen in this volume was 0.085 (F_{N_2}); therefore,

$$FRC = \frac{0.085 \times 22,000}{0.80} = 2,337 \text{ mL} \tag{17.2}$$

17.3 Physiologic Dead Space

The volume of ventilated lung that does not participate in gas exchange is the physiologic dead space (V_d). It is obvious that the physiologic dead space includes anatomic dead space, as well as the volume of any alveoli that are not perfused. In the lung, there are theoretically four types of alveoli, as shown in Figure 17.10. The normal alveolus (A) is both ventilated and perfused with blood. There are alveoli that are ventilated but not perfused (B); such alveoli contribute significantly to the physiologic dead space. There are alveoli that are not ventilated but perfused (C); such alveoli do not provide the exchange of respiratory gases. Finally, there are alveoli that are both poorly ventilated and poorly perfused (D); such alveoli contain high CO_2 and N_2 and low O_2. These alveoli are the last to expel their CO_2 and N_2 in washout tests.

Measurement of physiologic dead space is based on the assumption that there is almost complete equilibrium between alveolar pCO_2 and pulmonary capillary blood. Therefore, the arterial pCO_2 represents mean alveolar pCO_2 over many breaths when an arterial blood sample is drawn for analysis of pCO_2. The Bohr equation for physiologic dead space is

$$V_d = \left[\frac{paCO_2 - pECO_2}{paCO_2} \right] V_E \tag{17.3}$$

In this expression, $paCO_2$ is the partial pressure in the arterial blood sample which is withdrawn slowly during the test; $pECO_2$ is the partial pressure of CO_2 in the volume of expired air; V_E is the volume of expired air per breath (tidal volume).

In a typical test, the subject would breathe in room air and exhale into a collapsed (Douglas) bag. The test is continued for 3 min or more, and the number of breaths is counted in that period. An arterial blood sample is withdrawn during the collection period. The pCO_2 in the expired gas is measured, and

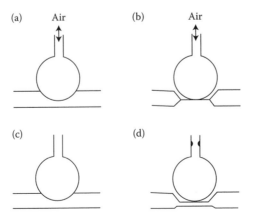

FIGURE 17.10 The four types of alveoli. (a) Ventilated and perfused. (b) Ventilated and not perfused. (c) Perfused and not ventilated. (d) Poorly perfused poorly ventilated.

then the volume of expired gas is measured by causing it to flow into a spirometer or flowmeter by collapsing the collecting bag.

In a typical 3-min test, the collected volume is 33 L, and the pCO_2 in the expired gas is 14.5 mm Hg. During the test, the pCO_2 in the arterial blood sample was 40 mm Hg. The number of breaths was 60; therefore, the average tidal volume was $33,000/60 = 550$ mL. The physiologic dead space (V_d) is

$$V_d = \left[\frac{40 - 14.5}{40} \right] 550 = 350 \text{ mL} \tag{17.4}$$

It is obvious that an elevated physiological dead space indicates lung tissue that is not perfused with blood.

References

Fry D.I., Hyatt R.E., and McCall C.B. 1957. Evaluation of three types of respiratory flowmeters. *Appl. Physiol.* 10: 210.

Silverman L. and Whittenberger J. 1950. Clinical pneumotachograph. *Meth. Med. Res.* 2: 104.

18

Mechanical Ventilation

Khosrow Behbehani
University of Texas

18.1 Introduction

This chapter provides an overview of the structure and function of mechanical ventilators. Mechanical ventilators, which are often also called respirators, are used to artificially ventilate the lungs of patients who are unable to breathe naturally from the atmosphere. In almost 105 years of development, many mechanical ventilators with different designs have been manufactured (Macintyre and Branson, 2009). Very early devices used bellows that were manually operated to inflate the lungs. Today's respirators employ an array of sophisticated components, such as microprocessors, fast-response servo valves, and precision transducers to mechanically ventilate the incapacitated patients. Large varieties of ventilators are now available for short-term treatment of acute respiratory dysfunction as well as long-term therapy for chronic respiratory conditions.

It is reasonable to broadly classify today's ventilators into two groups. The first and indeed the largest class is the critical care respirators used primarily in hospitals to treat patients for acute pulmonary disorders or following certain surgical procedures. The second class of mechanical ventilators includes less complicated machines that are primarily used at home to treat patients with chronic respiratory disorders.

The level of design complexity and engineering needed for the critical care ventilators is higher than the ventilators used for chronic treatment. However, many of the engineering concepts employed in designing critical care ventilators can also be applied in the simpler chronic care units. Therefore, this chapter focuses on the design of intensive care ventilators. Hence, the terms respirator, mechanical ventilator, or ventilator will be used from this point to refer to the intensive care unit respirators.

From the beginning, the designers of mechanical ventilators realized that in the vast majority of cases, the main task of a respirator is to ventilate the lungs in a manner as close to natural respiration

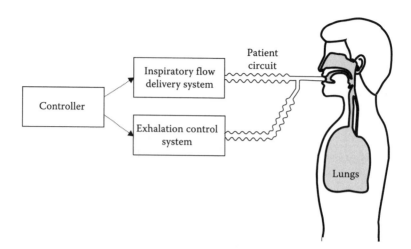

FIGURE 18.1   A simplified diagram of the functional blocks of a positive-pressure ventilator.

as possible. Since natural inspiration is a result of negative pressure in the pleural cavity generated by the distention of the diaphragm, designers initially developed ventilators that created the same effect. These ventilators are called negative-pressure ventilators. However, almost all modern ventilators use pressures greater than atmospheric pressures to ventilate the lungs and therefore they are known as positive-pressure ventilators. Owing to the overwhelming prevalence of positive-pressure ventilators in treating patients, this chapter describes only the positive-pressure ventilators.

18.2 Positive-Pressure Ventilators

Positive-pressure ventilators generate the inspiratory flow by applying a positive pressure (greater than the atmospheric pressure) to the airways. Figure 18.1 shows a simplified block diagram of a positive-pressure ventilator. During inspiration, the inspiratory flow delivery system creates a positive pressure in the tubes connected to the patient's airway, called *patient circuit,* and the exhalation control system closes a valve at the outlet of the tubing to the atmosphere. When the ventilator switches to exhalation, the inspiratory flow delivery system stops the positive pressure and the exhalation valve opens to the atmosphere. The use of a positive pressure gradient in creating the flow allows treating patients with high lung resistance and low compliance. As a result, positive-pressure ventilators have been very successful in treating a variety of breathing disorders, such as chronic obstructive pulmonary disorder, lung edema, and obstructed airways.

Positive-pressure ventilators have been employed to treat patients of all ages ranging from neonates to the elderly. Owing to anatomical differences between various patient populations, the ventilators and their modes of treating infants are different from those for adults. Nonetheless, their fundamental engineering design principles are similar. Adult ventilators comprise a larger percentage of ventilators manufactured and used in clinics. Therefore, the emphasis here is on the description of adult positive-pressure ventilators. Specifically, the concepts presented will be illustrated using a microprocessor-based design example, as almost all modern ventilators use microprocessor for the control of breath delivery.

18.3 Ventilation Modes

Since the advent of respirators, clinicians have devised various strategies to ventilate the lungs based on patient's conditions. As a result, two main categories of ventilation modes have been defined:

mandatory and spontaneous. *Mandatory mode* refers to the strategy for treating patients who need the respirator to completely take over the task of ventilating their lungs. However, some patients are able to exert the respiratory effort needed to breathe on their own, but may need to remain on the ventilator to receive oxygen-enriched air flow or slightly elevated airway pressure. When a ventilator delivers a breath to the patient according to the level of effort exerted by the patient, it is said that the ventilator operates in *spontaneous mode*. In many cases, it is necessary to first treat the patient with mandatory ventilation and as the patient's condition improves, spontaneous ventilation is introduced to wean the patient from mandatory breathing and restore natural breathing. For this purpose, several schemes for combining mandatory and spontaneous breathing have been established. For instance, when a patient is able to generate the needed effort for few breaths, but not sufficient for completely proper ventilation, mandatory breaths are added intermittently to supplement the patient's spontaneous breathing. Such a scheme is simply referred to as *synchronized intermittent mandatory ventilation* (SIMV).

18.3.1 Mandatory Ventilation

Responding to the clinicians' needs, biomedical engineers have employed two rather distinct approaches for delivering mandatory breaths: *volume-* and *pressure-controlled ventilation*. Volume-controlled ventilation refers to delivering a specified tidal volume to the patient during the inspiratory phase. Pressure-controlled ventilation refers to raising the airway pressure to a desired level (set by the therapist) during the inspiratory phase of each breath. Regardless of the type, a ventilator operating in mandatory mode must control all aspects of breathing, such as tidal volume, respiration rate, inspiratory flow pattern, and oxygen concentration of the breath. This is often labeled as *controlled mandatory ventilation* (CMV), a term that encompasses both volume- as well as pressure-controlled ventilation.

Figure 18.2 shows the flow and pressure waveforms for volume-controlled ventilation. In this illustration, the inspiratory flow waveform is chosen to be a half sine wave. In Figure 18.2a, t_i is the inspiration duration, t_e the exhalation period, and Q_i the amplitude of inspiratory flow. The ventilator delivers a tidal volume equal to the area under the flow waveform in Figure 18.2a at regular intervals $(t_i + t_e)$ set by the therapist. The resulting pressure waveform is shown in Figure 18.2b. It is noted that during volume-controlled ventilation, the ventilator attempts to deliver the desired volume of breath, irrespective of the patient's respiratory mechanics. However, the resulting pressure waveform, such as the one shown in Figure 18.2b, will be different depending on the patient's respiratory mechanics. Of course, for safety

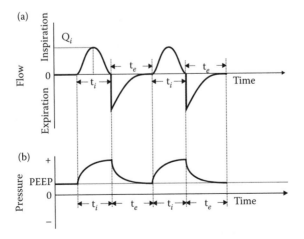

FIGURE 18.2 (a) Inspiratory flow for a mandatory volume-controlled ventilation breath and (b) airway pressure resulting from the breath delivery with a nonzero PEEP.

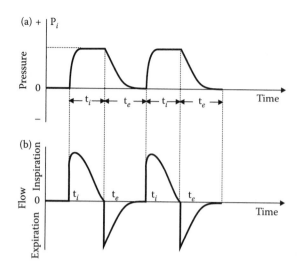

FIGURE 18.3   (a) Inspiratory pressure pattern for a mandatory pressure-controlled ventilation breath and (b) airway flow pattern resulting from the breath delivery. Note that PEEP is zero.

purposes, the ventilator must limit the maximum applied airway pressure according to the therapist's setting.

As can be seen in Figure 18.2b, the airway pressure at the end of exhalation may not end at atmospheric pressure (zero gauge). The *positive end expiratory pressure* or PEEP is sometimes used to prevent the alveoli from collapsing during expiration (Pierce, 2007). In other cases, the expiration pressure is allowed to return to the atmospheric level.

Figure 18.3 shows a plot of the pressure and flow during a mandatory pressure-controlled ventilation. In this case, the respirator raises the airway pressure and maintains it at the desired level, P_i, which is set by the therapist, independent of the patient's respiratory mechanics. Although the ventilator maintains the same pressure trajectory for patients with different respiratory mechanics, the resulting flow trajectory, shown in Figure 18.3b, will depend on the respiratory mechanics of each patient. As in the case of mandatory volume-controlled ventilation, the total volume of delivered breaths is monitored to ensure that patients receive adequate ventilation.

Owing to the need for monitoring both pressure and volume, in more recent years, new modes that combine several aspects of the volume- and pressure-controlled ventilation are devised. These modes are generally referred to as dual-control modes. Although these modes are relatively new and not all of their clinical outcomes are known, they utilize more of the power and flexibility that new ventilator hardware and software offer (Lellouche and Brochard, 2009). Two dual-control modes are described below.

18.3.2 Adaptive Pressure Control

This new mode is a form of pressure-controlled ventilation that simultaneously keeps track of the delivered tidal volume. Figure 18.4 shows characteristic changes of pressure, volume, and flow of inspiratory flow in this mode. As shown in the top panel of Figure 18.4, for each breath, (a) through (e), the ventilator controls the inspiratory pressure to a level that may vary from breath to breath. Specifically, the ventilator controls the pressure, but also monitors the delivered tidal volume and compares it with the desired tidal volume. If the actual delivered tidal volume matches the desired level, such as in (a), then the level of controlled pressure for the next breath will be the same. However, if the next breath produced a larger than desired tidal volume, such as in (b), then the controlled pressure will be reduced in the next breath (c). Similarly, if the tidal volume falls short, such as in (d), then the controlled pressure in the next breath, (e), will be raised to

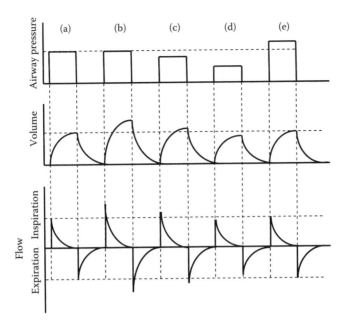

FIGURE 18.4   Patterns respiratory desired pressure and resulting volume and flow for adaptive pressure control ventilation mode. Breath illustration (a) through (e) shows how the applied inspiratory pressure is automatically adjusted to achieve the desired tidal volume.

a higher level to achieve the desired volume. Hence, the ventilator seeks delivering the desired tidal volume at fixed pressures that are adjusted from breath to breath. It is noted that in this mode of ventilation, while the pressure remains constant within the inspiratory interval, the level of inspiratory pressure is varied from one breath to the next by the ventilator to achieve the desired level of tidal volume.

18.3.3 Adaptive Support Ventilation

This new mode of ventilation aims to minimize the work of breathing as was proposed by Otis in 1950 (Otis et al., 1950), while accommodating changes in the patient's respiratory mechanics (Brunner and Iotti, 2002). A major point of distinction for this mode of ventilation is that it takes into account the respiratory mechanics of the patient (i.e., resistance and elastance of the combined airway and air-delivery system). Hence, it may be considered as one of the first closed-loop ventilators that adapts to the patient's condition. Adaptive support ventilation (ASV) can be applied as both a mandatory ventilation and a spontaneous ventilation. In this chapter, we describe only the mandatory ventilation form of ASV. A description of ASV in spontaneous breathing may be found in Wu et al. (2010) and Mireles-Cabodevila et al. (2009). When ASV is used to ventilate the patient in mandatory ventilation mode, the clinician inputs the ideal body weight (IBW) for the patient (based on height, gender, age, etc.). Using IBW, an (assumed) ideal minute volume is obtained by multiplying the IBW by 100 mL/min/kg. As the name implies, *minute volume* refers to the total inspiratory volume that a patient receives in 1 min. Additionally, the clinician needs to enter another parameter called percent of minute volume (PMV). The PMV indicates how the desired minute volume for the patient compares with the minute volume computed from IBW. For instance, a PMV of 100% means that the desired minute volume for the patient is the same as the minute volume computed from IBW. Alternatively, a PMV of 110% indicates that the desired minute volume is 10% above what is computed from the IBW. Once, the operator enters the IBW and PMV, the ASV algorithm determines an optimized respiration rate and tidal volume to minimize the work of breathing according to the principles proposed by Otis (Brunner and Iotti, 2002).

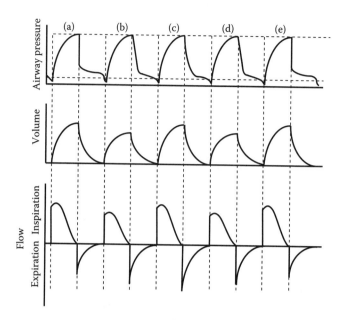

FIGURE 18.5 Patterns of respiratory pressure, volume, and flow for adaptive support ventilation mode. Breath illustrations (a) through (d) demonstrate how the respiratory frequency and volume are adjusted to minimize the work of breathing.

Figure 18.5 shows an illustration of the ASV breath delivery. In this illustration, the ventilator attempts to maintain the same airway pressure and PMV while respiratory mechanics vary. Specifically, breath (b) in Figure 18.5 has the same peak airway pressure as in (a), but a reduced peak inspiratory flow and lower respiration rate. This typifies the response of ASV to an increase in the respiratory impedance resulting in a lower peak flow to achieve the same peak airway pressure. Breath (c) in Figure 18.5 illustrates the ASV's ability to restore the flow and rate to the level of breath (a) if the patient's airway impedance goes back to the level equal to the one for breath (a). Breath (d) illustrates that if the impedance rises to the level of (b), the ASV algorithm will again adjust the flow and respiration rate accordingly.

18.3.4 Spontaneous Ventilation

An important phase in providing respiratory care to a recovering pulmonary patient is weaning the patient from the respirator. As the patient recovers and regains the ability to breathe independently, the spontaneous mode of ventilation allows the patient to initiate a breath and control the breath rate, flow rate, and the tidal volume. Ideally, when a respirator is functioning in the spontaneous mode, it should allow the patient take breaths with the same ease as breathing from the atmosphere. This, however, is difficult to achieve because the respirator does not have an infinite gas supply or an instantaneous response. In practice, the patient generally has to exert more effort to breathe in spontaneous mode than from the atmosphere. However, patient's effort is reduced as the ventilator response speed increases (Chatburn, 2004). Spontaneous ventilation is often used in conjunction with mandatory ventilation because the patient may still need breaths that are delivered entirely by the ventilator. Alternatively, when a patient can completely breathe on his own but needs oxygen-enriched breath or elevated airway pressure, spontaneous ventilation alone may be used.

As in the case of mandatory ventilation, several modes of spontaneous ventilation have been devised by therapists. Two of the most important and popular spontaneous breath delivery modes are described below.

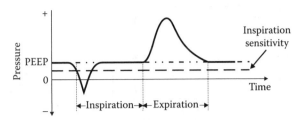

FIGURE 18.6 Airway pressure during a CPAP spontaneous breath delivery.

18.3.5 Continuous Positive Airway Pressure in Spontaneous Mode

In this mode, the ventilator maintains a positive pressure at the airway as the patient attempts to inspire. Figure 18.6 illustrates a typical airway pressure waveform during continuous positive airway pressure (CPAP) breath delivery. The therapist sets the sensitivity level lower than PEEP. The sensitivity is the pressure level that the patient has to attain by making an effort to breathe. This, in turn, triggers the ventilator to deliver a spontaneous breath by supplying air (or a mixture of air and oxygen) to raise the pressure back to the PEEP level. Typically, the PEEP and sensitivity levels are selected such that the patient will be impelled to exert effort to breathe independently. As in the case of the mandatory mode, when the patient exhales, the ventilator shuts off the flow of gas and opens the exhalation valve to allow the patient to exhale into the atmosphere.

18.3.6 Pressure Support in Spontaneous Mode

This mode is similar to the CPAP mode with the exception that during the inspiration the ventilator attempts to maintain the patient's airway pressure at a level above PEEP, called pressure support level. In fact, CPAP may be considered a special case of pressure support ventilation in which the support level is fixed at the atmospheric level.

Figure 18.7 shows a typical airway pressure waveform during the delivery of a *pressure support* breath. In this mode, when the patient's airway pressure drops below the therapist-set sensitivity line, the breath delivery system raises the airway pressure to the pressure support level (>PEEP), selected by the therapist. The ventilator stops the inspiratory gas flow when the patient starts to exhale and controls the exhalation valve to achieve the set PEEP level.

18.3.7 Breath Delivery Control

In a microprocessor-based ventilator, the mechanisms for delivering mandatory volume- and pressure-controlled ventilation have mostly common components. The primary difference lies in the control algorithms governing the delivery of breaths to the patient.

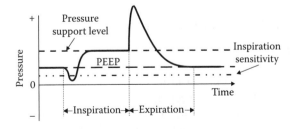

FIGURE 18.7 Airway pressure during a pressure support spontaneous breath delivery.

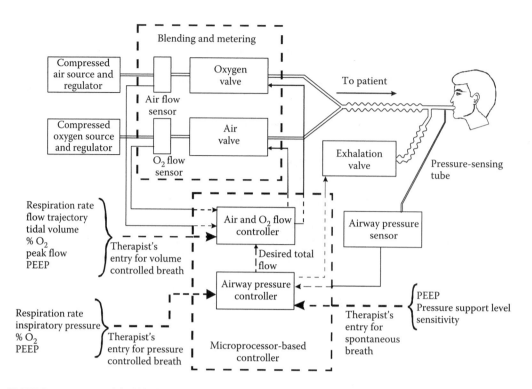

FIGURE 18.8　A simplified block diagram of a control structure for mandatory and spontaneous breath delivery.

Figure 18.8 shows a simplified block diagram for delivering mandatory and spontaneous ventilation. Compressed air and oxygen are normally stored in high pressure tanks ($\cong$1400 kPa) that are attached to the inlets of the ventilator. In some ventilators, an air compressor is used in place of a compressed air tank. Manufacturers of mechanical respirators have designed a variety of blending and metering devices (Chatburn, 2004). The primary purpose of the device is to enrich the inspiratory air flow with proper levels of oxygen and deliver a tidal volume according to the therapist's specifications. Since nearly two decades, the microprocessors are used to control the metering and blending of the breath delivery (Puritan-Bennett, 1990). In Figure 18.8, the air and oxygen valves are placed in closed feedback loops with the air and oxygen flow sensors. The microprocessor controls the valves to deliver the desired inspiratory air and oxygen flows for mandatory and spontaneous ventilation. During inhalation, the exhalation valve is closed to direct all of the delivered flows to the lungs. When exhalation begins, the microprocessor actuates the exhalation valve to achieve the desired PEEP level. The airway pressure sensor, shown on the right side of Figure 18.8, generates the feedback signal necessary for maintaining the desired PEEP (in both mandatory and spontaneous modes) and airway pressure during inspiratory breath delivery.

18.3.8　Mandatory Volume-Controlled Inspiratory Flow Delivery

In a microprocessor-controlled ventilator (Figure 18.8), the electronically actuated valves open from a closed position to allow the flow of blended gases to the patient. The control of flow through each valve depends on the therapist's specification for the mandatory breath. That is, the clinician must specify the following parameters for the delivery of volume-controlled mandatory ventilation breaths: (1) respiration rate; (2) flow waveform; (3) tidal volume; (4) oxygen concentration (of the delivered breath); (5) peak flow; and (6) PEEP, as shown in the lower left side of Figure 18.8. It is noted that the PEEP selected by the therapist in the mandatory mode is only used for the control of exhalation flow; this will be described later in this chapter. The microprocessor uses the first five of the above parameters to compute the total desired inspiratory flow trajectory. To illustrate this point, consider the delivery of a tidal volume using a half sine wave as shown in Figure 18.3. If the therapist selects a tidal volume of V_t (L), a respiration rate of n breaths per minute (bpm), the amplitude of the respirator flow, Q_i (L/s), then the total desired inspiratory flow, $Q_d(t)$, for a single breath, can be computed from the following equation:

$$Q_d(t) = \begin{cases} Q_i \sin\left(\dfrac{\pi t}{t_i}\right) & 0 \le t < t_i \\ 0 & t < t \le t_e \end{cases} \tag{18.1}$$

where t_i signifies the duration of inspiration and is computed from the following relationship:

$$t_i = \frac{\pi V_t}{2Q_i} \tag{18.2}$$

The duration of expiration in seconds is obtained from

$$t_e = \frac{60}{n} - t_i \tag{18.3}$$

The ratio of the inspiratory to expiratory period of a mandatory breath is often used for adjusting the respiration rate. This ratio is represented by I:E *(ratio)* and computed as follows. First, the inspiratory and expiratory periods are normalized with respect to t_i. Hence, the normalized inspiratory period becomes unity and the normalized expiratory period is given by $R = (t_e/t_i)$. Then, I:E ratio is simply expressed as 1:R.

To obtain the desired oxygen concentration in the delivered breath, the microprocessor computes the discrete form of $Q_d(t)$ as $Q_d(k)$, where k signifies the sample interval. Then, the total desired flow, $Q_d(k)$, is partitioned using the following relationships:

$$Q_{da}(k) = \frac{(1 - m)Q_d(k)}{(1 - c)} \tag{18.4}$$

and

$$Q_{dx}(k) = \frac{(m - c)Q_d(k)}{(1 - c)} \tag{18.5}$$

where $Q_{da}(k)$ is the desired air flow (the subscript *da* stands for desired air), $Q_{dx}(k)$ is the desired oxygen flow (the subscript *dx* stands for desired oxygen), m is the desired oxygen concentration, and c is the oxygen concentration of the ventilator air supply.

Several control design strategies may be appropriate for the control of air and oxygen flow delivery valves. A simple controller is the proportional plus integral controller that can be readily implemented in a microprocessor. For example, the controller for the air valve has the following form:

$$I(k) = K_p E(k) + K_i A(k) \tag{18.6}$$

where $E(k)$ and $A(k)$ are given by

$$E(k) = Q_{da}(k) - Q_{sa}(k) \tag{18.7}$$

$$A(k) = A(k-1) + E(k) \tag{18.8}$$

where $I(k)$ is the input (voltage or current) to the air valve at the kth sampling interval, $E(k)$ the error in the delivered flow, $Q_{da}(k)$ the desired air flow, $Q_{sa}(k)$ the sensed or actual air flow (the subscript sa stands for sensed air flow), $A(k)$ the integral (rectangular integration) part of the controller, and Kp and Ki are the controller design parameters. It is noted that Equations 18.6 through 18.8 are applicable to the control of either air or oxygen valve. For the control of oxygen flow valve, $Q_{dx}(k)$ replaces $Q_{da}(k)$ and $Q_{sx}(k)$ replaces $Q_{sa}(k)$, where $Q_{sx}(k)$ represents the sensed oxygen flow (the subscript sx stands for sensed oxygen flow).

The control structure shown in Figure 18.8 provides the flexibility of quickly adjusting the percent oxygen in the enriched breath gases. That is, the controller can regulate both the total flow and the percent oxygen delivered to the patient. Because the internal volume of the flow control valve is usually small (<50 mL), the desired change in the oxygen concentration of the delivered flow can be achieved within one inspiratory period. In actual clinical applications, rapid change of percent oxygen from one breath to another is often desirable, as it reduces the waiting time for the delivery of the desired oxygen concentration. A design similar to the one shown in Figure 18.8 has been successfully implemented in a microprocessor-based ventilator (Behbehani, 1984) and deployed in hospitals around the world.

18.3.9 Pressure-Controlled Inspiratory Flow Delivery

The therapist entry for pressure-controlled ventilation is shown in Figure 18.8 (lower left-hand side). In contrast to the volume-controlled ventilation, where $Q_d(t)$ was computed directly from operators' entry (Equations 18.1 through 18.3), the total desired flow is generated by the closed-loop airway pressure controller shown in Figure 18.8. This controller uses the therapist-selected inspiratory pressure, respiration rate, and the I:E ratio to compute the desired inspiratory pressure trajectory. The trajectory serves as the controller reference input. The controller then computes the flow necessary to make the actual airway pressure track the reference input. Assuming a proportional-plus-integral controller, the governing equations are

$$Q_d(k) = C_p E_p(k) + C_i A_p(k) \tag{18.9}$$

where Q_d is the computed desired flow, C_p and C_i are the controller design parameters, k represents the sample interval, and $E_p(k)$ and $A_p(k)$ are computed using the following equations:

$$E_p(k) = P_d(k) - P_s(k) \tag{18.10}$$

$$A_p(k) = A_p(k-1) + E_p(k) \tag{18.11}$$

where $E_p(k)$ is the difference between the desired pressure trajectory, $P_d(k)$, and the sensed airway pressure, $P_s(k)$, the parameter $A_p(k)$ represents the integral portion of the controller. Using Q_d from Equation 18.9, the control of air and O_2 valves is accomplished in the same manner as in the case of volume-controlled ventilation described earlier (Equations 18.4 through 18.8).

18.3.10 Expiratory Pressure Control in Mandatory Mode

It is often desirable to keep the patient's lungs inflated at the end of expiration at a pressure greater than the atmospheric level (Pierce, 2007). That is, rather than allowing the lungs to deflate during the exhalation, the controller closes the exhalation valve when the airway pressure reaches the PEEP level. When expiration begins, the ventilator terminates flow to the lungs. Hence, the regulation of the airway pressure is achieved by controlling the flow of patient-exhaled gases through the exhalation valve.

In a microprocessor-based ventilator, an electronically actuated valve can be employed that has adequate dynamic response (≈20 ms rise time) to regulate PEEP. For this purpose, the pressure in the patient's breath delivery circuit is measured using a pressure transducer (Figure 18.8). The microprocessor initially opens the exhalation valve completely to minimize resistance to expiratory flow. At the same time, it samples the pressure transducer's output and begins to close the exhalation valve as the pressure begins to approach the desired PEEP level. Because the patient's exhaled flow is the only source of pressure, if the airway pressure drops below PEEP, it cannot be brought back up until the next inspiratory period. Hence, an overrun (i.e., a drop to a level below PEEP) in the closed-loop control of PEEP should be avoided.

18.3.11 Spontaneous Breath Delivery Control

The small diameter (≅5 mm) pressure sensing tube, shown on the right side of Figure 18.8, pneumatically transmits the pneumatic pressure signal from the patient's airway to a pressure transducer placed in the ventilator. The output of the pressure transducer is amplified, filtered, and then sampled by the microprocessor. The controller receives the therapist's inputs regarding the spontaneous breath characteristics, such as the PEEP, sensitivity, and oxygen concentration, as shown in the lower right-hand side of Figure 18.8. The desired airway pressure is computed from the therapist entries of PEEP, pressure support level, and sensitivity. The multiple-loop control structure shown in Figure 18.8 is used to deliver a CPAP or a pressure support breath. The sensed proximal airway pressure is compared with the desired airway pressure. The airway pressure controller computes the total inspiratory flow level required to raise the airway pressure to the desired level. This flow level serves as the reference input or total desired flow for the flow control loop. Hence, in general, the desired total flow trajectory for the spontaneous breath delivery may be different for each inspiratory cycle. If the operator has specified oxygen concentration greater than 21.6% (the oxygen concentration of the ventilator air supply), the controller will partition the total required flow into the air and oxygen flow rates using Equations 18.4 and 18.5. The flow controller then uses the feedback signals from air and oxygen flow sensors and actuates the air and oxygen valves to deliver the desired flows.

For a microprocessor-based ventilator, the control algorithm for regulating the airway pressure can also be a proportional plus integral controller (Behbehani, 1984; Behbehani and Watanabe, 1986). In this case, the governing equations are identical to Equations 18.9 through 18.11.

18.4 Summary

Modern positive-pressure mechanical ventilators have been quite successful in treating patients with pulmonary disorders. Two major categories of breath delivery modes for these ventilators are mandatory and spontaneous. The volume- and pressure-controlled mandatory breath delivery and the governing control equations for these modes are presented in this chapter. Similarly, CPAP and support pressure modes of spontaneous breath delivery are described. Recent development of dual control modes that allow simultaneous monitoring and control of airway pressure and minute volume are also presented.

Defining Terms

Continuous positive airway pressure (CPAP): A spontaneous ventilation mode in which the ventilator maintains a constant positive pressure, near or below PEEP level, in the patient's airway while the patient breathes at will.

Controlled mandatory ventilation (CMV): A term that encompasses both pressure- and volume-controlled ventilation modes. It reflects that the ventilator controls all parameters of ventilating the patient.

I:E ratio: The ratio of normalized inspiratory interval to normalized expiratory interval of a mandatory breath. Both intervals are normalized with respect to the inspiratory period. Hence, the normalized inspiratory period is always unity.

Mandatory mode: A mode of mechanically ventilating the lungs, in which the ventilator controls all breath delivery parameters, such as tidal volume, respiration rate, flow waveform, and so on.

Minute volume: Total inspiratory volume delivered to a patient in 1 min.

Patient circuit: A set of tubes connecting the patient's airway to the outlet of a respirator.

Positive end expiratory pressure (PEEP): A therapist-selected patient's airway pressure level that the ventilator maintains at the end of expiration in either mandatory or spontaneous breathing.

Pressure support: A spontaneous breath delivery mode during which the ventilator applies a positive pressure greater than PEEP to the patient's airway during inspiration.

Pressure support level: Refers to the pressure level, above PEEP, that the ventilator maintains during the spontaneous inspiration.

Pressure-controlled ventilation: A mandatory mode of ventilation where during the inspiration phase of each breath a constant pressure is applied to the patient's airway independent of the patient's respiratory mechanics.

Spontaneous mode: A ventilation mode in which the patient initiates and breathes from the ventilator-supplied gas at will.

Synchronized intermittent mandatory ventilation: A mandatory mode of ventilation that is combined with a spontaneous mode and allows the patient to initiate and breathe spontaneously while monitoring the total volume of spontaneously delivered breaths and supplementing with mandatory breaths as needed.

Volume-controlled ventilation: A mandatory mode of ventilation where the volume of each breath is set by the therapist and the ventilator delivers that volume to the patient independent of the patient's respiratory mechanics.

References

Behbehani, K. 1984. PLM-Implementation of a multiple closed-loop control strategy for a microprocessor-controlled respirator. *Proceedings of the ACC Conference,* 574–576.

Behbehani, K. and Watanabe, N.T. 1986. A new application of digital computer simulation in the design of a microprocessor-based respirator. *Summer Simulation Conference,* 415–420.

Brunner, J.X. and Iotti, G.A. 2002. Adaptive support ventilation. *Minerva Anestesiol,* 68(5):365–368.

Chatburn, R.L. 2004. *Mechanical Ventilation,* 1st ed., Mandu Press Ltd., Cleveland Heights, Ohio.

Lellouche, F. and Brochard, L. 2009. Advanced closed loops during mechanical ventilation (PAV, NAVA, ASV, SmartCare). *Best Practice and Research Clinical Anesthesiology* 23:81–93.

MacIntyre, N.R. and Branson, R.D. 2009. *Mechanical Ventilation,* 2nd ed., Saunders Elsevier, St. Louis, Missouri.

Mireles-Cabodevila, E., Diaz-Guzman, E., Heresi, G.A., and Chaburn, R.L. 2009. Alternative modes of mechanical ventilation: A review for the hospitalist. *Cleveland Clinic Journal of Medicine* 76(7): 417–430.

Otis, A.B., Fenn, W.O., and Rahn H. 1950. Mechanics of breathing in man. *Journal of Applied Physiology* 2:592–607.

Pierce, L.N.B. 2007. *Management of the Mechanically Ventilated Patients*, 2nd ed., Saunders Elsevier, St. Louis, Missouri.

Puritan-Bennett 7200 Ventilator System Series. Ventilator, Options and Accessories, Part. No. 22300A, Carlsbad, California, September 1990.

Wu, C., Lin, H., Perng, W., Yang, S., Chen, C., Huang, Y.T., and Huang, K. 2010. Correlation between the % min vol setting and work of breathing during adaptive support ventilation in patients with respiratory failure. *Respiratory Care*, 55(3):334–341.

19

Essentials of Anesthesia Delivery

A. William Paulsen
Quinnipiac University

19.1 Introduction

This chapter will provide an introduction to the practice of anesthesiology and to the technology currently employed. Limitations on the length of this chapter, considering the enormous size of the topic, requires that this chapter relies on other elements within this handbook and other texts cited as general references for many of the details that inquisitive minds desire and deserve. References by Dorsch and Dorsch (2008), Gallagher and Issenberg (2007), Kofke and Nadkarni (2007), Kyle and Murray (2008), and Loeb (1993) give additional information regarding the topics in this chapter.

19.2 Components of Anesthesia Care

Anesthesia care usually begins with preoperative evaluation and assessment of the patient days before they enter the hospital or surgery center for surgery. Preoperative care begins when the patient enters the holding area before surgery where they are evaluated again and their medical history is reviewed as venous access is established and preoperative medication administered. The patient is transported to the operating room and all the monitoring systems are applied. When everyone is ready, anesthesia is induced and the surgery begins. Following the completion of surgery, the patient moves to the recovery room where they are monitored by the postanesthesia recovery unit nurses.

The practice of anesthesia includes more than just providing relief from pain; in fact, pain relief can be considered a secondary facet of the specialty. In actuality, the modern concept of the safe and efficacious delivery of anesthesia requires consideration of three fundamental tenets and is ordered here by relative importance:

1. Maintenance of vital organ function
2. The relief of pain
3. The maintenance of the "internal milieu"

The first, maintenance of vital organ function, is concerned with preventing damage to cells and organ systems that could result from inadequate supply of oxygen and other metabolic substrates. The delivery of blood and cellular substrates is often referred to as perfusion of the cells or tissues. During the delivery of an anesthetic, the patient's "vital signs" are monitored in an attempt to prevent inadequate tissue perfusion. However, the surgery itself, the patient's existing pathophysiology, drugs given for the relief of pain, or even the management of blood pressure may compromise tissue perfusion. There is a great need for a patient monitoring system to provide direct information concerning adequacy of perfusion. Why is adequate perfusion of tissues a higher priority than providing relief of pain for which anesthesia is named? A rather obvious extreme example is that without cerebral perfusion or perfusion of the spinal cord, delivery of an anesthetic is not necessary. Damage to other organ systems may result in a range of complications from delaying the patient's recovery to diminishing their quality of life or to premature death.

In other words, the primary purpose of anesthesia care is to maintain adequate delivery of required substrates to each organ and cell, which will hopefully preserve cellular function throughout the body. Surgical retraction may result in diminished blood flow to organ systems, again demonstrating the need to monitor adequacy of perfusion.

The second principle of anesthesia is to relieve the pain caused by surgery. The first use of ether for surgical anesthesia occurred in March of 1842 in Georgia by a surgeon named Crawford Long. More than 4 years later in October of 1846, there was a public demonstration of ether anesthesia for the relief of pain from a surgical procedure at the Massachusetts General Hospital. The use of ether and chloroform to render a patient unconscious spread quickly to England and Europe.

The field of treating chronic pain and suffering caused by many disease states is now managed by a subspecialty within anesthesia, called pain management. However, many pain services are multidisciplinary relying on neurologists, anesthesiologists, as well as other physician specialists.

The third principle of anesthesia is the maintenance of the internal environment of the body. For example, the regulation of electrolytes (sodium, potassium, chloride, magnesium, calcium, etc.), acid–base balance, and a host of supporting functions on which cellular function and organ system communications rest.

19.3 Who Delivers Anesthesia?

The person delivering anesthesia may be

- An anesthesiologist (physician specializing in anesthesiology)
- An anesthesiology physician assistant (a person trained in a medical school at the masters level to administer anesthesia as a member of the care team led by an anesthesiologist)
- Or a nurse anesthetist (a nurse with intensive care unit experience who has additional training in nurse anesthesia at the master's level)

19.4 Types of Anesthesia

There are three major categories of anesthesia provided to patients: (1) general anesthesia, (2) conduction anesthesia, and (3) monitored anesthesia care. General anesthesia typically includes the intravenous injection of anesthetic drugs (hypnotics such as propofol) that render the patient unconscious, followed by delivery of inhalation anesthetic drugs, intravenous analgesics, and often drugs that paralyze skeletal muscles. Immediately following drug administration, a plastic tube is inserted into the trachea and the patient is connected to an electropneumatic system to maintain ventilation of the lungs. All inhalation anesthetics are provided as liquids that require vaporizers to convert the liquid into a breathable vapor. In some cases, nitrous oxide is also administered along with the inhalation agent or other intravenous anesthetic drugs to maintain anesthesia for surgical procedures. When combinations of inhalation agents and intravenous agents are used together to provide anesthesia, it is called a balanced anesthetic.

Conduction anesthesia refers to blocking the conduction of pain and possibly motor nerve impulses traveling along specific nerves. This is also called regional anesthesia because it affects only a specific region of the body. The common forms of conduction anesthesia include spinal and epidural anesthesia, as well as specific nerve blocks, for example, axillary nerve blocks that are used to facilitate surgery of the forearm and hand. To achieve a successful conduction anesthetic, local anesthetic agents, such as lidocaine are injected into the proximity of specific nerves to block the conduction of electrical impulses. In addition, sedation may be provided intravenously to keep the patient comfortable while they are lying still for the surgery.

Monitored anesthesia care refers to monitoring and managing the patient's vital signs while administering sedatives and analgesics to keep the patient comfortable. Also, the anesthesia team is available to treat complications related to the surgical procedure. Typically, the surgeon administers topical or local anesthetics to alleviate regional pain. Throughout the hospital and in outlying locations, nurses, physician assistants, and others are providing what is called conscious sedation for patients. Conscious sedation can be very helpful in gastrointestinal laboratories, radiology, and other areas where patients need to be sedated but not anesthetized. Unfortunately, sedation is part of a continuum that spans local anesthesia only without much sedation, to general anesthesia. A person who administers a propofol infusion to make the patient comfortable may inadvertently cause the patient to stop breathing from the side effects of propofol. Without proper monitoring, the knowledge to recognize and effectively interpret the monitored data, and the skills required to manage a general anesthetic, the outcomes may be less than desired. There are many patient safety issues here that could benefit from improved technology and better drugs.

To provide the range of support required, from the paralyzed mechanically ventilated patient to the patient receiving monitored anesthesia care, a versatile anesthesia delivery system must be available to the anesthesia care team. Today's anesthesia delivery system comprises six major elements (Figure 19.1):

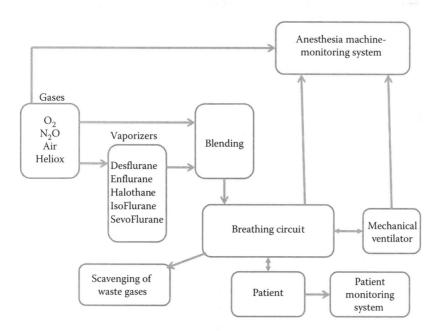

FIGURE 19.1 Block diagram of the basic components of the anesthesia delivery system.

(1) the primary and secondary sources of gases (O_2, air, N_2O, vacuum, gas scavenging, and possibly CO_2 and helium); (2) the gas blending and vaporization system; (3) the breathing circuit (including methods for manual and mechanical ventilation); (4) the excess gas scavenging system that minimizes potential pollution of the operating room by anesthetic gases; (5) instruments and equipment to monitor the function of the anesthesia delivery system; and (6) patient monitoring instrumentation and equipment. Newer additions to the anesthesia machine include the control of infusion pumps for the delivery of total intravenous anesthesia (TIVA), and closed-loop control of the patient's carbon dioxide concentrations and inhalation anesthetic levels (released in Europe, but not yet approved by the Food and Drug Administration (FDA) for use in the United States).

19.5 Gases Used during Anesthesia and Their Sources

Most inhaled anesthetic agents are liquids that are vaporized in a device within the anesthesia delivery system. The exception is xenon that is a naturally occurring gas and worthy of mention because it is an almost perfect inhalational anesthetic—except for one thing, cost. While it can provide general anesthesia, it is prohibitively expensive to produce because its concentration in the atmosphere is only 0.0000087% by volume.

The vaporized agents are then blended with other breathing gases before flowing into the breathing circuit and being administered to the patient. The most commonly administered form of anesthesia is called a balanced general anesthetic and is a combination of inhalation agent plus intravenous analgesic drugs. Intravenous drugs often require electromechanical devices to administer an appropriately controlled flow of drug to the patient.

Gases needed for the delivery of anesthesia are generally limited to oxygen (O_2), air, nitrous oxide (N_2O), and possibly helium (He). Vacuum and gas scavenging systems are also required. There needs to be secondary sources of these gases in the event of primary failure or questionable contamination. Typically, primary sources are those supplied from a hospital distribution system at 345 kPa (50 psig) through gas columns or wall outlets. The secondary sources of gas are cylinders hung on yokes on the anesthesia delivery system.

Oxygen provides an essential metabolic substrate for all human cells, but it is not without dangerous side effects. Prolonged exposure to high concentrations of oxygen may result in toxic effects within the lung that decrease diffusion of gas into and out of the blood. In neonates, the return to breathing air following prolonged exposure to elevated O_2 concentrations may result in a debilitating explosive blood vessel growth.

Oxygen is usually delivered to the hospital in liquid form (boiling point of −183°C), stored in cryogenic tanks, vaporized, and supplied to the hospital piping system as a gas. The reason for liquid storage is efficiency, since 1 L of liquid becomes 860 L of gas at standard temperature and pressure. The secondary source of oxygen within an anesthesia delivery system is usually one or more *E* cylinders filled with gaseous oxygen at a pressure of 15.2 MPa (2200 psig).

19.5.1 Air (78% N_2, 21% O_2, 0.9% Ar, and 0.1% Other Gases)

The primary use of air during anesthesia is as a diluent to decrease the inspired oxygen concentration. The typical primary source of medical air (there is an important distinction between "air" and "medical air" related to the quality and the requirements for periodic testing) is a special compressor that avoids hydrocarbon-based lubricants for purposes of medical air purity. Dryers are employed to rid the compressed air of water before distribution throughout the hospital. Medical facilities with limited need for medical air may use banks of *H* cylinders of dry medical air. A secondary source of air may be available on the anesthesia machine as an *E* cylinder containing dry gas at 15.2 MPa.

Nitrous oxide is a colorless, odorless, and nonirritating gas that does not support human life. Breathing more than 85% N_2O may be fatal. N_2O is not an anesthetic (except under hyperbaric conditions), rather, it is an analgesic and an amnestic. There are many reasons for administering N_2O during the course of

TABLE 19.1 Physical Properties of Gases Used during Anesthesia

Gas	Molecular Wt	Density (g/L)	Viscosity (cp)	Specific Heat (kJ/kg°C)
Oxygen	31.999	1.326	0.0203	0.917
Nitrogen	28.013	1.161	0.0175	1.040
Air	28.975	1.200	0.0181	1.010
Nitrous oxide	44.013	1.836	0.0144	0.839
Carbon dioxide	44.01	1.835	0.0148	0.850
Helium	4.003	0.1657	0.0194	5.190

an anesthetic including enhancing the speed of induction and emergence from anesthesia, decreasing the concentration requirements of potent inhalation anesthetics (i.e., halothane, isoflurane, etc.), and as an essential adjunct to narcotic analgesics. N_2O is supplied to anesthetizing locations from banks of *H* cylinders that are filled with 90% liquid at a pressure of 5.1 MPa (745 psig). Secondary supplies are available on the anesthesia machine in the form of *E* cylinders, again containing 90% liquid. Continual exposure to low levels of N_2O in the workplace has been implicated in several medical problems, including spontaneous abortion, infertility, birth defects, cancer, liver and kidney disease, and others. Although there is no conclusive evidence to support most of these implications, there is a recognized need to scavenge all waste anesthetic gases and periodically sample N_2O levels in the workplace to maintain the lowest possible levels consistent with reasonable risk to the operating room personnel and cost to the institution (Dorsch and Dorsch, 2008).

Carbon dioxide is colorless, odorless, but very irritating to breathe in higher concentrations. CO_2 is a by-product of human cellular metabolism and is not a life-sustaining gas. CO_2 influences many physiologic processes either directly or through the action of hydrogen ions by the reaction $CO_2 + H_2O \leftrightarrow H_2CO_3 \leftrightarrow H^+ + HCO_3^-$. Although not very common in the United States today, in the past, CO_2 was administered during anesthesia to stimulate respiration that was depressed by anesthetic agents and to cause increased blood flow in otherwise compromised vasculature during certain surgical procedures. Like N_2O, CO_2 is supplied as a liquid in *H* cylinders and then vaporized for distribution in pipeline systems or as a liquid in *E* cylinders that are located on the anesthesia machine. CO_2 may be used during cardiopulmonary bypass procedures while artificially oxygenating the blood.

Helium is a colorless, odorless, and nonirritating gas that does not support life. The primary use of helium in anesthesia is to enhance gas flow through small orifices as in asthma, airway trauma, or tracheal stenosis. The viscosity of helium is not different from other anesthetic gases (refer to Table 19.1) and is therefore not beneficial when the airway flow is laminar. However, in the event that ventilation must be performed through abnormally narrow orifices or tubes that create turbulent flow conditions, helium is the preferred carrier gas. Resistance to turbulent flow is proportional to the density rather than viscosity of the gas and helium is an order of magnitude less dense than other gases. A secondary advantage of helium is that it has a large specific heat relative to other anesthetic gases and, therefore, can carry the heat from laser surgery out of the airway more effectively than air, oxygen, or nitrous oxide, although this has never been demonstrated to be clinically significant. Helium is usually supplied as a mixture with oxygen (heliox, 25% O_2, and 75% helium).

19.5.2 Gas Blending and Vaporization System

The basic anesthesia machine utilizes primary low-pressure gas sources of 345 kPa (50 psig) available from wall or ceiling column outlets, and secondary high-pressure gas sources located on the machine. Oxygen may come from either the low-pressure source or from the 15.2 MPa (2200 psig) high-pressure yokes via cylinder pressure regulators. All anesthesia machines are required to have a safety system for limiting the minimum concentration of oxygen that can be delivered to the patient to 25%. Most currently available anesthesia machines are microprocessor based and of varying levels of electronic

TABLE 19.2   Physical Properties of Currently Available Volatile Anesthetic Agents

Agent Generic Name	Boiling Point (°C at 760 mmHg)	Vapor Pressure (mmHg at 20°C)	Liquid Density (g/mL)	MAC[a] (%)
Halothane	50.2	243	1.86	0.75
Enflurane	56.5	175	1.517	1.68
Isoflurane	48.5	238	1.496	1.15
Desflurane	23.5	664	1.45	6.0
Sevoflurane	58.5	160	1.51	2.0

[a] Minimum alveolar concentration is the percent of the agent required to provide surgical anesthesia to 50% of the population in terms of a cumulative dose–response curve. The lower the MAC, the more potent is the agent.

sophistication. Some machines use mechanical needle valves to control gas flows and employ electronic flow sensors for display purposes rather than use rotameter glass flow tubes. Other more sophisticated machines use electronic flow controllers instead of mechanical needle valves. Some machines even use microprocessor control of vaporization managing and measuring the flow of gas flowing through the vaporization chamber and the bypass line.

The physical properties of inhalational anesthetics are provided in Table 19.2. Note that desflurane, compared to other agents, has a boiling point that is close to normal room temperature and a vapor pressure that is close to atmospheric pressure at sea level. These properties dictated a new type of vaporizer that heats the agent to 39°C in order to meter the flow of desflurane vapor into the gas flow stream. The minimum alveolar concentration (MAC) of halothane, from Table 19.2 indicates that the agent is the most potent of the agents available today with desflurane as the least potent.

Microprocessors with their measurement and control functions provide means for integration of monitoring and assuring proper operation of the machine, but not proper use by the clinician. Anesthesia machines are becoming more like automobiles in that the microprocessors that monitor and control the engine performance have now eliminated the ability of the users to identify and locate problems. The machines have become so sophisticated that clinicians are no longer able to troubleshoot or find workarounds for problems that occur during use. Even the factory service personnel have become so specialized that hospitals that own several models of anesthesia delivery systems have different service personnel for different machines. Local service provided by clinical engineering departments to anesthesia equipment is becoming similar to how these departments handle patient monitoring. Clinical engineering departments stock printed circuit boards and modules that can be exchanged rather than troubleshooting to the component level. The advantages of all electronic anesthesia machines are to monitor proper function of complex electronics, integrate alarm functions to create smart alarms, and begin to implement control functions such as closed-loop control of ventilatory parameters. The downside to all electronic machines is the creation of numerous complex catastrophic failure modes.

Currently, most anesthesia machines in the United States use calibrated flow through vaporizers, meaning that all the gases from the various flowmeters are mixed in the manifold before entering the vaporizer. Any given vaporizer has a calibrated control knob that once set to the desired concentration for a specific agent will deliver that concentration to the patient. Some form of interlock system must be provided such that only one vaporizer may be activated at any given time. Figure 19.2 schematically illustrates the operation of a purely mechanical vaporizer with temperature compensation. This simple flow-over design permits a fraction of the total gas flow to pass into the vaporizing chamber where it becomes saturated with vapor before being added back to the total gas flow. Mathematically, this is approximated by

$$F_A = \frac{Q_{VC} * P_A}{P_B * (Q_{VC} + Q_G) - P_A * Q_G}$$

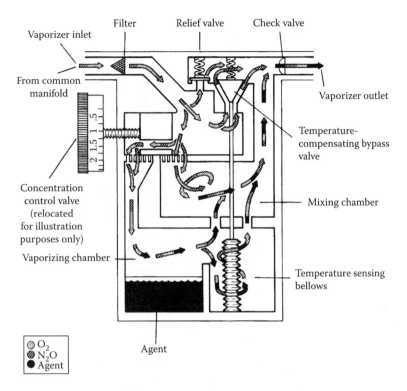

FIGURE 19.2 Schematic diagram of a calibrated in-line vaporizer that uses the flow-over technique for adding anesthetic vapor to the breathing-gas mixture.

where F_A is the fractional concentration of agent at the outlet of the vaporizer, Q_G the total flow of gas entering the vaporizer, Q_{VC} the amount of Q_G that is diverted into the vaporization chamber, P_A the vapor pressure of the agent, and P_B the barometric pressure. From Figure 19.2, the temperature compensator would decrease Q_{VC} as temperature increased because vapor pressure is proportional to temperature. The concentration accuracy over a range of clinically expected gas flows and temperatures is approximately ±15%. Because vaporization is an endothermic process, anesthetic vaporizers must have sufficient thermal mass and conductivity to permit the vaporization process to proceed independently of the rate at which the agent is being used.

The vaporizer for desflurane is in many cases unique in that it is electronic, and as Figure 19.3 illustrates, the liquid agent is heated and injects the desflurane vapor into the breathing gas. The electronics are all analog for safety reasons.

19.5.3 Breathing Circuits

The concept behind an effective breathing circuit is to provide an adequate volume of a controlled concentration of gas to the patient during inspiration and to carry the exhaled gases away from the patient during exhalation. There are several forms of breathing circuits that can be classified into two basic types: (1) open circuit, meaning no rebreathing of any gases and no CO_2 absorber present and (2) closed circuit, indicating the presence of CO_2 absorber and some rebreathing of other gases. Open circuits are rarely used because of the expense of delivering high gas flows as there is a great potential for the patient to rebreathe their own exhaled gases unless the fresh gas inflow is 2–3 times the patient's minute volume. The open circuits do have the advantage that their time constant for changing concentrations of oxygen or anesthetic agents is significantly less than a closed or semiclosed breathing system. Figure 19.4 illustrates the most popular

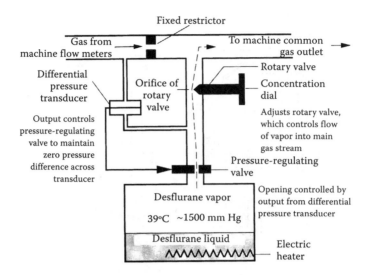

FIGURE 19.3   Schematic diagram of the TEC 6 electronic vaporizer for the administration of desflurane.

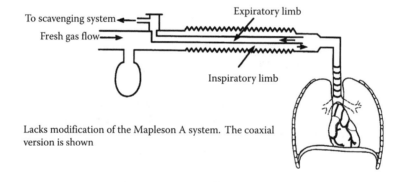

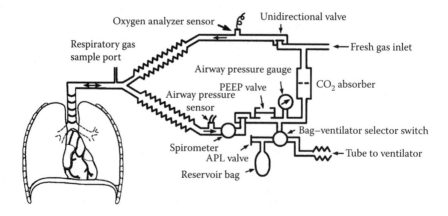

FIGURE 19.4   Diagram of a closed-circuit circle breathing system with unidirectional valves, inspired oxygen sensor, pressure sensor, and CO_2 absorber.

form of breathing circuit, the circle system, with oxygen monitor, circle pressure gage, volume monitor (spirometer), and airway pressure sensor. The circle is a closed system or semiclosed when the fresh gas inflow exceeds the patient's requirements. Excess gas evolves into the scavenging device and some of the exhaled gas is rebreathed after having the CO_2 removed. The inspiratory and expiratory valves in the circle system guarantee that gas flows to the patient from the inspiratory limb and away from the patient through the exhalation limb. In the event of a failure of either or both of these valves, the patients will rebreathe exhaled gas that contains CO_2, which is a potentially dangerous situation.

There are two forms of mechanical ventilation used during anesthesia: volume ventilation where the volume of gas delivered to the patient remains constant regardless of pressure that is required and pressure ventilation where the ventilator provides sufficient volume to the patient that is required to produce some desired pressure in the breathing circuit. Volume ventilation is the most popular because the volume delivered remains theoretically constant despite changes in lung compliance. Pressure ventilation is useful when compliance losses in the breathing circuit are high relative to the volume delivered to the lungs. Pressure ventilation also permits the alveoli with longer time constants ($\tau = R \times C$, R is airway resistance, C is alveolar compliance) to fill more completely.

There are multiple variations in these two methods of ventilation now available on anesthesia delivery systems:

1. Volume-controlled ventilation—the patient receives a specific volume of gas delivered to the lungs at set time intervals with pressure limit.
2. Pressure-controlled ventilation—a constant pressure applied to the airway and the lungs fill according to their compliance and the set pressure (volume = compliance × pressure).
3. Pressure-controlled ventilation with volume guarantee—a set pressure is delivered to the breathing circuit, but that pressure is altered by the ventilator until the set tidal volume is achieved.
4. Pressure-assist ventilation—this mode permits the patient to trigger a breath delivered by the ventilator assisting the patient's breathing.
5. Synchronous intermittent mandatory ventilation (SIMV)—this mode permits the patient to breathe on their own (spontaneous ventilation), but supplements the volume that the patient breathes according to a set breathing rate. For example, the SIMV rate may be set to 4 breaths per minute while the patient is breathing low volumes at a rate of 20 breaths/min. Every 12 s, the ventilator will assist a patient-triggered breath and deliver an adequate tidal volume. If the patient stops breathing, then the ventilator will deliver a set volume of gas 4 times/min.

Humidification is an important adjunct to the breathing circuit because it maintains the integrity of the cilia that line the airways and promote the removal of mucus and particulate matter from the lungs. Humidification of dry breathing gases can be accomplished by simple passive heat and moisture exchangers inserted into the breathing circuit at the level of the endotracheal tube connectors, or by elegant dual-servo electronic humidifiers that heat a reservoir filled with water and also heat a wire in the gas-delivery tube to prevent rainout of the water before it reaches the patient. Electronic safety measures must be included in these active devices because of the potential for burning the patient and the fire hazard.

19.5.4 Gas Scavenging Systems

The purpose of scavenging exhaled and excess anesthetic agents is to reduce or eliminate the potential hazard to employees who work in the environment where anesthetics are administered, including operating rooms, obstetrical areas, special-procedure areas, physician's offices, dentist's offices, and veterinarian's surgical suites. Typically, more gas is administered to the breathing circuit than is required by the patient, resulting in the necessity to remove excess gas from the circuit. The scavenging system must be capable of collecting gas from all components of the breathing circuit, including adjustable pressure level valves, ventilators, and sample-withdrawal type gas monitors, without

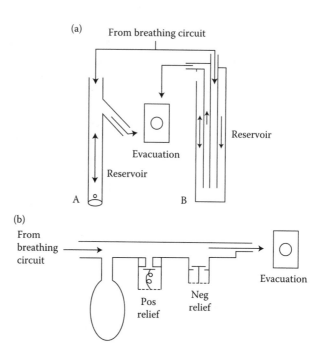

FIGURE 19.5   Examples of open- and closed-gas scavenger interfaces. The closed interface requires relief valves in the event of scavenging flow failure.

altering characteristics of the circuit, such as pressure or gas flow to the patient. There are two broad types of scavenging systems as illustrated in Figure 19.5: the open interface is a simple design that requires a large physical space for the reservoir volume, and the closed interface with an expandable reservoir bag that must include relief valves for handling the cases of no scavenged flow and great excess of scavenged flow.

    Trace-gas analysis must be performed to guarantee the efficacy of the scavenging system. The National Institutes of Occupational Safety and Health (NIOSH) recommends that trace levels of nitrous oxide must be maintained at or below 25 ppm time-weighted average and that halogenated anesthetic agents remain below 2 ppm.

19.6 Monitoring the Function of the Anesthesia Delivery System

The anesthesia machine can produce a single or combinations of catastrophic events, any one of which could be fatal to the patient: (1) delivery of a hypoxic gas mixture to the patient; (2) the inability to adequately ventilate the lungs by not producing positive pressure in the patient's lungs, not delivering an adequate volume of gas to the lungs, or by improper breathing circuit connections that permit the patient's lungs to receive only rebreathed gases; and (3) the delivery of an overdose of an inhalational anesthetic agent. The necessary monitoring equipment to guarantee proper function of the anesthesia delivery system includes at least

- Inspired oxygen concentration monitor with absolute low-level alarm of 19%
- Airway pressure monitor with alarms for
  - Low pressure indicative of inadequate breathing volume and possibly a leak
  - Sustained elevated pressures that could compromise cardiovascular function
  - High pressures that could cause pulmonary barotrauma
  - Subatmospheric pressure that could cause collapse of the lungs

- Exhaled gas volume monitor
- Carbon dioxide monitor (capnography)
- Inspired and exhaled concentration of anesthetic agents

Sound monitoring principles require: (1) the earliest possible detection of untoward events (before they result in physiologic derangements) and (2) specificity that results in rapid identification and resolution of the problem. An extremely useful rule to always consider is *"never monitor the anesthesia delivery system performance through the patient's physiologic responses."* That is, never intentionally use a device, such as a pulse oximeter, to detect a breathing circuit disconnection because the warning is very late and there is no specific information provided that leads to rapid resolution of the problem.

19.7 Monitoring the Patient

The anesthetist's responsibilities to the patient include providing relief from pain and preserving all existing normal cellular function of all organ systems. Currently, the latter obligation is fulfilled by monitoring essential physiologic parameters and correcting any substantial derangements that occur before they are translated to permanent cellular damage. The inadequacy of current monitoring methods can be appreciated by realizing that most monitoring modalities only indicate damage after an insult has occurred, at which point the hope is that it is reversible or that further damage can be prevented.

Standards for basic intraoperative monitoring of patients undergoing anesthesia, which were developed and adopted by the American Society of Anesthesiologists, became effective in 1990 and were last revised in 2005. Standard I concerns the responsibilities of anesthesia personnel, whereas standard II requires that the patient's oxygenation, ventilation, circulation, and temperature must be evaluated continually during all anesthetics. The following list includes patient monitoring options that are available to anesthesia providers:

- *Electrocardiogram*
- *Pulse oximetry*
- Urine output
- Cardiac output
- Electroencephalogram (EEG)
- Evoked potentials
- *Noninvasive or invasive blood pressure*
- *Temperature*
- Nerve stimulators
- Mixed venous oxygen saturation
- Transesophageal echo cardiography (TEE)
- Coagulation status
- Blood gases and electrolytes (P_{O_2}, P_{CO_2}, pH, BE, Na^+, K^+, Cl^-, Ca^{2+}, and glucose)
- Capnography and breathing gas analysis (O_2, CO_2, N_2O, anesthetic agents)
- BiSpectral index or entropy monitoring systems

19.7.1 Control of Patient Temperature

Anesthesia alters the thresholds for temperature regulation and the patient becomes unable to maintain normal body temperature. As the patient's temperature falls even a few degrees toward room temperature, several physiologic derangements occur: (1) drug action is prolonged, (2) blood coagulation is impaired, and (3) postoperative infection rate increases. On the positive side, cerebral protection from inadequate perfusion is enhanced by just a few degrees of cooling. Proper monitoring of core body temperature and forced hot air warming of the patient is essential.

19.7.2 Monitoring the Depth of Anesthesia

There are two very unpleasant experiences that patients may have while undergoing an inadequate anesthetic: (1) the patient is paralyzed and unable to communicate their state of discomfort, they are feeling the pain of surgery, and are aware of their surroundings; (2) the patient may be paralyzed, unable to communicate, and is aware of their surroundings, but is not feeling any pain. The ability to monitor the depth of anesthesia would provide a safeguard against these unpleasant experiences; however, despite numerous instruments and approaches to the problem, it remains elusive. Brain stem auditory-evoked responses have come closest to the depth of anesthesia monitoring, but it is difficult to perform, expensive, and not possible to perform during many types of surgery. A promising technology, called bispectral index (BIS monitoring) is purported to measure the level of patient hypnosis through multivariate analysis of a single channel of the EEG.

19.7.3 Anesthesia Computer-Aided Record Keeping

Conceptually, every anesthetist desires an automated anesthesia record-keeping system. Anesthesia care can be improved through the feedback provided by correct record keeping, but today's systems have an enormous overhead associated with their use when compared to standard paper record keeping. No doubt that automated anesthesia record keeping reduces the drudgery of routine recording of vital signs, but to enter drugs and drips and their dosages, fluids administered, urine output, blood loss, and other data require much more time and machine interaction than the current paper system. Despite attempts to use every input/output device ever produced by the computer industry from keyboards to bar codes to voice and handwriting recognition, no solution has been found that meets wide acceptance. The tenants of a successful system must include

1. The concept of a user-transparent system, which is ideally defined as no required communication between the computer and the clinician (far beyond the concept of user friendly), and therefore that is intuitively obvious to use even to the most casual users.
2. Recognition of the fact that educational institutions have very different requirements from private practice institutions.
3. Real-time hard copy of the record produced at the site of anesthetic administration that permits real-time editing and notation.
4. Ability to interface with a great variety of patient and anesthesia delivery system monitors from various suppliers.
5. Ability to interface with a large number of hospital information systems.
6. Inexpensive to purchase and maintain.

19.7.4 Alarms

Vigilance is the key to effective risk management but maintaining a vigilant state is not easy. The practice of anesthesia has been described as moments of shear terror connected by times of intense boredom. Alarms can play a significant role in redirecting one's attention during the boredom to the most important event regarding patient safety but only if false alarms can be eliminated, alarms can be prioritized, and all alarms concerning anesthetic management can be displayed in a single clearly visible location. Alarms should be integrated through multiple monitoring modalities to provide a sensitivity of one and specificity of one. The areas of patient and equipment alarms are a fertile ground for research.

19.7.5 Ergonomics

The study of ergonomics attempts to improve performance by optimizing the relationship between people and their work environment. Ergonomics has been defined as a discipline that investigates and applies information about human requirements, characteristics, abilities, and limitations to the design, development, and testing of equipment, systems, and jobs (Loeb, 1993). This field of study applied to anesthesia is only in its infancy and examples of poor ergonomic design abound in the anesthesia workplace.

19.7.6 Simulation in Anesthesia

Almost all anesthesia academic training institutions have simulators that are used for teaching anesthesia-related skills, critical thinking, assessing knowledge and clinical judgment, and for rehearsing team-based crisis management (Gallagher and Issenberg, 2007; Kofke and Nadkarni, 2007; Kyle and Murray, 2008). Complete patient simulators are hands-on high-fidelity realistic simulators that interface with physiologic monitoring equipment to simulate patient responses to equipment malfunctions, operator errors, and drug therapies. There are also crisis management simulators for coordinating team activities such as cardiac arrest, malignant hyperthermia, and triage following large-scale disasters. Simulators are currently being explored for certification and continued demonstration of qualifications for anesthesiologists and anesthetists. Several commercially available high-fidelity patient simulators dominate the simulation landscape in anesthesia. The best method of training is a combination of simulation and direct patient care. Haptic simulators are useful for teaching skills and specific procedures.

19.7.7 Reliability

The design of an anesthesia delivery system is unlike the design of most other medical devices because it is a life-support system. As such, its core elements deserve all the considerations of the latest fail-safe technologies. Too often, in today's quest to apply microprocessor technology to everything, trade-offs are made among reliability, cost, and engineering elegance. There is an ongoing debate concerning the advantages of microprocessor-based machines with numbers of catastrophic failure modes versus simple ultrareliable mechanical systems with an absolute minimum of catastrophic failure modes. There is a phase in the development cycle in which electronic controls are added with no real advantage over simple ultrareliable machines. The next phase is closing the loop and providing many advantages that make the delivery of anesthesia safer. However, the inclusion of microprocessors can enhance the safety of anesthesia delivery if they are implemented without adding catastrophic failure modes.

References

Dorsch, J.A., Dorsch, S.E. 2008. *Understanding Anesthesia Equipment*, 5th ed. Wolters Kluwer/Lippincott Williams & Wilkins, Philadelphia, PA.

Gallagher, C.J., Issenberg, S.B. 2007. *Simulation in Anesthesia*, Saunders Elsevier, Philadelphia.

Kofke, W.A., Nadkarni, V.M. 2007. New vistas in patient safety and simulation. *Anesthesiology Clinics* 25(2).

Kyle, R.R., Murray, W.B. 2008. *Clinical Simulation; Operations, Engineering and Management*. Academic Press, Elsevier, Inc., Burlington, MA.

Loeb, R. 1993. Ergonomics of the anesthesia workplace. *STA Interface* 4(3):18.

20

Electrosurgical Devices

20.1 Introduction

An electrosurgical unit (ESU) passes high-frequency electric current through biological tissues to achieve surgical modification of the tissue, such as cutting, coagulation, desiccation, ablation, lesioning, shrinkage, sealing, or fusion. Electrosurgery is also known as high-frequency (HF) surgery or surgical diathermy. The fundamental frequency of electrosurgical waveforms is generally above 200 kHz to minimize the potential for neuromuscular stimulation. Various forms of electrosurgery have been in practice since the 1920s to cut tissue effectively while at the same time controlling the amount of bleeding. Cutting is achieved primarily with a continuous sinusoidal waveform, whereas coagulation is achieved with a series of sinusoidal wave packets. The surgeon selects either one of these waveforms or a blend of them to suit the surgical needs. Electrosurgical current may be delivered using several methods with the most widely used being the monopolar and bipolar modes. The most noticeable difference between these two modes is the manner in which the electrical current enters and leaves the tissue. In the monopolar mode, the current flows from a small active electrode into the surgical site, spreads through the body, and returns to a large dispersive electrode on the skin. The high current density in the vicinity of the active electrode achieves the desired tissue effect, such as cutting or coagulation, whereas the low current density under the dispersive electrode causes no tissue damage. The monopolar mode may be used for cutting, coagulating, ablating, or lesioning tissue. In the bipolar mode, the current flows only through the tissue in contact with the bipolar electrodes. The most common type of bipolar instrument is in the form of forceps. The bipolar mode may be used for coagulation, desiccation, tissue ablation, vessel sealing, or tissue fusion.

The following sections describe in detail the theoretical and technological design details of ESUs, including their modes of operation, typical applications, and potential hazards.

20.2 Theory of Operation

In principle, electrosurgery is based on rapid heating of the tissue. To better understand the thermodynamic events during electrosurgery, it helps to know the general effects of heat on biological tissue.

Consider a tissue volume that experiences a temperature increase from normal body temperature to 45°C within a few seconds. Although the cells in this tissue volume show neither microscopic nor macroscopic changes, some cytochemical changes do in fact occur. However, these changes are reversible and the cells return to their normal function when the temperature returns to normal values. Above 45°C, irreversible changes take place that inhibit normal cell functions and lead to cell death. First, between 45°C and 60°C, the proteins in the cell lose their quaternary configuration and solidify into a glutinous substance that resembles the white of a hard-boiled egg. This process, termed coagulation, is accompanied by tissue blanching. Further, increasing the temperature up to 100°C leads to tissue drying, that is, the aqueous cell contents evaporate. This process is called desiccation. If the temperature is increased beyond 100°C, the solid contents of the tissue reduce to carbon, a process referred to as carbonization. Tissue damage not only depends on temperature, however, but also on the length of exposure to heat. Thus, the overall temperature-induced tissue damage is an integrative effect between temperature and time that is expressed mathematically by the Arrhenius relationship, where an exponential function of temperature is integrated over time [1].

In the monopolar mode, the active electrode either touches the tissue directly or is held a few millimeters above the tissue. When the electrode is held above the tissue, the electric current bridges the air gap by creating an electric discharge arc. A visible arc forms when the electric field strength exceeds 1 kV/mm in the gap and disappears when the field strength drops below a certain threshold level.

When the active electrode touches the tissue and the current flows directly from the electrode into the tissue without forming an arc, the rise in tissue temperature follows the bioheat equation

$$T - T_o = \frac{1}{\sigma \rho c} J^2 t \tag{20.1}$$

where T and T_o are the final and initial temperatures (K), σ is the electrical conductivity (S/m), ρ the tissue density (kg/m³), c the specific heat of the tissue (J/kg K), J the current density (A/m²), and t the duration (s) of heat application [1]. The bioheat equation is valid for short application times where secondary effects, such as heat transfer to surrounding tissues, blood perfusion, and metabolic heat, can be neglected. According to Equation 20.1, the surgeon has primarily three means of controlling the cutting or coagulation effect during electrosurgery: the contact area between the active electrode and tissue, the electrical current density, and the activation time. In most commercially available electrosurgical generators, the only output variables that can be adjusted are power and waveform (mode). The power setting as well as the type and size of the active electrode allows the surgeon some control over the current. Table 20.1 lists typical output power and mode settings for various surgical procedures. Table 20.2 lists some typical tissue impedance ranges seen during the use of an ESU in surgery. The values are shown as ranges because the impedance increases as the tissue dries out, and at the same time the output power of the ESU decreases.

20.3 Monopolar Mode

A continuous sinusoidal waveform, of sufficient voltage, cuts the tissue with very little hemostasis. This waveform is simply called cut or pure cut. During each positive and negative swing of the sinusoidal waveform, a new discharge arc forms and disappears at essentially the same tissue location. The electric current concentrates at this tissue location causing a sudden increase in temperature because of resistive heating. The rapid rise in temperature then vaporizes intracellular fluids, increases cell pressure, and ruptures the cell membrane, thereby parting the tissue. This chain of events is confined to the vicinity of the arc, because from there the electric current spreads to a much larger tissue volume and the current density is no longer sufficiently high to cause resistive heating damage. Typical output values for ESUs, in cut and other modes, are shown in Table 20.3.

TABLE 20.1   Typical ESU Power Settings for Various Surgical Procedures

Power-Level Range	Procedures
Low power	
<30 W cut	Neurosurgery
<30 W coag	Dermatology
	Plastic surgery
	Oral surgery
	Laparoscopic sterilization
	Vasectomy
Medium power	
30 W–150 W cut	General surgery
30 W–70 W coag	Laparotomies
	Head and neck surgery (ENT)
	Major orthopedic surgery
	Major vascular surgery
	Routine thoracic surgery
	Polypectomy
High power	
>150 W cut	Transurethral resection procedures
>70 W coag	(TURPs)
	Thoracotomies
	Ablative cancer surgery
	Mastectomies

Note: Ranges assume the use of a standard blade-type electrode; The use of a needle electrode, or other small current concentrating electrode, allows lower settings to be used; Users are urged to use the lowest setting that provides the desired clinical results.

TABLE 20.2   Typical Tissue Impedance Ranges during Electrosurgery

	Impedance Range (Ω)
Cut Mode Application	
Prostate tissue	400–1700
Oral cavity	1000–2000
Liver tissue	
Muscle tissue	
Gall bladder	1500–2400
Skin tissue	1700–2500
Bowel tissue	2500–3000
Periosteum	
Mesentery	3000–4200
Omentum	
Adipose tissue	3500– 4500
Scar tissue	
Adhesions	
Coag mode application	
Contact coagulation to stop bleeding	100–1000

TABLE 20.3 Typical Output Characteristics of ESUs

	Output Voltage Range Open Circuit, $V_{peak-peak}$ (V)	Output Power Range (W)	Frequency (kHz)	Crest Factor $\left(\dfrac{V_{peak}}{V_{rms}}\right)$	Duty Cycle (%)
Monopolar Modes					
Cut	200–5000	1–400	300–1750	1.4–2.1	100
Blend	1500–5800	1–300	300–1750	2.1–6.0	25–80
Desiccate	400–6500	1–200	240–800	3.5–6.0	50–100
Fulgurate/spray	6000–12,000	1–200	300–800	6.0–20.0	10–70
Bipolar mode					
Coagulate/ desiccate	200–1000	1–70	300–1050	1.6–12.0	25–100

Experimental observations have increasingly shown that hemostasis is achieved when cutting with an interrupted sinusoidal waveform or amplitude-modulated continuous waveform. These waveforms are typically called blend or blended cut. Some ESUs offer a choice of blend waveforms to allow the surgeon to select the degree of hemostasis desired.

When a continuous or interrupted waveform is used while the electrode is in direct contact with the tissue and the output voltage is too low to cause arcing, desiccation of the tissue occurs. Some ESUs have a distinct mode for this purpose called desiccation or contact coagulation.

In noncontact coagulation, the duty cycle of an interrupted waveform and the crest factor (ratio of peak voltage to rms voltage) influence the degree of hemostasis. Although a continuous waveform reestablishes the arc at essentially the same tissue location concentrating the heat there, an interrupted waveform causes the arc to reestablish itself at different tissue locations. The arc seems to dance from one location to the other, raising the temperature of the top tissue layer to coagulation levels. These noncontact coagulation waveforms are also called fulguration or spray. Because the current inside the tissue spreads very quickly from the point where the arc strikes, the heat concentrates in the top layer, primarily desiccating the tissue and causing some carbonization.

The most widely used monopolar active electrode is a small flat blade with symmetrical leading and trailing edges that is embedded at the tip of an insulated handle. The edges of the blade are shaped to easily initiate discharge arcs and to help the surgeon manipulate the incision; they cannot mechanically cut the tissue. Because the surgeon holds the handle in his hands like a pencil, it is often referred to as the "pencil." Many pencils contain one or more switches in their handle to control the electrosurgical waveform, primarily to switch between cutting and coagulation. Other active electrodes include needle electrodes, loop electrodes, ball electrodes, and laparoscopic electrodes. Needle electrodes are used for coagulating small tissue volumes like in neurosurgery or plastic surgery. Loop electrodes are used to resect nodular structures, such as polyps or to excise tissue samples for pathological analysis. An example would be the large loop excision of the transformation zone (LLETZ) procedure in which the transition zone of the cervix is excised. Electrosurgery at the tip of an endoscope or laparoscope requires yet another set of active electrodes and specialized training of the surgeon.

Besides the traditional uses described above, there are many new applications that use monopolar energy. Tissue may be ablated or lesions created to selectively kill undesired cells. Examples are soft tissue ablation that uses a rigid monopolar electrode introduced into a tumor and cardiac ablation, which uses a flexible catheter to create a lesion in the heart to treat an arrhythmia. The delivery of monopolar energy may also be enhanced by the addition of a controlled column of argon gas in the path between the active electrode and the tissue. The flow of argon gas assists in clearing the surgical site of fluid and improves visibility. When used in the coagulation mode, the argon gas is turned into a plasma, allowing tissue damage and smoke to be reduced, and producing a thinner, more flexible eschar. When used with the cut mode, lower power levels may be used.

20.4 Dispersive Electrodes

Dispersive electrodes are also called plate electrodes, passive electrodes, return electrodes, neutral electrodes, or grounding pads. The main purpose of the dispersive electrode is to return the monopolar high-frequency current to the ESU without causing harm to the patient. This is usually achieved by attaching a large-surface-area electrode to the patient's skin at some point away from the surgical site. The large electrode area and low contact impedance reduce the current density to levels where tissue heating is minimal. Because the ability of a dispersive electrode to avoid tissue heating and burns is of primary importance, dispersive electrodes are often characterized by their "heating factor." The heating factor describes the energy dissipated under the dispersive electrode and is equal to I^2t, where I is the rms current and t the time of exposure in seconds. During surgery, a typical value for the heating factor is 3 A^{2}s, but factors of up to 9 A^{2}s may occur during certain procedures [2].

Two types of dispersive electrodes are in common use today, the resistive type and the capacitive type. In disposable form, both electrodes have a similar structure and appearance. A thin, rectangular metallic foil has an insulating layer on the outside, connects to a gel-like material on the patient side and may be surrounded by adhesive foam. In the resistive type, the gel-like material is made of adhesive conductive gel, whereas in the capacitive type, it is made of dielectric nonconductive material. The adhesive foam and adhesive gel layer ensure that both electrodes maintain good skin contact to the patient, even if the electrode gets stressed mechanically from pulls on the electrode cable or some moisture develops under the electrode pad. Both types have specific advantages and disadvantages. Electrode failures and subsequent patient injury can be attributed mostly to improper application, electrode dislodgment, and electrode defects rather than to electrode design. There also exists a reusable capacitive dispersive electrode with an extra large, nonadhesive surface that is placed between the patient and the operating room table.

20.5 Bipolar Mode

The bipolar mode concentrates the current flow between two electrodes or two groups of electrodes, requiring considerably less power for achieving the same coagulation effect than the monopolar mode. For example, consider coagulating a small blood vessel with 3 mm external diameter and 2 mm internal diameter, a tissue resistivity of 360 Ωcm, a contact area of 2 $\times$ 4 mm, and a distance between the forceps tips of 1 mm. The tissue resistance between the forceps is 450 Ω as calculated from $R = \rho L/A$, where ρ is the resistivity, L the distance between the forceps, and A the contact area. Assuming a typical current density of 200 mA/cm^2, a small current of 16 mA, a voltage of 7.2 V, and a power level of 0.12 W suffice to coagulate this small blood vessel. In contrast, during monopolar coagulation, current levels of 200 mA and power levels of 100 W or more are not uncommon to achieve the same surgical effect. The temperature increase in the vessel tissue follows the bioheat Equation 20.1. If the specific heat of the vessel tissue is 4.2 J/kg K and the tissue density is 1 g/cm^3, then the temperature of the tissue between the forceps increases from 37°C to 57°C in 5.83 s. When the active electrode touches the tissue, less tissue damage occurs during coagulation because the charring and carbonization that accompany fulguration are avoided.

Surgeons may select among different sizes and shapes of forceps to further refine the desired clinical result. Fine-tipped forceps are frequently used in neurosurgery where very low power levels result in very small areas of tissue coagulation. Some hardware manufacturers have an autobipolar mode, which automatically turns the bipolar energy on when a tissue is grasped and automatically turns the energy off when a selectable level of coagulation is reached. This gives the surgeon a consistent level of coagulation, reduces tissue sticking, and greatly reduces fatigue in long procedures.

Advanced bipolar technologies include the sealing of blood vessels, fusion of tissue, tissue ablation, and bipolar cutting. Vessel sealing and tissue fusion uses special instruments and control algorithms to fuse the collagen within tissue. The most common use of this technology is to permanently seal blood vessels.

Tissue ablation utilizes bipolar or multipolar electrodes and specialized output waveforms to ablate soft or connective tissue. A tonsillectomy is an example of a procedure that may be performed using this bipolar method. Bipolar cutting does the same job as monopolar cutting but with the active and return electrodes in the same instrument. This allows lower powers to be used and a dispersive electrode is not required.

20.6 ESU Hazards

Improper use of electrosurgery may expose both the patient and the surgical staff to various hazards. By far, the most frequent hazard is an undesired burn. Less frequent are undesired neuromuscular stimulation, interference with pacemakers, or other devices, fires, and gas explosions [1,3].

Monopolar current returns to the ESU through the dispersive electrode. If the contact area of the dispersive electrode is large and the current exposure time short, then the skin temperature under the electrode does not rise above 45°C, which has been shown to be the maximum safe temperature [4]. However, to include a safety margin, the skin temperature should not rise more than 6°C above the normal surface temperature of 29–33°C [5]. The current density at any point under the dispersive electrode has to be significantly below the recognized burn threshold of 100 mA/cm² for 10 s. This means that the contact area between the electrode and the patient is the most important factor in preventing a dispersive electrode burn.

To avoid burns under dispersive electrodes, the IEC Standard for HF Surgical Devices [5] requires that "HF surgical equipment having a rated output power of more than 50 W shall be provided with a continuity monitor or contact quality monitor …." The most common of these is the contact quality monitor. A contact quality monitor consists of a circuit to measure the impedance between the two sides of a split dispersive electrode and the skin. This impedance is inversely proportional to the actual area of contact between the patient and the dispersive electrode. A small high-frequency current flows from one section of the dispersive electrode through the skin to the second section of the dispersive electrode. If the impedance between these two sections exceeds a certain threshold, or increases by a certain percentage, the patient contact area has unacceptably decreased, an audible alarm sounds, and the ESU output is disabled. The cable continuity monitor is less common. Unlike the contact quality monitor, this monitor only checks the continuity of the cable between the ESU and the dispersive electrode and sounds an alarm if the resistance in that conductor is greater than 1 Ω.

There are other sources of undesired burns. Active electrodes become hot when they are used. After use, the active electrode should be placed in a protective holster, if available, or on a suitable surface to isolate it from the patient and surgical staff [6]. The correct placement of an active electrode will also prevent the patient and/or surgeon from being injured, if an inadvertent activation of the ESU occurs (e.g., someone accidentally stepping on a foot pedal). Some surgeons use a practice called "buzzing the hemostat" in which a small bleeding vessel is grasped with a clamp or hemostat and the active electrode touched to the clamp while activating. Because of the high voltages involved and the stray capacitance to ground, the surgeon's glove may be compromised. This results in an instantaneous burn to the surgeon's finger, which feels like an electrical shock. If the surgical staff cannot be convinced to eliminate the practice of buzzing hemostats, the probability of burns can be reduced by using a cut waveform instead of a coagulation waveform (lower voltage), by maximizing contact between the surgeon's hand and the clamp, and by not activating until the active electrode is firmly touching the clamp.

Although it is commonly assumed that neuromuscular stimulation ceases or is insignificant at frequencies above 10 kHz, such stimulation has been observed in anesthetized patients undergoing certain electrosurgical procedures. This undesirable side effect of electrosurgery is generally attributed to nonlinear events that occur during the electric arcing between the active electrode and tissue [1]. These nonlinear events may rectify the high-frequency current leading to both dc and low-frequency ac components. These current components can reach magnitudes that stimulate nerve and muscle cells. To minimize the probability of unwanted neuromuscular stimulation, most ESUs incorporate in their output circuit a high-pass filter that suppresses dc and low-frequency ac components.

The use of electrosurgery means the presence of electric discharge arcs. This presents a potential fire hazard in an operating room where oxygen and flammable gases may be present. These flammable gases may be introduced by the surgical staff (anesthetics or flammable cleaning solutions), or may be generated within the patient themselves (bowel gases). The use of disposable paper drapes and dry surgical gauze also provides a flammable material that may be ignited by sparking or by contact with a hot active electrode. Therefore, prevention of fires and explosions depends primarily on the prudence and judgment of the ESU operator [7].

20.7 ESU Design

Modern ESUs contain building blocks that are also found in other medical devices, such as microprocessors, power supplies, enclosures, cables, indicators, displays, and alarms. The main building blocks unique to ESUs are control input switches, the high-frequency power amplifier, and the safety monitor.

Input control switches include front panel controls, footswitch controls, and handswitch controls. To make operating an ESU more uniform between models and manufacturers, and to reduce the possibility of operator error, the ANSI/AAMI/IEC 60601-2-2 standard [6] makes specific recommendations concerning the physical construction of ESUs and prescribes mechanical and electrical performance standards. For instance, front panel controls need to have their function identified by a permanent label and their output indicated on alphanumeric displays or on graduated scales; the pedals of foot switches need to be labeled and respond to a specified activation force; and if the active electrode handle incorporates two finger switches, their positions have to correspond to specific functions. Additional recommendations can be found in Reference 6.

Currently, three basic high-frequency power amplifiers are in use: the parallel connection of a bank of bipolar power transistors, the hybrid connection of parallel bipolar power transistors cascaded with metal oxide silicon field effect transistors (MOSFETs), and the bridge connection of MOSFETs. Each has unique properties and represents a stage in the evolution of ESUs.

In those devices that use a parallel bank of bipolar power transistors, the transistors are arranged in a Class A configuration. The bases, collectors, and emitters are all connected in parallel, and the collective base node is driven through a current-limiting resistor. A feedback resistor capacitor (RC) network between the base node and the collector node stabilizes the circuit. The collectors are usually fused individually before connecting to the common node, and through the primary coil of the step-up transformer to the high-voltage power supply. A capacitor and resistor in parallel to the primary coil create a resonant tank circuit that generates the output waveform at a specific frequency. Additional elements may be switched in and out of the primary parallel resistor inductor capacitor (RLC) circuit to alter the output power and waveform for various electrosurgical modes. Small-value resistors between the emitters and ground improve the current sharing between transistors. This configuration sometimes requires the use of matched sets of high-voltage power transistors.

A similar arrangement exists in amplifiers using parallel bipolar power transistors cascaded with a power MOSFET. This arrangement is called a hybrid cascode amplifier. In this type of amplifier, the collectors of a group of bipolar transistors are connected, via protection diodes, to one side of the primary of the step-up transformer. The other side of the primary is connected to the high-voltage power supply. The emitters of two or three bipolar transistors are connected, via current-limiting resistors, to the drain of an enhancement mode MOSFET. The source of the MOSFET is connected to ground and the gate of the MOSFET is connected to a voltage-snubbing network driven by a fixed-amplitude pulse created by a high-speed MOS driver circuit. The bases of the bipolar transistors are connected, via current control RC networks, to a common variable base voltage source. Each collector and base is separately fused. In cut modes, the gate drive pulse is at a fixed frequency and the base voltage is varied according to the power setting. In the coagulation modes, the base voltage is fixed, and the pulse width driving the MOSFET is varied. This changes the conduction time of the amplifier and controls the amount of energy imparted to the output transformer and its load. In the coagulation and the high-power cut modes, the bipolar power transistors are saturated and the voltage across the bipolar/MOSFET combination is low. This translates to high efficiency and low power dissipation.

The most common high-frequency power amplifier in use is a bridge connection of MOSFETs. In this configuration, the drains of a series of power MOSFETs are connected, via protection diodes, to one side of the primary of the step-up output transformer. The drain protection diodes protect the MOSFETs against the negative voltage swings of the transformer primary. The other side of the transformer primary is connected to the high-voltage power supply. The sources of the MOSFETs are connected to ground. The gate of each MOSFET has a resistor connected to ground and one to its driver circuitry. The resistor to ground speeds up the discharge of the gate capacitance when the MOSFET is turned on while the gate series resistor eliminates turn off oscillations. Various combinations of capacitors and/or inductor capacitor (LC) networks can be switched across the primary of the step-up output transformer to obtain different waveforms. In cut modes, the output power is controlled by varying the high-voltage power supply. In coagulation modes, the output power is controlled by varying the on time of the gate drive pulse.

Many manufacturers have begun to include sophisticated computer-based systems in their ESUs that not only simplify the use of the device but also increase the safety of patient and operator [8]. Some devices offer a so-called power-peak system that delivers a very short power peak at the beginning of electrosurgical cutting to start the cutting arc. Other modern devices use continuous monitoring of current and voltage levels to make automatic power adjustments and provide a smooth cutting action from the beginning of the incision to its end. Increased computing power, more sophisticated evaluation of voltage and current waveforms, and the addition of miniaturized sensors will continue to make ESUs more user friendly and safer.

Defining Terms

Active electrode: Electrode used for achieving desired surgical effect.
Coagulation: Solidifying proteins through the use of high-frequency currents that elevate the temperature of the tissue and reduce or terminate bleeding.
Desiccation: Drying of the tissue due to evaporation of intracellular fluids.
Dispersive electrode: Return electrode at which no electrosurgical effect is intended.
Fulguration: Random discharge of sparks between active electrode and tissue surface to achieve coagulation and/or desiccation.
Spray: Another term for fulguration. Sometimes, this waveform has a higher crest factor than fulguration.

References

1. Pearce, J.A., *Electrosurgery*, John Wiley & Sons, New York, 1986.
2. Overmyer, K.M., J.A. Pearce, and D.P. DeWitt, Measurements of temperature distributions at electro-surgical dispersive electrode sites, *J. Biomech.*, 101:66–72, 1972.
3. Francis G.G., *Unexplained Patient Burns: Investigating Iatrogenic Injuries*, Quest Publishing, Brea, CA, 1988.
4. Pearce, J.A., L.A. Geddes, J.F. Van Vleet, K. Foster, and J. Allen, Skin burns from electrosurgical current, *Med. Instrum.*, 17(3):225–231, 1983.
5. International Standard, Medical Electrical Equipment, Part 2: Particular requirements for the basic safety and essential performance of high frequency surgical equipment and high frequency surgical accessories, IEC 60601-2-2, 5th ed., 2009, International Electrotechnical Commission, Geneva, Switzerland.
6. Reed, A., Preventing thermal burns from electrosurgical instruments, *Infect. Control Today*, July 2001.

7. Podnos, Y.D. and R.A. Williams, Fires in the operating room, *Bull. Am. Coll. Surg.*, 82:8:14–17, 1997.
8. Haag, R. and A. Cuschieri, Recent advances in high-frequency electrosurgery: Development of automated systems, *J. R. Coll. Surg. Ednb.*, 38:354–364, 1993.

Further Information

American National Standard, Medical Electrical Equipment, Part 1: General requirements for basic safety and essential performance, ANSI/AAMI ES60601-1, 2005, Association for the Advancement of Medical Instrumentation, Arlington, VA.

American National Standard, Medical Electrical Equipment, Part 2: Particular requirements for the basic safety and essential performance of high frequency surgical equipment and high frequency surgical accessories, ANSI/AAMI/IEC 60601-2-2, 5th ed., 2009, Association for the Advancement of Medical Instrumentation, Arlington, VA.

International Standard, Medical Electrical Equipment, Part 1: General requirements for basic safety and essential performance, IEC 601-1, 3rd ed., 2005, International Electrotechnical Commission, Geneva, Switzerland.

21

Biomedical Lasers

Millard M. Judy
Baylor Research Institute

Approximately 20 years ago the CO_2 laser was introduced into surgical practice as a tool to photothermally ablate, and thus to incise and to debulk, soft tissues. Subsequently, three important factors have led to the expanding biomedical use of laser technology, particularly in surgery. These factors are (1) the increasing understanding of the wavelength selective interaction and associated effects of *ultraviolet-infrared (UV–IR) radiation* with biologic tissues, including those of acute damage and long-term healing, (2) the rapidly increasing availability of lasers emitting (essentially monochromatically) at those wavelengths that are strongly absorbed by molecular species within tissues, and (3) the availability of both optical fiber and lens technologies as well as of endoscopic technologies for delivery of the laser radiation to the often remote internal treatment site. Fusion of these factors has led to the development of currently available biomedical laser systems.

This chapter briefly reviews the current status of each of these three factors. In doing so, each of the following topics will be briefly discussed:

1. The physics of the interaction and the associated effects (including clinical efforts) of UV–IR radiation on biologic tissues
2. The fundamental principles that underlie the operations and construction of all lasers
3. The physical properties of the optical delivery systems used with the different biomedical lasers for delivery of the laser beam to the treatment site

4. The essential physical features of those biomedical lasers currently in routine use ranging over a number of clinical specialties, and brief descriptions of their use
5. The biomedical uses of other lasers used surgically in limited scale or which are currently being researched for applications in surgical and diagnostic procedures and the photosensitized inactivation of cancer tumors

In this review, effort is made in the text and in the last section to provide a number of key references and sources of information for each topic that will enable the reader's more in-depth pursuit.

21.1 Interaction and Effects of UV–IR Laser Radiation on Biologic Tissues

Electromagnetic radiation in the UV–IR spectral range propagates within biologic tissues until it is either scattered or absorbed.

21.1.1 Scattering in Biologic Tissue

Scattering in matter occurs only at the boundaries between regions having different optical refractive indices and is a process in which the energy of the radiation is conserved (Van de Hulst, 1957). Since biologic tissue is structurally inhomogeneous at the microscopic scale, for example, both subcellular and cellular dimensions, and at the macroscopic scale, for example, cellular assembly (tissue) dimensions, and predominantly contains water, proteins, lipids, and all different chemical species, it is generally regarded as a scatterer of UV–IR radiation. The general result of scattering is deviation of the direction of propagation of radiation. The deviation is strongest when wavelength and scatterer are comparable in dimension (Mie scattering) and when wavelength greatly exceeds particle size (Rayleigh scattering) (Van de Hulst, 1957). This dimensional relationship results in the deeper penetration into biologic tissues of those longer wavelengths which are not absorbed appreciably by pigments in the tissues. This results in the relative transparency of nonpigmented tissues over the visible and near-IR wavelength ranges.

21.1.2 Absorption in Biologic Tissue

Absorption of UV–IR radiation in matter arises from the wavelength-dependent resonant absorption of radiation by molecular electrons of optically absorbing molecular species (Grossweiner, 1989). Because of the chemical inhomogeneity of biologic tissues, the degree of absorption of incident radiation strongly depends upon its wavelength. The most prevalent or concentrated UV–IR absorbing molecular species in biologic tissues are listed in Table 21.1 along with associated high-absorbance wavelengths. These species include the peptide bonds; the phenylalanine, tyrosine, and tryptophan residues of proteins, all of which absorb in the UV range; oxy- and deoxyhemoglobin of blood which absorb in the visible to near-IR range; melanin, which absorbs throughout the UV to near-IR range, which decreases absorption occurring with increasing wavelength; and water, which absorbs maximally in the mid-IR range (Hale and Querry, 1973; Miller and Veitch, 1993; White et al., 1968). Biomedical lasers and their emitted radiation wavelength values also are tabulated in Table 21.1. The correlation between the wavelengths of clinically useful lasers and wavelength regions of absorption by constituents of biological tissues is evident. Additionally, exogenous light-absorbing chemical species may be intentionally present in tissues. These include:

1. Photosensitizers, such as porphyrins, which upon excitation with UV–visible light initiate photochemical reactions which are cytotoxic to the cells of the tissue, for example, a cancer which concentrates the photosensitizer relative to surrounding tissues (Spikes, 1989).
2. Dyes such as indocyanine green which, when dispersed in a concentrate fibrin protein gel can be used to localize 810 nm *GaAlAs* diode laser radiation and the associated heating to achieve

TABLE 21.1 UV–IR-Radiation-Absorbing Constituent of Biological Tissues and Biomedical Laser Wavelengths

Constituent	Tissue Type	Optical Absorption Wavelength[a] (nm)	Relative[b] Strength	Laser Type	Wavelength (nm)
Proteins	All				
Peptide bond		<220 (r)	++++++	ArF	193
Amino acid					
Residues					
Tryptophan		220–290 (r)	+		
Tyrosine		220–290 (r)	+		
Phenylalanine		220–2650 (r)	+		
Pigments					
Oxyhemoglobin	Blood	414 (p)	+++	Ar ion	488–514.5
	Vascular tissues	537 (p)	++	Frequency	532
		575 (p)	++	Doubled	
		970 (p)	+	Nd:YAG	
		690–1100 (r)		Diode	810
				Nd:YAG	1064
Deoxyhemoglobin	Blood	431 (p)	+++	Dye	400–700
	Vascular tissues	554 (p)	++	Nd:YAG	1064
Melanin	Skin	220–1000 (r)	++++	Ruby	693
Water	All	2.1 (p)	+++	Ho:YAG	2100
		3.02 (p)	++++++	Er:YAG	2940
		>2.94 (r)	++++	CO_2	10,640

[a] (p): Peak absorption wavelength; (r): wavelength range.
[b] The number of +signs qualitatively ranks the magnitude of the optical absorption.

localized thermal denaturation and bonding of collagen to affect joining or welding of tissue (Bass et al., 1992; Oz et al., 1989).

3. Tattoo pigments including graphite (black) and black, blue, green, and red organic dyes (Fitzpatrick, 1994; McGillis et al., 1994).

21.2 Penetration and Effects of UV–IR Laser Radiation into Biologic Tissue

Both scattering and absorption processes affect the variations of the intensity of radiation with propagation into tissues. In the absence of scattering, absorption results in an exponential decrease of radiation intensity described simply by Beers law (Grossweiner, 1989). With appreciable scattering present, the decrease in incident intensity from the surface is no longer monotonic. A maximum in local internal intensity is found to be present due to efficient back-scattering, which adds to the intensity of the incoming beam as shown, for example, by Miller and Veitch (1993) for visible light penetrating into the skin and by Rastegar et al. (1992) for 1.064 μm *Nd:YAG* laser radiation penetrating into the prostate gland. Thus, the relative contributions of absorption and scattering of incident laser radiation will stipulate the depth in a tissue at which the resulting tissue effects will be present. Since the absorbed energy can be released in a number of different ways including thermal vibrations, fluorescence, and resonant electronic energy transfer according to the identity of the absorber, the effects on tissue are in general different. Energy release from both hemoglobin and melanin pigments and from water is by molecular vibrations resulting in a local temperature rise. Sufficient continued energy absorption and release can result in local temperature increases which, as energy input increases, result in protein denaturation (41–65°C), water evaporation and boiling (up to ≈ 300°C under confining pressure of tissue), thermolysis of proteins, generation of gaseous decomposition products and of carbonaceous residue or char (≥300°C). The generation of residual char is minimized by sufficiently rapid energy input to support rapid gasification reactions. The clinical effect of this chain of thermal events is tissue ablation. Much smaller values of energy input result in coagulation of tissues due to protein denaturation.

Energy release from excited exogenous photosensitizing dyes is via formation of free-radical species or energy exchange with itinerant dissolved molecular oxygen (Spikes, 1989). Subsequent chemical reactions following free-radical formation or formation of an activated or more reactive form of molecular oxygen following energy exchange can be toxic to cells with takeup of the photosensitizer.

Energy release following absorption of *visible (VIS) radiation* by fluorescent molecular species, either endogenous to tissue or exogenous, is predominantly by emission of longer wavelength radiation (Lakowicz, 1983). Endogenous fluorescent species include tryptophan, tyrosine, phenylalanine, flavins, and metal-free porphyrins. Comparison of measured values of the intensity of fluorescence emission from hyperplastic (transformed precancerous) cervical cells to cancerous cervical cells with normal cervical epithelial cells shows a strong potential for diagnostic use in the automated diagnosis and staging of cervical cancer (Mahadevan et al., 1993).

21.3 Effects of Mid-IR Laser Radiation

Because of the very large absorption by water of radiation with wavelength in the IR range ≥2.0 µm, the radiation of *Ho:YAG, Er:YAG,* and CO_2 lasers is absorbed within a very short distance of the tissue surface, and scattering is essentially unimportant. Using published values of the water absorption coefficient (Hale and Querry, 1973) and assuming an 80% water content and that the decrease in intensity is exponential with distance, the depth in the "average" soft tissue at which the intensity has decreased to 10% of the incident value (the optical penetration depth) is estimated to be 619, 13, and 170 µm, respectively, for Ho:YAG, Er:YAG, and CO_2 laser radiation. Thus, the absorption of radiation from these laser sources and thermalization of this energy results essentially in the formation of a surface heat source. With sufficient energy input, tissue ablation through water boiling and tissue thermolysis occur at the surface. Penetration of heat to underlying tissues is by diffusion alone; thus, the depth of coagulation of tissue below the surface region of ablation is limited by competition between thermal diffusion and the rate of descent of the heated surface impacted by laser radiation during ablation of tissue. Because of this competition, coagulation depths obtained in soft biologic tissues with use of mid-IR laser radiation are typically ≤205–500 µm, and the ability to achieve sealing of blood vessels leading to hemostatic ("bloodless") surgery is limited (Judy et al., 1992; Schroder et al., 1987).

21.4 Effects of Near-IR Laser Radiation

The 810-nm and 1064-µm radiation, respectively, of the GaAlAs diode laser and Nd:YAG laser penetrate more deeply into biologic tissues than the radiation of longer-wavelength IR lasers. Thus, the resulting thermal effects arise from absorption at greater depth within tissues, and the depths of coagulation and degree of hemostasis achieved with these lasers tend to be greater than with the longer-wavelength IR lasers. For example, the optical penetration depths (10% incident intensity) for 810-nm and 1.024-µm radiation are estimated to be 4.6 and ≃8.6 mm, respectively, in canine prostate tissue (Rastegar et al., 1992). Energy deposition of 3600 J from each laser onto the urethral surface of the canine prostate results in maximum coagulation depths of 8 and 12 mm, respectively, using diode and Nd:YAG lasers (Motamedi et al., 1993). Depths of optical penetration and coagulation in porcine liver, a more vascular tissue than prostate gland, of 2.8 and ≃9.6 mm, respectively, were obtained with a Nd:YAG laser beam, and of 7 and 12 mm, respectively, with an 810-nm diode laser beam (Rastegar et al., 1992). The smaller penetration depth obtained with 810-nm diode radiation in liver than in prostate gland reflects the effect of greater vascularity (blood content) on near-IR propagation.

21.5 Effects of Visible-Range Laser Radiation

Blood and vascular tissues very efficiently absorb radiation in the visible wavelength range due to the strong absorption of hemoglobin. This absorption underlies, for example, the use of

1. The argon ion laser (488–514.5 nm) in the localized heating and thermal coagulation of the vascular choroid layer and adjacent retina, resulting in the anchoring of the retina in treatment of retinal detachment (Katoh and Peyman, 1988).
2. The argon ion laser (488–514.5 nm), frequency-doubled Nd:YAG laser (532 nm), and dye laser radiation (585 nm) in the coagulative treatment of cutaneous vascular lesions such as port wine stains (Mordon et al., 1993).
3. The argon ion (488–514.5 nm) and frequency-doubled Nd:YAG lasers (532 nm) in the ablation of pelvic endometrial lesions which contain brown iron-containing pigments (Keye et al., 1983).

Because of the large absorption by hemoglobin and iron-containing pigments, the incident laser radiation is essentially absorbed at the surface of the blood vessel or lesion, and the resulting thermal effects are essentially local (Miller and Veitch, 1993).

21.6 Effects of UV Laser Radiation

Whereas exposure of tissue to IR and visible-light-range laser energy result in removal of tissue by thermal ablation, exposure to *argon fluoride* (*ArF*) laser radiation of 193-nm wavelength results predominantly in ablation of tissue initiated by a photochemical process (Garrison and Srinivasan, 1985). This ablation arises from repulsive forces between like-charged regions of ionized protein molecules that result from ejection of molecular electrons following UV photon absorption (Garrison and Srinivasan, 1985). Because the ionization and repulsive processes are extremely efficient, little of the incident laser energy escapes as thermal vibrational energy, and the extent of thermal coagulation damage adjacent to the site of incidence is very limited (Garrison and Srinivasan, 1985). This feature and the ability to tune very finely the fluence emitted by the ArF laser so that micrometer depths of tissue can be removed have led to ongoing clinical trials to investigate the efficiency of the use of the ArF laser to selectively remove tissue from the surface of the human cornea for correction of short-sighted vision to eliminate the need for corrective eyewear (Van Saarloos and Constable, 1993).

21.7 Effects of Continuous and Pulsed IR–Visible Laser Radiation and Associated Temperature Rise

Heating following absorption of IR–visible laser radiation arises from molecular vibration during loss of the excitation energy and initially is manifested locally within the exposed region of tissue. If incidence of the laser energy is maintained for a sufficiently long time, the temperature within adjacent regions of biologic tissue increases due to heat diffusion. The mean squared distance $\langle X^2 \rangle$ over which appreciable heat diffusion and temperature rise occur during exposure time t can be described in terms of the thermal diffusion time τ by the equation:

$$\langle X^2 \rangle = \tau t \tag{21.1}$$

where τ is defined as the ratio of the thermal conductivity to the product of the heat capacity and density. For soft biologic tissues τ is approximately $1 \times 10^3 \ \mathrm{cm^2\,s^{-1}}$ (Meijering et al., 1993). Thus, with continued energy input, the distance over which thermal diffusion and temperature rise occurs increases. Conversely, with use of pulsed radiation, the distance of heat diffusion can be made very small; for example, with exposure to a 1-μs pulse, the mean thermal diffusion distance is found to be approximately 0.3 μm, or about 3–10% of a biologic cell diameter. If the laser radiation is strongly absorbed and the ablation of tissues is efficient, then little energy diffuses away from the site of incidence, and lateral thermally induced coagulation of tissue can be minimized with pulses of short duration. The effect of limiting lateral thermal damage is desirable in the cutting of cornea (Hibst et al., 1992) and sclera of the eye (Hill et al., 1993), and joint cartilage (Maes and Sherk, 1994), all of which are avascular (or nearly so, with cartilage), and the hemostasis arising from lateral tissue coagulation is not required.

21.8 General Description and Operation of Lasers

Lasers emit a beam of intense electromagnetic radiation that is essentially monochromatic or contains at most a few nearly monochromatic wavelengths and is typically only weakly divergent and easily focused into external optical systems. These attributes of laser radiation depend on the key phenomenon which underlies laser operation, that of light amplification by stimulated emission of radiation, which in turn gives rise to the acronym *LASER*.

In practice, a laser is generally a generator of radiation. The generator is constructed by housing a light-emitting medium within a cavity defined by mirrors which provide feedback of emitted radiation through the medium. With sustained excitation of the ionic or molecular species of the medium to give a large density of excited energy states, the spontaneous and attendant stimulated emission of radiation from these states by photons of identical wavelength (a lossless process), which is amplified by feedback due to photon reflection by the cavity mirrors, leads to the generation of a very large photon density within the cavity. With one cavity mirror being partially transmissive, say 0.1–1%, a fraction of the cavity energy is emitted as an intense beam. With suitable selection of a laser medium, cavity geometry, and peak wavelengths of mirror reflection, the beam is also essentially monochromatic and very nearly collimated.

Identity of the lasing molecular species or laser medium fixes the output wavelength of the laser. Laser media range from gases within a tubular cavity, organic dye molecules dissolved in a flowing inert liquid carrier and heat sink, to impurity-doped transparent crystalline rods (solid state lasers) and semiconducting diode junctions (Lengyel, 1971). The different physical properties of these media in part determine the methods used to excite them into lasing states.

Gas-filled, or gas lasers are typically excited by dc or rf electric current. The current either ionizes and excites the lasing gas, for example, argon, to give the electronically excited and lasing Ar+ ion, or ionizes a gaseous species in a mixture also containing the lasing species, for example, N_2, which by efficient energy transfer excites the lasing molecular vibrational states of the CO_2 molecule.

Dye lasers and so-called solid-state lasers are typically excited by intense light from either another laser or from a flashlamp. The excitation light wavelength range is selected to ensure efficient excitation at the absorption wavelength of the lasing species. Both excitation and output can be continuous, or the use of a pulsed flashlamp or pulsed exciting laser to pump a solid-state or dye laser gives pulsed output with high peak power and short pulse duration of 1 μs to 1 ms. Repeated excitation gives a train of pulses. Additionally, pulses of higher peak power and shorter duration of approximately 10 ns can be obtained from solid lasers by intracavity Q-switching (Lengyel, 1971). In this method, the density of excited states is transiently greatly increased by impeding the path between the totally reflecting and partially transmitting mirror of the cavity interrupting the stimulated emission process. Upon rapid removal of the impeding device (a beam-interrupting or -deflecting device), stimulated emission of the very large population of excited lasing states leads to emission of an intense laser pulse. The process can give single pulses or can be repeated to give a pulse train with repetition frequencies typically ranging from 1 Hz to 1 kHz.

Gallium–aluminum (GaAlAs) lasers are, as are all semiconducting diode lasers, excited by electrical current which creates excited hole-electron pairs in the vicinity of the diode junction. Those carrier pairs are the lasing species which emit spontaneously and with photon stimulation. The beam emerges parallel to the function with the plane of the function forming the cavity and thin-layer surface mirrors providing reflection. Use of continuous or pulsed excitation current results in continuous or pulsed output.

21.9 Biomedical Laser Beam Delivery Systems

Beam delivery systems for biomedical lasers guide the laser beam from the output mirror to the site of action on tissue. Beam powers of up to 100 W are transmitted routinely. All biomedical lasers incorporate a coaxial aiming beam, typically from a HeNe laser (632.8 nm) to illuminate the site of incidence on tissue.

Usually, the systems incorporate two different beam-guiding methods, either (1) a flexible fused silica (SiO_2) optical fiber or light guide, generally available currently for laser beam wavelengths between $\approx$400 nm and $\approx$2.1 μm, where SiO_2 is essentially transparent and (2) an articulated arm having beam-guiding mirrors for wavelengths greater than circa 2.1 μm (e.g., CO_2 lasers), for the Er:YAG and for pulsed lasers having peak power outputs capable of causing damage to optical fiber surfaces due to ionization by the intense electric field (e.g., pulsed ruby). The arm comprises straight tubular sections articulated together with high-quality power-handling dielectric mirrors at each articulation junction to guide the beam through each of the sections. Fused silica optical fibers usually are limited to a length of 1–3 m and to wavelengths in the visible-to-low midrange IR (<2.1 μm), because longer wavelengths of IR radiation are absorbed by water impurities (<2.9 μm) and by the SiO_2 lattice itself (wavelengths > 5 μm), as described by Levi (1980).

Since the flexibility, small diameter, and small mechanical inertia of optical fibers allow their use in either flexible or rigid endoscopes and offer significantly less inertia to hand movement, fibers for use at longer IR wavelengths are desired by clinicians. Currently, researchers are evaluating optical fiber materials transparent to longer IR wavelengths. Material systems showing promise are fused Al_2O_3 fibers in short lengths for use with near-3-μm radiation of the Er:YAG laser and *Ag halide* fibers in short lengths for use with the CO_2 laser emitting at 10.6 μm (Merberg, 1993). A flexible hollow Teflon waveguide 1.6 mm in diameter having a thin metal film overlain by a dielectric layer has been reported recently to transmit 10.6 μm CO_2 radiation with attenuation of 1.3 and 1.65 dB/m for straight and bent (5-mm radius, 90-degree bend) sections, respectively (Gannot et al., 1994).

21.9.1 Optical Fiber Transmission Characteristics

Guiding of the emitted laser beam along the optical fiber, typically of uniform circular cross-section, is due to total internal reflection of the radiation at the interface between the wall of the optical fiber core and the cladding material having refractive index n_1 less than that of the core n_2 (Levi, 1980). Total internal reflection occurs for any angle of incidence θ of the propagating beam with the wall of the fiber core such that $\theta > \theta_c$ where

$$\sin \theta_c = \left(\frac{n_1}{n_2} \right) \tag{21.2}$$

or in terms of the complementary angle α_c

$$\cos \alpha_c = \left(\frac{n_1}{n_2} \right) \tag{21.3}$$

For a focused input beam with apical angle α_m incident upon the flat face of the fiber as shown in Figure 21.1, total internal reflection and beam guidance within the fiber core will occur (Levi, 1980) for

$$NA = \sin(\alpha_m/2) \leq [n_2^2 - n_1^2]^{0.5} \tag{21.4}$$

where NA is the numerical aperture of the fiber.

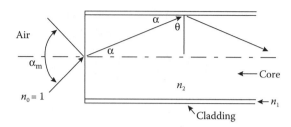

FIGURE 21.1   Critical reflection and propagation within an optical fiber.

This relationship ensures that the critical angle of incidence of the interface is not exceeded and that total internal reflection occurs (Levi, 1980). Typical values of NA for fused SiO_2 fibers with polymer cladding are in the range of 0.36–0.40. The typical values of $\alpha_m = 14°$ used to insert the beam of the biomedical laser into the fiber is much smaller than those values ($\simeq 21$–$23°$) corresponding to typical NA values. The maximum value of the propagation angle α typically used in biomedical laser systems is $\simeq 4.8°$.

Leakage of radiation at the core–cladding interface of the fused SiO_2 fiber is negligible, typically being 0.3 dB/m at 400 nm and 0.01 dB/m at 1.064 µm. Bends along the fiber length always decrease the angle of the incidence at the core–cladding interface. Bends do not give appreciable losses for values of the bending radius sufficiently large that the angle of incidence θ of the propagating beam in the bent core does not become less than θ_c at the core–cladding interface (Levi, 1980). The relationship given by Levi (1980) between the bending radius r_b, the fiber core radius r_o, the ratio (n_2/n_1) of fiber core to cladding refractive indices, and the propagation angle α in Figure 21.1 which ensures that the beam does not escape is

$$\frac{n_1}{n_2} > \frac{1-\rho}{1+\rho}\cos\alpha \tag{21.5}$$

where $\rho = (r_o/r_b)$. The inequality will hold for all $\alpha \le \alpha_c$ provided that

$$\frac{n_1}{n_2} \le \frac{1-\rho}{1+\rho} \tag{21.6}$$

Thus, the critical bending radius r_{bc} is the value of r_b such that Equation 21.6 is an equality. Use of Equation 21.6 predicts that bends with radii ≥ 12, 18, and 30 mm, respectively, will not result in appreciable beam leakage from fibers having 400–, 600–, and 1000-µm diameter cores, which are typical in biomedical use. Thus, use of fibers in flexible endoscopes usually does not compromise beam guidance.

Because the integrity of the core–cladding interface is critical to beam guiding, the clad fiber is encased typically in a tough but flexible protective fluoropolymer buffer coat.

21.9.2 Mirrored Articulated Arm Characteristics

Typically two or three relatively long tubular sections or arms of 50–80 cm length make up the portion of the articulated arm that extends from the laser output fixturing to the handpiece, endoscope, or operating microscope stage used to position the laser beam onto the tissue proper. Mirrors placed at the articulation of the arms and within the articulated handpiece, laparoscope, or operating microscope stage maintain the centration of the trajectory of the laser beam along the length of the delivery system. Dielectric multilayer mirrors (Levi, 1980) are routinely used in articulated devices. Their low–high reflectivity $\le 99.9 + \%$ and power-handling capabilities ensure efficient power transmission down the arm. Mirrors in articulated devices typically are held in kinetically adjustable mounts for rapid stable alignment to maintain beam concentration.

21.9.3 Optics for Beam Shaping on Tissues

Since the rate of heating on tissue, and hence rates of ablation and coagulation, depend directly on energy input per unit volume of tissue, selection of ablation and coagulation rates of various tissues is achieved through control of the energy density (J/cm^2 or $W\ s/cm^2$) of the laser beam. This parameter is readily achieved through use of optical elements such as discrete focusing lenses placed on the handpiece or rigid endoscope which controls the spot size upon the tissue surface or by affixing a so-called contact tip to the end of an optical fiber. These are conical or spherical in shape with diameters ranging from 300 to 1200 μm and with very short focal lengths. The tip is placed in contact with the tissue and generates a submillimeter-sized focal spot in tissue very near the interface between the tip and tissue. One advantage of using the contact tip over a focused beam is that ablation proceeds with small lateral depth of attendant coagulation (Judy et al., 1993a). This is because the energy of the tightly focused beam causes tissue thermolysis essentially at the tip surface and because the resulting tissue products strongly absorb the beam resulting in energy deposition and ablation essentially at the tip surface. This contrasts with the radiation penetrating deeply into tissue before thermolysis which occurs with a less tightly focused beam from a free lens or fiber. An additional advantage with the use of contact tips in the perception of the surgeon is that the kinesthetics of moving a contact tip along a resisting tissue surface more closely mimics the "touch" encountered in moving a scalpel across the tissue surface.

Recently a class of optical fiber tips has been developed which laterally directs the beam energy from a silica fiber (Judy et al., 1993b). These tips, either a gold reflective micromirror or an angled refractive prism, offer a lateral angle of deviation ranging from 35 to 105° from the optical fiber axis (undeviated beam direction). The beam reflected from a plane micromirror is unfocused and circular in cross-section, whereas the beam from a concave mirror and refractive devices is typically elliptical in shape, fused with distal diverging rays. Fibers with these terminations are currently finding rapidly expanding, large-scale application in coagulation (with 1.064-μm Nd:YAG laser radiation) of excess tissue lining the urethra in treatment of benign prostatic hypertrophy (Costello et al., 1992). The capability for lateral beam direction may offer additional utility of these terminated fibers in other clinical specialties.

21.9.4 Features of Routinely Used Biomedical Lasers

Currently four lasers are in routine large-scale clinical biomedical use to ablate, dissect, and to coagulate soft tissue. Two, the carbon dioxide (CO_2) and argon ion (Ar-ion) lasers, are gas-filled lasers. The other two employ solid-state lasing media. One is the Neodymium–yttrium–aluminum–garnet (Nd:YAG) laser, commonly referred to as a solid-state laser, and the other is the gallium–aluminum arsenide (GaAlAs) semiconductor diode laser. Salient features of the operating characteristics and biomedical applications of those lasers are listed in Tables 21.2 through 21.5. The operational descriptions are

TABLE 21.2 Operating Characteristics of Principal Biomedical Lasers

Characteristics	Ar Ion Laser	CO$_2$ Laser
Cavity medium	Argon gas, 133 Pa	10% CO_2, 10% Ne, and 80% He; 1330 Pa
Lasing species	Ar + ion	CO_2 molecule
Excitation	Electric discharge, continuous	Electric discharge, continuous, pulsed
Electric input	208 V_{AC}, 60 A	110 V_{AC}, 15 A
Wall plug efficiency	≈0.06%	≈10%
Characteristics	Nd:YAG laser	GaAlAs diode laser
Cavity medium	Nd-doped YAG	n–p junction, GaAlAs diode
Lasing species	Nd3t in YAG lattice	Hole-electron pairs at diode junction
Excitation	Flashlamp, continuous, pulsed	Electric current, continuous pulsed
Electric input	208/240 V_{AC}, 30 A continuous	110 V_{AC}, 15 A
	110 V_{AC}, 10 A pulsed	
Wall plug efficiency	≈1%	≈23%

TABLE 21.3   Output Beam Characteristics of Ar Ion and CO_2 Biomedical Lasers

Output Characteristics	Argon Laser	CO_2 Laser
Output power	2–8 W, continuous	1–100 W, continuous
Wavelength (s)	Multiple lines (454.6–528.7 nm), 488, 514.5, dominant	10.6 μm
Electromagnetic wave propagation mode	TEM_∞	TEM_∞
Beam guidance, shaping	Fused-silica optical fiber with contact tip or flat ended for beam emission, lensed handpiece. Slit lamp with ocular lens	Flexible articulated arm with mirrors; lensed handpiece or mirrored-microscope platen

TABLE 21.4   Output Beam Characteristics of Nd:YAG and GaAlAs Diode Biomedical Lasers

Output Characteristics	Nd:YAG Lasers	GaAlAs Diode Laser
Output power	1–100 W continuous at 1.064 millimicron 1–36 W continuous at 532 nm (frequency doubled with KTP)	1–25 W continuous
Wavelength (s)	1.064 μm/532 nm	810 nm
Electromagnetic wave propagation modes	Mixed modes	Mixed modes
Beam guidance and shaping	Fused SiO_2 optical fiber with contact tip directing mirrored or refracture tip	Fused SiO_2 optical fiber with contact tip or laterally directing mirrored or refracture tip

TABLE 21.5   Clinical Uses of Principal Biomedical Lasers

Ar Ion Laser	CO_2 Laser
Pigmented (vascular) soft-tissue ablation in gynecology, general and oral surgery, otolaryngology, vascular lesion coagulation in dermatology, and retinal coagulation in ophthalmology	Soft-tissue ablation–dissection and bulk tissue removal in dermatology; gynecology; general, oral, plastic, and neurosurgery; otolaryngology; podiatry; urology

Nd:YAG Laser	GaAlAs Diode Laser
Soft tissue, particularly pigmented vascular tissue, ablation–dissection, and bulk tissue removal—in dermatology; gastroenterology; gynecology; general, arthroscopic, neuroplastic, and thoracic surgery; urology; posterior capsulotomy (ophthalmology) with pulsed 1.064 millimicron and ocular lens	Pigmented (vascular) soft-tissue ablation–dissection and bulk removal in gynecology; gastroenterology, general, surgery, and urology; FDA approval for otolaryngology and thoracic surgery pending

typical of the lasers currently available commercially and do not represent the product of any single manufacturer.

21.9.5 Other Biomedical Lasers

Some important biomedical lasers have smaller-scale use or currently are being researched for biomedical application. The following four lasers have more limited scales of surgical use:

The Ho:YAG (Holmium:YAG) laser, emitting pulses of 2.1 μm wavelength and up to 4 J in energy, used in soft tissue ablation in arthroscopic (joint) surgery (FDA approved).

The Q-switched Ruby ($Cr:Al_2O_3$) laser, emitting pulses of 694-nm wavelength and up to 2 J in energy is used in dermatology to disperse black, blue, and green tattoo pigments and melanin in pigmented lesions (not melanoma) for subsequent removal by phagocytosis by macrophages (FDA approved).

The flashlamp pumped pulsed dye laser emitting 1- to 2-J pulses at either 577- or 585-nm wavelength (near the 537–577 absorption region of blood) is used for treatment of cutaneous vascular lesions and melanin pigmented lesions except melanoma. Use of pulsed radiation helps to localize the thermal damage to within the lesions to obtain low damage of adjacent tissue.

The following lasers are being investigated for clinical uses:

1. The Er:YAG laser, emitting at 2.94 μm near the major water absorption peak (OH stretch), is currently being investigated for ablation of tooth enamel and dentin (Li et al., 1992).
2. Dye lasers emitting at 630–690 nm are being investigated for application as light sources for exciting dihematoporphyrin ether or benzoporphyrin derivatives in investigation of the efficacy of these photosensitives in the treatment of esophageal, bronchial, and bladder carcinomas for the FDA approved process.

Defining Terms

Biomedical Laser Radiation Ranges

Infrared (IR) radiation: The portion of the electromagnetic spectrum within the wavelength range 760 nm–1 mm, with the regions 760 nm–1.400 μm and 1.400–10.00 μm, respectively, called the near- and mid-IR regions.

Ultraviolet (UV) radiation: The portion of the electromagnetic spectrum within the wavelength range 100–400 nm.

Visible (VIS) radiation: The portion of the electromagnetic spectrum within the wavelength range 400–760 nm.

Laser Medium Nomenclature

Argon fluoride (ArF): Argon fluoride eximer laser (an eximer is a diatomic molecule which can exist only in an excited state).

Ar ion: Argon ion.

CO_2: Carbon dioxide.

$Cr:Al_2O_3$: Ruby laser.

Er:YAG: Erbium–yttrium–aluminum–garnet.

GaAlAs: Gallium–aluminum laser.

HeNe: Helium–neon laser.

Ho:YAG: Holmium–yttrium–aluminum–garnet.

Nd:YAG: Neodymium–yttrium–aluminum–garnet.

Optical Fiber Nomenclature

Ag halide: Silver halide, halide ion, typically bromine (Br) and chlorine (Cl).

Fused silica: Fused SiO_2.

References

Bass L.S., Moazami N., Pocsidio J. et al. 1992. Change in type I collagen following laser welding. *Lasers Surg. Med.* 12: 500.

Costello A.J., Johnson D.E., and Bolton D.M. 1992. Nd:YAG laser ablation of the prostate as a treatment for benign prostate hypertrophy. *Lasers Surg. Med.* 12: 121.

Fitzpatrick R.E. 1993. Comparison of the Q-switched Ruby, Nd:YAG, and alexandrite lasers in tattoo removal. *Lasers Surg. Med.* (Suppl.) 6: 52.

Gannot I., Dror J., Calderon S. et al. 1994. Flexible waveguides for IR laser radiation and surgery applications. *Lasers Surg. Med.* 14: 184.

Garrison B.J. and Srinivasan R. 1985. Laser ablation of organic polymers: Microscopic models for photochemical and thermal processes. *J. Appl. Physiol.* 58: 2909.

Grossweiner L.I. 1989. Photophysics. In: K.C. Smith (ed.), *The Science of Photobiology*, pp. 1–47. New York, Plenum.

Hale G.M. and Querry M.R. 1973. Optical constants of water in the 200 nm to 200 μm wavelength region. *Appl. Opt.* 12: 555.

Hibst R., Bende T., and Schröder D. 1992. Wet corneal ablation by Er:YAG laser radiation. *Lasers Surg. Med.* (Suppl.) 4: 56.

Hill R.A., Le M.T., Yashiro H. et al. 1993. Ab-interno erbium (Er:YAG) laser sclerostomy with iridotomy in Dutch cross rabbits. *Lasers Surg. Med.* 13: 559.

Judy M.M., Matthews J.L., Aronoff B.L. et al. 1993a. Soft tissue studies with 805 nm diode laser radiation: Thermal effects with contact tips and comparison with effects of 1064 nm. Nd:YAG laser radiation. *Lasers Surg. Med.* 13: 528.

Judy M.M., Matthews J.L., Gardetto W.W. et al. 1993b. Side firing laser–fiber technology for minimally invasive transurethral treatment of benign prostate hyperplasia. *Proc. Soc. Photo-Opt. Instr. Eng. (SPIE)* 1982: 86.

Judy M.M., Matthews J.L., Goodson J.R. et al. 1992. Thermal effects in tissues from simultaneous coaxial CO_2 and Nd:YAG laser beams. *Lasers Surg. Med.* 12: 222.

Katoh N. and Peyman G.A. 1988. Effects of laser wavelengths on experimental retinal detachments and retinal vessels. *Jpn. J. Ophthalmol.* 32: 196.

Keye W.R., Matson G.A., and Dixon J. 1983. The use of the argon laser in treatment of experimental endometriosis. *Fertil. Steril.* 39: 26.

Lakowicz J.R. 1983. *Principles of Fluorescence Spectroscopy.* New York, Plenum.

Lengyel B.A. 1971. *Lasers.* New York, John Wiley.

Levi L. 1980. *Applied Optics*, Vol. 2. New York, John Wiley.

Li Z.Z., Code J.E., and Van de Merve W.P. 1992. Er:YAG laser ablation of enamel and dentin of human teeth: Determination of ablation rates at various fluences and pulse repetition rates. *Lasers Surg. Med.* 12: 625.

Maes K.E. and Sherk H.H. 1994. Bone and meniscal ablation using the erbium YAG laser. *Lasers Surg. Med.* (Suppl.) 6: 31.

Mahadevan A., Mitchel M.F., Silva E. et al. 1993. Study of the fluorescence properties of normal and neoplastic human cervical tissue. *Lasers Surg. Med.* 13: 647.

McGillis S.T., Bailin P.L., Fitzpatrick R.E. et al. 1994. Successful treatments of blue, green, brown and reddish-brown tattoos with the Q-switched alexandrite laser. *Laser Surg. Med.* (Suppl.) 6: 52.

Meijering L.J.T., VanGermert M.J.C., Gijsbers G.H.M. et al. 1993. Limits of radial time constants to approximate thermal response of tissue. *Lasers Surg. Med.* 13: 685.

Merberg G.N. 1993. Current status of infrared fiberoptics for medical laser power delivery. *Lasers Surg. Med.* 13: 572.

Miller I.D. and Veitch A.R. 1993. Optical modeling of light distributions in skin tissue following laser irradiation. *Lasers Surg. Med.* 13: 565.

Mordon S., Beacco C., Rotteleur G. et al. 1993. Relation between skin surface temperature and minimal blanching during argon, Nd:YAG 532, and cw dye 585 laser therapy of port-wine stains. *Lasers Surg. Med.* 13: 124.

Motamedi M., Torres J.H., Cammack T. et al. 1993. Thermodynamics of cw laser interaction with prostatic tissue: Effects of simultaneous cooling on lesion size. *Lasers Surg. Med.* (Suppl.) 5: 64.

Oz M.C., Chuck R.S., Johnson J.P. et al. 1989. Indocyanine green dye-enhanced welding with a diode laser. *Surg. Forum* 40: 316.

Rastegar S., Jacques S.C., Motamedi M. et al. 1992. Theoretical analysis of high-power diode laser (810 nm) and Nd:YAG laser (1064 nm) for coagulation of tissue: Predictions for prostate coagulation. *Proc. Soc. Photo-Opt. Instr. Eng. (SPIE)* 1646: 150.

Schroder T., Brackett K., and Joffe S. 1987. An experimental study of effects of electrocautery and various lasers on gastrointestinal tissue. *Surgery* 101: 691.

Spikes J.D. 1989. Photosensitization. In: K.C. Smith (ed.), *The Science of Photobiology*, 2nd ed., pp. 79–110. New York, Plenum.

Van de Hulst H.C. 1957. *Light Scattering by Small Particles*. New York, John Wiley.

Van Saarloos P.P. and Constable I.J. 1993. Improved eximer laser photorefractive keratectomy system. *Lasers Surg. Med.* 13: 189.

White A., Handler P., and Smith E.L. 1968. *Principles of Biochemistry*, 4th ed. New York, McGraw-Hill.

Further Information

Current research on the optical, thermal, and photochemical interactions of radiation and their effect on biologic tissues, are published routinely in the journals: *Laser in Medicine and Surgery, Lasers in the Life Sciences,* and *Photochemistry Photobiology* and to a lesser extent in *Applied Optics and Optical Engineering.*

Clinical evaluations of biomedical laser applications appear in *Lasers and Medicine and Surgery* and in journals devoted to clinical specialties such as *Journal of General Surgery, Journal of Urology, and Journal of Gastroenterological Surgery.*

The annual symposium proceedings of the biomedical section of the *Society of Photo-Optical Instrumentation Engineers (SPIE)* contain descriptions of new and current research on application of lasers and optics in biomedicine.

The book *Lasers* (a second edition by Bela A. Lengyel), although published in 1971, remains a valuable resource on the fundamental physics of lasers—gas, dye, solid-state, and semiconducting diode. A more recent book, *The Laser Guidebook* by Jeffrey Hecht, published in 1992, emphasizes the technical characteristics of the gas, diode, solid-state, and semiconducting diode lasers.

The Journal of Applied Physics, Physical Review Letters, and *Applied Physics Letters* carry descriptions of the newest advances and experimental phenomena in lasers and optics.

The book *Safety with Lasers and Other Optical Sources* by David Sliney and Myron Wolbarsht, published in 1980, remains a very valuable resource on matters of safety in laser use.

Laser safety standards for the United States are given for all laser uses and types in the American National Standard (ANSI) Z136.1-1993, Safe Use of Lasers.

22

Measuring Cellular Traction Forces at the Micro- and Nanoscale

Nathan J. Sniadecki
University of Washington

Christopher S. Chen
University of Pennsylvania

22.1 Introduction

Individual cells exert forces that are essential to the development and function of tissue in an organism. The tension produced by actin and myosin proteins produce traction forces that allow cells to migrate from one locality to another in an organism. These forces are also used by cells to contract in order to change the shape of a tissue or to provide rigidity to its structure. In this chapter, we will discuss the techniques and assays that have been developed to measure traction forces during migration and contraction. These tools have helped to understand how these forces are regulated and the role they play in the biological function of cells.

Traction forces are important at all stages of life because it provides a mechanism for a cell to move to areas of need and repair the integrity of a tissue. At the early stage of an organism, the process of gastrulation drives the movement of cells from positions on the periphery of an embryo to the inside to create the layers that become the ectoderm, mesoderm, and endoderm. Morphogenesis continues the process of folding, movements, and cellular contractility to reach the final form of an organism. Once a final stage of the architecture is reached, the repair and maintenance of the tissue requires further coordinated cell movement. White blood cells exit from the blood stream and crawl through nearby tissue to patrol for pathogens, mutated cells, and debris from dead cells. Cellular locomotion is important in healing the regions where cells have been scrapped away or damaged. Replacement cells migrate into a wound site from adjacent regions to restore the integrity of a tissue's boundary and rebuild the surrounding extracellular matrix.

The movement of cells can also have pathological effects as in the case of cancer where angiogenesis drives the sprouting of endothelial cells to form new blood vessel in the direction of a tumor. New vessels speed up the growth of the tumor by increasing its nutritional supply. However, a more dire consequence of cell locomotion arises when cancer cells migrate away from a tumor and metastasize into other vital tissue, overwhelming the tissue's ability to function properly and thereby possibly causing the organism to die.

The measurement of cellular forces is a difficult task because cells are living entities and are responsive to physical stimuli through a process known as mechanotransduction, which can be defined as a biological response to forces or mechanical properties of the microenvironment.[1,2] Mechanotransduction has been implicated to play a role in proliferation, differentiation, migration, and morphogenesis. In particular to traction forces, a cell is able to adjust the assembly of actin and myosin at different regions within its cytoplasm to change its direction of migration or contraction in response to a physical cue. Perhaps one of the most fascinating and simultaneously challenging aspects of studying traction forces is that they can change in response to the tool itself. If one puts a force transducer on a cell, the cell will adjust its traction forces in proportion to the mechanical stiffness of the transducer. The adaptability of cells to the tools used makes it difficult to characterize the natural state of cells. Thus, one of the major goals of cell mechanics is not only to measure cellular traction forces, but also to identify the mechanism by which cells sense, interpret, and respond to physical stimuli.

22.2 Contractile Apparatus of Cells

As previously introduced, the behavior and function of a cell's contractile apparatus is dependent on two major proteins—actin and myosin. These proteins serve as the contractile machinery that generates strain within a cell's cytoskeleton to produce traction forces. An actin filament is made up of globular monomers known as G-actin that organize into a double-helical strand known as F-actin (Figure 22.1a). Because all actin monomers are orientated in the same direction along the double helix, there is polarity in the filament. Unique properties are associated with the positive "barbed end" and the negative "pointed end" by the different proteins that bind to actin. Actin grows its length by the polymerization of free monomers at either end, but the growth rate at the positive end is significantly larger. Within a cell, actin filaments can be found as bundles of fibers, interwoven meshes, three-dimensional (3D) gels, or intermediaries of the three. These structures form the cytoskeleton that provides mechanical support to the structure of a cell. Actin is a very strong polymer, having a modulus of elasticity between 1 and 2 GPa, and plays an essential role in locomotion by pushing the membrane of a cell forward. However, the role it plays in conjunction with myosin is of major importance to traction forces.

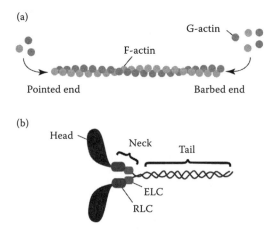

FIGURE 22.1 Actin and myosin proteins. (a) Actin forms a double-helix filament structure known as F-actin. Individual monomers known as G-actin are added at either end of the filament, but the rate of polymerization at the positive barbed end is significantly greater. (b) Myosin has a head region that binds to actin, a neck region that contains essential light chains (ELC) and regulatory light chains (RLC), and the tail region that is a coiled-coil structure.

Myosin converts chemical energy into mechanical work that slides actin filaments past each other to shorten the length of a cell. The structure of myosin has two heads, two necks, and a coiled-coil tail region (Figure 22.1b). Each head of myosin has an actin-binding site and utilizes ATP hydrolysis to move myosin toward the positive end of actin. The conformational change that arise from catalyzing ATP into ADP during ATP hydrolysis causes myosin's head to rotate about a fulcrum point in the neck region (Figure 22.2). The release of energy from ATP hydrolysis causes the head to cock forward to start the power stroke. When the head binds to actin, the phosphate dissociated from ATP is released and elastic energy stored in the cocked head is transferred to actin to complete the power stroke. The neck region plays a role as a stiff rod that increases the fulcrum action of myosin's head with each power stroke. Individual heads of myosin can deliver between 2 and 4 pN of force per power stroke.[3] The tail region of myosin interacts with the tail of another myosin to form a dimer, causing each myosin to be aligned antiparallel to the other. Multiple myosin dimers can self-assemble together into a myosin filament, which has a bipolar structure due to the myosin heads positioned at either end of the filament. The bipolar orientation of myosin filaments allows the heads to move actin filaments in opposite directions, or to create tension in the filaments when actin is restrained from sliding.

In the case of muscle, actin and myosin are arranged as parallel filaments that form a contractile unit called a sarcomere. Actin composes the thin filaments of the sarcomere and myosin forms the thick filaments (Figure 22.3a). Within each sarcomere unit, the positive ends of actin are anchored at the Z-disk by α-actinin, an actin cross-linking protein. Thin filaments are found at either side of the Z-disk and are aligned like the bristles of a hairbrush. Thick filaments are found interdigitated between thin filaments and their bipolar structure allows them to connect opposing thin filaments. Overall, this arrangement forms a structural sequence: Z-disk, thin filaments, thick filaments, thin filaments, Z-disk, and so on. Thin filaments are oriented with their negative ends facing each other and their positive ends at the Z-disk. When activated, myosin heads walk toward the positive ends of actin at both ends of the thick filament. This movement shortens the distance between opposing Z-disks by sliding actin filaments closer together. The structural sequence of the sarcomere is repeated along the length of a muscle cell and determines the overall distance the muscle can shorten.

The contractile apparatus in nonmuscle cells has many of the same proteins found in sarcomeres. Bundles of actin and myosin are known as stress fibers, which provide the cytoskeletal tension required for migration or contraction. Stress fibers are composed of bundles of actin filaments that are held

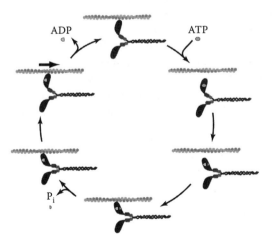

FIGURE 22.2 Actin–myosin power stroke cycle. At the top of the cycle, myosin releases from actin when ATP becomes bound. Myosin ATPase activity causes the dissociation of ATP into ADP and P_i, which changes the conformation of myosin for the power stroke. When myosin binds to actin, P_i is released and the head of myosin pulls on actin to impart a force on actin. The remaining ADP is then released and the power stroke cycle begins anew.

(a)

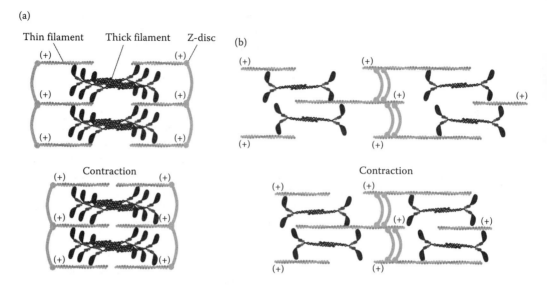

FIGURE 22.3 Contractile apparatus in cells. (a) A sarcomere is a highly organized contractile unit in muscle cells that uses actin thin filaments and myosin thick filaments to shorten the length of a muscle. (b) A stress fiber is a loosely organized contractile structure in nonmuscle cells that is essential for migration and contraction.

together by α-actinin and myosin (Figure 22.3b). The bands of α-actinin and myosin are observed to be periodic along the length of a stress fiber and the bands alternate with each other. In order for stress fibers to be contractile, the positive ends of actin cannot be oriented in the same direction or else myosin would simply walk along the filaments instead of sliding them past one another. Instead, actin filaments in a stress fiber need to have antiparallel alignment for the fiber to contract its length. The ends of a stress fiber are bound to adhesion sites with the extracellular matrix that allow the cell to deliver traction forces from the tension in the fiber.

For a cell to move, it requires the formation of new adhesions at its front end and the release of old adhesions at its back end. A useful conceptualization is that migration is a cycle of front protrusion, new adhesions, contraction, and release at the rear. A cell extends its membrane forward by actin polymerization to find new ligands for its integrin receptors to form a focal complex. Integrins are transmembrane receptors that mediate adhesion by binding to ligands in the extracellular matrix. On the cytoplasmic side, focal adhesion proteins connect integrins to the contractile apparatus of the cytoskeleton. Tension applied at a focal complex produces a traction force that pulls a cell forward. The tension also causes the complex to grow in size by recruiting additional focal adhesion proteins. These larger adhesion structures are referred to as focal adhesions and are found to be more stable than focal complexes, likely because of the abundant focal adhesion proteins that are able to aggregate additional integrins together to reinforce the bond strength to the extracellular matrix. To complete the migration step, a cell moves its body forward by contracting its length so as to create high force at its rear, breaking the bonds of a focal adhesion or contributing to its disassembly.

22.3 Design Consideration for Traction Force Assays

The difficulty in measuring traction forces arise because integrin-mediated adhesions can be as small as 100 nm in diameter and so the sensors must be able to resolve forces at a similar length scale. It is easy to see that this excludes most conventional force transducers, for instance, strain gages and metal springs. However, the same principles of elasticity that govern these tools are used to measure a cell's traction forces. To state simply, the strength of a force on a material is proportional to its deformation. Using this concept, known as Hooke's law, researchers have employed materials and techniques that have the appropriate physics and dimensions for measuring traction forces.

At the length scale of cells, the ratio of forces relative to each other is rather nonintuitive. In scaling down to the nanometer scale, a body force has a smaller effect on an object than a surface force. The former scales with length to the third power (L^3), whereas the latter scales with length to the second power (L^2). It is even more dramatic when one considers forces that scale only with length (L^1). To illustrate, an ant can lift up to a hundred times its own weight (L^3) because the strength of its muscles scale with their cross-sectional area (L^2), due to the number of thick filaments. However, an ant is easily trapped inside a droplet of water because of its surface tension, which scales with the length of the air–water interface (L^1). The implications of scaling laws for assaying traction forces is apparent when one considers that the weight of a cell with a 10 µm diameter is approximately 5 nN, yet the force at one of its focal adhesions can be larger than 100 nN.

The materials used in conventional force transducers and springs are not very feasible at the length scale of a cell. A typical metal has an elastic modulus that is greater than 50 GPa and so the shear strain for an area the size of a focal complex under the load of a traction force would be at most a few tenths of a percent. Given that a focal complex is already a difficult nanoscale structure to resolve with high-powered microscopy, the prospect of detecting a physical distortion that is a very small fraction of its size is nearly impossible. Therefore, softer structures are used instead of those that have low elastic moduli (Section 22.4.2) or slender dimensions (Section 22.4.3) because they can adequately measure a traction force by their larger degree of deformation.

To make slender objects for transducing traction forces, as in the case of cantilever force sensors, it is important to have control over the manufacturing dimensions. For this reason, nanotechnology and microfabrication have been used to construct the measurement devices. For example, cantilever beams have been built so thin and slender that although the elastic modulus of the materials are between 1 MPa and 100 GPa, the spring constant of the structure is in the range of 1–100 nN/µm. The structural flexibility allows the beam to deflect a few micrometers under the load of a traction force, which is an amount that is readily measured under a high-powered microscope.

The use of nanotechnology and microfabrication has also allowed thousands to millions of traction forces sensors to be manufactured at the same time. Large-scale production of the sensors is a major advantage in biological experiments. Cells within a culture or tissue are not identical. They have different degrees of metabolic activities, signaling reactions, cell cycle states, and differentiation cues due to stochastic processes. To overcome the "noise" in biological systems, large data sets are often required to make conclusions that are statistically significant. A supply of traction forces sensors that are plentiful and easy to prepare is a major benefit.

Not only must the mechanics of the new tools be tailored to the range of traction forces to be measured, but how to resolve the deflections must also be considered. Using a microscope to observe the deflection of a tool is a relatively noninvasive technique. Microscopy does require that the substrate be optically transparent, which limits materials available for fabrication. Additionally, one must consider whether to observe the forces exerted by one cell with high spatial and temporal accuracy, but with a limited data population, or whether to interrogate a large number of cells at a low magnification but with less measurement sensitivity. Overall, these considerations should act as a simple warning that one must treat each new system with a degree of guarded optimism on what kind of studies are possible because of the limits in its performance.

22.4 Traction Force Assays for Cells

To investigate traction forces and their role in physiology and pathology, tools have been made from materials that are biocompatible with cells and functionalized with proteins that allow cells to adhere through their integrin receptors. In general, studying traction forces involves culturing them on flexible substrates that physically deform under the applied load. Traction forces assays owe much to the work of Robert Hooke. In 1665, he was the first to use the term "cell" based on his observations with an early microscope and it is his theory of elasticity that is used predominantly to measure their forces.

22.4.1 Silicone Membrane Wrinkling

In the early 1980s, Albert Harris pioneered the first method for measuring traction forces.[4] His technique used a thin membrane of silicone rubber that wrinkled from the traction forces of a cell (Figure 22.4a). To create the silicone membrane, a film of liquid prepolymer was spread on a glass coverslip and briefly exposed to an open flame. The heat treatment created a thin skin of cured silicone rubber on top of the remaining silicone liquid. The skin was approximately 1 μm in thickness and the underlying silicone liquid served as a lubricant layer between the coverslip and the skin. Cells seeded onto the silicone membrane slowly pulled on the skin with a tangential force, producing wrinkles that were observed easily under an optical microscope. This technique was a breakthrough in that traction forces had been hypothesized previously, but had not been confirmed experimentally.

Albert Harris' technique could assess where there were regions of compression and tension beneath a cell by the shape and pattern of the wrinkles, which was useful in understanding the structures cells use to crawl. It was observed that the wrinkles were different between cell types, but there was no means to measure the strength of the traction forces that produced them, except to compare which cells produced more or less wrinkles than others. This tool also made major impact in assessing the enzymes and regulatory proteins that regulate traction forces by comparing the amount of wrinkles between different treatments or inhibitors given to cells.[5–9] Paradoxically, traction forces were found to be weakest among cell types that had the fastest migration speeds.[10] What was more puzzling was that fibroblasts were observed to have traction forces that were far larger than was required for cell migration. From this observation, traction forces were newly considered as factors in morphogenesis because fibroblasts were observed to pull matrix fibers into alignment, which bore a striking resemblance to the fiber arrangements seen in ligaments and tendons.

The silicone membrane wrinkling technique was later improved upon with an additional fabrication step to drastically reduce the stiffness of the substrate and provide a semiquantitative way to measure traction forces (Figure 22.4b). After flame curing, UV irradiation was used to weaken the elasticity of the silicone skin.[11,12] To calibrate the softer membranes, a known force from a glass pipette was applied to the surface and the length of the wrinkles that formed was measured. It was found that the length of a wrinkle increased linearly with the applied tip force. The improved wrinkling assay was used to study the change in contractility during cytokinesis, where daughter cells form by cleavage of the cytoplasm

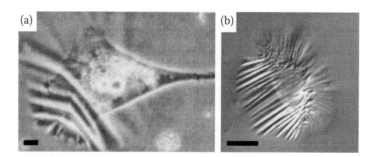

FIGURE 22.4 Silicone wrinkling membrane. (a) Fibroblast exerts traction forces that are strong enough to wrinkle the silicone rubber membrane. (Reproduced from Harris, A. K., Stopak, D. and Wild, P. *Nature* **290**, 249–251, 1981.) (b) Keratocyte produces significantly more wrinkles on silicone membranes made softer by UV irradiation. (Reproduced from Burton, K., Park, J. H. and Taylor, D. L. *Mol Biol Cell* **10**, 3745–3769, 1999.) Scale bars, 10 μm.

and then pull apart from each other. The increased number of wrinkles on the softer membranes allowed for assessing the different subcellular forces that occur during migration. At the lamellipodia of a migrating keratocyte, the wrinkles were radial and remain anchored to spots, possibly focal adhesion, as the cell advanced forward. Once these spots were translocated to the boundary between the lamellipodia and cell body, the wrinkles transitioned to compressive wrinkles. Overall, the improved spatial resolution of traction forces revealed that migration is a coordination of pulling forces at the front and detachment forces at the rear.

22.4.2 Traction Force Microscopy

Traction force microscopy is a technique that employs an elastic substrate, but instead of using wrinkles to indicate how strong a cell is as it distorts a substrate, beads or markers are embedded on the substrate to quantify traction forces by their displacement. The early approach developed in traction force microscopy was similar to Albert Harris' in that a thin silicone membrane on a liquid layer was used to detect traction forces, but micrometer-sized latex beads were stuck on the film and the membrane was kept taut so as to not wrinkle (Figure 22.5a). This approach had improved accuracy because traction forces could be measured quantitatively by the displacement of the beads.[13–15] The rigidity of the silicone membranes was rather high and so the technique was limited to analyzing cell types that were very contractile, like fibroblasts or keratocytes. Polyacrylamide gels were later adopted as the elasticity of the gels could be adjusted by the amount of bis-acrylamide cross-linker, so that a wider range of cell types could be studied.[16] Fluorescent beads were mixed into the polyacrylamide gel during the synthesis to act as markers of displacement and only those near the top surface of the gel were used for measuring traction forces (Figure 22.5b).

To compute traction forces, the positions of the beads are subtracted from their positions once the cell has been removed.[15,16] The subtraction creates a vector field that describes the deformation of the substrate from equilibrium. The displacements can then be used to solve for the traction forces by assuming that the membrane is an elastic material. Specifically, the membrane can be regarded as a semi-infinite half-space of an incompressible, elastic material with tangential forces applied only at the boundary

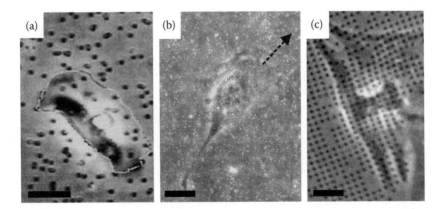

FIGURE 22.5 Traction force microscopy. (a) Keratocyte migrated on silicone membrane airbrushed with latex beads (scale bar, 20 μm). (Reproduced from Oliver, T., Dembo, M. and Jacobson, K. *Cell Motil Cytoskeleton* **31**, 225–240, 1995.) (b) Traction forces from a migrating fibroblast (arrow indicts direction of migration) are measured from the displacement of fluorescent beads embedded in a polyacrylamide gel (scale bar, 20 μm). (Reproduced from Munevar, S., Wang, Y. and Dembo, M. *Biophys J* **80**, 1744–1757, 2001.) (c) Contracting fibroblast distorts the regular array of micropatterned markers used to measure traction forces (scale bar, 20 μm). (Reproduced from Balaban, N. Q. et al. *Nat Cell Biol* **3**, 466–472, 2001.)

plane. Under these assumptions, the displacement vector field of the beads from the traction force vector field T is related by an integral relation:

$$u_i(x, y) = \iint G_{ij}(x - r, y - s)T_j(r, s)drds \tag{22.1}$$

where (x, y) is the position of bead and (s, r) is the position of the point-force. The problem is confined to the displacement of beads on the top surface of the substrate, so a two-dimensional (2D) solution is expected, where $1 \le i, j \le 2$ are the directional indices. Green's function G_{ij} relates the displacements u to the traction forces T beneath a cell. Because traction forces are discrete points, the integral becomes a set of linear equations $u_i = G_{ij}T_j$ which is inverted to solve for T_j. If one makes the assumption that Poisson's ratio is 0.5 because the substrate is incompressible, then Green's function has the form:

$$G_{ij}(\bar{x}) = \frac{3}{4\pi E}\left(\frac{\delta_{ij}}{|\bar{x}|} + \frac{x_i x_j}{|\bar{x}|^3}\right) \tag{22.2}$$

where E is the modulus of elasticity of the substrate and δ_{ij} is the Kronecker delta.

What may not be apparent in Equations 22.1 and 22.2 is that the beads embedded in the substrate do not move as an ideal elastic spring, in which their displacement is linearly proportional to an applied force. Instead, a single traction force displaces a bead proportionally to the stiffness E of the gel but also inversely to the distance $|\bar{x}|$ between them. The system of linear equations indicates that a bead is moved from the combined effect of multiple traction forces acting nearby. What is not certain in the experiments is how many points of force a cell exerts. This implies that the length of T could be greater than u, and so inverting the system of linear equations is not straightforward. To address this problem, regularization schemes are used that apply additional criteria on what range of solutions are feasible. These criteria include incorporating the constraint that the sum of all of the traction forces must balance because of equilibrium, the least complex solution be used, and whenever possible, traction forces are only applied at points where focal adhesions are detected.

If focal adhesions are not assessed for the last criterion, a grid-meshing approximation is superimposed on the area of cell during the calculation to solve for the traction forces at all regions beneath a cell. Because the beads are randomly seeded in the gel, there can be insufficient displacement information within regions of a cell to make an accurate estimation of the traction forces. The placement of mesh grids in these sparser areas leads to an ill-posed problem in solving for the force map because often more traction forces are assumed than there are displacement markers beneath a cell's area. To address this detection limitation, microfabricated regular arrays of fluorescent beads have been imprinted onto the elastomeric substrate for improved force tracking (Figure 22.5c).[17,18] The deformation of the marker pattern on the substrate is readily observed under a microscope. The patterns are formed with 800 nm or smaller spots that were spaced at 2 μm intervals. The calculation for the force mapping is similar to the random seeding but with significant reduction in the number of possible solutions due to the uniform density of displacement markers throughout the cell area.

The technique has led to various insights in cell mechanics. It has been shown that cells are able to adjust the strength of their traction forces in response to physical cues like rigidity or adhesivity of their environment.[19,20] How a cell responds to its physical environment with its traction forces has been implicated as a hallmark of cancer.[21–23] The technique has been used in combination with nanoscale manipulations like magnetic beads, laser nanoscissors, and nanoindentation to examine the mechanics of the cytoskeleton to verify different theories about its solidity or fluidity.[24–26] Overall, traction force microscopy is a relatively popular technique for measuring traction forces because the polyacrylamide gels are able to be fabricated with equipment commonly available in most laboratories.

22.4.3 Microfabricated Cantilever Force Sensors

In the previous methods, the use of a continuous membrane for measuring cell forces has the disadvantage that the traction forces are convoluted by the observed bead displacements. Because the calculation is not direct, constraints or assumptions are required to solve the inverse problem. A technique to transduce individual traction forces comes from the use of microfabricated cantilevers. The first demonstration of these sensors was a horizontal silicon cantilever that was made with microfabrication techniques (Figure 22.6a).[27,28] As a cell migrates across the surface, it bends the cantilever under the load of the traction force. Because the sensor is mechanically decoupled from the substrate, the deflection of the cantilever directly reports only the local force. The simple spring equation relates the deflection of the cantilever beam δ to the cellular traction force:

$$F = K\delta \tag{22.3}$$

where K is the measured spring constant for the cantilever (≈ 75 nN/μm). The fabrication steps involved in manufacturing the device were rather labor-intensive and expensive so these devices were reused between experiments. Although this technique could directly calculate a cell's traction force, it could only detect force at one point beneath a migrating cell. The beam could also defect only in its transverse direction and was very stiff in the longitudinal direction. Because of this, deflection was not due to the full strength of the traction force but to a portion of the traction force in the transverse direction. It was assumed that a cells' traction force acted in the same direction as its migration. This led to the calculation of traction forces by dividing by the sine of the angle between the migration direction and longitudinal axis of the beam.

A new approach was developed afterwards that modified the force sensor design by using vertical cantilevers.[29,30] With each cantilever placed perpendicular to the surface of the substrate, the spacing between force sensors could be significantly reduced and made it possible to have a high-density array of force sensors. This arrangement improved both the spatial resolution and the scope of possible experiments. Like Albert Harris' approach, the force sensor arrays were made from silicone rubber, but used a new manufacturing approach known as soft lithography.[31] Master templates for the cantilevers were

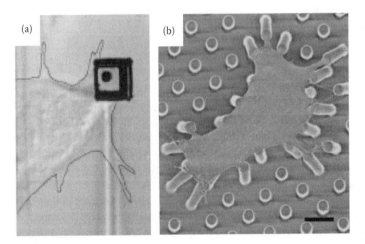

(a)

(b)

FIGURE 22.6 Microfabricated cantilever force sensors. (a) A silicon cantilever is constructed underneath a substrate. Its deflection is used to measure the traction force of a migrating fibroblast. (Reproduced from Galbraith, C. G. and Sheetz, M. P. *Proc Natl Acad Sci USA* **94**, 9114–9118, 1997.) (b) Local traction forces of a smooth muscle cell a measured with an array of vertical cantilever posts made from silicone elastomer (scale bar, 10 μm). (Reproduced from Tan, J. L. et al. *Proc Natl Acad Sci USA* **100**, 1484–1489, 2003.)

made from silicon or photoresist using microfabrication techniques.[32] Silicone rubber was then poured onto the masters, cured, and then peeled to create a replica of the master. The cost per device is inexpensive once the master has been built and many replicates can be made from the same master.

The deflection of a cantilever post is detectable under an optical microscope. As with the horizontal design, the deflection of a post is related by a simple cantilever beam relationship between force and displacement:

$$F = \left(\frac{3ED^4}{64L^3} \right) \delta \tag{22.4}$$

where E is the modulus of elasticity of the silicone, D the diameter of the cantilever post, and L its length. Unlike the horizontal cantilever devices, the deflection of the post are not limited to one axis, but can bend in all directions and so the deflection observed is a true vector quantity with which to gauge traction forces.

With the close proximity between sensors, the array of vertical cantilevers can examine traction forces at a higher density than previous methods and examine the forces at individual focal adhesions. Because the spring constant of these structure can be tailored by changing the length or diameter of the array (1–200 nN/μm), it has been possible to further examine the changes that a cell's contractile apparatus has with the stiffness of its microenvironment.[33–35] Another advantage is that each cantilever can deflect independently, which means that each array has millions of isolated sensors. This allows for studies that were not readily possible with previous techniques, like assessing the traction forces of large monolayers of cells as well as the tugging force between adjacent cells.[36–38] The array of cantilevers does have a nonphysiological topology, which may provide unique physical stimuli to the cells. However, fabrication technology allows the cantilevers to approach nanoscale dimensions, which makes it possible to have a higher density of force sensors that closely mimic a continuous substrate for a cell.[39]

22.5 Conclusion

The mechanical forces that cells generate through actin and myosin directly affect the function of tissue. The use of deformable substrates to measure traction forces has made it possible to better understand the proteins and structures associated with these forces. They have also begun to illuminate the mechanism that cells use to detect and respond to physical cues in their environment. The tools and techniques continue to improve both accuracy and precision as new approaches are incorporated from engineering and physics. Each new design comes closer to matching the length scale of cells, and with it brings a giant step in understanding the mechanisms of cell migration and contraction.

As the field moves forward, several issues need to be addressed to improve these techniques further. First, the reactions that cells have to the environments that the tools present should be considered. Topology, rigidity, and adhesivity of the tool can cause a mechanotransduction response that is independent of the response tested. On one hand, some would argue that these stimuli are nonphysiological and so little insight into the inner mechanisms of a cell is possible when using the tools. However, it should be noted that a plastic tissue culture dish is a rigid, planar environment that has little resemblance to an *in vivo* environment, yet the insights into cell biology from standard tissue culture have been immense. A stronger emphasis, however, should be made in building tools that can replicate mechanical cues so as to better analyze traction forces and to understand the role of mechanotransduction in cell biology. Second, because the devices used in measuring traction forces are built in-house, it is likely that they were calibrated in the early phase of their development, but subsequent tests and checks on their accuracy are sporadic. There are also major deviations in how the techniques are implemented in other laboratories. It is hard to compare the findings between studies if the methods used were widely different. It would be more advantageous if standard protocols were adopted or tools were made widely available so that a healthy degree of congruency and verification could be made in the field. Lastly, construction of these devices needs to be simple enough so that widespread use is possible. By reducing the barrier to use these tools, a larger effort can be directed at studying the numerous protein interactions that occur during traction force generation. Understanding the interactions between mechanical forces and biological response, how cells migrate, and how cells change the structure–function relations of tissues can provide valuable insight in the treatment of diseased states.

To achieve these goals, there are many future directions that the techniques described can be advanced. Foremost is the integration of traction force assays with other powerful microscopy techniques, such as fluorescent recovery after photobleaching (FRAP), GFP protein-labeling, fluorescent resonant emission transfer (FRET), super-resolution fluorescence microscopy, and 3D microscopy. These optical techniques allow one to detect proteins at the single molecular level, and in combination with traction force assays, provide a correlation between molecular activity and cell mechanics. To some degree, this direction has already been pursued.[17,40] Yet, there are still insights to be gained on the assembly of focal adhesions during migration and the interactions that myosin has with actin. Incorporating nanotechnology materials or devices may provide powerful new sensors that improve both spatial resolution and force measurement.[41] Because the size of an adhesion is hundreds of nanometers and the range of forces for single myosin motor is a few piconewtons, the ability to resolve these structures would provide greater insight into the mechanical behavior of cells. Additionally, the constructions of 3D measurement techniques, such as with gels or more complex sensing devices, would extend the current 2D understanding of traction forces into an environment more pertinent to cellular interactions in living tissue. Early attempts have been made that provide some understanding of 3D forces, but the substrates are still planar and constrain how the cell organizes its cytoskeleton and adhesions along those planes.[42,43] Lastly, strong exploration into the development of devices or techniques that are usable for *in vivo* studies of traction forces would open new areas of treatment for diseases in the cardiovascular and skeletal systems. From the activity and improvements so far, there is good reason to anticipate significant developments to come in understanding traction forces and cell mechanics.

Acknowledgments

NJS acknowledge support in part from grants from the National Science Foundation's CAREER Award and the National Institutes of Health (HL097284). CSC acknowledges support in part by grants from the National Institutes of Health (EB00262, EB08396, HL73305, HL90747, GM74048).

References

1. Sniadecki, N. J., Desai, R. A., Ruiz, S. A. and Chen, C. S. Nanotechnology for cell-substrate interactions. *Ann Biomed Eng* **34**, 59–74, 2006.
2. Chen, C. S. Mechanotransduction—A field pulling together? *J Cell Sci* **121**, 3285–3292, 2008.
3. Finer, J. T., Simmons, R. M. and Spudich, J. A. Single myosin molecule mechanics: Piconewton forces and nanometre steps. *Nature* **368**, 113–119, 1994.
4. Harris, A. K., Wild, P. and Stopak, D. Silicone rubber substrata: A new wrinkle in the study of cell locomotion. *Science* **208**, 177–179, 1980.
5. Chrzanowska-Wodnicka, M. and Burridge, K. Rho-stimulated contractility drives the formation of stress fibers and focal adhesions. *J Cell Biol* **133**, 1403–1415, 1996.
6. Helfman, D. M., Levy, E. T., Berthier, C., Shtutman, M., Riveline, D., Grosheva, I., Lachish-Zalait, A., Elbaum, M. and Bershadsky, A. D. Caldesmon inhibits nonmuscle cell contractility and interferes with the formation of focal adhesions. *Mol Biol Cell* **10**, 3097–3112, 1999.
7. Danowski, B. A., Imanaka-Yoshida, K., Sanger, J. M. and Sanger, J. W. Costameres are sites of force transmission to the substratum in adult rat cardiomyocytes. *J Cell Biol* **118**, 1411–1420, 1992.

8. Hinz, B., Celetta, G., Tomasek, J. J., Gabbiani, G. and Chaponnier, C. Alpha-smooth muscle actin expression upregulates fibroblast contractile activity. *Mol Biol Cell* **12**, 2730–2741, 2001.

9. Bogatcheva, N. V., Verin, A. D., Wang, P., Birukova, A. A., Birukov, K. G., Mirzopoyazova, T., Adyshev, D. M., Chiang, E. T., Crow, M. T. and Garcia, J. G. Phorbol esters increase MLC phosphorylation and actin remodeling in bovine lung endothelium without increased contraction. *Am J Physiol Lung Cell Mol Physiol* **285**, L415–426, 2003.

10. Harris, A. K., Stopak, D. and Wild, P. Fibroblast traction as a mechanism for collagen morphogenesis. *Nature* **290**, 249–251, 1981.

11. Burton, K. and Taylor, D. L. Traction forces of cytokinesis measured with optically modified elastic substrata. *Nature* **385**, 450–454, 1997.

12. Burton, K., Park, J. H. and Taylor, D. L. Keratocytes generate traction forces in two phases. *Mol Biol Cell* **10**, 3745–3769, 1999.

13. Lee, J., Leonard, M., Oliver, T., Ishihara, A. and Jacobson, K. Traction forces generated by locomoting keratocytes. *J Cell Biol* **127**, 1957–1964, 1994.

14. Oliver, T., Dembo, M. and Jacobson, K. Traction forces in locomoting cells. *Cell Motil Cytoskeleton* **31**, 225–240, 1995.

15. Dembo, M., Oliver, T., Ishihara, A. and Jacobson, K. Imaging the traction stresses exerted by locomoting cells with the elastic substratum method. *Biophys J* **70**, 2008–2022, 1996.

16. Dembo, M. and Wang, Y. L. Stresses at the cell-to-substrate interface during locomotion of fibroblasts. *Biophys J* **76**, 2307–2316, 1999.

17. Balaban, N. Q., Schwarz, U. S., Riveline, D., Goichberg, P., Tzur, G., Sabanay, I., Mahalu, D., Safran, S., Bershadsky, A., Addadi, L. and Geiger, B. Force and focal adhesion assembly: A close relationship studied using elastic micropatterned substrates. *Nat Cell Biol* **3**, 466–472, 2001.

18. Schwarz, U. S., Balaban, N. Q., Riveline, D., Bershadsky, A., Geiger, B. and Safran, S. A. Calculation of forces at focal adhesions from elastic substrate data: The effect of localized force and the need for regularization. *Biophys J* **83**, 1380–1394, 2002.

19. Wang, H. B., Dembo, M., Hanks, S. K. and Wang, Y. Focal adhesion kinase is involved in mechanosensing during fibroblast migration. *Proc Natl Acad Sci U S A* **98**, 11295–11300, 2001.

20. Reinhart-King, C. A., Dembo, M. and Hammer, D. A. The dynamics and mechanics of endothelial cell spreading. *Biophys J* **89**, 676–689, 2005.

21. Munevar, S., Wang, Y. and Dembo, M. Traction force microscopy of migrating normal and H-ras transformed 3T3 fibroblasts. *Biophys J* **80**, 1744–1757, 2001.

22. Paszek, M. J., Zahir, N., Johnson, K. R., Lakins, J. N., Rozenberg, G. I., Gefen, A., Reinhart-King, C. A. et al. Tensional homeostasis and the malignant phenotype. *Cancer Cell* **8**, 241–254, 2005.

23. Ghosh, K., Thodeti, C. K., Dudley, A. C., Mammoto, A., Klagsbrun, M. and Ingber, D. E. Tumor-derived endothelial cells exhibit aberrant Rho-mediated mechanosensing and abnormal angiogenesis in vitro. *Proc Natl Acad Sci U S A* **105**, 11305–11310, 2008.

24. Wang, N., Naruse, K., Stamenovic, D., Fredberg, J. J., Mijailovich, S. M., Tolic-Norrelykke, I. M., Polte, T., Mannix, R. and Ingber, D. E. Mechanical behavior in living cells consistent with the tensegrity model. *Proc Natl Acad Sci U S A* **98**, 7765–7770, 2001.

25. Kumar, S., Maxwell, I. Z., Heisterkamp, A., Polte, T. R., Lele, T. P., Salanga, M., Mazur, E. and Ingber, D. E. Viscoelastic retraction of single living stress fibers and its impact on cell shape, cytoskeletal organization, and extracellular matrix mechanics. *Biophys J* **90**, 3762–3773, 2006.

26. Krishnan, R., Park, C. Y., Lin, Y. C., Mead, J., Jaspers, R. T., Trepat, X., Lenormand, G. et al. Reinforcement versus fluidization in cytoskeletal mechanoresponsiveness. *PLoS One* **4**, e5486, 2009.

27. Galbraith, C. G. and Sheetz, M. P. A micromachined device provides a new bend on fibroblast traction forces. *Proc Natl Acad Sci U S A* **94**, 9114–9118, 1997.

28. Galbraith, C. G. and Sheetz, M. P. Keratocytes pull with similar forces on their dorsal and ventral surfaces. *J Cell Biol* **147**, 1313–1324, 1999.

29. Tan, J. L., Tien, J., Pirone, D. M., Gray, D. S., Bhadriraju, K. and Chen, C. S. Cells lying on a bed of microneedles: An approach to isolate mechanical force. *Proc Natl Acad Sci U S A* **100**, 1484–1489, 2003.

30. du Roure, O., Saez, A., Buguin, A., Austin, R. H., Chavrier, P., Siberzan, P. and Ladoux, B. Force mapping in epithelial cell migration. *Proc Natl Acad Sci U S A* **102**, 2390–2395, 2005.

31. Xia, Y. and Whitesides, G. M. Soft Lithography. *Annu Rev Mater Sci* **28**, 153–184, 1998.

32. Sniadecki, N. J. and Chen, C. S. Microfabricated silicone elastomeric post arrays for measuring traction forces of adherent cells. *Methods Cell Biol* **83**, 313–328, 2007.

33. Saez, A., Buguin, A., Silberzan, P. and Ladoux, B. Is the mechanical activity of epithelial cells controlled by deformations or forces? *Biophys J* **89**, L52–54, 2005.

34. Saez, A., Ghibaudo, M., Buguin, A., Silberzan, P. and Ladoux, B. Rigidity-driven growth and migration of epithelial cells on microstructured anisotropic substrates. *Proc Natl Acad Sci U S A* **104**, 8281–8286, 2007.

35. Ghibaudo, M., Saez, A., Trichet, L., Xayaphoummine, A., Browaeys, J., Silberzan, P., Buguin, A. and Ladoux, B. Traction forces and rigidity sensing regulate cell functions. *Soft Matter* **4**, 1836–1843, 2008.

36. Nelson, C. M., Jean, R. P., Tan, J. L., Liu, W. F., Sniadecki, N. J., Spector, A. A. and Chen, C. S. Emergent patterns of growth controlled by multicellular form and mechanics. *Proc Natl Acad Sci U S A* **102**, 11594–11599, 2005.

37. Ruiz, S. A. and Chen, C. S. Emergence of patterned stem cell differentiation within multicellular structures. *Stem Cells* **26**, 2921–2927, 2008.

38. Liu, Z., Tan, J. L., Cohen, D. M., Yang, M. T., Sniadecki, N. J., Ruiz, S. A., Nelson, C. M. and Chen, C. S. Mechanical tugging force regulates the size of cell-cell junctions. *Proc Natl Acad Sci U S A* **107**, 9944–9949, 2010.

39. Yang, M. T., Sniadecki, N. J. and Chen, C. S. Geometric considerations of micro- to nanoscale elastomeric post arrays to study cellular traction forces. *Adv Mater* **19**, 3119–3123, 2007.

40. Kong, H. J., Polte, T. R., Alsberg, E. and Mooney, D. J. FRET measurements of cell-traction forces and nano-scale clustering of adhesion ligands varied by substrate stiffness. *Proc Natl Acad Sci U S A* **102**, 4300–4305, 2005.

41. Sniadecki, N. J., Anguelouch, A., Yang, M. T., Lamb, C. M., Liu, Z., Kirschner, S. B., Liu, Y., Reich, D. H. and Chen, C. S. Magnetic microposts as an approach to apply forces to living cells. *Proc Natl Acad Sci U S A* **104**, 14553–14558, 2007.

42. Beningo, K. A., Dembo, M. and Wang, Y. L. Responses of fibroblasts to anchorage of dorsal extracellular matrix receptors. *Proc Natl Acad Sci U S A* **101**, 18024–18029, 2004.

43. Maskarinec, S. A., Franck, C., Tirrell, D. A. and Ravichandran, G. Quantifying cellular traction forces in three dimensions. *Proc Natl Acad Sci U S A* **106**, 22108–22113, 2009.

23

Blood Glucose Monitoring

David D.
Cunningham
Eastern Kentucky University

The availability of blood glucose monitoring devices for home use has significantly impacted the treatment of diabetes with the American Diabetes Association currently recommending that Type 1 insulin-dependent diabetic individuals perform blood glucose testing four times per day. Grave health issues are associated with high and low blood glucose levels. Injection of too much insulin without enough food lowers blood sugar into the hypoglycemic range, glucose below 60 mg/dL, resulting in mild confusion or in more severe cases loss of consciousness, seizure, and coma. On the other hand, long-term high blood sugar levels lead to diabetic complications such as eye, kidney, heart, nerve, or blood vessel disease (Diabetes Control and Complications Trial Research Group 1993). Complications were tracked in a large clinical study showing that an additional 5 years of life, 8 years of sight, 6 years free from kidney disease, and 6 years free of amputations can be expected for a diabetic following tight glucose control versus the standard regimen (Diabetes Control and Complications Trial Research Group 1996).

Glucose monitoring and control in the perioperative setting also has a significant effect on patient outcomes since a large percentage of nondiabetic patients, as well as diabetic patients, become hyperglycemic during induction with anesthesia, throughout surgery, and several hours postsurgery. A study published in 2001 showed critically ill patients intensively controlled to between 80 and 110 mg/dL glucose had fewer complications and a 34% lower in-hospital mortality than conventionally managed patients where treatment was initiated when glucose was >215 mg/dL and maintained between 180 and 200 mg/dL (van den Berghe et al. 2001). Subsequently, in 2006, a standard of care for critically ill patients, recommending glucose be kept as close to 110 mg/dL as possible and generally <140 mg/dL, was widely adopted. Unfortunately, additional studies of intensive control in the ICU generally found an increased incidence of hypoglycemia and failed to confirm the initial found benefit in survival, so the guidelines were withdrawn in 2008 (NICE-SUGAR Study Investigators 2009). The accuracy required of the glucose measurements to allow tight glucose control and avoid hypoglycemia received relatively little attention during the studies discussed above, but the painful experience of resetting treatment guidelines has brought the subject of glucose measurement into sharp focus among clinical researchers (Rice et al. 2010).

TABLE 23.1 Landmarks in Glucose Monitoring

1941—Effervescent tablet test for glucose in urine
1956—Dip and read test strip for glucose in urine
1964—Dry reagent blood glucose test strip requiring timing, wash step, and visual comparison to a color chart
1970—Meter to read reflected light from a test strip, designed for use in the doctor's office
1978—Major medical literature publications on home blood glucose monitoring with portable meters
1981—Finger lancing device automatically lances and retracts tip
1987—Electrochemical test strip and small meter in the form of a pen
1997—Multiple test strip package for easy loading into meter
2001—Alternate-site blood sampling for virtually painless testing

The current Food and Drug Administration (FDA) and ISO guidelines on the accuracy of self-monitoring blood glucose systems have been in place since 1996 and state that 95% of the readings must be within 20% of a reference method value for glucose values ≥75 mg/dL and within 15 mg/dL of reference values for glucose values <75 mg/dL. In June 2009, an initiative was launched by ISO with strong support by the FDA to tighten the requirements so that 95% of the readings are within 15% of a reference method value for glucose values ≥75 mg/dL and within 10 mg/dL of reference values for glucose values <75 mg/dL, with implementation by 2012. While industry will certainly meet any government-mandated standard, the cost of the systems may rise and new features such as faster time to result and lower blood sample requirements may not advance as rapidly. The continued need for simple, accurate glucose measurements has led to continuous improvements in sample test strips, electronic meters, sample acquisition techniques, and more recently, continuous monitoring systems.

Self-monitoring blood glucose systems based on single-use test strips are available from a number of companies through pharmacy and mail order; however, the more recently introduced continuous monitoring systems require a prescription. Some of the landmarks in glucose testing are shown in Table 23.1. The remainder of the chapter comprises a history of technical developments with an explanation of the principles behind optical and electrochemical sensing, including examples of the biochemical reactions used in commercial products.

23.1 Historical Methods of Glucose Monitoring

Diabetes is an ancient disease that was once identified by the attraction of ants to the urine of an affected individual. Later, physicians would often rely on the sweet taste of the urine in diagnosing the disease. Once the chemical-reducing properties of glucose were discovered, solutions of a copper salt and dye, typically *o*-toluidine, were used for laboratory tests, and by the 1940s the reagents had been formulated into tablets for use in test tubes of urine. More specific tests were developed using glucose oxidase, which could be impregnated on a dry paper strip. The reaction of glucose with glucose oxidase produces hydrogen peroxide that can subsequently react with a colorless dye precursor in the presence of hydrogen peroxide to form a visible color (see Equation 23.3). The first enzyme-based test strips required addition of the sample to the strip for 1 min and subsequent washing of the strip. Visual comparison of the color on the test strip to the color on a chart was required to estimate the glucose concentration. However, the measurement of glucose in urine is not adequate since only after the blood glucose level is very high for several hours does glucose "spill-over" into the urine. Other physiological fluids such as sweat and tears are not suitable because the glucose level is much lower than in blood.

Whole blood contains hemoglobin inside the red blood cells that can interfere with the measurement of color on a test strip. To prevent staining of the test strip with red blood cells, an ethyl cellulose layer was applied over the enzyme and dye-impregnated paper on a plastic support (Mast 1967). In another early commercially available test strip, the enzymes and dye were incorporated into a homogeneous water-resistant film that prevented penetration of red blood cells into the test strips and enable their easy removal upon washing (Rey et al. 1971). Through various generations of products, the formulations of the strips were improved to eliminate the washing/wiping steps and electronic meters were developed to measure the color.

23.2 Development of Colorimetric Test Strips and Optical Reflectance Meters

Optically based strips are generally constructed with various layers that provide a support function, a reflective function, an analytical function, and a sample-spreading function as illustrated in Figure 23.1. The support function serves as a foundation for the dry reagent and may also contain the reflective function. Otherwise, insoluble reflective or scattering materials such as TiO_2, $BaSO_4$, MgO, or ZnO are added to the dry reagent formulation. The analytical function contains the active enzyme. The reaction schemes used in several commercial products are described in greater detail later. The spreading function must rapidly disperse the sample laterally after application and quickly form a uniform sample concentration on the analytically active portion of the strip. Swellable films and semipermeable membranes, particularly glass fiber fleece has been used to spread and separate plasma from whole blood. Upon formation of the colored reaction product, the amount of diffuse light reflected from the analytical portion of the strip decreases according to the following equation:

$$\%R = (I_u/I_s)\, R_s \tag{23.1}$$

where I_u is the reflected light from the sample, I_s is the reflected light from a standard, and R_s is the percent reflectivity of the standard. The Kubelka–Munk equation gives the relationship in a more useful form:

$$C \propto K/S = (1 - R)^2/2R \tag{23.2}$$

where C is the concentration, K is the absorption coefficient, S is the scattering coefficient, and R is the percent reflectance divided by 100.

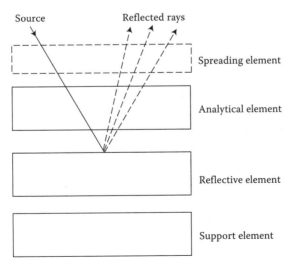

FIGURE 23.1   Basic functions of a reflectance-based test strip. (From Henning TP and Cunningham DD. Biosensors for personal diabetes management. In: *Commercial Biosensors*, pp. 3–46, 1998. Copyright Wiley-VCH Verlag GmbH & Co. KGaA. Reproduced with permission.)

The analytical function of the strip is based on an enzyme reaction with glucose and subsequent color-forming reactions. Although the most stable enzymes are chosen for product development, some loss in activity occurs during manufacturing due to factors such as pH, temperature, physical sheer stress, organic solvents, and various other denaturing actions or agents. Additional inactivation occurs during the storage of the product. In general, sufficient enzyme and other reagents are incorporated into the strip so that the assay reactions near completion in a conveniently short time. Reagent formulations often include thickening agents, builders, emulsifiers, dispersion agents, pigments, plasticizers, pore formers, wetting agents, and the like. These materials provide a uniform reaction layer required for good precision and accuracy. The cost of the materials in the strip must be low since it is used only once.

Many color-forming reactions have been developed into commercial products as indicated in the following examples. Manufacturers often use the same chemistry across multiple brands of strips and meters as indicated by the brief description of the active ingredients given in the test strip package insert. The glucose oxidase/peroxidase reaction scheme used in the Lifescan OneTouch™ (Phillips et al. 1990) and SureStep™ test strips is mentioned later. Glucose oxidase catalyzes the oxidation of glucose forming gluconic acid and hydrogen peroxide. The oxygen concentration in blood (ca. 0.3 mM) is much lower than the glucose concentration (3–35 mM), so oxygen from the atmosphere must diffuse into the test strip to bring the reaction to completion. Peroxidase catalyzes the reaction of the hydrogen peroxide with 3-methyl-2-benzothiazolinone hydrazone (MBTH) and 3-dimethylaminobenzoic acid (DMAB). A naphthalene sulfonic acid salt replaces DMAB in the SureStep strip.

$$\text{Glucose} + \text{oxygen} \xrightarrow{\text{GOx}} \text{gluconic acid} + H_2O_2$$
$$H_2O_2 + \text{MBTH} + \text{DMA} \xrightarrow{\text{peroxidase}} \text{BMBTH-DMAB (blue)}$$

(23.3)

The hexokinase reaction scheme used in the Bayer GLUCOMETER ENCORE™ test strip is shown later. Hexokinase, ATP, and magnesium react with glucose to produce glucose-6-phosphate. The glucose-6-phosphate reacts with glucose-6-phosphate dehydrogenase and NAD^+ to produce NADH. The NADH then reacts with diaphorase and reduces the tetrazolium indicator to produce a brown compound (formazan). The reaction sequence requires three enzymes but is insensitive to oxygen.

$$\text{Glucose} + \text{ATP} \xrightarrow[Mg^{+2}]{\text{HK}} \text{G-6-P} + \text{ADP}$$
$$\text{G-6-P} + NAD^+ \xrightarrow{\text{G-6-PDH}} \text{6-PG} + \text{NADH} + H^+$$
$$\text{NADH} + \text{tetrazolium} \xrightarrow{\text{diaphorase}} \text{formazan (brown)} + NAD^+$$

(23.4)

The reaction scheme originally used in the Roche Accu-Chek™ Instant™ test strip is shown later (Hoenes et al. 1995). Bis-(2-hydroxy-ethyl)-(4-hydroximinocyclohex-2,5-dienylidene) ammonium chloride (BHEHD) is reduced by glucose to the corresponding hydroxylamine derivative and further to the corresponding diamine under the catalytic action of glucose oxidase. Note that while oxygen is not required in the reaction, oxygen in the sample may compete with the intended reaction creating an oxygen dependency. The diamine reacts with a 2,18 phosphomolybdic acid salt to form molybdenum blue. More recent forms of the Accu-Chek Instant, Compact™, and Integra™ brand test strips were formulated with the oxygen-independent enzyme glucose dehydrogenase containing pyrroloquinoline quinine (GDH-PQQ) and the same reagents used to form molybdenum blue.

$$\text{Glucose} + \text{BHEHD} \xrightarrow{\text{GOx}} \text{diamine}$$
$$P_2Mo_{18}O_{62}^{-6} + \text{diamine} \longrightarrow MoO_{2.0}(OH) \text{ to } MoO_{2.5}(OH)_{0.5} \text{ (molybdenum blue)}$$

(23.5)

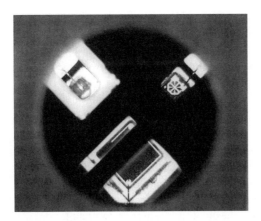

FIGURE 23.2 Photograph of light-emitting diodes and photodetector on the OneTouch meter. Photodetector at bottom, 635 nm light-emitting diode at top left, 700 nm light-emitting diode at top right. Optics viewed through the 4.5 mm hole in the strip after removal of the test strip reagent membrane. (Courtesy of John Grace.)

The reaction scheme used in the Roche Accu-Chek Easy™ test strip is shown later (Freitag 1990). Glucose oxidase reacts with ferricyanide and forms potassium ferric ferrocyanide (Prussian Blue). Again, oxygen is not required but may compete with the intended reaction.

$$\text{Glucose} + \text{GOx (ox)} \rightarrow \text{GOx (red)} \tag{23.6}$$

$$\text{GOx (red)} + [\text{Fe(CN)}_6]^{-3} \rightarrow \text{GOx (ox)} + [\text{Fe(CN)}_6]^{-4}$$

$$3[\text{Fe(CN)}_6]^{-4} + 4\text{FeCl}_3 \rightarrow \text{Fe}_4[\text{Fe(CN)}_6]_3 \text{ Prussian blue}$$

Current optical test strips and reflectance meters typically require 1.5–10 μL of blood and read out an answer in 10–30 s. A significant technical consideration in the development of a product is the measurement of samples spanning the range of red blood cell concentrations (percent hematocrit) typically found in whole blood. Common hematocrit and glucose ranges are 30–55% and 40–500 mg/dL (2.2–28 mM), respectively. The Lifescan OneTouch meter contains two light-emitting diodes (635 and 700 nm), which allows measurement of the color due to red blood cell and the color due to the dye. Reflectance measurements from both LEDs are measured with a single photodetector as shown in Figure 23.2. All glucose meters measure the detector signal at various timepoints and if the curve shape is not within reasonable limits an error message is generated. Some meters measure and correct for ambient temperature. Of course, optical systems are subject to interference from ambient light conditions and may not work in direct sunlight. Optical systems have gradually lost market share to electrochemical systems that were introduced commercially in 1987. Optical test strips generally require a larger blood sample and take longer to produce the result than electrochemical strips. Presently, optical reflectance meters are more costly to manufacture, require larger batteries, and are more difficult to calibrate than electrochemical meters.

23.3 Emergence of Electrochemical Strips

Electrochemical systems are based on the reaction of an electrochemically active mediator with an enzyme. The mediator is oxidized at a solid electrode with an applied positive potential. Electrons will flow between the mediator and electrode surface when a minimum energy is attained. The energy of the electrons in the mediator is fixed based on the chemical structure but the energy of the electrons in the solid electrode can be changed by applying a voltage between the working electrode and a second electrode. The rate of the electron transfer reaction between the mediator and a working electrode surface is given by the Butler–Volmer equation (Bard and Faulkner 1980). When the potential is large enough all the mediator reaching the electrode reacts rapidly and the reaction becomes diffusion controlled. The current from a diffusion-limited reaction follows the Cottrell equation:

$$i = (nFAD^{1/2}C)/(\pi^{1/2}t^{1/2}) \tag{23.7}$$

where i is the current, n is the number of electrons, F is Faraday's constant, A is the electrode area, C is the concentration, D is the diffusion coefficient, and t is the time. The current from a diffusion-controlled electrochemical reaction will decay away as the reciprocal square root of time. This means that the maximum electrochemical signal occurs at short times as opposed to color-forming reactions where the color becomes more intense with time. The electrochemical method relies on measuring the current from the electron transfer between the electrode and the mediator. However, when a potential is first applied to the electrode, the dipole moments of solvent molecules will align with the electric field on the surface of the electrode causing a current to flow. Thus, at very short times, this charging current interferes with the analytical measurement. Electrochemical sensors generally apply a potential to the electrode surface and measure the current after the charging current has decayed sufficiently. With small volumes of sample, coulometric analysis can be used to measure the current required for complete consumption of glucose (Feldman et al. 2000).

The reaction scheme used in the first commercial electrochemical test strip from MediSense (now Abbott Diabetes Care) is shown later. Electron transfer rates between the reduced form of glucose oxidase and ferricinium ion derivatives are very rapid compared with the unwanted side reaction with oxygen (Cass et al. 1984; Forrow et al. 2002). The Abbott Diabetes Care Precision QID™ strip includes the 1,1′-dimethyl-3-(2-amino-1-hydroxyethyl) ferrocene mediator, which has the desirable characteristics of high solubility in water, fast electron-shuttling (bimolecular rate constant of 4.3×10^5 M^{-1} s^{-1}), stability, and pH independence of the redox potential (Heller and Feldman 2008). Electrochemical oxidation of the ferrocene derivative is performed at 0.6 V. Oxidation of interferences, such as ascorbic acid and acetaminophen present in blood, are corrected for by measuring the current at a second electrode on the strip that does not contain glucose oxidase.

$$\text{Glucose} + \text{GOx (oxidized)} \rightarrow \text{gluconolactone} + \text{GOx (reduced)}$$

$$\text{GOx (reduced)} + \text{ferricinium}^+ \rightarrow \text{GOx (oxidized)} + \text{ferrocene} \tag{23.8}$$

$$\text{Ferrocene} \rightarrow \text{ferricinium}^+ + \text{electron (reaction at solid electrode surface)}$$

Several electrochemical test strips use ferricyanide rather than ferrocene as the electrochemical mediator although the potential required for oxidation is higher than for ferrocene derivatives. The LifeScan OneTouch FastTake™ and Ultra™ brand test strips include glucose oxidase and either 11 or 22 μg ferricyanide per strip. The strip readout is reduced from 15 to 5 s with the larger amount of ferricyanide mediator. Many Roche Accu-Chek strips, including the Comfort Curve™, Compete™, Advantage™, Aviva™, and Active™, are formulated with the oxygen-independent enzyme GDH-PQQ and ferricyanide as the mediator. An organic mediator, nitrosoanaline is used with GDH-PQQ in the Roche Accu-Chek Performa™ test strip.

The reaction scheme used in the Abbott Diabetes Care Precision-Xtra™ and Sof-Tact™ test strips is shown later. The GDH enzyme does not react with oxygen and the phenanthroline quinine mediator can be oxidized at 0.2 V, which is below the oxidation potential of most interfering substances.

$$\text{Glucose} + \text{GDH/NAD}^+ \rightarrow \text{GDH/NADH} + \text{gluconolactone}$$

$$\text{GDH/NADH} + \text{PQ} \rightarrow \text{GDH/NAD}^+ + \text{PQH}_2 \tag{23.9}$$

$$\text{PQH}_2 \rightarrow \text{PQ} + \text{electrons (reaction at solid electrode surface)}$$

The working electrode on most commercially available electrochemical strips is made by screen printing a conductive carbon ink on a plastic substrate; however, more expensive noble metal electrodes are also used. Historically, test strips have been manufactured, tested, and assigned a calibration code. The calibration code provided with each package of strips is sometimes manually entered into the meter by the user but other systems automatically read the calibration code from the strips. Meters designed for use in the hospital often have bar code readers to download calibration, quality control, and patient information. Test strips are supplied in bottles or individual foil wrappers to protect them from moisture over their shelf-life, typically about 1 year. The task of opening and inserting individual test strip into the meter has been minimized by packaging multiple test strips in the form of a disk-shaped cartridge or a drum that is placed into the meter. Disks or drums typically contain 10–17 test strips.

23.4 Enzyme Selectivity and Falsely Elevated Readings

Formulations containing GDH-PQQ became popular due to the lack of oxygen interference and the high catalytic activity of the enzyme relative to glucose oxidase (5000 U/mg vs 300 U/mg). However, GDH-PQQ oxidizes a wide range of sugars with reaction rates generally in the order: glucose (100%), maltose (58%), lactose (58%), galactose (10%), mannose (10%), and xylose (10%). Normally, the concentration of the other sugars is so much lower than the glucose concentration in blood that there is little interference. Until recently, it was not appreciated that patients receiving peritoneal dialysis using the osmotic agent icodextrin absorb and metabolize the icodextrin to shorter polysaccharides, mainly maltose, causing erroneously high glucose measurements. In addition, some injected drug products contain maltose as a part of the formulation, which also leads to high glucose readings. To address this issue, the FDA recently issued a public health notification recommending against the use of GDH-PQQ in glucose test strips (FDA Public Health Notification 2009). Research studies have shown that site-directed mutagenesis of GDH-PQQ can reduce the reactivity to maltose to about 10% that of glucose but cannot achieve the selectivity of either glucose oxidase or NADH-dependent glucose dehydrogenase (Igarashi et al. 2004). Besides adequate activity and selectivity, any new enzyme developed for use in test strips must have good thermal stability. Protein engineering approaches for improving enzyme stability include increasing the hydrophobic interaction in the interior core region of the protein, reducing the water-accessible hydrophobic surface area, and stabilizing the dipoles of the helical structure.

23.5 Improvements in User Interactions with the System and Alternate Site Testing

Both Type 1 and Type 2 diabetic individuals do not currently test as often as recommended by physicians, so systems developed in the last few years have aimed to improve compliance with physician recommendations while maintaining accuracy. Historically, the biggest source of errors in glucose testing involved interaction of the user with the system. Blood is typically collected by lancing the edge of the end of the finger to a depth of about 1.5 mm. Squeezing or milking is required to produce a hanging drop of blood. The target area on test strips is clearly identified by design. A common problem is smearing a drop of blood on top of a strip resulting in a thinner than normal layer of blood over part of the strip and a low reading. Many strips now require that the blood drop be applied to the end or side of the strip where capillary action is used to fill the strip. Partial filling can be detected electrochemically or by observation of the fill window on the strip. The small capillary space in the Abbott Diabetes Care Freestyle™ electrochemical strip requires only 300 nL of blood.

Progressively thinner diameter lancets have come to the market with current sizes typically in the 28–31 gauge range. Most lancets are manufactured with three grinding steps to give a tri-bevel point. After loading the lancet into the lancing device, a spring system automatically lances and retracts the point. The depth of lancing is commonly adjustable through the use of several settings on the device or use of a different end-piece cap. Unfortunately, the high density of nerve endings on the finger makes the process painful and some diabetic individuals do not test as often as they should due to the pain and residual soreness caused by fingersticks. Recently, lancing devices have been designed to lance and apply pressure on the skin of body sites other than the finger, a process termed "alternate site testing." The use of alternate site sampling lead to the realization that capillary blood from alternate sites can have slightly different glucose and hematocrit values than blood from a fingerstick due to the more arterial nature of blood in the fingertips. The pain associated with lancing alternate body sites is typically rated as painless a majority of the time and less painful than a fingerstick over 90% of the time. A low-volume test strip, typically 1 μL or less, is required to measure the small blood samples obtained from alternate sites. Some care and technique is required to obtain an adequate amount of blood and transfer it into the strips when using small blood samples.

Significant insight into blood collection from the skin was uncovered during the development of an alternative site device, the Abbott Diabetes Care Sof-Tact meter, which automatically extracts and trans-fers blood to the test strip (see Figure 23.3). The device contains a vacuum pump, a lancing device, and a test strip that is automatically indexed over the lancet wound after lancing. The vacuum turns off after sufficient blood enters the strip to make an electrical connection. The key factors and practical limits of blood extraction using vacuum combined with skin stretching were investigated to assure that sufficient blood could be obtained for testing (Cunningham et al. 2002). The amount of blood extracted increases with the application of heat or vacuum prior to lancing, the level of vacuum, the depth of lancing, the time of collection, and the amount of skin stretching (see Figure 23.4). Particularly important is the diameter and height that skin is allowed to stretch into a nosepiece after the application of vacuum as shown in Figure 23.5. Vacuum combined with skin stretching increases blood extraction by increasing the lancet wound opening, increasing the blood available for extraction by vasodilatation, and reducing the venous return of blood through the capillaries. The electrochemical test strip used with the meter can be inserted into a secondary support and used with a fingerstick sample when the battery is low.

The size of a meter is often determined by the size of the display although electrochemical meters can be made smaller than reflectance meters. The size and shape of one electrochemical meter, with a

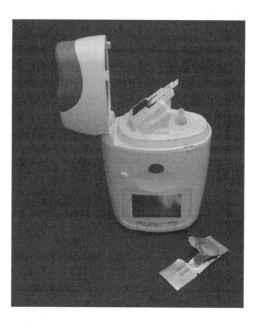

FIGURE 23.3 Sof-Tact meter with cover opened to load test strip and lancet. Test strip is inserted into an electri-cal connector. The hole in the opposite end of the test strip allows the lancet to pass through. The white cylindrical lancet is loaded into the lancet tip holder in the housing. To perform a test, the cover is closed, the gray area of the cover placed against the skin and the front button depressed.

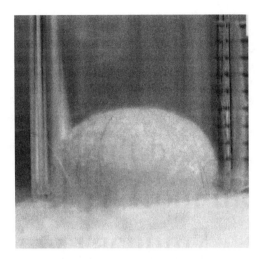

FIGURE 23.4 Photograph of skin on the forearm stretching up into a glass tube upon application of vacuum. Markings on tube at right in 1 mm increments. (Courtesy of Douglas Young.)

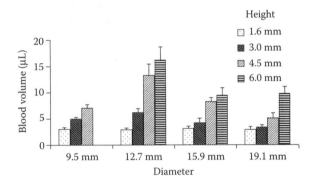

FIGURE 23.5 Effect of skin stretching by vacuum on blood volume extracted from lancet wounds on the forearm. Mean blood volume ± SE in 30 s with –7.5 psig vacuum for nosepieces of different inner diameter and inside step height. (From Cunningham et al., 2002. *J Appl Physiol* 92: 1089–1096. With permission.)

relatively small display, is indistinguishable from a standard ink pen. All meters store recent test results in memory and many allow downloading of the results to a computer. The variety of meters available in the market is mainly driven by the need to satisfy the desires of various customer segments that are driven by different factors, such as cost, ease of use, or incorporation of a specific design or functional feature. Advanced software functions are supplied with some meters to allow entry of exercise, food, and insulin doses, and a personal digital assistant–meter combination was brought to market.

23.6 Continuous Glucose Sensors

All the currently marketed continuous glucose-sensing systems in the United States have similar components. The sensor is contained within a sharp metal housing that is inserted through the skin, then the metal portion is retracted leaving the sensor in the skin. The sensor has a glucose oxidase working electrode portion located under the skin and electrical contacts that are connected to a battery-operated electrochemical potentiostat outside the skin. The electrical components often wirelessly transmit data to a remote display unit where the most recent glucose result and trend data are available. After insertion into the skin, the sensor is calibrated using blood glucose test strips, so a test strip meter is often incorporated into the system for this purpose. Initial calibration and recalibration requirements of the systems has become progressively less demanding over the past several years, but insertion of the sensor into the body changes the sensitivity of present-day sensors enough that some calibration is required. Mechanistic studies of the body's reaction to sensor insertion and testing of more biocompatible coatings is a very active area of investigation both in academia and in industry. However, limited information is available on advances in the area of biocompatible coatings, due to the proprietary nature of the work. Sensors are currently approved for use for up to 7 days, with the risk of infection at the insertion site becoming a concern at longer times.

The sensors marketed by Medtronic and Dexcom are based on a first-generation scheme where the working electrode oxidizes hydrogen peroxide generated by the reaction of glucose and oxygen as catalyzed by glucose oxidase. The working electrode must be covered with a material that is more permeable to oxygen than to glucose since the typical 0.1–0.3 mM concentration of oxygen in the body is much lower than the 2–30 mM concentration of glucose. The Medtronic sensor is a three-electrode system with a working, counter, and reference electrode, so the reference electrode area can be fairly small since no current passes through the reference electrode. The electrodes are fabricated on a thin flexible piece of plastic apparently using thin-film deposition techniques with a membrane polymer coating composed of a diisocyanate, a diamino silane, and a diol, which forms a polyurethane polyurea polymer (VanAntwerp 1999; Henning 2010). The Dexcom sensor is a two-electrode system consisting of a thin platinum wire and a larger silver wire with a silver chloride coating on the outside. During the oxidation of the hydrogen peroxide at about 0.6 V, the silver chloride is reduced. The glucose-limiting membrane is apparently a hydrophilic block copolymer of polyethylene glycol and a polyurethane mixed with a hydrophobic polyurethane polymer (Tapsak et al. 2007). Both the Medtronic and Dexcom sensors are inserted about 12 mm into the skin at a 45° angle but the form of the inserter and the method of electrical contact are of different design (Henning 2010).

The Abbott Diabetes Care sensor is based on a second-generation scheme where an exogenous mediator, in this case an osmium redox polymer, rather than oxygen reacts with the glucose oxidase (Feldman et al. 2003). The mediator can be added at higher effective concentrations than oxygen, eliminating the problem of low oxygen concentration. The sensor is a three-electrode design screen printed on a plastic substrate as shown in Figure 23.6. The reduced mediator is oxidized at a low potential, 0.04 V, so common electrochemical interferences in blood such as acetaminophen and ascorbic acid will not react at the working electrode. The current density of second-generation sensors can be much higher than in the first-generation system since the diffusion of glucose does not have to be reduced to below that of oxygen. The Abbott Diabetes Care sensor is inserted about 5 mm into the skin at a 90° angle.

The GlucoDay™ system based on microdialysis sampling of interstitial fluid was developed in Europe and introduced commercially by Menarini Diagnostics (Poscia et al. 2003). A microdialysis fiber 5 mm

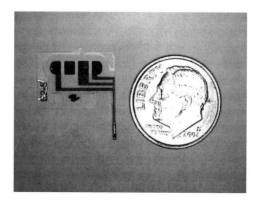

FIGURE 23.6 Abbott Diabetes Care sensor showing size relative to a U.S. dime. (Courtesy of Abbott Diabetes Care.)

long is inserted through the skin by a medical professional, perfused with a buffer solution at a flow rate of ~10 μL/min using a micropump, and the glucose content of the solution measured with a first-generation glucose sensor. The system is calibrated with a blood glucose test strip and the monitoring conducted for up to 48 h, after which the fiber is removed. At present, the high level of professional medical personnel involvement is a significant commercial limitation of the technology.

One 12-h device, the Cygnus GlucoWatch™ based on transdermal reverse iontophoresis (Kurnik et al. 1998) gained FDA approval but the acceptance of the device in the market was poor due to the need to calibrate the device with multiple fingersticks and poor precision and accuracy. The device is no longer commercially available.

23.7 Future Directions

Advances in self-monitoring glucose test strips and meters are difficult to predict given the already highly refined nature of the products in terms of cost of manufacture, size, reliability, ease of use, and time-to-result. Accuracy may be improved through the use of more advanced electrochemical measurements with improved signal-processing strategies or the use of redundant arrays of electrodes on a single strip. Emerging fabrication technologies such as nanoimprint lithography and electrochemical or electrode-less deposition of metals are capable of producing very fine detail without the use of expensive masks. The significant international investment in nanotechnology is producing a wide variety of advanced materials that prove useful in new products. Newly engineered enzymes and electron transfer chemistries may emerge to address selectivity, activity, stability, and other crucial factors. In this regard, several methods have already been reported to electrically connect the glucose oxidase catalytic center to an electrode, gold nanoparticle, or carbon nanotube (Cunningham and Stenken 2010).

The performance of continuous glucose monitoring systems has been rapidly improving and should soon reach the state where the signal is reliable enough to provide input into an insulin infusion pump to produce a "closed-loop" system. However, development of an appropriate algorithm to translate the glucose value into the correct insulin infusion pump setting is quite challenging. A strictly hardware-based system is ignorant of many important factors affecting future blood glucose levels, such as the size of the meal the patient will eat, the amount of exercise planned, or the level of daily stress encountered. So, systems allowing user input of information or "open-loop" control systems may prove more successful. Long-term sensing may involve surgical implantation of a battery-operated unit although many issues remain with the long-term stability of the sensor, miniaturization of the sensing electronics, and data transmitter and biocompatibility of the various materials of construction.

Many fluorescence-based sensing approaches have been investigated by academic and industrial groups. Perhaps the most interesting system involves the injection of glucose-sensitive fluorescent microspheres into the skin to create a "tattoo." The glucose measurement is then made by placing an appropriately designed intensity or time-based fluorometer over the skin area. Many reversible glucose-binding fluorescent systems have been reported with boronic acid derivatives, lectins, or glucose-binding proteins serving as the glucose-selective agent and fluorescent dyes, preferably with absorbance wavelengths above that of hemoglobin, serving as the reporter (McShane and Stein 2010). The *in vivo* stability of the glucose-selective agent and fluorescent dye will likely become more apparent as results from ongoing animal trials are published. Additional work may be needed to overcome the host response to the microspheres and to decrease the immunogenicity of the protein component, if used.

A number of noninvasive spectroscopic approaches have been investigated; however, the amount of clinical data reported to date is very limited. Near-infrared spectroscopy has received the most focused attention with careful analysis of instrumental capabilities and calculation of the net analytical signal indicating currently available hardware can generate glucose-specific information from physiological levels of glucose in body tissue. Additional work is needed to show how this information can be obtained in a reliable and practical manner. Raman spectroscopy and surface-enhanced Raman spectroscopic approaches have advanced through initial animal studies demonstrating partial proof-of-principle.

Likewise, the optical rotation of polarized light by glucose has been utilized to measure glucose particularly in the accessible portion of the aqueous humor of the eye.

Glucose changes also affect the osmotic strength of interstitial fluid, and sensors based on chemical swelling or shrinking of polymers, optical changes in the refractive index, and osmotic effects on electrochemical capacitance have been refined through *in vitro* studies. Prospective clinical trials are needed to more clearly identify the potential of these approaches.

Glucose monitoring of alternative body fluids such as sweat, saliva, gingival crevicular, or tear fluid has been investigated but these fluids generally have a lower glucose concentration than blood and the glucose content of these samples, obtained using traditional methods, does not change in a fixed proportion to the blood glucose concentration. Future studies may explore the possibility that acquisition of smaller physiological samples may show better correlation with blood glucose levels due to the lower anatomical and physiological stress required to obtain smaller volumes of fluid. Further miniaturization and refinement in the design of devices for the collection of small blood or interstitial fluid samples as well as insertion of sensing components into or through the skin is anticipated. Overall, the future of blood glucose monitoring looks very challenging and exciting.

Defining Terms

Alternate site testing: Lancing sites other than the finger to obtain blood in a less painful manner. The small volume of blood obtained from alternate sites requires use of a test strip requiring 1 µL or less of blood.

Type 1 Diabetes: The immune system destroys insulin-producing islet cells in the pancreas, usually in children and young adult, so regular injections of insulin are required (also referred to as juvenile diabetes).

Type 2 Diabetes: A complex disease based on gradual resistance to insulin and diminished production of insulin. Treatment often progresses from oral medications to insulin injections as disease progresses. Also referred to as adult onset diabetes and non-insulin-dependent diabetes mellitus (NIDDM).

References

Bard AJ and Faulkner LR. 1980. *Electrochemical Methods*. New York: John Wiley & Sons. pp. 103, 143.

Cass A, Davis G, Francis G, Hill H, Aston W, Higgins I, Plotkin E, Scott L, and Turner A. 1984. Ferrocene-mediated enzyme electrode for amperometric determination of glucose. *Anal Chem* 56:667–671.

Cunningham DD, Henning T, Shain E, Hannig J, Barua E, and Lee R. 2002. Blood extraction from lancet wounds using vacuum combined with skin stretching. *J Appl Phys* 92:1089–1096.

Cunningham DD and Stenken JA (eds), 2010. *In Vivo Glucose Sensing*. New York: John Wiley & Sons.

Diabetes Control and Complications Trial Research Group. 1993. The effect of intensive treatment of diabetes on the development and progression of long-term complications in insulin-dependent diabetes mellitus. *N Eng J Med* 329:977–986.

Diabetes Control and Complications Trial Research Group. 1996. Lifetime benefits and costs of Intensive therapy as practiced in the diabetes control and complications Trial. *JAMA* 276:1409–1415.

FDA Public Health Notification issued August 13, 2009: Potentially Fatal Errors with GDH-PQQ* Glucose Monitoring Technology. http://www.fda.gov/MedicalDevices/Safety/AlertsandNotices/PublicHealthNotifications/ucm176992.htm, accessed April 15, 2010.

Feldman B, Brazg R, Schwartz S, and Weinstein R. 2003. A continuous glucose sensor based on wired enzyme technology—Results from a 3-day trial in patients with type 1 diabetes. *Diabetes Technol Ther* 5:769–779.

Feldman B, McGarraugh G, Heller A, Bohannon N, Skyler J, DeLeeuw E, and Clarke D. 2000. FreeStyle: A small-volume electrochemical glucose sensor for home blood glucose testing. *Diabetes Technol Ther* 2:221–229.

Forrow NJ, Sanghera GS, and Walters SJ. 2002. The influence of structure in the reaction of electrochemically generated ferrocenium derivatives with reduced glucose oxidase. *J Chem Soc Dalton Trans* 3187.

Freitag H. 1990. Method and reagent for determination of an analyte via enzymatic means using a ferricyanide/ferric compound system. *United States Patent* 4,929,545.

Heller A and Feldman B. 2008. Electrochemical glucose sensors and their applications in diabetes management. *Chem Rev* 108:2482–2505.

Henning TP. 2010. Commercially available continuous glucose monitoring systems. In: *In Vivo Glucose Sensing*, eds D Cunningham and J Stenken, pp. 113–156. New York: John Wiley & Sons.

Henning TP and Cunningham DD 1998. Biosensors for personal diabetes management. In: *Commercial Biosensors*, ed. G. Ramsey, pp. 3–46. New York: John Wiley & Sons.

Hoenes J, Wielinger H, and Unkrig V. 1995. Use of a soluble salt of a heteropoly acid for the determination of an analyte, a corresponding method of determination as well as a suitable agent thereof. *United States Patent* 5,382,523.

Igarashi S, Hirokawa T, and Sode K. 2004. Engineering PQQ glucose dehydrogenase with improved substrate specificity: Site-directed mutagenesis studies on the active center of PQQ glucose dehydrogenase. *Biomol Eng* 21:81–89

Kurnik RT, Berner B, Tamada J, and Potts RO, 1998. Design and simulation of a reverse iontophoretic glucose monitoring device. *J Electrochem Soc* 145:4119–4125.

Mast RL. 1967. Test article for the detection of glucose. *United States Patent* 3,298,789.

McShane M and Stein E. 2010. Fluorescence-based glucose sensors. In: *In Vivo Glucose Sensing*, eds D Cunningham and J Stenken, pp. 113–156. New York: John Wiley & Sons.

NICE-SUGAR Study Investigators. 2009. Intensive versus conventional glucose control in critically ill patients. *N Engl J Med* 360:1283–1297.

Phillips R, McGarraugh G, Jurik F, and Underwood R. 1990. Minimum procedure system for the determination of analytes. *United States Patent* 4,935,346.

Poscia A, Mascini M, Moscone D et al. 2003. A microdialysis technique for continuous subcutaneous glucose monitoring in diabetic patients. *Biosens Bioelectron* 18:891–898.

Rey H, Rieckman P, Wiellager H, and Rittersdorf W. 1971. Diagnostic agent. *United States Patent* 3,630,957.

Rice MJ, Pitkin AD, and Coursin DB. 2010. Glucose measurement in the operating room: More complicated than it seems. *Anesth Analg* 110:1056–65.

Tapsak MA, Rhodes RK, Rathbun K, Shults MC, and McClure JD. 2007. Techniques to improve polyurethane membranes for implantable glucose sensors. *United States Patent* 7,226,978.

VanAntwerp WP. 1999. Polyurethane/polyurea compositions containing silicon for biosensor membranes. *United States Patent* 5,882,494.

Van den Berghe G, Wouters P, Weekers F et al. 2001. Intensive insulin therapy in the critically ill patients. *N Engl J Med* 345:1359–67.

Further Information

Test results of glucose meters are often compared with results from a reference method and presented in the form of a Clarke error grid that defines zones with different clinical implications. Clarke, WL, Cox, DC, Gonder-Frederick, LA, Carter, W, and Pohl, SL. 1987. Evaluating clinical accuracy of systems for self-monitoring of blood glucose. *Diabetes Care* 10: 622–628.

Error grid analysis has recently been extended for the evaluation of continuous glucose monitoring sensors. Kovatchev BP, Gonder-Frederick LA, Cox DJ, and Clarke WL. 2004. Evaluating the accuracy of continuous glucose-monitoring sensors. *Diabetes Care* 27:1922–1928.

Reviews and descriptions of many marketed products are available online at: www.childrenwithdiabetes.com.

Interviews of several people involved with the initial development of blood glucose meters are available online at: www.mendosa.com/history.htm.

24

Atomic Force Microscopy: Opportunities and Challenges for Probing Biomolecular Interactions

Gary C.H. Mo
University of Toronto

Christopher M. Yip
University of Toronto

24.1 Introduction

Discerning and understanding structure–function relationships is often predicated on our ability to measure these properties over a range of relevant length scales. A key concept in the fields of nanoscience and nanotechnology is that directly manipulating atomic and molecular interactions in matter can ultimately control a material's macroscopic physical, chemical, and electronic properties. This is often a consequence of understanding how complex molecular architectures, be they organic, inorganic, or biological, are derived from their constituent building blocks. To study phenomena at such a basic level, tools capable of performing functional measurements, in real time, over critical length scales are required. Such tools would enable researchers to visualize complex biomolecular structures, ideally in their native context, while simultaneously mapping their functional properties.

Powerful functional imaging tools such as single molecule fluorescence and nonlinear optical microscopies, such as coherent anti-Raman Stokes (CARS) and second-harmonic generation (SHG), through to the various electron microscopies (SEM/TEM/STEM) provide a suite of tools for characterizing phenomena under a vast range of conditions and situations. Indeed recent advances in these established techniques provide ample evidence of their continued evolution, including the exciting new development of super-resolution optical imaging [1–6] and live cell electron microscopies [7]. An exceptionally powerful complement to these conventional imaging techniques has been atomic force microscopy (AFM), or scanning probe microscopy (SPM), which, since its inception in the mid-1980s, has developed into one of the most useful tools for characterizing molecular-scale phenomena and interactions, and directly mapping their contribution to macroscopic mechanical properties, structures, and ultimately function.

This chapter explores some of the recent advances in SPM where it has been applied to the study of biomolecular structures and functions—from single molecules to large aggregates and complexes to live cells—and introduce some new innovations in the field of correlated imaging tools designed to address many of the key limitations of this family of techniques.

24.2 Background

SPM is founded on a simple fundamental principle: Direct mapping of the interactions between a nominally atomically sharp raster-scanning tip and a surface can be used to generate real-space images of surfaces. One can reasonably describe these images as isosurfaces of a parameter as a function of (x,y,z) space. Notably, these isosurfaces can be interpreted as maps of a diverse set of interactions, ranging from repulsive or attractive forces to local variations in temperature, adhesion, viscoelasticity, and even charge. SPM has become a well-accepted and established technique for characterizing surfaces and interfacial processes with atomic or molecular-scale resolution [8–11]. It has made a tremendous impact in the biological sciences and the fields of cellular and molecular biophysics [12], due in large part to its unique ability to resolve molecular structures and interaction forces in real time and often *in situ* [13–20]. This growth has been fostered by a continually evolving suite of SPM-based imaging modes, including intermittent contact or tapping mode [21], force volume mapping [22–28], and even spatially resolved nanomechanical property measurements [29]. These attributes are particularly compelling for the study of protein–protein and protein–substrate interactions, including both model and live cell membranes [30], and investigations of cellular dynamics and structures.

24.3 SPM Basics

The family of scanning probe microscopes arguably emerged from early efforts by Young on the "Topographiner" [31]; however, the scanning tunneling microscope (STM), which operates on the principle of measuring the tunneling current between two conducting surfaces separated by a very small distance [32], is often viewed as the forefather of the field. For biology, a more useful variant is AFM, which maps local variations in the inter-molecular and inter-atomic forces between a tip and a surface [33]. By moving the tip relative to the sample surface in the x–y plane, a surface contour map that reflects relative differences in interaction intensity as a function of surface position can be generated. The high spatial and force resolution afforded the atomic force or scanning probe microscope (SPM) is a consequence of the precise control maintained over the tip–sample separation distance through the use of piezoelectric scanners and sophisticated feedback control schemes. In a conventional SPM, the surface is scanned with a nominally atomically sharp tip mounted on the underside of an extremely sensitive cantilever. The spatial resolution of the SPM is a consequence of the sample itself, with near-atomic scale resolution often achievable on atomically flat surfaces, such as a crystal. On softer, more compliant surfaces, such as cells or surfaces with significant variations in surface structure, the resolution can be somewhat reduced. Similarly, although the theoretical force sensitivity of these tips is on the order of 10^{-14} Newtons (N), practical limitations reduce this value to ~10^{-10} N.

The relative motion of the tip and sample is controlled through the use of piezoelectric crystal scanners. The user sets the desired applied force or amplitude dampening in the case of the intermittent contact imaging. Deviations from these set point values are detected as *error* signals on a four-quadrant position-sensitive photodetector (PSPD), and then fed into the main computer (Figure 24.1). The error signal provided to the instrument is then used to generate a feedback signal that is used as the input to the feedback control software. The tip–sample separation distance is then dynamically changed in real

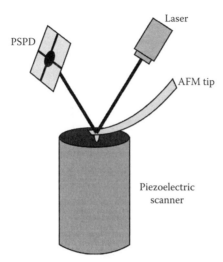

FIGURE 24.1 Schematic representation of the atomic force microscope. In this configuration, the sample would be mounted on the scanner and scanned under a fixed AFM tip. The laser is focused on the AFM tip and the position of the reflected laser spot is monitored on a position-sensitive photodetector (PSPD).

time and adjusted to return to the desired set point force. It is the amount of motion required to return to the desired set point value that is then converted into the observed isosurface. Although tip deflection is the simplest feedback signal, there are a host of other signals that could be used to control the tip–sample mapping, including tip oscillation (amplitude/phase), friction, surface charge, and even temperature.

24.4 Imaging Mechanisms

24.4.1 Contact

During imaging, the AFM tracks gradients in interaction force(s), either attractive or repulsive, between the tip and the surface (Figure 24.2). Similar to how the STM mapped out local variations in tip–sample tunneling current, the AFM uses this force gradient to generate an iso-force surface image. In contact mode imaging, the tip–sample interaction is maintained at a specific, user-defined load. This operating mode arguably provides the best resolution for imaging of surfaces and structures. It also provides direct access to the so-called friction force imaging where transient twisting of the cantilever during scanning can be used to develop maps of relative surface friction [34,35]. The ability to quantify such data is limited because of challenges in determining the torsional stiffness of the cantilevers, a problem exacerbated by the geometry of the cantilever. In contact mode the image represents a constant attractive (or repulsive) tip–sample force that is chosen by the user. Incorrect selection of this load results in sample damage (excessive force) or poor tracking (insufficient force). Subtle manipulation of these imaging forces affords the user the unique ability to both probe local structure and determine the response of the structure to the applied force.

24.4.2 Noncontact

In noncontact mode imaging, the AFM tip is actively oscillated near its resonance frequency at a distance of tens to hundreds of Angströms away from sample surface. The resulting image represents an isosurface corresponding to regions of constant amplitude dampening. As the forces between the tip and the surface are very small, noncontact mode AFM is ideally suited for imaging softer samples, such as proteins, surfactants, or membranes. In this mode, one often uses cantilevers with a higher spring

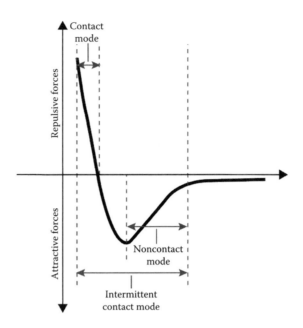

FIGURE 24.2 Schematic representation of the interaction forces between the AFM tip and an arbitrary surface as a function of separation distance. The schematic illustrates the regions of attractive and repulsive forces and the domains of AFM operation (contact/intermittent contact/noncontact).

constant than those employed during normal contact mode imaging. The net result is a very small feedback signal, which can make instrument control difficult and imaging challenging [36,37].

24.4.3 Intermittent Contact

This method, in which the tip alternates from the repulsive to the attractive regions of the tip–sample interaction curve, has become the method of choice currently for most AFM imaging. In early contact mode work, it was quickly realized that poorly adhering molecules could be rapidly displaced by the sweeping motion of the AFM cantilever. This "snow-plow" effect has been largely ameliorated by vertically oscillating the tip during imaging, which removes the lateral forces present during contact mode imaging. As the vertical oscillations occur at a drive frequency that is several orders of magnitude higher than the raster-scanning frequency, it is possible to obtain comparable lateral and vertical resolution as the continuous contact techniques. Because one detects the relative damping of the tip's free vertical oscillation during imaging, an intermittent contact mode AFM image can be viewed as an iso-energy dissipation landscape. Intermittent contact imaging provides access to other imaging modes, including phase imaging, which measures the phase shift between the applied and detected tip oscillations. This derivative signal is particularly useful for tracking spatial distributions of the relative modulus, viscoelasticity, and adhesive characteristics of surfaces, and has proven to be very powerful for studying polymeric materials [26,34,35,38–50]. Phase imaging is particularly useful for studying biological and biomimetic systems, including adsorbed proteins and supported lipid bilayers, even in the absence of topographic contrast [45,51–54].

In intermittent contact imaging, the cantilever can be oscillated either acoustically or magnetically. In the former, the cantilever is vertically oscillated by a piezoelectric crystal typically mounted under the cantilever at a characteristic resonant frequency. In air, this is typically a single value, determined largely by the stiffness of the cantilever. In fluid, mechanical coupling of the cantilever motion with the fluid, and the fluid cell, can result in a complex power spectrum with multiple apparent resonant peaks. In this case, choosing the appropriate peak to operate with can be difficult and experience is often the best guide. Selection of the appropriate cantilever for intermittent contact imaging will depend on the physical imaging environment (air/fluid). In air, one typically uses the so-called "diving board" tips, which have a relatively high resonance peak of approximately 250 kHz (depending on the manufacturer). In fluid, viscous coupling between the tip and the surrounding fluid results in an increase in the apparent resonant frequency of the tip. This allows the use of the conventional V-shaped contact-mode cantilevers. In magnetic mode, a magnetic AFM tip/cantilever assembly is placed in an oscillating magnetic field [55–57]. It is the interaction of the magnetic tip with the field that induces the tip oscillations. This is a fundamentally simpler approach with arguably finer control over the drive amplitude; however, this approach can be complicated by issues such as the quality of the coating and the nature of the sample.

24.4.3.1 Applications

The breadth of possible applications for SPM seems almost endless. As has been described earlier, the concepts underlying the instrument are simple and the technology itself has effectively become turnkey. This does not mean that SPM is a very transparent tool—it is critical that the user has a good grasp of the physical principles that underpin the generation of an SPM image. Similarly, the user must have a good understanding of the nature of their samples, and how they might behave during imaging—an aspect that is of particular interest to those investigating cellular phenomena. Recent reviews by Bottomley et al., and others provide an excellent perspective on the diverse range of topics that are being studied by this and related techniques [9–11,13,58]. In the following sections, we will explore how *in situ* SPM/AFM-based investigations have provided novel insights into the structure and function of biomolecular assemblies. SPM has made in-roads in several different arenas, which can be separated into several key areas: [1] imaging; [2] force spectroscopy; and [3] nanomechanical property measurement. We will focus in a few specific areas, rather than attempting to cover the whole scope of the field.

24.5 Imaging

The real-space imaging capabilities, coupled with the ability to simultaneously display derivative images, such as phase (viscoelasticity), friction, and temperature, are perhaps the most attractive attributes of the SPM. In the case of biomolecules, it is the ability to perform such imaging but in buffer media, under a variety of solution conditions and temperatures, in real time that has really powered the acceptance of this technique by the biomedical community [59–63]. Such capabilities are allowing researchers to gain a glimpse of the mechanics and dynamics of protein assembly and function, and the role of extrinsic factors, such as pH, temperature, or other ligands on these processes [64]. For example, *in situ* SPM has been used successfully to visualize and characterize voltage and pH-dependent conformational changes in two-dimensional arrays of OmpF [21], whereas several groups have used *in situ* SPM to characterize transcription and DNA-complex formation and individual proteins [65–73].

The raster-scanning action of the tip does, however, complicate *in situ* imaging. Processes occurring faster than the raster-scanning acquisition time of the SPM can be missed, or worse, create an artifact associated with the motion of the object. The magnitude of this problem obviously depends on the kinetics of the processes under study. This is particularly important when one is viewing live cell data in which conventional raster-scanning rates are necessarily slow (~1 Hz) [74–76]. Advances in tip and controller technology help to improve the stability of the SPM under fast-scan conditions. Strategies may include tips with active piezoelectric elements [77] smaller cantilevers with high-quality factors, or faster data acquisition and control hardware [78]. A particularly useful and low-cost option for improving time resolution is to simply *disable* one of the scanning directions so that the AFM image is a compilation of line scans taken at the same location as a function of time [79]. This would, therefore, generate an isosurface wherein one image axis reflects time and not position. This approach has been used quite successfully to examine single molecule dynamics in a study of the chaperonin GroES–GroEL complex [80].

Although recent efforts have resulted in particularly compelling new hardware and software implementations for faster biological AFM imaging, including live cells and protein dynamics [76,78,81–85], they continue to rely on a single cantilever probe to perform the imaging. A particularly compelling albeit challenging from the fabrication and control perspectives approach may be to consider the use of multiple imaging tips. Such a strategy would effectively parallelize the imaging process. The potential of such an approach remains largely unproven to date although SPM tip arrays have been developed for data storage applications and sensor applications [86–89].

24.6 Crystallography

In situ SPM has been used with great success to study the mechanisms associated with crystal growth [90], from amino acids [91], to zeolite crystallization [92], and biomineralization [93–95]. For protein crystals, studies have ranged from early investigations of lysozyme [96], to insulin [97], antibodies [98,99], and recently the mechanisms of protein crystal repair [99]. The advantages of SPM for characterizing protein crystallization have been very well discussed in reviews by McPherson and Vekilov [100,101]. Ordered crystalline materials formed through chemical cross-linking are also amenable to high-resolution imaging [102]. It is worth mentioning that the high spatial and temporal resolution capabilities of the SPM are ideal for examining and measuring the thermodynamic parameters for these processes. These range from local variations in free energy and their correlation with conventional models of crystal growth to relating step advancement rates to the product of the density of surface kink sites and the frequency of attachment [103]. Recently, Guo et al. [104] probed the nanomechanical properties of insulin crystals by AFM, providing intriguing insights into inter-planar strength and the local compressibility of the protein within its crystalline lattice in direct comparison with data obtained on insulin fibrils.

A particular challenge for SPM studies of crystal growth is that interpreting the data paradoxically often requires that one already has a known crystal structure or a related isoform for comparison of packing motifs and molecular orientation. *De novo* determination of two-dimensional crystal packing motifs can be readily achieved; however, extrapolations to possible space group symmetries are much more difficult [105–107]. Recently, the focus has shifted toward understanding the growth process. The ability to perform extended duration *in situ* imaging presents the crystallographer with the unique opportunity of directly determining the mechanisms and kinetics of crystal nucleation and growth [99,100,103,106,108–118]. Unlike x-ray approaches, the SPM cannot readily report on atomic-level details of the crystal and the molecular units. Rather, it provides details on crystal and molecular packing motifs with the individual molecules appearing as amorphous blob to the AFM, even when packed into a lattice, making it difficult to assign a specific secondary structure to the protein. Despite these challenges, *in situ* AFM studies of molecular and protein crystals have proven to be quite enlightening. Recent work by Danesh et al., resolved the difference between various crystal polymorphs including face-specific dissolution rates for drug candidates [119–121] while Guo et al. examined the effect of specific proteins on the crystallization of calcium oxalate monohydrate [122]. In a particularly interesting study, Frincu et al., investigated cholesterol crystallization from bile solutions using calcite as a model substrate [123]. In this work, the authors were able to use *in situ* SPM to characterize the role of specific substrate interactions in driving the initial nucleation events associated with cholesterol crystallization. Extended-duration imaging allowed the researchers to characterize the growth rates and the onset of Ostwald ripening under physiological conditions. They were able to confirm their observations and models by calculating the interfacial energies associated with the attachment of the cholesterol crystal to the calcite substrate. In their comprehensive review of the thermodynamics and kinetics of calcium phosphate biomineralization, Wang and Nancollas explored how AFM can be used to directly extract novel insights into the initial nucleation steps associated with crystal growth and phase formation [124]. Biomineralization and its health implications have stimulated numerous studies of calcium oxalate crystallization as it relates to kidney stones and strategies of their remediation [125–127]. These include studies of strategies for modifying the kinetics and habit of calcium oxalate crystals with small peptides, as reported by Wang et al. [128]. Milhiet et al. used detergent-disrupted bilayers to form two-dimensional crystals of several membrane proteins, enabling them to directly probe the structure of the exposed extracellular domains [129]. In our own work, we demonstrated that the self-assembly of small molecule dye aggregates into crystalline arrays with unique, structure-dependent spectroscopic properties on phospholipid bilayers was dependent on both electrostatic effects as well as substrate packing [130]. This work was particularly interesting as it revealed the role of the nucleating interface in controlling the structure, orientation, and packing of the dye aggregate nuclei, portending the design of other structured interfaces for controlling aggregate orientation, size, and properties. It is this powerful combination of *in situ* real-time characterization with theoretical modeling that has made *in situ* SPM particularly compelling for studying molecular self-assembly at interfaces.

24.6.1 Protein Aggregation and Fibril Formation

In a related context, the self-assembly of proteins into fibrillar motifs has been an area of active research for many years, owing in large part to the putative links to diseases such as Alzheimer's, Huntington's, and even diabetes in the context of *in vitro* insulin fibril formation [131,132]. A particular challenge for the field of protein aggregation lies in the complex map of association pathways and structures. Determining what are on- and off-pathway aggregates and their relationship to the disease pathology has proven to be quite difficult, owing in large part to the numerous intermolecular interactions that drive these self-assembly mechanisms. Directly identifying these pathways, tracking biomolecular self-association, and finding a causal link to a particular disease would be a tremendous asset for the design of drug inhibitors. Because *in situ* SPM can easily acquire real-space information on dynamic molecular-scale processes and structures that are difficult to assay clinically, it is ideal for *in situ* studies of protein aggregation and fibrillogenesis. These have included investigations of collagen [133–137], human stefin B [138], spider silk [139–142], insulin amyloid polypeptide (IAPP), amylin, β-amyloid, and synuclein [143–152]. *In situ* observation of Aβ assemblies has enabled direct observation of low molecular weight oligomers [153], whereas high-resolution imaging of islet amyloid polypeptide has been performed using frequency-modulation techniques [154]. In an intriguing study, Friedrichs et al. captured the reorientation of collagen fibrils in cells *in vitro* using AFM [155].

Perhaps, driven more by an applied technology perspective, *in situ* SPM has provided unique chemical insights not only into the process of fibrillization [156,157], but also the role of the nucleating substrate on directing the kinetics, orientation, and structure of the emerging fibril [158,159]. As noted by Kowalewski in their investigation of β-amyloid formation on different surfaces chemically and/or structural dissimilar substrate may in fact facilitate growth biasing the apparent kinetics and orientation of the aggregate [160]. Because SPM imaging requires a supporting substrate, there is often a tacit assumption that this surface is passive and would not adversely influence the aggregation or growth process. However, what has become immediately obvious from a number of studies is that these surfaces can, and do, alter the nucleation and growth patterns [161,162]. Characterization, either theoretical or experimental using the *in situ* capabilities of the SPM, will, in principle, identify how the local physical/electronic/chemical nature of the surface drives fibril formation [163]. One must ensure that appropriate controls were in place, or performed, so that the aggregate as seen by the SPM is clearly the responsible agent for nucleation. All of this certainly brings up the questions of [1] is the aggregate observed by these *in situ* tools truly the causative agent; [2] what role is the substrate playing in the aggregation or assembly pathway. The first point is a particularly compelling one when it concerns the studies of protein adsorption and assembly. Although the SPM can certainly resolve nanometer-sized objects on the substrate, the adsorption of the smallest species cannot be guaranteed. Correlating solution with surface self-assembly mechanisms and structures, especially in the context of biomolecular complexes and phenomena, can be challenging and often one must resort to complementary, corroborative tools such as light scattering.

24.6.2 Membrane Protein Structure and Assemblies

One area in which SPM has made a significant impact has been in the structural characterization of membrane dynamics and protein–membrane interactions and assembly. Supported planar lipid bilayers (SPB) are particularly attractive as model cell membranes [164] and recent work has provided very detailed insights of their local dynamics and structure [165–171], as well as the dynamics of domain formation [172–175]. Exploiting the *in situ* high-resolution imaging capabilities of the SPM and the conformal nature of supported bilayers, workers have been able to follow thermal phase transitions (gel-fluid) in supported bilayers [174,176,177] and Langmuir–Blodgett films [178]. Thermal transitions in mixed composition supported bilayers have been studied by *in situ* SPM [174,179], where the so-called ripple phase domains were seen to form as the system entered the gel–fluid coexistence regime [180]. These structural studies not only enrich our understanding on bilayers themselves, but also of their interactions with other biological systems.

In situ SPM has been particularly useful for investigating the dynamics of the so-called lipid rafts, which are small lipid heterogeneities thought to facilitate membrane protein function. With nanometer-scale topographical resolution, AFM observations showed that many membrane lipids and mixtures contain such lipid domains [181]. For example, Rinia et al., investigated the role of cholesterol in the formation of rafts using a complex mixture of dioleoylphosphatidylcholine (DOPC), sphingomyelin (SpM), and cholesterol as the model membrane [182]. In the absence of cholesterol, the mixture phase separates into gel-state SpM and fluid-state DOPC domains. As the cholesterol content increased, the authors reported the formation of SpM/cholesterol-rich domains or "lipid rafts" within the (DOPC) fluid domains. In related work, Van Duyl et al. (2003) observed similar domain formation for (1:1) SpM/DOPC SPBs containing 30 mol% cholesterol [183]. With cholesterol, the formation of these domains is not restricted to liquid–liquid coexistence phases [179]. The effect of dynamically changing the cholesterol levels on raft formation and structure was reported by Lawrence et al. [184]. By adding either water-soluble cholesterol or methyl-β-cyclodextrin (Mβ-CD), a cholesterol-sequestering agent, the authors were able to directly resolve the effect of adding or removing cholesterol on domain structure and dynamics, including a biphasic response to cholesterol level that was seen as a transient formation of raft domains as the cholesterol level was reduced. The *in situ* imaging capabilities of the SPM have provided direct evidence of domain formation for cardiolipin, a lipid enriched in the mitochondria that form domains only in the presence of phosphatidylethanolamine and not phosphatidylcholine [185]. *In situ* AFM was used to confirm that clustering of galactosylceramides on the extracellular membrane leaflet, a mechanism thought to facilitate virus adhesion, was a cholesterol-dependent process [186]. Our AFM-based studies of the late endosomal lipid bis-(monoacylglycero)-phosphoate (BMP), thought to cause multivesicular morphology through domain formation [187–189] confirmed this mechanism through coupled AFM phase and fluorescence imaging methods.

Using supported planar bilayers as a model substrate has been particularly useful for the study of membrane-associated molecules by AFM. Polycationic dendrimers were found to induce large, 15–40 nm diameter holes in the zwitterionic bilayers and remove fluid-phase lipids from the alveoli-mimicking Survanta bilayers [190,191]. Anesthetics, such as dibucaine and halothane, were found to compromise membrane structure and elasticity [168,184,192–206]. Several studies explored the interactions between membrane-active and membrane-associated proteins and membrane surfaces. For example, *in situ* SPM has revealed that the association of peptides with membranes can lead to dramatic changes in membrane morphology and membrane disruption. This was seen to be the case for the amphipathic peptides: filipin, amphotericin B, mellitin, and amylin [207–210]. In related work, the N-terminal domain of the capsid protein cleavage product of the flock house virus (FHV), has found to cause the formation of interdigitated lipid membrane domains [211]. We have seen similar effects in our studies of peptide-membrane interactions, including antimicrobial peptides and toxins [212–216]. Tilted peptides were found to cause hole formation while leaving the membrane morphology largely intact [217]. In contrast, the protein synaptotagmin can leave indentations but does not produce defects in anionic lipid bilayers

[218]. In related work, AFM studies revealed how membranes of Gram-negative bacteria disintegrate through to the action of antibacterial Sushi peptides [219]. The relative ease with which SPBs can be formed prompted studies of reconstituted membrane proteins, including ion channels and transmembrane receptors [194–203,220] and enzymes, such as ATP synthase and phosphatases [221,222]. The ease of forming complex model membranes from an SPB suspension helped drive investigations of reconstituted membrane protein functionality [16]. For example, *in situ* AFM has been used to examine the role of divalent ions, such as calcium in facilitating membrane protein insertion while inhibiting detergent interdigitation [223]. However, it is worth noting that because model membrane formation is typically performed by simple vesicle fusion, it is difficult to know *a priori* the orientation of a transmembrane protein in the final supported bilayer as protein reconstitution into the vesicle occurs via freeze-thaw or sonication [168,204–206]. The lipid-to-protein ratios can be manipulated to yield the ideal density or to investigate the structural differences caused by steric factors [224]. Ideally, there is a distinct difference in the size and/or shape of the extra- and intra-cellular domains, and statistical analysis of local surface topographies can be employed to at least infer a molecular orientation.

Peptide-membrane interactions are also thought to be critical to the mechanism of neurodegenerative diseases, such as Alzheimer's (AD) and Parkinson's (PD). For example, studies of α-synuclein with supported lipid bilayers revealed the gradual formation and growth of defects within the SPB [225]. Interestingly, the use of a mutant form of α-synuclein revealed a qualitatively slower rate of bilayer disruption. We conducted an analogous experiment to investigate the interaction between the β-amyloid (Aβ) peptide with SPBs prepared from a total brain lipid mixture [226]. *In situ* SPM revealed that the association of monomeric Aβ1-40 peptide with the SPBs resulted in rapid formation of fibrils followed by membrane disruption. Control experiments performed with pure component DMPC bilayers revealed similar membrane disruption; however, the mechanism was qualitatively different with the formation of amorphous aggregates rather than well-formed fibrils. Others have examined similar membrane-induced aggregation and self-assembly phenomena using a diverse range of model membrane compositions and peptides [190,227–229]. What is particularly compelling about these studies, aside from the ability to provide direct visualization of the effect of the interactions in real-time using the SPM, is the ease with which one can reliably fabricate model membranes of quite complex mixtures, ranging from simple homogeneous gel- or fluid-state bilayers through to complex heterogeneous mimics of bacterial and fungal membranes.

24.7 Force Spectroscopy

24.7.1 Fundamentals

By disabling the x- and y-scan directions and monitoring the tip deflection in the z-direction, the AFM is capable of measuring protein–protein and ligand-receptor binding forces, often with sub-picoNewton resolution. The ability to detect such low forces is because of the low spring constant of the AFM cantilever (0.60–0.06 N/m). In these AFM force curve measurements, the tip is modeled as a Hookian spring whereby the amount of tip deflection (Δz) is directly related to the attractive/repulsive forces (F) acting on the tip through the tip spring constant (k). At the start of the force curve, the AFM tip is held at a null position of zero deflection out of contact with the sample surface. The tip–sample separation distance is gradually reduced and then enlarged using a triangular voltage cycle applied to the piezoelectric scanner. This will bring the tip into and out of contact with the sample surface. As the piezo extends, the sample surface contacts the AFM tip causing the tip to deflect upward until a maximum applied force is reached and the scanner then begins to retract. We should note that when the gradient of the attractive force between the tip and sample exceeds the spring constant of the tip, the tip will "jump" into contact with the sample surface. As the scanner retracts, the upward tip deflection is reduced until it reaches the null position. As the sample continues to move away from the tip, attractive forces between the tip and the surface hold the tip in contact with the surface and the tip begins to deflect in the opposite direction. The tip continues to deflect downwards until the restoring force of the tip cantilever overcomes the attractive forces and the tip jumps out of contact with the sample surface (E), thereby providing us with an estimate of the tip–sample unbinding force, given as:

$$F = -k\Delta z$$

This force spectroscopy approach has found application ranging from mapping effect of varying ionic strength on the interactions between charged surfaces [230–245], to studying electrostatic forces at crystal surfaces [246,247].

24.7.1.1 Single Molecule Force Spectroscopy

Specific intermolecular interactions can be measured in single molecule force spectroscopy using ligand-modified SPM tips [248]. In principle, if we can measure the forces associated with the binding of a ligand to its complementary receptor, we may be able to correlate these forces with association energies [249]. By tethering a ligand of interest, in the correct orientation, to the force microscope tip and bringing the now-modified tip into contact with an appropriately functionalized surface, one can now conceivably directly measure the attractive and repulsive intermolecular forces between single molecules as a function of the tip–sample separation distance. The vertical tip jump during pull-off can be used to estimate the interaction force, which can be related to the number of binding sites, adhesive contact area, and the molecular packing density of the bound molecules. In the case of biomolecular systems, multiple intermolecular interactions exist and both dissociation and (re)association events may occur on the time scale of the experiment resulting in broad retraction curve with discrete, possibly quantized, pull-off events. This approach has been used to investigate biomolecular [22,56,250–252] and DNA-nucleotide interactions, along with the local mechanical properties of biomolecules [20,253–261]. Although estimates of the adhesive interaction forces may be obtained from the vertical tip excursions during the retraction phase of the force curve, during pull-off, the width and shape of the retraction curve reflects entropically unfavourable molecular unfolding and elongation processes.

Although simple in principle, it was soon recognized that the force spectroscopy experiment was highly sensitive to sampling conditions. For example, it is currently well recognized that the dynamics of the measurement will significantly influence the shape of the unbinding curve. It is well known that the rate of ligand-receptor dissociation increases with force resulting in a logarithmic dependence of the unbinding force with rate [262], and studies have shown that single molecule techniques, such as AFM, clearly sample an interaction energy landscape [263]. It is, therefore, evident that forces measured by the AFM cannot be trivially related to binding affinities [264]. Beyond these simple sampling rate dependence relationships, we must also be aware of the dynamics of the tip motion during the acquisition phase of the measurement. In particular, when these interactions are mapped in fluid media, one must consider the hydrodynamic drag associated with the (rapid) motion of the tip through the fluid [265]. This drag effect can be considerable when factored into the interaction force determination.

Another key consideration is that, in single molecule force spectroscopy, the ligands of interest are necessarily immobilized at force microscope tips and sample surfaces. In principle, this approach will allow one to directly measure or evaluate the spatial relationship between the ligand and its corresponding receptor site. For correct binding to occur, the ligands of interest must be correctly oriented, have the appropriate secondary and tertiary structure, and be sufficiently flexible (or have sufficiently high unrestricted mobility) that they can bind correctly. An appropriate immobilization strategy would, therefore, require *a priori* information about the ligand's sequence, conformation, and the location of the binding site(s) [266,267]. Strategies that have worked in the past include *N*-nitrilo-triacetic acid linkages [268], His-tags to preferentially orient ligands at surface [269,270], and, most recently, a rather interesting series of tripodal ligands [271–273]. Thiolated peptides can similarly be immobilized on gold-coated tips [274]. The critical consideration in all of these designs is the ability to robustly orient the ligand of interest appropriately. A particularly robust and reliable approach has been to rely on polyethylene glycol tethers to help extend the ligands away from the tip [252,275–281]. Force spectroscopy is not limited to patterned and model surfaces but can be performed on live cell surfaces. Alsteens et al. performed unfolding experiments directly on live cells [282]. Microbial surface ultrastructure and nanomechanical properties can be visualized [283]. Protein binding and AFM force spectroscopy on live cell membranes can be coupled to downstream processes, potentially revealing the mechanical role that the protein has in eliciting a response [284]. This type of *in situ*, pathway-specific biochemistry is often impossible to approach using more conventional techniques. Perhaps more compelling is the ability to perform such experiments under a range of conditions thus allowing the researcher to consider different, suboptimal conditions to examine induced stresses [285].

Recently, efforts have been underway to measure aggregate forces at intact biological interfaces, including bacterial biofilms on metal [286]. Microbeads were used to measure the adhesion and viscoelasticity of bacterial biofilms [287]. In addition to imaging or single molecular pulling/unfolding experiments, AFM has been used as a microscopic manipulator to dissect or deform bacteria cells [288,289]. As with single molecule force spectroscopy, the immobilization of cells becomes important in these studies. One approach is to engineer patterns and grow patches of single cells [290,291].

24.7.1.2 Force Volume

Acquiring force curves at each point on an image plane provides a means of acquiring the so-called force volume maps, a data-intensive imaging approach capable of providing a map of relative adhesion forces and charge densities across surfaces [23,292–294]. This approach has been used successfully to examine polymer surfaces and surfaces under fluid [295,296], as well as live cells [26,292,297]. Increasingly, force volume methodologies have been applied to live cell surfaces to spatially map interaction forces. These include efforts to investigate adhesin [298], polysaccharides [299,300], thiol-monolayers [301] interactions with bacterial or fungal surfaces to better understand the polarity and localization of specific processes. Not unexpectedly, these efforts have shown that specific antigen–antibody interactions are spatially concentrated in domains within the membrane [302].

24.7.1.3 Pulsed Force Mode

As indicated previously, force volume measurements are very time-consuming and this has led to the development of pulsed force mode imaging [303]. Capable of rapidly acquiring topographic, elasticity, and adhesion data, pulsed force mode operates by sampling selected regions of the force–distance curve during contact-mode imaging. During image scanning, an additional sinusoidal oscillation imparted to the tip brings the tip in and out of contact with the surface at each point of the image. Careful analysis of the pulsed force spectrum can yield details about surface elasticity and adhesion [304–309]. Compared with the ~ Hz sample rates present in conventional force volume imaging, in pulsed force mode, spectra are acquired on kHz sampling rates. Although this helps to resolve the issue related to the speed of data acquisition, one must clearly consider the possibilities associated (possible) with rate dependence of the adhesion forces, and as indicated in the previous section, the hydrodynamic forces would play a larger role.

24.7.2 Binding Forces

As discussed earlier, force spectroscopy samples regions of an energy landscape wherein the strength of a bond (and its lifetime) is highly dependent on the rate with which the spectra are collected [263,310]. At low loading rates, intermolecular bonds have long lifetimes but exhibit small unbinding forces, whereas at high loading rates, the same bonds have shorter lifetimes and larger unbinding forces. In the case of biomolecular complexes because multiple interactions are involved in stabilizing the binding interface, the dissociation pathway of a ligand-receptor complex will exhibit several unbinding energy barriers. This would suggest that one could in fact sample any number of dissociation pathways, each with its own set of transitional bonding interactions. Intriguingly, it was recently argued that the free-energy surface of a protein is significantly distorted during a force spectroscopy experiment and that such a distortion can result in certain complexities when one is considering a single molecule event [311]. The influence of experimental instrument parameters, such as loading rate, and their contribution to accurate modeling and interpretation of the rupture forces obtained from the force spectroscopy experiments has been well documented and described in a series of reports by the Akhremitchev group [312,313].

For the majority of single molecule force microscopy studies, individual ligands have been either randomly adsorbed or directly attached to the AFM tip through covalent bond formation. Covalent binding of a molecule to the tip offers a more stable "anchor" during force measurements as a covalent bond is ~10 times stronger than a typical ligand-receptor bond [314]. Covalent binding also facilitates oriented attachment of the ligand as compared to random adsorption where the orientation of the ligand on the tip surface must be statistically inferred. These advantages are tempered with the challenges present in immobilizing molecules to surfaces such as the AFM tip. As mentioned earlier, oriented ligands have been tethered covalently to AFM tips through use of flexible poly(ethylene-glycol) (PEG)-linkers [252]. In this manner, the peptide or ligand is extended away from the tip surface, which provides it with sufficient flexibility and conformational freedom for it to reorient and sample conformational space. Heterobifunctional PEG derivatives have provided the necessary synthetic flexibility for coupling a host of different ligands to the AFM tips [252,276,277,279,280,315–317]. Indeed, this approach remains a complex technical challenge as it requires due consideration of not only these factors but even seemingly mundane aspects such as the tip geometry and tilt, as was discussed in a recent publication by Rivera et al. [318].

Force spectroscopy pertains to mapping or measuring forces between discrete molecules. For example, several groups have investigated antibody–antigen interactions [319,320] and have shown that these unbinding forces may correlate with thermal dissociation rates [321]. Force spectroscopy has been used to study the energetics of protein adsorption [322]. Although the high force sensitivity of this approach is exceptionally attractive, it is equally important to recognize key experimental considerations, including the use of appropriate controls. Recently, various computational approaches, including steered molecular dynamics [323–328], Monte Carlo simulations [329,330], and graphical energy function analyses [331] have been used to simulate these dissociation and unfolding experiments. It has been particularly impressive to see the strong correlation between the structural changes resolved by these computational approaches and the experimentally determined unbinding events although much work remains to be done in terms of determining appropriate computational schemes for extending the simulation times to best match the experimental time frames and instrument parameters.

Force spectroscopy is also being applied to study protein unfolding pathways. It was recognized in early work that during the retraction phase of the AFM force curve, the molecule is subjected to a high tensile stress, and can undergo reversible elongation and unfolding. Careful control over the applied load (and the degree of extension) will allow one to probe molecular elasticity and the energetics involved in the unfolding/folding process [60,142,265,332–347]. Past studies have included investigations of titin [348], IgG phenotypes [349], various polysaccharides [350], and spider silk proteins [351]. The forces associated with protein fibril formation have been studied using force spectroscopy, including studies of the proteins involved in Parkinson's [352], Alzheimer's, and diabetes [353–355]. The Ikai group has done pioneering work with force spectroscopy of cell surface proteins, both using proteins adsorbed to a surface as well as natively presented on the membrane [356,357].

By bringing the AFM tip into contact with the surface-adsorbed molecules, and carefully controlling the rate and extent of withdrawal from the surface, it is now possible to resolve transitions that may be ascribed to unfolding of individual protein domains. Others have employed this "forced unfolding" approach to look at spectrin [358,359], lysozyme [360], and DNA [361]. Caution needs to be exercised during such experiments. Often the protein of interest is allowed to simply absorb to the substrate to form a film. Force curves performed on these films are then conducted in random locations and the retraction phase of the curve analyzed for elongation and unbinding events. This is a highly statistical approach and somewhat problematic. The general premise is that the tip will bind to the protein somewhere and that if sufficient samples are acquired, there will be a statistically relevant number of curves that will exhibit the anticipated number of unbinding and/or unfolding events. What is fundamentally challenging here is that there is no *a priori* means of knowing where the tip will bind to the protein, which would obviously affect its ability to under extension, and it is difficult to assess the interactions between the protein and the supporting substrate, or possibly other entangled proteins. To simplify the optimization and improve the statistical nature of the force spectroscopy experiment, efforts have been made by several groups to develop automated force spectroscopy systems [362].

Where single molecule imaging comes to the forefront is in the combination of imaging and single-molecule force spectroscopy. In the past, force spectroscopy has relied heavily on random sampling of the immobilized proteins, often without direct imaging of the selected protein. Recently, Raab et al. combined dynamic force microscopy, wherein a magnetically coated AFM tip is oscillated in close proximity to a surface by an alternating magnetic field. This enabled the researchers to apply what they termed "recognition imaging" to facilitate mapping of individual molecular recognition sites on a surface [279]. In recognition imaging, specific binding events are detected through dampening of the amplitude of oscillation of the ligand-modifed tip due to specific binding of the antibody on the tip to an antigen on the surface. The resulting AFM antibody-antigen recognition image will display regions of enhanced contrast that can be identified as possible binding sites or domains. In an excellent demonstration of the coupled imaging and force spectroscopy, Oesterhelt et al., studied the unfolding of bacteriorhodopsin by directly adsorbing native purple membrane to a surface, imaging the trimeric structure of the BR, and then carefully pulling on a selected molecule [60]. This allowed them to resolve the force required to destabilize the BR helices from the membrane and by reimaging the same area, show that extraction occurred two helices at a time. Computationally, these phenomena are most often modeled as freely jointed or worm-like chain systems [363]. To assess what exactly "forced unfolding" involves, Paci and Karplus examined the role of topology and energetics on protein unfolding via externally applied forces and compared it against the more traditional thermal unfolding pathways [364].

24.7.2.1 Mechanical properties

The use of the AFM/SPM as a nanomechanical tester has certainly blossomed. During the past 10 years, AFM-based nanoindentation has been used to determine the elastic modulus of polymers [365], biomolecules [366–371], cellular and tissue surfaces [372–380], pharmaceutical solids [381], and even teeth [382]. What is particularly challenging in these applications is the need for careful consideration when extrapolating bulk moduli against the nanoindentation data. Often the classical models need to be adjusted to compensate for the small (nanometer) contact areas involved in the indentation [383]. A particularly important consideration with AFM-based nanoindentation is the sampling geometry. Although traditional indentation instrumentation applies a purely vertical load on the sample, by virtue of the cantilever arrangement of the AFM system, there is also a lateral component to the indentation load. This leads to an asymmetry in the indentation profile. This asymmetry can make it difficult to compare AFM-based nanoindentation with traditional approaches using a center-loaded system. Often this effect is nullified by the use of a spherical tip with a well-defined geometry; however, this entails a further compromise in the ability to perform imaging before the indentation process. This effect has been extensively covered in the literature, especially in the context of polymer blends and composite materials [384–389]. Other considerations include the relative stiffness of the AFM cantilever, the magnitude of the applied load, tip shape which plays a significant role in the indentation process, and possibly the dwell-time. In many cases, the relatively soft cantilever will allow one to perform more precise modulus measurements including the ability to image before, and immediately after, an indentation measurement. At an even more pragmatic level, determining the stiffness both in-plane and torsional, of the cantilever can be challenging, with approaches ranging from the traditional end mass to new techniques based on thermal noise and resonant frequency shifts [390–392]. Accurate determination of these values is essential in order for the correct assessment of the local stiffness to be made.

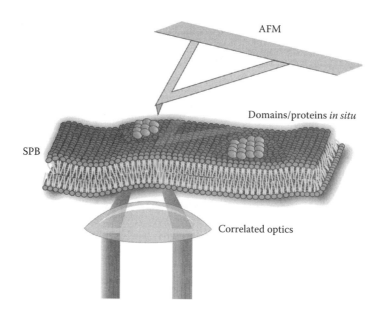

FIGURE 24.3 Schematic representation of a combinatorial AFM-fluorescence microscopy experiment, depicting AFM imaging of a supported planar lipid bilayer (SPB) containing membrane domains and/or proteins.

24.7.2.2 Coupled Imaging

Although AFM/SPM is certainly a powerful tool for following structure and dynamics at surfaces under a wide variety of conditions, it can only provide relative information within a given imaging frame. It similarly cannot confirm (easily) that the structure being imaged is in fact the protein of interest. A confirmation step can involve some *in situ* control, which might be a change in pH or T, or introduction of another ligand or reagent that would cause a change in the same that could be resolved by the SPM. Absent an *in situ* control, or in fact as an adjunct, careful shape/volume analysis is often conducted to characterize specific features in a sample. Image analysis and correlation tools and techniques are often exploited for postacquisition analysis. There has always been an obvious need for techniques or tools that can provide this complementary information, ideally in a form that could be readily integrated into the SPM.

Optical imaging represents perhaps the best tool for integration with SPM. This is motivated by the realization that there are a host of very powerful single molecule optical imaging techniques capable of addressing many of the key limitations of SPM, such as the ability to resolve dynamic events on millisecond time scales. Recent advances in confocal laser scanning (CLSM) and total internal reflection fluorescence (TIRFM) techniques have enabled single molecule detection with subdiffraction limited images [393–402] (Figure 24.3).

24.7.3 Near-Field: SNOM/NSOM

In the family of scanning probe microscopes, perhaps the best example of an integrated optical-SPM system are the scanning near-field (or near-field scanning) optical microscopes (NSOMs) which use near-field excitation of the sample to obtain subdiffraction limited images with spatial resolution comparable to conventional scanning probe microscopes [403–407]. NSOM has been used successfully in single molecule studies of dyes [408], proteins [409–411], and the structure of lignin and ion channels [412,413]. NSOM imaging has also provided insights into ligand-induced clustering of the ErbB2 receptor, a member of the epidermal growth factor (EGF) receptor tyrosine kinase family, in the membrane of live cells [414–416]. Fluorescence lifetime imaging by NSOM has been used to examine the energy and electron-transfer processes of the light harvesting complex (LHC II) [415,416] in intact photosynthetic membranes [417]. NSOM has also been used to monitor the fluorescence resonance energy transfer (FRET) between single pairs of donor and acceptor fluorophores on dsDNA molecules [418]. Challenges that face the NSOM community arguably lie in the robust design of the imaging tips [419,420]. However, NSOM as a tool is enjoying a resurgence of interest of late with recent efforts in polarized NSOM providing detailed insights into protein fibril structure [412,421] and lipid bilayer domains [422–424].

24.7.4 Evanescent Wave: TIRF

Time-resolved single-molecule imaging can be difficult and in the case of the AFM, one may question whether the local phenomena imaged by the AFM are specific to that particular imaging location. This is especially true for studies of dynamic phenomena because the scanning action of the AFM tip effectively acts to increase mass transfer into the imaging volume. Recently, combined AFM/TIRF techniques have been used to study force transmission [373] and single-particle manipulation [425] in cells. These studies helped to address a particularly challenging aspect of SPM, which was that SPM/AFM can only (realistically) infer data about the upper surface of structures and that data on the underside of a structure, for instance the focal adhesions of a cell, are largely invisible to the SPM tip. In the case of cell adhesion, one might be interested in how a cell responds to a local stress applied to its apical surface by monitoring changes in focal adhesion density and size. Using a combined AFM–TIRF system, it then becomes possible to directly interrogate the basal surface of the cell (by TIRF) while applying a load or examining the surface topography of the cell by *in situ* AFM. We recently reported on the design and use of an AFM-objective-based TIRF-based instrument for the study of supported bilayer systems [216,426,427]. By coupling these two instruments together, we were able to identify unequivocally the gel and fluid domains in a mixed dPOPC/dPPC system. What was particularly compelling was the observation of approximately 10–20% difference in the lateral dimension of the features as resolved by TIRF and AFM. Although this likely reflects the inherent diffraction limited nature of TIRFM, we can in fact use the AFM data to confirm the real-space size of the structures that are responsible for the fluorescence image contrast. This combined system also provided another interesting insight. The nonuniform fluorescence intensity across the domains resolved by TIRF may reflect a nonuniform distribution of NBD-PC within dPOPC. It may also be linked to the time required to capture a TIRF image relative to the AFM imaging. At a typical scan rate of 2 Hz, it would require approximately 4 min to capture a conventional 512×512 pixel AFM image, compared with the approximately 30 frame/s video imaging rate of the TIRF camera system. As such the TIRFM system represents an excellent means of visualizing, and capturing, data that occur on time scales faster than what can be readily resolved by the AFM. This further suggests that the differences in fluorescence intensity may reflect real-time fluctuations in the structure of the lipid bilayer that are not detected (or detectable) by AFM imaging. In a particularly intriguing experiment that used TIRF as an excitation source rather than in an imaging mode, Hugel and others were able to measure the effect of a conformational change on the relative stiffness of a photosensitive polymer [428]. By irradiating the sample *in situ*, they were able to initiate a *cis–trans* conformational change that resulted in a change in the backbone conformation of the polymer. Actin/titin in live cells can be followed by a combined TIRF and AFM strategy, simultaneously allowing one to dynamically stimulate the cytoskeleton while recording its fluorescence and mechanical response [429].

24.7.5 Confocal Fluorescence

The functional integration of confocal fluorescence with AFM microscopy is a particularly powerful approach. A complement to TIRF-AFM imaging, the confocal approach provides the added advantage of being able to section through the sample along the optical axis. Fluorescently labeled DNA and polystyrene beads have been correlated using fluorescence and AFM to both locate the features and analyze the laser excitation profile of the microscope [430]. Shaw and Yip have investigated dye partitioning and mechanisms of antimicrobial peptide action in model membranes using this correlated confocal-AFM approach [214,431,432]. What was particularly intriguing was the realization, perhaps not unexpectedly but now with direct spatial confirmation, that the addition of an extrinsic fluorophore to a molecule can dramatically affect its chemical properties. In the context of membrane-associated molecules, the addition of a large hydrophobic chromophore can alter the parent molecule's partitioning behavior in the member, possibly affecting its domain specificity and interactions. Our use of the coupled confocal-AFM platform provided direct evidence of this altered domain specificity and also a cautionary note for those who rely solely on fluorescence as a mechanism for identifying membrane structures.

Correlated functional assays also hold great promise for live cell imaging and force microscopy [433]. Confocal fluorescence has been employed to locate regions of focal adhesion before AFM ultrastructural imaging [434]. Two-photon confocal fluorescence was used to confirm the functionality and location of chloroplast grana, and AFM subsequently provided nanometer-scale structural details [435]. Yu et al. [436] performed force spectroscopy of transforming growth factor beta 1 and its receptor on live cell surfaces by locating these receptors through fluorescence, whereas others have taken advantage of sophisticated optical techniques such as Förster resonance energy transfer (FRET) in combined spectroscopic confocal-SPM imaging of biological systems [437,438]. In a particularly compelling approach, Trache et al. have integrated spinning disc confocal, TIRF, and AFM to provide a uniquely powerful platform for studying real-time cellular dynamics, mechanotransduction and signaling using the AFM platform as a nano-stimulator [439–441].

24.8 Summary

As can be readily seen in the brief survey of the SPM field, it is clearly expanding both in terms of techniques and range of applications. The systems are becoming more ubiquitous and certainly more approachable by the general user; however, what is clearly important is that care must be taken in data interpretation, instrument control, and sample preparation. For example, early studies of intermolecular forces often did not exercise the same level of control over their sampling conditions as is commonplace today and this clearly impacts critical analysis of the resulting force spectra. Recognizing the limitations of the tools and hopefully developing strategies that help to overcome these limitations represent a key goal for many SPM users.

As we have seen, fluorescence imaging, either as NSOM/TIRF/CSLM, when coupled with SPM provides an excellent *in situ* tool for characterizing biomolecular interactions and phenomena. Unfortunately, such a scheme requires specific labeling strategies, and it would be preferable to effect such measurements in the absence of a label. Indeed, as we have already presented, the use of extrinsic fluorophores can affect the behavior (folding, partitioning, distribution) of the parent molecule. Recent work has focused on near-field vibrational microscopy to acquire both IR and Raman spectra on nanometer length scales [442–444], whereas a combined Raman–SPM system was used to characterize the surface of an insect compound eye [443]. Indeed, the integration of vibrational spectroscopy with AFM has had a long history, starting with the pioneering work of Knoll and Keilman in 1999 with their tip-based scattering system and now its application to the study of polymer blends [445,446], efforts that have been adopted by various other groups with good results [447,448]. Other approaches to the functional integration of IR with AFM include the innovative exploitation of the photothermal effect with the AFM tip acting as an acousto-optic sensor [449,450]. This intriguing design has enabled submicron scale mapping of both topography and vibrational spectra of polymer domains and viruses and bacteria, portending its broader application in biophysical research. The integration of AFM with ATR-IR has also shown particular promise for tracking crystal growth, electrochemical phenomena as well as phase transitions and protein insertion in lipid bilayers [451–454]. It is critical to note that there is a clear difference in these coupled approaches. The tip-based scattering approaches and, to a lesser extent the photothermal technique, while providing spatial resolution that is on the order of the size of the tip, are inherently linked to the tip–sample interaction, the raster-scanning motion of the tip and the tunability of the IR excitation beam. This latter represents a particular challenge in that obtaining spectral information over a range of wavelengths would require either multiple tip scans, each at a different excitation wavelength, or modulation of the excitation wavelength while the tip is positioned at a specific location. Both of these are time-consuming strategies. These approaches may also not be particularly well suited for examining samples in solution where scattering effects may be difficult to reconcile. The integration of AFM with conventional ATR-IR provides for a completely decoupled approach with the AFM providing topographical insights while the ATR-IR system runs independently. Although this affords full access to all the spectral scanning capabilities of the IR system, it does sacrifice direct correlation of spectral details to a specific topographic feature. This is largely a consequence of the large, micron-sized, sampling region afforded the ATR configuration, especially in a multi-bounce configuration.

It is evident that the creative approaches to both the application of SPM for biology and to address its key challenges as a tool and technique will continue to provide biologists and biophysicist with unique new perspectives on long-standing research questions. This chapter has hopefully provided the reader with some interesting new perspectives on where this technique has been, and where it is headed. We see these new innovations in integrated single molecule correlated functional imaging as enabling tools and clear evidence of the continued evolution of the SPM field and its application to the study of biomolecular interactions.

References

1. Hsu, T. H., Liao, W. Y., Yang, P. C., Wang, C. C., Xiao, J. L., and Lee, C. H. 2007. Dynamics of cancer cell filopodia characterized by super-resolution bright-field optical microscopy, *Opt Express 15*, 76–82.
2. Huang, B., Wang, W., Bates, M., and Zhuang, X. 2008. Three-dimensional super-resolution imaging by stochastic optical reconstruction microscopy, *Science 319*, 810–813.
3. Egner, A., Jakobs, S., and Hell, S. W. 2002. Fast 100-nm resolution three-dimensional microscope reveals structural plasticity of mitochondria in live yeast, *Proc Natl Acad Sci USA 99*, 3370–3375.
4. Shroff, H., White, H., and Betzig, E. 2008. Photoactivated localization microscopy (palm) of adhesion complexes, *Curr Protoc Cell Biol Chapter 4*, Unit 4 21.
5. Shroff, H., Galbraith, C. G., Galbraith, J. A., and Betzig, E. 2008. Live-cell photoactivated localization microscopy of nanoscale adhesion dynamics, *Nat Methods 5*, 417–423.
6. Manley, S., Gillette, J. M., Patterson, G. H., Shroff, H., Hess, H. F., Betzig, E., and Lippincott-Schwartz, J. 2008. High-density mapping of single-molecule trajectories with photoactivated localization microscopy, *Nat Methods 5*, 155–157.
7. de Jonge, N., Peckys, D. B., Kremers, G. J., and Piston, D. W. 2009. Electron microscopy of whole cells in liquid with nanometer resolution, *Proc Natl Acad Sci USA 106*, 2159–2164.
8. Hansma, P. K., Elings, V., Marti, O., and Bracker, C. E. 1988. Scanning tunneling microscopy and atomic force microscopy: Application to biology and technology, *Science 242*, 209–216.
9. Lillehei, P. T., and Bottomley, L. A. 2000. Scanning probe microscopy, *Anal Chem 72*, 189R–196R.
10. Poggi, M. A., Bottomley, L. A., and Lillehei, P. T. 2002. Scanning probe microscopy, *Anal Chem 74*, 2851–2862.
11. Poggi, M. A., Gadsby, E. D., Bottomley, L. A., King, W. P., Oroudjev, E., and Hansma, H. 2004. Scanning probe microscopy, *Anal Chem 76*, 3429–3444.
12. Engel, A., and Muller, D. J. 2000. Observing single biomolecules at work with the atomic force microscope, *Nat Struct Biol 7*, 715–718.
13. Francis, L. W., Lewis, P. D., Wright, C. J., and Conlan, R. S. 2010. Atomic force microscopy comes of age, *Biol Cell 102*, 133–143.
14. Ikai, A. 2010. A review on: Atomic force microscopy applied to nano-mechanics of the cell, *Adv Biochem Eng Biotechnol 119*, 47–61.
15. Goksu, E. I., Vanegas, J. M., Blanchette, C. D., Lin, W. C., and Longo, M. L. 2009. AFM for structure and dynamics of biomembranes, *Biochim Biophys Acta 1788*, 254–266.

16. Frederix, P. L., Bosshart, P. D., and Engel, A. 2009. Atomic force microscopy of biological membranes, *Biophys J 96*, 329–338.

17. Muller, D. J. 2008. AFM: A nanotool in membrane biology, *Biochemistry 47*, 7986–7998.

18. Lamontagne, C. A., Cuerrier, C. M., and Grandbois, M. 2008. AFM as a tool to probe and manipulate cellular processes, *Pflugers Arch 456*, 61–70.

19. Dufrene, Y. F. 2008. Towards nanomicrobiology using atomic force microscopy, *Nat Rev Microbiol 6*, 674–680.

20. Hinterdorfer, P., and Dufrene, Y. F. 2006. Detection and localization of single molecular recognition events using atomic force microscopy, *Nat Methods 3*, 347–355.

21. Moller, C., Allen, M., Elings, V., Engel, A., and Muller, D. J. 1999. Tapping-mode atomic force microscopy produces faithful high-resolution images of protein surfaces, *Biophys J 77*, 1150–1158.

22. Florin, E. L., Moy, V. T., and Gaub, H. E. 1994. Adhesion forces between individual ligand–receptor pairs, *Science 264*, 415–417.

23. Heinz, W. F., and Hoh, J. H. 1999. Spatially resolved force spectroscopy of biological surfaces using the atomic force microscope, *Trends Biotechnol 17*, 143–150.

24. Rief, M., Oesterhelt, F., Heymann, B., and Gaub, H. E. 1997. Single molecule force spectroscopy on polysaccharides by atomic force microscopy, *Science 275*, 1295–1297.

25. Oesterfelt, F., Rief, M., and Gaub, H. E. 1999. Single molecule force spectroscopy by AFM indicates hleical structure of poly(ethylene-glycol) in water, *New J Phys 1*, 6.1–6.11.

26. Walch, M., Ziegler, U., and Groscurth, P. 2000. Effect of streptolysin o on the microelasticity of human platelets analyzed by atomic force microscopy, *Ultramicroscopy 82*, 259–267.

27. A-Hassan, E., Heinz, W. F., Antonik, M., D'Costa, N. P., Nageswaran, S., Schoenenberger, C.-A., and Hoh, J. H. 1998. Relative microelastic mapping of living cells by atomic force microscopy, *Biophys J 74*, 1564–1578.

28. Brown, H. G., and Hoh, J. H. 1997. Entropic exclusion by neurofilament sidearms: A mechanism for maintaining interfilament spacing, *Biochemistry 36*, 15035–15040.

29. Sahin, O., Magonov, S., Su, C., Quate, C. F., and Solgaard, O. 2007. An atomic force microscope tip designed to measure time-varying nanomechanical forces, *Nat Nanotechnol 2*, 507–514.

30. Pelling, A. E., Sehati, S., Gralla, E. B., Valentine, J. S., and Gimzewski, J. K. 2004. Local nanomechanical motion of the cell wall of saccharomyces cerevisiae, *Science 305*, 1147–1150.

31. Young, R., Ward, J., and Scire, F. 1971. The topografiner: An instrument for measuring surface microtopography, *Rev Sci Instr 43*, 999.

32. Binnig, G., Rohrer, H., Gerber, C., and Weibel, E. 1982. Tunneling through a controllable vacuum gap, *Rev Mod Phys 59*, 178–180.

33. Binnig, G., Quate, C. F., and Gerber, C. 1986. Atomic force microscope, *Phys Rev Lett 56*, 930–933.

34. Magonov, S. N., and Reneker, D. H. 1997. Characterization of polymer surfaces with atomic force microscopy, *Ann Rev Mater Sci 27*, 175–222.

35. Paige, M. F. 2003. A comparison of atomic force microscope friction and phase imaging for the characterization of an immiscible polystyrene/poly(methyl methacrylate) blend film, *Polymer 44*, 6345–6352.

36. Dinte, B. P., Watson, G. S., Dobson, J. F., and Myhra, S. 1996. Artefacts in non-contact mode force microscopy: The role of adsorbed moisture, *Ultramicroscopy 63*, 115–124.

37. Lvov, Y., Onda, M., Ariga, K., and Kunitake, T. 1998. Ultrathin films of charged polysaccharides assembled alternately with linear polyions, *J Biomater Sci Polym Ed 9*, 345–355.

38. Magonov, S. N., Elings, V., and Whangbo, M.-H. 1997. Phase imaging and stiffness in tapping mode AFM, *Surface Sci 375*, L385–L391.

39. Magonov, S. and Heaton, M. G. 1998. Atomic force microscopy, part 6: Recent developments in AFM of polymers, *Am Lab 30*(10), 9.

40. Magonov, S. and Godovsky, Y. 1999. Atomic force microscopy, part 8: Visualization of granular nanostructure in crystalline polymers, *Am Lab April 1999*, 52–58.

41. Hansma, H. G., Kim, K. J., Laney, D. E., Garcia, R. A., Argaman, M., Allen, M. J., and Parsons, S. M. 1997. Properties of biomolecules measured from atomic force microscope images: A review, *J Struct Biol 119*, 99–108.
42. Fritzsche, W. and Henderson, E. 1997. Mapping elasticity of rehydrated metaphase chromosomes by scanning force microscopy, *Ultramicroscopy 69*, 191–200.
43. Noy, A., Sanders, C. H., Vezenov, D. V., Wong, S. S., and Lieber, C. M. 1998. Chemically-sensitive imaging in tapping mode by chemical force microscopy: Relationship between phase lag and adhesion, *Langmuir 14*, 1508–1511.
44. Nagao, E. and Dvorak, J. A. 1999. Phase imaging by atomic force microscopy: Analysis of living homoiothermic vertebrate cells, *Biophys J 76*, 3289–3297.
45. Holland, N. B. and Marchant, R. E. 2000. Individual plasma proteins detected on rough biomaterials by phase imaging AFM, *J Biomed Mater Res 51*, 307–315.
46. Czajkowsky, D. M., Allen, M. J., Elings, V., and Shao, Z. 1998. Direct visualization of surface charge in aqueous solution, *Ultramicroscopy 74*, 1–5.
47. Brandsch, R., Bar, G., and Whangbo, M.-H. 1997. On the factors affecting the contrast of height and phase images in tapping mode atomic force microscopy, *Langmuir 13*, 6349–6353.
48. Winkler, R. G., Spatz, J. P., Sheiko, S., Moller, M., Reineker, P., and Marti, O. 1996. Imaging material properties by resonant tapping-force microscopy: A model investigation, *Phys Rev B 54*, 8908–8912.
49. Opdahl, A., Hoffer, S., Mailhot, B., and Somorjai, G. A. 2001. Polymer surface science, *Chem Rec 1*, 101–122.
50. Scott, W. W. and Bhushan, B. 2003. Use of phase imaging in atomic force microscopy for measurement of viscoelastic contrast in polymer nanocomposites and molecularly thick lubricant films, *Ultramicroscopy 97*, 151–169.
51. Krol, S., Ross, M., Sieber, M., Kunneke, S., Galla, H. J., and Janshoff, A. 2000. Formation of three-dimensional protein-lipid aggregates in monolayer films induced by surfactant protein b, *Biophys J 79*, 904–918.
52. Deleu, M., Nott, K., Brasseur, R., Jacques, P., Thonart, P., and Dufrene, Y. F. 2001. Imaging mixed lipid monolayers by dynamic atomic force microscopy, *Biochim Biophys Acta 1513*, 55–62.
53. Argaman, M., Golan, R., Thomson, N. H., and Hansma, H. G. 1997. Phase imaging of moving DNA molecules and DNA molecules replicated in the atomic force microscope, *Nucleic Acids Res 25*, 4379–4384.
54. Sitterberg, J., Ozcetin, A., Ehrhardt, C., and Bakowsky, U. 2010. Utilising atomic force microscopy for the characterisation of nanoscale drug delivery systems, *Eur J Pharm Biopharm 74*, 2–13.
55. Han, W., Lindsay, S. M., and Jing, T. 1996. A magnetically driven oscillating probe microscope for operation in liquids, *Appl Phys Lett 69*, 4111–4113.
56. Florin, E.-L., Radmacher, M., Fleck, B., and Gaub, H. E. 1994. Atomic force microscope with magnetic force modulation, *Rev Sci Instrum 65*, 639–643.
57. Lindsay, S. M., Lyubchenko Yu, L., Tao, N. J., Li, Y. Q., Oden, P. I., Derose, J. A., and Pan, J. 1993. Scanning tunneling microscopy and atomic force microscopy studies of biomaterials at a liquid-solid interface, *J Vac Sci Technol A 11*, 808–815.
58. Lillehei, P. T. and Bottomley, L. A. 2001. Scanning force microscopy of nucleic acid complexes, *Methods Enzymol 340*, 234–251.
59. Conway, K. A., Harper, J. D., and Lansbury, P. T., Jr. 2000. Fibrils formed *in vitro* from alpha-synuclein and two mutant forms linked to Parkinson's disease are typical amyloid, *Biochemistry 39*, 2552–2563.
60. Oesterhelt, F., Oesterhelt, D., Pfeiffer, M., Engel, A., Gaub, H. E., and Muller, D. J. 2000. Unfolding pathways of individual bacteriorhodopsins, *Science 288*, 143–146.
61. Rochet, J. C., Conway, K. A., and Lansbury, P. T., Jr. 2000. Inhibition of fibrillization and accumulation of prefibrillar oligomers in mixtures of human and mouse alpha-synuclein, *Biochemistry 39*, 10619–10626.

62. Moradian-Oldak, J., Paine, M. L., Lei, Y. P., Fincham, A. G., and Snead, M. L. 2000. Self-assembly properties of recombinant engineered amelogenin proteins analyzed by dynamic light scattering and atomic force microscopy, *J Struct Biol 131*, 27–37.

63. Trottier, M., Mat-Arip, Y., Zhang, C., Chen, C., Sheng, S., Shao, Z., and Guo, P. 2000. Probing the structure of monomers and dimers of the bacterial virus phi29 hexamer RNA complex by chemical modification, *RNA 6*, 1257–1266.

64. Thompson, J. B., Paloczi, G. T., Kindt, J. H., Michenfelder, M., Smith, B. L., Stucky, G., Morse, D. E., and Hansma, P. K. 2000. Direct observation of the transition from calcite to aragonite growth as induced by abalone shell proteins, *Biophys J 79*, 3307–3312.

65. Rivetti, C., Vannini, N., and Cellai, S. 2003. Imaging transcription complexes with the atomic force microscope, *Ital J Biochem 52*, 98–103.

66. Seong, G. H., Yanagida, Y., Aizawa, M., and Kobatake, E. 2002. Atomic force microscopy identification of transcription factor NFkappab bound to streptavidin-pin-holding DNA probe, *Anal Biochem 309*, 241–247.

67. Mukherjee, S., Brieba, L. G., and Sousa, R. 2002. Structural transitions mediating transcription initiation by T7 RNA polymerase, *Cell 110*, 81–91.

68. Hun Seong, G., Kobatake, E., Miura, K., Nakazawa, A., and Aizawa, M. 2002. Direct atomic force microscopy visualization of integration host factor- induced DNA bending structure of the promoter regulatory region on the Pseudomonas tol plasmid, *Biochem. Biophys. Res. Commun. 291*, 361–366.

69. Tahirov, T. H., Sato, K., Ichikawa-Iwata, E., Sasaki, M., Inoue-Bungo, T., Shiina, M., Kimura, K. et al. 2002. Mechanism of c-myb-c/ebp beta cooperation from separated sites on a promoter, *Cell 108*, 57–70.

70. Neaves, K. J., Huppert, J. L., Henderson, R. M., and Edwardson, J. M. 2009. Direct visualization of g-quadruplexes in DNA using atomic force microscopy, *Nucleic Acids Res 37*, 6269–6275.

71. Limanskaya, O. Y., and Limanskii, A. P. 2008. Imaging compaction of single supercoiled DNA molecules by atomic force microscopy, *Gen Physiol Biophys 27*, 322–337.

72. Lohr, D., Bash, R., Wang, H., Yodh, J., and Lindsay, S. 2007. Using atomic force microscopy to study chromatin structure and nucleosome remodeling, *Methods 41*, 333–341.

73. Sorel, I., Pietrement, O., Hamon, L., Baconnais, S., Cam, E. L., and Pastre, D. 2006. The Ecori-DNA complex as a model for investigating protein-DNA interactions by atomic force microscopy, *Biochemistry 45*, 14675–14682.

74. Jena, B. P. 2002. Fusion pore in live cells, *News Physiol Sci 17*, 219–222.

75. Cho, S. J., Quinn, A. S., Stromer, M. H., Dash, S., Cho, J., Taatjes, D. J., and Jena, B. P. 2002. Structure and dynamics of the fusion pore in live cells, *Cell Biol Int 26*, 35–42.

76. Ma, H., Snook, L. A., Tian, C., Kaminskyj, S. G. W., and Dahms, T. E. S. 2006. Fungal surface remodelling visualized by atomic force microscopy, *Mycol Res 110*, 879–886.

77. Rogers, B., Manning, L., Sulchek, T., and Adams, J. D. 2004. Improving tapping mode atomic force microscopy with piezoelectric cantilevers, *Ultramicroscopy 100*, 267–276.

78. Fantner, G. E., Schitter, G., Kindt, J. H., Ivanov, T., Ivanova, K., Patel, R., Holten-Andersen, N. et al. 2006. Components for high speed atomic force microscopy, *Ultramicroscopy 106*, 881–887.

79. Petsev, D. N., Thomas, B. R., Yau, S., and Vekilov, P. G. 2000. Interactions and aggregation of apoferritin molecules in solution: Effects of added electrolytes, *Biophys J 78*, 2060–2069.

80. Viani, M. B., Pietrasanta, L. I., Thompson, J. B., Chand, A., Gebeshuber, I. C., Kindt, J. H., Richter, M., Hansma, H. G., and Hansma, P. K. 2000. Probing protein–protein interactions in real time, *Nat Struct Biol 7*, 644–647.

81. Casuso, I., Kodera, N., Le Grimellec, C., Ando, T., and Scheuring, S. 2009. Contact-mode high-resolution high-speed atomic force microscopy movies of the purple membrane, *Biophys J 97*, 1354–1361.

82. Miyagi, A., Tsunaka, Y., Uchihashi, T., Mayanagi, K., Hirose, S., Morikawa, K., and Ando, T. 2008. Visualization of intrinsically disordered regions of proteins by high-speed atomic force microscopy, *ChemPhysChem 9*, 1859–1866.

83. Ando, T., Uchihashi, T., Kodera, N., Yamamoto, D., Miyagi, A., Taniguchi, M., and Yamashita, H. 2008. High-speed AFM and nano-visualization of biomolecular processes, *Pflugers Arch 456*, 211–225.

84. Ando, T., Kodera, N., Naito, Y., Kinoshita, T., Furuta, K., and Toyoshima, Y. Y. 2003. A high-speed atomic force microscope for studying biological macromolecules in action, *ChemPhysChem 4*, 1196–1202.

85. Fantner, G. E., Barbero, R. J., Gray, D. S., and Belcher, A. M. 2010. Kinetics of antimicrobial peptide activity measured on individual bacterial cells using high-speed atomic force microscopy, *Nat Nanotechnol 5*, 280–285.

86. Archibald, R., Datskos, P., Devault, G., Lamberti, V., Lavrik, N., Noid, D., Sepaniak, M., and Dutta, P. 2007. Independent component analysis of nanomechanical responses of cantilever arrays, *Anal Chim Acta 584*, 101–105.

87. Loui, A., Ratto, T. V., Wilson, T. S., McCall, S. K., Mukerjee, E. V., Love, A. H., and Hart, B. R. 2008. Chemical vapor discrimination using a compact and low-power array of piezoresistive microcantilevers, *Analyst 133*, 608–615.

88. Kim, S., Rahman, T., Senesac, L. R., Davison, B. H., and Thundat, T. 2009. Piezoresistive cantilever array sensor for consolidated bioprocess monitoring, *Scanning 31*, 204–210.

89. Kelling, S., Paoloni, F., Huang, J., Ostanin, V. P., and Elliott, S. R. 2009. Simultaneous readout of multiple microcantilever arrays with phase-shifting interferometric microscopy, *Rev Sci Instrum 80*, 093101.

90. Ward, M. D. 2001. Bulk crystals to surfaces: Combining x-ray diffraction and atomic force microscopy to probe the structure and formation of crystal interfaces, *Chem Rev 2001*, 1697–1725.

91. Manne, S., Cleveland, J. P., Stucky, G. D., and Hansma, P. K. 1993. Lattice resolution and solution kinetics on surfaces of amino acid crystals: An atomic force microscope study, *J. Crystal Growth 130*, 333–340.

92. Agger, J. R., Hanif, N., Cundy, C. S., Wade, A. P., Dennison, S., Rawlinson, P. A., and Anderson, M. W. 2003. Silicalite crystal growth investigated by atomic force microscopy, *J Am Chem Soc 125*, 830–839.

93. Teng, H. H., Dove, P. M., Orme, C. A., and De Yoreo, J. J. 1998. Thermodynamics of calcite growth: Baseline for understanding biomineral formation, *Science 282*, 724–727.

94. Costa, N. and Maquis, P. M. 1998. Biomimetic processing of calcium phosphate coating, *Med Eng Phys 20*, 602–606.

95. Wen, H. B., Moradian-Oldak, J., Zhong, J. P., Greenspan, D. C., and Fincham, A. G. 2000. Effects of amelogenin on the transforming surface microstructures of bioglass in a calcifying solution, *J Biomed Mater Res 52*, 762–773.

96. Durbin, S. D. and Feher, G. 1996. Protein crystallization, *Annu Rev Phys Chem 47*, 171–204.

97. Yip, C. M., Brader, M. L., Frank, B. H., DeFelippis, M. R., and Ward, M. D. 2000. Structural studies of a crystalline insulin analog complex with protamine by atomic force microscopy, *Biophys J 78*, 466–473.

98. Kuznetsov, Y. G., Malkin, A. J., Lucas, R. W., and McPherson, A. 2000. Atomic force microscopy studies of icosahedral virus crystal growth, *Colloids Surf B Biointerfaces 19*, 333–346.

99. Plomp, M., McPherson, A., and Malkin, A. J. 2003. Repair of impurity-poisoned protein crystal surfaces, *Proteins 50*, 486–495.

100. McPherson, A., Malkin, A. J., and Kuznetsov Yu, G. 2000. Atomic force microscopy in the study of macromolecular crystal growth, *Annu Rev Biophys Biomol Struct 29*, 361–410.

101. Vekilov, P. G. 2005. Kinetics and mechanisms of protein crystallization at the molecular level, *Methods Mol Biol 300*, 15–52.

102. Barrera, N. P., Ormond, S. J., Henderson, R. M., Murrell-Lagnado, R. D., and Edwardson, J. M. 2005. Atomic force microscopy imaging demonstrates that p2x[2] receptors are trimers but that p2x[6] receptor subunits do not oligomerize, *J Biol Chem 280*, 10759–10765.

103. Yau, S., Thomas, B. R., and Vekilov, P. G. 2000. Molecular mechanisms of crystallization and defect formation, *Phys Rev Lett 85*, 353–356.

104. Guo, S. and Akhremitchev, B. B. 2008. Investigation of mechanical properties of insulin crystals by atomic force microscopy, *Langmuir 24*, 880–887.

105. Larson, S. B., Kuznetsov, Y. G., Day, J., Zhou, J., Glaser, S., Braslawsky, G., and McPherson, A. 2005. Combined use of AFM and x-ray diffraction to analyze crystals of an engineered, domain-deleted antibody, *Acta Crystallogr D Biol Crystallogr 61*, 416–422.

106. Ko, T. P., Kuznetsov, Y. G., Malkin, A. J., Day, J., and McPherson, A. 2001. X-ray diffraction and atomic force microscopy analysis of twinned crystals: Rhombohedral canavalin, *Acta Crystallogr D Biol Crystallogr 57*, 829–839.

107. Yip, C. M., DeFelippis, M. R., Frank, B. H., Brader, M. L., and Ward, M. D. 1998. Structural and morphological characterization of ultralente insulin crystals by atomic force microscopy: Evidence of hydrophobically driven assembly, *Biophys J 75*, 1172–1179.

108. Malkin, A. J., Plomp, M., and McPherson, A. 2002. Application of atomic force microscopy to studies of surface processes in virus crystallization and structural biology, *Acta Crystallogr D Biol Crystallogr 58*, 1617–1621.

109. Plomp, M., Rice, M. K., Wagner, E. K., McPherson, A., and Malkin, A. J. 2002. Rapid visualization at high resolution of pathogens by atomic force microscopy: Structural studies of Herpes Simplex Virus-1, *Am J Pathol 160*, 1959–1966.

110. McPherson, A., Malkin, A. J., Kuznetsov, Y. G., and Plomp, M. 2001. Atomic force microscopy applications in macromolecular crystallography, *Acta Crystallogr D Biol Crystallogr 57*, 1053–1060.

111. Kuznetsov, Y. G., Larson, S. B., Day, J., Greenwood, A., and McPherson, A. 2001. Structural transitions of satellite tobacco mosaic virus particles, *Virology 284*, 223–234.

112. Kuznetsov, Y. G., Malkin, A. J., Lucas, R. W., Plomp, M., and McPherson, A. 2001. Imaging of viruses by atomic force microscopy, *J Gen Virol 82*, 2025–2034.

113. Lucas, R. W., Kuznetsov, Y. G., Larson, S. B., and McPherson, A. 2001. Crystallization of brome mosaic virus and t = 1 brome mosaic virus particles following a structural transition, *Virology 286*, 290–303.

114. Day, J., Kuznetsov, Y. G., Larson, S. B., Greenwood, A., and McPherson, A. 2001. Biophysical studies on the RNA cores of satellite tobacco mosaic virus, *Biophys J 80*, 2364–2371.

115. Kuznetsov, Y. G., Malkin, A. J., and McPherson, A. 2001. Self-repair of biological fibers catalyzed by the surface of a virus crystal, *Proteins 44*, 392–396.

116. Yau, S. T., Thomas, B. R., Galkin, O., Gliko, O., and Vekilov, P. G. 2001. Molecular mechanisms of microheterogeneity-induced defect formation in ferritin crystallization, *Proteins 43*, 343–352.

117. Yau, S. T. and Vekilov, P. G. 2000. Quasi-planar nucleus structure in apoferritin crystallization, *Nature 406*, 494–497.

118. Chen, K. and Vekilov, P. G. 2002. Evidence for the surface-diffusion mechanism of solution crystallization from molecular-level observations with ferritin, *Phys Rev E Stat Nonlin Soft Matter Phys 66*, 021606.

119. Danesh, A., Connell, S. D., Davies, M. C., Roberts, C. J., Tendler, S. J., Williams, P. M., and Wilkins, M. J. 2001. An *in situ* dissolution study of aspirin crystal planes [100] and [001] by atomic force microscopy, *Pharm Res 18*, 299–303.

120. Danesh, A., Chen, X., Davies, M. C., Roberts, C. J., Sanders, G. H., Tendler, S. J., Williams, P. M., and Wilkins, M. J. 2000. The discrimination of drug polymorphic forms from single crystals using atomic force microscopy, *Pharm Res 17*, 887–890.

121. Danesh, A., Chen, X., Davies, M. C., Roberts, C. J., Sanders, G. H. W., Tendler, S. J. B., and Williams, P. M. 2000. Polymorphic discrimination using atomic force microscopy: Distinguishing between two polymorphs of the drug cimetidine, *Langmuir 16*, 866–870.

122. Guo, S., Ward, M. D., and Wesson, J. A. 2002. Direct visualization of calcium oxalate monohydrate crystallization and dissolution with atomic force microscopy and the role of polymeric additives, *Langmuir 18*, 4282–4291.

123. Frincu, M. C., Fleming, S. D., Rohl, A. L., and Swift, J. A. 2004. The epitaxial growth of cholesterol crystals from bile solutions on calcite substrates, *J Am Chem Soc 126*, 7915–7924.

124. Wang, L. and Nancollas, G. H. 2009. Pathways to biomineralization and biodemineralization of calcium phosphates: The thermodynamic and kinetic controls, *Dalton Trans*, 2665–2672.

125. Wesson, J. A. and Ward, M. D. 2006. Role of crystal surface adhesion in kidney stone disease, *Curr Opin Nephrol Hypertens 15*, 386–393.

126. Sheng, X., Jung, T., Wesson, J. A., and Ward, M. D. 2005. Adhesion at calcium oxalate crystal surfaces and the effect of urinary constituents, *Proc Natl Acad Sci USA 102*, 267–272.

127. Sheng, X., Ward, M. D., and Wesson, J. A. 2005. Crystal surface adhesion explains the pathological activity of calcium oxalate hydrates in kidney stone formation, *J Am Soc Nephrol 16*, 1904–1908.

128. Wang, L., Qiu, S. R., Zachowicz, W., Guan, X., Deyoreo, J. J., Nancollas, G. H., and Hoyer, J. R. 2006. Modulation of calcium oxalate crystallization by linear aspartic acid-rich peptides, *Langmuir 22*, 7279–7285.

129. Milhiet, P. E., Gubellini, F., Berquand, A., Dosset, P., Rigaud, J. L., Le Grimellec, C., and Levy, D. 2006. High-resolution AFM of membrane proteins directly incorporated at high density in planar lipid bilayer, *Biophys J 91*, 3268–3275.

130. Mo, G. C. H. and Yip, C. M. 2009. Supported lipid bilayer templated J-aggregate growth: Role of stabilizing cation-pi interactions and headgroup packing, *Langmuir 25*, 10719–10729.

131. Waugh, D. F., Thompson, R. E., and Weimer, R. J. 1950. Assay of insulin *in vitro* by fibril elongation and precipitation, *J Biol Chem 185*, 85–95.

132. Foster, G. E., Macdonald, J., and Smart, J. V. 1951. The assay of insulin *in vitro* by fibril formation and precipitation, *J Pharm Pharmacol 3*, 897–904.

133. Baselt, D. R., Revel, J. P., and Baldeschwieler, J. D. 1993. Subfibrillar structure of Type I collagen observed by atomic force microscopy, *Biophys J 65*, 2644–2655.

134. Cotterill, G. F., Fergusson, J. A., Gani, J. S., and Burns, G. F. 1993. Scanning tunnelling microscopy of collagen I reveals filament bundles to be arranged in a left-handed helix, *Biochem Biophys Res Commun 194*, 973–977.

135. Gale, M., Pollanen, M. S., Markiewicz, P., and Goh, M. C. 1995. Sequential assembly of collagen revealed by atomic force microscopy, *Biophys J 68*, 2124–2128.

136. Watanabe, M., Kobayashi, M., Fujita, Y., Senga, K., Mizutani, H., Ueda, M., and Hoshino, T. 1997. Association of Type VI collagen with d-periodic collagen fibrils in developing tail tendons of mice, *Arch Histol Cytol 60*, 427–434.

137. Taatjes, D. J., Quinn, A. S., and Bovill, E. G. 1999. Imaging of collagen type III in fluid by atomic force microscopy, *Microsc Res Tech 44*, 347–352.

138. Zerovnik, E., Skarabot, M., Skerget, K., Giannini, S., Stoka, V., Jenko-Kokalj, S., and Staniforth, R. A. 2007. Amyloid fibril formation by human stefin b: Influence of pH and TFE on fibril growth and morphology, *Amyloid-J Protein Folding Disord 14*, 237–247.

139. Miller, L. D., Putthanarat, S., Eby, R. K., and Adams, W. W. 1999. Investigation of the nanofibrillar morphology in silk fibers by small angle x-ray scattering and atomic force microscopy, *Int J Biol Macromol 24*, 159–165.

140. Li, S. F., McGhie, A. J., and Tang, S. L. 1994. New internal structure of spider dragline silk revealed by atomic force microscopy, *Biophys J 66*, 1209–1212.

141. Gould, S. A., Tran, K. T., Spagna, J. C., Moore, A. M., and Shulman, J. B. 1999. Short and long range order of the morphology of silk from *Latrodectus hesperus* (black widow. as characterized by atomic force microscopy, *Int J Biol Macromol 24*, 151–157.

142. Oroudjev, E., Soares, J., Arcdiacono, S., Thompson, J. B., Fossey, S. A., and Hansma, H. G. 2002. Segmented nanofibers of spider dragline silk: Atomic force microscopy and single-molecule force spectroscopy, *Proc Natl Acad Sci USA 99 Suppl 2*, 6460–6465.

143. Harper, J. D., Lieber, C. M., and Lansbury, P. T., Jr. 1997. Atomic force microscopic imaging of seeded fibril formation and fibril branching by the Alzheimer's disease amyloid-beta protein, *Chem Biol 4*, 951–959.

144. Harper, J. D., Wong, S. S., Lieber, C. M., and Lansbury, P. T. 1997. Observation of metastable Ab amyloid protofibrils by atomic force microscopy, *Chem Biol 4*, 119–125.

145. Yang, D. S., Yip, C. M., Huang, T. H., Chakrabartty, A., and Fraser, P. E. 1999. Manipulating the amyloid-beta aggregation pathway with chemical chaperones, *J Biol Chem 274*, 32970–32974.

146. Huang, T. H., Yang, D. S., Plaskos, N. P., Go, S., Yip, C. M., Fraser, P. E., and Chakrabartty, A. 2000. Structural studies of soluble oligomers of the alzheimer beta-amyloid peptide, *J Mol Biol 297*, 73–87.

147. Roher, A. E., Baudry, J., Chaney, M. O., Kuo, Y. M., Stine, W. B., and Emmerling, M. R. 2000. Oligomerizaiton and fibril asssembly of the amyloid-beta protein, *Biochim Biophys Acta 1502*, 31–43.

148. Parbhu, A., Lin, H., Thimm, J., and Lal, R. 2002. Imaging real-time aggregation of amyloid beta protein [1–42] by atomic force microscopy, *Peptides 23*, 1265–1270.

149. Yip, C. M., Darabie, A. A., and McLaurin, J. 2002. Abeta42-peptide assembly on lipid bilayers, *J Mol Biol 318*, 97–107.

150. Gorman, P. M., Yip, C. M., Fraser, P. E., and Chakrabartty, A. 2003. Alternate aggregation pathways of the Alzheimer beta-amyloid peptide: Abeta association kinetics at endosomal pH, *J Mol Biol 325*, 743–757.

151. McLaurin, J., Darabie, A. A., and Morrison, M. R. 2002. Cholesterol, a modulator of membrane-associated abeta-fibrillogenesis, *Ann N Y Acad Sci 977*, 376–383.

152. Jansen, R., Dzwolak, W., and Winter, R. 2005. Amyloidogenic self-assembly of insulin aggregates probed by high resolution atomic force microscopy, *Biophys J 88*, 1344–1353.

153. Mastrangelo, I. A., Ahmed, M., Sato, T., Liu, W., Wang, C. P., Hough, P., and Smith, S. O. 2006. High-resolution atomic force microscopy of soluble Ab 42 oligomers, *J Mol Biol 358*, 106–119.

154. Fukuma, T., Mostaert, A. S., Serpell, L. C., and Jarvis, S. P. 2008. Revealing molecular-level surface structure of amyloid fibrils in liquid by means of frequency modulation atomic force microscopy, *Nanotechnology 19*(38), 384010.

155. Friedrichs, J., Taubenberger, A., Franz, C. M., and Muller, D. J. 2007. Cellular remodelling of individual collagen fibrils visualized by time-lapse AFM, *J Mol Biol 372*, 594–607.

156. Zheng, J., Jang, H., Ma, B., and Nussinov, R. 2008. Annular structures as intermediates in fibril formation of Alzheimer Ab[17–42], *J Phys Chem B 112*, 6856–6865.

157. Marek, P., Abedini, A., Song, B. B., Kanungo, M., Johnson, M. E., Gupta, R., Zaman, W., Wong, S. S., and Raleigh, D. P. 2007. Aromatic interactions are not required for amyloid fibril formation by islet amyloid polypeptide but do influence the rate of fibril formation and fibril morphology, *Biochemistry 46*, 3255–3261.

158. Ha, C., Ryu, J., and Park, C. B. 2007. Metal ions differentially influence the aggregation and deposition of Alzheimer's beta-amyloid on a solid template, *Biochemistry 46*, 6118–6125.

159. Elliott, J. T., Woodward, J. T., Umarji, A., Mei, Y., and Tona, A. 2007. The effect of surface chemistry on the formation of thin films of native fibrillar collagen, *Biomaterials 28*, 576–585.

160. Kowalewski, T. and Holtzman, D. M. 1999. *In situ* atomic force microscopy study of Alzheimer's beta-amyloid peptide on different substrates: New insights into mechanism of beta-sheet formation, *Proc Natl Acad Sci USA 96*, 3688–3693.

161. Wang, Z., Zhou, C., Wang, C., Wan, L., Fang, X., and Bai, C. 2003. AFM and STM study of beta-amyloid aggregation on graphite, *Ultramicroscopy 97*, 73–79.

162. Yang, G., Woodhouse, K. A., and Yip, C. M. 2002. Substrate-facilitated assembly of elastin-like peptides: Studies by variable-temperature *in situ* atomic force microscopy, *J Am Chem Soc 124*, 10648–10649.

163. Sherrat, M. J., Holmes, D. F., Shuttleworth, C. A., and Kielty, C. M. 2004. Substrate-dependent morphology of supramolecular assemblies: Fibrillin and type-IV collagen microfibrils, *Biophys J 86*, 3211–3222.

164. Sackmann, E. 1996. Supported membranes: Scientific and practical applications, *Science 271*, 43–48.

165. Richter, R., Mukhopadhyay, A., and Brisson, A. 2003. Pathways of lipid vesicle deposition on solid surfaces: A combined QCM-D and AFM study, *Biophys J 85*, 3035–3047.

166. Leonenko, Z. V., Carnini, A., and Cramb, D. T. 2000. Supported planar bilayer formation by vesicle fusion: The interaction of phospholipid vesicles with surfaces and the effect of gramicidin on bilayer properties using atomic force microscopy, *Biochim Biophys Acta 1509*, 131–147.

167. Dufrene, Y. F. and Lee, G. U. 2000. Advances in the characterization of supported lipid films with the atomic force microscope, *Biochim Biophys Acta 1509*, 14–41.

168. Jass, J., Tjarnhage, T., and Puu, G. 2000. From liposomes to supported, planar bilayer structures on hydrophilic and hydrophobic surfaces: An atomic force microscopy study, *Biophys J 79*, 3153–3163.

169. Blanchette, C. D., Orme, C. A., Ratto, T. V., and Longo, M. L. 2008. Quantifying growth of symmetric and asymmetric lipid bilayer domains, *Langmuir 24*, 1219–1224.

170. Fukuma, T., Higgins, M. J., and Jarvis, S. P. 2007. Direct imaging of individual intrinsic hydration layers on lipid bilayers at Angstrom resolution, *Biophys J 92*, 3603–3609.

171. Richter, R. P. and Brisson, A. R. 2005. Following the formation of supported lipid bilayers on mica: A study combining AFM, QCM-D, and ellipsometry, *Biophys J 88*, 3422–3433.

172. McKiernan, A. E., Ratto, T. V., and Longo, M. L. 2000. Domain growth, shapes, and topology in cationic lipid bilayers on mica by fluorescence and atomic force microscopy, *Biophys J 79*, 2605–2615.

173. Rinia, H. A., Demel, R. A., van der Eerden, J. P., and de Kruijff, B. 1999. Blistering of Langmuir–Blodgett bilayers containing anionic phospholipids as observed by atomic force microscopy, *Biophys J 77*, 1683–1693.

174. Giocondi, M.-C., Vie, V., Lesniewska, E., Milhiet, P.-E., Zinke-Allmang, M., and Le Grimellec, C. 2001. Phase topology and growth of single domains in lipid bilayers, *Langmuir 17*, 1653–1659.

175. Yuan, C., Chen, A., Kolb, P., and Moy, V. T. 2000. Energy landscape of streptavidin–biotin complexes measured by atomic force microscopy, *Biochemistry 39*, 10219–10223.

176. Tokumasu, F., Jin, A. J., and Dvorak, J. A. 2002. Lipid membrane phase behaviour elucidated in real time by controlled environment atomic force microscopy, *J Electron Microsc (Tokyo) 51*, 1–9.

177. Muresan, A. S., Diamant, H., and Lee, K. Y. 2001. Effect of temperature and composition on the formation of nanoscale compartments in phospholipid membranes, *J Am Chem Soc 123*, 6951–6952.

178. Nielsen, L. K., Bjornholm, T., and Mouritsen, O. G. 2000. Fluctuations caught in the act, *Nature 404*, 352.

179. Giocondi, M. C. and Le Grimellec, C. 2004. Temperature dependence of the surface topography in dimyristoylphosphatidylcholine/distearoylphosphatidylcholine multibilayers, *Biophys J 86*, 2218–2230.

180. Leidy, C., Kaasgaard, T., Crowe, J. H., Mouritsen, O. G., and Jorgensen, K. 2002. Ripples and the formation of anisotropic lipid domains: Imaging two-component supported double bilayers by atomic force microscopy, *Biophys J 83*, 2625–2633.

181. Jensen, M. H., Morris, E. J., and Simonsen, A. C. 2007. Domain shapes, coarsening, and random patterns in ternary membranes, *Langmuir 23*, 8135–8141.

182. Rinia, H. A. and de Kruijff, B. 2001. Imaging domains in model membranes with atomic force microscopy, *FEBS Lett 504*, 194–199.

183. van Duyl, B. Y., Ganchev, D., Chupin, V., de Kruijff, B., and Killian, J. A. 2003. Sphingomyelin is much more effective than saturated phosphatidylcholine in excluding unsaturated phosphatidylcholine from domains formed with cholesterol, *FEBS Lett 547*, 101–106.

184. Lawrence, J. C., Saslowsky, D. E., Edwardson, J. M., and Henderson, R. M. 2003. Real-time analysis of the effects of cholesterol on lipid raft behavior using atomic force microscopy, *Biophys J 84*, 1827–1832.

185. Domenech, O., Sanz, F., Montero, M. T., and Hernandez-Borrell, J. 2006. Thermodynamic and structural study of the main phospholipid components comprising the mitochondrial inner membrane, *Biochim Biophys Acta-Biomembranes 1758*, 213–221.

186. Blanchette, C. D., Lin, W. C., Ratto, T. V., and Longo, M. L. 2006. Galactosylceramide domain microstructure: Impact of cholesterol and nucleation/growth conditions, *Biophys J 90*, 4466–4478.

187. Kobayashi, T., Startchev, K., Whitney, A. J., and Gruenberg, J. 2001. Localization of lysobisphosphatidic acid-rich membrane domains in late endosomes, *Biol Chem 382*, 483–485.

188. Hayakawa, T., Makino, A., Murate, M., Sugimoto, I., Hashimoto, Y., Takahashi, H., Ito, K., Fujisawa, T., Matsuo, H., and Kobayashi, T. 2007. pH-dependent formation of membranous cytoplasmic body-like structure of ganglioside G(m1)/bis(monoacylglycero)phosphate mixed membranes, *Biophys J 92*, L13–L15.

189. Frederick, T. E., Chebukati, J. N., Mair, C. E., Goff, P. C., and Fanucci, G. E. 2009. Bis(monoacylglycero) phosphate forms stable small lamellar vesicle structures: Insights into vesicular body formation in endosomes, *Biophys J 96*, 1847–1855.

190. Mecke, A., Lee, D. K., Ramamoorthy, A., Orr, B. G., and Banaszak Holl, M. M. 2005. Membrane thinning due to antimicrobial peptide binding: An atomic force microscopy study of MSI-78 in lipid bilayers, *Biophys J 89*, 4043–4050.

191. Erickson, B., DiMaggio, S. C., Mullen, D. G., Kelly, C. V., Leroueil, P. R., Berry, S. A., Baker, J. R., Orr, B. G., and Holl, M. M. B. 2008. Interactions of poly(amidoamine) dendrimers with Survanta lung surfactant: The importance of lipid domains, *Langmuir 24*, 11003–11008.

192. Lorite, G. S., Nobre, T. M., Zaniquelli, M. E. D., de Paula, E., and Cotta, M. A. 2009. Dibucaine effects on structural and elastic properties of lipid bilayers, *Biophys Chem 139*, 75–83.

193. Leonenko, Z., Finot, E., and Cramb, D. 2006. AFM study of interaction forces in supported planar DPPC bilayers in the presence of general anesthetic halothane, *Biochim Biophys Acta-Biomembranes 1758*, 487–492.

194. Yuan, C. and Johnston, L. J. 2001. Atomic force microscopy studies of ganglioside GM1 domains in phosphatidylcholine and phosphatidylcholine/cholesterol bilayers, *Biophys J 81*, 1059–1069.

195. Fotiadis, D., Jeno, P., Mini, T., Wirtz, S., Muller, S. A., Fraysse, L., Kjellbom, P., and Engel, A. 2001. Structural characterization of two aquaporins isolated from native spinach leaf plasma membranes, *J Biol Chem 276*, 1707–1714.

196. Puu, G., Artursson, E., Gustafson, I., Lundstrom, M., and Jass, J. 2000. Distribution and stability of membrane proteins in lipid membranes on solid supports, *Biosens Bioelectron 15*, 31–41.

197. Puu, G., Gustafson, I., Artursson, E., and Ohlsson, P. A. 1995. Retained activities of some membrane proteins in stable lipid bilayers on a solid support, *Biosens Bioelectron 10*, 463–476.

198. Rinia, H. A., Kik, R. A., Demel, R. A., Snel, M. M. E., Killian, J. A., van Der Eerden, J. P. J. M., and de Kruijff, B. 2000. Visualization of highly ordered striated domains induced by transmembrane peptides in supported phosphatidylcholine bilayers, *Biochemistry 39*, 5852–5858.

199. Bayburt, T. H., Carlson, J. W., and Sligar, S. G. 1998. Reconstitution and imaging of a membrane protein in a nanometer-size phospholipid bilayer, *J Struct Biol 123*, 37–44.

200. Neff, D., Tripathi, S., Middendorf, K., Stahlberg, H., Butt, H. J., Bamberg, E., and Dencher, N. A. 1997. Chloroplast f0f1 atp synthase imaged by atomic force microscopy, *J Struct Biol 119*, 139–148.

201. Takeyasu, K., Omote, H., Nettikadan, S., Tokumasu, F., Iwamoto-Kihara, A., and Futai, M. 1996. Molecular imaging of *Escherichia coli* F0F1-ATPase in reconstituted membranes using atomic force microscopy, *FEBS Lett 392*, 110–113.

202. Lal, R., Kim, H., Garavito, R. M., and Arnsdorf, M. F. 1993. Imaging of reconstituted biological channels at molecular resolution by atomic force microscopy, *Am J Physiol 265*, C851–856.

203. Slade, A., Luh, J., Ho, S., and Yip, C. M. 2002. Single molecule imaging of supported planar lipid bilayer—Reconstituted human insulin receptors by *in situ* scanning probe microscopy, *J Struct Biol 137*, 283–291.

204. Puu, G. and Gustafson, I. 1997. Planar lipid bilayers on solid supports from liposomes—Factors of importance for kinetics and stability, *Biochim Biophys Acta 1327*, 149–161.

205. Reviakine, I. and Brisson, A. 2000. Formation of supported phospholipid bilayers from unilamellar vesicles investigated by atomic force microscopy, *Langmuir 16*, 1806–1815.

206. Radler, J., Strey, H., and Sackmann, E. 1995. Phenomenology and kinetics of lipid bilayer spreading on hydrophilic surfaces, *Langmuir 11*, 4539–4548.
207. Santos, N. C., Ter-Ovanesyan, E., Zasadzinski, J. A., Prieto, M., and Castanho, M. A. 1998. Filipin-induced lesions in planar phospholipid bilayers imaged by atomic force microscopy, *Biophys J 75*, 1869–1873.
208. Milhaud, J., Ponsinet, V., Takashi, M., and Michels, B. 2002. Interactions of the drug amphotericin b with phospholipid membranes containing or not ergosterol: New insight into the role of ergosterol, *Biochim Biophys Acta 1558*, 95–108.
209. Steinem, C., Galla, H.-J., and Janshoff, A. 2000. Interaction of melittin with solid supported membranes, *Phys Chem Chem Phys 2*, 4580–4585.
210. Green, J. D., Kreplak, L., Goldsbury, C., Blatter, X. L., Stolz, M., Cooper, G. S., Seelig, A., Kist-Ler, J., and Aebi, U. 2004. Atomic force microscopy reveals defects within mica supported lipid bilayers induced by the amyloidogenic human amylin peptide, *J Mol Biol 342*, 877–887.
211. Janshoff, A., Bong, D. T., Steinem, C., Johnson, J. E., and Ghadiri, M. R. 1999. An animal virus-derived peptide switches membrane morphology: Possible relevance to nodaviral transfection processes, *Biochemistry 38*, 5328–5336.
212. Shaw, J. E., Epand, R. F., Hsu, J. C., Mo, G. C., Epand, R. M., and Yip, C. M. 2008. Cationic peptide-induced remodelling of model membranes: Direct visualization by *in situ* atomic force microscopy, *J Struct Biol 162*, 121–138.
213. Oreopoulos, J., Epand, R. F., Epand, R. M., and Yip, C. M. 2010. Peptide-induced domain formation in supported lipid bilayers: Direct evidence by combined atomic force and polarized total internal reflection fluorescence microscopy, *Biophys J 98*, 815–823.
214. Shaw, J. E., Epand, R. F., Sinnathamby, K., Li, Z., Bittman, R., Epand, R. M., and Yip, C. M. 2006. Tracking peptide–membrane interactions: Insights from *in situ* coupled confocal-atomic force microscopy imaging of NAP-22 peptide insertion and assembly, *J Struct Biol 155*, 458–469.
215. Alattia, J. R., Shaw, J. E., Yip, C. M., and Prive, G. G. 2006. Direct visualization of saposin remodelling of lipid bilayers, *J Mol Biol 362*, 943–953.
216. Slade, A. L., Schoeniger, J. S., Sasaki, D. Y., and Yip, C. M. 2006. *in situ* scanning probe microscopy studies of tetanus toxin-membrane interactions, *Biophys J 91*, 4565–4574.
217. El Kirat, K., Burton, I., Dupres, V., and Dufrene, Y. F. 2005. Sample preparation procedures for biological atomic force microscopy, *J Microsc 218*, 199–207.
218. Shahin, V. and Barrera, N. P. 2008. Providing unique insight into cell biology via atomic force microscopy, *Int Rev Cytol 265*, 227–252.
219. Li, A., Lee, P. Y., Ho, B., Ding, J. L., and Lim, C. T. 2007. Atomic force microscopy study of the antimicrobial action of sushi peptides on Gram negative bacteria, *Biochimica Biophysica Acta-Biomembranes 1768*, 411–418.
220. Jang, K. E. and Ye, J. C. 2007. Single channel blind image deconvolution from radially symmetric blur kernels, *Opt Express 15*, 3791–3803.
221. Arechaga, I. and Fotiadis, D. 2007. Reconstitution of mitochondrial ATP synthase into lipid bilayers for structural analysis, *J Struct Biol 160*, 287–294.
222. Giocondi, M. C., Seantier, B., Dosset, P., Milhiet, P. E., and Le Grimellec, C. 2008. Characterizing the interactions between GPI-anchored alkaline phosphatases and membrane domains by AFM, *Pflugers Arch 456*, 179–188.
223. Berquand, A., Levy, D., Gubellini, F., Le Grimellec, C., and Milhiet, P. E. 2007. Influence of calcium on direct incorporation of membrane proteins into in-plane lipid bilayer, *Ultramicroscopy 107*, 928–933.
224. Goncalves, R. P., Busselez, J., Levy, D., Seguin, J., and Scheuring, S. 2005. Membrane insertion of rhodopseudomonas acidophila light harvesting complex 2 investigated by high resolution AFM, *J Struct Biol 149*, 79–86.
225. Jo, E., McLaurin, J., Yip, C. M., St George-Hyslop, P., and Fraser, P. E. 2000. α-synuclein membrane interactions and lipid specificity, *J Biol Chem 275*, 34328–34334.

226. Yip, C. M. and McLaurin, J. 2001. Amyloid-beta peptide assembly: A critical step in fibrillogenesis and membrane disruption, *Biophys J 80*, 1359–1371.
227. Hane, F., Drolle, E., and Leonenko, Z. 2010. Effect of cholesterol and amyloid-beta peptide on structure and function of mixed-lipid films and pulmonary surfactant BLES. An atomic force microscopy study, *Nanomedicine. 6(6)*, 808–814.
228. Choucair, A., Chakrapani, M., Chakravarthy, B., Katsaras, J., and Johnston, L. J. 2007. Preferential accumulation of Ab[1–42] on gel phase domains of lipid bilayers: An AFM and fluorescence study, *Biochim Biophys Acta 1768*, 146–154.
229. Lam, K. L., Ishitsuka, Y., Cheng, Y., Chien, K., Waring, A. J., Lehrer, R. I., and Lee, K. Y. 2006. Mechanism of supported membrane disruption by antimicrobial peptide protegrin-1, *J Phys Chem B 110*, 21282–21286.
230. Butt, H. 1991. Measureing electrostatic, Van der Waals, and hydration forces in electrolyte solutions with an atomic force microscope, *Biophys J 60*, 1438–1444.
231. Ducker, W. A., Senden, T. J., and Pashley, R. M. 1991. Direct measurement of colloidal forces using an atomic force microscope, *Nature 353*, 239–241.
232. Senden, T. J., and Drummond, C. J. 1995. Surface chemistry and tip–sample interactions in atomic force microscopy, *Colloids and Surfaces 94(1)*, 29–51.
233. Bowen, W. R., Hilal, N., Lovitt, R. W., and Wright, C. J. 1998. Direct measurement of interactions between adsorbed protein layers using an atomic force microscope, *J Colloid Interface Sci 197*, 348–352.
234. Lokar, W. J. and Ducker, W. A. 2004. Proximal adsorption at glass surfaces: Ionic strength, pH, chain length effects, *Langmuir 20*, 378–388.
235. Mosley, L. M., Hunter, K. A., and Ducker, W. A. 2003. Forces between colloid particles in natural waters, *Environ Sci Technol 37*, 3303–3308.
236. Lokar, W. J. and Ducker, W. A. 2002. Proximal adsorption of dodecyltrimethylammonium bromide to the silica-electrolyte solution interface, *Langmuir 18*, 3167–3175.
237. Liu, J.-F., Min, G., and Ducker, W. A. 2001. AFM study of cationic surfactants and cationic polyelectrolytes at the silica–water interface, *Langmuir 17*, 4895–4903.
238. Tulpar, A., Subramaniam, V., and Ducker, W. A. 2001. Decay lengths in double-layer forces in solutions of partly associated ions, *Langmuir 17*, 8451–8454.
239. Butt, H.-J., Jaschke, M., and Ducker, W. 1995. Measuring surface forces in aqueous electrolyte solution with the atomic force microscopy, *Bioelectrochem. Bioenergetics 38*, 191–201.
240. Ducker, W. A. Xu, Z., and Israelachvili, J. N. 1994. Measurements of hydrophobic and DLVO forces in bubble-surface interactions in aqueous solutions, *Langmuir 10*, 3279–3289.
241. Ducker, W. A., and Cook, R. F. 1990. Rapid measurement of static and dynamic surface forces, *Appl Phys Lett 56*, 2408–2410.
242. Manne, S. and Gaub, H. E. 1997. Force microscopy: Measurement of local interfacial forces and surface stresses, *Curr Opin Colloid Interface Sci 2*, 145–152.
243. Toikka, G. and Hayes, R. A. 1997. Direct measurement of colloidal forces between mica and silica in aqueous electrolyte, *J Colloid Interface Sci 191*, 102–109.
244. Zhang, J., Uchida, E., Yuama, Y., and Ikada, Y. 1997. Electrostatic interaction between ionic polymer grafted surfaces studied by atomic force microscopy, *J Colloid Interf Sci 188*, 431–438.
245. Hodges, C. S. 2002. Measuring forces with the AFM: Polymeric surfaces in liquids, *Adv Colloid Interface Sci 99*, 13–75.
246. Muster, T. H. and Prestidge, C. A. 2002. Face specific surface properties of pharmaceutical crystals, *J Pharm Sci 91*, 1432–1444.
247. Danesh, A., Davies, M. C., Hinder, S. J., Roberts, C. J., Tendler, S. J., Williams, P. M., and Wilkins, M. J. 2000. Surface characterization of aspirin crystal planes by dynamic chemical force microscopy, *Anal Chem 72*, 3419–3422.

248. Noy, A., Frisbie, C. D., Rozsnyai, L. F., Wrighton, M. S., and Leiber, C. M. 1995. Chemical force microscopy: Exploiting chemically-modified tips to quantify adhesion, friction, and functional group distributions in molecular assemblies., *J Am Chem Soc 117*, 7943–7951.

249. Leckband, D. 2000. Measuring the forces that control protein interactions, *Annu Rev Biophys Biomol Struct 29*, 1–26.

250. Rief, M., Gautel, M., Oesterhelt, F., Fernandez, J. M., and Gaub, H. E. 1997. Reversible unfolding of individual titin immunoglobulin domains by AFM, *Science 276*, 1109–1112.

251. Smith, D. A. and Radford, S. E. 2000. Protein folding: Pulling back the frontiers, *Curr Biol 10*, R662–R664.

252. Hinterdorfer, P., Baumgartner, W., Gruber, H. J., and Schilcher, K. 1996. Detection and localization of individual antibody–antigen recognition events by atomic force microscopy, *Proc Natl Acad Sci USA 93*, 3477–3481.

253. Lee, G. U., Chrisey, L. A., and Colton, R. J. 1994. Direct measurement of the forces between complementary strands of DNA, *Science 266*, 771–773.

254. Helenius, J., Heisenberg, C. P., Gaub, H. E., and Muller, D. J. 2008. Single-cell force spectroscopy, *J Cell Sci 121*, 1785–1791.

255. Linke, W. A. and Grutzner, A. 2008. Pulling single molecules of titin by AFM—Recent advances and physiological implications, *Pflugers Arch 456*, 101–115.

256. Kienberger, F., Ebner, A., Gruber, H. J., and Hinterdorfer, P. 2006. Molecular recognition imaging and force spectroscopy of single biomolecules, *Acc Chem Res 39*, 29–36.

257. Greulich, K. O. 2005. Single-molecule studies on DNA and RNA, *ChemPhysChem 6*, 2458–2471.

258. Alegre-Cebollada, J., Perez-Jimenez, R., Kosuri, P., and Fernandez, J. M. 2010. Single-molecule force spectroscopy approach to enzymatic catalysis, *J Biol Chem. 285*(25), 18961–18966.

259. Carrion-Vazquez, M., Oberhauser, A. F., Fisher, T. E., Marszalek, P. E., Li, H., and Fernandez, J. M. 2000. Mechanical design of proteins studied by single-molecule force spectroscopy and protein engineering, *Prog Biophys Mol Biol 74*, 63–91.

260. Fisher, T. E., Carrion-Vazquez, M., Oberhauser, A. F., Li, H., Marszalek, P. E., and Fernandez, J. M. 2000. Single molecular force spectroscopy of modular proteins in the nervous system, *Neuron 27*, 435–446.

261. Fisher, T. E., Marszalek, P. E., and Fernandez, J. M. 2000. Stretching single molecules into novel conformations using the atomic force microscope, *Nat Struct Biol 7*, 719–724.

262. Bell, G. I. 1978. Models for the specific adhesion of cells to cells, *Science 200*, 618–627.

263. Strunz, T., Oroszlan, K., Schumakovitch, I., Guntherodt, H. J., and Hegner, M. 2000. Model energy landscapes and the force-induced dissociation of ligand–receptor bonds, *Biophys J 79*(3), 1206–1212.

264. Merkel, R., Nassoy, P., Leung, A., Ritchie, K., and Evans, E. 1999. Energy landscapes of receptor-ligand bonds explored with dynamic force spectroscopy, *Nature 397*, 50–53.

265. Janovjak, H., Struckmeier, J., and Muller, D. J. 2005. Hydrodynamic effects in fast AFM single-molecule force measurements, *Eur Biophys J. 34*(1), 91–96.

266. Wagner, P. 1998. Immobilization strategies for biological scanning probe microscopy, *FEBS Lett 430*, 112–115.

267. Wadu-Mesthrige, K., Amro, N. A., and Liu, G. Y. 2000. Immobilization of proteins on self-assembled monolayers, *Scanning 22*, 380–388.

268. Schmitt, L., Ludwig, M., Gaub, H. E., and Tampe, R. 2000. A metal-chelating microscopy tip as a new toolbox for single-molecule experiments by atomic force microscopy, *Biophys J 78*, 3275–3285.

269. Ill, C. R., Keivens, V. M., Hale, J. E., Nakamura, K. K., Jue, R. A., Cheng, S., Melcher, E. D., Drake, B., and Smith, M. C. 1993. A COOH-terminal peptide confers regiospecific orientation and facilitates atomic force microscopy of an IGG1, *Biophys J 64*, 919–924.

270. Thomson, N. H., Smith, B. L., Almqvist, N., Schmitt, L., Kashlev, M., Kool, E. T., and Hansma, P. K. 1999. Oriented, active *Escherichia coli* RNA polymerase: An atomic force microscope study, *Biophys J 76*, 1024–1033.

271. Li, Q., Rukavishnikov, A. V., Petukhov, P. A., Zaikova, T. O., Jin, C., and Keana, J. F. 2003. Nanoscale tripodal 1,3,5,7-tetrasubstituted adamantanes for AFM applications, *J Org Chem 68*, 4862–4869.

272. Drew, M. E., Chworos, A., Oroudjev, E., Hansma, H., and Yamakoshi, Y. 2010. A tripod molecular tip for single molecule ligand–receptor force spectroscopy by AFM, *Langmuir 26*, 7117–7125.

273. Mukherjee, P. S., Das, N., and Stang, P. J. 2004. Self-assembly of nanoscopic coordination cages using a flexible tripodal amide containing linker, *J Org Chem 69*, 3526–3529.

274. Ganchev, D. N., Rijkers, D. T. S., Snel, M. M. E., Killian, J. A., and de Kruijff, B. 2004. Strength of integration of transmembrane alpha-helical peptides in lipid bilayers as determined by atomic force spectroscopy, *Biochemistry 43*, 14987–14993.

275. Stroh, C. M., Ebner, A., Geretschlager, M., Freudenthaler, G., Kienberger, F., Kamruzzahan, A. S., Smith-Gill, S. J., Gruber, H. J., and Hinterdorfer, P. 2004. Simultaneous topography and recognition imaging using force microscopy, *Biophys J 87*, 1981–1990.

276. Nevo, R., Stroh, C., Kienberger, F., Kaftan, D., Brumfeld, V., Elbaum, M., Reich, Z., and Hinterdorfer, P. 2003. A molecular switch between alternative conformational states in the complex of Ran and importin beta1, *Nat Struct Biol 10*, 553–557.

277. Kada, G., Blayney, L., Jeyakumar, L. H., Kienberger, F., Pastushenko, V. P., Fleischer, S., Schindler, H., Lai, F. A., and Hinterdorfer, P. 2001. Recognition force microscopy/spectroscopy of ion channels: Applications to the skeletal muscle Ca2+ release channel (ryr1), *Ultramicroscopy 86*, 129–137.

278. Schmidt, T., Hinterdorfer, P., and Schindler, H. 1999. Microscopy for recognition of individual biomolecules, *Microsc Res Tech 44*, 339–346.

279. Raab, A., Han, W., Badt, D., Smith-Gill, S. J., Lindsay, S. M., Schindler, H., and Hinterdorfer, P. 1999. Antibody recognition imaging by force microscopy, *Nat Biotechnol 17*, 901–905.

280. Baumgartner, W., Hinterdorfer, P., Ness, W., Raab, A., Vestweber, D., Schindler, H., and Drenckhahn, D. 2000. Cadherin interaction probed by atomic force microscopy, *Proc Natl Acad Sci USA 97*, 4005–4010.

281. Baumgartner, W., Hinterdorfer, P., and Schindler, H. 2000. Data analysis of interaction forces measured with the atomic force microscope, *Ultramicroscopy 82*, 85–95.

282. Alsteens, D., Dague, E., Verbelen, C., Andre, G., Dupres, V., and Dufrene, Y. F. 2009. Nanoscale imaging of microbial pathogens using atomic force microscopy, *Wiley Interdiscip Rev Nanomed Nanobiotechnol 1*, 168–180.

283. Pelling, A. E., Li, Y. N., Shi, W. Y., and Gimzewski, J. K. 2005. Nanoscale visualization and characterization of *Myxococcus Xanthus* cells with atomic force microscopy, *Proc Natl Acad Sci, USA 102*, 6484–6489.

284. Puchner, E. M., Alexandrovich, A., Kho, A. L., Hensen, U., Schafer, L. V., Brandmeier, B., Grater, F., Grubmuller, H., Gaub, H. E., and Gautel, M. 2008. Mechanoenzymatics of titin kinase, *Proc Natl Acad Sci, USA 105*, 13385–13390.

285. Gaboriaud, F., Gee, M. L., Strugnell, R., and Duval, J. F. L. 2008. Coupled electrostatic, hydrodynamic, and mechanical properties of bacterial interfaces in aqueous media, *Langmuir 24*, 10988–10995.

286. Sheng, X. X., Ting, Y. P., and Pehkonen, S. O. 2007. Force measurements of bacterial adhesion on metals using a cell probe atomic force microscope, *J Colloid Interface Sci 310*, 661–669.

287. Lau, P. C. Y., Dutcher, J. R., Beveridge, T. J., and Lam, J. S. 2009. Absolute quantitation of bacterial biofilm adhesion and viscoelasticity by microbead force spectroscopy, *Biophys J 96*, 2935–2948.

288. Nussio, M. R., Oncins, G., Ridelis, I., Szili, E., Shapter, J. G., Sanz, F., and Voelcker, N. H. 2009. Nanomechanical characterization of phospholipid bilayer islands on flat and porous substrates: A force spectroscopy study, *J Phys Chem B 113*, 10339–10347.

289. Gaboriaud, F., Parcha, B. S., Gee, M. L., Holden, J. A., and Strugnell, R. A. 2008. Spatially resolved force spectroscopy of bacterial surfaces using force–volume imaging, *Colloids Surfaces B-Biointerfaces 62*, 206–213.

290. Kang, S. and Elimelech, M. 2009. Bioinspired single bacterial cell force spectroscopy, *Langmuir 25*, 9656–9659.

291. Cerf, A., Cau, J. C., Vieu, C., and Dague, E. 2009. Nanomechanical properties of dead or alive single-patterned bacteria, *Langmuir 25*, 5731–5736.

292. Gad, M., Itoh, A., and Ikai, A. 1997. Mapping cell wall polysaccharides of living microbial cells using atomic force microscopy, *Cell Biol Int 21*, 697–706.

293. Radmacher, M. 1997. Measuring the elastic properties of biological samples with the AFM, *IEEE Eng Med Biol Mag 16*, 47–57.

294. Shellenberger, K. and Logan, B. E. 2002. Effect of molecular scale roughness of glass beads on colloidal and bacterial deposition, *Environ Sci Technol 36*, 184–189.

295. van der Werf, K. O., Putman, C. A., de Grooth, B. G., and Greve, J. 1994. Adhesion force imaging in air and liquid by adhesion mode atomic force microscopy, *Appl Phys Lett 65*, 1195–1197.

296. Mizes, H. A., Loh, K.-G., Miller, R. J. D., Ahujy, S. K., and Grabowski, G. A. 1991. Submicron probe of polymer adhesion wtih atomic force microscopy. Dependence on topography and material inhomogenities, *Appl Phys Lett 59*, 2901–2903.

297. Nagao, E. and Dvorak, J. A. 1998. An integrated approach to the study of living cells by atomic force microscopy, *J Microsc 191 (Pt 1)*, 8–19.

298. Dupres, V., Menozzi, F. D., Locht, C., Clare, B. H., Abbott, N. L., Cuenot, S., Bompard, C., Raze, D., and Dufrene, Y. F. 2005. Nanoscale mapping and functional analysis of individual adhesins on living bacteria, *Nat Methods 2*, 515–520.

299. Francius, G., Alsteens, D., Dupres, V., Lebeer, S., De Keersmaecker, S., Vanderleyden, J., Gruber, H. J., and Dufrene, Y. F. 2009. Stretching polysaccharides on live cells using single molecule force spectroscopy, *Nat Protoc 4*, 939–946.

300. Francius, G., Lebeer, S., Alsteens, D., Wildling, L., Gruber, H. J., Hols, P., De Keersmaecker, S., Vanderleyden, J., and Dufrene, Y. F. 2008. Detection, localization, and conformational analysis of single polysaccharide molecules on live bacteria, *Acs Nano 2*, 1921–1929.

301. Dufrene, Y. F. and Hinterdorfer, P. 2008. Recent progress in AFM molecular recognition studies, *Pflugers Arch 456*, 237–245.

302. Hu, M., Wang, J., Cai, J., Wu, Y., and Wang, X. 2008. Nanostructure and force spectroscopy analysis of human peripheral blood CD4+ t cells using atomic force microscopy, *Biochem Biophys Res Commun 374*, 90–94.

303. Rosa-Zeiser, A., Weilandt, E., Hild, S., and Marti, O. 1997. The simultaneous measurement of elastic, electrostatic and adhesive properties by scanning force microscopy: Pulsed force mode operation, *Meas Sci Technol 8*, 1333–1338.

304. Okabe, Y., Furugori, M., Tani, Y., Akiba, U., and Fujihira, M. 2000. Chemical force microscopy of microcontact-printed self-assembled monolayers by pulsed-force-mode atomic force microscopy, *Ultramicroscopy 82*, 203–212.

305. Fujihira, M., Furugori, M., Akiba, U., and Tani, Y. 2001. Study of microcontact printed patterns by chemical force microscopy, *Ultramicroscopy 86*, 75–83.

306. Zhang, H., Grim, P. C. M., Vosch, T., Wiesler, U.-M., Berresheim, A. J., Mullen, K., and De Schryver, F. C. 2000. Discrimination of dendrimer aggregates on mica based on adhesion force: A pulsed mode atomic force microscopy study, *Langmuir 16*, 9294–9298.

307. Schneider, M., Zhu, M., Papastavrou, G., Akari, S., and Mohwald, H. 2002. Chemical pulsed-force microscopy of single polyethyleneimine molecules in aqueous solution, *Langmuir 18*, 602–606.

308. Kresz, N., Kokavecz, J., Smausz, T., Hopp, B., Csete, A., Hild, S., and Marti, O. 2004. Investigation of pulsed laser deposited crystalline PTFE thin layer with pulsed force mode AFM, *Thin Solid Films 453–454*, 239–244.

309. Stenert, M., Döring, A., and Bandermann, F. 2004. Poly(methyl methacrylate)-block-polystyrene and polystyrene-block-poly(*n*-butyl acrylate) as compatibilizers in PMMA/PNBA blends, *e-Polymers 15*, 1–16.

310. Evans, E. and Ritchie, K. 1999. Strength of a weak bond connecting flexible polymer chains, *Biophys J 76*, 2439–2447.

311. Dudko, O. K., Hummer, G., and Szabo, A. 2006. Intrinsic rates and activation free energies from single-molecule pulling experiments, *Phys Rev Lett 96*, 108101.

312. Ray, C., Guo, S., Brown, J., Li, N., and Akhremitchev, B. B. 2010. Kinetic parameters from detection probability in single molecule force spectroscopy, *Langmuir 26*(14), 11951–11957.

313. Li, N., Guo, S., and Akhremitchev, B. B. 2010. Apparent dependence of rupture force on loading rate in single-molecule force spectroscopy, *ChemPhysChem 11*(10), 2096–2098.

314. Grandbois, M., Beyer, M., Rief, M., Clausen-Schaumann, H., and Gaub, H. E. 1999. How strong is a covalent bond? *Science 283*, 1727–1730.

315. Haselgrubler, T., Amerstorfer, A., Schindler, H., and Gruber, H. J. 1995. Synthesis and applications of a new poly(ethylene glycol. derivative for the crosslinking of amines with thiols, *Bioconjug Chem 6*, 242–248.

316. Willemsen, O. H., Snel, M. M., van der Werf, K. O., de Grooth, B. G., Greve, J., Hinterdorfer, P., Gruber, H. J., Schindler, H., van Kooyk, Y., and Figdor, C. G. 1998. Simultaneous height and adhesion imaging of antibody–antigen interactions by atomic force microscopy, *Biophys J 75*, 2220–2228.

317. Wielert-Badt, S., Hinterdorfer, P., Gruber, H. J., Lin, J. T., Badt, D., Wimmer, B., Schindler, H., and Kinne, R. K. 2002. Single molecule recognition of protein binding epitopes in brush border membranes by force microscopy, *Biophys J 82*, 2767–2774.

318. Rivera, M., Lee, W., Ke, C., Marszalek, P. E., Cole, D. G., and Clark, R. L. 2008. Minimizing pulling geometry errors in atomic force microscope single molecule force spectroscopy, *Biophys J 95*, 3991–3998.

319. Ros, R., Schwesinger, F., Anselmetti, D., Kubon, M., Schafer, R., Pluckthun, A., and Tiefenauer, L. 1998. Antigen binding forces of individually addressed single-chain fv antibody molecules, *Proc Natl Acad Sci USA 95*, 7402–7405.

320. Allen, S., Davies, J., Davies, M. C., Dawkes, A. C., Roberts, C. J., Tendler, S. J., and Williams, P. M. 1999. The influence of epitope availability on atomic-force microscope studies of antigen-antibody interactions, *Biochem J 341 (Pt 1)*, 173–178.

321. Schwesinger, F., Ros, R., Strunz, T., Anselmetti, D., Guntherodt, H. J., Honegger, A., Jermutus, L., Tiefenauer, L., and Pluckthun, A. 2000. Unbinding forces of single antibody-antigen complexes correlate with their thermal dissociation rates, *Proc Natl Acad Sci USA 97*, 9972–9977.

322. Gergely, C., Voegel, J., Schaaf, P., Senger, B., Maaloum, M., Horber, J. K., and Hemmerle, J. 2000. Unbinding process of adsorbed proteins under external stress studied by atomic force microscopy spectroscopy, *Proc Natl Acad Sci USA 97*, 10802–10807.

323. Guzman, D. L., Randall, A., Baldi, P., and Guan, Z. 2010. Computational and single-molecule force studies of a macro domain protein reveal a key molecular determinant for mechanical stability, *Proc Natl Acad Sci USA 107*, 1989–1994.

324. Sharma, D., Perisic, O., Peng, Q., Cao, Y., Lam, C., Lu, H., and Li, H. 2007. Single-molecule force spectroscopy reveals a mechanically stable protein fold and the rational tuning of its mechanical stability, *Proc Natl Acad Sci USA 104*, 9278–9283.

325. Kim, T., Rhee, A., and Yip, C. M. 2006. Force-induced insulin dimer dissociation: A molecular dynamics study, *J Am Chem Soc 128*, 5330–5331.

326. Gao, M., Wilmanns, M., and Schulten, K. 2002. Steered molecular dynamics studies of titin i1 domain unfolding, *Biophys J 83*, 3435–3445.

327. Gao, M., Craig, D., Vogel, V., and Schulten, K. 2002. Identifying unfolding intermediates of FN-III[10] by steered molecular dynamics, *J Mol Biol 323*, 939–950.

328. Isralewitz, B., Gao, M., and Schulten, K. 2001. Steered molecular dynamics and mechanical functions of proteins, *Curr Opin Struct Biol 11*, 224–230.

329. Clementi, C., Carloni, P., and Maritan, A. 1999. Protein design is a key factor for subunit–subunit association, *Proc Natl Acad Sci USA 96*, 9616–9621.

330. Eom, K., Makarov, D. E., and Rodin, G. J. 2005. Theoretical studies of the kinetics of mechanical unfolding of cross-linked polymer chains and their implications for single-molecule pulling experiments, *Phys Rev E Stat Nonlin Soft Matter Phys 71*, 021904.

331. Qian, H. and Shapiro, B. E. 1999. Graphical method for force analysis: Macromolecular mechanics with atomic force microscopy, *Proteins 37*, 576–581.

332. Fisher, T. E., Marszalek, P. E., Oberhauser, A. F., Carrion-Vazquez, M., and Fernandez, J. M. 1999. The micro-mechanics of single molecules studied with atomic force microscopy, *J Physiol 520 Pt 1*, 5–14.

333. Vesenka, J., Manne, S., Giberson, R., Marsh, T., and Henderson, E. 1993. Collidal gold particles as an incompressible atomic force microscope imaging standard for assessing the compressibility of biomolecules, *Biochem J 65*, 992–997.

334. Engel, A., Gaub, H. E., and Muller, D. J. 1999. Atomic force microscopy: A forceful way with single molecules, *Curr Biol 9*, R133–136.

335. Fotiadis, D., Scheuring, S., Muller, S. A., Engel, A., and Muller, D. J. 2002. Imaging and manipulation of biological structures with the AFM, *Micron 33*, 385–397.

336. Muller, D. J., Fotiadis, D., and Engel, A. 1998. Mapping flexible protein domains at subnanometer resolution with the atomic force microscope, *FEBS Lett 430*, 105–111.

337. Schwaiger, I., Kardinal, A., Schleicher, M., Noegel, A. A., and Rief, M. 2004. A mechanical unfolding intermediate in an actin-crosslinking protein, *Nat Struct Mol Biol 11*, 81–85.

338. Williams, P. M., Fowler, S. B., Best, R. B., Toca-Herrera, J. L., Scott, K. A., Steward, A., and Clarke, J. 2003. Hidden complexity in the mechanical properties of titin, *Nature 422*, 446–449.

339. Kellermayer, M. S., Bustamante, C., and Granzier, H. L. 2003. Mechanics and structure of titin oligomers explored with atomic force microscopy, *Biochim Biophys Acta 1604*, 105–114.

340. Hertadi, R., Gruswitz, F., Silver, L., Koide, A., Koide, S., Arakawa, H., and Ikai, A. 2003. Unfolding mechanics of multiple ospa substructures investigated with single molecule force spectroscopy, *J Mol Biol 333*, 993–1002.

341. Carrion-Vazquez, M., Li, H., Lu, H., Marszalek, P. E., Oberhauser, A. F., and Fernandez, J. M. 2003. The mechanical stability of ubiquitin is linkage dependent, *Nat Struct Biol 10*(9), 738–743.

342. Rief, M. and Grubmuller, H. 2002. Force spectroscopy of single biomolecules, *ChemPhysChem 3*, 255–261.

343. Oberhauser, A. F., Badilla-Fernandez, C., Carrion-Vazquez, M., and Fernandez, J. M. 2002. The mechanical hierarchies of fibronectin observed with single-molecule afm, *J Mol Biol 319*, 433–447.

344. Muller, D. J., Kessler, M., Oesterhelt, F., Moller, C., Oesterhelt, D., and Gaub, H. 2002. Stability of bacteriorhodopsin alpha-helices and loops analyzed by single-molecule force spectroscopy, *Biophys J 83*, 3578–3588.

345. Best, R. B. and Clarke, J. 2002. What can atomic force microscopy tell us about protein folding?, *Chem Commun (Camb) Feb 7*,(3), 183–192.

346. Rief, M., Gautel, M., and Gaub, H. E. 2000. Unfolding forces of titin and fibronectin domains directly measured by AFM, *Adv Exp Med Biol 481*, 129–136; discussion 137–141.

347. Zhang, Y., Cui, F. Z., Wang, X. M., Feng, Q. L., and Zhu, X. D. 2002. Mechanical properties of skeletal bone in gene-mutated stopsel(dtl28d) and wild-type zebrafish (*Danio rerio*) measured by atomic force microscopy-based nanoindentation, *Bone 30*, 541–546.

348. Oberhauser, A. F., Hansma, P. K., Carrion-Vazquez, M., and Fernandez, J. M. 2001. Stepwise unfolding of titin under force-clamp atomic force microscopy, *Proc Natl Acad Sci USA 98*, 468–472.

349. Carrion-Vazquez, M., Marszalek, P. E., Oberhauser, A. F., and Fernandez, J. M. 1999. Atomic force microscopy captures length phenotypes in single proteins, *Proc Natl Acad Sci USA 96*, 11288–11292.

350. Marszalek, P. E., Lu, H., Li, H., Carrion-Vazquez, M., Oberhauser, A. F., Schulten, K., and Fernandez, J. M. 1999. Mechanical unfolding intermediates in titin modules, *Nature 402*, 100–103.

351. Becker, N., Oroudjev, E., Mutz, S., Cleveland, J. P., Hansma, P. K., Hayashi, C. Y., Makarov, D. E., and Hansma, H. G. 2003. Molecular nanosprings in spider capture-silk threads, *Nat Mater 2*, 278–283.

352. Yu, J., Malkova, S., and Lyubchenko, Y. L. 2008. Alpha-synuclein misfolding: Single molecule AFM force spectroscopy study, *J Mol Biol 384*, 992–1001.

353. Guo, S. and Akhremitchev, B. B. 2006. Packing density and structural heterogeneity of insulin amyloid fibrils measured by AFM nanoindentation, *Biomacromolecules 7*, 1630–1636.

354. Osada, T., Itoh, A., and Ikai, A. 2003. Mapping of the receptor-associated protein (RAP) binding proteins on living fibroblast cells using an atomic force microscope, *Ultramicroscopy 97*, 353–357.

355. Smith, J. F., Knowles, T. P., Dobson, C. M., Macphee, C. E., and Welland, M. E. 2006. Characterization of the nanoscale properties of individual amyloid fibrils, *Proc Natl Acad Sci USA 103*, 15806–15811.

356. Yan, C., Yersin, A., Afrin, R., Sekiguchi, H., and Ikai, A. 2009. Single molecular dynamic interactions between glycophorin A and lectin as probed by atomic force microscopy, *Biophys Chem 144*, 72–77.

357. Lesoil, C., Nonaka, T., Sekiguchi, H., Osada, T., Miyata, M., Afrin, R., and Ikai, A. 2010. Molecular shape and binding force of mycoplasma mobile's leg protein gli349 revealed by an afm study, *Biochem Biophys Res Commun 391*, 1312–1317.

358. Rief, M., Pascual, J., Saraste, M., and Gaub, H. E. 1999. Single molecule force spectroscopy of spectrin repeats: Low unfolding forces in helix bundles, *J Mol Biol 286*, 553–561.

359. Lenne, P. F., Raae, A. J., Altmann, S. M., Saraste, M., and Horber, J. K. 2000. States and transitions during forced unfolding of a single spectrin repeat, *FEBS Lett 476*, 124–128.

360. Yang, G., Cecconi, C., Baase, W. A., Vetter, I. R., Breyer, W. A., Haack, J. A., Matthews, B. W., Dahlquist, F. W., and Bustamante, C. 2000. Solid-state synthesis and mechanical unfolding of polymers of t4 lysozyme, *Proc Natl Acad Sci USA 97*, 139–144.

361. Clausen-Schaumann, H., Rief, M., Tolksdorf, C., and Gaub, H. E. 2000. Mechanical stability of single DNA molecules, *Biophys J 78*, 1997–2007.

362. Struckmeier, J., Wahl, R., Leuschner, M., Nunes, J., Janovjak, H., Geisler, U., Hofmann, G., Jahnke, T., and Muller, D. J. 2008. Fully automated single-molecule force spectroscopy for screening applications, *Nanotechnology 19*(38), 384020.

363. Zhang, B., and Evans, J. S. 2001. Modeling AFM-induced PEVK extension and the reversible unfolding of Ig/Fn III domains in single and multiple titin molecules, *Biophys J 80*, 597–605.

364. Paci, E. and Karplus, M. 2000. Unfolding proteins by external forces and temperature: The importance of topology and energetics, *Proc Natl Acad Sci USA 97*, 6521–6526.

365. Weisenhorn, A. L., Khorsandi, M., Kasas, S., Gotzos, V., and Butt, H.-J. 1993. Deformation and height anomaly of soft surfaces studied with an AFM, *Nanotechnology 4*, 106–113.

366. Vinckier, A., Dumortier, C., Engelborghs, Y., and Hellemans, L. 1996. Dynamical and mechanical study of immobilized microtubules with atomic force microscopy, *J Vac Sci Technol 14*, 1427–1431.

367. Laney, D. E., Garcia, R. A., Parsons, S. M., and Hansma, H. G. 1997. Changes in the elastic properties of cholinergic synaptic vesicles as measured by atomic force microscopy, *Biophys J 72*, 806–813.

368. Lekka, M., Laidler, P., Gil, D., Lekki, J., Stachura, Z., and Hrynkiewicz, A. Z. 1999. Elasticity of normal and cancerous human bladder cells studied by scanning force microscopy, *Eur Biophys J 28*, 312–316.

369. Parbhu, A. N., Bryson, W. G., and Lal, R. 1999. Disulfide bonds in the outer layer of keratin fibers confer higher mechanical rigidity: Correlative nano-indentation and elasticity measurement with an AFM, *Biochemistry 38*, 11755–11761.

370. Suda, H., Sasaki, Y. C., Oishi, N., Hiraoka, N., and Sutoh, K. 1999. Elasticity of mutant myosin subfragment-1 arranged on a functional silver surface, *Biochem Biophys Res Commun 261*, 276–282.

371. Cuenot, S., Demoustier-Champagne, S., and Nysten, B. 2000. Elastic modulus of polypyrrole nanotubes, *Phys Rev Lett 85*, 1690–1693.

372. Alhadlaq, A., Elisseeff, J. H., Hong, L., Williams, C. G., Caplan, A. I., Sharma, B., Kopher, R. A. et al. 2004. Adult stem cell driven genesis of human-shaped articular condyle, *Ann Biomed Eng 32*, 911–923.

373. Mathur, A. B., Truskey, G. A., and Reichert, W. M. 2000. Atomic force and total internal reflection fluorescence microscopy for the study of force transmission in endothelial cells, *Biophys J 78*, 1725–1735.
374. Velegol, S. B. and Logan, B. E. 2002. Contributions of bacterial surface polymers, electrostatics, and cell elasticity to the shape of AFM force curves, *Langmuir 18*, 5256–5262.
375. Touhami, A., Nysten, B., and Dufrene, Y. F. 2003. Nanoscale mapping of the elasticity of microbial cells by atomic force microscopy, *Langmuir 19*, 1745–1751.
376. Shroff, S. G., Saner, D. R., and Lal, R. 1995. Dynamic micromechanical properties of cultured rat atrial myocytes measured by atomic force microscopy, *Am J Physiol 269*, C286–292.
377. Ebenstein, D. M. and Pruitt, L. A. 2004. Nanoindentation of soft hydrated materials for application to vascular tissues, *J Biomed Mater Res 69A*, 222–232.
378. Thurner, P. J. 2009. Atomic force microscopy and indentation force measurement of bone, *Wiley Interdiscip Rev Nanomed Nanobiotechnol 1*, 624–649.
379. Grant, C. A., Brockwell, D. J., Radford, S. E., and Thomson, N. H. 2009. Tuning the elastic modulus of hydrated collagen fibrils, *Biophys J 97*, 2985–2992.
380. Lee, B., Han, L., Frank, E. H., Chubinskaya, S., Ortiz, C., and Grodzinsky, A. J. 2010. Dynamic mechanical properties of the tissue-engineered matrix associated with individual chondrocytes, *J Biomech 43*, 469–476.
381. Liao, X. and Wiedmann, T. S. 2004. Characterization of pharmaceutical solids by scanning probe microscopy, *J Pharm Sci 93*, 2250–2258.
382. Balooch, G., Marshall, G. W., Marshall, S. J., Warren, O. L., Asif, S. A., and Balooch, M. 2004. Evaluation of a new modulus mapping technique to investigate microstructural features of human teeth, *J Biomech 37*, 1223–1232.
383. Landman, U., Luedtke, W. D., Burnham, N. A., and Colton, R. J. 1990. Atomistic mechanisms and dynamics of adhesion, nanoindentation, and fracture, *Science 248*, 454–461.
384. Van Landringham, M. R., McKnight, S. H., Palmese, G. R., Bogetti, T. A., Eduljee, R. F., and Gillespie, J. W. J. 1997. Characterization of interphase regions using atomic force microscopy, *Mat Res Soc Symp Proc 458*, 313–318.
385. Van Landringham, M. R., McKnight, S. H., Palmese, G. R., Eduljee, R. F., Gillespie, J. W. J., and McCullough, R. L. 1997. Relating polymer indentation behavior to elastic modulus using atomic force microscopy, *Mat Res Soc Symp Proc 440*, 195–200.
386. Van Landringham, M. R., McKnight, S. H., Palmese, G. R., Huang, X., Bogetti, T. A., Eduljee, R. F., and Gillespie, J. W. J. 1997. Nanoscale indentation of polymer systems using the atomic force microscope, *J Adhesion 64*, 31–59.
387. Van Landringham, M. R., Dagastine, R. R., Eduljee, R. F., McCullough, R. L., and Gillespie, J. W. J. 1999. Characterization of nanoscale property variations in polymer composite systems: Part 1—experimental results, *Composites Part A 30*(1), 75–83.
388. Bogetti, T. A., Wang, T., Van Landringham, M. R., Eduljee, R. F., and Gillespie, J. W. J. 1999. Characterization of nanoscale property variations in polymer composite systems: Part 2—finite element modeling, *Composites Part A 30*, 85–94.
389. Bischel, M. S., Van Landringham, M. R., Eduljee, R. F., Gillespie, J. W. J., and Schultz, J. M. 2000. On the use of nanoscale indentation with the AFM in the identification of phases in blends on linear low density polyethylene and high density polyethylene, *J Mat Sci 35*, 221–228.
390. Cleveland, J. P., Manne, S., Bocek, D., and Hansma, P. K. 1993. A nondestructive method for determining the spring constant of cantilevers for scanning force microscopy, *Rev Sci Instrum 64*, 403–405.
391. Bogdanovic, G., Meurk, A., and Rutland, M. W. 2000. Tip friction—Torsional spring constant determination, *Colloids Surf B Biointerfaces 19*, 397–405.
392. Hutter, J. L. and Bechhoefer, J. 1993. Calibration of atomic-force microscope tips, *Rev Sci Instrum 64*, 1868–1873.
393. Sako, Y., Hibino, k., Miyauchi, T., Miyamoto, Y., Ueda, M., and Yanagida, T. 2000. Single-molecule imaging of signaling molecules in living cells, *Single Mol 2*, 159–163.

394. Sako, Y., Minoghchi, S., and Yanagida, T. 2000. Single-molecule imaging of egfr signalling on the surface of living cells, *Nat Cell Biol 2*, 168–172.

395. Ambrose, W. P., Goodwin, P. M., and Nolan, J. P. 1999. Single-molecule detection with total internal reflectance excitation: Comparing signal-to-background and total signals in different geometries, *Cytometry 36*, 224–231.

396. Osborne, M. A., Barnes, C. L., Balasubramanian, S., and Klenerman, D. 2001. Probing DNA surface attachment and local environment using single molecule spectroscopy, *J Phys Chem B 105*, 3120–3126.

397. Wakelin, S. and Bagshaw, C. R. 2003. A prism combination for near isotropic fluorescence excitation by total internal reflection, *J Microsc 209*, 143–148.

398. Michalet, X., Kapanidis, A. N., Laurence, T., Pinaud, F., Doose, S., Pflughoefft, M., and Weiss, S. 2003. The power and prospects of fluorescence microscopies and spectroscopies, *Annu Rev Biophys Biomol Struct 32*, 161–182.

399. Cannone, F., Chirico, G., and Diaspro, A. 2003. Two-photon interactions at single fluorescent molecule level, *J Biomed Opt 8*, 391–395.

400. Borisenko, V., Lougheed, T., Hesse, J., Fureder-Kitzmuller, E., Fertig, N., Behrends, J. C., Woolley, G. A., and Schutz, G. J. 2003. Simultaneous optical and electrical recording of single gramicidin channels, *Biophys J 84*, 612–622.

401. Sako, Y. and Uyemura, T. 2002. Total internal reflection fluorescence microscopy for single-molecule imaging in living cells, *Cell Struct Funct 27*, 357–365.

402. Ludes, M. D. and Wirth, M. J. 2002. Single-molecule resolution and fluorescence imaging of mixed-mode sorption of a dye at the interface of c18 and acetonitrile/water, *Anal Chem 74*, 386–393.

403. Harris, C. M. 2003. Shedding light on nsom, *Anal Chem 75*, 223A–228A.

404. Sekatskii, S. K., Shubeita, G. T., and Dietler, G. 2000. Time-gated scanning near-field optical microscopy, *Appl Phys Lett 77*, 2089–2091.

405. Muramatsu, H., Chiba, N., Umemoto, T., Homma, K., Nakajima, K., Ataka, T., Ohta, S., Kusumi, A., and Fujihira, M. 1995. Development of near-field optic/atomic force microscope for biological materials in aqueous solutions, *Ultramicroscopy 61*, 265–269.

406. Edidin, M. 2001. Near-field scanning optical microscopy, a siren call to biology, *Traffic 2*, 797–803.

407. de Lange, F., Cambi, A., Huijbens, R., de Bakker, B., Rensen, W., Garcia-Parajo, M., van Hulst, N., and Figdor, C. G. 2001. Cell biology beyond the diffraction limit: Near-field scanning optical microscopy, *J Cell Sci 114*, 4153–4160.

408. Betzig, E. and Chichester, R. J. 1993. Single molecules observed by near-field scanning optical microscopy, *Science 262*, 1422–1425.

409. Garcia-Parajo, M. F., Veerman, J. A., Segers-Nolten, G. M., de Grooth, B. G., Greve, J., and van Hulst, N. F. 1999. Visualising individual green fluorescent proteins with a near field optical microscope, *Cytometry 36*, 239–246.

410. van Hulst, N. F., Veerman, J. A., Garcia-Parajo, M. F., and Kuipers, J. 2000. Analysis of individual (macro)molecules and proteins using near-field optics, *J Chem Phys 112*, 7799–7810.

411. Moers, M. H., Ruiter, A. G., Jalocha, A., and van Hulst, N. F. 1995. Detection of fluorescence *in situ* hybridization on human metaphase chromosomes by near-field scanning optical microscopy, *Ultramicroscopy 61*, 279–283.

412. Micic, M., Radotic, K., Jeremic, M., Djikanovic, D., and Kammer, S. B. 2004. Study of the lignin model compound supramolecular structure by combination of near-field scanning optical microscopy and atomic force microscopy, *Colloids Surf B Biointerfaces 34*, 33–40.

413. Ianoul, A., Street, M., Grant, D., Pezacki, J., Taylor, R. S., and Johnston, L. J. 2004. Near-field scanning fluorescence microscopy study of ion channel clusters in cardiac myocyte membranes, *Biophys J 87*(5), 3525–3535.

414. Nagy, P., Jenei, A., Kirsch, A. K., Szollosi, J., Damjanovich, S., and Jovin, T. M. 1999. Activation-dependent clustering of the Erbb2 receptor tyrosine kinase detected by scanning near-field optical microscopy, *J Cell Sci 112 (Pt 11)*, 1733–1741.

415. Sommer, A. P. and Franke, R. P. 2002. Near-field optical analysis of living cells *in vitro*, *J Proteome Res 1*, 111–114.
416. Hosaka, N., and Saiki, T. 2001. Near-field fluorescence imaging of single molecules with a resolution in the range of 10 nm, *J Microsc 202*, 362–364.
417. Dunn, R. C., Holtom, G. R., Mets, L., and Xie, X. S. 1994. Near-field imaging and fluorescence life-time measurement of light harvesting complexes in intact photosynthetic membranes, *J Phys Chem 98*, 3094–3098.
418. Ha, T., Enderle, T., Ogletree, D. F., Chemla, D. S., Selvin, P. R., and Weiss, S. 1996. Probing the interaction between two single molecules: Fluorescence resonance energy transfer between a single donor and a single acceptor, *Proc Natl Acad Sci USA 93*, 6264–6268.
419. Prikulis, J., Murty, K. V., Olin, H., and Kall, M. 2003. Large-area topography analysis and near-field Raman spectroscopy using bent fibre probes, *J Microsc 210*, 269–273.
420. Burgos, P., Lu, Z., Ianoul, A., Hnatovsky, C., Viriot, M. L., Johnston, L. J., and Taylor, R. S. 2003. Near-field scanning optical microscopy probes: A comparison of pulled and double-etched bent NSOM probes for fluorescence imaging of biological samples, *J Microsc 211*, 37–47.
421. Kitts, C. C., and Vanden Bout, D. A. 2009. Near-field scanning optical microscopy measurements of fluorescent molecular probes binding to insulin amyloid fibrils, *J Phys Chem B 113*, 12090–12095.
422. Tokumasu, F., Hwang, J., and Dvorak, J. A. 2004. Heterogeneous molecular distribution in supported multicomponent lipid bilayers, *Langmuir 20*, 614–618.
423. Vobornik, D., Rouleau, Y., Haley, J., Bani-Yaghoub, M., Taylor, R., Johnston, L. J., and Pezacki, J. P. 2009. Nanoscale organization of beta2-adrenergic receptor-venus fusion protein domains on the surface of mammalian cells, *Biochem Biophys Res Commun 382*, 85–90.
424. Ianoul, A. and Johnston, L. J. 2007. Near-field scanning optical microscopy to identify membrane microdomains, *Methods Mol Biol 400*, 469–480.
425. Nishida, S., Funabashi, Y., and Ikai, A. 2002. Combination of AFM with an objective-type total internal reflection fluorescence microscope (TIRFM) for nanomanipulation of single cells, *Ultramicroscopy 91*, 269–274.
426. Shaw, J. E., Slade, A., and Yip, C. M. 2003. Simultaneous *in situ* total internal reflectance fluorescence/atomic force microscopy studies of DPPC/DPOPC microdomains in supported planar lipid bilayers, *J Am Chem Soc 125*, 111838–111839.
427. Oreopoulos, J. and Yip, C. M. 2008. Combined scanning probe and total internal reflection fluorescence microscopy, *Methods 46*, 2–10.
428. Hugel, T., Holland, N. B., Cattani, A., Moroder, L., Seitz, M., and Gaub, H. E. 2002. Single-molecule optomechanical cycle, *Science 296*, 1103–1106.
429. Kellermayer, M. S. Z., Karsai, A., Kengyel, A., Nagy, A., Bianco, P., Huber, T., Kulcsar, A., Niedetzky, C., Proksch, R., and Grama, L. 2006. Spatially and temporally synchronized atomic force and total internal reflection fluorescence microscopy for imaging and manipulating cells and biomolecules, *Biophys J 91*, 2665–2677.
430. Kolodny, L. A., Willard, D. M., Carillo, L. L., Nelson, M. W., and Van Orden, A. 2001. Spatially correlated fluorescence/AFM of individual nanosized particles and biomolecules, *Anal Chem 73*, 1959–1966.
431. Shaw, J. E., Alattia, J. R., Verity, J. E., Prive, G. G., and Yip, C. M. 2006. Mechanisms of antimicrobial peptide action: Studies of indolicidin assembly at model membrane interfaces by *in situ* atomic force microscopy, *J Struct Biol 154*, 42–58.
432. Shaw, J. E., Epand, R. F., Epand, R. M., Li, Z., Bittman, R., and Yip, C. M. 2006. Correlated fluorescence-atomic force microscopy of membrane domains: Structure of fluorescence probes determines lipid localization, *Biophys J 90*, 2170–2178.
433. Deng, Z., Lulevich, V., Liu, F. T., and Liu, G. Y. 2010. Applications of atomic force microscopy in biophysical chemistry of cells, *J Phys Chem B 114*, 5971–5982.
434. Franz, C. M., and Muller, D. J. 2005. Analyzing focal adhesion structure by atomic force microscopy, *J Cell Sci 118*, 5315–5323.

435. Gradinaru, C. C., Martinsson, P., Aartsma, T. J., and Schmidt, T. 2004. Simultaneous atomic-force and two-photon fluorescence imaging of biological specimens *in vivo*, *Ultramicroscopy 99*, 235–245.

436. Yu, J. P., Wang, Q., Shi, X. L., Ma, X. Y., Yang, H. Y., Chen, Y. G., and Fang, X. H. 2007. Single-molecule force spectroscopy study of interaction between transforming growth factor beta 1 and its receptor in living cells, *J Phys Chem B 111*, 13619–13625.

437. Sun, Z., Juriani, A., Meininger, G. A., and Meissner, K. E. 2009. Probing cell surface interactions using atomic force microscope cantilevers functionalized for quantum dot-enabled Förster resonance energy transfer, *J Biomed Opt 14*(4), 040502.

438. Trache, A. and Meininger, G. A. 2005. Atomic force-multi-optical imaging integrated microscope for monitoring molecular dynamics in live cells, *J Biomed Opt 10*(6), 064023.

439. Trache, A. and Lim, S. M. 2009. Integrated microscopy for real-time imaging of mechanotransduction studies in live cells, *J Biomed Opt 14*, 034024.

440. Na, S., Trache, A., Trzeciakowski, J., Sun, Z., Meininger, G. A., and Humphrey, J. D. 2008. Time-dependent changes in smooth muscle cell stiffness and focal adhesion area in response to cyclic equibiaxial stretch, *Ann Biomed Eng 36*, 369–380.

441. Trache, A. and Meininger, G. A. 2005. Atomic force-multi-optical imaging integrated microscope for monitoring molecular dynamics in live cells, *J Biomed Opt 10*, 064023.

442. Hillenbrand, R., Taubner, T., and Keilmann, F. 2002. Phonon-enhanced light matter interaction at the nanometre scale, *Nature 418*, 159–162.

443. Anderson, M. S. and Gaimari, S. D. 2003. Raman-atomic force microscopy of the ommatidial surfaces of dipteran compound eyes, *J Struct Biol 142*, 364–368.

444. Knoll, A., Magerle, R., and Krausch, G. 2001. Tapping mode atomic force microscopy on polymers: Where is the true sample surface?, *Macromolecules 34*, 4159–4165.

445. Raschke, M. B., Molina, L., Elsaesser, T., Kim, D. H., Knoll, W., and Hinrichs, K. 2005. Apertureless near-field vibrational imaging of block-copolymer nanostructures with ultrahigh spatial resolution, *ChemPhysChem 6*, 2197–2203.

446. Knoll, B. and Keilmann, F. 1999. Mid-infrared scanning near-field optical microscope resolves 30 nm, *J Microsc 194*, 512–515.

447. Paulite, M., Fakhraai, Z., Akhremitchev, B. B., Mueller, K., and Walker, G. C. 2009. Assembly, tuning and use of an apertureless near field infrared microscope for protein imaging, *J Vis Exp Nov 25*, (33).

448. Mueller, K., Yang, X., Paulite, M., Fakhraai, Z., Gunari, N., and Walker, G. C. 2008. Chemical imaging of the surface of self-assembled polystyrene-b-poly(methyl methacrylate) diblock copolymer films using apertureless near-field IR microscopy, *Langmuir 24*, 6946–6951.

449. Dazzi, A., Prazeres, R., Glotin, F., Ortega, J. M., Al-Sawaftah, M., and de Frutos, M. 2008. Chemical mapping of the distribution of viruses into infected bacteria with a photothermal method, *Ultramicroscopy 108*, 635–641.

450. Dazzi, A., Prazeres, R., Glotin, F., and Ortega, J. M. 2007. Analysis of nano-chemical mapping performed by an AFM-based ("AFMIR") acousto-optic technique, *Ultramicroscopy 107*, 1194–1200.

451. Brucherseifer, M., Kranz, C., and Mizaikoff, B. 2007. Combined *in situ* atomic force microscopy-infrared-attenuated total reflection spectroscopy, *Anal Chem 79*, 8803–8806.

452. Wang, L., Kowalik, J., Mizaikoff, B., and Kranz, C. 2010. Combining scanning electrochemical microscopy with infrared attenuated total reflection spectroscopy for *in situ* studies of electrochemically induced processes, *Anal Chem 82*, 3139–3145.

453. Wang, L., Kranz, C., and Mizaikoff, B. 2010. Monitoring scanning electrochemical microscopy approach curves with mid-infrared spectroscopy: Toward a novel current-independent positioning mode, *Anal Chem 82*, 3132–3138.

454. Verity, J. E., Chhabra, N., Sinnathamby, K., and Yip, C. M. 2009. Tracking molecular interactions in membranes by simultaneous ATR-FTIR-AFM, *Biophys J 97*, 1225–1231.

25

Parenteral Infusion Devices

Gregory I. Voss
IVAC Corporation

Robert D.
Butterfield
IVAC Corporation

The circulatory system is the body's primary pathway for both the distribution of oxygen and other nutrients and the removal of carbon dioxide and other waste products. Since the entire blood supply in a healthy adult completely circulates within 60 s, substances introduced into the circulatory system are distributed rapidly. Thus intravenous (IV) and intraarterial access routes provide an effective pathway for the delivery of fluid, blood, and medicants to a patient's vital organs. Consequently, about 80% of hospitalized patients receive infusion therapy. Peripheral and central veins are used for the majority of infusions. Umbilical artery delivery (in neonates), enteral delivery of nutrients, and epidural delivery of anesthetics and analgesics comprise smaller patient populations. A variety of devices can be used to provide flow through an intravenous catheter. An intravenous delivery system typically consists of three major components: (1) fluid or drug reservoir, (2) catheter system for transferring the fluid or drug from the reservoir into the vasculature through a venipuncture, and (3) device for regulation and/or generating flow (see Figure 25.1).

This chapter is separated into five sections. Section 25.1 describes the clinical needs associated with intravenous drug delivery that determine device performance criteria. Section 25.2 reviews the principles of flow through a tube; Section 25.3 introduces the underlying electromechanical principles for flow regulation and/or generation and their ability to meet the clinical performance criteria. Section 25.4 reviews complications associated with intravenous therapy, and Section 25.5 concludes with a short list of articles providing more detailed information.

25.1 Performance Criteria for IV Infusion Devices

The IV pathway provides an excellent route for continuous drug therapy. The ideal delivery system regulates drug concentration in the body to achieve and maintain a desired result. When the drug's effect cannot be monitored directly, it is frequently assumed that a specific blood concentration or infusion

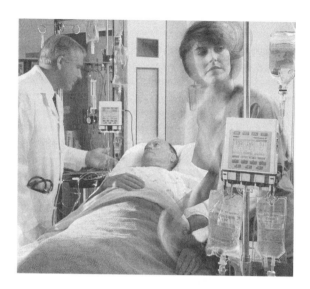

FIGURE 25.1 Typical IV infusion system.

rate will achieve the therapeutic objective. Although underinfusion may not provide sufficient therapy, overinfusion can produce even more serious toxic side effects.

The therapeutic range and risks associated with under- and overinfusion are highly drug and patient dependent. Intravenous delivery of fluids and electrolytes often does not require very accurate regulation. Low-risk patients can generally tolerate well infusion rate variability of ±30% for fluids. In some situations, however, specifically for fluid-restricted patients, prolonged under- or overinfusion of fluids can compromise the patient's cardiovascular and renal systems.

The infusion of many drugs, especially potent cardioactive agents, requires high accuracy. For example, postcoronary-artery-bypass-graft patients commonly receive sodium nitroprusside to lower arterial blood pressure. Hypertension, associated with underinfusion, subjects the graft sutures to higher stress with an increased risk for internal bleeding. Hypotension associated with overinfusion can compromise the cardiovascular state of the patient. Nitroprusside's potency, short onset delay, and short half-life (30–180 s) provide for very tight control, enabling the clinician to quickly respond to the many events that alter the patient's arterial pressure. The fast response of drugs such as nitroprusside creates a need for short-term flow uniformity as well as long-term accuracy.

The British Department of Health employs *Trumpet curves* in their Health Equipment Information reports to compare flow uniformity of infusion pumps. For a prescribed flow rate, the trumpet curve is the plot of the maximum and minimum measured percentage flow rate error as a function of the accumulation interval (Figure 25.2). Flow is measured gravimetrically in 30-s blocks for 1 h. These blocks are summed to produce 120-s, 300-s, and other longer total accumulation intervals. Though the 120-s window may not detect flow variations important in delivery of the fastest acting agents, the trumpet curve provides a helpful means for performance comparison among infusion devices. Additional statistical information such as standard deviations may be derived from the basic trumpet flow measurements.

The short half-life of certain pharmacologic agents and the clotting reaction time of blood during periods of stagnant flow require that fluid flow be maintained without significant interruption. Specifically, concern has been expressed in the literature that the infusion of sodium nitroprusside and other short half-life drugs occur without interruption exceeding 20 s. Thus, minimization of false alarms and rapid detection of occlusions are important aspects of maintaining a constant vascular concentration. Accidental occlusions of the IV line due to improper positioning of stopcocks or clamps, kinked tubing, and clotted catheters are common.

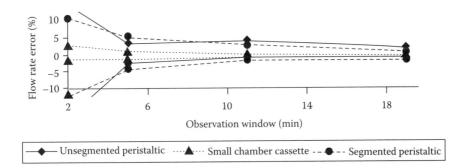

FIGURE 25.2 Trumpet curve for several representative large-volume infusion pumps operated at 5 mL/h. Note that peristaltic pumps were designed for low-risk patients.

Occlusions between pump and patient present a secondary complication in maintaining serum drug concentration. Until detected, the pump will infuse, storing fluid in the delivery set. When the occlusion is eliminated, the stored volume is delivered to the patient in a bolus. With concentrated pharmaceutic agents, this bolus can produce a large perturbation in the patient's status.

Occlusions of the pump intake also interrupt delivery. If detection is delayed, inadequate flow can result. During an intake occlusion, in some pump designs removal of the delivery set can produce abrupt aspiration of blood. This event may precipitate clotting and cause injury to the infusion site.

The common practice of delivering multiple drugs through a single venous access port produces an additional challenge to maintaining uniform drug concentration. Although some mixing will occur in the venous access catheter, fluid in the catheter more closely resembles a first-in/first-out digital queue: during delivery, drugs from the various infusion devices mix at the catheter input, an equivalent fluid volume discharges from the outlet. Rate changes and flow nonuniformity cause the mass flow of drugs at the outlet to differ from those at the input. Consider a venous access catheter with a volume of 2 mL and a total flow of 10 mL/h. Due to the digital queue phenomenon, an incremental change in the intake flow rate of an individual drug will not appear at the output for 12 min. In addition, changing flow rates for one drug will cause short-term marked swings in the delivery rate of drugs using the same access catheter. When the delay becomes significantly larger than the time constant for a drug that is titrated to a measurable patient response, titration becomes extremely difficult leading to large oscillations.

As discussed, the performance requirements for drug delivery vary with multiple factors: drug, fluid restriction, and patient risk. Thus the delivery of potent agents to fluid-restricted patients at risk requires the highest performance standards defined by flow rate accuracy, flow rate uniformity, and ability to minimize risk of IV-site complications. These performance requirements need to be appropriately balanced with the device cost and the impact on clinician productivity.

25.2 Flow through an IV Delivery System

The physical properties associated with the flow of fluids through cylindrical tubes provide the foundation for understanding flow through a catheter into the vasculature. Hagen–Poiseuille's equation for laminar flow of a Newtonian fluid through a rigid tube states

$$Q = \pi \cdot r^4 \cdot \frac{(P_1 - P_2)}{8 \cdot \eta \cdot L} \tag{25.1}$$

where Q is the flow; P_1 and P_2 are the pressures at the inlet and outlet of the tube, respectively; L and r are the length and internal radius of the tube, respectively; and η is fluid viscosity. Although many drug delivery systems do not strictly meet the flow conditions for precise application of the laminar flow

TABLE 25.1 Resistance Measurements for Catheter Components Used for Infusion

Component	Length, cm	Flow Resistance, Fluid ohm, mmHg/(L/h)
Standard administration set	91–213	4.3–5.3
Extension tube for CVP monitoring	15	15.5
19-gauge epidural catheter	91	290.4–497.1
18-gauge needle	6–9	14.1–17.9
23-gauge needle	2.5–9	165.2–344.0
25-gauge needle	1.5–4.0	525.1–1412.0
Vicra Quick-Cath 18-gauge catheter	5	12.9
Extension set with 0.22 µm air-eliminating filter		623.0
0.2 µm filter		555.0

Note: Mean values are presented over a range of infusions (100, 200, and 300 mL/h) and sample size ($n = 10$).

equation, it does provide insight into the relationship between flow and pressure in a catheter. The fluid analog of Ohms Law describes the resistance to flow under constant flow conditions:

$$R = \frac{P_1 - P_2}{Q} \tag{25.2}$$

Thus, resistance to flow through a tube correlates directly with catheter length and fluid viscosity and inversely with the fourth power of catheter diameter. For steady flow, the delivery system can be modeled as a series of resistors representing each component, including administration set, access catheter, and circulatory system. When dynamic aspects of the delivery system are considered, a more detailed model including catheter and venous compliance, fluid inertia, and turbulent flow is required. Flow resistance may be defined with units of mm Hg/(L/h), so that 1 fluid ohm = 4.8×10^{-11} Pa s/m^3. Studies determining flow resistance for several catheter components with distilled water for flow rates of 100, 200, and 300 mL/h appear in Table 25.1.

25.3 Intravenous Infusion Devices

From Hagen–Poiselluie's equation, two general approaches to intravenous infusion become apparent. First, a hydrostatic pressure gradient can be used with adjustment of delivery system resistance controlling flow rate. Complications such as partial obstructions result in reduced flow which may be detected by an automatic flow monitor. Second, a constant displacement flow source can be used. Now complications may be detected by monitoring elevated fluid pressure and/or flow resistance. At the risk of overgeneralization, the relative strengths of each approach will be presented.

25.3.1 Gravity Flow/Resistance Regulation

The simplest means for providing regulated flow employs gravity as the driving force with a roller clamp as controlled resistance. Placement of the fluid reservoir 60–100 cm above the patient's right atrium provides a hydrostatic pressure gradient P_h equal to 1.34 mm Hg/cm of elevation. The modest physiologic mean pressure in the veins, P_v, minimally reduces the net hydrostatic pressure gradient. The equation for flow becomes

$$Q = \frac{P_h - P_v}{R_{mfr} + R_n} \tag{25.3}$$

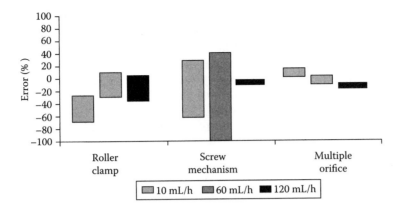

FIGURE 25.3 Drift in flow rate (mean ± standard deviation) over a 4-h period for three mechanical flow regulators at initial flow rates of 10, 60, and 120 mL/h with distilled water at constant hydrostatic pressure gradient.

where R_{mfr} and R_n are the resistance to flow through the mechanical flow regulator and the remainder of the delivery system, respectively. Replacing the variables with representative values for an infusion of 5% saline solution into a healthy adult at 100 mL/h yields

$$100 \text{ mL/h} = \frac{(68 - 8) \text{ mmHg}}{(550 + 50) \text{ mmHg/(L/h)}} \tag{25.4}$$

Gravity flow cannot be used for arterial infusions since the higher vascular pressure exceeds available hydrostatic pressure.

Flow stability in a gravity infusion system is subject to variations in hydrostatic and venous pressure as well as catheter resistance. However, the most important factor is the change in flow regulator resistance caused by viscoelastic creep of the tubing wall (see Figure 25.3). Caution must be used in assuming that a preset flow regulator setting will accurately provide a predetermined rate. The clinician typically estimates flow rate by counting the frequency of drops falling through an in-line drip-forming chamber, adjusting the clamp to obtain the desired drop rate. The cross-sectional area of the drip chamber orifice is the major determinant of drop volume. Various manufacturers provide minidrip sets designed for pediatric (e.g., 60 drops/mL) and regular sets designed for adult (10–20 drops/mL) patients. Tolerances on the drip chamber can cause a 3% error in minidrip sets and a 17% error in regular sets at 125 mL/h flow rate with 5% dextrose in water. Mean drop size for rapid rates increased by as much as 25% over the size of drops which form slowly. In addition, variation in the specific gravity and surface tension of fluids can provide an additional large source of drop size variability.

Some mechanical flow regulating devices incorporate the principle of a Starling resistor. In a Starling device, resistance is proportional to hydrostatic pressure gradient. Thus, the device provides a negative feedback mechanism to reduce flow variation as the available pressure gradient changes with time.

Mechanical flow regulators comprise the largest segment of intravenous infusion systems, providing the simplest means of operation. Patient transport is simple, since these devices require no electric power. Mechanical flow regulators are most useful where the patient is not fluid restricted and the acceptable therapeutic rate range of the drug is relatively wide with minimal risk of serious adverse sequelae. The most common use for these systems is the administration of fluids and electrolytes.

25.3.2 Volumetric Infusion Pumps

Active pumping infusion devices combine electronics with a mechanism to generate flow. These devices have higher performance standards than simple gravity flow regulators. The Association for the

Advancement of Medical Instrumentation (AAMI) recommends that long-term rate accuracy for infusion pumps remain within ±10% of the set rate for general infusion and, for the more demanding applications, that long-term flow remains within ±5%. Such requirements typically extend to those agents with narrow therapeutic indices and/or low flow rates, such as the neonatal population or other fluid-restricted patients. The British Department of Health has established three main categories for hospital-based infusion devices: neonatal infusions, high-risk infusions, and low-risk infusions. Infusion control for neonates requires the highest performance standards, because their size severely restricts fluid volume. A fourth category, ambulatory infusion, pertains to pumps worn by patients.

25.3.3 Controllers

These devices automate the process of adjusting the mechanical flow regulator. The most common controllers utilize sensors to count the number of drops passing through the drip chamber to provide flow feedback for automatic rate adjustment. Flow rate accuracy remains limited by the rate and viscosity dependence of drop size. Delivery set motion associated with ambulation and improper angulation of the drip chamber can also hinder accurate rate detection.

An alternative to the drop counter is a volumetric metering chamber. A McGaw Corporation controller delivery set uses a rigid chamber divided by a flexible membrane. Instrument-controlled valves allow fluid to fill one chamber from the fluid reservoir, displacing the membrane driving the fluid from the second chamber toward the patient. When inlet and outlet valves reverse state, the second chamber is filled while the first chamber delivers to the patient. The frequency of state change determines the average flow rate. Volumetric accuracy demands primarily on the dimensional tolerances of the chamber. Although volumetric controllers may provide greater accuracy than drop-counting controllers, their disposables are inherently more complex, and maximum flow is still limited by head height and system resistance.

Beyond improvements in flow rate accuracy, controllers should provide an added level of patient safety by quickly detecting IV-site complications. The IVAC Corporation has developed a series of controllers employing pulsed modulated flow providing for monitoring of flow resistance as well as improved accuracy.

The maximum flow rate achieved by gravimetric based infusion systems can become limited by R_n and by concurrent infusion from other sources through the same catheter. In drop-counting devices, flow rate uniformity suffers at low flow rates from the discrete nature of the drop detector.

In contrast with infusion controllers, pumps generate flow by mechanized displacement of the contents of a volumetric chamber. Typical designs provide high flow rate accuracy and uniformity for a wide rate range (0.1–1000.0 mL/h) of infusion rates. Rate error correlates directly with effective chamber volume, which, in turn, depends on both instrument and disposable repeatability, precision, and stability under varying load. Stepper or servo-controlled dc motors are typically used to provide the driving force for the fluid. At low flow rates, dc motors usually operate in a discrete stepping mode. On average, each step propels a small quanta of fluid toward the patient. Flow rate uniformity therefore is a function of both the average volume per quanta and the variation in volume. Mechanism factors influencing rate uniformity include: stepping resolution, gearing and activator geometries, volumetric chamber coupling geometry, and chamber elasticity. When the quanta volume is not inherently uniform over the mechanism's cycle, software control has been used to compensate for the variation.

25.3.4 Syringe Pumps

These pumps employ a syringe as both reservoir and volumetric pumping chamber. A precision lead-screw is used to produce constant linear advancement of the syringe plunger. Except for those ambulatory systems that utilize specific microsyringes, pumps generally accept syringes ranging in size from 5 to 100 mL. Flow rate accuracy and uniformity are determined by both mechanism displacement characteristics and tolerance on the internal syringe diameter. Since syringe mechanisms can generate a specified linear travel with less than 1% error, the manufacturing tolerance on the internal cross-sectional area of the syringe largely determines flow rate accuracy. Although syringes can be manufactured to tighter tolerances, standard plastic syringes provide long-term accuracy of ±5%. Flow rate uniformity, however, can benefit from the ability to select syringe size (see Figure 25.4). Since many syringes have similar stroke length, diameter variation provides control of volume. Also the linear advancement per step is typically fixed. Therefore selection of a lower-volume syringe provides smaller-volume quanta. This allows tradeoffs among drug concentration, flow rate, and duration of flow per syringe. Slack in the gear train and drive shaft coupling as well as plunger slip cause rate inaccuracies during the initial stages of delivery (see Figure 25.5a).

Since the syringe volumes are typically much smaller than reservoirs used with other infusion devices, syringe pumps generally deliver drugs in either fluid-restricted environments or for short duration. With high-quality syringes, flow rate uniformity in syringe pumps is generally superior to that accomplished by other infusion pumps. With the drug reservoir enclosed within the device, syringe pumps manage patient transport well, including the operating room environment.

Cassette pumps conceptually mimic the piston type action of the syringe pump but provide an automated means of repeatedly emptying and refilling the cassette. The process of refilling the cassette in single piston devices requires an interruption in flow (see Figure 25.5b). The length of interruption relative to the drug's half-life determines the impact of the refill period on hemodynamic stability. To eliminate the interruption caused by refill, dual piston devices alternate refill and delivery states, providing nearly continuous output. Others implement cassettes with very small volumes which can refill in less than a second (see Figure 25.2). Tight control of the internal cross-sectional area of the pumping chamber provides exceptional flow rate accuracy. Manufacturers have recently developed remarkably small cassette pumps that can still generate the full spectrum of infusion rate (0.1–999.0 mL/h). These systems combine pumping chamber, inlet and outlet valving, pressure sensing, and air detection into a single complex component.

Peristaltic pumps operate on a short segment of the IV tubing. Peristaltic pumps can be separated into two subtypes. Rotary peristaltic mechanisms operate by compressing the pumping segment against the rotor housing with rollers mounted on the housing. With rotation, the rollers push fluid from the container through the tubing toward the patient. At least one of the rollers completely occludes the tubing against the housing at all times precluding free flow from the reservoir to the patient. During a portion of the revolution, two rollers trap fluid in the intervening pumping segment. The captured volume between the rollers determines volumetric accuracy. Linear peristaltic pumps hold the pumping segment in a channel pressed against a rigid backing plate. An array of cam-driven actuators sequentially occlude the segment starting with the section nearest the reservoir forcing fluid toward the patient with a sinusoidal wave action. In a typical design using uniform motor step intervals, a characteristic flow wave resembling a positively biased sine wave is produced (see Figure 25.5c).

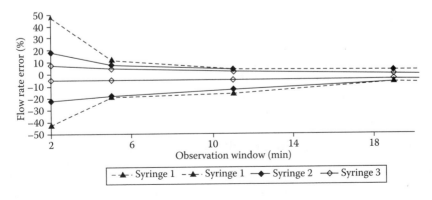

FIGURE 25.4 Effect of syringe type on trumpet curve of a syringe pump at 1 mL/h.

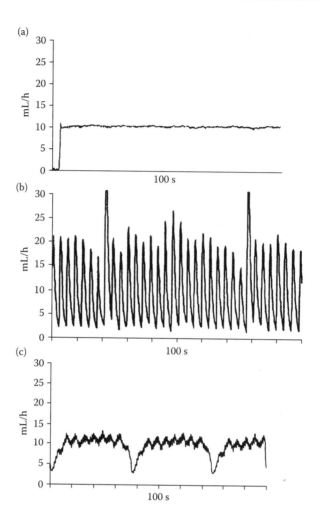

FIGURE 25.5 Continuous flow pattern for a representative, (a) syringe, (b) cassette, and (c) linear peristaltic pump at 10 mL/h.

Infusion pumps provide significant advantages over both manual flow regulators and controllers in several categories. Infusion pumps can provide accurate delivery over a wide range of infusion rates (0.1–999.0 mL/h). Neither elevated system resistance nor distal line pressure limit the maximum infusion rate. Infusion pumps can support a wider range of applications including arterial infusions, spinal and epidural infusions, and infusions into pulmonary artery or central venous catheters. Flow rate accuracy of infusion pumps is highly dependent on the segment employed as the pumping chamber (see Figure 25.2). Incorporating special syringes or pumping segments can significantly improve flow rate accuracy (see Figure 25.6). Both manufacturing tolerances and segment material composition significantly dictate flow rate accuracy. Time- and temperature-related properties of the pumping segment further impact long-term drift in flow rate.

25.4 Managing Occlusions of the Delivery System

One of the most common problems in managing an IV delivery system is the rapid detection of occlusion in the delivery system. With a complete occlusion, the resistance to flow approaches infinity. In this condition, gravimetric-based devices cease to generate flow. Mechanical flow regulators have no

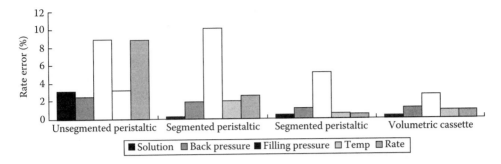

FIGURE 25.6 Impact of five variables on flow rate accuracy in four different infusion pumps. Variables tested included solution: Distilled water and 25% dextrose in water, back pressure: −100 and 300 mm Hg, pumping segment filling pressure: −30 inches of water and +30 inches of water, temperature: 10°C and 40°C, and infusion rate: 5 mL/h and 500 mL/h. Note: First and second peristaltic mechanism qualified for low-risk patients, while the third peristaltic device qualified for high-risk patients.

mechanism for adverse event detection and thus must rely on the clinician to identify an occlusion as part of routine patient care. Electronic controllers sense the absence of flow and alarm in response to their inability to sustain the desired flow rate.

The problem of rapidly detecting an occlusion in an infusion pump is more complex. Upstream occlusions that occur between the fluid reservoir and the pumping mechanism impact the system quite differently than downstream occlusions which occur between the pump and the patient. When an occlusion occurs downstream from an infusion pump, the pump continues to propel fluid into the section of tubing between the pump and the occlusion. The time rate of pressure rise in that section increases in direct proportion to flow rate and inversely with tubing compliance (compliance, C, is the volume increase in a closed tube per mm Hg pressure applied). The most common approach to detecting downstream occlusion requires a pressure transducer immediately below the pumping mechanism. These devices generate an alarm when either the mean pressure or rate of change in pressure exceeds a threshold. For pressure-limited designs, the time to downstream alarm (TTA) may be estimated as

$$\text{TTA} = \frac{P_{\text{alarm}} \cdot C_{\text{delivery-set}}}{\text{flow rate}} \tag{25.5}$$

Using a representative tubing compliance of 1 μL/mm Hg, flow rate of 1 mL/h, and a fixed alarm threshold set of 500 mm Hg, the time to alarm becomes

$$\text{TTA} = \frac{500_{\text{mmHg}} \cdot 1000 \text{ mL/mmHg}}{1 \text{ mL/h}} = 30 \text{ min} \tag{25.6}$$

where TTA is the time from occlusion to alarm detection. Pressure-based detection algorithms depend on accuracy and stability of the sensing system. Lowering the threshold on absolute or relative pressure for occlusion alarm reduces the TTA, but at the cost of increasing the likelihood of false alarms. Patient movement, patient-to-pump height variations, and other clinical circumstances can cause wide perturbations in line pressure. To optimize the balance between fast TTA and minimal false alarms, some infusion pumps allow the alarm threshold to be set by the clinician or be automatically shifted upward in response to alarms; other pumps attempt to optimize performance by varying pressure alarm thresholds with flow rate.

A second approach to detection of downstream occlusions uses motor torque as an indirect measure of the load seen by the pumping mechanism. Although this approach eliminates the need for a pressure sensor, it introduces additional sources for error including friction in the gear mechanism or pumping mechanism that requires additional safety margins to protect against false alarms. In syringe pumps, where the coefficient of static friction of the syringe bung (rubber end of the syringe plunger) against the syringe wall can be substantial, occlusion detection can exceed 1 h at low flow rates.

Direct, continuous measurement of downstream flow resistance may provide a monitoring modality which overcomes the disadvantages of pressure-based alarm systems, especially at low infusion rates. Such a monitoring system would have the added advantage of performance unaffected by flow rate, hydrostatic pressure variations, and motion artifacts.

Upstream occlusions can cause large negative pressures as the pumping mechanism generates a vacuum on the upstream tubing segment. The tube may collapse and the vacuum may pull air through the tubing walls or form cavitation bubbles. A pressure sensor situated above the mechanism or a pressure sensor below the mechanism synchronized with filling of the pumping chamber can detect the vacuum associated with an upstream occlusion. Optical or ultrasound transducers, situated below the mechanism, can detect air bubbles in the catheter, and air-eliminating filters can remove air, preventing large air emboli from being introduced into the patient.

Some of the most serious complications of IV therapy occur at the venipuncture site; these include extravasation, postinfusion phlebitis (and thrombophlebitis), IV-related infections, ecchymosis, and hematomas. Other problems that do not occur as frequently include speed shock and allergic reactions.

Extravasation (or infiltration) is the inadvertent perfusion of infusate into the interstitial tissue. Reported percentage of patients to whom extravasation has occurred ranges from 10% to over 25%. Tissue damage does not occur frequently, but the consequences can be severe, including skin necrosis requiring significant plastic and reconstructive surgery and amputation of limbs. The frequency of extravasation injury correlates with age, state of consciousness, and venous circulation of the patient as well as the type, location, and placement of the intravenous cannula. Drugs that have high osmolality, vessicant properties, or the ability to induce ischemia correlate with frequency of extravasation injury. Neonatal and pediatric patients who possess limited communication skills, constantly move, and have small veins that are difficult to cannulate require superior vigilance to protect against extravasation.

Since interstitial tissue provides a greater resistance to fluid flow than the venous pathway, infusion devices with accurate and precise pressure monitoring systems have been used to detect small pressure increases due to extravasation. To successfully implement this technique requires diligence by the clinician, since patient movement, flow rate, catheter resistance, and venous pressure variations can obscure the small pressure variations resulting from the extravasation. Others have investigated the ability of a pumping mechanism to withdraw blood as indicative of problems in a patent line. The catheter tip, however, may be partially in and out of the vein such that infiltration occurs yet blood can be withdrawn from the patient. A vein might also collapse under negative pressure in a patent line without successful blood withdrawal. Techniques currently being investigated which monitor infusion impedance (resistance and compliance) show promise for assisting in the detection of extravasation.

When a catheter tip wedges into the internal lining of the vein wall, it is considered positional. With the fluid path restricted by the vein wall, increases in line resistance may indicate a positional catheter. With patient movement, for example wrist flexation, the catheter may move in and out of the positional state. Since a positional catheter is thought to be more prone toward extravasation than other catheters, early detection of a positional catheter and appropriate adjustment of catheter position may be helpful in reducing the frequency of extravasation.

Postinfusion phlebitis is acute inflammation of a vein used for IV infusion. The chief characteristic is a reddened area or red streak that follows the course of the vein with tenderness, warmth, and edema at the venipuncture site. The vein, which normally is very compliant, also hardens. Phlebitis positively correlates with infusion rate and with the infusion of vesicants.

Fluid overload and speed shock result from the accidental administration of a large fluid volume over a short interval. Speed shock associates more frequently with the delivery of potent medications, rather than fluids. These problems most commonly occur with manually regulated IV systems, which do not provide the safety features of instrumented lines. Many IV sets designed for instrumented operation will free flow when the set is removed from the instrument without manual clamping. To protect against this possibility, some sets are automatically placed in the occluded state on disengagement. Although an apparent advantage, reliance on such automatic devices may create a false sense of security and lead to manual errors with sets not incorporating these features.

25.5 Summary

Intravenous infusion has become the mode of choice for delivery of a large class of fluids and drugs both in hospital and alternative care settings. Modern infusion devices provide the clinician with a wide array of choices for performing intravenous therapy. Selection of the appropriate device for a specified application requires understanding of drug pharmacology and pharmacokinetics, fluid mechanics, and device design and performance characteristics. Continuing improvements in performance, safety, and cost of these systems will allow even broader utilization of intravenous delivery in a variety of settings.

References

Association for the Advancement of Medical Instrumentation. 1992. *Standard for Infusion Devices.* Arlington.

Bohony J. 1993. Nine common intravenous complications and what to do about them. *Am. J. Nurs.* 10: 45.

British Department of Health. 1990. *Evaluation of Infusion Pumps and Controllers.* HEI Report #198.

Glass P.S.A., Jacobs J.R., Reves J.G. 1991. Technology for continuous infusions in anesthesia. Continuous infusions in anesthesia. *Int. Anesthesiol. Clin.* 29: 39.

MacCara M. 1983. Extravasation: A hazard of intravenous therapy. *Drug Intell. Clin. Pharm.* 17: 713.

Further Information

Peter Glass provides a strong rationale for intravenous therapy including pharmacokinetic and pharmaco-dynamic bases for continuous delivery. Clinical complications around intravenous therapy are well summarized by MacCara (1983) and Bohony (1993). The AAMI Standard for Infusion Devices provides a comprehensive means of evaluating infusion device technology, and the British Department of Health OHEI Report #198 provides a competitive analysis of pumps and controllers.

26

Clinical Laboratory: Separation and Spectral Methods

Richard L. Roa
Baylor University Medical Center

26.1 Introduction

The purpose of the clinical laboratory is to analyze body fluids and tissues for specific substances of interest and to report the results in a form which is of value to clinicians in the diagnosis and treatment of disease. A large range of tests has been developed to achieve this purpose. Four terms commonly used to describe tests are *accuracy, precision, sensitivity,* and *specificity*. An accurate test, on average, yields true values. Precision is the ability of a test to produce identical results upon repeated trials. Sensitivity is a measure of how small an amount of substance can be measured. Specificity is the degree to which a test measures the substance of interest without being affected by other substances which may be present in greater amounts.

The first step in many laboratory tests is to separate the material of interest from other substances. This may be accomplished through extraction, filtration, and centrifugation. Another step is derivatization, in which the substance of interest is chemically altered through addition of reagents to change it into a substance which is easily measured. For example, one method for measuring glucose is to add otoluidine which, under proper conditions, forms a green-colored solution with an absorption maximum at 630 nm. Separation and derivatization both improve the specificity required of good tests.

26.2 Separation Methods

Centrifuges are used to separate materials on the basis of their relative densities. The most common use in the laboratory is the separation of cells and platelets from the liquid part of the blood. This requires a relative centrifugal force (RCF) of roughly 1000*g* (1000 times the force of gravity) for a period of 10 min.

Relative centrifugal force is a function of the speed of rotation and the distance of the sample from the center of rotation as stated in Equation 26.1

$$\text{RCF} = (1.12 \times 10^{-5}) \, r(\text{rpm})^2 \qquad (26.1)$$

where RCF is the relative centrifugal force in g, and r is the radius in cm.

Some mixtures require higher g-loads in order to achieve separation in a reasonable period of time. Special rotors contain the sample tubes inside a smooth container, which minimizes air resistance to allow faster rotational speeds. Refrigerated units maintain the samples at a cool temperature throughout long high-speed runs which could lead to sample heating due to air friction on the rotor. Ultracentrifuges operate at speeds on the order of 100,000 rpm and provide relative centrifugal forces of up to 600,000g. These usually require vacuum pumps to remove the air which would otherwise retard the rotation and heat the rotor.

26.3 Chromatographic Separations

Chromatographic separations depend upon the different rates at which various substances moving in a stream (mobile phase) are retarded by a stationary material (stationary phase) as they pass over it. The mobile phase can be a volatilized sample transported by an inert carrier gas such as helium or a liquid transported by an organic solvent such as acetone. Stationary phases are quite diverse depending upon the separation being made, but most are contained within a long, thin tube (column). Liquid stationary phases may be used by coating them onto inert packing materials. When a sample is introduced into a chromatographic column, it is carried through it by the mobile phase. As it passes through the column, the substances which have greater affinity for the stationary phase fall behind those with less affinity. The separated substances may be detected as individual peaks by a suitable detector placed at the end of the chromatographic column.

26.4 Gas Chromatography

The most common instrumental chromatographic method used in the clinical laboratory is the gas–liquid chromatograph. In this system the mobile phase is a gas, and the stationary phase is a liquid coated onto either an inert support material, in the case of a packed column, or the inner walls of a very thin tube, in the case of a capillary column. Capillary columns have the greatest resolving power but cannot handle large sample quantities. The sample is injected into a small heated chamber at the beginning of the column, where it is volatilized if it is not already a gaseous sample. The sample is then carried through the column by an inert carrier gas, typically helium or nitrogen. The column is completely housed within an oven. Many gas chromatographs allow for the oven temperature to be programmed to slowly increase for a set time after the sample injection is made. This produces peaks which are spread more uniformly over time.

Four detection methods commonly used with gas chromatography are thermal conductivity, flame ionization, nitrogen/phosphorous, and mass spectrometry. The thermal conductivity detector takes advantage of variations in thermal conductivity between the carrier gas and the gas being measured. A heated filament immersed in the gas leaving the chromatographic column is part of a Wheatstone bridge circuit. Small variations in the conductivity of the gas cause changes in the resistance of the filament, which are recorded. The flame ionization detector measures the current between two plates with a voltage applied between them. When an organic material appears in the flame, ions which contribute to the current are formed. The NP detector, or nitrogen/phosphorous detector, is a modified flame ionization detector (see Figure 26.1) which is particularly sensitive to nitrogen- and phosphorous-containing compounds.

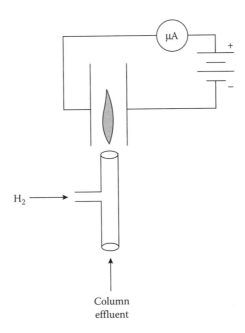

FIGURE 26.1 Flame ionization detector. Organic compounds in the column effluent are ionized in the flame, producing a current proportional to the amount of the compound present.

Mass spectrometry (MS) provides excellent sensitivity and selectivity. The concept behind these devices is that the volatilized sample molecules are broken into ionized fragments which are then passed through a mass analyzer that separates the fragments according to their mass/charge (m/z) ratios. A mass spectrum, which is a plot of the relative abundance of the various fragments versus m/z, is produced. The mass spectrum is characteristic of the molecule sampled. The mass analyzer most commonly used with gas chromatographs is the quadrupole detector, which consists of four rods that have dc and RF voltages applied to them. The m/z spectrum can be scanned by appropriate changes in the applied voltages. The detector operates in a manner similar to that of a photomultiplier tube except that the collision of the charged particles with the cathode begins the electron cascade, resulting in a measurable electric pulse for each charged particle captured. The MS must operate in a high vacuum, which requires good pumps and a porous barrier between the GC and MS that limits the amount of carrier gas entering the MS.

26.5 High-Performance Liquid Chromatography

In liquid chromatography, the mobile phase is liquid. High-performance liquid chromatography (HPLC) refers to systems which obtain excellent resolution in a reasonable time by forcing the mobile phase at high pressure through a long thin column. The most common pumps used are pistons driven by asymmetrical cams. By using two such pumps in parallel and operating out of phase, pressure fluctuations can be minimized. Typical pressures are 350–1500 psi, though the pressure may be as high as 10,000 psi. Flow rates are in the 1–10 mL/min range.

A common method for placing a sample onto the column is with a loop injector, consisting of a loop of tubing which is filled with the sample. By a rotation of the loop, it is brought in series with the column, and the sample is carried onto the column. A UV/visible spectrophotometer is often used as a detector for this method. A mercury arc lamp with the 254-nm emission isolated is useful for detection of aromatic compounds, while diode array detectors allow a complete spectrum from 190 to 600 nm in 10 ms.

This provides for detection and identification of compounds as they come off the column. Fluorescent, electrochemical, and mass analyzer detectors are also used.

26.6 Basis for Spectral Methods

Spectral methods rely on the absorption or emission of electromagnetic radiation by the sample of interest. Electromagnetic radiation is often described in terms of frequency or wavelength. Wavelengths are those obtained in a vacuum and may be calculated with the formula

$$\lambda = c/\nu$$

(26.2)

where λ is the wavelength in meters, c the speed of light in vacuum (3×10^8 m/s), and ν the frequency in Hz.

The frequency range of interest for most clinical laboratory work consists of the visible (390–780 nm) and the ultraviolet or UV (180–390 nm) ranges. Many substances absorb different wavelengths preferentially. When this occurs in the visible region, they are colored. In general, the color of a substance is the complement of the color it absorbs, for example, absorption in the blue produces a yellow color. For a given wavelength or bandwidth, transmittance is defined as

$$T = \frac{I_t}{I_i}$$

(26.3)

where T is the transmittance ratio (often expressed as %), I_i the incident light intensity, and I_t the transmitted light intensity. Absorbance is defined as

$$A = -\log_{10} 1/T$$

(26.4)

Under suitable conditions, the absorbance of a solution with an absorbing compound dissolved in it is proportional to the concentration of that compound as well as the path length of light through it. This relationship is expressed by Beer's law:

$$A = abc$$

(26.5)

where A is the absorbance, a a constant, b the path length, and c the concentration.

A number of situations may cause deviations from Beer's law, such as high concentration or mixtures of compounds which absorb at the wavelength of interest. From an instrumental standpoint, the primary causes are stray light and excessive spectral bandwidth. Stray light refers to any light reaching the detector other than light from the desired pass-band which has passed through sample. Sources of stray light may include room light leaking into the detection chamber, scatter from the cuvette, and undesired *fluorescence*.

A typical spectrophotometer consists of a light source, some form of wavelength selection, and a detector for measuring the light transmitted through the samples. There is no single light source that covers the entire visible and UV spectrum. The source most commonly used for the visible part of the spectrum is the tungsten–halogen lamp, which provides continuous radiation over the range of 360–950 nm. The deuterium lamp has become the standard for much UV work. It covers the range from 220 to 360 nm. Instruments which cover the entire UV/visible range use both lamps with a means for switching from one lamp to the other at a wavelength of approximately 360 nm (Figure 26.2).

Wavelength selection is accomplished with filters, prisms, and diffraction gratings. Specially designed interference filters can provide bandwidths as small as 5 nm. These are useful for instruments which do

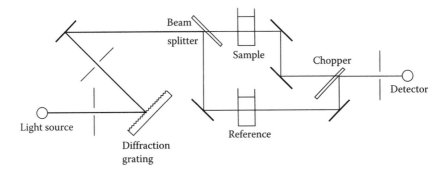

FIGURE 26.2 Dual-beam spectrophotometer. The diffraction grating is rotated to select the desired wavelength. The beam splitter consists of a half-silvered mirror which passes half the light while reflecting the other half. A rotating mirror with cut-out sections (chopper) alternately directs one beam and then the other to the detector.

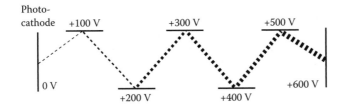

FIGURE 26.3 Photomultiplier tube. Incident photons cause the photocathode to emit electrons which collide with the first dynode which emits additional electrons. Multiple dynodes provide sufficient gain to produce an easily measurable electric pulse from a single photon.

not need to scan a range of wavelengths. Prisms produce a nonlinear dispersion of wavelengths with the longer wavelengths closer together than the shorter ones. Since the light must pass through the prism material, they must be made of quartz for UV work. Diffraction gratings are surfaces with 1000–3000 grooves/mm cut into them. They may be transmissive or reflective; the reflective ones are more popular since there is no attenuation of light by the material. They produce a linear dispersion. By proper selection of slit widths, pass bands of 0.1 nm are commonly achieved.

The most common detector is the photomultiplier tube, which consists of a photosensitive cathode that emits electrons in proportion to the intensity of light striking it (Figure 26.3). A series of 10–15 dynodes, each at 50–100 V greater potential than the preceding one, produce an electron amplification of 4–6 per stage. Overall gains are typically a million or more. Photomultiplier tubes respond quickly and cover the entire spectral range. They require a high voltage supply and can be damaged if exposed to room light while the high voltage is applied.

26.7 Fluorometry

Certain molecules absorb a photon's energy and then emit a photon with less energy (longer wavelength). When the reemission occurs in less than 10^{-8} s, the process is known as fluorescence. This physical process provides the means for assays which are 10–100 times as sensitive as those based on absorption measurements. This increase in sensitivity is largely because the light measured is all from the sample of interest. A dim light is easily measured against a black background, while it may be lost if added to an already bright background.

Fluorometers and spectrofluorometers are very similar to photometers and spectrophotometers but with two major differences. Fluorometers and spectrofluorometers use two monochrometers, one for

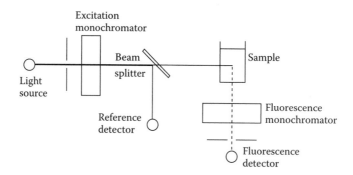

FIGURE 26.4   Spectrofluorometer. Fluorescence methods can be extremely sensitive to the low background interference. Since the detector is off-axis from the incident light and a second monochromator blocks light of wavelengths illuminating the sample, virtually no signal reaches the detector other than the desired fluorescence.

excitation light and one for emitted light. By proper selection of the bandpass regions, all the light used to excite the sample can be blocked from the detector, assuring that the detector sees only fluorescence. The other difference is that the detector is aligned off-axis, commonly at 90°, from the excitation source. At this angle, scatter is minimal, which helps ensure a dark background for the measured fluorescence. Some spectrofluorometers use polarization filters both on the input and output light beams, which allows for fluorescence polarization studies (Figure 26.4). An intense light source in the visible-to-UV range is desirable. A common source is the xenon or mercury arc lamps, which provide a continuum of radiation over this range.

26.8 Flame Photometry

Flame photometry is used to measure sodium, potassium, and lithium in body fluids. When these elements are heated in a flame they emit characteristic wavelengths of light. The major emission lines are 589 nm (yellow) for sodium, 767 nm (violet) for potassium, and 671 nm (red) for lithium. An atomizer introduces a fine mist of the sample into a flame. For routine laboratory use, a propane and compressed air flame is adequate. High-quality interference filters with narrow pass bands are often used to isolate the major emission lines. The narrow band pass is necessary to maximize the signal-to-noise ratio. Since it is impossible to maintain stable aspiration, atomization, and flame characteristics, it is necessary to use an internal standard of known concentration while making measurements of unknowns. In this way the ratio of the unknown sample's emission to the internal standard's emission remains stable even as the total signal fluctuates. An internal standard is usually an element which is found in very low concentration in the sample fluid. By adding a high concentration of this element to the sample, its concentration can be known to a high degree of accuracy. Lithium, potassium, and cesium all may be used as internal standards depending upon the particular assay being conducted.

26.9 Atomic Absorption Spectroscopy

Atomic absorption spectroscopy is based on the fact that just as metal elements have unique emission lines, they have identical absorption lines when in a gaseous or dissociated state. The atomic absorption spectrometer takes advantage of these physical characteristics in a clever manner, producing an instrument with approximately 100 times the sensitivity of a flame photometer for similar elements. The sample is aspirated into a flame, where the majority of the atoms of the element being measured remain in the ground state, where they are capable of absorbing light at their characteristic wavelengths. An intense source of exactly these wavelengths is produced by a hollow cathode lamp. These lamps are constructed so that the cathode is made from the element to be measured, and the lamps are filled with a low pressure of argon or neon gas. When a current is passed through the lamp, metal atoms are sputtered off the cathode and collide with the argon or neon in the tube, producing emission of the characteristic wavelengths. A monochromator and photodetector complete the system.

Light reaching the detector is a combination of that which is emitted by the sample (undesirable) and light from the hollow cathode lamp which was not absorbed by the sample in the flame (desirable). By pulsing the light from the lamp either by directly pulsing the lamp or with a chopper, and using a detector which is sensitive to ac signals and insensitive to dc signals, the undesirable emission signal is eliminated. Each element to be measured requires a lamp with that element present in the cathode. Multielement lamps have been developed to minimize the number of lamps required. Atomic absorption spectrophotometers may be either single beam or double beam; the double-beam instruments have greater stability.

There are various flameless methods for atomic absorption spectroscopy in which the burner is replaced with a method for vaporizing the element of interest without a flame. The graphite furnace which heats the sample to 2700° consists of a hollow graphite tube which is heated by passing a large current through it. The sample is placed within the tube, and the light beam is passed through it while the sample is heated.

26.10 Turbidimetry and Nephelometry

Light scattering by particles in solution is directly proportional to both concentration and molecular weight of the particles. For small molecules the scattering is insignificant, but for proteins, immunoglobulins, immune complexes, and other large particles, light scattering can be an effective method for the detection and measurement of particle concentration. For a given wavelength λ of light and particle size d, scattering is described as Raleigh ($d < \lambda/10$), Raleigh–Debye ($d \approx \lambda$), or Mie ($d > 10\,\lambda$). For particles that are small compared to the wavelength, the scattering is equal in all directions. However, as the particle size becomes larger than the wavelength of light, it becomes preferentially scattered in the forward direction. Light-scattering techniques are widely used to detect the formation of antigen–antibody complexes in immunoassays.

When light scattering is measured by the attenuation of a beam of light through a solution, it is called *turbidimetry*. This is essentially the same as absorption measurements with a photometer except that a large passband is acceptable. When maximum sensitivity is required a different method is used—direct measurement of the scattered light with a detector placed at an angle to the central beam. This method is called *nephelometry*. A typical nephelometer will have a light source, filter, sample cuvette, and detector set at an angle to the incident beam (Figure 26.5).

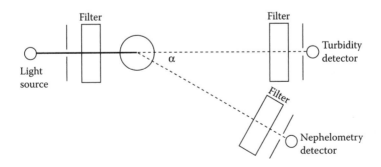

FIGURE 26.5 Nephelometer. Light scattered by large molecules is measured at an angle α away from the axis of incident light. The filters select the wavelength range desired and block undesired fluorescence. When $\alpha = 0$, the technique is known as turbidimetry.

Defining Terms

Accuracy: The degree to which the average value of repeated measurements approximate the true value
being measured.

Fluorescence: Emission of light by an atom or molecule following absorption of a photon by greater
energy. Emission normally occurs within 10^{-8} of absorption.

Nephelometry: Measurement of the amount of light scattered by particles suspended in a fluid.

Precision: A measure of test reproducibility.

Sensitivity: A measure of how small an amount or concentration of an analyte can be detected.

Specificity: A measure of how well a test detects the intended analyte without being "fooled" by other
substances in the sample.

Turbidimetry: Measurement of the attenuation of a light beam due to light lost to scattering by particles
suspended in a fluid.

References

1. Burtis C.A. and Ashwood E.R. (Eds.) 1994. *Tietz Textbook of Clinical Chemistry*, 2nd ed., Philadelphia,
W.B. Saunders.
2. Hicks M.R., Haven M.C., and Schenken J.R. et al. (Eds.) 1987. *Laboratory Instrumentation*, 3rd ed.,
Philadelphia, Lippincott.
3. Kaplan L.A. and Pesce A.J. (Eds.) 1989. *Clinical Chemistry: Theory, Analysis, and Correlation*, 2nd
ed., St. Louis, Mosby.
4. Tietz N.W. (Ed.) 1987. *Fundamentals of Clinical Chemistry*, 3rd ed., Philadelphia, W.B. Saunders.
5. Ward J.M., Lehmann C.A., and Leiken A.M. 1994. *Clinical Laboratory Instrumentation and
Automation: Principles, Applications, and Selection*, Philadelphia, W.B. Saunders.

27

Clinical Laboratory: Nonspectral Methods and Automation

Richard L. Roa
Baylor University Medical Center

27.1 Particle Counting and Identification

The Coulter principle was the first major advance in automating blood cell counts. The cells to be counted are drawn through a small aperture between two fluid compartments, and the electric impedance between the two compartments is monitored (see Figure 27.1). As cells pass through the aperture, the impedance increases in proportion to the volume of the cell, allowing large numbers of cells to be counted and sized rapidly. Red cells are counted by pulling diluted blood through the aperture. Since red cells greatly outnumber white cells, the contribution of white cells to the red cell count is usually neglected. White cells are counted by first destroying the red cells and using a more concentrated sample.

Modern cell counters using the Coulter principle often use *hydrodynamic focusing* to improve the performance of the instrument. A sheath fluid is introduced which flows along the outside of a channel with the sample stream inside it. By maintaining laminar flow conditions and narrowing the channel, the sample stream is focused into a very thin column with the cells in single file. This eliminates problems with cells flowing along the side of the aperture or sticking to it and minimizes problems with having more than one cell in the aperture at a time.

Flow cytometry is a method for characterizing, counting, and separating cells which are suspended in a fluid. The basic flow cytometer uses hydrodynamic focusing to produce a very thin stream of fluid containing cells moving in single file through a quartz flow chamber (Figure 27.2). The cells are characterized on the basis of their scattering and fluorescent properties. This simultaneous measurement of scattering and fluorescence is accomplished with a sophisticated optical system that detects light from the sample both at the wavelength of the excitation source (scattering) as well as at longer wavelengths (fluorescence) at more than one angle. Analysis of these measurements produces parameters related

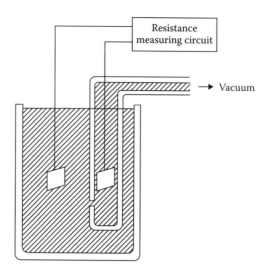

FIGURE 27.1 Coulter method. Blood cells are surrounded by an insulating membrane, which makes them non-conductive. The resistance of electrolyte-filled channel will increase slightly as cells flow through it. This resistance variation yields both the total number of cells which flow through the channel and the volume of each cell.

to the cells' size, granularity, and natural or tagged fluorescence. High-pressure mercury or xenon arc lamps can be used as light sources, but the argon laser (488 nm) is the preferred source for high-performance instruments.

One of the more interesting features of this technology is that particular cells may be selected at rates that allow collection of quantities of particular cell types adequate for further chemical testing. This is accomplished by breaking the outgoing stream into a series of tiny droplets using piezoelectric vibration. By charging the stream of droplets and then using deflection plates controlled by the cell analyzer, the cells of interest can be diverted into collection vessels.

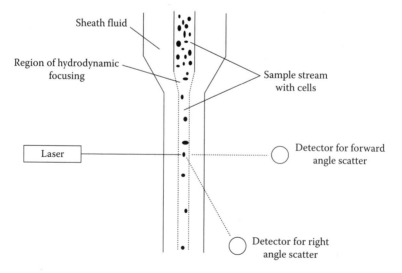

FIGURE 27.2 Flow cytometer. By combining hydrodynamic focusing, state-of-the-art optics, fluorescent labels, and high-speed computing, large numbers of cells can be characterized and sorted automatically.

The development of monoclonal antibodies coupled with flow cytometry allows for quantitation of T and B cells to assess the status of the immune system as well as characterization of leukemias, lymphomas, and other disorders.

27.2 Electrochemical Methods

Electrochemical methods are increasingly popular in the clinical laboratory, for measurement not only of electrolytes, blood gases, and pH but also of simple compounds such as glucose. *Potentiometry* is a method in which a voltage is developed across electrochemical cells as shown in Figure 27.3. This voltage is measured with little or no current flow.

Ideally, one would like to measure all potentials between the reference solution in the indicator electrode and the test solution. Unfortunately there is no way to do that. Interface potentials develop across any metal–liquid boundary, across liquid junctions, and across the ion-selective membrane. The key to making potentiometric measurements is to ensure that all the potentials are constant and do not vary with the composition of the test solution except for the potential of interest across the ion-selective membrane. By maintaining the solutions within the electrodes constant, the potential between these solutions and the metal electrodes immersed in them is constant. The liquid junction is a structure which severely limits bulk flow of the solution but allows free passage of all ions between the solutions. The reference electrode commonly is filled with saturated KCl, which produces a small, constant liquid-junction potential. Thus, any change in the measured voltage (V) is due to a change in the ion concentration in the test solution for which the membrane is selective.

The potential which develops across an ion-selective membrane is given by the Nernst equation:

$$V = \left(\frac{RT}{zF}\right)\ln\frac{a_2}{a_1}$$

(27.1)

where R is the gas constant = 8.314 J/K mol, T = the temperature in K, z = the ionization number, F = the Faraday constant = 9.649×10^4 C/mol, a_n = the activity of ion in solution n. When one of the solutions is a reference solution, this equation can be rewritten in a convenient form as

$$V = V_0 + \frac{N}{z}\log_{10} a$$

(27.2)

where V_0 is the constant voltage due to reference solution and N the Nernst slope ≈ 59 mV/decade at room temperature. The actual Nernst slope is usually slightly less than the theoretical value. Thus, the typical

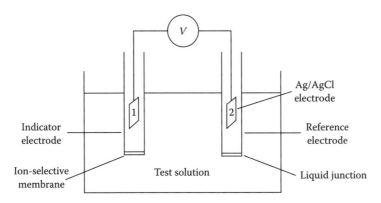

FIGURE 27.3 Electrochemical cell.

pH meter has two calibration controls. One adjusts the offset to account for the value of V_0, and the other adjusts the range to account for both temperature effects and deviations from the theoretical Nernst slope.

27.3 Ion-Specific Electrodes

Ion-selective electrodes use membranes which are permeable only to the ion being measured. To the extent that this can be done, the specificity of the electrode can be very high. One way of overcoming a lack of specificity for certain electrodes is to make multiple simultaneous measurement of several ions which include the most important interfering ones. A simple algorithm can then make corrections for the interfering effects. This technique is used in some commercial electrolyte analyzers. A partial list of the ions that can be measured with ion-selective electrodes includes H^+ (pH), Na^+, K^+, Li^+, Ca^{2+}, Cl^-, F^-, NH_4^+, and CO_2.

NH_4^+, and CO_2 are both measured with a modified ion-selective electrode. They use a pH electrode modified with a thin layer of a solution (sodium bicarbonate for CO_2 and ammonium chloride for NH_4^+) whose pH varies depending on the concentration of ammonium ions or CO_2 it is equilibrated with. A thin membrane holds the solution against the pH glass electrode and provides for equilibration with the sample solution. Note that the CO_2 electrode in Figure 27.4 is a combination electrode. This means that both the reference and indicating electrodes have been combined into one unit. Most pH electrodes are made as combination electrodes.

The Clark electrode measures pO_2 by measuring the current developed by an electrode with an applied voltage rather than a voltage measurement. This is an example of *amperometry*. In this electrode a voltage of approximately -0.65 V is applied to a platinum electrode relative to an Ag/AgCl electrode in an electrolyte solution. The reaction

$$O_2 + 2H^+ + 2e^- \rightarrow H_2O_2$$

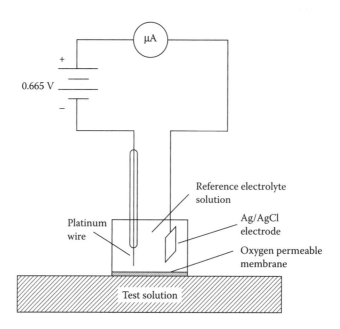

FIGURE 27.4 Clark electrode.

proceeds at a rate proportional to the partial pressure of oxygen in the solution. The electrons involved in this reaction form a current which is proportional to the rate of the reaction and thus to the pO_2 in the solution.

27.4 Radioactive Methods

Isotopes are atoms which have identical atomic number (number of protons) but different atomic mass numbers (protons + neutrons). Since they have the same number of electrons in the neutral atom, they have identical chemical properties. This provides an ideal method for labeling molecules in a way that allows for detection at extremely low concentrations. Labeling with radioactive isotopes is extensively used in radioimmunoassays where the amount of antigen bound to specific antibodies is measured. The details of radioactive decay are complex, but for our purposes there are three types of emission from decaying nuclei: *alpha, beta,* and *gamma radiation*. Alpha particles are made up of two neutrons and two protons (helium nucleus). Alpha emitters are rarely used in the clinical laboratory. Beta emission consists of electrons or positrons emitted from the nucleus. They have a continuous range of energies up to a maximum value characteristic of the isotope. *Beta radiation* is highly interactive with matter and cannot penetrate very far in most materials. Gamma radiation is a high-energy form of electromagnetic radiation. This type of radiation may be continuous, discrete, or mixed depending on the details of the decay process. It has greater penetrating ability than beta radiation (see Figure 27.5).

The kinetic energy spectrum of emitted radiation is characteristic of the isotope. The energy is commonly measured in electron volts (eV). One electron volt is the energy acquired by an electron falling through a potential of 1 V. The isotopes commonly used in the clinical laboratory have energy spectra which range from 18 keV to 3.6 MeV.

The activity of a quantity of radioactive isotope is defined as the number of disintegrations per second which occur. The usual units are the curie (Ci), which is defined as 3.7×10^{10} dps, and the becquerel (Bq), defined as 1 dps. Specific activity for a given isotope is defined as activity per unit mass of the isotope.

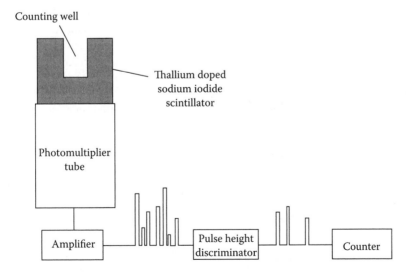

FIGURE 27.5 Gamma counted. The intensity of the light flash produced when a gamma photon interacts with a scintillator is proportional to the energy of the photon. The photomultiplier tube converts these light flashes into electric pulses which can be selected according to size (gamma energy) and counted.

The rate of decay for a given isotope is characterized by the decay constant λ, which is the proportion of the isotope which decays in unit time. Thus, the rate of loss of radioactive isotope is governed by the equation

$$\frac{dN}{dt} = -\lambda N \tag{27.3}$$

where N is the amount of radioactive isotope present at time t. The solution to this differential equation is

$$N = N_0 \, e^{-\lambda t} \tag{27.4}$$

It can easily be shown that the amount of radioactive isotope present will be reduced by half after time

$$t_{1/2} = \frac{0.693}{\lambda} \tag{27.5}$$

This is known as the half-life for the isotope and can vary widely; for example, carbon-14 has a half-life of 5760 years, and iodine-131 has a half-life of 8.1 days.

The most common method for detection of radiation in the clinical laboratory is by *scintillation*. This is the conversion of radiation energy into photons in the visible or near-UV range. These are detected with photomultiplier tubes.

For gamma radiation, the scintillating crystal is made of sodium iodide doped with about 1% thallium, producing 20–30 photons for each electron-volt of energy absorbed. The photomultiplier tube and amplifier circuit produce voltage pulses proportional to the energy of the absorbed radiation. These voltage pulses are usually passed through a pulse-height analyzer which eliminates pulses outside a preset energy range (window). Multichannel analyzers can discriminate between two or more isotopes if they have well-separated energy maxima. There generally will be some spill down of counts from the higher-energy isotope into the lower-energy isotope's window, but this effect can be corrected with a simple algorithm. Multiple well detectors with up to 64 detectors in an array are available which increase the throughput for counting systems greatly. Counters using the sodium iodide crystal scintillator are referred to as gamma counters or well counters.

The lower energy and short penetration ability of beta particles requires a scintillator in direct contact with the decaying isotope. This is accomplished by dissolving or suspending the sample in a liquid fluor. Counters which use this technique are called beta counters or liquid scintillation counters.

Liquid scintillation counters use two photomultiplier tubes with a coincidence circuit that prevents counting of events seen by only one of the tubes. In this way, false counts due to chemiluminescence and noise in the phototube are greatly reduced. Quenching is a problem in all liquid scintillation counters. Quenching is any process which reduces the efficiency of the scintillation counting process, where efficiency is defined as

$$\text{Efficiency} = \text{counts per minute/decays per minute} \tag{27.6}$$

A number of techniques have been developed that automatically correct for quenching effects to produce estimates of true decays per minute from the raw counts. Currently there is a trend away from beta-emitting isotopic labels, but these assays are still used in many laboratories.

27.5 Coagulation Timers

Screening for and diagnosis of coagulation disorders is accomplished by assays that determine how long it takes for blood to clot following initiation of the clotting cascade by various reagents. A variety of instruments have been designed to automate this procedure. In addition to increasing the speed and throughput of such testing, these instruments improve the reproducibility of such tests. All the instruments provide precise introduction of reagents, accurate timing circuits, and temperature control. They differ in the method for detecting clot formation. One of the older methods still in use is to dip a small metal hook into the blood sample repeatedly and lift it a few millimeters above the surface. The electric resistance between the hook and the sample is measured, and when fibrin filaments form, they produce a conductive pathway which is detected as clot formation. Other systems detect the increase in viscosity due to fibrin formation or the scattering due to the large polymerized molecules formed. Absorption and fluorescence spectroscopy can also be used for clot detection.

27.6 Osmometers

The *colligative properties* of a solution are a function of the number of solute particles present regardless of size or identity. Increased solute concentration causes an increase in osmotic pressure and boiling point and a decrease in vapor pressure and freezing point. Measuring these changes provides information on the total solute concentration regardless of type. The most accurate and popular method used in clinical laboratories is the measurement of freezing point depression. With this method, the sample is supercooled to a few degrees below 0°C while being stirred gently. Freezing is then initiated by vigorous stirring. The heat of fusion quickly brings the solution to a slushy state where an equilibrium exists between ice and liquid, ensuring that the temperature is at the freezing point. This temperature is measured. A solute concentration of 1 osmol/kg water produces a freezing point depression of 1.858°C. The measured temperature depression is easily calibrated in units of milliosmols/kg water.

The vapor pressure depression method has the advantage of smaller sample size. However, it is not as precise as the freezing point method and cannot measure the contribution of volatile solutes such as ethanol. This method is not used as widely as the freezing point depression method in clinical laboratories.

Osmolality of blood is primarily due to electrolytes such as Na^+ and Cl^-. Proteins with molecular weights of 30,000 or more atomic mass units (amu) contribute very little to total osmolality due to their smaller numbers (a single Na^+ ion contributes just as much to osmotic pressure as a large protein molecule). However, the contribution to osmolality made by proteins is of great interest when monitoring conditions leading to pulmonary edema. This value is known as colloid osmotic pressure, or oncotic pressure, and is measured with a membrane permeable to water and all molecules smaller than about 30,000 amu. By placing a reference saline solution on one side and the unknown sample on the other, an osmotic pressure is developed across the membrane. This pressure is measured with a pressure transducer and can be related to the true colloid osmotic pressure through a calibration procedure using known standards.

27.7 Automation

Improvements in technology coupled with increased demand for laboratory tests as well as pressures to reduce costs have led to the rapid development of highly automated laboratory instruments. Typical automated instruments contain mechanisms for measuring, mixing, and transport of samples and reagents, measurement systems, and one or more microprocessors to control the entire system. In addition to system control, the computer systems store calibration curves, match test results to specimen IDs, and generate reports. Automated instruments are dedicated to complete blood counts, coagulation studies, microbiology assays, and immunochemistry, as well as high-volume instruments used in clinical chemistry laboratories. The chemistry analyzers tend to fall into one of four classes: continuous flow, centrifugal, pack-based, and dry-slide-based systems. The continuous flow systems pass successive samples and reagents through a single set of tubing, where they are directed to appropriate mixing, dialyzing, and measuring stations. Carry-over from one sample to the next is minimized by the introduction of air bubbles and wash solution between samples.

Centrifugal analyzers use plastic rotors which serve as reservoirs for samples and reagents and also as cuvettes for optical measurements. Spinning the plastic rotor mixes, incubates, and transports the test solution into the cuvette portion of the rotor, where the optical measurements are made while the rotor is spinning.

Pack-based systems are those in which each test uses a special pack with the proper reagents and sample preservation devices built-in. The sample is automatically introduced into as many packs as tests required. The packs are then processed sequentially.

Dry chemistry analyzers use no liquid reagents. The reagents and other sample preparation methods are layered onto a slide. The liquid sample is placed on the slide, and after a period of time the color developed is read by reflectance photometry. Ion-selective electrodes have been incorporated into the same slide format.

There are a number of technological innovations found in many of the automated instruments. One innovation is the use of fiberoptic bundles to channel excitation energy toward the sample as well as transmitted, reflected, or emitted light away from the sample to the detectors. This provides a great deal of flexibility in instrument layout. Multiwavelength analysis using a spinning filter wheel or diode array detectors is commonly found. The computers associated with these instruments allow for innovative improvements in the assays. For instance, when many analytes are being analyzed from one sample, the interference effects of one analyte on the measurement of another can be predicted and corrected before the final report is printed.

27.8 Trends in Laboratory Instrumentation

Predicting the future direction of laboratory instrumentation is difficult, but there seem to be some clear trends. Decentralization of the laboratory functions will continue with more instruments being located in or around ICUs, operating rooms, emergency rooms, and physician offices. More electrochemistry-based tests will be developed. The flame photometer is already being replaced with ion-selective electrode methods. Instruments which analyze whole blood rather than *plasma* or *serum* will reduce the amount of time required for sample preparation and will further encourage testing away from the central laboratory. Dry reagent methods increasingly will replace wet chemistry methods. Radioimmunoassays will continue to decline with the increasing use of methods for performing immunoassays that do not rely upon radioisotopes such as enzyme-linked fluorescent assays. Books by Burtis and Ashwood (1994), Hicks et al. (1987), Kaplan and Pesce (1989), and Tietz (1987) give an overview of the concepts in this chapter.

Defining Terms

Alpha radiation: Particulate radiation consisting of a helium nucleus emitted from a decaying a nucleus.
Amperometry: Measurements based on current flow produced in an electrochemical cell by an applied voltage.
Beta radiation: Particulate radiation consisting of an electron or positron emitted from a decaying nucleus.
Colligative properties: Physical properties that depend on the number of molecules present rather than on their individual properties.
Gamma radiation: Electromagnetic radiation emitted from an atom undergoing nuclear decay.
Hydrodynamic focusing: A process in which a fluid stream is first surrounded by a second fluid and then narrowed to a thin stream by a narrowing of the channel.
Isotopes: Atoms with the same number of protons but differing numbers of neutrons.
Plasma: The liquid portion of blood.
Potentiometry: Measurement of the potential produced by electrochemical cells under equilibrium conditions with no current flow.

Scintillation: The conversion of the kinetic energy of a charged particle or photon to a flash of light.
Serum: The liquid portion of blood remaining after clotting has occurred.

References

Burtis C.A. and Ashwood E.R. (Eds.) 1994. *Tietz Textbook of Clinical Chemistry,* 2nd ed., Philadelphia, Saunders Company.

Hicks M.R., Haven M.C., Schenken J.R. et al. (Eds.) 1987. *Laboratory Instrumentation,* 3rd ed., Philadelphia, Lippincott Company, 1987.

Kaplan L.A. and Pesce A.J. (Eds.) 1989. *Clinical Chemistry: Theory, Analysis, and Correlation,* 2nd ed., St. Louis, Mosby.

Tietz N.W. (Ed.). 1987. *Fundamentals of Clinical Chemistry,* 3rd ed., Philadelphia, W.B. Saunders.

Ward J.M., Lehmann C.A., and Leiken A.M. 1994. *Clinical Laboratory Instrumentation and Automation: Principles, Applications, and Selection,* Philadelphia, W.B. Saunders.

28

Noninvasive Optical Monitoring

Ross Flewelling
Nellcor Inc.

28.1 Introduction

Optical measures of physiologic status are attractive because they can provide a simple, noninvasive, yet real-time assessment of medical condition. Noninvasive optical monitoring is taken here to mean the use of visible or near-infrared light to directly assess the internal physiologic status of a person without the need of extracting a blood of tissue sample or using a catheter. Liquid water strongly absorbs ultraviolet and infrared radiation, and thus these spectral regions are useful only for analyzing thin surface layers or respiratory gases, neither of which will be the subject of this review. Instead, it is the visible and near-infrared portions of the electromagnetic spectrum that provide a unique "optical window" into the human body, opening new vistas for noninvasive monitoring technologies.

Various molecules in the human body possess distinctive spectral absorption characteristics in the visible or near-infrared spectral regions and therefore make optical monitoring possible. The most strongly absorbing molecules at physiologic concentrations are the hemoglobins, myoglobins, *cytochromes*, melanins, carotenes, and bilirubin (see Figure 28.1 for some examples). Perhaps less appreciated are the less distinctive and weakly absorbing yet ubiquitous materials possessing spectral characteristics in the near-infrared: water, fat, proteins, and sugars. Simple optical methods are now available to quantitatively and noninvasively measure some of these compounds directly in intact tissue. The most successful methods to date have used hemoglobins to assess the oxygen content of blood, cytochromes to assess the respiratory status of cells, and possibly near-infrared to assess endogenous concentrations of metabolites, including glucose.

28.2 Oximetry and Pulse Oximetry

Failure to provide adequate oxygen to tissues—*hypoxia*—can in a matter of minutes result in reduced work capacity of muscles, depressed mental activity, and ultimately cell death. It is therefore of considerable interest to reliably and accurately determine the amount of oxygen in blood or tissues. *Oximetry* is

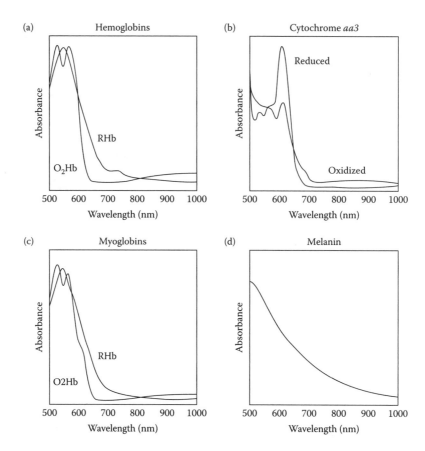

FIGURE 28.1 Absorption spectra of some endogenous biologic materials: (a) hemoglobins, (b) cytochrome *aa3*, (c) myoglobins, and (d) melanin.

the determination of the oxygen content of blood of tissues, normally by optical means. In the clinical laboratory the oxygen content of whole blood can be determined by a bench-top cooximeter or blood gas analyzer. But the need for timely clinical information and the desire to minimize the inconvenience and cost of extracting a blood sample and later analyze it in the lab has led to the search for alternative noninvasive optical methods. Since the 1930s, attempts have been made to use multiple wavelengths of light to arrive at a complete spectral characterization of a tissue. These approaches, although somewhat successful, have remained of limited utility owing to the awkward instrumentation and unreliable results.

It was not until the invention of *pulse oximetry* in the 1970s and its commercial development and application in the 1980s that noninvasive oximetry became practical. Pulse oximetry is an extremely easy-to-use, noninvasive, and accurate measurement of real-time arterial oxygen saturation. Pulse oximetry is now used routinely in clinical practice, has become a standard of care in all U.S. operating rooms, and is increasingly used wherever critical patients are found. The explosive growth of this new technology and its considerable utility led John Severinghaus and Poul Astrup (1986, p. 287) in an excellent historical review to conclude that pulse oximetry was "arguably the most significant technological advance ever made in monitoring the well-being and safety of patients during anesthesia, recovery and critical care."

28.2.1 Background

The partial pressure of oxygen (pO_2) in tissues need only be about 3 mmHg to support basic metabolic demands. This tissue level, however, requires capillary pO_2 to be near 40 mmHg, with a corresponding arterial pO_2 of about 95 mmHg. Most of the oxygen carried by blood is stored in red blood cells reversibly bound to hemoglobin molecules. Oxygen saturation (SaO_2) is defined as the percentage of hemoglobin-bound oxygen compared to the total amount of hemoglobin available for reversible oxygen binding. The relationship between the oxygen partial pressure in blood and the oxygen saturation of blood is given by the hemoglobin oxygen dissociation curve as shown in Figure 28.2. The higher the pO_2 in blood, the higher the SaO_2. But due to the highly cooperative binding of four oxygen molecules to each hemoglobin molecule, the oxygen binding curve is sigmoidal, and consequently the SaO_2 value is particularly sensitive to dangerously low pO_2 levels. With a normal arterial blood pO_2 above 90 mmHg, the oxygen saturation should be at least 95%, and a pulse oximeter can readily verify a safe oxygen level. If oxygen content falls, say to a pO_2 below 40 mmHg, metabolic needs may not be met, and the corresponding oxygen saturation will drop below 80%. Pulse oximetry therefore provides a direct measure of oxygen sufficiency and will alert the clinician to any danger of imminent hypoxia in a patient.

Although endogenous molecular oxygen is not optically observable, hemoglobin serves as an oxygen-sensitive "dye" such that when oxygen reversibly binds to the iron atom in the large heme prosthetic group, the electron distribution of the heme is shifted, producing a significant color change. The optical absorption of hemoglobin in its oxygenated and deoxygenated states is shown in Figure 28.1. Fully oxygenated blood absorbs strongly in the blue and appears bright red; deoxygenated blood absorbs through the visible region and is very dark (appearing blue when observed through tissue due to light scattering effects). Thus the optical absorption spectra of oxyhemoglobin (O_2Hb) and "reduced" deoxyhemoglobin (RHb) differ substantially, and this difference provides the basis for spectroscopic determinations of the proportion of the two hemoglobin states. In addition to these two normal functional hemoglobins, there are also *dysfunctional hemoglobins*—carboxyhemoglobin, methemoglobin, and sulfhemoglobin—which are spectroscopically distinct but do not bind oxygen reversibly. Oxygen saturation is therefore defined in Equation 28.1 only in terms of the *functional saturation* with respect to O_2Hb and RHb:

$$SaO_2 = \frac{O_2Hb}{RHb + O_2Hb} \times 100\% \qquad (28.1)$$

Cooximeters are bench-top analyzers that accept whole blood samples and utilize four or more wavelengths of monochromatic light, typically between 500 and 650 nm, to spectroscopically determine the various individual hemoglobins in the sample. If a blood sample can be provided, this spectroscopic method is accurate and reliable. Attempts to make an equivalent quantitative analysis noninvasively

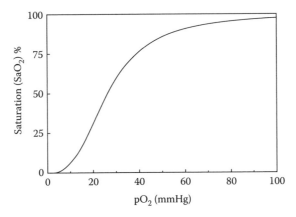

FIGURE 28.2 Hemoglobin oxygen dissociation curve showing the sigmoidal relationship between the partial pressure of oxygen and the oxygen saturation of blood. The curve is given approximately by $\%SaO_2 = 100\%/[1 + P_{50}/pO_2^n]$, with $n = 2.8$ and $P_{50} = 26$ mmHg.

through intact tissue have been fraught with difficulty. The problem has been to contend with the wide variation in scattering and nonspecific absorption properties of very complex heterogeneous tissue. One of the more successful approaches, marketed by Hewlett–Packard, used eight optical wavelengths transmitted through the pinna of the ear. In this approach a "bloodless" measurement is first obtained by squeezing as much blood as possible from an area of tissue; the arterial blood is then allowed to flow back, and the oxygen saturation is determined by analyzing the change in the spectral absorbance characteristics of the tissue. While this method works fairly well, it is cumbersome, operator dependent, and does not always work well on poorly perfused or highly pigmented subjects.

In the early 1970s, Takuo Aoyagi recognized that most of the interfering nonspecific tissue effects could be eliminated by utilizing only the change in the signal during an arterial pulse. Although an early prototype was built in Japan, it was not until the refinements in implementation and application by Biox (now Ohmeda) and Nellcor Incorporated in the 1980s that the technology became widely adopted as a safety monitor for critical care use.

28.2.2 Theory

Pulse oximetry is based on the fractional change in light transmission during an arterial pulse at two different wavelengths. In this method the fractional change in the signal is due only to the arterial blood itself, and therefore the complicated nonpulsatile and highly variable optical characteristics of tissue are eliminated. In a typical configuration, light at two different wavelengths illuminating one side of a finger will be detected on the other side, after having traversed the intervening vascular tissues (Figure 28.3). The transmission of light at each wavelength is a function of the thickness, color, and structure of the skin, tissue, bone, blood, and other material through which the light passes. The absorbance of light by a sample is defined as the negative logarithm of the ratio of the light intensity in the presence of the sample (I) to that without (I_0): $A = -\log(I/I_0)$. According to the *Beer–Lambert law*, the absorbance of a sample at a given wavelength with a molar absorptivity (ε) is directly proportional to both the concentration (c) and pathlength (l) of the absorbing material: $A = \varepsilon c l$. (In actuality, biologic tissue is highly scattering, and the Beer–Lambert law is only approximately correct; see the references for further elaboration). Visible or near-infrared light passing through about one centimeter of tissue (e.g., a finger) will be attenuated by about one or two orders of magnitude for a typical emitter–detector geometry, corresponding to an effective optical density (OD) of 1–2 OD (the detected light intensity is decreased by one order of magnitude for each OD unit). Although hemoglobin in the blood is the single strongest absorbing molecule, most of the total attenuation is due to the scattering of light away from the detector by the highly heterogeneous tissue. Since human tissue contains about 7% blood, and since

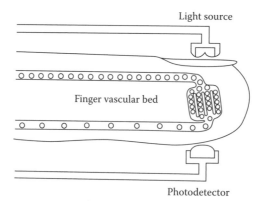

FIGURE 28.3 Typical pulse oximeter sensing configuration on a finger. Light at two different wavelengths is emitted by the source, diffusely scattered through the finger, and detected on the opposite side by a photodetector.

blood contains typically about 14 g/dL hemoglobin, the effective hemoglobin concentration in tissue is about 1 g/dL (~150 μM). At the wavelengths used for pulse oximetry (650–950 nm), the oxy- and deoxyhemoglobin molar absorptivities fall in the range of 100–1000 $M^{-1}cm^{-1}$, and consequently hemoglobin accounts for less than 0.2 OD of the total observed optical density. Of this amount, perhaps only 10% is pulsatile, and consequently pulse signals of only a few percent are ultimately measured, at times even one-tenth of this.

A mathematical model for pulse oximetry begins by considering light at two wavelengths, λ_1 and λ_2, passing through tissue and being detected at a distant location as in Figure 28.3. At each wavelength the total light attenuation is described by four different component absorbances: oxyhemoglobin in the blood (concentration c_o, molar absorptivity ε_o, and effective pathlength l_o), "reduced" deoxyhemoglobin in the blood (concentration c_r, molar absorptivity ε_r, and effective pathlength l_r), specific variable absorbances that are not from the arterial blood (concentration c_x, molar absorptivity ε_x, and effective pathlength l_x), and all other nonspecific sources of optical attenuation, combined as A_y, which can include light scattering, geometric factors, and characteristics of the emitter and detector elements. The total absorbance at the two wavelengths can then be written:

$$\begin{cases} A_{\lambda_1} = \varepsilon_{o_1} c_o l_o + \varepsilon_{r_1} c_r l_r + \varepsilon_{x_1} c_x l_x + A_{y_1} \\ A_{\lambda_2} = \varepsilon_{o_2} c_o l_o + \varepsilon_{r_2} c_r l_r + \varepsilon_{x_2} c_x l_x + A_{y_2} \end{cases} \tag{28.2}$$

The blood volume change due to the arterial pulse results in a modulation of the measured absorbances. By taking the time rate of change of the absorbances, the two last terms in each equation are effectively zero, since the concentration and effective pathlength of absorbing material outside the arterial blood do not change during a pulse [$d(c_x l_x)/dt = 0$], and all the nonspecific effects on light attenuation are also effectively invariant on the time scale of a cardiac cycle ($dA_y/dt = 0$). Since the extinction coefficients are constant, and the blood concentrations are constant on the time scale of a pulse, the time-dependent changes in the absorbances at the two wavelengths can be assigned entirely to the change in the blood pathlength (dl_o/dt and dl_r/dt). With the additional assumption that these two blood pathlength changes are equivalent (or more generally, their ratio is a constant), the ratio R of the time rate of change of the absorbance at wavelength 1 to that at wavelength 2 reduces to the following:

$$R = \frac{dA_{\lambda_1}/dt}{dA_{\lambda_2}/dt} = \frac{-d\log(I_1/I_o)/dt}{-d\log(I_2/I_o)/dt} = \frac{(\Delta I_1/I_1)}{(\Delta I_2/I_2)} = \frac{\varepsilon_{o_1} c_o + \varepsilon_{r_1} c_r}{\varepsilon_{o_2} c_o + \varepsilon_{r_2} c_r} \tag{28.3}$$

Observing that functional oxygen saturation is given by $S = c_o/(c_o + c_r)$, and that $(1 - S) = c_r/(c_o + c_r)$, the oxygen saturation can then be written in terms of the ratio R as follows

$$S = \frac{\varepsilon_{r1} - \varepsilon_{r2}R}{(\varepsilon_{r1} - \varepsilon_{o1}) - (\varepsilon_{r2} - \varepsilon_{o2})R} \tag{28.4}$$

Equation 28.4 provides the desired relationship between the experimentally determined ratio R and the clinically desired oxygen saturation S. In actual use, commonly available LEDs are used as the light sources, typically a red LED near 660 nm and a near-infrared LED selected in the range 890–950 nm. Such LEDs are not monochromatic light sources, typically with bandwidths between 20 and 50 nm, and therefore standard molar absorptivities for hemoglobin cannot be used directly in Equation 28.4. Further, the simple model presented above is only approximately true; for example, the two wavelengths do not necessarily have the exact same pathlength changes, and second-order scattering effects have

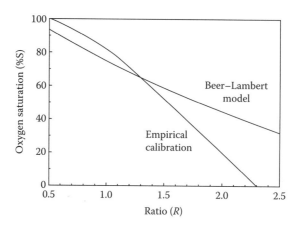

FIGURE 28.4 Relationship between the measured ratio of fractional changes in light intensity at two wavelengths, R, and the oxygen saturation S. Beer–Lambert model is from Equation 28.4 with $\varepsilon_{o1} = 100$, $\varepsilon_{o2} = 300$, $\varepsilon_{r1} = 800$, and $\varepsilon_{r2} = 200$. Empirical calibration is based on $\%S = 100\% \times (a - bR)/(c - dR)$ with $a = 1000$, $b = 550$, $c = 900$, and $d = 350$, with a linear extrapolation below 70%.

been ignored. Consequently the relationship between S and R is instead determined empirically by fitting the clinical data to a generalized function of the form $S = (a - bR)/(c - dR)$. The final empirical calibration will ultimately depend on the details of an individual sensor design, but these variations can be determined for each sensor and included in unique calibration parameters. A typical empirical calibration for R vs. S is shown in Figure 28.4, together with the curve that standard molar absorptivities would predict.

In this way the measurement of the ratio of the fractional change in signal intensity of the two LEDs is used along with the empirically determined calibration equation to obtain a beat-by-beat measurement of the arterial oxygen saturation in a perfused tissue—continuously, noninvasively, and to an accuracy of a few percent.

28.2.3 Application and Future Directions

Pulse oximetry is now routinely used in nearly all operating rooms and critical care areas in the United States and increasingly throughout the world. It has become so pervasive and useful that it is now being called the "fifth" vital sign (for an excellent review of practical aspects and clinical applications of the technology see Kelleher (1989)).

The principal advantages of pulse oximetry are that it provides continuous, accurate, and reliable monitoring of arterial oxygen saturation on nearly all patients, utilizing a variety of convenient sensors, reusable as well as disposable. Single-patient-use adhesive sensors can easily be applied to fingers for adults and children and to arms for legs or neonates. Surface reflectance sensors have also been developed based on the same principles and offer a wider choice for sensor location, though they tend to be less accurate and prone to more types of interference.

Limitations of pulse oximetry include sensitivity to high levels of optical or electric interference, errors due to high concentrations of dysfunctional hemoglobins (methemoglobin or carboxyhemoglobin) or interference from physiologic dyes (such as methylene blue). Other important factors, such as total hemoglobin content, fetal hemoglobin, or sickle cell trait, have little or no effect on the measurement except under extreme conditions. Performance can also be compromised by poor signal quality, as may occur for poorly perfused tissues with weak pulse amplitudes or by motion artifact.

Hardware and software advances continue to provide more sensitive signal detection and filtering capabilities, allowing pulse oximeters to work better on more ambulatory patients. Already some pulse oximeters incorporate ECG synchronization for improved signal processing. A pulse oximeter for use in labor and delivery is currently under active development by several research groups and companies. A likely implementation may include use of a reflectance surface sensor for the fetal head to monitor the adequacy of fetal oxygenation. This application is still in active development, and clinical utility remains to be demonstrated.

28.3 Nonpulsatile Spectroscopy

28.3.1 Background

Nonpulsatile optical spectroscopy has been used for more than half a century for noninvasive medical assessment, such as in the use of multiwavelength tissue analysis for oximetry and skin reflectance measurement for bilirubin assessment in jaundiced neonates. These early applications have found some limited use, but with modest impact. Recent investigations into new nonpulsatile spectroscopy methods for assessment of deep-tissue oxygenation (e.g., cerebral oxygen monitoring), for evaluation of respiratory status at the cellular level, and for the detection of other critical analytes, such as glucose, may yet prove more fruitful. The former applications have led to spectroscopic studies of cytochromes in tissues, and the latter has led to considerable work into new approaches in near-infrared analysis of intact tissues.

28.3.2 Cytochrome Spectroscopy

Cytochromes are electron-transporting, heme-containing proteins found in the inner membranes of mitochondria and are required in the process of oxidative phosphorylation to convert metabolites and oxygen into CO_2 and high-energy phosphates. In this metabolic process the cytochromes are reversibly oxidized and reduced, and consequently the oxidation–reduction states of cytochromes c and aa_3 in particular are direct measures of the respiratory condition of the cell. Changes in the absorption spectra of these molecules, particularly near 600 and 830 nm for cytochrome aa_3, accompany this shift. By monitoring these spectral changes, the cytochrome oxidation state in the tissues can be determined (see, e.g., Jöbsis 1977 and Jöbsis et al. 1977). As with all nonpulsatile approaches, the difficulty is to remove the dependence of the measurements on the various nonspecific absorbing materials and highly variable scattering effects of the tissue. To date, instruments designed to measure cytochrome spectral changes can successfully track relative changes in brain oxygenation, but absolute quantitation has not yet been demonstrated.

28.3.3 Near-Infrared Spectroscopy and Glucose Monitoring

Near-infrared (NIR), the spectral region between 780 and 3000 nm, is characterized by broad and overlapping spectral peaks produced by the overtones and combinations of infrared vibrational modes. Figure 28.5 shows typical NIR absorption spectra of fat, water, and starch. Exploitation of this spectral region for *in vivo* analysis has been hindered by the same complexities of nonpulsatile tissue spectroscopy described above and is further confounded by the very broad and indistinct spectral features characteristic of the NIR. Despite these difficulties, NIR spectroscopy has garnered considerable attention, since it may enable the analysis of common analytes.

Karl Norris and coworkers pioneered the practical application of NIR spectroscopy, using it to evaluate water, fat, and sugar content of agricultural products (see Burns and Cuirczak 1992; Osborne et al. 1993). The further development of sophisticated *multivariate analysis* techniques, together with new scattering models (e.g., Kubelka–Munk theory) and high-performance instrumentation, further extended the application of NIR methods. Over the past decade, many research groups and companies have touted the use of NIR techniques for medical monitoring, such as for determining the relative fat, protein, and water content of tissue, and more recently for noninvasive glucose measurement. The body

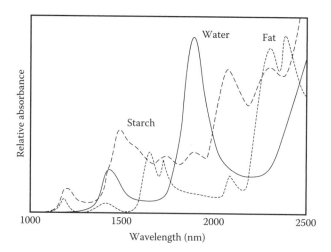

FIGURE 28.5 Typical near-infrared absorption spectra of several biologic materials.

composition analyses are useful but crude and are mainly limited to applications in nutrition and sports medicine. Noninvasive glucose monitoring, however, is of considerable interest.

More than 2 million diabetics in the United States lance their fingers three to six times a day to obtain a drop of blood for chemical glucose determination. The ability of these individuals to control their glucose levels, and the quality of their life generally, would dramatically improve if a simple, noninvasive method for determining blood glucose levels could be developed. Among the noninvasive optical methods proposed for this purpose are optical rotation, NIR analysis, and Raman spectroscopy. The first two have received the most attention. Optical rotation methods aim to exploit the small optical rotation of polarized light by glucose. To measure physiologic glucose levels in a 1-cm thick sample to an accuracy of 25 mg/dL would require instrumentation that can reliably detect an optical rotation of at least 1 millidegree. Finding an appropriate *in vivo* optical path for such measurements has proved most difficult, with most approaches looking to use either the aqueous humor or the anterior chamber of the eye (Coté et al., 1992; Rabinovitch et al., 1982). Although several groups have developed laboratory analyzers that can measure such a small effect, so far *in vivo* measurement has not been demonstrated, due both to unwanted scattering and optical activity of biomaterials in the optical path and to the inherent difficulty in developing a practical instrument with the required sensitivity.

NIR methods for noninvasive glucose determination are particularly attractive, although the task is formidable. Glucose has spectral characteristics near 1500 nm and in the 2000–2500 nm band where many other compounds also absorb, and the magnitude of the glucose absorbance in biologic samples is typically two orders of magnitude lower than those of water, fat, or protein. The normal detection limit for NIR spectroscopy is on the order of one part in 10^3, whereas a change of 25 mg/dL in glucose concentration corresponds to an absorbance change of 10^{-4}–10^{-5}. In fact, the temperature dependence of the NIR absorption of water alone is at least an order of magnitude greater than the signal from glucose in solution. Indeed, some have suggested that the apparent glucose signature in complex NIR spectra may actually be the secondary effect of glucose on the water.

Sophisticated chemometric (particularly multivariate analysis) methods have been employed to try to extract the glucose signal out of the noise (for methods reviews see Martens and Næs (1989) and Haaland (1992)). Several groups have reported using multivariate techniques to quantitate glucose in whole blood samples, with encouraging results (Haaland et al., 1992). And despite all theoretical disputations to the contrary, some groups claim the successful application of these multivariate analysis methods to noninvasive *in vivo* glucose determination in patients (Robinson et al., 1992). Yet even with the many groups working in this area, much of the work remains unpublished, and few if any of the reports have been independently validated.

28.3.4 Time-Resolved Spectroscopy

The fundamental problem in making quantitative optical measurements through intact tissue is dealing with the complex scattering phenomena. This scattering makes it difficult to determine the effective pathlength for the light, and therefore attempts to use the Beer–Lambert law, or even to determine a consistent empirical calibration, continue to be thwarted. Application of new techniques in time-resolved spectroscopy may be able to tackle this problem. Thinking of light as a packet of photons, if a single packet from a light source is sent through tissue, then a distant receiver will detect a photon distribution over time—the photons least scattered arriving first and the photons most scattered arriving later. In principle, the first photons arriving at the detector passed directly through the tissue. For these first photons the distance between the emitter and the detector is fixed and known, and the Beer–Lambert law should apply, permitting determination of an *absolute* concentration for an absorbing component. The difficulty in this is, first, that the measurement time scale must be on the order of the photon transit time (subnanosec), and second, that the number of photons getting through without scattering will be extremely small, and therefore the detector must be exquisitely sensitive. Although these considerable technical problems have been overcome in the laboratory, their implementation in a practical instrument applied to a real subject remains to be demonstrated. This same approach is also being investigated for noninvasive optical imaging, since the unscattered photons should produce sharp images (see Chance et al. 1988, Chance 1991, and Yoo and Alfano 1989).

28.4 Conclusions

The remarkable success of pulse oximetry has established noninvasive optical monitoring of vital physiologic functions as a modality of considerable value. Hardware and algorithm advances in pulse oximetry are beginning to broaden its use outside the traditional operating room and critical care areas. Other promising applications of noninvasive optical monitoring are emerging, such as for measuring deep tissue oxygen levels, determining cellular metabolic status, or for quantitative determination of other important physiologic parameters such as blood glucose. Although these latter applications are not yet practical, they may ultimately impact noninvasive clinical monitoring just as dramatically as pulse oximetry.

Defining Terms

Beer–Lambert law: Principle stating that the optical absorbance of a substance is proportional to both the concentration of the substance and the pathlength of the sample.

Cytochromes: Heme-containing proteins found in the membranes of mitochondria and required for oxidative phosphorylation, with characteristic optical absorbance spectra.

Dysfunctional hemoglobins: Those hemoglobin species that cannot reversibly bind oxygen (carboxyhemoglobin, methemoglobin, and sulfhemoglobin).

Functional saturation: The ratio of oxygenated hemoglobin to total nondysfunctional hemoglobins (oxyhemoglobin plus deoxyhemoglobin).

Hypoxia: Inadequate oxygen supply to tissues necessary to maintain metabolic activity.

Multivariate analysis: Empirical models developed to relate multiple spectral intensities from many calibration samples to known analyte concentrations, resulting in an optimal set of calibration parameters.

Oximetry: The determination of blood or tissue oxygen content, generally by optical means.

Pulse oximetry: The determination of functional oxygen saturation of pulsatile arterial blood by ratiometric measurement of tissue optical absorbance changes.

References

Burns, D.A. and Ciurczak, E.W. (Eds.). 1992. *Handbook of Near-Infrared Analysis*. New York, Marcel Dekker.

Chance, B. 1991. Optical method. *Annu. Rev. Biophys. Biophys. Chem.* 20: 1.

Chance, B., Leigh, J.S., Miyake, H. et al. 1988. Comparison of time-resolved and -unresolved measurements of deoxyhemoglobin in brain. *Proc. Natl Acad. Sci. USA* 85: 4971.

Coté G.L., Fox M.D., and Northrop, R.B. 1992. Noninvasive optical polarimetric glucose sensing using a true phase measurement technique. *IEEE Trans. Biomed. Eng.* 39: 752.

Haaland, D.M. 1992. Multivariate calibration methods applied to the quantitative analysis of infrared spectra. In P.C. Jurs (Ed.), *Computer-Enhanced Analytical Spectroscopy*, Vol. 3, pp. 1–30. New York, Plenum Press.

Haaland, D.M., Robinson, M.R., Koepp, G.W. et al. 1992. Reagentless near-infrared determination of glucose in whole blood using multivariate calibration. *Appl. Spectros.* 46: 1575.

Jöbsis, F.F. 1977. Noninvasive, infrared monitoring of cerebral and myocardial oxygen sufficiency and circulatory parameters. *Science* 198: 1264.

Jöbsis, F.F., Keizer, L.H., LaManna, J.C. et al. 1977. Reflectance spectrophotometry of cytochrome aa_3 in vivo. *J. Appl. Physiol.* 43: 858.

Kelleher, J.F. 1989. Pulse oximetry. *J. Clin. Monit.* 5: 37.

Martens, H. and Næs, T. 1989. *Multivariate Calibration*. New York, John Wiley & Sons.

Osborne, B.G., Fearn, T., and Hindle, P.H. 1993. *Practical NIR Spectroscopy with Applications in Food and Beverage Analysis*. Essex, England, Longman Scientific & Technical.

Payne, J.P. and Severinghaus, J.W. (Eds.). 1986. *Pulse Oximetry*. New York, Springer-Verlag.

Rabinovitch, B., March, W.F., and Adams, R.L. 1982. Noninvasive glucose monitoring of the aqueous humor of the eye: Part I. Measurement of very small optical rotations. *Diabetes Care* 5: 254.

Robinson, M.R., Eaton, R.P., Haaland, D.M. et al. 1992. Noninvasive glucose monitoring in diabetic patients: A preliminary evaluation. *Clin. Chem.* 38: 1618.

Severinghaus, J.W. and Astrup, P.B. 1986. History of blood gas analysis. VI. Oximetry. *J. Clin. Monit.* 2: 135.

Severinghaus, J.W. and Honda, Y. 1987a. History of blood gas analysis. VII. Pulse oximetry. *J. Clin. Monit.* 3: 135.

Severinghaus, J.W. and Honda, Y. 1987b. Pulse oximetry. *Int. Anesthesiol. Clin.* 25: 205.

Severinghaus, J.W. and Kelleher, J.F. 1992. Recent developments in pulse oximetry. *Anesthesiology* 76: 1018.

Tremper, K.K. and Barker, S.J. 1989. Pulse oximetry. *Anesthesiology* 70: 98.

Wukitsch, M.W., Petterson, M.T., Tobler, D.R. et al. 1988. Pulse oximetry: Analysis of theory, technology, and practice. *J. Clin. Monit.* 4: 290.

Yoo, K.M. and Alfano, R.R. 1989. Photon localization in a disordered multilayered system. *Phys. Rev. B* 39: 5806.

Further Information

Two collections of papers on pulse oximetry include a book edited by J.P. Payne and J.W. Severinghaus, *Pulse Oximetry* (New York, Springer-Verlag, 1986), and a journal collection—*International Anesthesiology Clinics* (25, 1987). For technical reviews of pulse oximetry, see J.A. Pologe's, 1987 "Pulse Oximetry" (*Int. Anesthesiol. Clin.* 25: 137), Kevin K. Tremper and Steven J. Barker's, 1989 "Pulse Oximetry" (*Anesthesiology* 70: 98), and Michael W. Wukitsch, Michael T. Patterson, David R. Tobler, and coworkers' 1988 "Pulse Oximetry: Analysis of Theory, Technology, and Practice" (*J. Clin. Monit.* 4: 290).

For a review of practical and clinical applications of pulse oximetry, see the excellent review by Joseph K. Kelleher 1989 and John Severinghaus and Joseph F. Kelleher 1992. John Severinghaus and Yoshiyuki Honda have written several excellent histories of pulse oximetry (1987a, 1987b).

For an overview of applied near-infrared spectroscopy, see Donald A. Burns and Emil W. Ciurczak 1992 and B.G. Osborne, T. Fearn, and P.H. Hindle 1993. For a good overview of multivariate methods, see Harald Martens and Tormod Næs 1989.

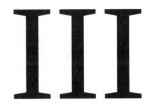

Human Performance Engineering

Donald R. Peterson
Texas A&M University

Preface

The ultimate goal of human performance engineering is the enhancement of performance and safety of humans in the execution of tasks. The more formalized conception of this field was initially fueled by military needs. It has steadily evolved to become an important component in industrial and other settings as well. In a biomedical engineering context, the scope of definition applied to the term "human" not only encompasses individuals with capabilities that differ from those of a typical healthy individual in many possible different ways (e.g., individuals who are disabled, injured, and unusually endowed) but also includes those who are simply "healthy" (e.g., health care professionals). Consequently, one finds a wide range of problems in which human performance engineering and associated methods are employed. A few examples include

- Evaluation of an individual's performance capacities to determine the efficacy of new therapeutic interventions or the so-called level of disability for the worker's compensation and other medical–legal purposes
- Design of assistive devices and work sites in such a way that a person with some deficiency in their performance resource profile will be able to accomplish a given task to a specified level of performance
- Design of operator interfaces for medical instruments that promote efficient, safe, and error-free use

But human performance engineering is not only concerned with situations that are directly linked to a medical context or motivated by a medical problem. Evaluation and optimization of performance in specific sport tasks, work tasks, playing musical instruments, and even education represent relevant application targets. Human performance engineering encompasses the exciting prospect of helping individuals achieve their personal best in selected endeavors. In general, the field encompasses applications in medical and nonmedical contexts.

In basic and most general terms, each of the representative application situations noted involves one or more of the following: (1) a human, (2) a task(s), and (3) the interface of a human to a task(s). Human performance engineering emphasizes concepts, methods, and tools that strive toward the treatment of each of these areas with the same engineering rigor that is routinely applied to artificial systems (e.g., mechanical and electronic). Importance is thus placed on models (a combination of cause and effect and statistical), measurements (of varying degrees of sophistication that are selected to fit needs of a particular circumstance), and diverse types of analyses. Many specialty areas within biomedical engineering begin with an emphasis on a specific subsystem and then proceed to deal with it at lower levels of detail (sometimes even at the molecular level) to determine how it functions and often why it malfunctions. One way of characterizing human performance engineering is to note that it emphasizes subsystems and their performance capacities (i.e., how well a system functions), the integration of these into a whole and their interactions, and their operation in the execution of tasks that are of ultimate concern to humans. These include tasks of daily living, work, and recreation. In recent years, there has been an increased concern within medical communities on issues such as quality of life, treatment outcome measures, and treatment cost-effectiveness. By linking human subsystems into the "whole" and discovering objective quantitative relationships between the human and tasks, human performance engineering can play a leading role in addressing these and other related concerns.

Human performance engineering combines knowledge, expertise, concepts, and methods from across many disciplines (e.g., biomechanics, neuroscience, psychology, physiology, and many others), which, in their overlapping aspect, essentially deal with similar types of problems. For the fourth edition of this section, a total of 11 chapters are presented, three of which (i.e., Chapters 79, 81, and 83) have been substantially updated and revised to ensure the presentation of modern viewpoints and developments. To capture the essence of the problems addressed by human performance engineering and the knowledge base that is unique to it, a conceptual framework is necessary. Few candidate frameworks exist even within the relevant disciplines. To serve this role, Chapter 75 presents the elemental resource model, which was introduced about two decades ago and includes the concepts of general systems performance theory. Its utility and appropriateness have been demonstrated in a variety of situations and has garnered wider acceptance than any other such framework known. In a further attempt to enhance continuity across this section, the authors were encouraged to consider the elemental resource model and to incorporate basic concepts and terms, where applicable. Chapters 76 through 78 look "toward the human" and focus on the measurement of performance capacities of specific groups of human subsystem and related issues. Owing to a combination of the complexity of the human system (even when viewed as a collection of rather high-level subsystems) and limited space available, the treatment is not comprehensive. For example, the measurement of sensory performance capacities (e.g., tactile, visual, and auditory) is not included. Both systems and tasks can be viewed at various hierarchical levels. Chapters 76 and 77 focus on a rather "low" systems level and discuss the basic functional units such as actuator, processor, and memory systems, while Chapter 78 moves to a more intermediate level, where speech, postural control, gait, and hand–eye coordination systems could be considered. The measurement of structural parameters, which play important roles in both performance measurement and many analyses, is also not allocated the separate chapter it deserves (as a minimum) due to space limitations. Chapters 79 and 80 then shift focus to consider the analysis of different types of tasks in a similar, representative fashion. Chapters 81 through 83 are included to provide insight into a representative selection of application types. Space constraints, the complexity of human performance, and the great variety of tasks that can be considered limit the level of detail with which such material can be reasonably presented. Work in all application areas is now benefiting from computer-based tools, which is the underlying theme of Chapter 84. The section concludes with Chapter 85, which is a look to the future and includes a summary of selected limitations, identification of some corresponding research and development needs, and speculation regarding the nature of the anticipated evolution of the field.

Many have contributed their talents to this exciting field in terms of both research and applications; yet, much remains to be done. Much appreciation goes to the authors, not only for their contributions and cooperation during the preparation of this section but also for their willingness to accept the burdens of communicating complex subject matter reasonably, selectively, and as accurately as possible within the imposed constraints.

George V. Kondraske
Original preface author, Third edition
University of Texas, Arlington
Arlington, Texas

Fourth edition preface edited by Donald R. Peterson
Texas A&M University
Texarkana, Texas

The Elemental Resource Model for Human Performance

George V. Kondraske
*University of Texas,
Arlington*

29.1 Introduction

Humans are complex *systems*. Our natural interest in things and ourselves that we do has given rise to the study of this complex system at every conceivable level ranging from genetic, through cellular and organ systems, to interactions of the total human with the environment in the conduct of purposeful activities. At each level, there are corresponding practitioners who attempt to discover and rectify or prevent problems at the respective level. Some practitioners are concerned with specific individuals, while others (e.g., biomedical scientists and product designers) address populations as a whole. Problems dealt with span medical and nonmedical contexts, often with interaction between the two. Models play a key role not only in understanding the key issues at each level, but also in describing relationships between various levels and in providing frameworks that allow practitioners to obtain reasonably predictable results in a systematic and efficient fashion. In this chapter, a working model for human system–*task* interfaces is presented. Any such model must, of course, consider not only the interface per se, but also representations of the human system and tasks. The model presented here, the Elemental Resource Model (ERM), represents the most recent effort in a relatively small family of models that attempt to address similar needs.

29.1.1 Background

The interface of a human to a task of daily living (e.g., work, recreation, or other) represents a level that is quite high in the hierarchy noted above. One way in which to summarize previous efforts directed at this level, across various application contexts, is to recognize two different lines along which study has evolved (1) bottom-up and (2) top-down. Taken together, these relative terms imply a focus of interest at a particular level of convergence, which, here, is the human–task interface level. It is emphasized that these terms are used here to characterize the general course of development and not specific approaches applied at a particular instant of time. A broad view is necessary to grapple with the many previous efforts that either are, or could be, construed to be pertinent.

The biomedical community has approached the human–task interface largely along the "bottom-up" path. This is not surprising given the historical evolution of interest first in anatomy (human structure) and then physiology (*function*). The introduction of chemistry, giving rise to biochemistry, and the refinement of the microscope provided motivations to include even lower hierarchical levels of inquiry and of a substantially different character. Models in this broad "bottom-up" category begin with *anatomical components* and include muscles, nerves, tendons (or subcomponents thereof), or subsets of organs (e.g., heart, lungs, vasculature, etc.). They often focus on relationships between components and exhibit a scope that stays within the confines of the human system. Many cause-and-effect models have been developed at these lower levels for specific purposes (e.g., to understand lines of action of muscle forces and their changes during motion about a given joint).

As a natural consequence of linkages that occur between hierarchical levels and our tendency to utilize that which exists, consideration of an issue at any selected level (in this case, the human–task interface level) brings into consideration *all lower levels* and all models that have been put forth with the stated purpose of understanding problems or behaviors at the original level of focus. The amount of detail that is appropriate or required at these original, lower levels results in great complexity when applied to the total human at the human–task interface level. In addition, many lower-level modeling efforts (even those which are quantitative) are aimed primarily at obtaining a basic scientific understanding of human physiology or specific pathologies (i.e., pertaining to *populations* of humans). In such circumstances, highly specialized, invasive, and cumbersome laboratory procedures for obtaining the necessary data to populate models are justified. However, it is difficult and sometimes impossible to obtain data describing *a specific individual* to be utilized in analyses when such models are extended to the human–task interface level. Another result of drawing lower-level models (and their approaches) into the human–task interface context is that the results have a specific and singular character (e.g., biomechanical vs. neuromuscular control vs. psychologic, etc.) (e.g., Card et al., 1986; Hemami, 1988; Schoner and Kelso, 1988; Gottlieb et al., 1989; Delp et al., 1990). Models that incorporate most or all of the multiple aspects of the human system or frameworks for integrating multiple lower-level modeling approaches have been lacking. Lower-level models that serve meaningful purposes at the original level of focus have provided and will continue to provide insights into specific issues related to human *performance* at multiple levels of consideration. However, their direct extension to serve general needs at the human–task interface level has inherent problems; a different approach is suggested.

A "top-down" progression can be observed over the major history in human factors/ergonomic (Taylor, 1911; Gilbreth and Gilbreth, 1917) and vocational assessment (e.g., Botterbusch, 1987) fields (although the former has more recently emphasized a "human-centered" concept with regard to design applications). In contrast to the bottom-up path in which anatomical components form the initial basis of modeling efforts, the focus along the top-down developmental path begins with consideration of the *task or job* which is to be performed by the total human. The great variety in the full breadth of activities in which humans can be engaged gives rise to one aspect of complexity at this level that pertains to taxonomies for job and task classification (e.g., Fleishman and Quaintance, 1984; Meister, 1989; U.S. Department of Labor, 1992). Another enigmatic aspect that quickly adds complexity with respect to modeling concerns the appropriate level to be used to dissect the items (e.g., jobs) at the highest level into lower level components (e.g., tasks and subtasks). In fact, the choice of level is complicated by the fact that no clear definition has evolved for a set of levels from which to choose.

After progressing through various levels at which all model elements represent tasks and are completely outside the confines of the human body, a level is eventually reached where one encounters the human. Attempts to go further have been motivated, for example, by desires to predict performance of a human in a given task (e.g., lifting an object, assembling a product, etc.) from a set of measures that characterizes the human. From the human–task interface, difficulty is encountered with regard to the strategy for approaching a system as complex, multifaceted, and multipurpose as a human (Fleishman and Quaintance, 1984; Wickens, 1984). In essence, the full scope of options that have emerged from the bottom-up development path are now encountered from the opposite direction. Options range from relatively gross analyses (e.g., estimates of the "fraction" of a task that is physical or mental) to those which are much more detailed and quantitative. The daunting prospect of considering a "comprehensive quantitative model" has led to approaches and models, argued to be "more practical," in which sets of parameters are often selected in a somewhat mysterious fashion based on experience (including previous research) and intuition. The selected parameters are then used to develop predictive models, most of which have been based primarily on statistical methods (i.e., regression models) (Fleishman, 1967; Fleishman and Quaintance, 1984). Although the basic modeling tools depend only on correlation, it is usually possible to envision a causal link between the independent variables selected (e.g., visual acuity) and the dependent variable to be predicted (e.g., piloting an aircraft). Models (one per task) are then tested in a given population and graded with regard to their prediction ability, the best of which have performed marginally (Kondraske and Beehler, 1994). Another characteristic associated with many of the statistically based modeling efforts from the noted communities is the almost exclusive use of healthy, "normal" subjects for model development (i.e., humans with impairments were excluded). Homogeneity is a requirement of such statistical models, leading to the need for one model per task per population (at best). Moreover, working with a mindset that considers only normal subjects can be observed to skew estimates regarding which of the many parameters that one might choose for incorporation in a model are "most important." The relatively few exceptions that employ cause-and-effect models (e.g., based on physical laws) at some level of fidelity (e.g., Chaffin and Andersson, 1991) often adopt methods that have emerged from the bottom-up path and are, as noted above, limited in character at the "total human" level (e.g., "biomechanical" in the example cited).

It is critical to note that the issue is *not* that no useful models have emerged from previous efforts but rather that no clear comprehensive strategy has emerged for modeling at the human–task interface level. A National Research Council panel on human performance modeling (Baron et al., 1990) considered the fundamental issues discussed here and also underscored needs for models at the human–task interface level. While it was concluded that an all-inclusive model might be desirable (i.e., high fidelity, in the sense that biomechanical, information processing, sensory and perceptual aspects, etc. are represented), such a model was characterized as being highly unlikely to achieve and perhaps ultimately not useful because it would be overly complex for many applications. The basic recommendation made by this panel was to pursue development of more limited scope submodels. The implication is that two or more submodels could be integrated to achieve a broader range of fidelity, with the combination selected to meet the needs of particular situations. The desire to divide efforts due to inherent complexity of the problem also surfaces within the histories of the bottom-up and top-down development paths discussed above. While a reasonable concept in theory, one component in the division of effort that has consistently been underrepresented is the part that ties together the so-called submodels. Without a conceptual framework for integration of relatively independent modeling efforts and a set of common modeling constructs, prospects for long-term progress are difficult to envision. This, along with the recognition that enough work had been undertaken in the submodel areas so that key issues and common denominators could be identified, motivated development of the ERM.

The broad objectives of the ERM are most like those of Fleishman and colleagues (Fleishman, 1966, 1972, 1982; Fleishman and Quaintance, 1984), whose efforts in human performance are generally well known in many disciplines. These are the only two efforts known that (1) focus on the total human in a task situation (i.e., directly address the human–task interface level); (2) consider tasks in general, and not only a specific task such as gait, lifting, reading, and so on; (3) incorporate all aspects of the total human system (e.g., sensory, biomechanical, information processing, etc.); and (4) aim at quantitative models.

There are also some similarities with regard to the incorporation of the ideas of "abilities" (of humans) and "requirements" (of tasks). The work of Fleishman and colleagues has thus been influential in shaping the ERM either directly or indirectly through its influence of others. However, there are several substantive conceptual differences that have resulted in considerably different end-points. Fleishman's work emerged from "the task" perspective and is rooted in psychology, whereas the ERM emerges from the perspective of "human system architecture" and is rooted in engineering methodology with regard to quantitative aspects of system performance and also incorporates psychology *and* physiology. Both approaches address humans *and* tasks and both efforts contain aspects identifiable with psychology and engineering, as they ultimately must. These different perspectives, however, may explain in part some of the major differences. Aspects unique to the ERM include (1) it is based on modeling and measurement of *all* aspects of a system's performance using *resource constructs*; (2) the use of cause-and-effect *resource economic principles* (i.e., the idea of threshold "costs" for achieving a given level of performance in any given high-level task); (3) the concept of monadology (i.e., the use of a finite set of "elements" to explain a complex phenomenon); and (4) a consistent strategy for identifying performance elements at different hierarchical levels.

The ERM attempts to provide a quantitative and relatively straightforward framework for characterizing the human system, tasks, and the interface of the human to tasks. It depends in large part on, and evolves directly from, a separate body of material collectively referred to as general systems performance theory (GSPT). GSPT was developed first and independently; that is, removed from the human system context. It incorporates resource constructs exclusively for modeling of the abstract idea of *system performance*, including specific rules for measuring performance resource availability, and resource economic principles to provide a cause-and-effect analysis of the interface of any system (e.g., humans) to tasks. The concept of a "performance model" is emphasized and distinguished from other model types.

29.2 Basic Principles

The history of the ERM and the context in which it was developed are described elsewhere (Kondraske, 1987a, 1990b, 1995). It is important to note that the ERM is derived from the combination of GSPT with the philosophy of monadology and their application to the human system. As such, these two constituents are briefly reviewed before presenting and discussing the actual ERM.

29.2.1 General Systems Performance Theory

The concept of "performance" now pervades all aspects of life, especially decision-making processes that involve both human and artificial systems. Yet, it has not been well-understood theoretically, and systematic techniques for modeling and its measurement have been lacking. While a considerable body of material applicable to general systems theory exists, the concept of performance has not been incorporated in it nor has performance been addressed in a general fashion elsewhere. Most of the knowledge that exists regarding performance and its quantitative treatment has evolved within individual application contexts, where generalizations can easily be elusive.

Performance is multifaceted, pertaining to how well a given system executes an intended function and the various factors that contribute to this. It differs from *behavior* of a system in that "the best of something" is implied. The broad objectives of GSPT are

1. To provide a common conceptual basis for defining and measuring all aspects of the performance of any *system*.
2. To provide a common conceptual basis for the analysis of any *task* in a manner that facilitates system–task interface assessments and decision making.
3. To identify cause-and-effect principles, or laws, that explain what occurs when any given system is used to accomplish any given task.

While GSPT was motivated by needs in situations where the human is "the system" of interest and it was first presented in this context (Kondraske, 1987a), application of it has been extended to the context of artificial systems. These experiences range from computer vision and sensor fusion (Yen and Kondraske, 1992) to robotics (Kondraske and Standridge, 1988; Kondraske and Khoury, 1992).

A succinct statement of GSPT designed to emphasize key constructs is presented below in a step-like format. The order of steps is intended to suggest how one might approach any system or system–task interface situation to apply GSPT. While somewhat terse and "to-the-point," it is nonetheless an essential prerequisite for a reasonably complete understanding of the ERM:

1. Within a domain of interest, select any level of abstraction and identify the system(s) of interest (i.e., the physical *structure*) and its *function* (i.e., purpose).
2. Consider "the system" and "the task" separately.
3. Use a *resource construct* to model the system's *performance*. First, consider the unique intangible qualities that characterize *how well a system executes its function*. Each of these is considered to represent a unique *performance resource* associated with a specific *dimension of performance* (e.g., speed, accuracy, stability, smoothness, "friendliness," etc.) of that system. Each performance resource is recognized as a *desirable* item (e.g., endurance vs. fatigue, accuracy vs. error, etc.) "possessed" by the system in a certain quantitative amount. Thus, one can consider *quantifying* the amount of given *quality* available. As illustrated, an important consequence of using the resource construct at this stage is that confusion associated with duality of terms is eliminated.
4. Looking toward the system, identify all "I" dimensions of performance associated with it. In situations where the system does not yet exist (i.e., design contexts), it is helpful to note that dimensions of performance of the system are the same as those of the task.
5a. Keeping the resource construct in mind, define a parameterized metric for each dimension of performance (e.g., speed, accuracy, etc.). If the resource construct is followed, values will be produced with these metrics that are always nonnegative. Furthermore, a larger numerical value will consistently represent *more* of a given resource and therefore *more performance capacity*.
5b. Measure system performance with the system *removed from* the specific intended task. This is a reinforcement of step (2). The general strategy is to *maximally stress* the system (within limits of comfort and/or safety, when appropriate) to define its *performance envelope*; or more specifically, the envelope that defines *performance resource availability*, $R_{AS}(t)$. Note that $R_{AS}(t)$ is a continuous surface in the system's nonnegative, multidimensional performance space. Also note that unless all dimensions of performance and parameterized metrics associated with each are defined using the resource construct, a performance envelope cannot be guaranteed. Addressing the issue of measurement more specifically, consider resource availability values, $R_{A_i}|_{Q_{i,k}}(t)$ for $i = 1 - I$, associated with each of the "I" dimensions of performance. Here, each $Q_{i,k}$ represents a unique condition, in terms of a set of values R_i along *other* identified dimensions of performance, under which a specific resource availability (R_{A_i}) is measured; that is, $Q_{i,k} = \{R_{1,k}, R_{2,k}, ..., R_{p,k}\}$ for all $p \neq i$ $(1 \geq p \geq I)$. The subscript "k" is used to distinguish several possible conditions under which a given resource availability (R_{A_i}) can be measured. These values are measured using a set of "test-tasks," each of which is designed to *maximally stress* the system (within limits of comfort and safety, when appropriate) (a) along each dimension of performance individually (where $Q_{i,k} = Q_{i,0} = \{0,0,...,0\}$), or (b) along selected subsets of dimensions of performance simultaneously (i.e., $Q_{i,k} = Q_{i,n}$, where each possible $Q_{i,n}$ has one or more nonzero elements). The points obtained $(R_{A_i}|_{Q_{i,k}}(t))$ provide the basis to estimate the performance envelope, $R_{As}(t)$. Note that if only on-axis points are obtained (e.g., maximally stress one specific performance resource availability with minimal or no stress on other performance resources, or the $Q_{i,0}$ condition), a rectangular or idealized performance envelope is obtained. A more accurate representation, which would be contained within the idealized envelope, can be obtained at the expense of making additional measurements or the use of known mathematical functions that define the shape of envelope in two or more dimensions.

5c. Define estimates of single-number *system figures-of-merit*, or *composite performance capacities*, as the mathematical product of all or any selected subset of $R_{A_i} |_{Q_{i,0}}(t)$. If more accuracy is desired and a sufficient number of data points is available from the measurement process described in (5b), composite performance capacities can be determined by integration over $R_{A_S}(t)$ to determine the volume enclosed by the envelope. The *composite performance capacity* is a measure of performance at a higher level of abstraction than any individual dimension of performance at the "system" level, representing the capacity of the system to perform tasks which place demands on *those performance resources availabilities included in the calculation*. Different composite performance capacities can be computed for a given system by selecting different combinations of dimensions of performance. Note that the definition of a composite performance capacity used here preserves dimensionality; for example, if speed and accuracy dimensions are included in the calculation, the result has units of speed × accuracy. (This step is used only when needed; e.g., when two general-purpose systems of the same type are to be compared. However, if decision making that involves the interface of a specific system to a specific task is the issue at hand, a composite performance capacity is generally not of any use.)

6. Assess the "need for detail." This amounts to a determination of the number of hierarchical levels included in the analysis. If the need is to determine whether the currently identified "system" can work in the given task or how well it can execute its function, go to step (7) now. If the need is to determine the *contribution of one or more constituent subsystems* or why a desired level of performance is not achieved at the system level, repeat 1 = >5 for all "J" functional units (subsystems), or a selected subset thereof based on need, that forms the system that was originally identified in step (1); that is, go to the next lowest hierarchical level.

7. At the "system" level, look toward the task(s) of interest. Measure, estimate, or calculate *demands* on system performance resources (e.g., the speed, accuracy, etc. required), $R_{D_i} |_{Q'_{i,k}}(t)$, where the notation here is analogous to that employed in step (5b). This represents the quantitative definition and communication of *goals*, or the set of values (P_{HLT}) representing level of performance (P) desired in a specific high-level task (HLT). Use a worst-case or other less-conservative strategy (with due consideration of the impact of this choice) to summarize variations over time. This will result in a set of "M" points (R_{D_m}, for m = 1–M) that lie in the multidimensional space defined by the set of "I" dimensions of performance. Typically, M ≥ I.

8. Use *resource economic principles* (i.e., require $R_A \geq R_D$ for "success") at the system level *and* at all system–task interfaces at the subsystem level (if included) to evaluate success/failure at each interface. More specifically, for a given system–task interface, all task–demand points (i.e., the set of R_{D_m} associated with a given task or subtask) must lie within the performance resource envelope, $R_{A_S}(t)$, of the corresponding system. This is the key law that governs system–task interfaces. If a two-level model is used (i.e., "system" and "subsystem" levels are incorporated), map system level demands to demands on constituent subsystems. That is, functional relationships between P_{HLT} and demands imposed on constituent subsystems (i.e., $R_{D_i}(t, P_{HLT})$) must be determined. The nature of these mappings depends on the type of systems in question (e.g., mechanical, information processing, etc.). The basic process includes application of step (7) to the subtasks associated with each subsystem. If *resource utilization flexibility* (i.e., redundancy in subsystems of similar types) exists, select the "best" or optimal subsystem configuration (handled in GSPT with the concept of *performance resource substitution*) and procedure (i.e., use of performance resources over time) as that which allows *accomplishment of goals* with *minimization of stress* on available performance resources across all subsystems and over the time of task execution. Thus, redundancy is addressed in terms of a constrained performance resource optimization problem. Stress on individual performance resources is defined as $0 \leq R_{D_{ij}}(t, P_{HLT})/R_{A_{ij}}(t) \leq 1$. It is also useful to define and take note of reserve capacity; that is, the margin between available and utilized performance resources.

The above statement is intended to reflect the true complexity that exists in systems, tasks, and their interfaces when viewed primarily from the perspective of performance. This provides a basis for the judicious decision making required to realize "the best" *practical implementation* in a given situation where many engineering trade-offs must be considered. While a two-level approach is described above, it should be apparent that it could be applied with any number of hierarchical levels by repeating the steps outlined in an iterative fashion starting at a different level each time. A striking feature of GSPT is the *threshold effect* associated with the resource economic principle. This nonlinearity has important implications in quantitative human performance modeling, as well as interesting ramifications in practical applications such as rehabilitation, sports, and education. Note also no distinction is made as to whether a given performance resource is derived from a human or artificial system; both types of systems, or subcomponents thereof, can be incorporated into models and analyses.

29.2.2 Monadology

Monadology dates back to 384 BC (Neel, 1977) but was formalized and its importance emphasized by Gottfried Wilhelm Leibniz, inventor of calculus, in his text *Monadologia* in 1714. This text presents what is commonly called *Leibniz's Monadology* and has been translated and incorporated into contemporary philosophy texts (Leibniz and Montgomery, 1992). It is essentially the idea of "basic elements" *vis a vis* chemistry, alphabets, genetic building blocks, etc. The concept is thus already well accepted as being vital to the systematic description of human systems from certain perspectives (i.e., chemical, genetic). Success associated with previous application of monadology, whether intentional or unwitting (i.e., discovered to be at play *after* a given taxonomy has emerged), compels its serious *a priori* consideration for other problems.

Insight into how monadology is applied to human performance modeling is perhaps more readily obtained with reference to a widely known example in which monadology is evident, such as chemistry. Prior to modern chemistry (i.e., prior to the introduction of the periodic table), alchemy existed. The world was viewed as being composed of an infinite variety of unique *substances*. The periodic table captured the notion that this infinite variety of substances could all be defined in terms of a finite set of basic elements. Substances have since been analyzed using the "language" of chemistry and organized into categories of various complexity, that is, elements, simple compounds, complex compounds, etc. Despite the fact that this transition occurred approximately 200 years ago, compounds remain, which have yet to be analyzed. Furthermore, the initial periodic table was incorrect and has undergone revision up to relatively recent times. Analogously, in the alchemy of human performance the world is viewed as being composed of an infinite variety of unique tasks. A "chemistry" can be envisioned that first starts with the identification of the "basic elements," or more specifically, *basic elements of performance*. Simple and complex tasks are thus analogous to simple and complex compounds, respectively. The analogy carries over to quantitative aspects of GSPT as well. Consider typical equations of chemical reactions with resources on the left and products (i.e., tasks) on the right. Simple compounds (tasks) are realized by drawing upon basic elements in the proper combination and amounts. The amount of "product" (level of performance in a high-level task) obtained depends on availability of the *limiting resource*.

Another informative aspect of this analogy is the issue of how to deal with the treatment of hierarchical level. Clearly, the chemical elements are made up of smaller particles (e.g., protons, neutrons, and electrons). Physicists have identified even smaller, more elusive entities such as bosons, quarks, and so on. Do we need to consider items at this lowest level of abstraction each time a simple compound such as hydrochloric acid is made? Likewise, the term "basic" in basic elements of performance is clearly relative and requires the choice of a particular hierarchical level of abstraction for the identification of systems or basic functional units; a level which is considered to be both natural and useful for the purpose at hand. Just as it is possible but not always necessary or practical to map chemical elements down to the atomic particle level, it is possible to consider mapping a basic element of performance (see latter) such as elbow flexor torque production capacity down to the level of muscle fibers, biochemical reactions at neuromuscular junctions, and so forth.

29.2.3 The Elemental Resource Model

The resource and resource economic constructs used in GSPT specifically to address performance have employed and have become well-established in some segments of the human performance field, specifically with regard to attention and information processing (Navon and Gopher, 1979; Wickens, 1984). However, in these cases the term "resource" is used mostly conceptually (in contrast to quantitatively), somewhat softly defined, and applied to refer in various instances to systems (e.g., different processing centers), broad functions (e.g., memory vs. processing), and sometimes to infer a particular aspect of performance (e.g., attentional resources). In the ERM, through the application of GSPT, these constructs are incorporated universally (i.e., applied to all human subsystems) and specifically to model "performance" at both conceptual and quantitative levels. In addition to the concept of monadology, the insights of others (Turvey et al., 1978; Schoner and Kelso, 1988) were valuable in reinforcing the basic "systems architecture" employed in the ERM and in refining description of more subtle, but important aspects.

As illustrated in Figure 29.1, the ERM contains multiple hierarchical levels. Specifically, three levels are defined (1) the basic element level, (2) the *generic intermediate level*, and (3) the high level. GSPT is to define performance measures at any hierarchical level. This implies that to measure performance, one must isolate the desired system and then stress it maximally along one dimension of performance (or more, if interaction effects are desired) to determine performance resource availability. For example, consider the human "posture stabilizing" system (at the generic intermediate level), which is stressed maximally along a stability dimension. As further illustrated below, the basic element level contains and represents measurable stepping-stones in the human system hierarchy between lower-level systems (i.e., ligaments, tendons, nerves, etc.) and higher-level tasks.

A summary representation emphasizing the basic element level of the ERM is depicted in Figure 29.2. While this figure is intended to be more or less self-explanatory, a brief walk-through is warranted.

29.2.3.1 Looking toward the Human

The entire human (lower portion of Figure 29.2) is modeled as a pool of elemental *performance resources*, which are grouped into one of the four different domains (1) life sustaining, (2) environmental interface (containing purely sensory and sensorimotor components), (3) the central processing, and (4) information. Within each of the first three domains, physical subsystems referred to as *functional units* are identified (see labels along horizontal aspect of grids) through application of fairly rigorous criteria (Kondraske, 1990b). GSPT is applied to each functional unit, yielding first a set of dimensions of performance (defined using a resource construct) for each unit. A single *Basic Element of Performance* (BEP) is defined by specifying two items (1) the basic functional unit and (2) one of its dimensions of performance. Within a domain, not every dimension of performance indicated in Figure 29.2 is applicable to every functional unit in that domain. However, there is an increasing degree of "likeness" among functional units (i.e., fewer fundamentally different types) in this regard as one moves from life sustaining, to environmental interface, to central processing domains. The fourth domain, the information domain, is substantially different from the other three. Whereas the first three represent physical systems and their intangible performance resources, the information domain simply represents information. Thus, while memory functional units are located within the central processing domain, the contents of memory (e.g., motor programs and associated reference information) are partitioned into the information domain. As illustrated, information is grouped but within each group there are many specific skills. The set of available performance resources $(R_{A_{ij}}(t)|_Q)$ consist of both BEPs (i = dimension of performance, j = functional unit) and information sets (e.g., type "i" within group "j"). Although

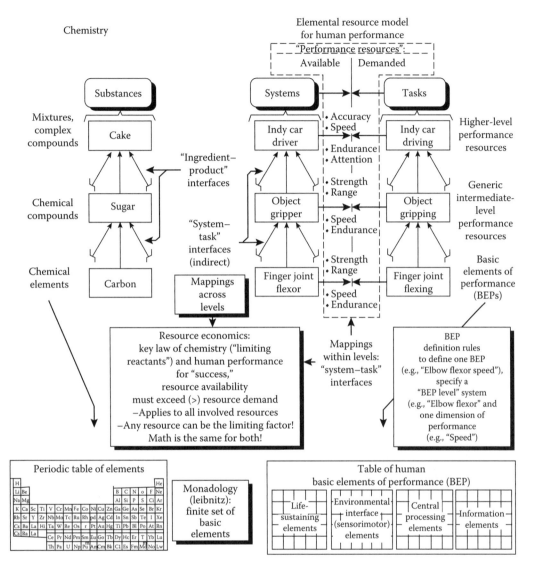

FIGURE 29.1 Elemental resource model contains multiple hierarchical levels. Performance resources (i.e., the basic elements) at the "basic element level" are finite in number, as dictated by the finite set of human subsystems and the finite set of their respective dimensions of performance. At higher levels, new "systems" can be readily created by configuration of systems at the basic element level. Consequently, there are in infinite number of performance resources (i.e., higher-level elements) at these levels. However, rules of general systems performance theory (refer to text) are applied at any level in the same way resulting in the identification of the system, its function, dimensions of performance, performance resource availabilities (system attributes), and performance resource demands (task attributes).

intrinsically different, both fit the resource construct. This approach permits even the most abstract items such as motivation and friendliness to be considered with the same basic framework as strength and speed.

Note that resource availability in GSPT and thus in the ERM is potentially a function of time, allowing quantitative modeling of dynamic processes such as child development, aging, disuse atrophy, and rehabilitation. The notation further implies that availability of a given resource must be evaluated at a

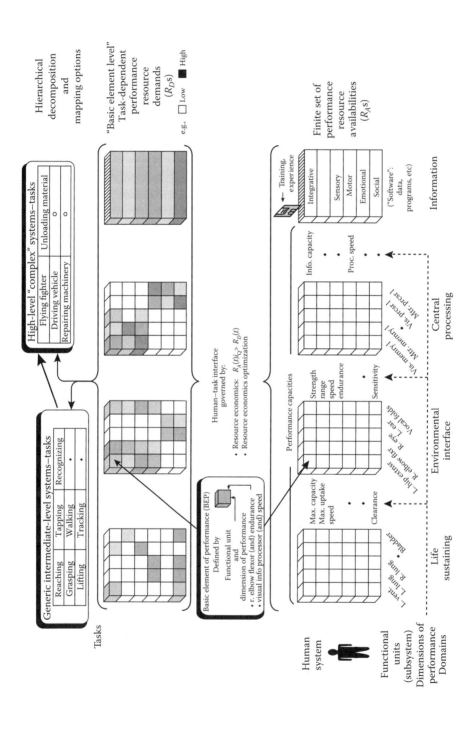

FIGURE 29.2 Summary of the major constructs of the elemental resource model, emphasizing the categorization of performance resources at the basic element level into four: life-sustaining, environmental interface, central-processing, and information domains.

specific operating point, denoted as Q. At least conceptually, many parameters can be used to characterize this Q point. In general, the goal of measurement when looking "toward the human" is to isolate functional units and maximally stress (safely) individual performance resources to determine availability. Such measures reflect performance capacities. The simplest Q point is one in which there is stress along only one dimension of performance (i.e., that corresponding to the resource being stressed). Higher fidelity representation is possible at the expense of additional measurements. The degree to which isolation can be achieved is of practical concern in humans. Nonetheless, it is felt that reasonable isolation can be achieved in most situations (Kondraske, 1990a,b). Moreover, this and similar issues of practical concern should be addressed as separate problems; that is, they should not be permitted to obfuscate or thwart efforts to explain phenomenon at the human–task interface.

29.2.3.2 Looking toward the Task

The mid-portion of Figure 29.2 suggests the representation of any given task in terms of the unique set of demands $(R_{D_{ij}}(t))$ imposed on the pool of BEPs and information resources; that is, this is the elemental level of task representation. Shading implies that demands can be represented quantitatively in terms of amount. The upper portion of the figure defines hierarchical mapping options, where mapping is the process of translating what happens in tasks typically executed by humans to the elemental level. Two such additional levels (for a total of three, including the elemental level) are included as part of the ERM (1) generic intermediate-level tasks, and (2) higher-level complex tasks. At all three levels (Figures 29.1 and 29.2) tasks are processes which occur over time and can be characterized by specific goals (e.g., in terms of speed, force, etc.) and related to systems at the same level that possess performance resources. Using established analytic techniques, even the most complex task can be divided into discrete task segments. Then mapping analyses, which take into account task procedures (e.g., a squatting subject with two hands on the side of a box …), are applied to each task segment to determine $R_{D_{ij}}(t)$. Once this is found, the worst case or a selected percentile point in the resource demand distribution (over a time period corresponding to a selected task segment) can be used to obtain a single numerical value representation of demand for a given resource *and* the conditions under which the given demand occurs; that is, the Q' point (e.g., at what speed and position angle does the worst-case demand on elbow flexor torque occur?). This reduction process requires parameterization algorithms that are similar to those used to process time-series data collected during tests designed to measure performance resource availability.

29.2.3.3 The Human–Task Interface

Using GSPT, success in achieving the goals of a given task segment is governed by resource economic principles requiring that $R_{A_{ij}}(t)|_Q \geq R_{D_{ij}}(t)$ for all *is* and *js* (i.e., $R_{A_{11}} \geq R_{D_{11}}$ AND $R_{A_{12}} \geq R_{D_{12}}$ AND $R_{A_{13}} \geq R_{D_{13}} \cdots$). In other words, all task demands, when translated to the individual subsystems involved, must fit within the envelopes that define performance resource availability. Adequacy associated with any one resource is a *necessary, but not sufficient condition* for success. Concepts and observations in human performance referred to as "compensation" or "redundancy" are explained in terms of *resource utilization flexibility,* which includes the possibility of substituting one performance resource (of the same dimensionality) for another (i.e., *resource substitution*). It has been hypothesized (Kondraske, 1990b) that an optimal performance resource utilization is achieved through learning. Furthermore, the optimization rule suggested by GSPT is that the human system is driven to accomplish task goals and use procedures that minimize performance resource stress (i.e., the fraction of available performance resources utilized) over the duration of a given task segment and across all BEPs involved. Minimizing stress is equivalent to maximizing the margin between available and utilized performance resources. Thus, optimization is highly dependent on the resource availability profile and it would be predicted, for instance, that two individuals with different resource availability profiles would not optimally accomplish the same task goals by using identical procedures.

29.3 Application Issues

Implications of the ERM and what it demonstrates regarding intrinsic demands imposed by nature and methods for creatively navigating these demands over both the short and long terms are considered. The ERM offers a number of flexibilities with regard to how it can be applied (e.g., "in whole" or "in part," "conceptually" or "rigorously," with "low-tech" or sophisticated "high-tech" tools, and to define performance measures or to develop predictive models). While immediate application is possible at a conceptual level of application, it also provides the motivation and potential to consider coordinated, collaborative developments that allow rigorous and efficient solutions to complex problems by practitioners without extraordinary training.

The ERM provides a basis for obtaining insight into the nature of routine tasks that clinicians and other practitioners are expected to perform; there are both "troublesome" and "promising" insights in this regard. Perhaps the most obvious troublesome aspect is that the ERM makes it painfully evident that *many* BEPs are typically called into play in tasks of daily living, work, or recreation and that resource insufficiency associated with *any one* of this subset of BEPs can be the factor which limits performance in the higher-level task. The further implication is that for rigorous application, one must know (via measurement and analyses) the availability and demand associated with each and every one of these unique resources. An additional complexity with which practitioners must cope is the high degree of specificity and complexity of resources in the information domain (i.e., the "software"). There is no simple, rapid way to probe into this domain of the ERM to determine if the information required for a given task is correct; it requires methods analogous to those used to debug software source code.

The aspects that hold promise are associated with (1) the nature of hierarchical systems; (2) the threshold mathematics of resource economics; and (3) the fact that when "*n*" resources combine to address a single task, the mathematics of logical combination is employed to arrive at an overall assessment. That is, the individual "$R_A \geq R_D$?" questions result in a set of "OK" or "Not OK" results that are combined with logical "AND" operations to obtain the final "OK" or "Not OK" assessment. (*Note*: the "OR" operator is used when resource substitution is possible.)

29.3.1 Conceptual, Low-Tech, Practical Application

The ERM description alone can be used simply to provide a common conceptual basis for discussing the wide range of concepts, measurements, methods, and processes of relevance in human performance or a particular application area (Frisch, 1993; Syndulko et al., 1988; Mayer and Gatchel, 1991). It can also be used at this level as a basis for structured assessment (Kondraske, 1988b, 1994b, 1995) of individuals in situations including therapy prescription, assistive device prescription, independent living, decision making (e.g., self-feeding, driving, etc.), age, or gender discrimination issues in work or recreational tasks, etc. At points in such processes, it is often more important to consider the full scope of different performance resources involved in a task using even a crude level of quantification than it is to consider just a select few in great depth. A "checklist" approach is recommended. The professional uses only his or her judgment and experience to consider both the specific individual and the specific task of interest to make quantitative but relatively gross assessments of resource adequacy using a triage-like categorization process (e.g., with "definitely limiting," "definitely not limiting," or "not sure" categories). This is feasible because of the threshold nature of the system–task interface; in cases where R_A and R_D are widely and separately instrumented, high resolution measurements are not required to determine if a given performance resource is limiting. Any resource(s) so identified as "definitely limiting" becomes an immediate focus of interest. If none is categorized as such, concern moves to those in the "not sure" category in which case more sensitive measurements may be required. Purely subjective methods of measuring resource availability and demands can be augmented with selected, more objective, and higher-resolution measurements in "hybrid applications."

29.3.2 Conceptual, Theoretical Application

The ERM can be used in its broadest conceptual sense as a basis for formulating context-dependent models for specific situations involving human performance. Dillon et al. (2000) utilized ERM constructs to propose approaches to deal with outcome assessment in engineering education, Chesky et al. (2002) applied the ERM as a basis for a conceptual understanding of medical problems of musicians, and Olson and Kondraske (2005) incorporated it into pain management.

It can also be employed in a theoretical fashion to reconsider previous work in human performance. For example, it can be employed to reason why Fleishman (Fleishman and Quaintance, 1984) (as well as others) achieve promising, but limited, success with statistically based predictions of performance in higher-level tasks using regression models with independent variables, which can now be viewed as representing lower-level performance resources (in most cases). Specifically, regression models rely fundamentally on an assumption that there exists some correlation between dependent and each independent variable, the latter of which typically represent scores from maximal performance tasks and therefore reflect resource availability (using GSPT and ERM logic). Brief reflection results in the realization that correlation is not to be anticipated between the level of performance attainable in a "higher-level task" and *availability* of one of the many performance resources essential to the task (e.g., if four cups of flour are needed for a given cake, having 40 cups available will not *alone* result in a larger cake of equal quality—availability of another ingredient may in fact be limiting). Rather, correlation *is* expected between high-level task performance and the amount of resource *utilization*. Unfortunately, as noted above, the independent variables used typically reflect resource availability. The incomplete labeling of performance variables in such studies reflects the general failure to distinguish between utilization and availability. Why not, then, just use measures of resource utilization in such statistical models? Resource availability measures are simple to obtain in the laboratory without requiring that the individual executes *the* high-level task of interest. Resource utilization measures can only be obtained experimentally by requiring the subject to execute the task in question, which is counterproductive with respect to the goal of using a set of laboratory measurements to extrapolate to performance in one or more higher-level task situations. Regression models based on linear combination of resource *availability* measures do not reflect the nonlinear threshold effect accounted for with resource economic, GSPT-based performance models. One potential alternative based on GSPT and termed nonlinear causal resource analysis (NCRA) has been proposed (Kondraske, 1988a; Vasta and Kondraske, 1994). NCRA application examples are cited in Section 29.3.4.

29.3.3 Application "In Part"

In this approach, whole domains (i.e., many BEPs) are assessed simultaneously resulting in an estimate or well-founded assumption, which states that "all performance resources in Domain X are nonlimiting in Task(s) Y." Such assumptions are often well justified. For example, it would be reasonable to assume that a young male with a sport-related knee injury would have only a reduction in performance resource availability in the environmental interface domain. More specifically, it is reasonable to assume that the scope of interest can be confined to a smaller subset of functional units, as in gait or speech. These can then be addressed with rigorous application. Examples of this level and manner of applying the ERM have been or are being developed for head/neck control in the context of assistive communication device prescription (Carr, 1989); workplace design (Kondraske, 1988c); evaluating worksites and individuals with disabilities for employment (Parnianpour and Marras, 1993); gait (Carollo and Kondraske, 1987); measurement of upper extremity motor control (Behbehani et al., 1988); speech production performance (Jafari, 1989a; Jafari et al., 1989b); and to illustrate changes in performance capacity associated with aging (Kondraske, 1989). Additionally, in some applications only the Generic Intermediate Level needs to be considered. For example, one may only need to know how well an individual can walk, lift, etc. While it is sometimes painfully clear just how complex is the execution of even a relatively simple task, it can also be recognized that relatively simple, justifiable, and efficient strategies can be developed to maintain a reasonable degree of utility in a given context.

29.3.4 Rigorous, High-Tech Application

While this path may offer the greatest potential for impact, it also presents the greatest challenge. The ultimate *goal* would be to capture the analytic and modeling capability (as implied by the above discussions) for a "total human" (single subject or populations) and "any task" in a desktop computer system (used along with synergistic "peripherals" that adopt the same framework, such as measurement tools (Kondraske, 1990a)). This suggests a long-term, collaborative effort. However, intermediate tools that provide significant utility are feasible (e.g., Vasta and Kondraske, 1994) and needed (Allard et al., 1994; Vasta and Kondraske, 1994). A promising example of such tools based directly on GSPT and the ERM is NCRA (Vasta and Kondraske, 1994; Kondraske et al., 1997). This inferential method has recently been used (Kondraske et al., 1997) to develop models that relate performance resource demands on various human subsystems to the level of performance attained in higher level mobility tasks (e.g., gait and stair climbing). In turn, these models have been used to predict level of performance in these higher level tasks with success that exceeds that which has been obtained with regression models. Furthermore, the NCRA method inherently provides not only a prediction of high-level task performance, but also identifies which performance resources are most likely to be preventing better performance (i.e., which ones are the "limiting performance resources"). Similar applications of NCRA have been used to develop models of laparoscopic surgical performance (Gettman et al., 2003; Johnson et al., 2004), driving performance (Fischer et al., 2002), and to understand falls in elderly subjects (Murphy, 2002). A special NCRA software package has been developed to facilitate model development and use. While such tools that are useful to practitioners are desirable, they are almost essential for the efficient conduct of in-depth experimental work with the ERM.

The issue of biologic variability and its influence on numerical analyses can be raised in the context of rigorous numerical application. In this regard, the methods underlying GSPT and the ERM (or any similar cause-and-effect model) are noted to be analogous with those used to design artificial systems. In recent years, conceptual approaches and mathematical tools widely known as Taguchi methods (Bendell et al., 1988) have shown to be effective for understanding and managing a very similar type of variability that surfaces in the manufacture of artificial systems (e.g., variability associated with performance of components of larger systems and the effect on aspects of performance of the final "product"). Such tools may prove useful in working through engineering problems such as those associated with variability.

29.4 Conclusion

The ERM is a step toward the goal of achieving an application-independent approach to modeling any human–task interface. It provides a systematic and generalizable (across all subsystem types) means of identifying performance measures that characterize human subsystems, as well as a consistent basis for performance measurement definition (and task analysis). It has also served to stimulate focus on a standardized, distinct set of variables, which facilitates clear communication of an individual's status among professionals.

After the initial presentation, refinements in both GSPT and the ERM were made. However, the basic approaches, terminology, and constructs used in each have remained quite stable. More recent work has focused on development of various components required for application of the ERM in nontrivial situations. This entails using GSPT and basic ERM concepts to guide a full "fleshing out" of the details of measurement parameterizations and models for different types of human subsystems, definition of standard conventions and notations, and development of computer-based tools. In addition, experimental studies designed to evaluate key constructs of the ERM and to demonstrate the various ways in which it can be applied are being conducted. A good portion of the developmental work is aimed at building a capability to conduct more complex, nontrivial experimental studies. Collaborations with other research groups have also emerged and are being supported to the extent possible. Experiences with it in various contexts and at various levels of application have been productive and encouraging.

The ERM is one, relatively young attempt at organizing and dealing with the complexity of some major aspects of human performance. There is no known alternative that, in a specific sense, attempts to accomplish the same goals as the working model presented here. Is it good enough? For what purposes? Is a completely different approach or merely refinement required? The process of revision is central to the natural course of the history of ideas. Needs for generalizations in human performance persist.

Defining Terms

Basic element of performance (BEP): A modeling item at the basic element level in the ERM is defined by identification of a specific system at this level and one of its dimensions of performance (e.g., functional unit = visual information processor, dimension of performance = speed, BEP = visual information processor speed).

Behavior: A general term that relates to what a human or artificial system does while carrying out its function(s) under given conditions. Often, behavior is characterized by measurement of selected parameters or identification of unique system states over time.

Composite performance capacity: A performance capacity at a higher level of abstraction, formed by combining two or more lower-level performance capacities (e.g., via integration to determine the area or volume within a performance envelope).

Dimension of performance: A unique quality that characterizes how well a system executes its function (e.g., speed, accuracy, and torque production); one of axes or the label associated with one of the axes in a multidimensional performance space.

Function: The purpose of a system. Some systems map to a single primary function (e.g., process visual information). Others (e.g., the human arm) map to multiple functions, although at any given time multifunction systems are likely to be executing a single function (e.g., polishing a car). Functions can be described and inventoried, whereas level of performance of a given function can be measured.

Generic intermediate level: One of three major hierarchical levels for systems and tasks identified in the elemental resource model. The generic intermediate level represents new systems (e.g., postural maintenance system, object gripper, object lifter, etc.) formed by the combination of functional units at the basic element level (e.g., flexors, extensors, processors, etc.). The term "generic" is used to imply the high frequency of use of systems at this level in tasks of daily life (i.e., items at the "high level" in the ERM).

Goal: A desired end-point (i.e., result) typically characterized by multiple parameters, at least one of which is specified. Examples include specified task goals (e.g., move an object of specified mass from point A to point B in 3 s) or estimated task performance (maximum mass, range, speed of movement obtainable given a specified elemental performance resource availability profile), depending on whether a reverse or forward analysis problem is undertaken. Whereas function describes the general process of a task, the goal directly relates to performance, and is quantitative.

Limiting resource: A performance resource at any hierarchical level (e.g., vertical lift strength and knee flexor speed) that is available in an amount that is less than the worst case demand imposed by a task. Thus, a given resource can only be "limiting" when considered in the context of a specific task.

Performance: Unique qualities of a human or artificial system (e.g., strength, speed, accuracy, and endurance) that pertain to how well that system executes its function.

Performance capacity: A quantity in finite availability that is possessed by a system or subsystem, drawn on during the execution of tasks, and limits some aspects (e.g., speed, force production, etc.) of a system's ability to execute tasks; or, the limit of that aspect itself.

Performance envelope: The surface in a multidimensional performance space, formed with a selected subset of a system's dimensions of performance, that defines the limits of a systems performance. Tasks represented by points which fall within this envelope can be performed by the system in question.

Performance resource: A unique quality of a system's performance modeled and quantified using a resource construct.

Performance resource substitution: The term used in GSPT to describe the manner in which intelligent systems, such as humans, utilize redundancy or adapt to unusual circumstances (e.g., injuries) to obtain optimal procedures for executing a task.

Procedure: A set of constraints placed on a system in which flexibility exists regarding how a goal (or set of goals) associated with a given function can be achieved. Procedure specification requires specification of initial, intermediate and final states, or conditions dictating how the goal is to be accomplished. Such specification can be thought of in terms of removing some degrees of freedom.

Resource construct: The collective set of attributes that define and uniquely characterize a resource. Usually, the term is applied to only tangible items. A resource is desirable, measurable in terms of amount (from zero to some finite positive value) in such a manner that a larger numerical value indicates a greater amount of the resource.

Resource economic principle: The principle, observable in many contexts, which states that the amount of a given resource that is available (e.g., money) must exceed the demand placed on it (e.g., cost of an item) if a specified goal (e.g., purchase of the item) is to be achieved.

Resource utilization flexibility: A term used in GSPT to describe situations in which there is more than one possible source of a given performance resource type, that is, redundant supplies exist.

Structure: Physical manifestation and attributes of a human or artificial system and the object of one type of measurements at multiple hierarchical levels.

Style: Allowance for variation within a procedure, resulting in the intentional incomplete specification of a procedure or resulting from either intentional or unintentional incomplete specification of procedure.

System: A physical structure, at any hierarchical level of abstraction, that executes one or more functions.

Task: That which results from (1) the combination of specified functions, goals and procedures, or (2) the specification of function and goals and the observation of procedures utilized to achieve the goals.

References

Allard, P., Stokes, I.A.F., and Blanchi, J.P. 1994. *Three-Dimensional Analysis of Human Movement*, Human Kinetics, Champaign, IL.

Baron, S., Kruser, D.S., and Huey, B.M., eds. 1990. *Quantitative Modeling of Human Performance in Complex, Dynamic Systems*, National Academy Press, Washington, DC.

Behbehani, K., Kondraske, G.V., and Richmond, J.R. 1988. Investigation of upper extremity visuomotor control performance measures. *IEEE Trans. Biomed. Eng.*, 35: 518–525.

Bendell, A., Disney, J., and Pridmore, W.A. 1988. *Taguchi Methods: Applications in World Industry*, IFS Publishing, London.

Botterbusch, K.F. *Vocational Assessment and Evaluation Systems: A Comparison*. Stout Vocational Rehabilitation Institute, University of Wisconsin, Menomonie, WI.

Card, S.K., Moran, T.P., and Newell, A. 1986. The model human processor. In: Boff, K.R., Kaufman, L., and Thomas, J.P. (eds.), *Handbook of Perception and Human Performance*, Vol. II, Wiley, New York, pp. 45.1–45.35.

Carollo, J.J. and Kondraske, G.V. 1987. The prerequisite resources for walking: Characterization using a task analysis strategy. In: Leinberger, J. (ed.), *Proceedings of the 9th Annual IEEE Engineering in Medical and Biological Society Conference*, p. 357.

Carr, B. 1989. *Head/Neck Control Performance Measurement and Task Interface Model.* MS thesis, University of Texas at Arlington, Arlington, TX.

Chaffin, D.B. and Andersson, G.B.J. 1991. *Occupational Biomechanics*, John Wiley and Sons, New York.

Chesky, K., Kondraske, G.V., Henoch, M., and Rubin, B. 2002. Musicians' health. In: Colwell, R. and Richardson, C. (eds.), *The New Handbook of Research on Music Teaching and Learning*, Oxford University Press, New York, pp. 1023–1039.

Delp, S.L., Loan, J.P., Hoy, M.G., Zajac, F.E., Topp, E.L., and Rosen, J.M. 1990. An interactive graphics-based model of the lower extremity to study orthopaedic surgical procedures. *IEEE Trans. Biomed. Eng.* 37: 757–767.

Dillon, W.E., Kondraske, G.V., Everett, L.J., and Volz, R.A. 2000. Performance theory based outcome measurement in engineering education and training. *IEEE Trans. Eng. Edu.* 43: 92–99.

Fischer, C.A., Kondraske, G.V., and Stewart, R.M. 2002. Prediction of driving performance using non-linear causal resource analysis. *CD-ROM Proceedings of the 24th International Conference on IEEE Engineering in Medicine and Biological Society*, Houston, October 23–26, pp. 2473–2474.

Fleishman, E.A. 1956. Psychomotor selection tests: Research and application in the United States Air Force. *Pers. Psychol.* 9: 449–467.

Fleishman, E.A. 1966. Human abilities and the acquisition of skill. In: Bilodeau, E.A. (ed.), *Acquisition of Skill*, Academic Press, New York, pp. 147–167.

Fleishman, E.A. 1967. Performance assessment based on an empirically derived task taxonomy. *Hum. Factors* 9: 349–366.

Fleishman, E.A. 1972. Structure and measurement of psychomotor abilities. In: Singer, R.N. (ed.), *The Psychomotor Domain: Movement Behavior*, Lea and Febiger, Philadelphia, pp. 78–106.

Fleishman, E.A. 1982. Systems for describing human tasks. *Am. Psychol.* 37: 821–824.

Fleishman, E.A. and Quaintance, M.K. 1984. *Taxonomies of Human Performance*, Academic Press, Orlando, FL.

Frisch, H.P. 1993. Man/machine interaction dynamics and performance analysis. In *Proceedings of the NATO-Army-NASA Advanced Study Institute on Concurrent Engineering Tools and Technologies for Mechanical System Design*, Springer-Verlag, New York.

Gettman, M.T., Kondraske, G.V., Traxer, O., Ogan, K., Napper, C., Jones, D.B., Pearle, M.S., and Cadeddu, J. 2003. Assessment of basic human performance resources predicts operative performance of laparoscopic surgery. *J. Am. Coll. Surg.* 197: 489–496.

Gilbreth, F.B. and Gilbreth, F.M. 1917. *Applied Motion Study.* Sturgis and Walton Co., New York.

Gottlieb, G.L., Corcos, D.M., and Agarwal, G.C. 1989. Strategies for the control of voluntary movements with one mechanical degree of freedom, *Behav. Brain Sci.* 12: 189–250.

Hemami, H. 1988. Modeling, control, and simulation of human movement, *CRC Crit. Rev. Bioeng.* 13: 1–34.

Jafari, M. 1989a. *Modeling and Measurement of Human Speech Performance toward Pathology Pattern Recognition*, Dissertation, the University of Texas at Arlington, Arlington, TX.

Jafari, M., Wong, K.H., Behbehani, K., and Kondraske, G.V. 1989b. Performance characterization of human pitch control system: An acoustic approach. *J. Acoust. Soc. Am.* 85: 1322–1328.

Johnson, D.B., Kondraske, G.V., Wilhelm, D.M., Jacomides, L., Ogan, K., Pearle, M.S., and Cadeddu, J.A. 2004. Assessment of basic human performance resources predicts performance of virtual ureterorenoscopy. *J. Urol.* 171: 80–84.

Kondraske, G.V. 1987a. Human performance: Science or art? In: Foster, K. (ed.), *Proceedings of 13th Northeast Bioengineering Conference*, pp. 44–47.

Kondraske, G.V. 1987b. Looking at the study of human performance. *SOMA: Eng. Hum. Body* (ASME) 2: 50.

Kondraske, G.V. 1988a. Experimental evaluation of an elemental resource model for human performance. In: Harris, G. and Walker, C. (eds.), *Proceedings of the 10th Annual IEEE Engineering in Medicine and Biological Society Conference*, IEEE, New York, pp. 1612–1613.

Kondraske, G.V. 1988b. Human performance measurement and task analysis, In: Enders, A. (ed.), *Technology for Independent Living Sourcebook*, 2nd ed., RESNA, Washington, DC.

Kondraske, G.V. 1988c. Workplace design: An elemental resource approach to task analysis and human performance measurements. *Proceedings of the International Conference on Association in Advances Rehabilitation Technology*, pp. 608–611.

Kondraske, G.V. 1989. Neuromuscular performance: Resource economics and product-based composite indices. *Proceedings of the 11th Annual IEEE Engineering in Medicine and Biological Society Conference*, IEEE, New York, pp. 1045–1046.

Kondraske, G.V. 1990a. A PC-based performance measurement laboratory system. *J. Clin. Eng.* 15: 467–477.

Kondraske, G.V. 1990b. Quantitative measurement and assessment of performance. In: Smith, R.V. and Leslie, J.H. (eds.), *Rehabilitation Engineering*, CRC Press, Boca Raton, FL, pp. 101–125.

Kondraske, G.V. 1993. *The HPI Shorthand Notation System for Human System Parameters*, Technical Report 92–001R V1.5, Human Performance Institute, The University of Texas at Arlington, Arlington, TX.

Kondraske, G.V. 1995. An elemental resource model for the human–task interface. *Int. J. Technol. Assess. Health Care* 11: 153–173.

Kondraske, G.V. 1995. Measurement tools and processes in rehabilitation engineering. In: Bronzino, J.D. (ed.), *Handbook of Biomedical Engineering*, CRC Press, Boca Raton, FL.

Kondraske, G.V. and Beehler, P.J.H. 1994. Applying general systems performance theory and the elemental resource model to gender-related issues in physical education and sport. *Women Sport Phys. Act. J.* 3: 1–19.

Kondraske, G.V., Beehler, P.J.H., Behbehani, K., Chwialkowski, M., Imrhan, S., Mooney, V., Pape, E., Richmond, J., Smith, S., and von Maltzahn, W. 1988. Measuring human performance: Concepts, methods, and application examples. *SOMA: Eng. Hum. Body (ASME)* Jan: 6–13.

Kondraske, G.V., Johnston, C., Pearson, A., and Tarbox, L. 1997. Performance prediction and limiting resource identification with nonlinear causal resource analysis. *Proceedings, 19th Annual Engineering in Medicine and Biology Society Conference*, pp. 1813–1816.

Kondraske, G.V. and Khoury, G.J. 1992. Telerobotic system performance measurement: Motivation and methods. In: *Cooperative Intelligent Robotics in Space III*, SPIE, Vol. 1829, pp. 161–172.

Kondraske, G.V. and Standridge, R. 1988. Robot performance: Conceptual strategies. In: *Conference of Digest IEEE Midcon/88 Technological Conference*, IEEE, New York, pp. 359–362.

Leibniz, G.W. and Montgomery, G.R. *Discourse on Metaphysics and the Monadology*. Prometheus Books, 1992.

Mayer, T.G. and Gatchel, R.J. 1991. *Functional Restoration for Spinal Disorders: The Sports Medicine Approach*, Lea & Febeger, Philadelphia, pp. 66–77.

Meister, D. 1989. *Conceptual Aspects of Human Performance*, The Johns Hopkins University Press, Baltimore.

Murphy, M. 2002. The fall factor. *Rehab. Manag.* 15: 34–38.

Navon, D. and Gopher, D. 1979. On the economy of the human processing system. *Psych. Rev.* 86: 214–253.

Neel, A. 1977. *Theories of Psychology: A Handbook*, Schenkman Publishing Co., Cambridge, MA.

Olson, S. and Kondraske, G.V. 2005, in press. Clinical applications of the elemental resource model and performance theory. In: Simmonds, M.J. (ed.), *Measuring and Managing Pain, Patients, and Practitioners. Assessment, Outcomes and Evidence*. Elsevier Press, New York.

Parnianpour, M. and Marras, W.S. 1993. Development of clinical protocols based on ergonomics evaluation in response to American Disability Act, 1992, In: *Rehabilitation Engineering Center Proposal to National Institute on Disability and Rehabilitation Research*, Ohio State University, Columbus, OH.

Schoner, G. and Kelso, J.A.S. 1988. Dynamic pattern generation in behavioral and neural systems. *Science* 239: 1513–1520.

Syndulko, K., Tourtellotte, W.W., and Richter, E. 1988. Toward the objective measurement of central processing resources. *Med. Biol. Soc. Mag.* 7: 17–20.

Taylor, F.W. 1911. *The Principles of Scientific Management*. Harper and Brothers, New York.

Turvey, M.T., Shaw, R.E., and Mace, W. 1978. Issues in the theory of action: Degrees of freedom, coordinative structures, and coalitions. In: Requin, J. (ed.), *Attention and Performance VII*, Lawrence Earlbaum Association, Hillsdale, NJ.

U.S. Department of Labor. 1992. *Dictionary of Occupation Titles*, 4th ed., Claitor's Publishing Division, Baton Rouge, LA, pp. 1401–1404.

Vasta, P.J. and Kondraske, G.V. 1994. Performance prediction of an upper extremity reciprocal task using non-linear causal resource analysis, In *Proceedings of 16th Annual IEEE Engineering in Medicine and Biology Society Conference*, IEEE, New York

Wickens, C.D. 1984. *Engineering Psychology and Human Performance*, Charles E. Merrill Publishing Co., Columbus, OH.

World Health Organization (WHO). 1980. International classification of impairments, disabilities, and handicaps. *WHO Chronicle* 34: 376.

Yen, S.S. and Kondraske, G.V. 1992. Machine shape perception: Object recognition based on need-driven resolution flexibility and convex-hull carving. In *Proceedings of the Conference of Intelligent Robots Computer Vision X: Algorithms Techniques*, SPIE, 1607: 176–187.

Further Information

General discussions of major issues associated with human performance modeling can be found in the following texts:

Fleishman, E.A. and Quaintance, M.K. 1984. *Taxonomies of Human Performance*, Academic Press, Orlando, FL.

Meister, D. 1989. *Conceptual Aspects of Human Performance*, The Johns Hopkins University Press, Baltimore.

Neel, A. 1977. *Theories of Psychology: A Handbook*, Schenkman Publishing Co., Cambridge, MA.

Requin, J. 1978. *Attention and Performance VII*, Lawrence Earlbaum Association, Hillsdale, NJ.

Wickens, C.D. 1984. *Engineering Psychology and Human Performance*, Charles E. Merrill Publishing Co., Columbus, OH.

More detailed information regarding general systems performance theory, the elemental resource model, and their application is available from the Human Performance Institute, PO Box 19180, University of Texas at Arlington, Arlington, TX 76019–0180 and at the HPI website: http://www-ee.uta.edu/hpi

30

Measurement of Neuromuscular Performance Capacities

Susan S. Smith
Texas Women's University

Movements allow us to interact with our environment, express ourselves, and communicate with each other. Life is movement. Movement is constantly occurring at many hierarchical levels including cellular and subcellular levels. By using the adjective "human" to clarify the term "movement," we are not only defining the species of interest, but also limiting the study to observable performance and its more overt causes. Study of human performance is of interest to a broad range of professionals including rehabilitation engineers, orthopedic surgeons, therapists, biomechanists, kinesiologists, psychologists, and so on. Because of the complexity of human performance and the variety of investigators, the study of human performance is conducted from several theoretical perspectives including (1) anatomical, (2) purpose or character of the movement (such as locomotion), (3) physiological, (4) biomechanical, (5) psychological, (6) socio-cultural, and (7) integrative. The elemental resource model (ERM), presented at the beginning of this section, is an integrative model that incorporates aspects of the other models into a singular system accounting for the human, the task, and the human–task interface (Kondraske, 2005).

The purposes of this chapter are to (1) provide reasons for measuring four selected variables of human performance: extremes/*range of motion*, strength, *speed of movement*, and *endurance*; (2) briefly define and discuss these variables; (3) overview selected instruments and methods used to measure these variables; and (4) discuss interpretation of performance for a given neuromuscular subsystem.

30.1 Neuromuscular Functional Units

While the theoretical perspectives listed previously may be useful within specific contexts or within specific disciplines, the broader appreciation of human performance and its control can be gained from the perspective of an integrative model such as the ERM (Kondraske, 2005). This model organizes performance resources into four different domains. Basic movements, such as elbow flexion, are executed by *neuromuscular functional units* in the environmental interface domain. Intermediate and complex tasks, such as walking and playing the piano, utilize multiple basic functional units. The human performing a movement operates the involved functional units along different dimensions of performance according to the demands of the task. Dimensions of performance are factors such as joint motion, strength, speed of movement, and endurance. Lifting a heavy box off the floor requires, among other things, a specific amount of strength associated with neuromuscular functional units of the back, legs, and arms according to the weight and size of the box. Reaching for a light-weight box from the top shelf of a closet requires that the shoulder achieve certain *extremes of motion* according to the height of the shelf.

Whereas four dimensions of performance are considered individually in this chapter, they are *highly interdependent*. For example, strength availability during a movement is partly dependent on joint angle. Despite interdependence, considering the variables as different dimensions is essential to studying human performance. The components limiting the human's ability to complete a task can only be identified and subsequently enhanced by determining, for example, that the reason the human cannot reach the box off the top shelf is not because of insufficient range of motion of the shoulder, but because of insufficient strength of the shoulder musculature required to lift the arm through the range of motion. Isolating the subsystems involved in a task and maximally stressing them along one or more "isolated" dimensions of performance is a key concept in the ERM. "Maximally stressing" the subsystems means that the maximum amount of the resource available is being determined. This differs from determining the amount of the resource that happened to be used while performing a particular task. Often the distinction between obtaining maximal performance from a human and submaximal performance is in the instructions given the subject. For example, when measuring speed, we say, "move as fast as you can."

30.1.1 Purposes of Measuring Selected Neuromuscular Performance Capacities

Range of motion, strength, speed of movement, and endurance can be measured for one or more of the following purposes:

1. To determine the amount of the resource available and to compare it to the normal value for that individual. "Normal" is frequently determined by comparisons with the opposite extremity or with normative data when available. This information can be used to develop goals and a program to change the performance.

2. To assist in determining the possible affects of insufficient or imbalanced amounts of the variable on a person's performance of activities of daily living, work, sport, and leisure pursuits. In this case the amount of the variable is compared to the demands of the task, rather than to norms or to the opposite extremity.
3. To assist in diagnosis of medical conditions and the nature of movement dysfunctions.
4. To reassess status in order to determine the effectiveness of a program designed to change the amount of the variable.
5. To motivate persons to comply with treatment or training regimes.
6. To document status and the results of treatment or training and to communicate with other involved persons.
7. To assist in ergonomically designed furniture, equipment, techniques, and environments.
8. To provide information that when combined with other measures of human performance can be used to predict functional capabilities.

30.2 Range of Motion and Extremes of Motion

Range of motion (ROM) is the amount of movement that occurs at a joint. ROM is typically measured by noting the *extremes of motion (EOM)*. The designated reference or zero position must be specified for measurements of the two extremes of motion. For example, to measure elbow (radiohumeral joint) flexion and extension, the preferred starting position is with the subject supine with the arm parallel to the lateral midline of the body with the palm facing upward (Norkin and White, 2003; Reese and Bandy, 2002). Measurements are taken with the elbow in the fully flexed position and with the elbow in the fully extended position.

30.2.1 Movement Terminology

Joint movements are described using a coordinate system with the human body in anatomical position. Anatomical position of the body is an erect position, face forward, arms at sides, palms facing forward, and fingers and thumbs in extension. The central coordinate system consists of three cardinal planes and axes with its origin located between the cornua of the sacrum (Panjabi et al., 1974). Figure 30.1 demonstrates the planes and axes of the central coordinate system. The same coordinate system can parallel the master system at any joint in the body by relocating the origin to any defined point.

The sagittal plane is the y, z plane; and the frontal (or coronal) plane is the y, x plane; and the horizontal (or transverse) plane is the x, z plane. Movements are described in relation to the origin of the coordinate system. The arrows indicate the positive direction of each axis. An anterior translation is $+z$; a posterior translation is $-z$. Clockwise rotations are $+\theta$, and counterclockwise rotations are $-\theta$.

Joints are described as having degrees of freedom (DOF) of movement; DOF, that is, the number of axes associated with a joint each of which allows motion in a plane in three-dimensional space. If a motion occurs in one plane and around one axis, the joint is defined as having one DOF. Joints with movements in two planes occurring around two different axes, have two DOF, and so on.

Angular movements refer to motions that cause an increase or decrease in the angle between the articulating bones. Angular movements are flexion, extension, abduction, adduction, and lateral flexion (see Table 30.1). Rotational movements generally occur around a longitudinal (or vertical) axis except for movements of the clavicle and scapula. The rotational movements occurring around the longitudinal axis (internal rotation, external rotation, opposition, horizontal abduction, and horizontal adduction) are described in Table 30.1. Rotation of the scapula is described in terms of the direction of the inferior angle. Movement of the inferior angle of the scapula toward the midline is a medial (or downward) rotation, and movement of the inferior angle away from the midline is lateral (or upward) rotation. In the extremities, the anterior surface of the extremity is used as the reference area. Because the head, neck, trunk, and pelvis rotate about a midsagittal, longitudinal axis, rotation of these parts is designated as right or left.

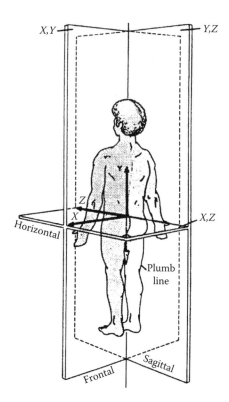

FIGURE 30.1   Planes and axes are illustrated in anatomical position. The central coordinate system with its origin between the cornua of the sacrum is shown. (From White III A.A. and Panjabi M.M. 1990. *Clinical Biomechanics of the Spine*, 2nd ed., p. 87. Philadelphia, JB Lippincott Company. With permission.)

A communications problem often exists in describing motion using the terms defined in Table 30.1. A body segment can be in a position such as flexion, but can be moving toward extension. This confusion is partially remedied by using the form of the word with the suffix, *-ion*, to indicate a static position and using the suffix, *-ing*, to denote a movement. Thus, an elbow can be in a position of 90° flex *ion* and also extend *ing*.

30.2.2 Factors Influencing ROM/EOM and ROM/EOM Measurements

The ROM and EOM available at a joint are determined by morphology and the soft tissues surrounding and crossing a joint, including the joint capsule, ligaments, tendons, and muscles. Other factors such as age, gender, swelling, muscle mass development, body fat, passive insufficiency (change in the ROM/EOM available at one joint in a two-joint muscle complex caused by the position of the other joint), and time of day (diurnal effect) also affect the amount of motion available. Some persons, because of posture, genetics, body type, or movement habits, normally demonstrate hypermobile or hypomobile joints. Dominance has not been found to significantly affect available ROM. See discussion in Miller (1985). The shapes of joint surfaces, which are designed to allow movement in particular directions, can become altered by disease, trauma, and posture, thereby increasing or decreasing the ROM/EOM. Additionally, the soft tissues crossing a joint can become short (contracted) or overstretched altering the ROM/EOM.

The type of movement, active or passive, also affects ROM/EOM. When measuring active ROM (AROM), the person voluntarily contracts muscles and moves the body part through the available motion. When measuring passive ROM (PROM), the examiner moves the body part through the ROM.

TABLE 30.1 Movement Terms, Planes, Axes, and Descriptions of Movements

Movement Term	Plane	Axis	Description of Movement
Flexion	Sagittal	Frontal	Bending of a part such that the anterior surfaces approximate each other. However, flexion of the knee, ankle, foot, and toes refers to movement in the posterior direction.
Extension	Sagittal	Frontal	Opposite of flexion; involves straightening a body part.
Abduction	Frontal	Sagittal	Movement away from the midline of the body or body part; abduction of the wrist is sometimes called *radial deviation*.
Adduction	Frontal	Sagittal	Movement toward the midline of the body or body part; adduction of the wrist is sometimes called *ulnar deviation*.
Lateral flexion	Frontal	Sagittal	Term used to denote lateral movements of the head, neck, and trunk.
Internal (medial) rotation	Horizontal	Longitudinal	Turning movement of the anterior surface of a part toward the midline of the body; internal rotation of the forearm is referred to as *pronation*.
External (lateral) rotation	Horizontal	Longitudinal	Turning movement of the anterior surface of a part away from the midline of the body; external rotation of the forearm is referred to as *supination*.
Opposition	Multiple	Multiple	Movement of the tips of the thumb and little finger toward each other.
Horizontal abduction	Horizontal	Longitudinal	Movement of the arm in a posterior direction away from the midline of the body with the shoulder joint in 90° of either flexion or abduction.
Horizontal adduction	Horizontal	Longitudinal	Movement of the arm in an anterior direction toward the midline of the body with the shoulder joint in 90° of either flexion or abduction.
Tilt	Depends on joint	Depends on joint	Term used to describe certain movements of the scapula and pelvis. In the scapula, an anterior tilt occurs when the coracoid process moves in an anterior and downward direction while the inferior angle moves in a posterior and upward direction. A posterior tilt of the scapula is the opposite of an anterior tilt. In the pelvis, an anterior tilt is rotation of the anterior superior spines (ASISs) of the pelvis in an anterior and downward direction; a posterior tilt is movement of the ASISs in a posterior and upward direction. A lateral tilt of the pelvis occurs when the pelvis is not in level from side to side, but one ASIS is higher than the other one.
Gliding	Depends on joint	Depends on joint	Movements that occur when one articulating surface slides on the opposite surface.
Elevation	Frontal		A gliding movement of the scapula in an upward direction as in shrugging the shoulders.
Depression	Frontal		Movement of the scapula downward in a direction reverse of elevation.

PROM is usually slightly greater than AROM due to the extensibility of the tissues crossing and comprising the joint. AROM can be decreased because of restricted joint mobility, muscle weakness, pain, unwillingness to move, or inability to follow instructions. PROM is assessed to clinically determine the integrity of the joint and the extent of structural limitation.

30.2.3 Instrumented Systems Used to Measure ROM/EOM

The most common instrument used to measure joint ROM/EOM is a goniometer. The universal goniometer, shown in Figure 30.2a, is most widely used clinically. A variety of universal goniometers have been developed for specific applications. Two other types of goniometers are also shown in Figure 30.2.

Table 30.2 lists and compares several goniometric instruments used to measure ROM/EOM. Choice of the instrument used to measure ROM/EOM depends upon the degree of accuracy required, time available to the examiner, the measurement environment, the body segment being measured, and the equipment available.

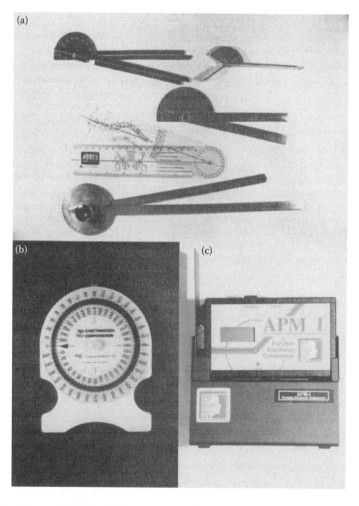

FIGURE 30.2 Three types of goniometric instruments used to measure range and extremes of motion are shown: (a) typical 180- and 360-degree universal goniometers of various sizes; (b) a fluid goniometer, which is activated by the effects of gravity; (c) an APM I digital electronic device that works similarly to a pendulum goniometer, but is not limited by gravity dependency.

TABLE 30.2 Comparison of Various Goniometers Commonly Used to Measure Joint Range and Extremes of Motion

Type of Goniometer	Advantages/Uses	Disadvantages/Limitations
Universal goniometer		
A protractor-like device with one arm considered movable and the other arm stationary; protractor can have a 180 or 360°(scale and is usually numbered in both directions; available in a range of sizes and styles to accommodate different joints (see Figure 30.2a)	Inexpensive; portable; familiar devices; size of the joint being measured determines size of the goniometer used; clear plastic goniometers have a line through the center of the arms to make alignment easier and more accurate; finger goniometers can be placed over the dorsal aspect of the joint being measured	Several goniometers of different sizes may be required, especially if digits are measured; full-circle models may be difficult to align when the subject is recumbent and axis alignment is inhibited by the protractor bumping the surface; the increments on the protractors may vary from 1, 2, or 5°; placement of the arms is a potential source of error
Fluid (or bubble) goniometer		
A device with a fluid-filled channel with a 360° scale that relies on the effects of gravity (see Figure 30.2b); dial turns allowing the goniometer to be "zeroed"; some models are strapped on and others must be held against the body part	Quick and easy to use because it is not usually aligned with bony landmarks; does not have to conform to body segments; useful for measuring neck and spinal movements; using a pair of fluid goniometers permits distinguishing regional spinal motion	More expensive than universal goniometers; using a pair of goniometers is awkward; useless for motions in the horizontal plane; error can be induced by slipping, skin movement, variations in amount of soft tissue owing to muscle contraction, swelling, or fat, and the examiner's hand pressure changing body segment contour; reliability may be sacrificed from lack of orientation to landmarks and difficulty with consistent realignment (Miller, 1985)
Pendulum goniometer		
A scaled, inclinometer-like device with a needle or pointer (usually weighted); some models are strapped on and others must be held against the body part (not shown)	Inexpensive; same advantages as for the fluid goniometer described above	Some models cannot be "zeroed"; useless for motions in the horizontal plane; same soft tissue error concerns as described above for the fluid goniometer
"Myrin" OB goniometer		
A fluid-filled, rotatable container consisting of compass needle that responds to the earth's magnetic field (to measure horizontal motion), a gravity-activated inclination needle (to measure frontal and sagittal motion), and a scale (not shown)	Can be strapped on the body part allowing the hands free to stabilize and move the body part; not necessary to align the goniometer with the joint axis; permits measurements in all three planes	Expensive and bulky compared with universal goniometer; not useful for measuring small joints of hand and foot; susceptible to magnetic fields (Clarkson, 2000); subject to same soft tissue error concerns described above under fluid goniometer
Arthrodial protractor		
A large, flat, clear plastic protractor without arms that has a level on the straight edge (not shown)	Does not need to conform to body segments; most useful for measuring joint rotation and axioskeletal motion	Not useful for measuring smaller joints, especially those with lesser ROMs; usually scaled in large increments only
APM I		
Computerized goniometer with digital sensing and electronics; can either perform continuous monitoring or calculate individual ROM/EOM from a compound motion function (see Figure 30.2c)	Easy to use; provides rapid digital read-out; measures angles in *any* plane of motion (by using an "inertial" type of sensor gravity dependency is eliminated allowing for easier measurement of rotary movements, such as trunk rotation); one hand is free to stabilize and move body segments; particularly easy for measuring regional spinal movements	Expensive compared to most other instruments described; device must be rotated perpendicular to the direction of segment motion only; unit must stabilize prior to measurement; excessive delays in recording must be avoided; subject to the same soft tissue error concerns as described above under fluid goniometer, unless the device is aligned along (versus on) the body segment

continued

TABLE 30.2 (continued)   Comparison of Various Goniometers Commonly Used to Measure Joint Range and Extremes of Motion

Type of Goniometer	Advantages/Uses	Disadvantages/Limitations
Electrogoniometer		
Arms of a goniometer are attached to a potentiometer and are strapped to the proximal and distal body parts; movement from the device causes resistance in the potentiometer, which measures the ROM (not shown)	More useful for dynamic ROM, especially for determining kinematic variables during activities such as gait; provides immediate data; some electrogoniometers permit measurement in one, two, or three dimensions	Aligning and attaching the device is time-consuming and not amenable to all body segments; device and equipment needed to use it are moderately expensive; essentially laboratory equipment; less accurate for measurement of absolute limb position; device itself is cumbersome and may alter the movement being studied

Non-goniometric methods of joint measurement are available. Tape measures, radiographs, photography, cinematography, videotape, and various optoelectric movement-monitoring systems can also be used to measure or calculate the motion available at various joints. These methods are beyond the scope of this chapter.

30.2.4 Key Concepts in Goniometric Measurement

Numerous textbooks (Palmer and Epler, 1998; Clarkson, 2000; Reese and Bandy, 2002; Norkin and White, 2003) are available that describe precise procedures for goniometric measurements of each joint. Unfortunately, there is a lack of standardization among these references.

In general, the anatomical position of zero degrees (*preferred starting position*) is the desired starting position for all ROM/EOM measurements except rotation at the hip, shoulder, and forearm. The arms of the goniometer are usually aligned parallel and lateral to the long axis of the moving and the fixed-body segments in line with the appropriate landmarks. In the past, some authors contended that placement of the axis of the goniometer should be congruent with the joint axis for accurate measurement (Wiechec and Krusen, 1939; West, 1945). However, the axis of rotation for joints changes as the body segment moves through its ROM; therefore, a goniometer cannot be placed in a position in line with the joint axis during movement. Robson (1966) described how variations in the placement of the goniometer's axis could affect the accuracy of ROM measurements. Miller (1985) suggested that the axis problem could be handled by ignoring the goniometer's axis and concentrating on the accurate alignment of the arms of the goniometer with the specified landmarks. Potentially some accuracy may be sacrificed, but the technique is simplified and theoretically more reproducible. When using devices such as the APM I, pictured in Figure 30.2c, the manufacturer's user's manual (Human Performance Measurement, Inc., 1998–2003) recommends placing the alignment guide of the device *along* the side of body segments vs. placing the device directly on body segments (as is frequently done when using the fluid goniometer pictured in Figure 30.2b). Placing the device along the body segment avoids minimizes procedural measurement noise caused by varying pressure on the soft tissue and interindividual differences in soft tissue structure (which can be relevant when establishing norms or comparing a given subject to norms). In any case, the subject's movement is observed during testing for unwanted motions that could result in inaccurate measurement. For example, a subject might attempt to increase forearm supination by laterally flexing the trunk.

30.2.5 Numerical Notation Systems

Three primary systems exist for expressing joint motion in terms of degrees. These are the *0–180 System*, the *180–0 System*, and the *360 System*. The 0–180 System is the most widely accepted system in medical applications and may be the easiest system to interpret. In the 0–180 System, the starting position for all movements is considered to be 0°, and movements proceed toward 180°. As the joint motion increases, the numbers on the goniometric scale increase. In the 180–0 System, movements toward flexion approach 0° and movements toward extension approach 180°. Different rules are used for the other planes of motion. The 360 System is similar to the 180–0 System, which movements are frequently performed from a starting position of 180°. Movements of extension or adduction, which go beyond the neutral position, approach 360°. Joint motion can be reported in tables, charts, graphs, or pictures. In the 0–180 System, the starting and ending ranges are recorded separately, as 0–130°. If a joint cannot be started in the 0° position, the actual starting position is recorded, as 10–130°.

30.3 Strength

Muscle strength implies the force or torque production capacity of muscles. However, to measure strength, the term must be operationally defined. One definition modified from Clarkson (2000) states that muscular strength is the maximal amount of torque or force that a muscle or muscle groups can voluntarily exert in one maximal effort, when type of muscle contraction, limb velocity, and joint angle(s) are specified.

30.3.1 Strength Testing and Muscle Terminology

Physiologically, skeletal muscle strength is the ability of muscle fibers to generate maximal tension for a brief time interval. A muscle's ability to generate maximal tension and to sustain tension for differing time intervals is dependent on the muscle's cross-sectional area (the larger the cross-sectional area, the greater the strength), geometry (including the muscle fiber arrangement, length, moment arm, and angle of pennation), and physiology. Characteristics of muscle fibers have been classified based on twitch tension and fatigability. Different fiber types have different metabolic traits. Different types of muscle fibers are differentially stressed depending on the intensity and duration of the contraction. Ideally, strength tests should measure the ability of the muscle to develop tension rapidly and to sustain the tension for brief time intervals. In order to truly measure muscle tension, a measurement device must be directly attached to the muscle or tendon. Whereas this direct procedure has been performed (Komi, 1990), it is hardly useful as a routine clinical measure. Indirect measures are used to estimate the strength of muscle groups performing a given function, such as elbow flexion.

Muscles work together in groups and may be classified according to the major role of the group in producing movement. The *prime mover*, or *agonist*, is a muscle or muscle group that makes the major contribution to movement at a joint. The *antagonist* is a muscle or muscle group that has an opposite action to the prime mover(s). The antagonist relaxes as the agonist moves the body part through the ROM. *Synergists* are accessory muscles that contract and work with the agonist to produce the desired movement. Synergists may work by stabilizing proximal joints, preventing unwanted movement, and joining with the prime mover to produce a movement that one muscle group acting alone could not produce.

A number of terms and concepts are important toward understanding the nature and scope of strength capacity testing. Several of these terms are defined below; however, there are no universally accepted definitions for these terms.

Dynamic contraction: The output of muscles moving body segments (Kroemer, 1991).
Isometric: Tension develops in a muscle, but the muscle length does not change and no movement occurs.
Static: Same as isometric.
Isotonic: A muscle develops constant tension against a load or resistance. Kroemer (1991) suggests the term, *isoforce*, more aptly describes this condition.
Concentric: A contraction in which a muscle develops internal force that exceeds the external force of resistance, the muscle shortens, and movement is produced (Gowitzke et al., 1980).

Eccentric: A contraction in which a muscle lengthens while continuing to maintain tension (Gowitzke et al., 1980).

Isokinetic: A condition where the angular velocity is held constant. Kroemer (1991) prefers the term, *isovelocity*, to describe this type of muscle exertion.

Isoinertial: A static or dynamic muscle contraction where the external load is held constant (Kroemer, 1983).

30.3.2 Factors Influencing Muscle Strength and Strength Measurement

In addition to the anatomical and physiological factors affecting strength, other factors must be considered when strength testing. The ability of a muscle to develop tension depends on the type of muscle contraction. Per unit of muscle, the greatest tension can be generated eccentrically, less can be developed isometrically, and the least can be generated concentrically. These differences in tension-generating capacity are so great that the type of contraction being strength-tested requires specification.

Additionally, strength is partially determined by the ability of the nervous system to cause more motor units to fire synchronously. As one trains, practices an activity, or learns test expectations, strength can increase. Therefore, strength is affected by previous training and testing. This is an important consideration in standardizing testing and in retesting.

A muscle's attachments define the angle of pull of the tendon on the bone and thereby the mechanical leverage at the joint center. Each muscle has a moment arm length, which is the length of a line normal to the muscle passing through the joint center. This moment arm length changes with the joint angle, which changes the muscle's tension output. Optimal tension is developed when a muscle is pulling at a 90° angle to the bony segment.

Changes in muscle length alter the force-generating capacity of muscle. This is called the *length–tension relationship*. *Active* tension decreases when a muscle is either lengthened or shortened relative to its resting length. However, applying a precontraction stretch, or slightly lengthening a muscle and the series elastic component (connective tissue), prior to a contraction causes a greater amount of *total* tension to be developed (Soderberg, 1992). Of course, excessive lengthening would reduce the tension-generating capacity.

A number of muscles cross over more than one joint. The length of these muscles may be inadequate to permit complete ROM of all joints involved. When a multijoint muscle simultaneously shortens at all joints it crosses, further effective tension development is prevented. This phenomenon is called *active insufficiency*. For example, when the hamstrings are tested as knee flexors with the hip extended, less tension can be developed than when the hamstrings are tested with the hip flexed. Therefore, when testing the strength of multijoint muscles, the position of all involved joints must be considered.

The *load–velocity relationship* is also important in testing muscle strength. A load–velocity curve can be generated by plotting the velocity of motion of the muscle lever arm against the external load. With concentric muscle contractions, the least tension is developed at the highest velocity of movement and vice versa. When the external load equals the maximal force that the muscle can exert, the velocity of shortening reaches zero and the muscle contracts isometrically. When the load is increased further, the muscle lengthens eccentrically. During eccentric contractions, the highest tension can be achieved at the highest velocity of movement (Komi, 1973).

The force generated by a muscle is proportional to the contraction time. The longer the contraction time, the greater the force development up to the point of maximum tension. Slower contraction leads to greater force production because more time is allowed for the tension produced in contractile elements to be transferred through the noncontractile components to the tendon. This is the *force–time relationship*. Tension in the tendon will reach the maximum tension developed by the contractile tissues only if the active contraction process is of adequate (even up to 300 ms) duration (Sukop and Nelson, 1974).

Subject effort or motivation, gender, age, fatigue, time of day, temperature, occupation, and dominance can also affect force or torque production capacity. Important additional considerations may be changes in muscle function as a result of pain, overstretching, immobilization, trauma, paralytic disorders, neurologic conditions, and muscle transfers.

30.3.3 Grading Systems and Parameters Measured

Clinically, the two most frequently used methods of strength testing are actually noninstrumented tests: the manual muscle test (MMT) and the functional muscle test (see Amundsen (1990) for more information on functional muscle tests). In each of these cases interval scaled grading criteria are operationally defined. However, a distinct advantage of using instruments to measure strength is that quantifiable units can be obtained.

Deciding whether to measure force (a translational quantity) or torque (a rotational quantity) is an important issue in testing strength. Even when the functional units of interest produce rotational motion, force measurement at some point along the moment arm is common. This is due to the evolution from manual muscle tests to the use of objective measurements where a force sensor replaces the human examiner sense of force resisted or generated. If d is the distance from the point of rotation to the point of force measurement and the force vector is tangent to the arc of motion, then

$$T = Fd \qquad (30.1)$$

Therefore, when force is measured, unless the measurement devices are applied at the same anatomical position for each test, force measurements can differ substantially even though the torque production capacity about the selected DOF is the same. Torque can be measured directly if the strength-testing device has an axis of rotation that can be aligned with the anatomical axis of rotation and a torque sensor is used, as in many isokinetic test devices. When this is not the case, the moment arm can be measured and torque calculated. Thus, for neuromuscular systems producing rotational motion, torque measures make the most sense and are preferred. The use of force measurements is the result of clinical traditional and these measures can be easily converted to torque units using knowledge of the applicable moment arm. Force measures are appropriate in whole-body exertions, such as lifting, where the motion is fundamentally translational. Another issue is whether to measure and record peak or averaged values. However, if strength is defined as maximum torque production capacity, peak values are implied.

In addition to single numerical values, some strength measurement systems display and print force or torque (vs. time) curves, angle-torque curves, and graphs. Computerized systems frequently compare the "involved" with the "uninvolved" extremity calculating "percent deficits." As strength is considered proportional to body weight (perhaps erroneously, see Delitto (1990)), force and torque measurements are frequently reported as a peak torque-to-body-weight ratio. This is seemingly to facilitate use of normative data where present, as the normalization results in a reduction in the variance of the data distribution.

30.3.4 Methods and Instruments Used to Measure Muscle Strength

There are two broad categories of testing force or torque production capacity: one category consists of measuring the capacity of defined, local muscle groups (e.g., elbow flexors); the second category of tests consists of measuring several muscle groups on a whole-body basis performing a higher-level task (e.g., lifting). The purpose of the test, required level of sensitivity, and expense are primary factors in selecting the method of strength testing. No single method has emerged as being clearly superior or more widely applicable. Like screwdrivers, different types and different sizes are needed depending upon job demands.

Many of the instrumented strength-testing techniques, which are becoming more standardized clinically and which are almost exclusively used in engineering applications, are based on the concepts and methods of MMT. Although not used for performance capacity tests, because of the ease, practicality, and speed of manual testing, it is still considered a useful tool, especially diagnostically to localize lesions and confirm weakness. Several MMT grading systems prevail. These differ in the actual test positions and premises upon which muscle grading is based. For example, the approach promoted by Kendall et al. (2005) tests a specific muscle (e.g., brachioradialis) rather than a motion. The Daniels and Worthingham method (Hislop and Montgomery, 2002) tests motions (e.g., elbow flexion) that involve all the agonists and synergists used to perform the movement. The latter is considered more functional and less time-consuming, but less specific. The reader is advised to consult these references directly for more information about MMT methods. Further discussion of noninstrumented tests is beyond the scope of this chapter.

An argument can be made for using isometric strength testing because the force or torque reflects actual muscle tension as the position of the body part is held constant and the muscle mechanics do not change. Additionally, good stabilization is easier to achieve, and muscle actions can be better isolated. However, some clinicians prefer dynamic tests, perceiving them as more reflective of function. An unfortunate fact is that neither static nor dynamic strength measurements alone can reveal whether strength is adequate for functional activities. However, strength measurements can be used with models and engineering analyses for such assessments.

Selected instrumented methods of measuring force or torque production capacity are listed and compared in Table 30.3. Table 30.3 is by no means comprehensive. More in-depth review and comparisons of various methods can be found in Amundsen (1990) and Mayhew and Rothstein (1985). Figure 30.3 illustrates three common instruments used to measure strength.

30.3.5 Key Concepts in Measuring Strength

Because of the number of factors influencing strength and strength testing (discussed in Section 30.3.2), one can become discouraged rather than challenged when faced with the need to measure strength. Optimally, strength testing would be based on the "worst-case" functional performance demands required by an individual in his or her daily life. "Worst-case" testing requires knowing the performance demands of tasks including the positions required, types of muscle contractions, and so on.

In the absence of such data, current strategy is to choose the instruments and techniques that maximally stress the system under a set of representative conditions that either (a) seem logical based on knowledge of the task, or (b) have been reported as appropriate and reliable for the population of interest. An attempt is made to standardize the testing in terms of contraction type, test administration instructions, feedback, warm-up, number of trials, time of day, examiner, duration of contraction (usually 4–6 s), method and location of application of force, testing order, environmental distractions, subject posture and position of testing, degree of stabilization, and rest intervals between exertions (usually 30 s to 2 min) (Chaffin, 1975; Smidt and Rogers, 1982). In addition, the subject must be observed for muscle group substitutions and "trick" movements.

30.4 Speed of Movement

Speed of movement refers to the rate of movement of the body or body segments. The maximum movement speed that can be achieved represents another unique performance capacity of an identified system that is responsible for producing motion. Everyday living, work, and sport tasks are commonly described in terms of the speed requirements (e.g., repetitions per minute or per hour). For physical tasks, such descriptions translate to translational motion speeds (e.g., as in lifting) as well as rotational motion speeds (i.e., movement about a DOF of the joint systems involved). Thus, there is important motivation to characterize this capacity.

TABLE 30.3 Comparison of Various Instrumented Methods Used to Measure Muscle Strength

Instrument/Method	Advantages/Uses	Disadvantages/Limitations
Repetition maximum		
Amount of weight a subject can lift a given number of times and no more; one determines either a one-repetition maximum (1-RM) or a ten-repetition maximum (10-RM). A 1-RM is the maximum amount of weight a subject can lift once; a 10-RM is the amount of weight a subject can lift 10 times; a particular protocol to determine RMs is defined (DeLorme and Watkins, 1948); measures dynamic strength in terms of weight (pounds or kilograms) lifted	Requires minimal equipment (weights); inexpensive and easy to administer; frequently used informally to assess progress in strength training	Uses serial testing of adding weights that may invalidate subsequent testing; no control for speed of contraction or positioning; minimal information available on the reliability and validity of this method
Hand-held dynamometer		
Device held in the examiner's hand used to test strength; devices use either hydraulics, strain gauges (load–cells), or spring systems (see Figure 30.3a); used with a "break test" (the examiner exerts a force against the body segment to be tested until the part gives way) or a "make test" (the examiner applies a constant force while the subject exerts a maximum force against it); "make tests" are frequently preferred for use with hand-held dynamometers (Smidt, 1984; Bohannon, 1990) measures force; unclear whether test measures isometric or eccentric force (this may depend on whether a "make test" or a "break test" is used)	Similar to manual muscle testing (MMT) in test positions and sites for load application; increased objectivity over MMT; portable; easy to administer; relatively inexpensive; commercially available from several suppliers; adaptable for a variety of test sites; provide immediate output; spring and hydraulic systems are nonelectrical; load–cell based systems provide more precise digital measurements	Stabilization of the device and body segment can be difficult; results can be affected by the examiner's strength; limited usefulness with large muscle groups; spring-based systems fatigue over time becoming inaccurate; range and sensitivity of the systems vary; shape of the unit grasped by the examiner and shape of the end-piece vary in comfort, and therefore the force a subject or examiner is willing to exert; more valuable for testing subjects with weakness than for less involved or healthy subjects due to range limits within the device (see discussion in Bohannon (1990))
Cable tensiometer		
One end of a cable is attached to an immovable object and the other end is attached to a limb segment; the tensiometer is placed between the sites of fixation; as the cable is pulled, it presses on the tensiometer's riser which is connected to a gauge (see discussion in Mayhew and Rothstein (1985)); measures isometric force	Mostly used in research settings; evidence presented on reliability when used with normal subjects (Clarke, 1952; Clarke et al., 1954); relatively inexpensive	Requires special equipment for testing; testing is time-consuming and some tests require two examiners; unfamiliar to most clinicians; not readily available; less sensitive at low force levels
Strain gauge		
Electroconductive material applied to metal rings or rods; a load applied to the ring or bar deforms the metal and a gauge; deformation of the gauge changes the electrical resistance of the gauge causing a voltage variation; this change can be converted and displayed using a strip chart recorder or digital display; measures isometric force	Mostly used in research settings; increased sensitivity for testing strong and weak muscles	Strain gauges require frequent calibration and are sensitive to temperature variations; to be accurate the body part must pull or push against the gauge in the same line that the calibration weights were applied; unfamiliar to most clinicians; not commercially available; difficult to interface the device comfortably with the subject

continued

TABLE 30.3 (continued) Comparison of Various Instrumented Methods Used to Measure Muscle Strength

Instrument/Method	Advantages/Uses	Disadvantages/Limitations
Isokinetic dynamometer		
Constant velocity loading device; several models marketed by a number of different companies; most consist of a movable lever arm controlled by an electronic servomotor that can be preset for selected angular velocities usually between 0 and 500° per second; when the subject attempts to accelerate beyond the pre-set machine speed, the machine resists the movement; a load cell measures the torque needed to prevent body part acceleration beyond the selected speed; computers provide digital displays and printouts (see typical device in Figure 30.3b); measures isokinetic-concentric (and in some cases, isokinetic-eccentric) and isometric strength; provides torque (or occasionally force) data; debate exists about whether data are ratio-scaled or not; accounting for the weight of the segment permits ratio-scaling (Winter et al., 1981)	Permits dynamic testing of most major body segments; especially useful for stronger movements; most devices provide good stabilization; measures reciprocal muscle contractions; widespread clinical acceptance; also records angular data, work, power, and endurance-related measures; provides a number of different reporting options; also used as exercises devices	Devices are large and expensive; need calibration with external weights or are "self-calibrating"; signal damping and "windowing" may affect data obtained; angle-specific measurements may not be accurate if a damp is used because torque readings do not relate to the goniometric measurements; joints must be aligned with the mechanical axis of the machine; inferences about muscle function in daily activities from isokinetic test results have not been validated; data obtained between different brands are not interchangeable; adequate stabilization may be difficult to achieve for some movements; may not usable with especially tall or short persons
Hand dynamometer		
Instruments to measure gripping or pinching strength specifically for the hand; usually use a spring scale or strain-gauge system (see typical grip strength testing device in Figure 30.3c); measures isometric force	Readily available from several suppliers; easy to use; relatively inexpensive; widespread use; some normative data available	Only useful for the hand; different brands not interchangeable; normative data only useful when reported for the same instrument and when measurements are taken with the same body position and instrument setting; must be recalibrated frequently

30.4.1 Speed of Movement Terminology

Speed of movement must be differentiated from *speed of contraction*. Speed of contraction refers to how fast a muscle generates tension. Two body parts may be moving through an arc with the same speed of movement; however, if one part has a greater mass, its muscles must develop more tension per unit of time to move the heavier body part at the same speed as the lighter body part.

Speed, velocity, and acceleration also can be distinguished. The terms velocity and speed are often used interchangeably; however, the two quantities are frequently not identical. Velocity means the rate of motion *in a particular direction. Acceleration* results from a change in velocity over time. General velocity and acceleration measurements are beyond the intent of this chapter. Reaction speed and response speed are other related variables also not considered.

30.4.2 Factors Influencing Speed of Movement and Speed of Movement Measurements

Muscles with larger moment arms, longer muscle fibers, and less pennation tend to be capable of generating greater speed. Many of the same factors influencing strength, discussed earlier, such as muscle

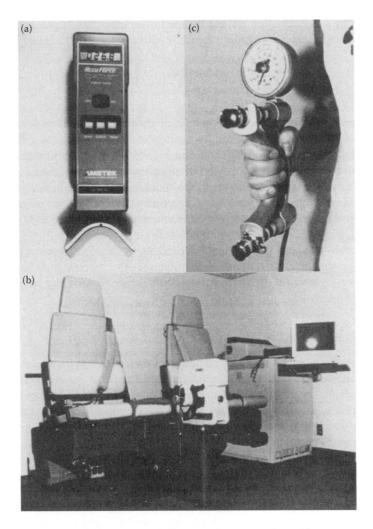

FIGURE 30.3 Three types of instrumented strength testing devices are shown (a) a representative example of a typical hand-held dynamometer; (b) an example of an isokinetic strength testing device; and (c) a hand dynamometer used to measure grip strength.

length, fatigue, and temperature affect the muscle's contractile rate. The load–velocity relationship is especially important when testing speed of movement. In addition to these and other physiological factors, speed can be reduced by factors such as friction, air resistance, gravity, unnecessary movements, and inertia (Jensen and Fisher, 1979).

30.4.3 Parameters Measured

Speed of movement can be measured as a linear quantity or as an angular quantity. Typically, if the whole body is moving linearly in space as in walking or running, a point such as the center of gravity is picked, and translational motion is measured. Also, when an identified point on a body segment (e.g., the tip of the index finger) is moved in space, translational movement is observed, and motion is measured in translational terms. If the speed of a rotational motion system (e.g., elbow flexors) is being measured, then the angular quantity is determined. As the focus here is on measuring isolated neuromuscular performance capacities, the angular metric is emphasized. Angular speed of a body segment is obtained by: angular speed = change in angular position/change in time,

$$\partial = \frac{\Delta\phi}{\Delta t}$$

(30.2)

Thus, speed of movement may be expressed in revolutions, degrees, or radians per unit of time, such as degrees per second (deg/s).

Another type of speed measure applies to well-defined (over fixed angle or distance) cyclic motions. Here repetitions per unit time or cycles per unit time measures are sometimes used. However, in almost every one of these situations, speed can be expressed in degrees per second or meters per second. The latter units are preferred because they allow easier comparison of speeds across a variety of tasks. The only occasion when this is difficult is when translation motion is not in a simple straight line, such as when a person is performing a complex assembly task with multiple subtasks.

The issue of whether to express speed as maximum, averaged, or instantaneous values must also be decided, based on which measure is a more useful indicator of the performance being measured. In addition to numerical reporting of speed data, time-history graphs of speed may be helpful in comparing some types of performance.

30.4.4 Instruments Used to Measure Speed of Movement

When movement time is greater than a few seconds and the distance is known, speed can be measured with a stopwatch or with switch plates, such as the time elapsed in moving between two points or over a specified angle. With rapid angular joint movements, switch plates or electrogoniometers with electronic timing devices are required. Speeds can also be computed from the distance or angle and time data available from cinematography, optoelectric movement monitoring systems, and videotape systems. Some dynamic strength testing devices involve presetting a load and measuring the speed of movement.

In addition, accelerometers can be used to measure acceleration directly, and speed can be derived through integration. However, piezoelectric models have no steady-state response and may not be useful for slower movements. Single accelerometers are used to measure linear motion. Simple rotatory motions require two accelerometers. Triaxial accelerometers are commercially available that contain three premounted accelerometers perpendicular to each other. Multiple accelerometer outputs require appropriate processing to resolve the vector component corresponding to the desired speed. Accelerometers are most appropriately used to measure acceleration when they are mounted on rigid materials. Accelerometers have the advantage of continuously and directly measuring acceleration in an immediately usable form. They can also be very accurate if well-mounted. Because they require soft tissue fixation and cabling or telemetry, they may alter performance and further error may be induced by relative motion of the device and tissues. The systems are moderately expensive (see discussion of accelerometers in Robertson and Sprigings (1987)).

30.4.5 Key Concepts in Speed of Movement Measurement

As discussed, maximum speed is determined when there is little stress on torque production resources. As resistance increases, speed will decrease. Therefore, the load must be considered and specified when testing speed. Because speed of movement data are calculated from displacement and temporal data, a key issue is minimizing error that might result from collecting this information. Error can result from inaccurate identification of anatomical landmarks, improper calibration, perspective error, instrument synchronization error, resolution, digitization error, or vibration. The sampling rate of some of the measurement systems may become an issue when faster movements are being analyzed. In addition, the dynamic characteristics of signal conditioning systems should be reported.

30.5 Endurance

Endurance is the ability of a system to sustain an activity for a prolonged time (static endurance) or to perform repeatedly (dynamic endurance). Endurance can apply to the body as a whole, a particular body system, or to specific neuromuscular functional units. High levels of endurance imply that a given level of performance can be continued for a long time period.

30.5.1 Endurance Terminology

General endurance of the body as a whole is traditionally considered cardiovascular endurance, or aerobic capacity. Cardiovascular endurance is most frequently viewed in terms of V_{O2max}. This chapter considers only endurance of neuromuscular systems. Although many central and peripheral anatomic sites and physiologic processes contribute to a loss of endurance, endurance of neuromuscular functional units is also referred to as *muscular endurance*.

Absolute muscle endurance is defined as the amount of time that a neuromuscular system can continue to accomplish a specified task against a constant resistance (load and rate) without relating the resistance to the muscle's strength. Absolute muscle endurance and strength are highly correlated. Conversely, strength and *relative muscle endurance* are inversely related. That is, when resistance is adjusted to the person's strength, a weaker person tends to demonstrate more endurance than a stronger person. Furthermore, the same relationships between absolute and relative endurance and strength are correlated by type of contraction; in other words, there is a strong positive correlation between isotonic strength and *absolute* isotonic endurance and vice versa for strength and *relative* isotonic endurance. The same types of relationships exist for isometric strength and isometric endurance (Jensen and Fisher, 1979).

30.5.2 Factors Influencing Neuromuscular Endurance and Measurement of Endurance

Specific muscle fiber types, namely fast-twitch fatigue-resistant fibers (FR), generate intermediate levels of tension and are resistant to short-term fatigue (a duration of about 2 min or intermittent stimulation). Slow-twitch fibers (S) generate low levels of tension slowly, and are highly resistant to fatigue. Muscle contractions longer than 10 s, but less than 2 min, will reflect local muscle endurance (Åstrand et al., 2003). For durations longer than 2 min, the S fibers will be most stressed. A submaximal isometric contraction to the point of voluntary fatigue will primarily stress the FR and S fibers (Thorstensson and Karlsson, 1976). Repetitive, submaximal, dynamic contractions continued for about 2–6 min will measure the capacity of FR and S fibers. Strength testing requires short duration and maximal contractions; therefore, to differentiate strength and endurance testing, the duration and intensity of the contractions must be considered.

Because strength affects endurance, all of the factors discussed previously as influencing strength, also influence endurance. In addition to muscle physiology and muscle strength, endurance is dependent upon the extensiveness of the muscle's capillary beds, the involved neuromuscular mechanisms, contraction force, load, and the rate at which the activity is performed.

Endurance time, or the time for muscles to reach fatigue, is a function of the contraction force or load (von Rohmert, 1960). As the load (or torque required) increases, endurance time decreases. Also, as speed increases, particularly with activities involving concentric muscle contractions, endurance decreases.

30.5.3 Parameters Measured

Endurance is *how long* an activity can be performed at the required load and rate level. Thus, the basic unit of measure is time. Time is the only measure of how long it takes to complete a task. If the focus is on a given variable (e.g., strength, speed, or endurance), it is necessary to either control or measure the others. When the focus is endurance, the other factors of force or torque, speed, and joint angle, can be described as conditions under which endurance is measured. Because of the interactions of endurance and load or endurance and time (as e.g.), a number of *endurance-related* measures have evolved. These endurance-related measures have clouded endurance testing.

One endurance-related measure uses either the number of repetitions that can be performed at 20%, 25%, or 50% of maximum peak torque or force. The units used to reflect endurance in this case are number of repetitions at a specified torque or force level. One difficulty with this definition has been described previously, that is, the issue of relative vs. absolute muscle endurance. Rothstein and Rose (1982) demonstrated that elderly subjects with selected muscle fiber type atrophy were able to maintain 50% of their peak torque longer than young subjects. However, if a high force level is required to perform the task, then the younger subject would have more endurance in that particular activity (Rothstein, 1982). Another difficulty is that the "repetition method" can be used only for dynamic activities. If isometric activities are involved, then the time an activity can be sustained at a specified force or torque level is measured. Why have different units of endurance? Time could be used in both cases. Furthermore, the issue of absolute vs. relative muscle endurance becomes irrelevant if the demands of the task are measured.

Yet another method used to reflect endurance is to calculate an endurance-related work ratio. Many isokinetic testing devices, such as the one shown in Figure 30.3b, will calculate work (integrate force or torque over displacement). In this case, the total amount of work performed in the first five repetitions is compared with the total amount of work performed in the last five repetitions of a series of repetitions (usually 25 or more). Work degradation *reflects* endurance and is reported as percentage. An additional limitation of using these endurance ratios is that work cannot be determined in isometric test protocols. Mechanically there is no movement, and no work is being performed.

Overall, the greatest limitation with most *endurance-related* approaches is that the measures obtained cannot be used to perform task-related assessments. In a workplace assessment, for example, one can determine how long a specific task (defined by the conditions of load, range, and speed) needs to be performed. Endurance-related metrics can be used to reflect changes over time in a subject's available endurance capacity; however, endurance-related metrics cannot be compared to the demands of the task. Task demands are measured in time or repetitions (e.g., 10 h) with a given rate (e.g., 1/0.5 h) from which total time (e.g., 5 h) can be calculated. A true endurance measure (vs. an endurance-related measure) can serve both purposes. Time reflects changes in endurance as the result of disease, disuse, training, or rehabilitation and also can be linked to task demands.

30.5.4 Methods and Instruments Used to Measure Neuromuscular Endurance

Selection of the method or instrument used to measure endurance depends on the purpose of the measurement and whether endurance or endurance-related measures will be obtained. As in strength testing, endurance tests can involve simple, low-level tasks or whole-body, higher-level activities. The simplest method of measuring endurance is to define a task in terms of performance criteria and then time the performance with a stopwatch. A subject is given a load and a posture and asked to hold it "as long as possible" or to move from one point to another point at a specific rate of movement for "as long as possible."

An example of a static endurance test is the Sorensen test used to measure endurance of the trunk extensors (Biering-Sorensen, 1984). This test measures how long a person can sustain his or her torso in a suspended prone posture. The individual is not asked to perform a maximal voluntary contraction, but an indirect calculation of load is possible (Smidt and Blanpied, 1987).

An example of a dynamic endurance test is either a standardized or nonstandardized, dynamic isoinertial (see description in Section 30.3.1 on strength testing) repetition test. In other words, the subject is asked to lift a known load with a specified body part or parts until defined conditions can no longer be met. Conditions such as acceleration, distance, method of performance, or speed may or may not be controlled. The more standardized of these tests, particularly those that involve lifting capacity, are reported and projections about performance capacity over time are estimated (Snook, 1978). Ergometers and some of the isokinetic dynamometers discussed earlier measure work, and several can calculate endurance-related ratios. These devices could be adapted to measure endurance in time units.

30.5.5 Key Concepts in Measuring Muscle Endurance

Of the four variables of human performance discussed in this chapter, endurance testing is the least developed and standardized. Except for test duration and rest intervals, attention to the same guidelines as described for strength testing is currently recommended.

30.6 Reliability, Validity, and Limitations in Testing

Space does not permit a complete review of these important topics. However, a few key comments are in order. First, it is important to note that reliability and validity are not inherent qualities of instruments, but exist in the measurements obtained only within the context in which they are tested. Second, reliability and validity are not either present or absent but are present or absent along a continuum. Third, traditional quantitative measures of reliability might indicate how much reliability a given measurement method demonstrates, but not how much reliability is actually needed. Fourth, technology has advanced to the extent that it is generally possible to measure physical variables such as time, force, torque, angles, and speed accurately, repeatably, and with high resolution. Finally, clinical generalizability of human performance capacity ultimately measures results from looking at the body of literature on reliability as a whole and not from single studies.

For these types of variables, results of reliability studies basically report that (1) if the instrumentation is good, and (2) if established, optimal procedures are carefully followed, then results of repeat testing will usually be in the range of about 5–20% of each other. This range of repeatability depends on (1) the particular variable being measured (i.e., repeated endurance measures will differ more than repeated measures of hinge joint EOM), and (2) the magnitude of the given performance capacity (i.e., errors are often in fixed amounts such as 3° for ROM; thus, 3° out of 180° is smaller percentage-wise than 3° out of 20°). One can usually determine an applicable working value (e.g., 5 or 20%) by careful review of the relevant reliability studies. Much of the difference obtained in test–retest is because of limitations in how well one can reasonably control procedures and the actual variability of the parameter being measured, even in the most ideal test subjects. Measurements should be used with these thoughts in mind. If a specific application requires extreme repeatability, then a reliability study should be conducted under conditions that most closely match those in which the need arises. Reliability discussions specific to the some of the focal measures of this chapter are presented in Amundsen (1990), Hellebrandt et al. (1949), Mayhew and Rothstein (1985), and Miller (1985).

Measurements can be reliable, but useless, without validity. Most validity studies have compared the results of one instrument to another instrument or to known quantities. This is the classical type of validity testing, which is an effort to determine whether the measurement reflects the variable being measured. In the absence of a "gold standard" this type of testing is of limited value. In addition to traditional studies of the validity of measurements, the issue of the *validity of the inferences* based on the measurements is becoming increasingly important (Rothstein and Echternach, 1993). That is, can the measurements be used to make inferences about human performance in real-life situations? Unfortunately, measurements that have not demonstrated more than content validity are frequently used as though they are predictive. The validity of the inferences made from human performance data needs to be rigorously addressed.

Specific measurement limitations were briefly addressed in Tables 30.2 and 30.3 and in the written descriptions of various measurement techniques and instruments. Other limitations have more to do with interpreting the data. A general limitation is that performance variables are not fixed human attributes. Another limitation is that population data are limited, and available normative data are, unfortunately, frequently extrapolated to women, older persons, and so on (Chaffin et al., 1999). Some normative data suggest the amount of resources, such as strength, ROM, speed of movement, and endurance, *required* for given activities; other data suggest the amount *available*. As previously mentioned, these are two different issues. Performance measurements may yield information about the current status of performance, but testing rarely indicates the *cause* or the nature of dysfunction. More definitive, diagnostic studies are used to answer these questions. While, considerable information exists with regard to measuring performance capacities of human systems, much less energy has been directed to understanding requirements of tasks. The link between functional performance in tasks and laboratory-acquired measurements is a critical question and a major limitation in interpreting test data. The ERM addresses several of these limitations by using a multidimensional, individualized, cause-and-effect model.

30.7 Performance Capacity Space Representations

In both the study and practice, performance of neuromuscular systems has been characterized along one or two dimensions of performance at a time. However, human subsystems function within a *multi-dimensional* performance space. ROM/EOM, strength, movement speed, and endurance capacities are not only interdependent, but may also vary uniquely within individuals. Multiple measurements are necessary to characterize a person's performance capacity space, and performance capacity is dependent on the task to be performed. Therefore, both the individual and the task must be considered when selecting measurement tools and procedures (Chaffin et al., 1999).

In many of the disciplines in which human performance is of interest, traditional thinking has often focused on single number measures of ROM, strength, speed, and so forth. More recent systems engineering approaches (Kondraske, 2005) emphasize consideration of the performance envelope of a given system and suggest ways to integrate single measurement points that define the limits of performance of a given system (Vasta and Kondraske, 1997). Figure 30.4 illustrates a three-dimensional performance envelope derived from torque, angle, and velocity data for the knee extensor system. The additional dimension of endurance can be represented by displaying this envelope after performing an activity for different lengths of time. A higher-level, composite performance capacity, as is sometimes needed,

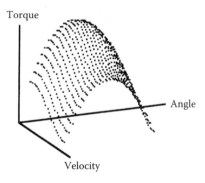

FIGURE 30.4 An example of a torque–angle–velocity performance envelope for the knee extensor system. (From Vasta P.J. and Kondraske G.V. 1994. Technical Report 94-001R p. 11. University of Texas at Arlington, Human Performance Institute, Arlington, Texas. With permission.)

could be derived by computing the volume enclosed by this envelope. Such representations also facilitate assessment of the given system in a specific task; that is, a task is defined as a point in this space that will either fall inside or outside the envelope.

30.8 Conclusion

In conclusion, human movement is so essential that it demands interest and awe from the most casual observer to the most sophisticated scientists. The complexity of performance is truly inspiring. We are challenged to understand it. We want to reduce it to comprehensible units and then enhance it, reproduce it, restore it, and predict it. To do so, we must be able to define and quantify the variables. Hence, an array of instruments and methods has emerged to measure various aspects of human performance. To date, measurement of neuromuscular performance capacities along the dimensions of ROM/EOM, strength, speed of movement, and endurance represents a giant stride but only the "tip of the iceberg." Progress in developing reliable, accurate, and valid instruments and in understanding the factors influencing the measurements cannot be permitted to discourage us from the larger issues of applying the measurements toward a purpose. Yet, single measurements will not suffice; multiple measurements of different aspects of performance will be necessary to fully characterize human movement.

Defining Terms

Endurance: The amount of time a body or body segments can sustain a specified static or repetitive activity.

Extremes of motion (EOM): The end ranges of motion at a joint measured in degrees.

Muscle strength: The maximal amount of torque or force production capacity that a muscle or muscle groups can voluntarily exert in one maximal effort, when type of muscle contraction, movement velocity, and joint angle(s) are specified.

Neuromuscular functional units: Systems (that is, the combination of nerves, muscles, tendons, ligaments, and so on) responsible for producing basic movements.

Range of motion (ROM): The amount of movement that occurs at a joint, typically measured in degrees. ROM is usually measured by noting the extremes of motion, or as the difference between the extreme motion and the reference position.

Speed of movement: The rate of movement of the body or body segments.

References

Amundsen L.R. 1990. *Muscle Strength Testing: Instrumented and Non-Instrumented Systems.* New York, Churchill Livingstone.

Åstrand P.-O., Rodahl K., Dahl H.A., and Stromme S.B. 2003. *Textbook of Work Physiology: Physiological Bases of Exercise,* 4th ed. Champaign, IL, Human Kinetics Publishers.

Biering-Sorensen F. 1984. Physical measurements as risk indicators for low back trouble over a one year period. *Spine* 9: 106–119.

Bohannon R.W. 1990. Muscle strength testing with hand-held dynamometers. In: L.R. Amundsen (Ed.), *Muscle Strength Testing: Instrumented and Non-Instrumented Systems,* pp. 69–88. New York, Churchill Livingstone.

Chaffin D.B. 1975. Ergonomics guide for the assessment of human strength. *Am. Ind. Hyg. J.* 36: 505–510.

Chaffin D.B., Andersson G.B.J., and Martin B.J. 1999. *Occupational Biomechanics,* 3rd ed. New York, Wiley-Interscience.

Clarke H.H. 1954. Comparison of instruments for recording muscle strength. *Res. Q.* 25: 398–411.

Clarke H.H., Bailey T.L., and Shay C.T. 1952. New objective strength tests of muscle groups by cable-tension methods. *Res. Q.* 23: 136–148.

Clarkson H.M. 2000. *Musculoskeletal Assessment: Joint Range of Motion and Manual Muscle Strength,* 2nd ed. Philadelphia, Lippincott, Williams & Wilkins.

Delitto, A. 1990. Trunk strength testing. In: L.R. Amundsen (Ed.), *Muscle Strength Testing: Instrumented and Non-Instrumented Systems,* pp. 151–162. New York, Churchill Livingstone.

DeLorme T.L. and Watkins A.L. 1948. Technics of progressive resistive exercise. *Arch. Phys. Med. Rehabil.* 29: 263–273.

Gowitzke B.A., Milner M., and O'Connel A.L., 1980. *Understanding the Scientific Bases of Human Movement,* 2nd ed. Baltimore, Williams & Wilkins.

Hellebrandt F.A., Duvall E.N., and Moore M.L. 1949. The measurement of joint motion: Part III—reliability of goniometry. *Phys. Ther. Rev.* 29: 302–307.

Hislop H.J. and Montgomery J. 2002. *Daniels and Worthingham's Muscle Testing: Techniques of Manual Examination,* 7th ed. Philadelphia, WB Saunders Company.

Human Performance Measurement, Inc. 1998–2003. *APM I Portable Electronic Goniometer: User's Manual.* PO Box 1996, Arlington, TX 76004-1996.

Jensen C.R. and Fisher A.G. 1979. *Scientific Basis of Athletic Conditioning,* 2nd ed. Philadelphia, Lea & Febiger.

Kendall F.P., McCreary E.K., Provance P.G., Rodgers M., and Romani W. 2005. *Muscles: Testing and Function with Posture and Pain.* Philadelphia, Lippincott, Williams & Wilkins.

Komi P.V. 1973. Measurement of the force–velocity relationship in human muscle under concentric and eccentric contractions. In: S. Cerquiglini, A. Venerando, and J. Wartenweiler (Eds.), *Biomechanics III,* pp. 224–229. Baltimore, University Park Press.

Komi P.V. 1990. Relevance of *in vivo* force measurements to human biomechanics. *J. Biomech.* 23: 23–34.

Kondraske G.V. 2005. A working model for human system–task interfaces. In: J.D. Bronzino (Ed.), *Biomedical Engineering Handbook,* 3rd ed. Boca Raton, FL, CRC Press, Inc.

Kroemer K.H.E. 1983. An isoinertial technique to assess individual lifting capability. *Hum. Factors* 25: 493–506.

Kroemer K.H.E. 1991. A taxonomy of dynamic muscle exertions. *J. Hum. Muscle Perform.* 1: 1–4.

Mayhew T.P. and Rothstein J.M. 1985. Measurement of muscle performance with instruments. In: J.M. Rothstein (Ed.), *Measurement in Physical Therapy,* pp. 57–102. New York, Churchill Livingstone.

Miller P.J. 1985. Assessment of joint motion. In: J.M. Rothstein (Ed.), *Measurement in Physical Therapy,* pp. 103–136. New York, Churchill Livingstone.

Norkin C.C. and White D.J. 2003. *Measurement of Joint Motion: A Guide to Goniometry,* 3rd ed. Philadelphia, FA Davis Company.

Palmer M.L. and Epler M.E. 1998. *Fundamentals of Musculoskeletal Assessment Techniques,* 2nd ed. Philadelphia, JB Lippincott Company.

Panjabi M.M., White III A.A., and Brand R.A. 1974. A note on defining body parts configurations. *J. Biomech.* 7: 385–387.

Reese N.B. and Bandy W.D. 2002. *Joint Range of Motion and Muscle Length Testing.* Philadelphia, WB Saunders Company.

Robertson G. and Sprigings E. 1987. Kinematics. In: D.A. Dainty and R.W. Norman (Eds.), *Standardizing Biomechanical Testing in Sport,* pp. 9–20. Champaign, IL, Human Kinetics Publishers, Inc.

Robson P. 1966. A method to reduce the variable error in joint range measurement. *Ann. Phys. Med.* 8: 262–265.

Rothstein J.M. 1982. Muscle biology: Clinical considerations. *Phys. Ther.* 62: 1823–1830.

Rothstein J.M. and Echternach J.L. 1993. *Primer on Measurement: An Introductory Guide to Measurement Issues.* Alexandria, VA, American Physical Therapy Association.

Rothstein J.M. and Rose S.J. 1982. Muscle mutability—part II: Adaptation to drugs, metabolic factors, and aging. *Phys. Ther.* 62: 1788–1798.

Smidt G.L. 1984. *Muscle Strength Testing: A System Based on Mechanics.* Iowa City IA, SPARK Instruments and Academics, Inc.

Smidt G.L. and Blanpied P.R. 1987. Analysis of strength tests and resistive exercises commonly used for low-back disorders. *Spine* 12: 1025–1034.

Smidt G.L and Rogers M.R. 1982. Factors contributing to the regulation and clinical assessment of muscular strength. *Phys. Ther.* 62: 1284–1290.

Snook S.H. 1978. The design of manual handling tasks. *Ergonomics* 21: 963–985.

Soderberg G.L. 1992. Skeletal muscle function. In: D.P. Currier and R.M. Nelson (Eds.), *Dynamics of Human Biologic Tissues*, pp. 74–96. Philadelphia, FA Davis Company.

Sukop J. and Nelson R.C. 1974. Effects of isometric training in the force-time characteristics of muscle contractions. In: R.C. Nelson, and C.A. Morehouse (Eds.), *Biomechanics IV*, pp. 440–447. Baltimore, University Park Press.

Thorstensson A. and Karlsson J. 1976. Fatiguability and fibre composition of human skeletal muscle. *Acta Physiol. Scand.* 98: 318–322.

Vasta P.J. and Kondraske G.V. 1994. A multi-dimensional performance space model for the human knee extensor, Technical Report 94-001R. University of Texas at Arlington, Human Performance Institute, Arlington, Texas.

Vasta P.J. and Kondraske G.V. 1997. An approach to estimating performance capacity envelopes: Knee extensor system example. *Proceedings of the 19th Annual Engineering in Medicine and Biology Society Conference*, pp. 1713–1716.

von Rohmert W. 1960. Ermittlung von erholungspausen fur statische arbeit des menschen. *Int. Z. Angew. Physiol.* 18: 123–124.

West C.C. 1945. Measurement of joint motion. *Arch. Phys. Med.* 26: 414–425.

White III A.A. and Panjabi M.M. 1990. *Clinical Biomechanics of the Spine*, 2nd ed. Philadelphia, JB Lippincott Company.

Wiechec F.J. and Krusen F.H. 1939. A new method of joint measurement and a review of the literature. *Am. J. Surg.* 43: 659–668.

Winter D.A., Wells R.P., and Orr G.W. 1981. Errors in the use of isokinetic dynamometers. *Eur. J. Appl. Physiol.* 46: 397–408.

Further Information

Journals: *Clinical Biomechanics, Journal of Biomechanics, Medicine and Science in Sports and Exercise, Physical Therapy.*

Smith S.S. and Kondraske G.V. 1987. Computerized system for quantitative measurement of sensorimotor aspects of human performance. *Phys. Ther.* 67: 1860–1866.

Task Force on Standards for Measurement in Physical Therapy. 1991. Standards for tests and measurements in physical therapy practice. *Phys. Ther.* 71: 589–622.

31

Measurement and Analysis of Sensory-Motor Performance: Tracking Tasks

Richard D. Jones
*New Zealand Brain
Research Institute*
University of Canterbury
University of Otago
*Canterbury District Health
Board*

31.1 Introduction

The human nervous system is capable of simultaneous, integrated, and coordinated control of 100–150 mechanical degrees of freedom of movement in the body via tensions generated by about 700 muscles. In its widest context, movement is carried out by a *sensory-motor system* (= sensorimotor system) comprising multiple sensors (visual, auditory, proprioceptive), multiple actuators (muscles and skeletal system), and an intermediary processor which can be summarized as a multiple-input multiple-output nonlinear dynamic adaptive control system. This grand control system comprises a large number of interconnected processors and sub-controllers at various sites in the central nervous system (CNS) of which the more important are the cerebral cortex, thalamus, basal ganglia, cerebellum, and spinal cord. It is capable of responding with remarkable accuracy, speed (when necessary), appropriateness, versatility, and adaptability to a wide spectrum of continuous and discrete stimuli and conditions. It also possesses considerable capabilities for learning new skills, for long-term improvement of performance with practice, and being able to switch quickly between quite different tasks. Certainly, by contrast, it is orders of magnitude more complex and sophisticated than the most advanced robotic systems currently available—although the latter can have superior and often highly desirable attributes such as precision and repeatability and a much greater immunity from factors such as fatigue, distraction, boredom, and lack of motivation!

This chapter has a primary focus on the sensory-motor control function. First, it introduces several important concepts relating to *sensory-motor control, accuracy of movement, a performance resource*, and *a performance capacity*. Second, it provides an overview of apparatuses and methods for the *measurement* and *analysis* of complex sensory-motor performance of the *upper-limbs* (cf. lower-limbs and oculomotor system) by means of *tracking tasks*.

31.2 Basic Principles

31.2.1 Sensory-Motor Control and Accuracy of Movement

The sensory-motor control system is a central component of the sensory-motor system and, from the perspective of Kondraske's *elemental resource model* of human performance (1995, 2006a), can be considered as a hierarchy of multiple interconnected sensory-motor controllers in the *central processing and skills domains* (cf. environmental interface domain, comprising sensors and actuators, and life-sustaining domains) of the elemental resource model. These controllers range from low-level elemental level controllers for control of movement around single joints, through intermediate-level controllers needed to generate integrated movements of an entire limb and involving multiple joints and degrees of freedom, and high-level controllers and processors to enable coordinated synergistic multi-limb movements and the carrying out of *central executive* functions concerned with allocation and switching of resources for execution of multiple tasks simultaneously.

Each of these controllers is considered to possess limited *performance resources*—or *performance capacities*—necessary to carry out their control functions. Performance resources are characterized by dimensions of performance, which for controllers are *accuracy of movement* (including steadiness and stability) and *speed of movement*. Accuracy is the most important of these and can be divided into four major classes:

1. Spatial accuracy—Required by tasks which are *self-paced* and for which time taken is of secondary or minimal importance and includes tracing (e.g., map-tracking), walking, reaching, grasping, and, in fact, many activities of daily living. Limitation in speed performance resources should have no influence on this class of accuracy.

2. Spatial accuracy with time constraints—Identical to "spatial accuracy" except that, in addition to accuracy, speed of execution of task is also of importance. Because maximal performance capacities for accuracy and speed of movement cannot, in general, be realized simultaneously, the carrying out of such tasks must necessarily involve speed-accuracy trade-offs (Fitts, 1954; Fitts and Posner, 1967; Murata and Iwase, 2001; Battaglia and Schrater, 2007; Jax et al., 2007; Bye and Neilson, 2008). The extent to which accuracy is sacrificed for increased speed of execution, or vice versa, is dependent on the actual or perceived relative importance of accuracy and speed.

3. Temporal accuracy—Required by tasks which place minimal demands on positional accuracy and includes single and multi-finger tapping and foot tapping.
4. Spatiotemporal accuracy—Required by tasks which place considerable demand on attainment of simultaneous spatial and temporal accuracy. This includes externally paced positional tasks such as tracking, driving a vehicle, flying a plane, ball games and sports, and video games. It should be stressed, however, that most self-paced tasks also involve a considerable interrelationship between space and time.

Tracking tasks are well established as able to provide one of the most accurate and flexible means for laboratory-based measurement of spatiotemporal accuracy and, thus, of the *performance capacity* of sensory-motor control or sensory-motor coordination. In addition, they provide an unsurpassed framework for studies of the underlying control mechanisms of motor function (Lynn et al., 1979; Cooper et al., 1989; Neilson et al., 1993, 1998; Davidson et al., 2000, 2002; Neilson and Neilson, 2002)—the potential for which was recognized as early as 1943 as seen in writings by Craik (1966). They have achieved this status through their (a) ability to maximally stress the accuracy *dimension of performance* and, hence, the corresponding control performance resource, (b) continuous nature and wide range of type and characteristics of input target signals they permit, (c) facility for a wide range of 1-D, 2-D, and 2-D sensors for measuring a subject's motor output, and (d) measure of continuous performance (cf. discrete tasks such as reaction time tests).

From this perspective, it will be of little surprise to find that tracking tasks are the primary thrust of this chapter.

31.2.2 Influence of Lower-Level Performance Resources on Higher-Level Control Performance Resources

By their very nature, tasks which enable one to measure spatiotemporal accuracy are complex or higher-level sensory-motor tasks. These place demands on a large number of lower-level performance resources such as visual acuity, visual perception, range of movement, strength, simple reaction times, acceleration/deceleration, static steadiness, dynamic steadiness, prediction, memory, open-loop movements, concentration span, central executive function (attention switching, divided attention, multitasking), utilization of preview, and learning.

It is, therefore, important to ask: If there are so many performance resources involved in tracking, can tracking performance provide an accurate estimate of sensory-motor control performance capacities? Or, if differences are seen in tracking performance between subjects, do these necessarily indicate comparable differences in control performance capacities? Yes, they can, but only if the control resource is the *only* resource being maximally stressed during the tracking task. Confirmation that the other performance resources are not also being maximally stressed for a particular subject can be ascertained by two means. First, by independently measuring the capacity of the other performance resources and confirming that these are considerably greater than that determined as necessary for the tracking task in question. For example, if the speed range for a certain reference group on a nontarget speed test is 650–1250 mm/s and the highest speed of a tracking target signal is 240 mm/s, then one can be reasonably confident that intra-group differences in performance on the tracking task are unrelated to intra-group differences in speed. Second, where this process is less straightforward or not possible, it may be possible to alter the demands imposed by the task on the performance resource in question. For example, one could see whether visual acuity was being maximally stressed in a tracking task (and, hence, be a significant limiting factor to the performance obtained) by increasing or decreasing the eye-screen distance. Similarly, one could look at strength in this context by altering the friction, damping, or inertia of the sensor, or at range of movement by altering the gain of the sensor.

The conclusion that a task and a performance resource are unrelated for a particular group does not, of course, mean that this can necessarily be extrapolated to some other group. For example, strength may be uncorrelated with tracking performance in healthy males yet be a factor responsible for poorer tracking performance in females (Jones et al., 1986) and the primary factor in the paretic arm of subjects who have suffered a stroke (Jones et al., 1989).

The foregoing discussion is based on the concept of an assumption that if a task requires less than the absolute maximum available of a particular performance resource, then performance on that task will be independent of that performance resource. Not surprisingly, the reality is unlikely to be this simplistic or clear-cut! If, for example, a tracking task places moderate sub-maximal demands on several performance resources, these performance resources will be stressed to varying levels such that the subject may tend to optimize the utilization of those resources (Kondraske, 1995, 2006a) so as to achieve an acceptable balance between accuracy, speed, stress/effort, and fatigue (physical and cognitive). Thus, although strength available maybe much greater than strength needed (i.e., Resource available >> Resource demand) for both male and female individuals, the differential in strength could well be responsible for male individuals performing better on tracking tasks than female individuals due to the higher acceleration performance resource in male individuals and, hence, ability to correct tracking errors faster (Jones et al., 1986).

31.3 Measurement of Sensory-Motor Performance

31.3.1 Techniques: An Overview

Tracking tasks are the primary methodological approach outlined in this chapter for measurement of sensory-motor control performance. There are, however, a large number of other approaches, each with their own set of apparatuses and methods, which can provide similar or different data on aspects of sensory-motor control performance. It is possible to give only a cursory mention of these other techniques in this chapter.

Hand and foot test boards comprising multiple touch-plate sensors provide measures of accuracy and speed of lateral reaching-tapping abilities (Kondraske et al., 1984, 1988).

Measurement of steadiness and tremor in an upper-limb, lower-limb, or segment of either, particularly when subtended, can be made using variable-size holes, accelerometers, or force transducers (Potvin et al., 1975). A dual-axis capacitive transducer developed by Kondraske et al. (1984) provides an improved means of quantifying steadiness and tremor due to it requiring no mechanical connection to the subject (i.e., no added inertia) and by providing an output of limb position as opposed to less informative measures of acceleration or force. Interestingly, tests of steadiness can be appropriately considered as a category of tracking tasks in which the target is static. The same is also true for measurement of postural stability using force balance platforms, whether for standing (Kondraske et al., 1984; Myklebust et al., 2009) or sitting (Riedel et al., 1992; Schilling et al., 2009).

While the primary focus in this chapter is on measuring tracking performance in the upper limbs, many of the tasks can equally be applied to measurement of oculomotor function, including random targets for assessing smooth pursuit function and predictable and unpredictable step targets for assessing saccadic function (MacAskill et al., 2002; Muir et al., 2003; Heitger et al., 2004, 2008, 2009).

31.3.2 Tracking Tasks: An Overview

A tracking task is a laboratory-based test apparatus characterized by a continuous input signal—the target—which a subject must attempt to match as closely as possible by his/her output response by controlling the position of (or force applied to) some sensor. It provides unequalled opportunities for wide-ranging experimental control over sensors, displays, target signals, dimensionality (degrees of freedom), control modes, controlled system dynamics, and sensor-display compatibility, as well as the application of a vast armamentarium of linear and nonlinear techniques for response signal analysis and systems identification. Because of this, the tracking task has proven to be *the* most powerful and versatile tool for assessing, studying, and modeling higher-level functioning of the human "black-box" sensory-motor system.

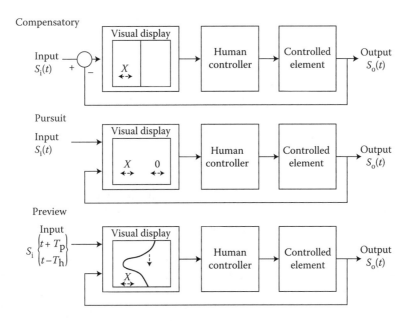

FIGURE 31.1 Modes of tracking. (i) Compensatory: subject aims to keep his error signal X (= input signal – output signal = $s_i(t) - s_o(t)$) on the stationary vertical line; (ii) pursuit: subject aims to keep his output signal X, $s_o(t)$, on the target input signal O, $s_i(t)$; (iii) preview: subject aims to keep his output signal X, $s_o(t)$, on the descending target input signal $[s_i(t + T_p)$ to $s_i(t - T_h)]$, where t = present time, T_p = preview time, T_h = history or postview time.

There are three basic categories of tracking tasks, differing primarily in their visual display and corresponding control system (Figure 31.1). The pursuit task displays both the present input and output signals, whereas the compensatory task displays only the difference or error signal between these. The preview task (Poulton, 1964; Welford, 1968; Jones and Donaldson, 1986; Jones et al., 1996; Klaver et al., 2004) (Figure 31.2) is similar to the pursuit task except that the subject can see in advance where the input signal is going to be and plan accordingly to minimize the resultant error signal. Tracing tasks (Driscoll, 1975; Stern et al., 1983; Hocherman and Aharon-Peretz, 1994; Gowen and Miall, 2006) are effectively self-paced 2-D preview tracking tasks. The input–output nature of tracking tasks has made them most suitable for analysis using engineering control theories. This has led to

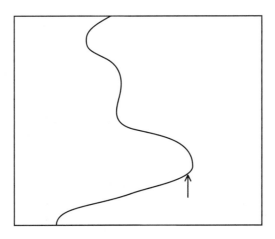

FIGURE 31.2 Visual display for random tracking with a preview of 8.0 s and postview of 1.1 s.

the common view of pursuit tracking as a task involving continuous negative feedback (Notterman et al., 1982) but there is evidence that tracking viewed as a series of discrete events is more appropriate (Bösser, 1984; Neilson et al., 1988a; Bye and Neilson, 2010). The inclusion of preview of the input signal greatly complicates characterization of the human controller and Sheridan (1966) suggested three models of preview control which employ the notions of constrained preview and nonuniform importance of input. Lynn et al. (1979) and Neilson et al. (1992) have also demonstrated how, by treating the neurologically impaired subject as a black-box, control analysis can lead to further information on underlying neurological control mechanisms. Davidson et al. (2000, 2002) and Ghous and Neilson (2002) have done likewise in their investigations of open-loop control mechanisms in healthy subjects.

Despite the widespread utilization and acceptance of tracking tasks as a powerful and versatile means for quantifying and studying sensory-motor control performance and capacities, there is little available on the market in this area. The most obvious exception to this is the photoelectric pursuit rotor which is ubiquitous in the motor behavior laboratories of university psychology departments and has been available since the 1950s (Welford, 1968; Schmidt, 1982; Siegel, 1985). It is a paced 2-D task with a target with the periodic on each revolution. Although inexpensive, the pursuit rotor is a crude tracking task allowing limited control over target signals and possessing a very gross performance analysis in terms of time on target. Thus, essentially all of the many and varied tracking tasks which have been used in countless experimental studies around the world, with some of these tasks having moved into clinical neurology and rehabilitation environments as objective and quantitative assessment tools, have been developed by the users themselves for their specific objectives. That is, surprisingly, there are essentially no computer-based tracking test systems commercially available. The need for such, including sensors for both upper- and lower-limbs, seems obvious as this would open up the possibility of a much broader and widespread use of tracking tasks. In particular, this would help facilitate much greater utilization of tracking tasks outside of traditional research areas and in more routine assessment applications in clinical, rehabilitative, vocational, sports, and other environments.

Whatever the reason(s) for needing a tracking task to quantify sensory-motor control performance or capacity, there are a number of options available and factors to be considered in choosing or designing a tracking task. These are discussed in Sections 31.3.3 through 31.3.14.

31.3.3 Sensors

Sensors for measuring a subject's motor output in 1-D tracking tasks can be categorized under (a) movements involving a single degree of freedom such as flexion–extension rotation around a single joint such as elbow (Lynn et al., 1977; Deuschl et al., 1996; O'Dwyer et al., 1996; Soliveri et al., 1997), wrist (Warabi et al., 1986; Gibson et al., 1987; Johnson et al., 1996; Liu et al., 1999; Feys et al., 2005; Notley et al., 2007), or a finger, or pronation–supination of the wrist (Evarts et al., 1981), and (b) movements involving two or more degrees of freedom of a body part (e.g., hand)—that is, coordinated movement at multiple joints—which are either 1-D, such as some form of linear transducer (Patrick and Mutlusoy, 1982; Baroni et al., 1984; van den Berg et al., 1987; Johnson et al., 1996) or 2-D, such as steering wheel (Buck, 1982; Ferslew et al., 1982; Jones and Donaldson, 1986; Jones et al., 1993, 2002; Davidson et al., 2000, 2002; Heitger et al., 2004, 2007; Peiris et al., 2006, 2011; Innes et al., 2007, 2009a; Hoggarth et al., 2010), stirring wheel (De Souza et al., 1980), position stick (i.e., 1-D joystick) (Potvin et al., 1977; Neilson and Neilson, 1980; Miall et al., 1985; O'Dwyer and Neilson, 1998; Watson and Jones, 1998), joystick (Kondraske et al., 1984; Anderson, 1986; Behbehani et al., 1988; Dalrymple-Alford et al., 1994; Watson et al., 1997; Watson and Jones, 1998; Gonzalez et al., 2000; Allen et al., 2007; Poudel et al., 2008, 2010b; Siengsukon and Boyd, 2009a), finger-controlled rotating knob (Neilson et al., 1993), light-pen (Neilson and Neilson, 1980), and MRI-compatible pneumatic squeeze bulb/ball (Oishi et al., 2011) (e.g., Current Designs—www.curdes.

com). Force sticks, utilizing strain-gauge transducers mounted on a cantilever, are also commonly used as sensors (Garvey, 1960; Potvin et al., 1977; Miller and Freund, 1980; Kondraske et al., 1984; Anderson, 1986; van den Berg et al., 1987; Barr et al., 1988; Stelmach and Worrington, 1988; Chelette et al., 1995; Van Orden et al., 2000; Allen et al., 2007; Jasper et al., 2010). Isometric integrated EMG (i.e., full-wave rectification and low-pass filtering of the raw EMG) can also be used to control the tracking response cursor, as was done by Neilson et al. (1990) to help show that impairment of sensory-motor learning is the primary cause of functional disability in cerebral palsy.

Sensors for 2-D tasks must, of course, be capable of moving with and recording two degrees of freedom. Joysticks are commonly used for this and range in size from small, for wrist/finger movement (Bloxham et al., 1984; Anderson, 1986; Frith et al., 1986; Neilson et al., 1998; Gonzalez et al., 2000; Allen et al., 2007), including MRI-compatible joysticks (Poudel, 2008, 2010b) (e.g., Current Designs—www.curdes.com), up to large floor-mounted joysticks for arm movements primarily involving shoulder and elbow function (Kondraske et al., 1984; Anderson, 1986; Behbehani et al., 1988; Jones et al., 1993; Dalrymple-Alford et al., 1994; Watson et al., 1997; Watson and Jones, 1998). Other 2-D task sensors include computer mouse (Korteling and Kaptein, 1996), computer track-ball (Petrilli et al., 2005), hand-held stylus for the photoelectric pursuit rotor (Schmidt, 1982; Siegel, 1985), plexiglass tracing (Driscoll, 1975; Stern et al., 1983; Hocherman and Aharon-Peretz, 1994; Gowen and Miall, 2006), touch-sensitive screen (Engel and Soechting, 2000), and tasks utilizing sonic digitizers (Stern, 1986; Viviani and Mounoud, 1990; Hocherman and Aharon-Peretz, 1994). Abend et al. (1982) and Flash and Hogan (1985) used a two-joint mechanical arm to restrict hand movements to the horizontal plane in the investigation of CNS control of two-joint (shoulder and elbow) movements in trajectory formation. Stern et al. (1983) simply used the subject's finger as the sensor for a tracing task on a vertical plexiglass screen; a video camera behind the screen recorded finger movements. Novel whole-body 2-D tracking is also possible by having subjects alter their posture while standing on a dual-axis force platform (Kondraske et al., 1984).

1-D sensors can also be used in 2-D tasks by way of bimanual tracking. For example, O'Dwyer and Neilson (1995) and Neilson and Neilson (2002) used two 1-D joysticks to investigate dynamic synergies between the right and left arms.

More recently, high spatial precision 3-D sensors have become available via infrared LED markers combined and camera system (e.g., Optotrak—www.ndigital.com/lifesciences/certus-motioncapture-system.php) or electromagnetic trackers (e.g., Polhemus—polhemus.com; Flock-of-Birds, trakSTAR—www.ascension-tech.com) and play an important role in 3-D virtual-environment systems (Mrotek et al., 2006; Myall et al., 2008).

31.3.4 Displays

In the early days of tracking, mechanical-based displays were used, such as a rotating smoked drum (Vince, 1948), the ubiquitous pursuit rotor, and a paper-strip preview task (Poulton, 1964; Welford, 1968). An oscilloscope was used in a large number of tracking tasks, initially driven by analog circuitry (Flowers, 1976; Anderson, 1986; Sheridan et al., 1987) but later by D/A outputs on digital computers (Kondraske et al., 1984; Miall et al., 1985; Sheridan et al., 1987; Cooper et al., 1989). Standard raster-based television screens have been used by some workers (Potvin et al., 1977; Beppu et al., 1984). Nonraster vector graphics displays, such as Digital Equipment's VT11 dynamic graphics unit, proved valuable during the PDP-era as a means for generating more complex dynamic stimuli such as squares (Neilson and Neilson, 1980; Frith et al., 1986) and preview (Jones and Donaldson, 1986) (Figure 31.2). More recently, raster-based color graphics boards have allowed impressive static displays and simple dynamic tracking displays to be generated on PCs. However, such boards are not, in general, immediately amenable for the generation of flawless dynamic displays involving more complex stimuli, such as required for preview tracking. Jones et al. (1993) overcame this drawback by the use of specially written high-speed assembly-language routines for driving their display. These generated a display of the target and the subject's response marker by considering the video memory (configured in EGA mode) as four overlapping planes, each switchable (via a mask), and each capable of displaying the background color and a single color from a palette. Two planes were used to display the target, with the remaining two being used to display the subject's pointer. The current target was displayed on one target plane, while the next view of the target, in its new position, was being drawn on the other nondisplayed target plane. The role of the two planes was reversed when the computer received a vertical synchronization interrupt from the graphics controller indicating the completion of a raster. Through a combination of a high update-rate of 60.34 Hz (i.e., the vertical interrupt frequency), assembly language, and dual display buffers, it was possible to obtain an extremely smooth dynamic color display. Their system for tracking and other quantitative sensory-motor assessments was further enhanced through its facility to generate dynamic color graphics on two high-resolution monitors simultaneously: one for the tracking display, and one for use by the assessor for task control and analysis. The monitors were driven by a ZX1000 graphic controller (Artist Graphics Inc.), at 800 × 600, and a standard VGA controller, respectively.

In contrast to the above CRT-based displays, Warabi et al. (1986) used a laser-beam spot to indicate a subject's hand position together with a row of LEDs for displaying a step target. Similarly, Gibson et al. (1987) used a galvanometer-controlled laser spot to display smooth and step stimuli on a curved screen together with a white-light spot controlled by subject. Leist et al. (1987), Viviani and Mounoud (1990), and Klockgether (1994) also used galvanometer-controlled spots but via back-projection onto a curved screen, transparent digitizing table, and plexiglass surface, respectively. Van den Berg et al. (1987) used two rows of 240 LEDs each to display target and response. 2-D arrays of LEDs have also been used to indicate step targets in 2-D tracking tasks (Abend et al., 1982; Flash and Hogan, 1985).

However, graphics and display technologies have moved on substantially from the above heady days. Flat-screen LED displays have mostly replaced CRT-based displays, and high-resolution dual-screen color graphics built into motherboards are near standard in desktop and laptop computers. Similarly, the availability of powerful (and often open-source) graphics development software packages and libraries has greatly simplified the task of generating real-time dynamic graphics needed for tracking task displays.

Full-immersion 3-D virtual environments, via red/green glasses and green (left eye) and red (right eye) images rear-projected onto a large vertical screen (Mrotek et al., 2006) or a half-silvered mirror and stereoscopic glasses approach (Myall, 2008), have more recently opened up opportunities and applications for 3-D tracking.

While strictly not tracking tasks, driving simulators are often used instead of tracking tasks to provide a more realistic real-world environment, especially when one of the aims is, not surprisingly, to simulate the on-road task and environment (Banks et al., 2004; Lin et al., 2005; Desai and Haque, 2006; Lee, 2006; Schultheis et al., 2006, 2007; Cadeddu and Kondraske, 2007; Golz et al., 2007; Anund et al., 2008; Boyle et al., 2008; Lowden et al., 2009; Sommer et al., 2009; Boyle and Lee, 2010; Golz and Sommer, 2010; Jung et al., 2010; Sommer and Golz, 2010; Vadeby et al., 2010; Martens et al., 2011; Mayhew et al., 2011; Calhoun and Pearlson, 2012). Other than their more complex simulated real-road displays, the presence of distractors, and sometimes the presence of multiple tasks, a major distinguishing feature of driving simulators from tracking tasks is their substantial dead-zone within which the subject is not penalized as long as they keep within the lane markings or sides of the road. In many situations (e.g., driving) this is reasonably valid but, conversely, driving simulation is more difficult to score, with, for example, smaller deviations being ignored and the confounding presence of self-pacing. Notwithstanding, driving simulators are a valuable tool in driving research and driving assessment.

31.3.5 Target Signals

Tracking targets cover a spectrum from smoothly changing (low-bandwidth) targets, such as sinusoidal and random, through constant velocity ramp targets, to abrupt changing step targets.

31.3.5.1 Sinusoidal Targets

The periodicity, constancy of task complexity (over cycles), and spectral purity of sine targets make them valuable for measurement of within-run changes in performance (e.g., learning, lapses in concentration) (Jones and Donaldson, 1981), the study of ability to make use of the periodicity to improve tracking performance (Jones and Donaldson, 1989), and the study of the human frequency response (Leist et al., 1987). Several other workers have also used sine targets in their tracking tasks (Potvin et al., 1977; Miller and Freund, 1980; Ferslew et al., 1982; Notterman et al., 1982; Johnson et al., 1996; Soliveri et al., 1997; Heitger et al., 2004; Innes et al., 2007, 2009a; Siengsukon and Boyd, 2009a; Hoggarth et al., 2010).

Bloxham et al. (1984) and Frith et al. (1986) extended the use of sinewaves into a 2-D domain by having subjects track a moving circle on the screen.

31.3.5.2 Random Targets

These are commonly generated via a sum-of-sines approach in which a number of harmonically or nonharmonically related sinusoids of random phase are superimposed (Cassell et al., 1973; Neilson and Neilson, 1980; Miall et al., 1985; Baddeley et al., 1986; Frith et al., 1986; van den Berg et al., 1987; Barr et al., 1988; Cooper et al., 1989; Jones et al., 1993, 1996, 2002; Dalrymple-Alford et al., 1994, 2003; Hufschmidt and Lücking, 1995; Makeig and Jolley, 1996; Backs, 1997; Watson et al., 1997; Watson and Jones, 1998; Davidson et al., 2000, 2002; Heitger et al., 2004, 2007; Oytam et al., 2005; Peiris et al., 2006, 2011; Innes et al., 2007, 2009b; Huang et al., 2008; Poudel et al., 2009, 2010a,b; Hoggarth et al., 2010). If harmonically related, this can effectively give a flat spectrum target out to whatever bandwidth is required. Thus, in Jones et al.'s systems (Jones et al., 1993; Watson et al., 1997; Davidson et al., 2000; Peiris et al., 2006; Poudel et al., 2008; Innes et al., 2009b) the random signal generation program asks the user for the required signal bandwidth and then calculates the number of equal amplitude harmonics that must be summed together to give this bandwidth, each harmonic being assigned a randomly selected phase from a uniform phase distribution. Each target comprises 4096 (2^{12}) or more samples, a duration of at least 68 s (4096 samples/60.34 Hz), and a fundamental frequency of 0.0147 Hz (i.e., period of 68 s). By this means it is possible to have several different pseudo-random target signals that are nonperiodic up to 68-s duration, have flat spectra within a user-specified bandwidth, no components above this bandwidth, and whose spectra can be accurately computed by FFT from any 68-s block of target (or response). Another common approach to the generation of random targets is to digitally filter a sequence of pseudo-random numbers (Lynn et al., 1977; Potvin et al., 1977; Kondraske et al., 1984; van den Berg et al., 1987; Neilson et al., 1993; Neilson and Neilson, 2002), although this method gives less control over the spectral characteristics of the target. Bösser (1984) summed a number of these filtered sequences in such a way as to generate a target having an approximate $1/f$ spectrum. Another smooth pursuit target was generated by linking together short segments of sinewaves with randomly selected frequencies up to some maximum (Gibson et al., 1987) and was thus effectively a hybrid sinusoidal-random target.

In studies of lapses of responsiveness (e.g., microsleeps, lapses of sustained attention, lapses of focused attention), a 1-D target and most 2-D targets have "flat-spots" during which it is not possible to say definitively that a flat-spot in the response was due to a lapse (Peiris et al., 2006; Davidson et al., 2007; Huang et al., 2008). Poudel et al. (2008, 2009, 2010a,b) overcame this deficiency by designing a 2-D tracking task in which the speed of the target never goes below 20 mm/s (Figure 31.3); hence, a flat-spot in the tracking response can only be attributed to a true lapse of responsiveness.

31.3.5.3 Ramp Targets

Ramp targets have been used in conjunction with sensory gaps of target or response to study predictive tracking and ability to execute smooth constant velocity movements in the absence of immediate visual cues in normal subjects (Flowers, 1978b) and subjects with cerebellar disorders (Beppu et al., 1987), stroke (Jones et al., 1989), and Parkinson's disease (Cooke et al., 1978; Flowers, 1978a; Liu et al., 1999).

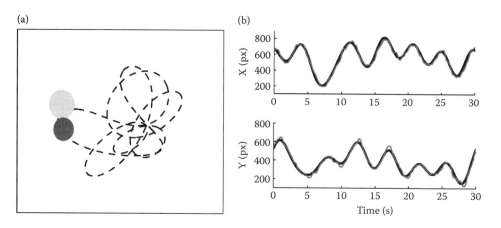

FIGURE 31.3   2-D random tracking task in which the speed of the target never goes below 20 mm/s, i.e., no flat-spots.

31.3.5.4 Step Targets

Step targets have been used in many applications and studies to measure and investigate abilities to predict, program, and execute ballistic (open-loop) movements. To enable this, spatial and temporal unpredictability have been incorporated into step tasks in various ways:

- *Temporal predictability*: The time of onset of steps has ranged from (a) explicitly predictable, with preview of the stimulus (Day et al., 1984; Jones et al., 1993), (b) implicitly predictable, with fixed interval between steps (Potvin et al., 1977; Cooke et al., 1978; Flowers, 1978b; Abend et al., 1982; Deuschl et al., 1996; Johnson et al., 1996; Sailer et al., 2002; Feys et al., 2005), to (c) unpredictable, with intervals between steps varied randomly over spans lying somewhere between 1.5 and 7.0 s (Angel et al., 1970; Flowers, 1978b; Kondraske et al., 1984; Anderson, 1986; Jones and Donaldson, 1986; Warabi et al., 1986; Gibson et al., 1987; Sheridan et al., 1987; Jones et al., 1993, 2002; Neilson et al., 1995; Watson et al., 1997; O'Dwyer and Neilson, 1998; Heitger et al., 2004; Allen et al., 2007; Innes et al., 2007, 2009a).
- *Amplitude predictability*: The amplitude of steps has ranged from (a) explicitly predictable, where the endpoint of the step is shown explicitly prior to the "Go" stimulus (Abend et al., 1982; Baroni et al., 1984; Sheridan et al., 1987; Jones et al., 1993; Deuschl et al., 1996; Watson et al., 1997; Feys et al., 2005), (b) implicitly predictable, where all steps have the same amplitude (Angel et al., 1970; Potvin et al., 1977; Cooke et al., 1978; Day et al., 1984; Kondraske et al., 1984; Anderson, 1986; Johnson et al., 1996; O'Dwyer and Neilson, 1998) or return-to-center steps in variable-amplitude step tasks (Flowers, 1976; Jones and Donaldson, 1986; Jones et al., 1993), to (c) unpredictable, with between 2 and 8 randomly distributed amplitudes (Flowers, 1976; Jones and Donaldson, 1986; Warabi et al., 1986; Gibson et al., 1987; Sheridan et al., 1987; Jones et al., 1993, 2002; Sailer et al., 2002; Heitger et al., 2004; Allen et al., 2007; Innes et al., 2007, 2009a).
- *Direction predictability*: Step tasks have had steps whose direction ranged from (a) all steps explicitly predictable, alternating between right and left (Flowers, 1976; Potvin et al., 1977; Cooke et al., 1978; Baroni et al., 1984; Kondraske et al., 1984; Johnson et al., 1996; O'Dwyer and Neilson, 1998; Sailer et al., 2002; Feys et al., 2005; Allen et al., 2007), or all in one direction (i.e., a series of discontinuous steps) (Sheridan et al., 1987), or between corners of an invisible square (Anderson, 1986), or having preview (Abend et al., 1982; Jones et al., 1993), (b) most steps predictable but with occasional "surprises" for studying anticipation (Flowers, 1978a), (c) a combination of unpredictable (outward) and predictable (back-to-center) steps (Angel et al.,

TABLE 31.1 Unpredictability in Step Tracking Tasks

		Temporal			Spatial-Amplitude			Spatial-Direction			Overall
		Full	Partial	None	Full	Partial	None	Full	Partial	None	Full
Angel et al. (1970)[a]	1-D	•				•		•		•	
Flowers (1976)[a]	1-D	•			•	•				•	
Potvin et al. (1977)	1-D		•			•				•	
Cooke et al. (1978)	1-D		•			•				•	
Flowers (1978a)	1-D		•			•			•		
Baroni et al. (1984)	1-D	•					•			•	
Day et al. (1984)	1-D			•		•		•			
Kondraske et al. (1984)	1-D	•				•				•	
Warabi et al. (1986)	1-D	•			•			•			•
Jones and Donaldson (1986)[a]	1-D	•			•	•		•		•	•
Gibson et al. (1987)	1-D	•			•			•			•
Sheridan et al. (1987)[a]	1-D	•			•		•			•	
Jones et al. (1993)[a]	1-D	•		•	•	•	•	•		•	•
Deuschl et al. (1996)	1-D		•				•			•	
Johnson et al. (1996)	1-D		•			•				•	
O'Dwyer and Neilson (1998)	1-D	•				•				•	
Sailor et al. (2002)	1-D		•			•				•	
Feys et al. (2005)	1-D		•				•			•	
Allen et al. (2007)[a]	1-D			•	•		•		•	•	
Abend et al. (1982)	2-D		•				•			•	
Anderson (1986)	2-D	•				•				•	
Watson et al. (1997)	2-D	•					•	•			
Ariff et al. (2002)	2-D		•			•			•		

[a] Several variations of unpredictability within one task or between multiple tasks.

1970; Jones and Donaldson, 1986; Jones et al., 1993; Watson et al., 1997), and (d) all steps unpredictable, with multiple endpoints (Warabi et al., 1986; Gibson et al., 1987) or resetting between single steps (Day et al., 1984).

The three elements of unpredictability can be combined in various ways to generate tasks ranging from completely predictable to completely unpredictable (Table 31.1). Several groups have implemented several variations of unpredictability both within and between step tracking tasks to investigate the possible loss of ability to use predictability to improve performance in, for example, Parkinson's disease (Flowers, 1978a; Sheridan et al., 1987; Watson et al., 1997). In addition to unpredictability, other characteristics can be built into step tasks including explicit target zones (Sheridan et al., 1987) and visual gaps in target (Flowers, 1976; Warabi et al., 1986).

An example of a 1-D step tracking task possessing full spatial and temporal unpredictability is that of Jones and colleagues (Jones and Donaldson, 1986; Jones et al., 1993; Heitger et al., 2004; Innes et al., 2007, 2009a) (Figure 31.4a). The task comprises 32 abrupt steps alternating between displacement from and return to center screen. In the nonpreview form, spatial unpredictability is present in the outward steps through four randomly distributed amplitude/direction movements (large and small steps requiring 90.0 and 22.5 deg on a steering wheel, respectively, and both to right and left of center) with temporal unpredictability achieved via four randomly distributed durations between steps (2.8, 3.4, 4.0, 4.6 s). This

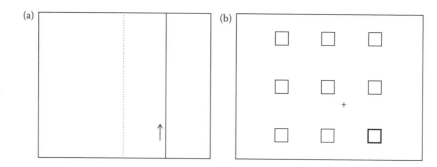

FIGURE 31.4 Visual displays for (a) 1-D step tracking task and (b) 2-D step tracking task (bottom-right square is current target).

task has been used, together with preview random tracking, to demonstrate deficits in sensory-motor control in the asymptomatic "good" arm of subjects who have had a unilateral stroke (Jones et al., 1989).

Watson et al. (1997) provided an example of a 2-D step tracking task with spatial and temporal unpredictability. In this task the subject must move a cross from within a central starting square to within one of eight 10-mm × 10-mm target squares that appear on the screen with temporal and spatial unpredictability (Figure 31.4b). The centers of the eight surrounding targets are positioned at the vertices and midway along the perimeter of an imaginary 100-mm × 100-mm square centered on the central square. To initiate the task, the subject places the cross within the perimeter of the central target. After a 2.0–5.0-s delay, one of the surrounding blue targets turns green and the subject moves the cross to within the green target square as quickly and as accurately as possible. After a further delay, the central target turns green indicating onset of the spatially predictive "back-to-center" target. The task, which comprises ten outward and ten return targets, was used to show that Parkinsonian subjects perform worse than matched controls on all measures of step tracking but are not impaired in their ability to benefit from spatial predictability to improve performance.

Step tasks with explicit target zones, in 1-D (Sheridan et al., 1987) or 2-D (Watson et al., 1997), provide the possibility of altering task difficulty by varying the size of the target. On the basis that subjects need only aim to get their marker somewhere within target zone (cf. close to center) then, according to Fitts's (1954) ratio rule, the difficulty of the primary movement is proportional to $\log_2(2A/W)$, where A is the amplitude of the movement and W is the width of the target.

31.3.5.5 Switching Targets

Jones et al. (1986, 1989, 1993) combined two quite different modes of tracking within a single task. Combination tracking involves alternating between preview random and nonpreview step tracking over 11-s cycles (Figure 31.5). Thus, while tracking the random target, the preview signal is abruptly and unpredictably replaced by a stationary vertical line at some distance from the random signal, and vice versa. Although the steps occur with a fixed fore-period (as with the step tasks listed above with implicit temporal predictability) of 7.3 s, subjects are not informed of this and, irrespective, Weber's law (Fitts and Posner, 1967) indicates the accuracy of prediction of steps with such a long pre-stimulus warning is very low. Combination tracking allows the study of ability to change *motor set* (Robertson and Flowers, 1990) between quite different modes of tracking and is analogous to having to quickly and appropriately respond to an unexpected obstacle, such as a child running onto the road, while driving a vehicle.

31.3.6 Dimensionality

The number of dimensions of a tracking task usually refers to the number of Cartesian coordinates in which the *target* moves, rather than those of the response marker or sensor handle, or the number of degrees of freedom of the target or of the upper limb. For example, (1) even with a 2-D joystick sensor

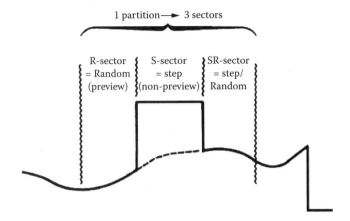

FIGURE 31.5 Section of input waveform in combination tracking in which the target alternates between preview-random and non-preview-step.

or light-pen, if the target moves in the vertical direction only (Neilson and Neilson, 1980; Kondraske et al., 1984; Miall et al., 1985; Jones et al., 1993), the task is only considered 1-D, irrespective of whether the response marker is confined to vertical movements on the screen or not; (2) if the target trajectory is a circle (Bloxham et al., 1984), the task is 2-D despite the target having only one degree of freedom (i.e., radius *r* is constant); and (3) a pursuit rotor is a 2-D task as it has a target which moves in two dimensions (whether Cartesian or polar) as well as doing so with two degrees of freedom (Welford, 1968).

Watson and Jones (1998) compared random 2-D with 1-D performance but in doing so scaled their 2-D target down so as to have an average displacement and velocity equal to that of its 1-D horizontal and vertical components. By this means they were able to unequivocally demonstrate that there is poorer performance on 2-D tasks and that this is due to both the increased dimensionality and increased position/speed demands of an unscaled 2-D task. Conversely, Oytam et al. (2005) showed that a 2-D tracking task has a response delay no longer than a 1-D task in healthy subjects.

Dual-axis tracking is a variant of 2-D tracking in which the 2-D task comprises two simultaneous orthogonal 1-D tasks in which one or more of the target, input device, control dynamics, and on-line feedback are different between the two axes. It has been used to investigate mechanisms and characteristics of 2-D tracking, and it has been shown that a 2-D task is indeed a single task rather than two separate orthogonal tasks (Navon et al., 1984; Fracker and Wickens, 1989).

More recently, virtual visuoperceptual environments combined with LED or electromagnetic 3-D trackers have provided a means for moving tracking tasks into the realm of 3-D (Mrotek et al., 2006; Myall et al., 2008).

31.3.7 Tracking Mode

The two primary modes of tracking—compensatory and pursuit—were introduced in Section 31.3.2 and Figure 31.1. Most tasks are of the pursuit type, which reflects its greater parallel with real-world sensory-motor tasks, but the compensatory task, in which the subject sees only the instantaneous value of the error signal, has proven valuable in several studies (Vince, 1948; Garvey, 1960; Potvin et al., 1977; Miller and Freund, 1980; Bösser, 1984; Barr et al., 1988; Makeig and Jolley, 1996; Backs, 1997; Huang et al., 2008; Gazes et al., 2010). The compensatory mode can be preferentially chosen for control-theory modeling due to its simpler set of defining equations (Potvin et al., 1977). Makeig and Jolly (1996) developed a novel variation to the standard compensatory tracking task by superimposing on the random target a second "force" equivalent to the force of gravity so as to cause the response disc to slip on an unseen slippery surface.

The preview task (Poulton, 1964; Welford, 1968; Potvin et al., 1977; Jones and Donaldson, 1986, 1989; Gianutsos, 1994; Jones et al., 1996, 2002; Kisacanin et al., 2000; Dalrymple-Alford et al., 2003; Heitger et al., 2004; Peiris et al., 2006; Innes et al., 2007, 2009a; Hoggarth et al., 2010) is an important variation of pursuit tracking in which a still greater correspondence with everyday tasks is achieved.

31.3.8 Controlled System Dynamics

It is well established that subjects can deal satisfactorily with a variety of tracking systems incorporating different control characteristics (Poulton, 1974; Neilson et al., 1995). Notwithstanding, the majority of tracking tasks have a zero-order controlled system in which the position of the response marker is proportional to the position of the sensor and the mechanical characteristics of friction, inertial mass, and velocity damping are simply those of the input device. Van den Berg et al. (1987) eliminated even these by feeding back a force signal from a strain gauge on the tracking handle to the power amplifier of a torque motor connected to their sensor. Conversely, Neilson et al. (1993) artificially introduced mechanical characteristics into the movement of their response marker by having a linear second-order filter as the controlled system; by an appropriate transfer function ($H(z) = 0.4060/(1 - 1.061z^{-1} + 0.4610z^{-2})$), they were able to introduce inertial lag and under-damping (resonant peak at 2.0 Hz). Miall et al. (1985) and Myall et al. (2008) introduced delays between their sensor and the displayed response so that they could study the effect of delayed visual feedback on performance. Soliveri et al. (1997) used both first-order (velocity) and zero-order (position) linear control dynamics to investigate differences in learning between parkinsonian and control subjects and between on- and off-medication. Navon et al. (1984) used a combination of velocity and acceleration control dynamics in their study on dual-axis tracking. Nonlinear transfer functions, such as second-order Volterra (fading memory) nonlinearities, have also been used in tracking controlled systems, primarily as a means for investigating adaptive inverse modeling mechanisms in the brain relating to voluntary movement (Davidson et al., 2000, 2002; Ghous and Neilson, 2002).

Controlled system dynamics can also be changed during a task. In "critical tracking," a novel variation of pursuit tracking conceived by Jex (1966), the delay of the controlled system increases during the task. There is no external target but instead the subject's own instability acts as an input to an increasingly unstable controlled system, $Y(s) = K\lambda/(s - \lambda)$, in which the level of instability, represented by the root λ ($= 1/T$), is steadily increased during the task until a preset error is exceeded. The task has been described as analogous to driving a truck with no brakes down a hill on a winding road (Potvin et al., 1977). The task has been applied clinically (Potvin et al., 1977; Kondraske et al., 1984; Behbehani et al., 1988) and shown to be a reliable measure of small changes in neurological function. Alternatively, gain-change step tracking (Neilson et al., 1995), in which the gain of the control-display relation is increased or decreased without warning, has been used to investigate adaptive mechanisms in healthy subjects (O'Dwyer and Neilson, 1998; Myall, 2010) and those with Parkinson's disease (Myall, 2010).

Having a torque motor as part of the sensor opens up several new possibilities. It can be operated as a "torque servo," in which applied torque is independent of position (Kondraske et al., 1984), or a "position servo," in which applied torque is proportional to position error (together with velocity damping if desired) (Thomas et al., 1976). By adding external force perturbations, it is possible to measure and study neuromuscular reflexes and limb transfer function (i.e., stiffness, viscosity, and inertia), such as by applying constant velocity movements (Kondraske et al., 1984) or pulsatile (van den Berg et al., 1987), sinusoidal (Gottlieb et al., 1984), or random (Kearney and Hunter, 1983; van den Berg et al., 1987) force perturbations. Alternatively, the torque motor can be used to alter controlled-system characteristics in tracking tasks for studies and/or improvement of voluntary movement. For example, van den Berg et al. (1987) cancelled unwanted controller characteristics. Chelette et al. (1995) used "force reflection" to improve tracking performance in both normal subjects and those with spasticity, and Johnson et al. (1996) used antiviscous loading to investigate the cause of poor tracking in patients with Parkinson's disease.

31.3.9 Sensor-Display Compatibility

It is generally accepted that the level of compatibility between sensor and display in continuous tracking tasks influences the accuracy of performance (Neilson and Neilson, 1980). The perfectly compatible sensor is the display marker itself (Poulton, 1974) where the subject holds and moves the response marker directly such as with a light-pen in tracking (Neilson and Neilson, 1980), rotary pursuit (Welford, 1968; Schmidt, 1982), handle on a two-joint mechanical arm (Abend et al., 1982), self-paced 2-D tracking tasks (Driscoll, 1975; Stern et al., 1984; Hocherman and Aharon-Peretz, 1994; Gowen and Miall, 2006; Reithler et al., 2006), direct 2-D tracking on a touch-sensitive screen (Engel and Soechting, 2000), or 3-D tracking tasks in a virtual environment (Mrotek et al., 2006; Myall et al., 2008). Similarly, van den Berg et al. (1987) achieved a high sensor-display compatibility by having the LED arrays for target and response displayed directly above a horizontally moving handle. However, the majority of tracking tasks have sensors which are quite separate from the response marker displayed on an oscilloscope or computer screen. Sensor-display compatibility can be maximized in this case by having the sensor physically close to the display, moving in the same direction as the marker, and with a minimum of controlled system dynamics (e.g., zero-order). In the case of a joystick in a 2-D task, for example, direct compatibility (*Left–Right → Left–Right*) is easier than inverse compatibility (*Left–Right → Right–Left*), which is easier than noncompatibility (*Left–Right → Up–Down*). In contrast, fore-aft movements on a joystick appear to possess bidirectional compatibility in that *Fore–aft → Up–Down* seems as inherently natural as *Fore–aft → Down–Up* (i.e., no obvious inverse).

Sensor-display compatibility may not, however, be overly critical to performance. For example, Neilson and Neilson (1980) found no decrement in performance on random tracking of overall error scores, such as mean absolute error, between a light pen and a 1-D joystick; nevertheless, the latter did result in a decrease in gain, an increase in phase lag, and an increase in the noncoherent response component. Conversely, normal subjects find incompatible 2-D tracking very difficult to perform, taking up to 4 h of practice to reach a level of performance equal to that seen on pre-practice 2-D compatible tracking (Neilson et al., 1998).

31.3.10 Response Sampling Rates

Although some workers have manually analyzed tracking data from multichannel analog chart recordings (Flowers, 1976; Beppu et al., 1984) or analog-processed results (Potvin et al., 1977), the majority have used computers, sometimes via a magnetic tape intermediary (Flowers, 1978a; Day et al., 1984; Miall et al., 1985), to digitize data for automated analyses. Sampling rates used have varied from 10 Hz (Neilson and Neilson, 1980), through 20 Hz (Cooper et al., 1989; Neilson et al., 1993, 1998), 28.6 Hz (Jones and Donaldson, 1986), 30.2 Hz (Watson et al., 1997; Watson and Jones, 1998), 40 Hz (Frith et al., 1986), 60 Hz (Viviani and Mounoud, 1990), 60.3 Hz (= screen's vertical interrupt rate) (Viviani and Mounoud, 1990; Jones et al., 1993; Poudel et al., 2008, 2010b), 66.7 Hz (O'Dwyer and Neilson, 1998), 100 Hz (Abend et al., 1982; Stern et al., 1984; Hocherman and Aharon-Peretz, 1994; Jasper et al., 2010), to as unnecessarily high as 240 Hz (Myall et al., 2008), 250 Hz (Day et al., 1984), and 500 Hz (Feys et al., 2005).

For the most part, a relatively low sampling rate is quite satisfactory for analysis of tracking performance as long as the Nyquist criterion is met and there is appropriate analog or digital low-pass filtering to prevent aliasing. Spectral analysis indicates that the fastest of voluntary arm movements have no power above about 8–7 Hz (Jones and Donaldson, 1986). This is very similar to the maximal voluntary oscillations of the elbow of 4–6 Hz (Neilson, 1972; Leist et al., 1987) and to maximum finger tapping rates of 6–7 Hz (Muir et al., 1995). The sampling rate can be reduced still further if the primary interest is only of *coherent* performance, whose bandwidth is only of the order of 2 Hz for both kinesthetic stimuli (Neilson, 1972) and visual stimuli (Leist et al., 1987; Neilson et al., 1993); that is, performance above 2 Hz must be open-loop and, hence, learned and pre-programmed (Neilson, 1972). Thus, from an information theory point of view, there is no need to sample tracking performance beyond, say, 20 Hz.

However, a higher rate may well be justified on the grounds of needing better temporal resolution than 50 ms for transient or cross-correlation analysis, unless one is prepared to regenerate the signal between samples by some form of interpolation (e.g., sinc, spline, polynomial).

31.3.11 Divided-Attention Tasks

Jones and Pollock (2004) developed a divided-attention task (or dual-task) in which the subject has to divide their attention between two simultaneously performed tasks: a continuous visuomotor *Preview-Random Tracking* task and an intermittent visuoperceptual *Arrows Perception* task (Figure 31.6). Prior to the dual task, the subject is tested separately on the tracking and arrows perception tasks so as to obtain baseline performance data from which degradation of performance on each of the tasks when performed concurrently can be quantified. This divided-attention task has proven of particular value as one of the tests in off-road driving assessment of healthy older subjects (Hoggarth et al., 2010) and persons with neurological disorders (Innes et al., 2007, 2009b; Hoggarth, 2011).

Other implementations of divided-attention tasks also have continuous random tracking as the primary task but with a concurrent memory task (van Eekelen and Kerkhof, 2003; Jasper et al., 2010), concurrent digit span task (Baddeley et al., 1986; Dalrymple-Alford et al., 1994), concurrent auditory odd-ball task (Backs, 1997), or an intermittent visual detection task (Gazes et al., 2010), the latter being used to investigate the existence of competition for a capacity-limited "bottle-neck" stage.

31.3.12 Other Measures

Several researchers have further extended the information which can be derived from upper-limb tracking performance by comparison with other simultaneously recorded biosignals. The most common of these is the EMG, particularly integrated EMG due to its close parallel to force of contraction (Neilson, 1972) and where the tracking movement is constrained to be around a single joint. The EMG has been used together with step tracking for fractionating reaction times into premotor and motor components

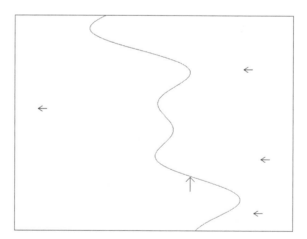

FIGURE 31.6 Divided-attention task (or dual-task) in which subjects have to divide their attention between two simultaneously performed tasks: a continuous *Preview-Random Tracking* task and an intermittent *Arrows Perception* task. While tracking the preview-random target (8.0-s preview) with a steering wheel, 12 consecutive sets of four arrows are displayed on the same screen (for 4.8 s, with 1.0 s between sets) and the subjects aim to maintain accurate tracking of the target while scanning the arrows and determining whether or not all 4 arrows are pointing in the same direction.

(Anson, 1987; Sheridan et al., 1987) and confirmation of open-loop primary movements (Sittig et al., 1985; Sheridan et al., 1987). In smooth tracking, correlation/cross-spectral analysis between the EMG and limb position has been used to study limb dynamics (Neilson, 1972; Barr et al., 1988).

In contrast, Cooper et al. (1989) measured the EEG at four sites during 2-D random tracking to show that slow changes in the EEG (equivalent to the Bereitschafts potential preceding self-paced voluntary movement), particularly at the vertex, are correlated with the absolute velocity of the target.

Simultaneous measurement of hand and eye movements has been undertaken by several researchers to investigate aspects of coupling between eye and hand movements. Eye movements were measured via electrooculography (horizontal only) (Warabi et al., 1986; Leist et al., 1987) or the infra-red limbus reflection technique (Gibson et al., 1987; Sailer et al., 2002; Feys et al., 2005). Interestingly, Leist et al. (1987) found that ocular pursuit and self-paced oscillations were limited to about 1.0 and 2.2 Hz, respectively, whereas the equivalent values for arm movements are 2 and 4–6 Hz, respectively.

31.3.13 Standard Assessment Procedures

Having designed and constructed a tracking task or set of tracking tasks with the characteristics necessary to allow measurement of the sensory-motor control performance under investigation, it is essential that this process be complemented by a well formulated set of standard assessment procedures. These must include (a) standard physical setup, in which positioning of subject, sensor, and screen are tightly specified and controlled, as well as factors such as screen brightness, room lighting, and so on and (b) standardized instructions. The latter are particularly important in tasks where speed-accuracy trade-off (Fitts, 1954; Agarwal and Logsdon, 1990; Murata and Iwase, 2001; Battaglia and Schrater, 2007; Jax et al., 2007; Helton et al., 2009; Bye and Neilson, 2010) is possible. This applies particularly to step tracking, in which leaving the tracking strategy completely up to subjects introduces the possibility of misinterpretation of differences in performance on certain measures, such as reaction time, rise time, and mean absolute error. For example, subjects need to know if it is more important to have the initial movement end up close to the target (i.e., emphasis on accuracy of primary movement) or to get within the vicinity of the target as soon as possible (i.e., emphasis on speed of primary movement); the latter results in greater under/overshooting but also tends to result in lower mean errors). The most common approach taken is to stress the importance of both speed and accuracy with an instruction to subjects of the form: "Follow the target as fast and as accurately as possible."

31.3.14 Test and Experimental Protocols

The design of appropriate test and experimental protocols is also a crucial component of the tracking task design process (Pitrella and Kruger, 1983). When comparisons are made between different subjects, tasks, and/or conditions, careful consideration needs to be given to the paramount factors of *matching* and *balancing* to minimize the possibility of significant differences being due to some bias or confounding variable other than that under investigation. Matching can be achieved between experimental and control subjects in an inter-subject design by having average or paired equivalence on age, gender, education, and so on, or through an intra-subject design in which the subjects act as their own control in, say, a study of dominant versus nondominant arm performance. Balancing is primarily needed to offset *order effects* due to learning which pervade much of sensory-motor performance (Welford, 1968; Poulton, 1974; Schmidt, 1982; Frith et al., 1986; Jones et al., 1990). A study by Jones and Donaldson (1989) provides a good example of the application of these principles. Their study, aimed at investigating the effect of Parkinson's disease on predictive motor planning, involved 16 Parkinsonian subjects and 16 age- and sex-matched control subjects. These were then divided into eight subgroups in a three-way randomized cross-over design so as to eliminate between- and within-session order effects in determining the effect of target type, target preview, and medication on tracking performance.

31.4 Analysis of Sensory-Motor Performance

Analyses of raw tracking data provide performance information which is objective and quantitative and which can be divided into two broad classes:

- Measures of global (or overall or integrated) accuracy of performance.
- Measures of characteristics of performance.

31.4.1 Measures of Global Accuracy of Performance

The most commonly used measure of global or overall accuracy is the *mean absolute error* (MAE) (Poulton, 1974; Jones and Donaldson, 1986), which indicates the average distance the subject was away from the target irrespective of side; it is also variously called average absolute error (Poulton, 1974), modulus mean error (Poulton, 1974), mean rectified error (Neilson and Neilson, 1980), and, simply, tracking error (Kondraske et al., 1984; Behbehani et al., 1988). In contrast, the mean error, or constant position error, is of little value as it simply indicates only the extent to which the response is more on one side of the target than the other (Poulton, 1974). Measures of overall performance which give greater weighting to larger errors include mean square error (Neilson et al., 1993), root mean square error (McRuer and Krendel, 1959; Poulton, 1974; Navon et al., 1984; O'Dwyer and Neilson, 1995), variance of error (Neilson and Neilson, 1980), and standard deviation of error (Poulton, 1974). Relative or normalized error score equivalents of these can be calculated by expressing the raw error scores as a percentage of the respective scores obtained had subject simply held the response marker stationary at the mean target position (Poulton, 1974; Neilson and Neilson, 1980; Day et al., 1984); that is, No-Response = 100%. Alternatively, the relative root mean square error, defined as the square root of the ratio of the mean square value of the error signal to the mean square value of the target signal expressed as a percentage, allows tracking errors to be compared across tests using different target signals (Neilson et al., 1998).

Overall coherence is an important alternative to the above measures when it is wished to assess the similarity between target and response waveforms but there is a substantial delay between them. It provides an estimate of the proportion of the response that is correlated with the target over all frequencies (O'Dwyer and Neilson, 1995; O'Dwyer et al., 1996).

An issue met in viewing error scores from the perspective of Kondraske's elemental resource model (1995, 2006a,b) is the unifying requirement of its associated *general systems performance theory* (*GSPT*) that all dimensions of performance must be in a form for which a higher numerical value indicates a superior performance. Thus, scores which state that a *smaller* score indicates a superior performance, including reaction times, movement times, and all error scores, need to be transformed into *performance scores*. For example:

- Central response speed = 1/(reaction time)
- Information processing speed = 1/(8-choice reaction time)
- Movement speed = 1/(movement time)
- Tracking accuracy = 1/(tracking error)

As transformation via inversion is nonlinear, the distributions of raw error scores and derived performance will be quite different. This has no effect on ordinal analyses, such as nonparametric statistics, but will have some effect on linear analyses, such as parametric statistics, linear regression/correlation, and so on, and may include improvements due to a possible greater normality of the distributions of derived performances. An alternative transformation which would retain a linear relationship with the error scores is

- Tracking accuracy (%) = 100 – Relative tracking error

However, while this gives a dimension of performance with the desired "bigger is better" characteristic, it also raises the possibility of negative values, implying an accuracy worse than zero!—the author can attest to some subjects ending up with error scores worse than the hands–off score. Irrespective of GSPT, there is no doubt that it is beneficial to deal conceptually and analytically with multiple performance measures when *all* measures are consistently defined in terms of "bigger is better."

Time on target is a much cruder measure of tracking performance than all of the above but it has been used reasonably widely due to it being the result obtained from the pursuit rotor. The crudeness generally reflects (a) a lack of spatiotemporal sampling during a task (i.e., simple summation of time on target only) preventing the possibility of further analysis of any form, and (b) a task's performance *ceiling* due to the target having a finite zone within which greater accuracy, relative to center of zone, is unrewarded. This latter factor can, however, be used to advantage for the case where the investigator wishes to have control over the *difficulty* of a task, to gain, for example, similar levels of task difficulty across subjects irrespective of individual ability. This attribute has been used very effectively with 2-D random tracking tasks to minimize the confounding effects of major differences in task load between experimental and control subjects in dual-task studies of impairment of central executive function in subjects with Alzheimer's disease (Baddeley et al., 1986) and Parkinson's disease (Dalrymple-Alford et al., 1994).

31.4.2 Measures of Characteristics of Performance

Measures of global accuracy of tracking performance can detect and quantify the presence of abnormal sensory-motor control performance capacities with considerable sensitivity. Conversely, they are unable to give any indication of which of the many subsystems or performance resources in the overall sensory-motor system are, or may be, responsible for the abnormal performance. Nor can they provide any particular insight into the underlying neuromuscular control mechanisms of normal or abnormal performance.

Four approaches can be taken to provide information necessary to help identify the sensory-motor subsystems and their properties responsible for the *characteristics* of observed normal and abnormal performance:

- *Batteries of neurologic sensory-motor tests*: These tests can be used to, at least ideally, isolate and quantify the various sensory, motor, cognitive, and integrative functions and subsystems involved in sensory-motor performance as measured globally by, for example, tracking tasks.
- *Functional decomposition*: Fractionation of the various performance resources contributing to tracking performance.
- *Traditional signal processing approaches*: Time domain (ballistic and nonballistic) and frequency domain techniques.
- *Graphical analysis*: This has primarily been developed for measurement and investigation of changes in performance and underlying performance resources over time.

31.4.3 Batteries of Neurologic Sensory-Motor Tests

Potvin and colleagues (1975, 1985), now led by Kondraske et al. (1984, 2006), have developed an impressively comprehensive battery of tests for quantitative evaluation of neurologic function, covering a number of sensory, motor, cognitive, and sensory-motor functions and performance resources. Similarly, Jones and colleagues (Jones et al., 1993, 2002; Heitger et al., 2007; Innes et al., 2009a) have developed a battery of computerized sensory-motor and cognitive tests (*SMCTests*™) which, in addition to several tracking tasks, includes tests of component performance resources including visuoperception, nontracking visuomotor ability (ballistic movements, static and dynamic steadiness), complex attention, visual search, decision making, impulse control, planning, and divided attention. Many of these tests have been specifically designed to isolate and quantify the various performance resources involved in tracking tasks and in driving. There is, therefore, a close resemblance between some of the component tests and the tracking tasks, and between several tests and on-road driving, so as to maximize the validity of inter-test comparisons.

31.4.4 Functional Decomposition of Tracking Performance

There are three main approaches whereby tracking performance can be fractionated or decomposed into its functional components: sensory, perceptual, cognitive, motor planning, and motor execution.

The first approach involves breaking the ballistic response in step tracking into reaction time, movement time, overshoot, and settling time (Flowers, 1976; Jones and Donaldson, 1986; Behbehani et al., 1988; Watson et al., 1997) (see Section 31.4.6). This allows indirect deductions about cognitive, motor planning, and motor execution functions, although the distinction between cognitive and motor elements is often unclear.

The second approach involves calculation of differentials in tracking performance from inter-trial alterations in target and/or controlled system dynamics. This has been successfully used to demonstrate and study deficits in Parkinson's disease with respect to predictive motor planning (Flowers, 1978c, 1978a; Stern et al., 1983; Bloxham et al., 1984; Day et al., 1984; Sheridan et al., 1987; Jones and Donaldson, 1989; Soliveri et al., 1997; Watson et al., 1997) and acquisition/modification of motor sets (Frith et al., 1986), and increased reliance on visual feedback (Flowers, 1976, 1978a; Cooke et al., 1978; Warabi et al., 1988; Klockgether and Dichgans, 1994; Liu et al., 1999). This approach has also been used successfully to demonstrate and investigate internal inverse models in the brain (see Section 31.5.5).

The third approach allows a more direct identification of the contribution of certain elemental resources to tracking performance during a specific tracking run. For example, by introducing the concept of a visuoperceptual buffer zone, it is possible to estimate the contribution of visuoperceptual function to tracking performance (Jones et al., 1996). This technique has been used to demonstrate that impaired visuoperceptual function in Parkinsonian subjects plays only a minor role in their poor tracking performance (Jones et al., 1996) but, conversely, that impaired tracking performance in stutterers is predominantly due to reduced dynamic visuospatial perception (Jones et al., 2002). Furthermore, the visuoperceptual function can itself be fractionated into visual acuity, static perception, and dynamic perception (Jones and Donaldson, 1995).

31.4.5 Time-Domain Analysis of Tracking Performance: Nonballistic

There are several run-averaged biases which can indicate the general form of errors being made, particularly when the tracking performance is subnormal. Positive *side of target* (%) and *direction of target* (%) biases reflect a greater proportion of errors occurring to the right of the target or while the target is moving to the right, respectively (Jones and Donaldson, 1986) which, if substantial, may indicate the presence of some visuoperceptual deficit. Similarly, the *side of screen* bias (assuming mean target position is mid-screen) (Jones and Donaldson, 1986) is identical to the mean error or constant position error.

Perhaps the single most important measure of performance, other than mean absolute or RMS error, for nontransient targets is that of the average time delay, or *lag*, of a subject's response with respect to the target signal. The lag is most commonly defined as being the shift τ corresponding to the peak of the cross-correlation function, calculated directly in the time domain or indirectly via the inverse of the cross-spectrum in the frequency domain. Although simulation studies indicate that these techniques are at least as accurate and as robust to noise/remnants as the alternatives listed below (Watson, 1994), one needs to be aware of a bias leading to underestimation of the magnitude of the lag (or lead) due to distortion of the standard cross-correlation function, but specifically of the peak toward zero shift. The distortion arises due to the varying overlap of two truncated signals (i.e., the target and the response) resulting in the multiplication of the cross-correlation function by a triangle (maximum at $\tau = 0$ and zero at $\tau = NT_s$, assuming signals of equal length NT_s. This effect is minimal as long as both signals have a mean value of zero. Temporal resolution is another factor deserving consideration. If desired, greater resolution than that of the sampling period can be obtained by interpolation of the points around the peak of the cross-correlation function by some form of curve fitting (e.g., inverse parabola).

An alternative estimate of the lag, which has proven accurate on simulated responses, can be gained from the *least squares time delay estimation* by finding the time shift between the response and target at which the mean square error is minimized (Fertner and Sjölund, 1986; Jones et al., 1993; Innes et al., 2009a). Another approach, *phase shift time delay* estimation, calculates lag from the gradient of the straight line providing a best least squares to the phase points in the cross-spectrum (Watson et al., 1997). This *phase-correlation* technique has, however, proven more robust to noncorrelated remnants in the response than the other procedures (Watson, 1994).

Several measures used to help characterize within-run variability in performance include variance of error (Neilson and Neilson, 1980), standard deviation of error (Poulton, 1974), and inconsistency (Jones and Donaldson, 1986).

31.4.6 Time-Domain Analysis of Tracking Performance: Ballistic

Irrespective of any of the above nonballistic analyses, evaluation of step tracking performance usually involves separate ballistic or transient analysis of each of the step responses. This generally takes the form of breaking up each response into three phases (Figure 31.7): (1) reaction time phase, or the time between onset of step stimulus and initiation of movement defined by exit from a visible or invisible reaction zone, (2) primary movement phase, or the open-loop ballistic movement made by most normal subjects aiming to get within the vicinity of the target as quickly as possible, the end of which is defined as the first stationary point, and (3) secondary correction phase, comprising one or more adjustments and the remaining time needed to enter and stay within target zone. The step measures from individual

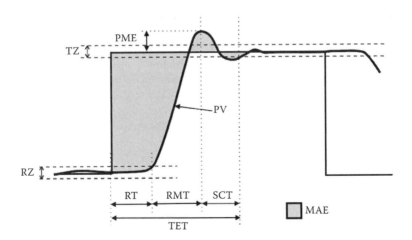

FIGURE 31.7 Transient response analysis. Tolerance zones: RZ is the reaction zone, and TZ is the target zone. Performance parameters: RT is the reaction time, PMT is the primary movement time, SCT is the secondary correction time, TET is the target entry time, PV is the peak velocity, PME is the primary movement error, and MAE is the mean absolute error over a fixed interval following stimulus.

steps can then be grouped into various step categories to allow evaluation of the effect of step size, spatial predictability, arm dominance, and so on, on transient performance.

Accuracy of the primary aimed movement can also be characterized in terms of a constant error and a variable error (standard deviation of error), which are considered to be indices of accuracy of central motor programming and motor execution, respectively (Guiard et al., 1983).

Phase-plane (velocity vs. position) plots provide an alternative means for displaying and examining the qualitative characteristics of step tracking responses. In particular, they have proven valuable for rapid detection of gross abnormalities (Potvin et al., 1985). Behbehani et al. (1988) introduced a novel quantitative element to phase-plane analysis by deriving an index of coordination [IN1] where V_m is the maximum velocity during an outward and return step and A is the area within the resultant loop on the phase-plane plot.

31.4.7 Frequency-Domain Analysis of Tracking Performance

Cross-correlation and spectral analysis have proven invaluable tools for quantifying the frequency-dependent characteristics of the human subject. The cross-spectral density function, or cross-spectrum $S_{xy}(f)$, can be obtained from the random target $x(t)$ and random response $y(t)$ by taking the Fourier transform of the cross-correlation function $r_{xy}(\tau)$, that is, $S_{xy}(f) = F[r_{xy}(\tau)]$, or in the frequency domain via $S_{xy}(f) = X(f)Y(f)^*$, or by a nonparametric system identification approach (e.g., "spa.m" in MATLAB®). The cross-spectrum provides estimates of the relative amplitude (i.e., gain) and phase-lag at each frequency. Gain, phase, and remnant frequency response curves provide objective measures of pursuit tracking behavior, irrespective of linearity, and are considered a most appropriate "quasi-linear" tool for obtaining a quantitative assessment of pursuit tracking behavior (Neilson and Neilson, 1980). From the cross-spectrum one can also derive the *coherence function* which gives the proportion of the response signal linearly related to the target at each frequency: $C_{xy}(f) = |S_{xy}(f)|^2/S_x(f)S_y(f)$, where $S_{xy}(f)$ is the cross-spectral density between $x(t)$ and $y(t)$, and $S_x(f)$ and $S_y(f)$ are the auto-spectral densities of $x(t)$ and $y(t)$, respectively. Lynn et al. (1977) emphasized, however, that one must be cognizant of the difficulty representing tracking performance by a quasi-linear time-invariant transfer function, especially if the run is of short duration or if the target waveform is of limited bandwidth, as the results can be so statistically unreliable as to make description by a second- or third-order transfer function quite unrealistic. Van den Berg et al. (1987) chose four parameters to characterize tracking performance: low-frequency performance via the mean gain of transfer function at the 3 lowest of 8 frequencies in target signal, high-frequency performance via the frequency at which the gain has dropped to less than 0.4, mean delay via shift of peak of the cross-correlation function, and remnant via power in frequencies introduced by subject relative to total power. Spectral and coherence analysis have been used to demonstrate (i) the human bandwidth is about 2 Hz for both kinesthetic tracking (Neilson, 1972) and visual tracking (Neilson et al., 1993), (ii) a much greater relative amplitude of the second harmonic in the response of cerebellar subjects in sine tracking (Miller and Freund, 1980), (iii) a near constant lag except at low frequencies in normal subjects (Cassell et al., 1973), (iv) adaptation to time-varying signals (Bösser, 1984), (v) formation of internal models of novel visuomotor relationships for feedforward control in the brain (Davidson et al., 2000) and confirmation, via simulations, of nonlinear control systems in the brain (Davidson et al., 2002), (vi) 2-D asymmetry in postural steadiness (Myklebust et al., 2009), and (vii) formation of non-dynamic and dynamic inter-limb synergies in a bimanual tracking task (O'Dwyer and Neilson, 1995).

31.4.8 Graphical Analysis of Tracking Performance

Most of the above analyses give quantitative estimates of some aspect of performance which is effectively assumed to be constant over time, other than for experimental and inter-session fluctuations. This is frequently not the case, especially for more complex sensory-motor tasks such as tracking. Changes in performance over time can be divided into two major classes:

- *Class I*—Owing to factors such as practice, fatigue, sleep deprivation, lapses of responsiveness, time of day, stimulants and depressants, lack of practice, and changes in task complexity, in which the underlying performance resources remain unchanged.
- *Class II*—Owing to factors in which there have been abrupt or gradual changes in underlying performance resources at one or more sites in the sensory-motor system due to aging, trauma, or pathology.

Studies of Class I factors using tracking tasks are complicated most by the intra-run *difficulty* of a task not being constant. Changes in tracking accuracy *during* a run can be viewed via graphs of target, response, and/or errors. The latter is particularly informative for sinusoidal targets for which the mean absolute errors can be calculated over consecutive epochs, corresponding to sine-wave cycles, and plotted both in a histogram form and as a smoothed version of this (Jones and Donaldson, 1981, 1986). As complexity of task is constant over short epochs (cf. random pursuit task), the error graph gives an accurate measure of a subject's time-dependent spatiotemporal accuracy that is not confounded by changes in task difficulty and, therefore, gives a true indication of changes in performance due to factors such as learning, fatigue, and lapses in concentration. However, the same can also be achieved for pseudo-random targets due to their periodicity over longer intervals, such as 128 s (Peiris et al., 2006) and 30 s (Poudel et al., 2008). This is of considerable value when time-on-task effects are required following extended continuous-tracking sessions, such as 60 min (Peiris et al., 2006) and 50 min (Poudel et al., 2010a).

Neilson et al. (1998) devised an alternative procedure for intra-run analysis, termed micro-movement analysis, based upon segmentation of the X and Y deflections of the response cursor on the basis of discontinuities, flat regions, and changes in direction of the response. They used this to identify changes in visuomotor coupling during the first 4 min of tracking on a 2-D compatible task following 4 h of practice on a 2-D incompatible task. They proposed that these changes are evidence of rapid switching between different sensory-motor models in the brain.

By comparison, as long as the task remains unchanged over successive runs, studies of class II factors using tracking tasks are complicated most by inter-run *learning*. Although most learning occurs over the first one or two runs or sessions, tracking performance can continue to improve over extended periods as evidenced by, for example, significant improvements still being made by normal subjects after nine weekly sessions (Jones and Donaldson, 1981). Consequently, a major difficulty met in the interpretation of serial measures of performance following acute brain damage is differentiation of neurologic recovery from normal learning. Furthermore, it is not simply a matter of subtracting off the degree of improved performance due to learning seen in normal control subjects. Jones et al. (1990) developed graphical analysis techniques which provide for the removal of the learning factor, as much as is possible, and which can be applied to generating recovery curves for individual subjects following acute brain damage such as stroke. They demonstrated that, for tracking, percentage improvement in performance (PIP) graphs give more reliable evidence of neurologic recovery than absolute improvement in performance (PIA) graphs due to the former's greater independence from what are often considerably different absolute levels of performance.

31.4.8 Statistical Analysis

Parametric statistics (*t*-tests, ANOVA, discriminant analysis) are by far the most commonly used in studies of sensory-motor/psychomotor performance due, in large part, to their ability to draw out interactions between dependent variables. However, there is often a strong case for using nonparametric statistics. For example, the Wilcoxon matched-pairs statistic may be preferable for both between-group and within-subject comparisons due to its greater robustness over its parametric paired *t*-test equivalent, with only minimal loss of power if data are parametric. This is important due to many sensory-motor measures having very skewed distributions as well as considerably different variances between normal and patient groups.

31.5 Applications

Tracking tasks provide objective and quantitative measures and characteristics of sensory-motor control performance and capacities which have proven invaluable in six main classes of applications:

- Clinical screening for sensory-motor deficits
- Neurology and rehabilitation research
- Human performance and factors research (healthy subjects)
- Vocational and recruitment screening
- Modeling and prediction of human performance
- Computational modeling of the human brain

31.5.1 Clinical Screening for Sensory-Motor Deficits

An excellent example of tracking tasks being used in clinical practice for the detection and/or quantification of sensory-motor deficits (arising from one or more lesions in one or more sites in the sensory-motor system) is that of providing objective measures in off-road driving assessment systems/programs (Jones et al., 1983; Croft and Jones, 1987; Gianutsos, 1994; Korteling and Kaptein, 1996; Fischer et al., 2002; Innes et al., 2007, 2011a; Hoggarth et al., 2010).

31.5.2 Neurology and Rehabilitation Research

Tracking tasks have been used extensively in research studies of neurological disorders and rehabilitation. They have been used to identify and/or quantify sensory-motor control deficits in:

- Parkinson's disease (Cassell et al., 1973; Cooke et al., 1978; Flowers, 1976, 1978a, 1978c; Stern et al., 1983; Baroni et al., 1984; Bloxham et al., 1984; Day et al., 1984; Frith et al., 1986; Stern, 1986; Warabi et al., 1986, 1988; Gibson et al., 1987; Sheridan et al., 1987; Behbehani et al., 1988, 1990; Stelmach and Worrington, 1988; Jones and Donaldson, 1989; Dalrymple-Alford et al., 1994; Hocherman and Aharon-Peretz, 1994; Klockgether and Dichgans, 1994; Watson, 1994; Hufschmidt and Lücking, 1995; Johnson et al., 1996; Soliveri et al., 1997; Watson et al., 1997; Gonzalez et al., 2000; Fischer et al., 2002; Allen et al., 2007)
- Stroke (Lynn et al., 1977; De Souza et al., 1980; Jones and Donaldson, 1981; Stelmach and Worrington, 1988; Jones et al., 1989, 1990; O'Dwyer et al., 1996; Fischer et al., 2002; Notley et al., 2007; Siengsukon and Boyd, 2009a,b)
- Traumatic brain injury (Jones and Donaldson, 1981; Korteling and Kaptein, 1996; Heitger et al., 2004, 2007; Innes et al., 2007)
- Cerebral palsy (Neilson et al., 1990, 1992)
- Cerebellar disorders (Beppu et al., 1984, 1987; Becker et al., 1991; Cody et al., 1993; Deuschl et al., 1996)
- Alzheimer's disease (Baddeley et al., 1986; Kisacanin et al., 2000; Hoggarth, 2011)
- Stuttering (Neilson, 1980; Neilson et al., 1992; Zebrowski et al., 1997; Jones et al., 2002)

There are also many examples of patients being assessed repeatedly on tracking tasks for periods up to 12 or more months. This has been done to quantify recovery following stroke (Lynn et al., 1977; De Souza et al., 1980; Jones and Donaldson, 1981; Jones et al., 1989, 1990) and traumatic brain injury (Jones and Donaldson, 1981; Heitger et al., 2004, 2007). Tracking tasks have also been used to quantify changes due to medication, such as in Parkinson's disease (Baroni et al., 1984; Johnson et al., 1996; Soliveri et al., 1997).

31.5.3 Human Performance and Factors Research

Tracking tasks have been used extensively in research studies of human performance in healthy subjects and, in particular, on *factors* having beneficial or detrimental effects on sensory-motor performance, such as:

- Learning by *practicing* the same task or similar tasks (Poulton, 1974; Notterman et al., 1982; Schmidt, 1982; Jones et al., 1986, 1990)
- Learning by *adapting* to major changes in the tracking task, such as in controlled system dynamics, sensor-display relationships, target signals, or visual display of target or response (O'Dwyer and Neilson, 1995; Backs, 1997; Foulkes and Miall, 2000; Davidson et al., 2002; Miall and Jackson, 2006)
- Age (Jones et al., 1986)
- Gender (Jones et al., 1986)
- Dimensionality (Watson and Jones, 1998)
- Time-of-day (Dalrymple-Alford et al., 2003; Jasper et al., 2010)
- Time-on-task (Welford, 1968; Potvin and Tourtellotte, 1975; Van Orden et al., 2000; Petrilli et al., 2005; Peiris et al., 2006; Poudel et al., 2010a)
- Alcohol (Dalrymple-Alford et al., 2003)
- Reduced alertness due to physical fatigue, mental fatigue, sleepiness, sleep deprivation, and/or trait propensity for excessive daytime sleepiness leading to impaired performance. Decrements in performance can range right from minimal (e.g., mildly drowsy) to complete lapses of responsiveness due to lapses of sustained attention, microsleeps (0.5–15 s), or nodding off (>15 s) (Makeig and Jolley, 1996; Peiris et al., 2006, 2011; Davidson et al., 2007; Huang et al., 2008; Poudel et al., 2008, 2010a; Jones et al., 2010)
- Loss of task-orientated attention due to distraction, which can be external or internal and voluntary or involuntary

31.5.4 Vocational and Recruitment Screening

The origin of tracking tasks actually goes back to World War II when they were developed and used to help screen and train aircraft pilots (Welford, 1968; Poulton, 1974). Since then, they have been used to a rather limited degree to determine suitability for recruitment into various vocations in terms of confirming a minimum level, or detecting a superior level, of sensory-motor performance capacity. There is considerable scope for much greater use of tracking tasks alongside psychometric tests as part of the recruitment process, particularly in the transport and defense sectors. They also have the potential to help identify persons with a trait for excessive daytime sleepiness and, even more so, a high propensity for microsleeps (Innes et al., 2010, 2011b) in occupations in which complete lapses of responsiveness can lead to fatal/multi-fatality accidents, such as in long-distance driving, aircraft piloting, air-traffic control, and train drivers.

31.5.5 Modeling and Prediction of Human Performance

Tracking tasks have played an important role in modeling and prediction of human performance. Thus, in contrast to fractionation of performance on a high-level task (e.g., tracking, driving) (see Section 31.4.4), Kondraske et al. (1995, 2006a, b, 2006) have developed techniques for the reverse process. They have shown how their hierarchical elemental resource model, together with *non-linear causal resource analysis* (NCRA), can be used to *predict* performance on high-level tasks from performance on a number of lower-level tasks (Vasta and Kondraske, 1994; Kondraske et al., 1997, 2002; Fischer et al., 2002; Gettman et al., 2003; Matsumoto et al., 2006; Kondraske and Stewart, 2009). This approach has considerable potential in application areas such as rehabilitation. For example, it has been used in driving assessment programs to predict on-road driving ability from performance on several key lower-level off-road/clinic-based tasks pertinent to driving, such as reaction time, visuospatial, cognitive, and tracking tasks (Fischer et al., 2002; Innes et al., 2007, 2009b; Hoggarth et al., 2010).

However, a caution: Innes et al. (2011a) compared the ability of six modeling approaches to predict driving ability (as assessed by driving occupational therapists blinded to off-road results) based on performance on a battery of sensory-motor and cognitive tests (*SMCTests*™) (see Section 31.4.3) in 501 people with brain disorders. At the classification level, they found that two kernel methods—support vector machine (SVM) and product kernel density (PK)—were substantially more accurate at classifying on-road pass or fail (SVM 99.6%, PK 99.8%) than the four other models—kernel product density (KP 81%), binary logistic regression (BLR 78%), discriminant analysis (DA 76%), and NCRA (74%). However, accuracy decreased substantially for all of the kernel models when cross-validation techniques were used to estimate prediction of on-road pass or fail in an independent referral group (SVM 76%, PK 73%, KP 72%) but decreased only slightly for BLR (76%) and DA (75%) (cross-validation of NCRA was not possible). From this, they concluded that, at least for this predictive problem, while kernel-based models are successful at modeling complex data at a classification level, this is likely to be due to overfitting of the data, which does not lead to an improvement in accuracy in independent data over and above the accuracy of other less complex modeling techniques.

31.5.6 Computational Modeling of the Human Brain

Through their continuous nature and versatility to incorporate different targets, different modes of tracking, different sensor-display compatibilities, control system dynamics, and so on, tracking tasks have proven a powerful experimental tool in helping develop, train, and validate computational models of the brain (Jex, 1966; Desmedt, 1978; Lynn et al., 1979; Bösser, 1984; Flash and Hogan, 1985; Neilson et al., 1992, 1998; Sriharan, 1997; Davidson et al., 1999, 2000, 2002; Engel and Soechting, 2000; Ariff et al., 2002; Ghous and Neilson, 2002; Neilson and Neilson, 2002, 2004; Miall and Jackson, 2006; Bye and Neilson, 2010). This includes experimental confirmation of the presence of internal inverse models (Davidson et al., 2000, 2002; Ghous and Neilson, 2002), investigations of intermittency (Vince, 1948; Miall et al., 1985; Neilson et al., 1988a; Foulkes and Miall, 2000; Oytam et al., 2005), investigations of the formation of synergies (O'Dwyer and Neilson, 1995; Neilson and Neilson, 2002; Oytam et al., 2005), and confirmation, rejection, or refinement of computational models of sensory-motor function (Neilson et al., 1988a, b, 1992, 1995, 1998; O'Dwyer and Neilson, 1995; Davidson et al., 2002; Ghous and Neilson, 2002; Miall and Reckess, 2002; Miall and Jackson, 2006).

Defining Terms

Accuracy of movement: The primary *dimension of performance* achieved by the *sensory-motor control* performance resource.

Basic element of performance: Defined by a *functional unit* and a *dimension of performance*, for example, right elbow flexor + speed.

Dimension of performance: A basic measure of performance such as speed, range of movement, strength, spatial perception, spatiotemporal accuracy.

Functional unit: A subsystem such as right elbow flexor, left eye, motor memory.

Performance capacity: The maximal level of performance possible on a particular dimension of performance.

Performance resource: One of a pool of elemental resources, from which the entire human is modeled (Kondraske, 2006a), and which is available for performing tasks. These resources can be subdivided into life sustaining, environmental interface, central processing, and skills domains, and have a parallel with *basic elements of performances.*

Sensor: [in context of tracking tasks] A device for measuring/transducing a subject's motor output.

Sensory-motor control: A primary *performance resource* responsible for overall sensory-motor performance and, in particular, the *dimension of performance* of *accuracy of movement*. The other performance resources on which accuracy of movement is also dependent are strength, reaction time, speed, steadiness, and so on.

Sensory-motor performance: Overall/integrated performance of the *sensory-motor system*, comprising multiple constituent performance resources and associated *dimensions of performance*, including strength, speed, reaction time, steadiness, visual acuity, visuoperception, and *sensory-motor control*.

Sensory-motor system: Comprises all performance resources responsible for all types of *sensory-motor performance*. Encompasses sensory systems (visual, auditory, proprioceptive, tactile), motor systems (muscles, neuromuscular pathways and reflexes, motor planning, motor execution and coordination), and many higher-level systems in the CNS (visuoperception, cognition, memory, central executive, arousal, attention, default mode, etc.).

Spatiotemporal accuracy: The class of accuracy most required by tasks which place considerable demand on attainment of simultaneous spatial and temporal accuracy. This refers particularly to *paced* tasks such as tracking, driving, ball games, and video games.

Tracking task: A laboratory apparatus and associated procedures which have proven one of the most versatile means for assessing and studying the human "black-box" *sensory-motor system* by providing a continuous record of a subject's response, via some *sensor*, to any one of a large number of continuous and well-controlled stimulus or target signals.

References

Abend, W., Bizzi, E., and Morasso, P. 1982. Human arm trajectory formation. *Brain* 105: 331–348.

Agarwal, G. C. and Logsdon, J. B. 1990. Optimal principles for skilled limb movements & speed accuracy tradeoff. *Proc. Ann. Int. Conf. IEEE Eng. Med. Biol. Soc.* 12: 2318–2319.

Allen, D. P., Playfer, J. R., Aly, N. M., Duffey, P., Heald, A., Smith, S. L., and Halliday, D. M. 2007. On the use of low-cost computer peripherals for the assessment of motor dysfunction in Parkinson's disease—Quantification of bradykinesia using target tracking tasks. *IEEE Trans. Neural Systems Rehab. Eng.* 15: 286–294.

Anderson, O. T. 1986. A system for quantitative assessment of dyscoordination and tremor. *Acta Neurol. Scand.* 73: 291–294.

Angel, R. W., Alston, W., and Higgins, J. R. 1970. Control of movement in Parkinson's disease. *Brain* 93: 1–14.

Anson, J. C. 1987. Fractionated simple reaction time as a function of movement direction and level of prestimulus muscle tension. *Int. J. Neurosci.* 35: 140.

Anund, A., Kecklund, G., Vadeby, A., Hjalmdahl, M., and Akerstedt, T. 2008. The alerting effect of hitting a rumble strip—A simulator study with sleepy drivers. *Accid. Anal. Prev.* 40: 1970–1976.

Ariff, G., Donchin, O., Nanayakkara, T., and Shadmehr, R. 2002. A real-time state predictor in motor control: Study of saccadic eye movements during unseen reaching movements. *J. Neurosci.* 22: 7721–7729.

Backs, R. W. 1997. Psychophysiological aspects of selective and divided attention during continuous manual tracking. *Acta Psychol. (Amst.)* 96: 167–191.

Baddeley, A., Logie, R., Bressi, S., Della Salla, S., and Spinnler, H. 1986. Dementia and working memory. *Q. J. Exp. Psychol.* 38A: 603–618.

Banks, S., Catcheside, P., Lack, L., Grunstein, R. R., and McEvoy, R. D. 2004. Low levels of alcohol impair driving simulator performance and reduce perception of crash risk in partially sleep deprived subjects. *Sleep* 27: 1063–1067.

Baroni, A., Benvenuti, F., Fantini, L., Pantaleo, T., and Urbani, F. 1984. Human ballistic arm abduction movements: Effects of L-dopa treatment in Parkinson's disease. *Neurology* 34: 868–876.

Barr, R. E., Hamlin, R. D., Abraham, L. D., and Greene, D. E. 1988. Electromyographic evaluation of operator performance in manual control tracking. *Proc. Ann. Int. Conf. IEEE Eng. Med. Biol. Soc.* 10: 1608–1609.

Battaglia, P. W. and Schrater, P. R. 2007. Humans trade off viewing time and movement duration to improve visuomotor accuracy in a fast reaching task. *J. Neurosci.* 27: 6984–6994.

Becker, W. J., Morrice, B. L., Clark, A. W., and Lee, R. G. 1991. Multi-joint reaching movements and eye–hand tracking in cerebellar incoordination: Investigation of a patient with complete loss of Purkinje cells. *Canad. J. Neurol. Sci.* 18: 476–487.

Behbehani, K., Kondraske, G. V., and Richmond, J. R. 1988. Investigation of upper extremity visuomotor control performance measures. *IEEE Trans. Biomed. Eng.* 35: 518–525.

Behbehani, K., Kondraske, G. V., Tintner, R., Tindall, R. A. S., and Imrhan, S. N. 1990. Evaluation of quantitative measures of upper extremity speed and coordination in healthy persons and in three patients populations. *Arch. Phys. Med. Rehabil.* 71: 106–111.

Beppu, H., Nagaoka, M., and Tanaka, R. 1987. Analysis of cerebellar motor disorders by visually-guided elbow tracking movement: 2. Contributions of the visual cues on slow ramp pursuit. *Brain* 110: 1–18.

Beppu, H., Suda, M., and Tanaka, R. 1984. Analysis of cerebellar motor disorders by visually-guided elbow tracking movement. *Brain* 107: 787–809.

Bloxham, C. A., Mindel, T. A., and Frith, C. D. 1984. Initiation and execution of predictable and unpredictable movements in Parkinson's disease. *Brain* 107: 371–384.

Bösser, T. 1984. Adaptation to time-varying signals and control-theory models of tracking behaviour. *Psychol. Res.* 46: 155–167.

Boyle, L. N. and Lee, J. D. 2010. Using driving simulators to assess driving safety. *Accid. Anal. Prev.* 42: 785–787.

Boyle, L. N., Tippin, J., Paul, A., and Rizzo, M. 2008. Driver performance in the moments surrounding a microsleep. *Transp. Res. Part F. Traffic Psychol. Behav.* 11: 126–136.

Buck, L. 1982. Location versus distance in determining movement accuracy. *J. Mot. Behav.* 14: 287–300.

Bye, R. T. and Neilson, P. D. 2008. The BUMP model of response planning: Variable horizon predictive control accounts for the speed-accuracy tradeoffs and velocity profiles of aimed movement. *Hum. Mov. Sci.* 27: 771–798.

Bye, R. T. and Neilson, P. D. 2010. The BUMP model of response planning: Intermittent predictive control accounts for 10 Hz physiological tremor. *Hum. Mov. Sci.* 29: 713–736.

Cadeddu, J. A. and Kondraske, G. V. 2007. Human performance testing and simulators. *J. Endourol.* 21: 300–304.

Calhoun, V. D. and Pearlson, G. D. 2012. A selective review of simulated driving studies: Combining naturalistic and hybrid paradigms, analysis approaches, and future directions. *NeuroImage* 59: 25–35.

Cassell, K., Shaw, K., and Stern, G. 1973. A computerised tracking technique for the assessment of Parkinsonian motor disabilities. *Brain* 96: 815–826.

Chelette, T. L., Repperger, D. W., and Phillips, C. A. 1995. Enhanced metrics for identification of forearm rehabilitation. *IEEE Trans. Rehab. Eng.* 3: 122–131.

Cody, F. W. J., Lovgreen, B., and Schady 1993. Increased dependence upon information of movement performance during visuo-motor tracking in cerebellar disorders. *Electroencephalogr. Clin. Neurophysiol.* 89: 399–407.

Cooke, J. D., Brown, J. D., and Brooks, V. B. 1978. Increased dependence on visual information for movement control in patients with Parkinson's disease. *Canad. J. Neurol. Sci.* 5: 413–415.

Cooper, R., McCallum, W. C., and Cornthwaite, S. P. 1989. Slow potential changes related to the velocity of target movement in a tracking task. *Electroencephalogr. Clin. Neurophysiol.* 72: 232–239.

Craik, K. J. W. 1966. The mechanism of human action. In: Sherwood, S. L. (Ed.) *The Nature of Psychology—A Selection of Papers, Essays, and Other Writings by the Late Kenneth J. W. Craik.* Cambridge University Press, Cambridge.

Croft, D. and Jones, R. D. 1987. The value of off-road tests in the assessment of driving potential of unlicensed disabled people. *Br. J. Occup. Ther.* 50: 357–361.

Dalrymple-Alford, J. C., Kalders, A. S., Jones, R. D., and Watson, R. W. 1994. A central executive deficit in patients with Parkinson's disease. *J. Neurol. Neurosurg. Psychiatry* 57: 360–367.

Dalrymple-Alford, J. C., Kerr, P. A., and Jones, R. D. 2003. The effects of alcohol on driving-related sensorimotor performance across four times of day. *J. Stud. Alc.* 64: 93–97.

Davidson, P. R., Jones, R. D., and Peiris, M. T. R. 2007. EEG-based lapse detection with high temporal resolution. *IEEE Trans. Biomed. Eng.* 54: 832–839.

Davidson, P. R., Jones, R. D., Sirisena, H. R., and Andreae, J. H. 2000. Detection of adaptive inverse models in the human nervous system. *Hum. Mov. Sci.* 19: 761–795.

Davidson, P. R., Jones, R. D., Sirisena, H. R., and Andreae, J. H. 2002. Simulating closed- and open-loop voluntary movement: A nonlinear control-systems approach. *IEEE Trans. Biomed. Eng.* 49: 1242–1252.

Davidson, P. R., Jones, R. D., Sirisena, H. R., Andreae, J. H., and Neilson, P. D. 1999. Evaluation of nonlinear generalizations of the Adaptive Model Theory. *Proc. Int. Conf. IEEE Eng. Med. Biol. Soc.* 21: 392.

Day, B. L., Dick, J. P. R., and Marsden, C. D. 1984. Patient's with Parkinson's disease can employ a predictive motor strategy. *J. Neurol. Neurosurg. Psychiatry* 47: 1299–1306.

Desai, A. V. and Haque, M. A. 2006. Vigilance monitoring for operator safety: A simulation study on highway driving. *J. Safety Res.* 37: 139–147.

Desmedt, J. E. 1978. *Cerebral Motor Control in Man: Long Loop Mechanisms*, Karger, Basel.

De Souza, L. H., Langton Hewer, R., Lynn, P. A., Mller, S., and Reed, G. A. L. 1980. Assessment of recovery of arm control in hemiplegic stroke patients: 2. Comparison of arm function tests and pursuit tracking in relation to clinical recovery. *Int. Rehab. Med.* 2: 10–16.

Deuschl, G., Toro, C., Zeffiro, T., Massaquoi, S., and Hallett, M. 1996. Adaptation motor learning of arm movements in patients with cerebellar disease. *J. Neurol. Neurosurg. Psychiatry* 60: 515–519.

Driscoll, M. C. 1975. Creative technological aids for the learning-disabled child. *Am. J. Occup. Ther.* 29: 102–105.

Engel, K. C. and Soechting, J. F. 2000. Manual tracking in two dimensions. *J. Neurophysiol.* 83: 3483–3496.

Evarts, E. V., Teräväinen, H., and Calne, D. B. 1981. Reaction time in Parkinson's disease. *Brain* 104: 167–186.

Ferslew, K. E., Manno, J. E., Manno, B. R., Vekovius, W. A., Hubbard, J. M., and Bairnsfather, L. E. 1982. Pursuit meter II, a computer-based device for testing pursuit-tracking performance. *Percep. Mot. Skills* 54: 779–784.

Fertner, A. and Sjölund, S. J. 1986. Comparison of various time delay estimation methods by computer simulation. *IEEE Trans. Acoust.* 34: 1329–1330.

Feys, P., Helsen, W. F., Liu, X., Nuttin, B., Lavrysen, A., Swinnen, S. P., and Ketelaer, P. 2005. Interaction between eye and hand movements in multiple sclerosis patients with intention tremor. *Mov. Disord.* 20: 705–713.

Fischer, C. A., Kondraske, G. V., and Stewart, R. M. 2002. Prediction of driving performance using nonlinear causal resource analysis. *Proc. Ann. Int. Conf. IEEE Eng. Med. Biol. Soc.* 24: 2473–2474.

Fitts, P. M. 1954. The information capacity of the human motor system in controlling the amplitude of movement. *J. Exp. Psychol.* 47: 381–391.

Fitts, P. M. and Posner, M. I. 1967. *Human Performance*, Brooks/Cole, California.

Flash, T. and Hogan, N. 1985. The coordination of arm movements: An experimentally confirmed mathematical model. *J. Neurosci.* 5: 1688–1703.

Flowers, K. A. 1976. Visual 'closed-loop' and 'open-loop' characteristics of voluntary movement in patients with Parkinsonism and intention tremor. *Brain* 99: 269–310.

Flowers, K. A. 1978a. Lack of prediction in the motor behaviour of Parkinsonism. *Brain* 101: 35–52.

Flowers, K. A. 1978b. The predictive control of behaviour: Appropriate and inappropriate actions beyond the input in a tracking task. *Ergonomics* 21: 109–122.

Flowers, K. A. 1978c. Some frequency response characteristics of Parkinsonism on pursuit tracking. *Brain* 101: 19–34.

Foulkes, A. J. and Miall, R. C. 2000. Adaptation to visual feedback delays in a human manual tracking task. *Exp. Brain Res.* 131: 101–110.

Fracker, M. L. and Wickens, C. D. 1989. Resources, confusions, and compatibility in dual-axis tracking: Displays, controls, and dynamics. *J. Exp. Psychol.* 15: 80–96.

Frith, C. D., Bloxham, C. A., and Carpenter, K. N. 1986. Impairments in the learning and performance of a new manual skill in patients with Parkinson's disease. *J. Neurol. Neurosurg. Psychiatry* 49: 661–668.

Garvey, W. D. 1960. A comparison of the effects of training and secondary tasks on tracking behavior. *J. App. Psychol.* 44: 370–375.

Gazes, Y., Rakitin, B. C., Steffener, J., Habeck, C., Butterfield, B., Ghez, C., and Stern, Y. 2010. Performance degradation and altered cerebral activation during dual performance: Evidence for a bottom-up attentional system. *Behav. Brain Res.* 210: 229–239.

Gettman, M. T., Kondraske, G. V., Traxer, O., Ogan, K., Napper, C., Jones, D. B., Pearle, M. S., and Cadeddu, J. A. 2003. Assessment of basic human performance resources predicts operative performance of laparoscopic surgery. *J. Am. Coll. Surg.* 197: 489–96.

Ghous, A. and Neilson, P. D. 2002. Evidence for internal representation of a static nonlinearity in a visual tracking task. *Hum. Mov. Sci.* 21: 847–879.

Gianutsos, R. 1994. Driving advisement with the Elemental Driving Simulator (EDS): When less suffices. *Behav. Res. Meth. Instrum. Comput.* 26: 183–186.

Gibson, J. M., Pimlott, R., and Kennard, C. 1987. Ocular motor and manual tracking in Parkinson's disease and the effect of treatment. *Neurology* 50: 853–860.

Golz, M. and Sommer, D. 2010. Monitoring of drowsiness and microsleep. *Proc. Ann. Int. Conf. IEEE Eng. Med. Biol. Soc.* 32: 1787.

Golz, M., Sommer, D., Chen, M., Trutschel, U., and Mandic, D. 2007. Feature fusion for the detection of microsleep events. *J. VLSI Signal Process. Syst.* 49: 329–342.

Gonzalez, J. G., Heredia, E. A., Rahman, T., Barner, K. E., and Arce, G. R. 2000. Optimal digital filtering for tremor suppression. *IEEE Trans. Biomed. Eng.* 47: 664–673.

Gottlieb, G. L., Agarwal, G. C., and Penn, R. 1984. Sinusoidal oscillation of the ankle as a means of evaluating the spastic patient. *J. Neurol. Neurosurg. Psychiatry* 41: 32–39.

Gowen, E. and Miall, R. C. 2006. Eye-hand interactions in tracing and drawing tasks. *Hum. Mov. Sci.* 25: 568–585.

Guiard, Y., Diaz, G., and Beaubaton, D. 1983. Left-hand advantage in right-handers for spatial constant error: Preliminary evidence in a unimanual ballistic aimed movement. *Neuropsychologia* 21: 111–115.

Heitger, M., Jones, R., and Anderson, T. 2008. A new approach to predicting postconcussion syndrome after mild traumatic brain injury based upon eye movement function. *Proc. Ann. Int. Conf. IEEE Eng. Med. Biol. Soc.* 30: 3570–3573.

Heitger, M. H., Anderson, T. J., Jones, R. D., Dalrymple-Alford, J. C., Frampton, C. M., and Ardagh, M. W. 2004. Eye movement and visuomotor arm movement deficits following mild closed head injury. *Brain* 127: 575–590.

Heitger, M. H., Jones, R. D., Dalrymple-Alford, J. C., Frampton, C. M., Ardagh, M. W., and Anderson, T. J. 2007. Mild head injury—A close relationship between motor function at 1 week post-injury and overall recovery at 3 and 6 months. *J. Neurol. Sci.* 253: 34–47.

Heitger, M. H., Jones, R. D., Macleod, A. D., Snell, D. L., Frampton, C. M., and Anderson, T. J. 2009. Impaired eye movements in post-concussion syndrome indicate suboptimal brain function beyond the influence of depression, malingering or intellectual ability. *Brain* 132: 2850–2870.

Helton, W. S., Kern, R. P., and Walker, D. R. 2009. Conscious thought and the sustained attention to response task. *Conscious. Cogn.* 18: 600–607.

Hocherman, S. and Aharon-Peretz, J. 1994. Two-dimensional tracing and tracking in patients with Parkinson's disease. *Neurology* 44: 111–116.

Hoggarth, P. 2011. Prediction of driving ability in healthy older adults and adults with Alzheimer's dementia or mild cognitive impairment. Doctoral dissertation, Psychology, University of Canterbury, Christchurch, New Zealand.

Hoggarth, P. A., Innes, C. R., Dalrymple-Alford, J. C., Severinsen, J. E., and Jones, R. D. 2010. Comparison of a linear and a non-linear model for using sensory-motor, cognitive, personality, and demographic data to predict driving ability in healthy older adults. *Accid. Anal. Prev.* 42: 1759–1768.

Huang, R.-S., Jung, T.-P., Delorme, A., and Makeig, S. 2008. Tonic and phasic electroencephalographic dynamics during continuous compensatory tracking. *NeuroImage* 39: 1896–1909.

Hufschmidt, A. and Lücking, C. 1995. Abnormalities of tracking behavior in Parkinson's disease. *Mov. Disord.* 10: 267–276.

Innes, C. R. H., Jones, R. D., Anderson, T. J., Hollobon, S. G., and Dalrymple-Alford, J. C. 2009a. Performance in normal subjects on a novel battery of driving-related sensory-motor and cognitive tests. *Behav. Res. Methods* 42: 284–294.

Innes, C. R. H., Jones, R. D., Dalrymple-Alford, J. C., Hayes, S., Hollobon, S., Severinsen, J., Smith, G., Nicholls, A., and Anderson, T. J. 2007. Sensory-motor and cognitive tests predict driving ability of persons with brain disorders. *J. Neurol. Sci.* 260: 188–198.

Innes, C. R. H., Jones, R. D., Dalrymple-Alford, J. C., and Severinsen, J. 2009b. Prediction of driving ability in people with dementia- and non-dementia-related brain disorders. *Proc. Int. Driv. Symp. Hum. Factors Driv. Assess. Train. Veh. Des.* 5: 342–348.

Innes, C. R. H., Lee, D., Chen, C., Ponder-Sutton, A. M., Melzer, T. R., and Jones, R. D. 2011a. Do complex models increase prediction of complex behaviours? Predicting driving ability in people with brain disorders. *Q. J. Exp. Psychol.* 64: 1714–1725.

Innes, C. R. H., Poudel, G. R., and Jones, R. D. 2011b. A paradoxical relationship between usual sleep efficiency and behavioural microsleep propensity following a single night of sleep restriction. (Abstract). *Sleep Biol. Rhythms* 9: 238–239.

Innes, C. R. H., Poudel, G. R., Signal, T. L., and Jones, R. D. 2010. Behavioural microsleeps in normally-rested people. *Proc. Ann. Int. Conf. IEEE Eng. Med. Biol. Soc.* 32: 4448–4451.

Jasper, I., Roenneberg, T., Haubler, A., Zierdt, A., Marquardt, C., and Hermsdorfer, J. 2010. Circadian rhythm in force tracking and in dual task costs. *Chronobiol. Int.* 27: 653–673.

Jax, S., Rosenbaum, D., and Vaughan, J. 2007. Extending Fitts' Law to manual obstacle avoidance. *Exp. Brain Res.* 180: 775–779.

Jex, H. R. 1966. A "critical" tracking task for manual control research. *IEEE Trans. Hum. Factors Electronics* 7: 138–145.

Johnson, M. T. V., Kipnis, A. N., Coltz, J. D., Gupta, A., Silverstein, P., Zwiebel, F., and Ebner, T. J. 1996. Effects of levodopa and viscosity on the velocity and accuracy of visually guided tracking in Parkinson's disease. *Brain* 119: 801–813.

Jones, R., Giddens, H., and Croft, D. 1983. Assessment and training of brain-damaged drivers. *Am. J. Occup. Ther.* 37: 754–760.

Jones, R. D. and Donaldson, I. M. 1981. Measurement of integrated sensory-motor function following brain damage by a preview tracking task. *Int. Rehab. Med.* 3: 71–83.

Jones, R. D. and Donaldson, I. M. 1986. Measurement of sensory-motor integrated function in neurological disorders: three computerised tracking tasks. *Med. Biol. Eng. Comput.* 24: 536–540.

Jones, R. D. and Donaldson, I. M. 1989. Tracking tasks and the study of predictive motor planning in Parkinson's disease. *Proc. Int. Conf. IEEE Eng. Med. Biol. Soc.* 11: 1055–1056.

Jones, R. D. and Donaldson, I. M. 1995. Fractionation of visuoperceptual dysfunction in Parkinson's disease. *J. Neurol. Sci.* 131: 43–50.

Jones, R. D., Donaldson, I. M., and Parkin, P. J. 1989. Impairment and recovery of ipsilateral sensory-motor function following unilateral cerebral infarction. *Brain* 112: 113–132.

Jones, R. D., Donaldson, I. M., Parkin, P. J., and Coppage, S. A. 1990. Impairment and recovery profiles of sensory-motor function following stroke: Single-case graphical analysis techniques. *Int. Disabil. Stud.* 12: 141–148.

Jones, R. D., Donaldson, I. M., and Sharman, N. B. 1996. A technique for the removal of the visuospatial component from tracking performance and its application to Parkinson's disease. *IEEE Trans. Biomed. Eng.* 43: 1001–1010.

Jones, R. D. and Pollock, T. S. 2004. *Symbols-Scanning Test and Symbols-and-Tracking Dual-Task Test.* Patent No. 520069, New Zealand.

Jones, R. D., Poudel, G. R., Innes, C. R. H., Davidson, P. R., Peiris, M. T. R., Malla, A. M., Signal, L., Carroll, G. J., Watts, R., and Bones, P. J. 2010. Lapses of responsiveness: Characteristics, detection, and underlying mechanisms. *Proc. Ann. Int. Conf. IEEE Eng. Med. Biol. Soc.* 32: 1788–1791.

Jones, R. D., Sharman, N. B., Watson, R. W., and Muir, S. R. 1993. A PC-based battery of tests for quantitative assessment of upper-limb sensory-motor function in brain disorders. *Proc. Int. Conf. IEEE Eng. Med. Biol. Soc.* 15: 1414–1415.

Jones, R. D., White, A. J., Lawson, K. H., and Anderson, T. J. 2002. Visuoperceptual and visuomotor deficits in developmental stutterers: An exploratory study. *Hum. Mov. Sci.* 21: 603–619.

Jones, R. D., Williams, L. R. T., and Wells, J. E. 1986. Effects of laterality, sex, and age on computerized sensory-motor tests. *J. Hum. Mot. Stud.* 12: 163–182.

Jung, T.-P., Huang, K.-C., Chuang, C.-H., Chen, J.-A., Ko, L.-W., Chiu, T.-W., and Lin, C.-T. 2010. Arousing feedback rectifies lapse in performance and corresponding EEG power spectrum. *Proc. Ann. Int. Conf. IEEE Eng. Med. Biol. Soc.* 32: 1792–1795.

Kearney, R. E. and Hunter, I. W. 1983. System identification of human triceps surae stretch reflex dynamics. *Exp. Brain Res.* 51: 117–127.

Kisacanin, B., Agarwal, G. C., Taber, J., and Hier, D. 2000. Computerised evaluation of cognitive and motor function. *Med. Biol. Eng. Comput.* 38: 68–73.

Klaver, P., Fell, J., Weis, S., de Greiff, A., Ruhlmann, J., Reul, J., Elger, C. E., and Fernandez, G. 2004. Using visual advance information: An event-related functional MRI study. *Cogn. Brain Res.* 20: 242–255.

Klockgether, T. and Dichgans, J. 1994. Visual control of arm movement in Parkinson's disease. *Mov. Disord.* 9: 48–56.

Kondraske, G. V. 1995. An elemental resource model for the human-task interface. *Int. J. Technol. Assess. Health Care* 11: 153–173.

Kondraske, G. V. 2006a. The elemental resource model for human performance. In: Bronzino, J. D. (Ed.) *The Biomedical Engineering Handbook—Biomedical Engineering Fundamentals.* 3rd ed, pp. 75: 1–19, CRC Press, Boca Raton, Florida.

Kondraske, G. V. 2006b. Measurement of information-processing subsystem performance capacities. In: Bronzino, J. D. (Ed.) *The Biomedical Engineering Handbook—Biomedical Engineering Fundamentals.* 3rd ed, pp. 78: 1–14, CRC Press, Boca Raton, Florida.

Kondraske, G. V., Behbehani, K., Chwialkowski, M., Richmond, R., and van Maltzahn, W. 1988. A system for human performance measurement. *IEEE Eng. Med. Biol. Mag.* March: 23–27.

Kondraske, G. V., Cadeddu, J. A., Napper, C., and Jones, D. B. 2002. Prediction of surgical skill and limitations from basic performance capacities using nonlinear causal resource analysis. *Proc. Ann. Int. Conf. IEEE Eng. Med. Biol. Soc.* 24: 2360–2361.

Kondraske, G. V., Johnson, C., Pearson, A., and Tarbox, L. 1997. Performance prediction and limited resource identification with nonlinear causal resource analysis. *Proc. Ann. Int. Conf. IEEE Eng. Med. Biol. Soc.* 19: 1813–1816.

Kondraske, G. V., Mulukutla, R., and Stewart, R. M. 2006. Investigation of a portable performance measurement system for neurologic screening in clinics. *Proc. Int. Conf. IEEE Eng. Med. Biol. Soc.* 28: 3962–3965.

Kondraske, G. V., Potvin, A. R., Tourtellotte, W. W., and Syndulko, K. 1984. A computer-based system for automated quantitation of neurologic function. *IEEE Trans. Biomed. Eng.* 31: 401–414.

Kondraske, G. V. and Stewart, R. M. 2009. New methodology for identifying hierarchical relationships among performance measures: Concepts and demonstration in Parkinson's disease. *Proc. Int. Conf. IEEE Eng. Med. Biol. Soc.* 31: 5279–5282.

Korteling, J. E. and Kaptein, N. A. 1996. Neuropsychological driving fitness tests for brain-damaged subjects. *Arch. Phys. Med. Rehabil.* 77: 138–146.

Lee, H. C. 2006. Virtual driving tests for older adult drivers? *Br. J. Occup. Ther.* 69: 138–141.

Leist, A., Freund, H. J., and Cohen, B. 1987. Comparative characteristics of predictive eye-hand tracking. *Hum. Neurobiol.* 6: 19–26.

Lin, C.-T., Wu, R.-C., Liang, S.-F., Chao, W.-H., Chen, Y.-J., and Jung, T.-P. 2005. EEG-based drowsiness estimation for safety driving using independent component analysis. *IEEE Trans. Circuits Systems* 52: 2726–2738.

Liu, X., Tubbesing, S. A., Aziz, T. Z., Miall, R. C., and Stein, J. F. 1999. Effects of visual feedback on manual tracking and action tremor in Parkinson's disease. *Exp. Brain Res.* 129: 477–481.

Lowden, A., Anund, A., Kecklund, G., Peters, B., and Akerstedt, T. 2009. Wakefulness in young and elderly subjects driving at night in a car simulator. *Accid. Anal. Prev.* 41: 1001–1007.

Lynn, P. A., Parker, W. R., Reed, G. A. L., Baldwin, J. F., and Pilsworth, B. W. 1979. New approaches to modelling the disable human operator. *Med. Biol. Eng. Comput.* 17: 344–348.

Lynn, P. A., Reed, G. A. L., Parker, W. R., and Langton Hewer, R. 1977. Some applications of human-operator research to the assessment of disability in stroke. *Med. Biol. Eng.* 15: 184–188.

MacAskill, M. R., Anderson, T. J., and Jones, R. D. 2002. Adaptive modification of saccades in Parkinson's disease. *Brain* 125: 1570–1582.

Makeig, S. and Jolley, K. 1996. *COMPTRACK—A Compensatory Tracking Task for Monitoring Alertness.* Naval Health Research Center, San Diego, CA.

Martens, M., Simons, R., and Ramaekers, J. 2011. Dexamphetamine and alcohol effects in simulated driving and cognitive task performance. *Proc. Int. Driv. Symp. Hum. Factors Driv. Assess. Train. Veh. Des.* 6: 52–58.

Matsumoto, E. D., Kondraske, G. V., Ogan, K., Jacomides, L., Wilhelm, D. M., Pearle, M. S., and Cadeddu, J. A. 2006. Assessment of basic human performance resources predicts performance of ureteroscopy. *Am. J. Surg.* 191: 817–820.

Mayhew, D. R., Simpson, H. M., Wood, K. M., Lonero, L., Clinton, K. M., and Johnson, A. G. 2011. On-road and simulated driving: Concurrent and discriminant validation. *J. Safety Res.* 42: 267–275.

McRuer, D. T. and Krendel, E. S. 1959. The human operator as a servo element. *J. Franklin Institute* 267: 381–403.

Miall, R. C. and Jackson, J. K. 2006. Adaptation to visual feedback delays in manual tracking: Evidence against the Smith Predictor model of human visually guided action. *Exp. Brain Res.* 172: 77–84.

Miall, R. C. and Reckess, G. Z. 2002. The cerebellum and the timing of coordinated eye and hand tracking. *Brain Cogn.* 48: 212–226.

Miall, R. C., Weir, D. J., and Stein, J. F. 1985. Visuomotor tracking with delayed visual feedback. *Neuroscience* 16: 511–520.

Miller, R. G. and Freund, H. J. 1980. Cerebellar dyssynergia in humans—A quantitative analysis. *Ann. Neurol.* 8: 574–579.

Mrotek, L., Gielen, C. C. A. M., and Flanders, M. 2006. Manual tracking in three dimensions. *Exp. Brain Res.* 171: 99–115.

Muir, S. R., Jones, R. D., Andreae, J. H., and Donaldson, I. M. 1995. Measurement and analysis of single and multiple finger tapping in normal and Parkinsonian subjects. *Parkinsonism Related Disord.* 1: 89–96.

Muir, S. R., MacAskill, M. R., Herron, D., Goelz, H., Anderson, T. J., and Jones, R. D. 2003. EMMA—An eye movement measurement and analysis system. *Australas. Phys. Eng. Sci. Med.* 26: 18–24.

Murata, A. and Iwase, H. 2001. Extending Fitts' law to a three-dimensional pointing task. *Hum. Mov. Sci.* 20: 791–805.

Myall, D. J. 2010. Investigations into motor adaptation and Parkinson's disease using virtual environments and computational frameworks. Doctoral dissertation, Medicine, University of Otago, Christchurch, New Zealand.

Myall, D. J., MacAskill, M. R., Davidson, P. R., Anderson, T. J., and Jones, R. D. 2008. Design of a modular and low-latency virtual-environment platform for applications in motor adaptation research, neurological disorders, and neurorehabilitation. *IEEE Trans. Neural Systems Rehab. Eng.* 16: 298–309.

Myklebust, J. B., Lovett, E. G., Myklebust, B. M., Reynolds, N., Milkowski, L., and Prieto, T. E. 2009. Two-dimensional coherence for measurement of asymmetry in postural steadiness. *Gait & Posture* 29: 1–5.

Navon, D., Gopher, D., Chillag, N., and Spitz, G. 1984. On separability of and interference between tracking dimensions in dual-axis tracking. *J. Mot. Behav.* 16: 364–391.

Neilson, M. D. 1980. *Stuttering and the control of speech: A systems analysis approach.* Doctoral dissertation, University of New South Wales, Sydney.

Neilson, P. D. 1972. Speed of response or bandwidth of voluntary system controlling elbow position in intact man. *Med. Biol. Eng.* 10: 450–459.

Neilson, P. D. and Neilson, M. D. 1980. Influence of control-display compatibility on tracking behaviour. *Q. J. Exp. Psychol.* 32: 125–135.

Neilson, P. D. and Neilson, M. D. 2002. Anisotropic tracking: Evidence for automatic synergy formation in a bimanual task. *Hum. Mov. Sci.* 21: 723–748.

Neilson, P. D. and Neilson, M. D. 2004. A new view on visuomotor channels: The case of the disappearing dynamics. *Hum. Mov. Sci.* 23: 257–283.

Neilson, P. D., Neilson, M. D., and O'Dwyer, N. J. 1988a. Internal models and intermittency: A theoretical account of human tracking behaviour. *Biol. Cybern.* 58: 101–112.

Neilson, P. D., Neilson, M. D., and O'Dwyer, N. J. 1992. Adaptive model theory: Application to disorders of motor control. In: Summers, J. J. (Ed.) *Approaches to the Study of Motor Control and Learning.* pp. 495–548, Elsevier, Amsterdam.

Neilson, P. D., Neilson, M. D., and O'Dwyer, N. J. 1993. What limits high speed tracking performance? *Hum. Mov. Sci.* 12: 85–109.

Neilson, P. D., Neilson, M. D., and O'Dwyer, N. J. 1995. Adaptive optimal control of human tracking. In: Glencross, D. J. and Piek, J. P. (Eds.) *Motor Control and Sensory-Motor Integration: Issues and Directions.* pp. 97–140, Elsevier Science, Amsterdam.

Neilson, P. D., Neilson, M. D. and O'Dwyer, N. J. 1998. Evidence for rapid switching of sensory-motor models. In: Piek, J. (Ed.) *Motor Control and Human Skill: A Multidisciplinary Perspective.* pp. 105–126, Human Kinetics, Champaign, IL.

Neilson, P. D., O'Dwyer, N. J., and Nash, J. 1990. Control of isometric muscle activity in cerebral palsy. *Devel. Med. Child Neurol.* 32: 778–788.

Neilson, P. D., O'Dwyer, N. J., and Neilson, M. D. 1988b. Stochastic prediction in pursuit tracking: An experimental test of adaptive model theory. *Biol. Cybern.* 58: 113–122.

Notley, S. V., Turk, R., Pickering, R., Simpson, D. M., and Burridge, J. H. 2007. Analysis of the quality of wrist movement during a simple tracking task. *Physiol. Meas.* 28: 881–895.

Notterman, J. M., Tufano, D. R., and Hrapsky, J. S. 1982. Visuo-motor organization: Differences between and within individuals. *Percep. Mot. Skills* 54: 723–750.

O'Dwyer, N. J. and Neilson, P. D. 1995. Learning a dynamic limb synergy. In: Glencross, D. J. and Piek, J. P. (Eds.) *Motor Control and Sensory-Motor Integration: Issues and Directions.* pp. 289–317, Elsevier Science, Amsterdam.

O'Dwyer, N. J. and Neilson, P. D. 1998. Adaptation to a changed sensory-motor relation: Immediate and delayed parametric modification. In: Piek, J. P. (Ed.) *Motor Behavior and Human Skill—A Multidisciplinary Approach.* pp. 75–104, Human Kinetic, Champaign, IL.

O'Dwyer, N. J., Ada, L., and Neilson, P. D. 1996. Spasticity and muscle contracture following stroke. *Brain* 119: 1737–1749.

Oishi, M. M., TalebiFard, P., and McKeown, M. J. 2011. Assessing manual pursuit tracking in Parkinson's disease via linear dynamical systems. *Ann. Biomed. Eng.* 39: 2263–2273.

Oytam, Y., Neilson, P. D., and O'Dwyer, N. J. 2005. Degrees of freedom and motor planning in purposive movement. *Hum. Mov. Sci.* 24: 710–730.

Patrick, J. and Mutlusoy, F. 1982. The relationship between types of feedback, gain of a display and feedback precision in acquisition of a simple motor task. *Q. J. Exp. Psychol.* 34A: 171–182.

Peiris, M. T. R., Davidson, P. R., Bones, P. J., and Jones, R. D. 2011. Detection of lapses in responsiveness from the EEG. *J. Neural Eng.* 8 (016003): 1–15.

Peiris, M. T. R., Jones, R. D., Davidson, P. R., Carroll, G. J., and Bones, P. J. 2006. Frequent lapses of responsiveness during an extended visuomotor tracking task in non-sleep-deprived subjects. *J. Sleep Res.* 15: 291–300.

Petrilli, R. M., Jay, S. M., Dawson, D., and Lamond, N. 2005. The impact of sustained wakefulness and time-of-day on OSPAT performance. *Ind Health* 43: 186–192.

Pitrella, F. D. and Kruger, W. 1983. Design and validation of matching tests to form equal groups for tracking experiments. *Ergonomics* 26: 833–845.

Potvin, A. R., Albers, J. W., Stribley, R. F., Tourtellotte, W. W., and Pew, R. W. 1975. A battery of tests for evaluating steadiness in clinical trials. *Med. Biol. Eng.* 13: 914–921.

Potvin, A. R., Doerr, J. A., Estes, J. T., and Tourtellotte, W. W. 1977. Portable clinical tracking-task instrument. *Med. Biol. Eng. Comput.* 15: 391–397.

Potvin, A. R. and Tourtellotte, W. W. 1975. The neurological examination: Advancement in its quantification. *Arch. Phys. Med. Rehabil.* 56: 425–442.

Potvin, A. R., Tourtellotte, W. W., Potvin, J. H., Kondraske, G. V., and Syndulko, K. 1985. *The Quantitative Examination of Neurologic Function*, CRC Press, Boca Raton, FL.

Poudel, G. R., Innes, C. R. H., Bones, P. J., and Jones, R. D. 2010a. The relationship between behavioural microsleeps, visuomotor performance and EEG theta. *Proc. Ann. Int. Conf. IEEE Eng. Med. Biol. Soc.* 32: 4452–4455.

Poudel, G. R., Jones, R. D., and Innes, C. R. H. 2008. A 2-D pursuit tracking task for behavioural detection of lapses. *Australas. Phys. Eng. Sci. Med.* 31: 528–529.

Poudel, G. R., Jones, R. D., Innes, C. R. H., Davidson, P. R., Watts, R., and Bones, P. J. 2010b. Measurement of BOLD changes due to cued eye-closure and stopping during a continuous visuomotor task via model-based and model-free approaches. *IEEE Trans. Neural Systems Rehab. Eng.* 18: 479–488.

Poudel, G. R., Jones, R. D., Innes, C. R. H., Watts, R., Signal, T. L., and Bones, P. J. 2009. fMRI correlates of behavioural microsleeps during a continuous visuomotor task. *Proc. Ann. Int. Conf. IEEE Eng. Med. Biol. Soc.* 31: 2919–2922.

Poulton, E. C. 1964. Postview and preview in tracking with complex and simple inputs. *Ergonomics* 7: 257–266.

Poulton, E. C. 1974. *Tracking Skill and Manual Control*, Academic Press, New York.

Reithler, J., Reithler, H., van den Boogert, E., Goebel, R., and van Mier, H. 2006. Resistance-based high resolution recording of predefined 2-dimensional pen trajectories in an fMRI setting. *J. Neurosci. Meth.* 152: 10–17.

Riedel, S. A., Harris, G. F., and Jizzine, H. A. 1992. An investigation of seated postural stability. *IEEE Eng. Med. Biol. Mag.* 11: 42–47.

Robertson, C. and Flowers, K. A. 1990. Motor set in Parkinson's disease. *J. Neurol. Neurosurg. Psychiatry* 53: 583–592.

Sailer, U., Eggert, T., Ditterich, J., and Straube, A. 2002. Global effect of a nearby distractor on targeting eye and hand movements. *J. Exp. Psychol. Hum. Percept. Perform.* 28: 1432–1446.

Schilling, R. J., Bollt, E. M., Fulk, G. D., Skufca, J. D., Al-Ajlouni, A. F., and Robinson, C. J. 2009. A quiet standing index for testing the postural sway of healthy and diabetic adults across a range of ages. *IEEE Trans. Biomed. Eng.* 56: 292–302.

Schmidt, R. A. 1982. *Motor Control and Learning: A Behavioral Emphasis*, Human Kinetics, Champagne, Illinois.

Schultheis, M. T., Rebimbas, J., Mourant, R., and Millis, S. R. 2007. Examining the usability of a virtual reality driving simulator. *Assist. Technol.* 19: 1–8.

Schultheis, M. T., Simone, L. K., Roseman, E., Nead, R., Rebimbas, J., and Mourant, R. 2006. Stopping behavior in a VR driving simulator: A new clinical measure for the assessment of driving. *Proc. Ann. Int. Conf. IEEE Eng. Med. Biol. Soc.* 28: 4921–4924.

Sheridan, M. R., Flowers, K. A., and Hurrell, J. 1987. Programming and execution of movement in Parkinson's disease. *Brain* 110: 1247–1271.

Sheridan, T. B. 1966. Three models of preview control. *IEEE Trans. Hum. Factors Electronics* 7: 91–102.

Siegel, D. 1985. Information processing abilities and performance on two perceptual-motor tasks. *Percep. Mot. Skills* 60: 459–466.

Siengsukon, C. and Boyd, L. A. 2009a. Sleep enhances off-line spatial and temporal motor learning after stroke. *Neurorehabil. Neural Repair* 23: 327–335.

Siengsukon, C. F. and Boyd, L. A. 2009b. Sleep to learn after stroke: Implicit and explicit off-line motor learning. *Neurosci. Lett.* 451: 1–5.

Sittig, A. C., Denier van der Gon, J. J., Gielen, C. C., and van Wilk, A. J. 1985. The attainment of target position during step-tracking movements despite a shift of initial position. *Exp. Brain Res.* 60: 407–410.

Soliveri, P., Brown, R. G., Jahanshahi, M., Caraceni, T., and Marsden, C. D. 1997. Learning manual pursuit tracking skills in patients with Parkinson's disease. *Brain* 120: 1325–1337.

Sommer, D. and Golz, M. 2010. Evaluation of PERCLOS based current fatigue monitoring technologies. *Proc. Ann. Int. Conf. IEEE Eng. Med. Biol. Soc.* 32: 4456–4459.

Sommer, D., Golz, M., Schnupp, T., Krajewski, J., Trutschel, U., and Edwards, D. 2009. A measure of strong driver fatigue. *Proc. Int. Driv. Symp. Hum. Factors Driv. Assess. Train. Veh. Des.* 5: 9–15.

Sriharan, A. 1997. Mathematical modelling of the human operator control system through tracking tasks. Masters thesis, University of New South Wales, Sydney, Australia.

Stelmach, G. E. and Worrington, C. J. 1988. The preparation and production of isometric force in Parkinson's disease. *Neuropsychologia* 26: 93–103.

Stern, Y. 1986. Patients with Parkinson's disease can employ a predictive motor strategy. *J. Neurol. Neurosurg. Psychiatry* 49: 107–108.

Stern, Y., Mayeux, R., and Rosen, J. 1984. Contribution of perceptual motor dysfunction to construction and tracing disturbances in Parkinson's disease. *J. Neurol. Neurosurg. Psychiatry* 47: 983–989.

Stern, Y., Mayeux, R., Rosen, J., and Ilson, J. 1983. Perceptual motor dysfunction in Parkinson's disease: A deficit in sequential and predictive voluntary movement. *J. Neurol. Neurosurg. Psychiatry* 46: 145–151.

Thomas, J. S., Croft, D. A., and Brooks, V. B. 1976. A manipulandum for human motor studies. *IEEE Trans. Biomed. Eng.* 23: 83–84.

Vadeby, A., Forsman, A., Kecklund, G., Akerstedt, T., Sandberg, D., and Anund, A. 2010. Sleepiness and prediction of driver impairment in simulator studies using a Cox proportional hazard approach. *Accid. Anal. Prev.* 42: 835–841.

van den Berg, R., Mooi, B., Denier van der Gon, J. J., and Gielen, C. C. A. M. 1987. Equipment for the quantification of motor performance for clinical purposes. *Med. Biol. Eng. Comput.* 25: 311–316.

van Eekelen, A. P. J. and Kerkhof, G. A. 2003. No interference of task complexity with circadian rhythmicity in a constant routine protocol. *Ergonomics* 46: 1578–1593.

Van Orden, K. F., Jung, T.-P., and Makeig, S. 2000. Combined eye activity measures accurately estimate changes in sustained visual task performance. *Biol. Psychol.* 52: 221–240.

Vasta, P. J. and Kondraske, G. V. 1994. Performance prediction of an upper extremity reciprocal task using non-linear causal resource analysis. *Proc. Int. Conf. IEEE Eng. Med. Biol. Soc.* 16: 305–306.

Vasta, P. J. and Kondraske, G. V. 2006. Human performance engineering design and analysis tools. In: Bronzino, J. D. (Ed.) *The Biomedical Engineering Handbook—Biomedical Engineering Fundamentals.* 3rd ed, pp. 84: 1–16, CRC Press, Boca Raton, Florida.

Vince, M. A. 1948. The intermittency of control movements and the psychological refractory period. *Brit. J. Psychol.* 38: 149–157.

Viviani, P. and Mounoud, P. 1990. Perceptuomotor compatibility in pursuit tracking of two-dimensional movements. *J. Mot. Behav.* 22: 407–443.

Warabi, T., Noda, H., Yanagisawa, N., Tashiro, K., and Shindo, R. 1986. Changes in sensorimotor function associated with the degree of bradykinesia of Parkinson's disease. *Brain* 109: 1209–1224.

Warabi, T., Yanagisawa, N., and Shindo, R. 1988. Changes in strategy of aiming tasks in Parkinson's disease. *Brain* 111: 497–505.

Watson, R. W. 1994. Advances in zero-based consistent deconvolution and Evaluation of human sensory-motor function. Doctoral Dissertation, University of Canterbury, Christchurch, New Zealand.

Watson, R. W. and Jones, R. D. 1998. A comparison of two-dimensional and one-dimensional tracking performance in normal subjects. *J. Mot. Behav.* 30: 359–366.

Watson, R. W., Jones, R. D., and Sharman, N. B. 1997. Two-dimensional tracking tasks for quantification of sensory-motor dysfunction and their application to Parkinson's disease. *Med. Biol. Eng. Comput.* 35: 141–145.

Welford, A. T. 1968. *Fundamentals of Skill,* Methuen, London.

Zebrowski, P. M., Moon, J. B., and Robin, D. A. 1997. Visuomotor tracking in children who stutter: A preliminary view. In: Hulstijn, W., Peters, H. and Van Lieshout, P. (Eds.) *Speech Production: Motor Control, Brain Research and Fluency Disorders.* pp. 579–584, Elsevier, Amsterdam.

32

Measurement of Information-Processing Subsystem Performance Capacities

George V. Kondraske
University of Texas,
Arlington

Paul J. Vasta
University of Texas,
Arlington

32.1 Introduction

The human brain has been the subject of much scientific research. While a tremendous amount of information exists and considerable progress has been made in unlocking its many mysteries, many gaps in understanding exist. However, it is not essential to understand in full detail how a given function of the brain is mediated in order to accept that it (i.e., the function) exists, or to understand how to maximally isolate, stress, and characterize at least selected attributes of its performance quantitatively. In this chapter, a systems view of major functional aspects of the brain is used as a basis for discussing methods employed to measure what can be termed central processing performance capacities. Central processing capacities are distinguished from the information that is processed. In humans, the latter can be viewed to represent the contents of *memory* (e.g., facts, "programs," etc.). Clearly, both the information itself and the characteristics of the systems that process it (i.e., the various capacities discussed below) combine to realize what are commonly observed as skills whether perceptual, motor, cognitive, or other.

Investigations of how humans process information have been performed within various fields including psychology, cognitive science, and information theory with the primary motivation being to better understand how human information-processing works and the factors that influence it. On the basis that it provided a rigorous definition for the measurement of information, it can be argued that

Shannon's information theory (Shannon, 1948) has been and continues to be one of the more important developments to influence both the science and engineering associated with human information processing. Several early attempts to apply it to human information processing (Hick, 1952; Hyman, 1953; Fitts, 1954) have stood the test of time and have provided the basis for subsequent efforts of both researchers and practitioners. These works are central to the material presented here. In addition, the work of Wiener (1955) is also noteworthy in that it began the process of viewing human and artificial information processing from a common perspective. Analogies between humans and computers have proven to be very useful up to certain limits.

While there is considerable overlap and frequent interchange, the roles of science and engineering are different. In the present context, the emphasis is on aspects of the latter. It has been necessary to engineer useful measurement tools and processes without complete science to serve a wide variety of purposes that have demanded *attention* in both clinical and nonclinical contexts. Whether purposeful or accidental, methods of systems engineering have been incorporated and have proven useful in dealing with the complexity of human brain structure and function. While scientific controversies continue to exist, much research has contributed to the now common view of separate (both in function and location) processing subsystems that make up the whole. Various versions of a general distributed, multiprocessor model of human brain function have been popularly sketched (Gazzaniga, 1985; Minsky, 1986; Ornstein, 1986). For example, it is widely known that the occipital lobe of the brain is responsible for visual information processing while other areas have been found to correspond to other functions. It is not possible to do justice here to the tremendous scope of work that has been put forth and therefore to the brain itself. Nonetheless, this compartmentalistic or systems approach, which stresses major functional systems that must exist based on overwhelming empirical evidence, has proven to be useful for explaining many normal and pathologic behavioral observations. This approach is essential to the development of meaningful and practical performance measurement strategies such as those described.

32.2 Basic Principles

Many of the past efforts in which performance-related measurements have played a significant role have been directed toward basic research. Furthermore, much of this research has been aimed at uncovering the general operational frameworks of normal human information processing and not the measurement of performance capacities and their use, either alone or in combination with other capacity metrics, to characterize humans of various types (e.g., normal, aged, handicapped, etc.). However, representative models and theories provide direction for, and are themselves shaped by, subsequent measurement efforts. While there are many principles and basic observations that have some relevance, the scope of material presented later is limited to topics that more specifically support the understanding of human information-processing *performance capacity* measurement.

32.2.1 Functional Model of Central Information Processing

A simplified, although quite robust, model that is useful within the context of human information processing is illustrated in Figure 32.1. With this figure, attention is called to systems, their functions, and major interconnectivities. At a functional level that is relatively high within the hierarchy of the human central nervous system, the central processing system can be considered to be composed of two types of subsystems: (1) *information processors* and (2) *memories*. As can be seen from the diagram, information from the environment is provided to the information-processing subsystems through human sensor subsystems. These not only include the obvious sensors (e.g., the eyes) that receive input from external sources but also those specifically designed to provide information regarding the internal environment, including proprioception and state of being. The capacity to process information input from multiple sources at a conscious level is finite. Overload is prevented by limiting the amount of information

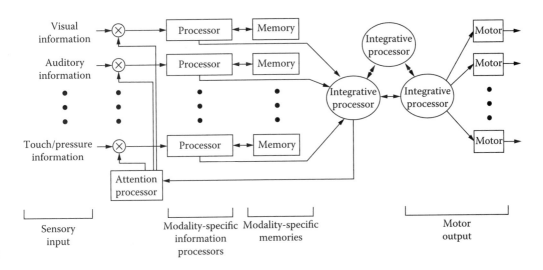

FIGURE 32.1 A functional systems-level block diagram of human information-processing description of the measurement of subsystem performance capacities.

simultaneously received; specific sensory information of high priority is controlled by what may be termed an *attention processor*. Information associated with a given sensor system is processed by a corresponding processor. The model further suggests that there are memory subsystems for each sensory modality in bidirectional communications with the associated processor. Thus, modality-specific information (e.g., visual, auditory, etc.) may be referenced and processed with new information. As information is received and processed at modality-specific levels it is combined at a higher level by integrative processors to generate situation-specific responses. These may be in the form of a musculoskeletal, cognitive, or attention-modifying events, as well as any combination of these.

General measurement issues of fidelity, validity, and reliability are natural concerns in measurement of information-processing performance capacities. Special issues emerge that increase the overall complexity of the problem when attempting to measure attributes that reflect *just* the information-processing subsystems. Unlike a computer where one may remove a memory module, place it in a special test unit, and determine its capacity, the accessibility of the subsystems within the human brain is such that it is impossible to perfectly isolate and directly measure any of the individual components. When measuring characteristics of human information-processing subsystems, it is necessary to address measurement goals that are similar to those applied to analogous artificial system within the constraint that human sensors and motoric subsystems must also be utilized (Table 32.1).

32.2.2 Performance Capacities

In considering the performance of human information-processing systems, the resource-based perspective represented by the Elemental Resource Model (Kondraske, 2000) is adopted here. This model for human performance encompasses all types of human subsystems and is the result of the application of a general theoretical framework for system performance to the human system and its subsystems. A central idea incorporated in this framework, universal to all types of systems, is that of *performance capacity*. This implies a finite availability of some quantity that thereby limits performance. A general two-part approach is used to identify unique performance capacities (e.g., visual information *processor speed*): (1) identify the system (e.g., visual information processor) and (2) identify the dimension of performance (e.g., speed). In this framework, system performance capacities are characterized by availability of performance resources along each of the identified dimensions. These *performance resources*

TABLE 32.1 The Combination of the Human Sensor Subsystem (Determined by Stimulus Source) and Responder Isolates Unique Subsystems

Capacity Types	Stimulus Type(s)	Responder[a]	Measurements
Attention	Visual Auditory	Upper extremity Vocal system	Length of time that a task can be performed to specification and accuracy (if appropriate for task) when subject is instructed to perform for "as long as possible"
Processor speed	Visual Visual Visual Auditory Auditory Auditory Vibrotactile	Upper extremity Lower extremity Vocal system Upper extremity Lower extremity Vocal system Upper extremity	Inverse of time required to react to stimulus (i.e., stimuli/s) when subject is instructed to respond "as quickly as possible"
Processor accuracy	Visual Visual Visual Auditory Auditory Auditory Vibrotactile	Upper extremity Lower extremity Vocal system Upper extremity Lower extremity Vocal system Upper extremity	Subject is asked to perform task (e.g., typically recognition of symbols from set with similar information content across symbols) "as accurately as possible" and without stress on speed of measures of accuracy. The correct percentage (out of a predetermined set size) is often used, although different accuracy measures have been proposed (Green and Swets, 1966; Wickelgren, 1977).
Processor speed–accuracy	Visual Visual Visual Auditory Auditory Auditory Vibrotactile	Upper extremity Lower extremity Vocal system Upper extremity Lower extremity Vocal system Upper extremity	Basically a combination of tests that stress speed and accuracy capacities individually, as well as both speed and accuracy measures are obtained as defined above to get off-axis data points in two-dimensional speed–accuracy space. Both speed and accuracy can be maximally stressed (e.g., by instructing subject to perform "as fast and accurately as possible") or accuracy can be measured at different speeds by varying time available for responses and stressing accuracy within this constraint
Memory storage capacity	Visual Visual Visual Auditory Auditory Auditory Vibrotactile	(Same options as above[b])	Maximum amount of information of type defined by stimulus that the subject is able to recall. Stimuli usually consist of sets of symbols of varying complexity in different sets (e.g., spatially distributed lights, alphanumeric characters, words, motions, etc.) but similar amount of information per symbol in a given set. Units of "bits" are ideal, but not often possible if number of bits per symbol is unknown. In such cases, units are often reported as "symbols," "chunks," or "items"

Note: A number of representative, but not exhaustive combinations are illustrated for each information-processing capacity type. Depending on objectives of the test task (as communicated to the subject under test) and metrics obtained, many different unique capacities are defined. In some applications (e.g., in evaluating a subject who has suffered a stroke in very localized region of the brain) the specificity is important. In others (e.g., in evaluating a neurologic disease with widespread generalized effects) the responder may be chosen for convenience.

[a] General terms are used in table to illustrate combination options. Very specific definition that controls the motoric functional units involved as precisely as possible should be used for any given capacity test. For example (1) upper extremity (shoulder flexor vs. elbow flexor vs. digit 2 flexor) and (2) vocal system (lingua-dental "ta" vs. labial "pa" response), etc.

[b] Unless motor memory capacities are being tested, the responder is typically chosen to minimize stress on motoric processing and, compared to processor performance measures, not to isolate a unique motor memory system.

are to be distinguished from less rigorously defined general processing resources described by others (e.g., Kahneman, 1973; Wickens, 1984). However, many of the important basic constructs associated with the idea of "a resource" are employed in a similar fashion in each of these contexts. For processors, key dimensions of performance are speed and accuracy. *Processor speed* and *processor accuracy* capacities are thus identified. For memory systems, key dimensions of performance are storage capacity, speed (e.g., retrieval) and accuracy (e.g., retrieval). Other important attributes of performance capacities are discussed in other sections of this chapter.

Many aspects of information-processing performance have been investigated resulting in discoveries that have provided insight to the capacities of subsystems as well as refinement to both system structure and function definitions (Lachman et al., 1979). One of the oldest studies in which the basic concept of information-processing performance capacity was recognized addressed "speed of mental processes" (Donders, 1868). The basic idea of capacity has been a central topic of interest in human information-processing research (Moray, 1967; Posner and Boies, 1971; Schneider and Shiffrin, 1977; Shiffrin and Schneider, 1977).

32.2.3 Stimulus–Response Scenario

The *stimulus–response scenario*, perhaps most often recognized in association with behavioral psychology, has emerged as a fundamental paradigm in psychology experiments (Neel, 1977). Aside from general utility in research, it is also an essential component of strategies for measurement of human information-processing performance capacities. A typical example is the well-known reaction time test in which the maximum speed (and sometimes accuracy) at which information can be processed is of interest. Here, a subject is presented a stimulus specific to some sensory modality (e.g., visual, auditory, and tactile) and is instructed to respond in a prescribed manner (e.g., lift a hand from a switch "as fast as possible" when the identified stimulus occurs). This general approach, which has become so popular and useful in psychology, can also be recognized as one that has been commonly employed in engineering to characterize artificial systems (e.g., amplifiers, motors, etc.). A specific known signal (stimulus) is applied to the system's input and the corresponding output (response) is observed. Specified, measurable attributes of the output, in combination with the known characteristics of the input, are used to infer various characteristics of the system under test. When the focus of interest is the performance limits of processing systems, these characteristics include processing speed, processing accuracy, memory storage capacity, etc.

In performance capacity tests, an important related component is the *prestimulus set*, or simply the way in which the system is "programmed to respond to the stimulus." This is usually accomplished by one or more components of the instructions given to the subject under test (e.g., respond "as quickly as possible," etc.) just prior to the execution of an actual test.

32.2.4 Measurement of Information (Stimulus Characterization)

Within a given sensory modality, it is easy to understand that different stimuli place different demands or "loads" on information-processing systems. Thus, in order to properly interpret results of performance tests, it is necessary to describe the stimulus. While this remains a topic of ongoing research with inherent controversies, some useful working constructs are available. At issue is not simply a qualitative description, but the *measurement* of stimulus content (or complexity). Shannon's information theory (1948), which teaches how to measure the amount of information associated with a generalized information source, has been the primary tool used in these efforts. Thus, a stimulus can be characterized in terms of the amount of information present in it. Simple stimuli (e.g., a light that is "on" or "off") possess less information than complex stimuli (e.g., a computer screen with menus, buttons, etc.). The best successes in attempts to quantitatively characterize stimuli have been achieved for simple discrete stimuli

(Hick, 1952; Hyman, 1953). From Shannon, the amount of information associated with a given symbol "i," selected from a source with "*n*" such symbols is given by:

$$I_i = \log_2(1/p_i) \qquad (32.1)$$

where p_i is the probability of occurrence of symbol "i" (within a finite symbol set) and the result has the units of "bits." Thus, high probability stimuli contain less information than low probability stimuli. It is a relatively straightforward matter to control the probabilities associated with symbols that serve as stimuli in test situations. The application of basic information theory to the characterization of stimuli that are more complex (i.e., multiple components, continuous stimuli) is challenging both theoretically and practically (e.g., large symbol sets, different sets with different probability distributions that must be controlled, etc.).

If stimuli are not or cannot be characterized robustly in terms of a measure with units of "bits," operationally defined units are frequently used (e.g., "items," "chunks," "stimuli," etc.). In addition, as many stimulus attributes as possible are identified and quantified and others are simply "described." This at least maximizes the opportunity for obtaining repeatable measurements. However, the additional implication is that the number of "bits per item" or "bits per chunk" is waiting to be delineated and perhaps a conversion could be substituted at a later time. While this state leaves much to be desired from a rigorous measurement perspective, it is nonetheless quite common in the evolution of measurement for many physical quantities and allows useful work to be conducted.

32.2.5 Speed–Accuracy Trade-Off

Fundamental to all human information-processing systems and tasks is the so-called *speed–accuracy trade-off*. This basic limitation can be observed in relatively high-level everyday tasks such as reading, writing, typing, listening to a lecture, etc. Psychologists (Wickelgren, 1977) have studied this trade-off in many different contexts. Fitts (1966) demonstrated a relationship between measures reflecting actual performance (reaction time and errors) to incentive-based task goals (i.e., were subjects attempting to achieve high speed or high accuracy). As shown in Figure 32.2, relationships that have been found suggest an upper limit to the combination of speed and accuracy available for information-processing tasks. In this figure, original reaction time measures have been transformed by simple inversion to obtain true

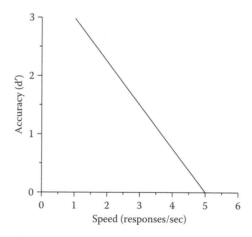

FIGURE 32.2 A typical information-processing performance envelope in two-dimensional speed–accuracy space. (Data from Wickelgren, W.A. 1977. *Acta Psychol.* 41, 67–85.)

speed measures, which also conform to the resource construct used in modeling performance capacities, as described in Section 32.2.2. The result then defines a two-dimensional (e.g., speed–accuracy) performance envelope for information-processing systems. The area within this envelope, given that each dimensions represents a resource-based performance capacity, represents a higher level or composite performance capacity metric (with units of speed × accuracy), analogous in some respects to a gain–bandwidth product or work (force × displacement) metric.

32.2.6 Divided Attention and Time Sharing

An approach sometimes used in a variety of measurement contexts incorporates a *dual-task or divided attention scenario* that is designed to require use of attention resources in two different simultaneously executed tasks (e.g., Wickens, 1984). For example, visual tracking (primary task) accuracy *and* speed of response to an embedded visual stimulus (secondary task) can be measured. Details of the potential time-sharing possibilities at play are quite complex (Schneider and Shiffrin, 1977; Shiffrin and Schneider, 1977).

In comparison to single-task performance test situations, in which the attention processor may not be working at capacity, the additional demand is designed to change (compared to a single-task baseline) and sometimes maximizes the stress on attention performance resources. Performance on both primary and secondary tasks, compared to levels attained when each task is independently performed, can provide an indirect measure of capacity associated with attention (Parasuraman and Davies, 1984). This approach has been useful in determining relative differences in demand imposed by two different primary tasks by comparison of results from respective tests in which a fixed secondary task is used with different primary tasks. Of more direct relevance to the present context, an appropriate secondary task can be used to control in part the conditions under which a given performance capacity (defined in a standard way and measured in association with the primary task) is measured, for example, visual information-processing speed can be measured with no additional attention load or with several different additional attention load levels. While it may be possible to rank order secondary tasks in terms of the additional load presented, there are no known methods to quantify attention load in absolute terms.

32.3 General Measurement Paradigms

Despite the complexity of human information-processing, a fairly small number of different measurement paradigms have emerged for quantification of the many unique human information-processing performance capacities. This is perhaps in part due to the limited number of system types (e.g., processors and memories). A good portion of the observed complexity can therefore be attributed to the number of different processors and memories, as well as the vastness and diversity of actual information that humans typically possess (i.e., facts, knowledge, skills, etc.). While most of the paradigms described below have been used for decades, it is helpful to recognize that they all conform to, or can be made to conform to, the more recently proposed (Kondraske, 1987, 1995) generalized strategy for measuring any aspect of performance for any human subsystem: (1) maximally isolate first the system of interest, (2) maximally isolate the dimensions of performance of interest, and (3) maximally stress (tempered by safety considerations when appropriate) the system along those dimensions.

32.3.1 Information-Processing Speed

The paradigm for measuring information-processing speed is commonly referred to as a reaction time test since the elapsed time (i.e., the processing time) between the onset of a given stimulus and the occurrence of a prescribed response is the basic measurable quantity. To obtain a processing speed measure, the stimulus content in "bits," "chunks," or simply "stimuli" is divided by the processing time to yield measures with units of bits, chunks, or stimuli. Choice of stimulus modality isolates a specific sensory processor, whereas choice of a responder (e.g., index finger, upper extremity motion caused primarily by shoulder flexors, etc.) isolates a motoric processor associated with generation of the response. Much research has addressed the allocation of portions of the total processing time to various subsystem components (Sternberg, 1966). The system of primary interest as presented here is the sensory processor. Processing times associated with the motoric processor involved in the response are substantially less in normal systems. However, it is recommended that a given processor speed capacity be identified not only by the sensor subsystem stressed, but also by the responder (e.g., visual shoulder flexor information processor speed). This identifies not only the test scenario employed but also the complete information path.

32.3.2 Information-Processing Accuracy and Speed–Accuracy Combinations

In contrast to processor speed capacity that describes limits on information rate, accuracy relates to the ability to resolve content. In general, paradigms for tests that include accuracy measures typically involve a finite set of symbols with a corresponding set of responses. Various stimulus presentation–response scenarios can be used. For example, a stimulus can be randomly selected from the set with the subject required to identify the stimulus presented. Alternately, a subset of stimuli can be presented and the subject asked to select the response corresponding to the symbol not in the subset (size of subsets should be small if it is desired to minimize stress on memory capacities). A key element is that, within a poststimulus–response window, the subject is forced to select one of the available responses. This allows accuracy of the response to be measured in any of a number of ways ranging from relatively simple to complex (Green and Swets, 1966; Wickelgren, 1977). The response window is either relatively open-ended, as short as possible and variable (based on the speed of the subject's response), or fixed at a given length of time. When only accuracy is stressed, subjects are instructed to perform as accurately as possible and the stress on speed is minimized (e.g., "take your time"). In a second type of speed–accuracy test, subjects are instructed to perform as fast and as accurately as possible, maximally stressing both dimensions while both accuracy and speed of responses are measured. In a variation of this general paradigm, a fixed-response window size is selected to challenge response speed. This provides a known point along the speed dimension of performance. In all three cases, measured response accuracy provides the second coordinate of a point in the two-dimensional speed–accuracy performance space. The combination of different paradigms can be used to determine the speed–accuracy performance envelope (see Section 32.2.5).

32.3.3 Memory Capacity

As used here, *memory capacity* refers to the amount of information that can be stored and recalled. It is well accepted that separate memory exists for different sensory modalities. Also, short-, medium-, and long-term memory systems have been identified (Crook et al., 1986). Thus, separate capacities can be identified for each. Higher level capacities can also be identified with processes that utilize memory, such as scanning (Sternberg, 1966). A comprehensive assessment of memory would require tasks that challenge the various memory systems to determine resources available, singly and along different combinations of their various modalities, most directly relevant to the individual's developmental stage (infant, youth, adolescent, young adult, middle aged adult, or older adult), and reflecting the diversity and depth of life experiences of that individual. No such comprehensive batteries are available. As noted by Syndulko et al. (1988), "Most typically, a variety of individual tests are utilized that evaluate selected aspects of memory systems under artificial conditions that relate best to college students." This general circumstance is in part due to the lack of generalized performance measurement strategies for memory. Despite such diversity, perhaps the most common variation of the many memory capacity tests involves providing a stimuli of the appropriate modality and requiring complete, accurate recall (i.e., a response) after some specified period of delay. The response window is selected to be relatively long so that processor speed is only minimally stressed. Typically, a test begins with a stimulus that has low information content (i.e., one that should be within capacity limits of the lowest one expects to encounter). If the response is correct, the information content of the stimuli is increased and another trial is administered. It is typically assumed that the amount of information added after each successful trial is fairly constant. Examples include: adding another light to a spatially distributed light pattern, adding another randomly selected digit (0–9) to a sequence of such digits, etc. By continuing this process of progressively increasing the amount of stimulus information until an inaccurate response is obtained, the isolated memory capacity is assumed to be maximally stressed. The result is simply the amount of information stored and recalled, in units of bits, chunks, or items.

32.3.4 Attention

Tests for basic attention capacity can be considered to be somewhat analogous to endurance capacity tests for neuromuscular systems. Simply put, the length of time over which a specified information-processing task can be executed provides a measure of attention capacity (or attention span). The test paradigm typically involves presentation at random time intervals of a randomly selected stimulus from a finite predefined symbol set for a relatively short, fixed time (e.g., 1 s). Within a predefined response window (with a maximum duration that is selected so that processing speed resources are minimally stressed), the subject must generate a response corresponding to the stimulus that occurred. Attention is maximally stressed by continuing this process until the subject either (1) makes no response within the allocated response window, or (2) produces an incorrect response (i.e., a response associated with a stimulus that was not presented). These criteria thus essentially define the point at which the specified task (i.e., recognize stimuli and respond correctly within a generous period of time allotted) can no longer be completed. Once again, choice of stimulus modality isolates a specific sensory processor (e.g., visual, auditory, tactile, etc.). Clearly, stimulus complexity is also important. Stress on higher-level cognitive resources can be minimized by choice of simple stimuli (e.g., lights, tones, etc.). Motoric processors associated with response generation are also involved. However, these are minimally stressed and as long as basic functionality is present the choice of responder should have little influence on results compared to, for example, the influence occurring during processor speed capacity measurements.

32.4 Measurement Instruments and Procedures

Given the above functional systems model for human information-processing (Figure 32.1) and review of measurement paradigms for information-processing subsystems, a general architecture for instruments capable of measuring information-processing performance capacities can be defined (Figure 32.3). It is interesting to observe that this architecture parallels the human information-processing system (i.e., compare Figures 32.1 and 32.3).

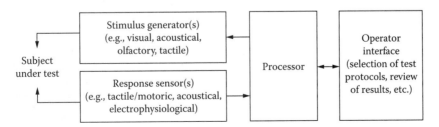

FIGURE 32.3 The general architecture for instruments used to measure human information-processing performance capacities.

Most such instruments are computer based, allowing for generation of stimuli with different contents, presentation of stimuli at precisely timed intervals, measurement of processing times (from which processing speeds are derived) with high accuracy (typically, to within 1 ms), and accurate recording of responses and determination of their correctness.

A typical desktop computer system fits the general architecture presented in Figure 32.3 and, as such, it has been widely exploited "as is" physically with appropriate software to conduct information-processing tests. This is adequate for tests for higher level, complex cognitive processing tasks due to the longer processing times involved. That is, screen refresh times and keyboard response times are smaller fractions of total times measured and contribute less error. However, for measurement of more basic performance capacities and to allow testing of subjects who do not possess normal physical performance capacities, custom test setups are essential. The general design goal for these stimuli generators and response sensors is to minimize the stress on human sensory, motor, and aspects of central processing resources that are not the target of the test. For example, the size of standard keyboard switches imposes demands on positioning accuracy when, for example, visual information-processing accuracy is being tested. According to Fitts' Law (Fitts, 1954), the task component involved with hitting the desired response key (i.e., the component that occurs after the visual information-processing component) requires longer processing times (associated with the motoric response task) for smaller targets. Thus, to minimize such influences, a relatively large target is suggested. Along the same lines of reasoning, these additional design guidelines are important (1) key stimulus attributes that are not related to information content should be well above normal minimum human sensing thresholds (e.g., relatively bright lights that do not stress visual sensitivity and large characters or symbols that do not stress visual acuity), (2) response speeds of stimulus generators and response sensors should be much faster than the fastest human response speed that is anticipated to be measured.

Even the many custom devices reported in the literature (as well as commercially available versions of some) have been devised to support research into fundamental aspects of information-processing and are used in studies that typically involve only healthy young college students. While such devices measure the stated or implied capacities well in this population, the often unstated assumption regarding other involved performance capacities (i.e., that they are available in "normal" amounts) is severely challenged when the subject under test is a member of a population with impairments (e.g., head injured, multiple sclerosis, Parkinson disease, etc.).

A representative instrument (Kondraske et al., 1984; Kondraske, 1990) is illustrated in Figure 32.4. This device incorporates 8 LEDs and 15 high-speed touch sensors ("home," A1–A8 and B1–B6) and a dedicated internal microprocessor to measure an array of different performance capacities associated with information-processing. Measures at the most basic hierarchical level (visual information-processing speed, visual–spatial memory capacity, visual attention span, etc.) and intermediate level (coordination tasks involving different sets of more basic functional units) are included.

For example, visual-upper extremity information-processing speed is measured in a paradigm whereby the test subject first places his/her hand on the "home" plate. A random time after an audible warning cue, one out of eight LEDs (e.g., LED 4) stimulates the subject to respond "as quickly as possible" by lifting his/her hand off the home plate and touching the sensor (e.g., A4) associated with the lighted LED. Each LED represents a binary (ON or OFF) information source. Since an equiprobable selection scheme is employed, the $\log_2$ (# choices) represents the number of bits of information to be processed when determining which LED is lighted. In this example, the number of choices is eight; prior to the test the subject was informed that any one of eight LEDs would be selected. Modes reflecting different information loads (1, 2, 4, or 8 choices) are available. Processing speed (in stimuli per sec) is obtained as a result from each trial by inverting the total processing time, measured as the time from presentation of the stimulus until the subject's hand is lifted off the home plate. By combining time measures from two or more tests with different information loads, a more direct measure of true processing speed in bits per second is obtained. For example, results from an 8-choice (3 bit load) test and a 1-choice test (0 bit load) are combined as follows: (3 bits − 0 bits)/$(t_3 − t_0)$, where t_n is the reaction time measured for an

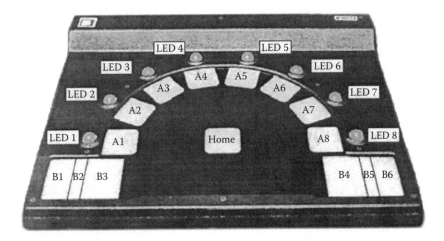

FIGURE 32.4 Major components of a specific microprocessor-based instrument (Human Performance Measurement, Inc. Model BEP I) for measurement of a selected subset of information-processing capacities incorporating high-intensity LEDs for visual stimuli and large contact area, fast touch sensors to acquire responses (made by the upper extremity) from the subject under test (semicircle radius is 15 cm).

"*n*" bit information load. This method removes transmission and other time delays not associated with the primary visual information-processing task. Multiple trials are performed (typically, 3 × number of choices, but no less than five trials for any mode) to improve test–retest reliability in the final measures, which are computed by averaging over a fraction (best 80%) of the trials. While even more trials might further improve repeatability of final capacity measures in some subjects, the overall test duration must be considered in light of the desire (from a test design perspective) to minimize stress on attention resources that could vary widely over potential test subjects. Careful trade-offs are necessary.

Visual–spatial memory capacity is measured using the same device. A random sequence of LEDs, beginning with a sequence length of "one," is presented to the subject. The subject responds by contacting (with their preferred hand) the subset of touch sensors (from A1 to A8) corresponding to the LEDs incorporated in a given stimulus presentation, in the same order as the LEDs sequence was presented. A correct response causes a new trial to be initiated automatically with the sequence length increased by one. The maximum length of this sequence (in items) that the subject can repeat without error is used as the measure of visual–spatial memory capacity. The better of two trials is used as a final score. The bright LEDs, relatively large contact area of the touch sensors (5 × 5 cm²), and a relatively long poststimulus–response window (up to 10 s) ensure that other performance resources are minimally stressed.

A measure of visual attention span is obtained with a task in which random LEDs are lighted for 1 s at random intervals ranging from 4 to 15 s. After each LED is lighted, a response window is entered (3 s maximum) during which the subject is required to indicate that a lighted LED was observed by contacting the corresponding touch sensor. The task continues until either the wrong touch sensor is contacted or no response is received within the defined response window. The time (in seconds) from the beginning of the test until an "end of test" criterion is met is used as the measure of visual attention performance capacity. The simple stimuli ensure that higher level cognitive resources are minimally stressed. This allows a wide range of populations to be tested, including young children. Some normal subjects can achieve very long attention spans (e.g., hours) with this specific scenario, while some head-injured subjects (for example) produce times less than 60 s.

One example of a more comprehensive, computer-based memory performance test battery is that developed by Crook and colleagues (1986). This battery is directed at older adults, evaluates memory in the visual and auditory modalities at each of the three temporal process levels, and utilizes challenges that relate well to the daily activities of the target group. The challenges (i.e., stimulus sets) are computer generated and controlled, administered by means of a color graphics terminal, and, in some cases, played from a videodisc player to provide as realistic of a stimulus representation as possible outside of using actors in the everyday environment of the subject. The battery takes 60–90 min to administer, and provides a profile of scores across the various measurement domains. Extensive age and gender norms are available to scale the scores in terms of percentiles. Despite its scope, it does not provide, nor was it intended to provide, information about modalities other than visual and auditory (e.g., tactile, kinesthetic, or olfactory). It also does not address long-term memory storage beyond about 45 min. (Consider the test administration complexities in doing so.) Nonetheless, it represents one of the most sophisticated memory performance measurement and assessment systems currently available.

32.5 Present Limitations

General methods and associated tools do not exist to quantify the information content of any arbitrary stimulus within a given modality (e.g., visual, auditory, etc.). Success has only been achieved for relatively simple stimuli (e.g., lights which are on or off, at fixed positions spatially, etc.). It can be said, however, that serious attempts to quantify complex stimuli even in one modality appear to be lacking. To the practitioner, this prevents standardization that could occur across many information-processing performance capacity metrics. For example, information-processing speed capacities cannot yet universally be expressed in terms of bits. Perhaps more significantly, this limitation not only impacts looking toward the human and the measurement of intrinsic performance capacities, but also the analysis of information-processing tasks in quantitative terms. This, in turn, has limited the way in which information-processing performance capacity measures can be utilized. Whereas one can measure grip strength available in a subject (a neuromuscular capacity) and also the worst-case grip force required to support turning a door knob, it is not yet possible to determine how much visual information one must process to reach out and find the door knob.

As was also noted, one cannot ideally isolate the systems under test. The required involvement of human sensory and motoric systems also requires the use of ancillary performance tests that establish at least some minimal levels of performance availabilities in these systems (e.g., visual acuity, etc.) in order to lend validity to measures of information-processing performance capacities. New imaging techniques and advanced electroencephalographic and magnetoencephalographic techniques such as brain mapping may offer the basis for new approaches that circumvent in part this limitation. While the cost and practicality of using these techniques routinely is likely to be prohibitive for the foreseeable future, the use of such techniques in research settings to optimize and establish validity of simpler methods can be anticipated.

Moray (1967) was one of many to use the analogy to data and program storage in a digital computer to facilitate understanding of a "limited capacity concept" with regard to human information-processing. In the material presented, emphasis has been placed on the components analogous to those within the realm of computer hardware (i.e., processors and memories). These have been dealt with at their most basic operational levels for testing purposes, attempting to intentionally limit stresses on the test subject's acquired skill (i.e., stored information itself). It has been implied and is argued that knowledge of these hardware system capacities is in itself quite useful (e.g., it is helpful to know whether your desktop computer's basic information-processing rate is 800 MHz or 2 GHz). However, many tasks that humans perform daily, which involve information-processing require not only processing and storage capacities, but also the use of *unique information* acquired in the past (i.e., training or "programs"). These software components, which like processor and memory performance capacities also represent a necessary but not sufficient resource for completion of the specific task at hand, present even greater challenges to evaluation. If the analogy to computer programs is used (or even musical scores, plans, scripts, etc.), it can be observed that even the smallest "programming error" can lead to a failure of the total system in accomplishing its intended purpose with the intended degree of performance. Checking the integrity of human "programs" can be envisioned to be relatively easy if the desired functionality is in fact found to be present. However, if functionality is not present and diagnostic data points to a "software problem," a more difficult challenge is at hand. Methods which can be employed to reveal the source of the error in the basic information itself (i.e., the contents of memory) can be expected to be just as tedious as checking the integrity of code written for digital computers.

Defining Terms

Attention: A performance capacity representing the length of time that an information-processing system can carry out a prescribed task when maximally stressed to do so. This is analogous to endurance in neuromuscular subsystems.

Dual-task scenario: A test paradigm characteristic by a primary and secondary task and measurement of subject performance in both.

Memory: One of two major subsystem types of the human information-processing system that performs the function of storage of information for possible later retrieval and use.

Performance capacity: A quantity in finite availability that is possessed by a system or subsystem, drawn on during the execution of tasks, and limits some aspect (e.g., speed, accuracy, etc.), a system's ability to execute tasks; or, the limit of that aspect itself.

Prestimulus set: The manner in which an human system is programmed to respond to an ensuing stimulus.

Processor: One of two major subsystems types within the human information-processing system that performs the general function of processing information. Multiple processors at different hierarchical levels can be identified (e.g., those specific to sensory modalities, integrative processors, etc.).

Processor accuracy: The aspect, quality, or dimension of performance of a processor that characterizes the ability to correctly process information.

Processor speed: The aspect, quality, or dimension of performance of an information processor that characterizes the rate at which information is processed.

Speed–accuracy trade-off: A fundamental limit of human information-processing systems at any level of abstraction that is most likely due to a more basic limit in channel capacity; that is, channel capacity can be used to achieve more accuracy at the expense of speed or to achieve more speed at the expense of accuracy.

References

Crook, T., Salama, M., and Gobert, J. 1986. A computerized test battery for detecting and assessing memory disorders. In *Senile Dementia: Early Detection*. Eds. Bes, A. et al., pp. 79–85. John Libbey Eurotext.

Donders, F.C. 1868–1869. Over de snelheid van psychische processen. Onderzoekingen gedaan in het Psyiologish Laboratorium der Utrechtsche Hoogeschooll. In *Attention and Performance II*. Ed. W.G. Koster. translated by W.G. Koster. *Acta Psychol.* 30: 412–31.

Fitts, P.M. 1954. The information capacity of the human motor system in controlling the amplitude of movement. *J. Exp. Psychol.* 47: 381–391.

Fitts, P.M. 1966. Cognitive aspects of information processing: III. Set for speed versus accuracy. *J. Exp. Psychol.* 71: 849–857.

Gazzaniga, M.S. *The Social Brain*. Basic Books, Inc., New York.

Green, D.M. and Swets, J.R. 1966. *Signal Detection Theory and Psychophysics*. John Wiley and Sons, Inc., New York.

Hick, W. 1952. On the rate of gain of information. *Q. J. Exp. Psychol.* 4: 11–26.

Hunt, E. 1986. Experimental perspectives: Theoretical memory models. In *Handbook for Clinical Memory Assessment of Older Adults*. Ed. Poon, L.W., pp. 43–54. American Psychological Assoc., Washington, D.C.

Hyman, R. 1953. Stimulus information as a determinant of reaction time. *J. Exp. Psychol.* 45: 423–432.

Kahneman, D. 1973. *Attention and Effort*. Prentice-Hall, Englewood Cliffs, NJ.

Kondraske, G.V. 1987. Human performance: Science or art. In *Proceedings of 13th Northeast Bioengineering Conference*. Ed. Foster, K.R., pp. 44–47. Institute of Electrical and Electronics Engineers, New York.

Kondraske, G.V. 1990. A PC-based performance measurement laboratory system. *J. Clin. Eng.* 15: 467–478.

Kondraske, G.V. 1995. A working model for human system–task interfaces. In *Handbook of Biomedical Engineering*. Ed. Bronzino, J.D., CRC Press, Inc., Boca Raton, FL.

Kondraske, G.V., Potvin, A.R., Tourtellotte, W.W., and Syndulko, K. 1984. A computer-based system for automated quantification of neurologic function. *IEEE Trans. Biomed. Eng.* 31: 401–414.

Lachman, R., Lachman, J.L., and Butterfield, E.C. 1979. *Cognitive Psychology and Information Processing: An Introduction*. Lawrence Erlbaum Assoc., Hillsdale, NJ.

Minsky, M. 1986. *The Society of Mind*. Simon & Schuster, New York.

Moray N. 1967. Where is capacity limited? A survey and a model. *Acta Psychol.* 27: 84–92.

Neel, A. 1977. *Theories of Psychology: A Handbook*. Schenkman Publishing Co., Cambridge, MA.

Ornstein, R. 1986. *Multimind*. Hougton Mifflin Co., Boston.

Parasuraman, R. and Davies, D.R., Eds. 1984. *Varieties of Attention*. Academic Press, Inc., Orlando, FL.

Posner, M.I. and Boies, S.J. 1971. Components of attention. *Psychol. Rev.* 78: 391–408.

Sanders, M.S. and McCormick, E.J. 1987. *Human Factors in Engineering and Design*. McGraw-Hill, New York.

Schneider, W. and Shiffrin, R.M. 1977. Controlled and automatic human information processing: I. Detection, search, and attention. *Psychol. Rev.* 84: 1–66.

Shannon, C.E. 1948. A mathematical theory of communication. *Bell Syst. Tech. J.* 27: 379–423.

Shiffrin, R.M. and Schneider, W. 1977. Controlled and automatic human information processing: II. Perceptual learning, automatic attending, and a general theory. *Psychol. Rev.* 84: 127–190.

Squire, L.R. and Butters, N. 1992. *Neuropsychology of Memory*. The Guilford Press, New York.

Sternberg, S. 1966. High-speed scanning in human memory. *Science* 153: 652–654.

Syndulko, K., Tourtellotte, W.W., and Richter, E. 1988. Toward the objective measurement of central processing resources. *IEEE Eng. Med. Biol. Soc. Mag.* 7: 17–20.

Wickens, C.D. 1984. *Engineering Psychology and Human Performance*. Charles E. Merrill Publishing, Columbus, OH.

Wickelgren, W.A. 1977. Speed–accuracy tradeoff and information processing dynamics. *Acta Psychol. (North-Holland)* 41: 67–85.

Wiener, N. 1955. *Cybernetics; or, Control and Communications in the Animal and the Machine*. Wiley, New York.

Further Information

A particularly informative, yet concise historical review of the major perspectives in psychology leading up to much of the more recent work involving quantitative measurements of information processing and determination of information-processing capacities is provided in Neel, A. 1977. *Theories of Psychology: A Handbook*, Schenkman Publishing Co., Cambridge, MA.

Human information processing has long been and continues to be a major topic of interest of the U.S. military. Considerable in-depth information and experimental results are available in the form of technical reports, many of which are unclassified. *CSERIAC Gateway*, published by the Crew System Ergonomics Information Analysis Center (CSERIAC), is distributed free of charge and provides timely information on scientific, technical, and engineering knowledge. For subscription information contact AL/CFH/CSERIAC, Bldg. 248, 2255 H St., Wright-Patterson Air Force Base, Ohio,

45433. Also, the North Atlantic Treaty Organization AGAARD (Advisory Group for Aerospace Research & Development) Aerospace Medical Panel Working Group 12, has worked on standards for a human performance test battery for military environments (much of which addresses information processing) and has defined data exchange formats. Documents can be obtained through the National Technical Information Service (NTIS), 5285 Port Royal Road, Springfield, VA 22161, USA.

Information regarding the design, construction, and evaluation of instrumentation (including quantitative attributes of stimuli, etc.) are often embedded in journal articles with titles that emphasis the major question of the study (i.e., not the instrumentation). Most appear in the many journals associated with the fields of psychology, neurology, and neuroscience.

33

High-Level Task Analysis: Using Cognitive Task Analysis in Human–Machine System Design

Ken Maxwell
IBM
MaxwellX

33.1 Introduction

Task analysis emerged prominently during World War II as a set of new methods applicable to analyzing the functions performed by human–machine systems and has persisted as an integral part of the engineering process (Hoffman and Militello 2009). Task analysis is a generic term that refers to methods for identifying, describing, and modeling task data to inform and guide system design and validation.

The continuing integration of information technology (IT) into communications, manufacturing, transportation, power, and medical systems has increasingly shifted human activity from manual to cognitive. Although cognitive components were never completely absent from task analyses, this shift bore the need for greater scrutiny of cognitive tasks and a deeper understanding of the nature of human activity in complex sociotechnical contexts. Cognitive task analysis (CTA) refers to the methods used to identify, describe, and model the cognitive, rather than manual, components of task requirements and performance.

This chapter presents a process and associated methods for analyzing cognitive tasks. It describes the use of CTA together with human cognitive processing and performance models in product design, and presents performance-based frameworks for guiding the design of human–machine systems. This chapter is not intended as a review. Selected techniques are presented to familiarize the reader with different major approaches that are currently applied to solving real-world engineering problems.

33.2 Fundamentals and New Directions

33.2.1 Tasks and Task Hierarchies

Tasks are goal-directed patterns of action performed to achieve human purposes. Tasks are delineated at different levels with respect to their defined goals and their contribution to satisfying a purpose. Low-level tasks combine to accomplish higher-level tasks. Figure 33.1 delineates two tasks at distinct levels: an application task and an interaction task.

In Figure 33.1, both the human and product functionally contribute to and work together in performing the application task. The functions and lower-level tasks needed to perform the application task are distributed between them. This distribution, known as allocation, is based on the capabilities and limitations each possesses. The allocation of function is a major factor in determining the interactions between the human and product that need to be performed.

Application tasks represent functions of the system or subsystem such as effectively monitoring the human's blood pressure (as in the e.g.), retrieving and reviewing a patient's medical history, delivering medications to various hospital departments using a robot, or planning a surgical procedure using simulation systems. Performing these functions contributes to satisfying the broader human purpose. Interaction tasks include the set of interactions between the human and product to collaboratively accomplish the application task.

Both application tasks and interaction tasks may be described at multiple levels. For example, the application task of reviewing a medical record may involve the lower-level application task of retrieving the record from an electronic database. The retrieval task, in turn, may entail a still lower-level

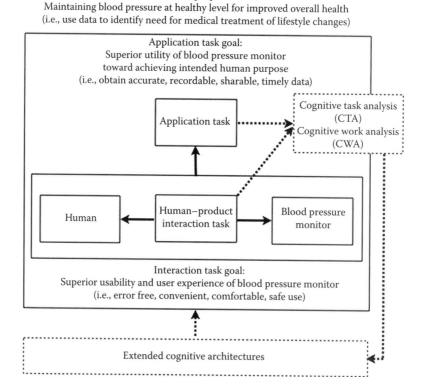

FIGURE 33.1   Task levels and task-to-design process flow.

search task. Each task level imposes cognitive demands on the task performers with regard to each performer's individual functional responsibilities and the need to interact with other performers or system components.

As an example, consider the application task of performing a surgical procedure. Performing the surgery depends on having task performers with applicable expertise about the patient, and using the available surgical instruments, facilities, and procedures. Differences in the capability and nature of the available personnel, tools, and other resources can dramatically change the distribution of functions between the human and machine components and the required interactions among them.

In one case, a surgeon may be interacting with a sophisticated robot that is actually performing the surgery. In a second case, the surgeon might also be in real-time consultation with a remote team of experts who can monitor the procedure and provide advice. In a third case, the surgeon might be using older less-capable equipment without much assistance from other health personnel. The surgeon's functional responsibilities in performing a successful surgery (the application task) vary greatly among these cases. In the first case, the surgeon may be primarily in a supervisory role, in the second case, decision making is shared and collaborative, and in the third case, the surgeon may need to perform many more manual tasks than in either of the previous cases. The required interactions the surgeon has with other personnel and components of the system also vary greatly among these different cases.

Performing tasks imposes sensory–perceptual, motor, cognitive, emotional, and social demands on the agents, that is, persons or machines, performing them. These demands result from the combination of (1) task complexity, (2) performance requirements, and (3) environmental factors. In cognitive tasks, cognitive demands predominate and variedly involve decision making, problem solving, interpretive reasoning, maintaining situation awareness (SA), prediction, and applying domain knowledge. When performed by teams, cognitive tasks also require collaborating and communicating among team members (Cooke and Gorman 2009).

Typically, lower-level tasks are procedural with low variability. However, higher-level tasks generally involve many information sources, complex processes and tools, and multiple agents with distributed and overlapping responsibilities. At higher levels, tasks increasingly require dynamic, nonlinear, flexible, or adaptive performance strategies and processes.

33.2.2 Scope of Analysis

For illustration purposes, Figure 33.1 includes one human interacting with one product. However, more complex systems may include many humans interacting among themselves and with many products of various types and capabilities. Table 33.1 presents a view of the complicated and varied relationships among major healthcare systems and entities and high-level healthcare activities. The variance described in the relationships depends on the design of the healthcare system taken as a whole. The table illustrates how practitioner, organizational, technological, and business resources can be differentially applied to the demands of healthcare consumers. The analysis methods, frameworks, and models presented in this chapter are means of determining those consumer needs and the ways in which available resources can be applied to satisfy them.

As more holistic perspectives on system design have become popular, the practice of task analysis has expanded toward analysis of higher-level integrated structures involving organizations of multiple performers working with one or more complex tools. This expansion has manifested in various forms.

In design, approaches to framing the design problem have extended beyond a singular human-centered focus to broader perspectives such as activities. Activity theory views *activities* as fundamental constructs that involve social and organizational factors, tools, agency, and context of use (Kaptelinin and Nardi 2006). Activities refer to complex composites of tasks that entail performing many simpler but interrelated actions in meaningful ways. From an activity theory perspective, there is benefit to modeling even the seemingly isolated use of a simple product by a single user within a larger context of interrelationships with other people, tools, and broader human purposes.

TABLE 33.1 Differential Applicability of Major Healthcare System Components to High-Level Healthcare Activities

Major Healthcare System Components	Monitor and Identify Need	Diagnose Condition	Determine Treatment/Care	Care Delivery	Follow-Up and On-Going Care
Access (e.g., insurance, Medicare)	Not used to facilitative	Not used to facilitative	Facilitative to major	Major	Not used to major
Support/information resources (e.g., social media, family/friends, and support groups)	Not used to major	Not used to major	Not used to major	Not used to facilitative	Not used to major
Care facilities (e.g., surgeries, assisted living)	Not used to major	Not used to major	Not used to major	Major	Not used to major
Treatment instruments (e.g., surgical tools and robots)	Not used to facilitative	Not used to facilitative	Not used to facilitative	Major	Not used to major
Communication and collaboration systems (e.g., telepresence)	Not used to major	Not used to major	Not used to major	Not used to major	Not used to major
Medical care providers (e.g., physicians, nurses)	Not used to major	Major	Major	Major	Not used to major
Medical knowledge systems (e.g., medical decision aids)	Not used to facilitative	Not used to major	Not used to major	Not used to facilitative	Not used to facilitative
Medical information systems (e.g., medical record databases)	Not used to facilitative	Major	Facilitative to major	Facilitative to major	Facilitative to major
Data-collection instruments (e.g., blood pressure monitor)	Major	Major	Not used to facilitative	Not used to major	Major

Illustrative of this emphasis on activity are approaches to designing human–machine systems such that they directly support high-level activities necessary to satisfying the system's purpose. For example, SA is a high-level dynamic, continuous, and critical activity necessary for the successful performance of human–machine systems across many application domains. Endsley developed a three-level model of the SA activity (perception, comprehension, and projection) and, with colleagues, developed the situation awareness-oriented design process (SAOD) consisting of three phases (SA requirements analysis, application of SA design principles, and SA measurement). The use of SAOD complements existing design considerations but considers additional factors that account for the dynamic and nonlinear aspects of performance in real-world contexts (Endsley 1995, Endsley and Hoffman 2002).

In analysis of cognitive task components, holistic perspectives have moved beyond using CTA alone to more general analyses of cognitive work. Cognitive work analysis (CWA) includes methods to describe and represent the functional work domain applicable to human–machine systems without specifying particular technologies to accomplish the work (Miller 2004, Lintern 2009, Vicente 1999).

In performance modeling, cognitive architectures have been extended models of cognitive mechanisms with a mix of control theory, queuing theory, machine learning and artificial intelligence, among others (Gray 2008). For example, the queuing network-model human processor (QN-MHP) extends the serial cognitive processing mechanisms in the MHP with queuing networks that enable concurrent modeling of system tasks (Liu et al. 2006). The adaptive control of thought-rational (ACT-R) model is a prominent cognitive architecture developed by Anderson (2007). The scent-based navigation and information foraging in the ACT cognitive architecture (SNIF-ACT) model extends ACT with a

Bayesian-satisfying model that incorporates perceived relevance in modeling navigation on the World-Wide Web (Fu and Pirolli 2007).

With consideration of these broader factors, the level of performance obtained on cognitive activities and tasks depends on

- The knowledge, expertise, experience, and cognitive skills of the agent or agents performing them (humans or intelligent machine agents).
- The social and organizational relationships among the agents.
- The environmental contexts in which the tasks are performed.
- The utility and usability of the tools used in performing the activities and tasks.

Since the successful use of biomedical products and systems is often critical, it is imperative that designers understand and accommodate the cognitive demands on and abilities of users not only with regard to use of specific tools but the broader activity and work context in which complex human–machine systems operate. This understanding and accommodation is achieved, in part, through the methods described below.

33.2.3 A General Analysis-to-Design Process Flow

In addition to depicting task relationships, Figure 33.1 depicts an analysis-to-design process in which the tasks and work domain are analyzed using CTA and CWA methods.

These data by themselves are of limited use in design because the task data address only requirements for resources. To be useful in design, task data must be analyzed along with the goals and performance capabilities of the task and work-performing agents (i.e., humans and machines). Therefore, with these data, human–machine-task models are created and evaluated using extended cognitive architectures. The models inform system design decisions, and as depicted in Figure 33.1, designs consistent with the model flow are developed. To the degree that the human–machine-task system model is coordinated by consistent, or at least relatable, constructs across all elements, its effectiveness in guiding good design concepts will increase. Further, the quality and precision of applied decisions are enhanced to the degree that these constructs are quantitative. The cognitive architectures described herein provide general frameworks for creating models of task performance that make quantitative predictions with various cognitive mechanisms.

Design is iterative. However, prototyping and evaluation processes that are essential to design refinement through iteration are not depicted in Figure 33.1. Also absent are user-profiling activities that should be performed early in the design process and that inform the human performance models included in the cognitive architectures.

33.3 CTA: Process and Methods

Figure 33.2 depicts the task-analysis process in four major steps. Before any data are collected, required data should be defined on the basis of the characteristics of the design decisions they need to support. Selection and use of data-collection methods, task models, and task metrics are later informed by these data requirements.

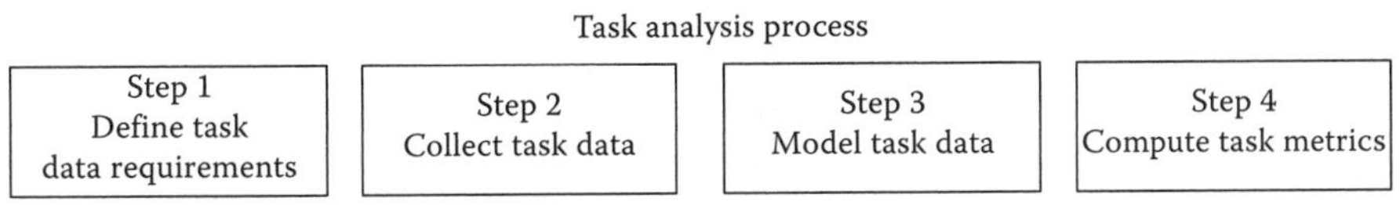

Task analysis process

Step 1 Define task data requirements	Step 2 Collect task data	Step 3 Model task data	Step 4 Compute task metrics

FIGURE 33.2 General analytic process for analyzing and modeling task data for design purposes.

33.3.1 Step 1: Define Task Data Requirements

In step 1, the task data required for the analysis are defined. The major factors involved in determining data needs are (1) the scope of design problems being addressed (i.e., the functional scope of the human–machine-task system being analyzed), (2) the point in the engineering process at which the analysis is conducted, and (3) the extent to which the product is new or being revised. Task analysis can be applied to existing systems or to proposed systems for which tasks themselves need to be defined.

33.3.1.1 Engineering Phase Considerations

Task data are applicable in all phases and iterations of product development. Different types of task data can be collected as the fidelity of system prototypes progresses and operational systems become available. These differences are apparent by examining three points in the system engineering process at which task analysis is of particular utility.

Predesign: Task data, together with data about human and technology availability and performance, are used to (1) define and allocate tasks, (2) develop procedures to accomplish the tasks, and (3) identify the needed human–machine interfaces. Note that the description of a task depends on the technology assumed. For example, a writing task would be accomplished differently with paper and pencil, a manual typewriter, or a computer with word-processing software.

Design: During the design phase, task scenarios, prototypes, and simulations are used to detail and refine the task procedures, task requirements, allocation decisions, and human–machine interface design.

Postdevelopment: Analyzing well-defined tasks performed by an operational system provides a detailed description of task procedures and resource requirements that can be used to improve task performance and the system design. For example, Rogers et al. (2001) were able to reveal many sources of errors and design recommendations from their task analysis of a consumer blood glucose meter. Suri (2000) used task and user analyses of an existing defibrillator to identify errors and safety concerns, and as a basis for a new design.

33.3.1.2 Engineering Design Decision Considerations

The design decisions that the task analysis will support have the greatest impact on what type of data are needed. Applications of task analysis vary greatly and include decisions that may or may not involve machines. Applications include, but are not limited to those described below.

Human–machine-task allocation: Allocation of tasks is a major systems-engineering decision. Task analysis is used to identify task load and performance requirements and contributes to assessing workload. Workload assessment provides a basis for assigning task responsibilities to humans and machines such that performance requirements can be satisfied and workload levels are not excessively low or high. These assessments augment qualitative allocation strategies (e.g., Fitts' lists) in which tasks are assigned on judgments of the relative performance capacities of humans and machines on generic tasks. Allocating tasks requires that the resource demands associated with each lower-level task are assessed and that the human and machine resources available can be matched against these at comparable levels of analysis.

In modern human–machine systems, task assignments may be adaptive or blended rather than strictly allocated. The information-processing capabilities of modern machines often include some form of task knowledge and reasoning capabilities that provide for an adaptive task allocation that shifts the task demands on the basis of contextual variables. Also, in many cases, human performance is augmented by (blended with) machine performance to accomplish a given task.

Task–technology trade-offs: Task analyses may be performed for systems that have yet to be developed but for which functional and performance requirements have been defined. In these cases, the analysis will be based on the defined requirements combined with data on human performance capacities and available machine technology. These analyses can be used to assess the workload, technology, and performance trade-offs expected with different human–machine system configurations.

Human–machine interface design: CTA provides not only a basis for allocating task responsibilities to humans and machines but also can be used to define display and control requirements for the interface between humans and machines.

Job design: The roles humans satisfy in complex systems and organizations (e.g., manager, operator, and maintainer) are generally designed to include many mental tasks. By identifying and describing the mental skills and resources required for task performance, task analysis provides a basis for optimizing job performance in new and existing systems.

Personnel selection and job fitness: CTA yields a specification of information-processing resources (e.g., speed, accuracy) required for task performance. This specification can be used in combination with measurements of the available resources an individual possesses. Assessing performance resource sufficiency provides a basis for selecting personnel and determining if injured, rehabilitated personnel are sufficiently recovered to safely return to work.

Training systems development: Task analysis identifies and characterizes the skills, knowledge, and mental capabilities that are necessary or sufficient for task performance. More specifically, it can be used to characterize differences in these abilities and in task performance between experts and novices. These differences serve as a basis for designing effective personnel training systems.

These applications of task analysis reduce to answering the following types of questions:

- What is the best way to structure the task procedures?
- Does a specific individual have the needed cognitive resources to perform the task?
- What knowledge or skills does an individual need to acquire to perform the task with a given technology?
- Can the task be modified to accommodate the special needs of individuals?

When biomedical products or other machines are involved:

- What human and machine combinations are most capable of performing the task?
- How should human and machine components interact in performing the task?

To answer these applied questions, the following data must be defined and described:

- The cognitive demands of the application task (e.g., knowledge, required information-processing activities, speed, and accuracy in performance actions).
- The cognitive capacities of humans in the system (e.g., knowledge, learning ability, processing speed, and processing accuracy).

If machines are involved:

- The information-processing capacities of machine components (e.g., knowledge, artificial intelligence, processing speed, algorithms, and data).
- The cognitive demands of the human–machine interaction task.
- The human–machine interaction capacities of the humans in the system.
- The human–machine interaction capacities of applicable machines.

33.3.2 Step 2: Collect Task Data

Once the required task data are determined, they need to be collected. Table 33.2 lists seven generic techniques for acquiring cognitive task data. The techniques are not mutually exclusive. For example, all techniques use some form of observation. Instrumented human–machine interface techniques and protocol analysis are used as knowledge-acquisition techniques. Each data-collection technique is described in more detail below.

Knowledge-acquisition and elicitation techniques: Knowledge acquisition refers to the activity of eliciting and obtaining the knowledge and reasoning processes needed to perform tasks from task performers.

TABLE 33.2 Task Data-Collection Techniques

Technique	Data Collected	Requirements	Engineering Phase
Knowledge acquisition	Knowledge requirements Strategies	Task performers Interaction instruments Prototypes and simulations	All
Interview	Procedures and strategies Information requirements and flow Knowledge requirements Workload Collaboration requirements	Task performers	All
Documentation review	Procedures and strategies Information requirements and flow Knowledge requirement Collaboration requirements	Design documents	All
Protocol analysis	Procedures and strategies Information requirements and flow Knowledge requirements Workload Collaboration requirements	Task performers Task scenarios	Design Postdevelopment
Instrumented human–machine interface	Procedures and strategies Performance Frequency Information requirements and flow	Task performers Applicable hardware and software	Design Postdevelopment
Observation	Procedures Information requirements and flow Workload Collaboration requirements	Task performers Prototypes or developed systems Monitoring instruments	Design Postdevelopment
Contextual inquiry	Procedures and strategies Information requirements and flow Knowledge requirements Workload Collaboration requirements	Real-world contexts Task performers	All
Ethnographic studies	Procedures and strategies Information requirements and flow Knowledge requirements Workload Collaboration requirements	Real-world contexts Task performers Documentation instruments (e.g., video recorder)	All

Knowledge-acquisition techniques became popular as means to elicit knowledge from experts for building knowledge-based systems. In knowledge-based systems, expert users are essential sources. Weiss and Shanteau (2003) have defined three categories of expertise: expert judges, prediction experts, and performance experts and an empirical assessment technique for determining experts. Knowledge-acquisition techniques are also often used to elicit cognitive task data in general (Lehto et al. 1992). Depending on the product or system being developed, the knowledge of novice and expert task performers may be applicable.

Knowledge-acquisition methods include

- Interviewing techniques
- Event-based knowledge elicitation (Fowlkes et al. 2000)
- Automatic inductive methods that infer and specify knowledge
- Protocol analysis (Ericsson and Simon 1984)

- Psychological scaling (Cooke and McDonald 1988)
- Repertory grids from personal construct psychology theory (Boose 1985)
- Observational techniques (Boy and Nuss 1988)

See Cooke (1994) for a review of knowledge-elicitation techniques.

Interview: Interviews can be conducted in a variety of ways from very structured and focused exploratory. Interviews can be performed with individuals or groups. Interviews can provide a wide variety of task data.

Documentation review: To the extent that design documentation is available, that documentation can be an important source of task data. Design documentation may include system, subsystem and component architectures, information flows, use cases, and user profiles among other information relevant to task analysis and design.

Protocol analysis: Protocol analysis refers to various techniques for collecting data in the form of verbal reports. In this methodology, persons generate thinking-aloud protocols of the unobservable (i.e., cognitive) activities they perform while accomplishing a task (Ericsson and Simon 1984). The verbal reports represent behavioral descriptions from which task strategies, requirements, procedures, and problem areas can be derived. Protocols provide data on the sequence in which tasks are performed and thus can be used to identify the strategies used by humans in accomplishing tasks that can be performed in multiple ways.

There are several issues that need to be considered about the validity of using verbal reports as data and inferring thought processes from them. Ericsson and Simon (1984) address these concerns by demonstrating how verbal protocols are distinct from retrospective responses and classical introspection by trained observers and detailing the methods for collecting and analyzing protocols.

Instrumented human–machine interface techniques: These techniques are used to passively and unobtrusively collect objective data on task performance and the procedures by building the data collection into the interface itself. These techniques are used to record the timing, sequences, and frequencies of explicit actions. These can, for example, model navigation through a website using search and hyperlink actions or the low-level actions that are done to accomplish the navigation such as keystrokes, button pushes, and mouse movements.

The data associated with actions can be used to infer workload and to study the frequency of actions, their temporal relationships, and human error. Although these data are objective, they are restricted to overt responses and, by themselves, do not provide a basis for analyzing cognitive components. Modeling the cognitive task components involves correlating these action data with data about the situations and system behavior that elicited the actions and the changes in the situations and system state caused by the actions, that is, knowledge of context is vital to properly interpret interactions.

Observation techniques: Observation is a generic term referring to many techniques that can use a wide range of instruments to monitor situations and the behavior of systems and task performers. Two types of observation are distinguished. In direct observation, a human observer is with the task performer as he or she performs the task. In indirect observation, a human observer monitors the task performer remotely with audio and visual monitoring systems. Indirect observation can be done as the task is being performed or after the fact by using a recording. Observation techniques may be unobtrusive or invasive, record subjective or objective data, and may be used in controlled testing or real-world environments.

Contextual inquiry: Contextual inquiry is a situated field interview (real-world use environment) method, related to ethnographic research, in which a researcher observes a user's interaction with and use of systems in real-world contexts. The researcher watches and periodically interviews the user and colleagues about the activities while they are being performed. The technique is less burdensome on the user because much of the time is devoted to direct observation of the user's actions. The combination of direct observation of users working in context together with probing users to articulate important aspects of their work leads the researcher to a deep understanding of the work.

Ethnographic studies: These are in-the-field studies that have been adopted from anthropology research. The researchers are embedded to some level with the users and garner data on how they interact in real life with the products or systems under study or similar products or systems or to identify the need for such products. In an ethnographic study of independent elders, Forlizzi et al. (2004) identified two groups of elders, well and declining based in part on cognitive factors identified during the study.

33.3.3 Steps 3 and 4: Model Task Data and Compute Task Metrics

Steps 3 and 4 are the actual analysis steps. The task data are modeled in accordance with a selected modeling method and cognitive architecture (as applicable). This model is used to compute various task metrics and performance predictions that will be used to inform design decisions.

33.3.3.1 Modeling Task Data

Table 33.3 lists eight major approaches for modeling cognitive task data. Each has been shown to be useful in applied decision making and each is described below.

Task-timeline analysis: Timeline analysis organizes and relates low-level tasks on the basis of their time of onset, duration, and concurrences in the context of performing a high-level task. Any task taxonomy or decomposition model can be used to define the lower-level tasks that will be mapped to the high-level task timeline. Generally, the task-timeline mapping is constructed by decomposing a high-level task in terms of specific scenarios because different scenarios can have very different task and time requirements.

TABLE 33.3   Analytic Techniques for Modeling Tasks

Technique	Modeled Dimensions/Characteristics	Analysis
Task timeline analysis	Temporal onset, duration, and concurrences	Task-load estimates Task complexity
GOMS, NGOMSL, CPM-GOMS, and keystroke-level analysis	Task and system knowledge required by task performers Overt low-level actions Procedures Temporal relationships CPM_GOMS incorporates critical paths with analysis of dependencies and relationships	Task Complexity Knowledge requirements Performance estimates from production rule simulation Serial and parallel task performance.
TAG	Task and system knowledge required by task performers Observable low-level actions Action sequences	Task complexity Task consistency Knowledge requirements
Fleishman and Quaintance's cognitive task taxonomy	Identifies 23 cognitive abilities underlying task performance. Tasks are modeled in terms of required abilities.	Cognitive ability requirements Performance requirements
Knowledge-representation techniques	Task and system knowledge required by task performers	Knowledge requirements
Elemental resource model	Mental resources needed to perform tasks Resources are defined in terms of function and performance requirements	Functional requirements Performance requirements
SA model and SAOD process	Models SA as a three-level process (perception, comprehension, and projection)	SA requirements SA design principles SA measurements
CWA	A family of interrelation methods forming a framework for analyzing the requirements of large human–machine systems	Work-domain analysis Organizational coordination Cognitive states, strategies, and modes

This technique is useful for analyzing workload, allocating tasks, and determining human and system performance requirements. When the resource requirements for each lower-level task are mapped to the timeline, the result is a dynamic task-demand profile.

Wickens (1984) discusses two limitations of timeline analysis. First, the technique often does not account for time-sharing capabilities in which the performance of multiple tasks can be accomplished efficiently when resource demands are low. Second, the technique is most effective when analyzing forced-pace activities. The more freedom the human has to schedule activities, the harder it is to construct a useful timeline.

GOMS, NGOMSL, and CPM-GOMS analysis: GOMS, an acronym for goals, operators, methods, and selection rules (Card et al. 1983, 1986) is an analytic technique for modeling (1) the knowledge about a task and a machine that a task performer must possess and (2) the operations that a task agent must execute to accomplish the task using the machine. On the basis of the work by Newell and Simon (1972) in human problem solving, the model was extended by Kieras (1988) into NGOMSL (for natural GOMS language), which affords a more detailed analysis and specification of tasks. CPM-GOMS (Cognitive, Perceptual, Motor GOMS) incorporates a critical path network that enables an analysis of parallel activity.

In GOMS and its variants, goals represent what a human is trying to accomplish. Operators are elementary, perceptual, cognitive, or motor acts that may be observable or unobservable. Methods are sequences of operations that accomplish a goal. Selection rules are criteria used to select one method to apply when many methods are available.

The NGOMSL analysis uses this model to predict quantitative measures of the complexity of the knowledge required to perform a task with a system. These measures include learning time, amount of transfer, and task execution time. To accomplish this, methods (i.e., procedural knowledge) are represented in the form of production rules. These are IF-THEN rules that describe knowledge in approximately equal-sized units. The number of rules needed to represent a task provides a measure of the complexity of that task. Time predictions are obtained by modeling the production rules in a computer program that stimulates the tasks being analyzed.

The keystroke-level task model is an abbreviated application of the GOMS analysis (Card et al. 1983) that models only the overt actions (i.e., the observable operators and methods) taken by the task performer. In this way, it does not require the inferences about mental processes required by the full GOMS approach. The model was developed with regard to a computer system and defines six operators: a keystroke or mouse button push, pointing using a mouse, moving the mouse, moving hands between the mouse and keyboard, mental preparation, and system response. Tasks are modeled by identifying the sequence of operators needed to perform the task.

Task-action grammar analysis: Task-action grammar (TAG) (Payne and Green 1986, Schiele and Green 1990) defines a formal structure for modeling the knowledge required to perform simple tasks with a given system. Task knowledge is represented as sequences of simple acts. Similarities in the syntactic representation of simple tasks are used to derive higher-level schemas that apply across tasks possessing a family resemblance. The ability to derive schemas is used to assess the consistency of the tasks performed with a given user interface and has implications for ease of learning and overall usability. In similarity with NGOMSL, the number of grammatical rules and schemas provides a quantitative measure of task and interface complexity.

Fleishman and Quaintance's cognitive task taxonomy: Task taxonomies classify tasks on the basis of various characteristics and properties. As such, they can serve a useful purpose in modeling tasks. Tasks of the same taxonomic classification will have similar characteristics and similar requirements. This inference provides a basis for efficiently creating models for analyzed tasks. Fleishman and Quaintance (1984) provide an extensive review of taxonomies of human performance and identify four classifications: (1) behavior descriptions, (2) behavior requirements, (3) ability requirements, and (4) task characteristics. They further detail a taxonomy of human abilities that identifies 23 cognitive factors underlying task performance. These factors were derived from an analysis of empirical performance data collected from a large number of diversified tasks and individuals. The factors constitute a structure for modeling cognitive tasks. That is, these factors can be mapped onto specific tasks and thus specify the cognitive abilities needed to perform the task.

Knowledge-representation techniques: Knowledge representation is a generic term that refers to several formalisms for modeling knowledge about tasks, systems, and the physical environment. Major representation schemes include production rules, frames, scripts, and cases. Production rules represent knowledge as a set of condition–consequence (i.e., IF-THEN) associations. The executive process-interactive control (EPIC) cognitive architecture incorporates a cognitive processor implemented as a production rule system with an associated working memory (Hornoff 2004, Kieras and Meyer 1997). Barnard and May (1999) present a unified cognitive architecture based on interacting cognitive subsystems. The architecture incorporates two approaches, one of which implements cognitive activity as a production rule system.

Frames, scripts, and cases are different forms of schemas that represent knowledge as typical stereotypical chunks. Rules and scripts generally represent procedural knowledge, whereas frames and cases represent declarative knowledge. By formally representing data acquired from knowledge-acquisition techniques, a model of the procedural and declarative knowledge required to perform a task is created.

Elemental resource analysis of tasks: The elemental resource model (ERM) (Kondraske 2006) defines human performance in terms of the performance and skill resources (capacities) that a human or system possesses and which can be brought to bear in performing tasks. Elemental resources are defined at a low level such that many of them may be required to perform a high-level task. In addition, intermediate-level resources are defined to provide task-analysis targets at a less-granular (i.e., higher hierarchical) level. In this model, a resource is defined as a paired construct consisting of a functional capability (e.g., visual word recognition) combined with a performance capability (e.g., recognition speed). Thus, even though the functional capability is the same, visual-word-recognition speed and visual-word-recognition accuracy are defined as two distinct resources because they model two distinct dimensions of performance. This model can be applied in task analysis by decomposing the mental components of a task in terms of the resources that a human or system performing them is required to process.

SA model and the SOAD process: The SA model and SAOD process, developed by Endsley (1995, 2002), were described earlier in this chapter. Taken together, the three-level SA model and multistep process for analyzing SA guide designs of systems that support superior SA operationally themselves provide a comprehensive framework for analysis and design. Pieces of the SOAD process drawn from CWA are discussed below.

CWA: CWA is not a specific method but a framework of interrelated methods for modeling work domains, the organizational coordination needs, and the cognitive processing states, strategies, and modes entailed by the work (Lintern 2009, Vicente 1999). It defines a multistage analytic process intended to specify a broad array of the requirements for large human–machine systems. Much of the foundational work in CWA draws from early work done by Rasmussen (1983, 1986; Rasmussen and Goodstein 1988).

A popular method of CWA is work-domain analysis in which a two-dimensional abstraction–decomposition space (ADS) of the system being analyzed is described (Miller 2004). On one dimension, various levels of functionality from basic physical form through functional purpose are specified. The second dimension decomposes the system into various levels of subsystems and components. Information pertinent to the combination of each abstraction level with each decomposition level is described.

33.3.3.2 Incorporating Cognitive Architectures

The analysis of task data by themselves is of limited use in making applied decisions because task data address only one side of the design problem, that is, requirements. For example, a task-timeline analysis provides a model from which a measure of task demand can be computed. However, this analysis does not indicate whether the task load is acceptable or how it could be optimally distributed among humans and machines. Making these judgments requires consideration of human and machine capabilities. Similarly, using the NGOMSL and TAG models, a measure of task complexity can be computed, indicating that one task or procedure is more complex than another. However, these judgments are solely based on the number of task steps and the amount of information needed to perform each step and do not consider how difficult each step is for a human or machine to perform.

Using these task models without referencing or incorporating human and machine models forces a general assumption that task difficulty is a linear function of complexity (modeled as more task steps or information requirements). Even with this assumption, the task model by itself provides no indication of the acceptability of the task complexity or expected human or machine performance. Human and machine processing and performance models inform both of these judgments. Therefore, task analysis is used in combination with human and machine models to make design decisions.

Using task, human, and machine models in concert is facilitated if the cognitive components being modeled are described in consistent, or at least relatable, terms across task, human, and machine entities. Further, the quality and precision of the decision will be enhanced to the degree that the task requirements and human and machine capabilities are described quantitatively.

Five models of human cognitive processes and performance are discussed below. These were selected because they (1) describe concepts that are generally applicable to a wide range of information-processing tasks and (2) are engineering-oriented models for use on applied problems.

33.3.3.2.1 The Model Human Processor

MHP (Card et al. 1983, 1986) defines three interacting processing subsystems: perceptual, cognitive, and motor. The perceptual and cognitive subsystems include memories. Within each subsystem, processing parameters (e.g., perceptual processor, long-term memory, visual-image memory, and eye movements) and metrics (e.g., capacity, speed, and decay rate) are defined. Using data from numerous empirical studies, the MHP defines typical range values for 19 parameters. To apply the model, processing parameters are associated with an analysis of the steps involved in accomplishing a task with a given system. Values for each parameter are assigned and summed, providing time estimates for task completion. An extension of MHP called QN-MHP that incorporates queuing networks to model concurrent performance was described earlier in this chapter (Liu et al. 2006).

33.3.3.2.2 ACT-R

The ACT-R architecture developed by Anderson is the basis for much work in cognitive modeling. See Anderson (2007) for an in-depth discussion of the model. It uses both procedural and declarative representations and incorporates many parameters that can be set to optimize the fit to cognitive task data. ACT-R can be used to model individual task performance as well as average performance (Rehling et al. 2004).

ACT-R is composed of perceptual–motor and memory modules implemented as production rules. Both declarative and procedural memory are modeled. A pattern-matching mechanism is used to select production rules applicable to the situation. Buffers are used to interact with and represent the state of modules. ACT-R is implemented as a computer language. Users create a program containing relevant task data to model the task and task performance. An extension of ACT called SNIF-ACT that incorporates a Bayesian navigation mechanism was described earlier in this chapter (Fu and Pirolli 2007).

33.3.3.2.3 SOAR

SOAR is an advanced cognitive architecture originally developed by Newell (1990) that has undergone many revisions and extensions performance (Laird 2008, Laird and Rosenbloom 1996). SOAR represents a theory of cognition with a set of explicit cognitive mechanisms. It provides scaffolding upon which cognitive task data can be modeled and used to evaluate design options and guide design decisions.

Its current implementation includes many learning, memory, and general processing mechanisms capable of modeling the performance of many varied complex tasks performed by human–machine systems. Learning mechanisms include chunking, reinforcement learning, episodic learning, and semantic learning. Memories have been extended to include procedural knowledge, episodic memory, and semantic memory. Cognitive processing mechanisms include, among others, decision making, reasoning, and planning. Modeling cognitive task performance is enabled with algorithms for acquiring, storing and retrieving information, and decision making.

33.3.3.2.4 CLARION

CLARION is an advanced cognitive architecture (Helie and Sun 2010, Sun 2009) that includes four main subsystems: action centered (e.g., decision making), nonaction centered (e.g., episodic and semantic memory), motivational (e.g., low-level drives, peer approval, and esteem), and metacognitive (knowledge about one's own cognition that influences the other subsystems). The action and nonaction-centered subsystems further distinguish between explicit and implicit representations that enable interactive dual processes for learning, decision making, and other cognitive tasks. The inclusion of both explicit and implicit processes and representations distinguishes CLARION from ACT-R and SOAR.

Additionally, CLARION includes both low- and high-level motivational processes that can impact the performance of cognitive tasks. Although CLARION (such as ACT-R and SOAR) models a single cognitive agent, the motivational processes capture important social aspects of task modeling that are important to higher-level more holistic perspectives on task analysis discussed earlier.

33.3.3.2.5 ERM of Human Performance

ERM (Kondraske 2006) was discussed briefly in the preceding section as a task-analysis technique. That discussion addressed how the ERM uses the same quantitative modeling construct (i.e., elemental performance resources) for task requirements and human capabilities. Major classes of resources include motor, environmental (i.e., sensing), central processing (i.e., perception and cognition), and skills (i.e., knowledge). Central processing and information (skill) resources are of interest in this chapter. When applied to humans or to machines (i.e., agents who perform tasks), the ERM describes the perceptual, cognitive, and knowledge resources available to the agent. If the agent has a deficiency in any of these elemental resources, the agent cannot complete a task requiring that resource. In this case, agents with sufficient resources need to be selected, agents with insufficient resources need to be trained, or the task goals or procedures need to be modified to accommodate the resources available to the agents targeted to perform the task. ERM derives from a broader theory of general systems performance (GSPT) developed by Kondraske.

Gettman et al. (2003) report an application of this performance model to laparoscopic surgery. In this study, the relationships between objective measures of human basic performance resources (BPRs) and laparoscopic performance were evaluated using nonlinear causal resource analysis (NCRA), a novel predictive and explanatory modeling approach based on GSPT. Results suggest promise in predicting laparoscopic performance, and thus the predictive power of applying such analysis and modeling strategies in design.

Defining Terms

Cognitive architecture: A generic model and framework consisting of cognitive processing mechanisms within which data, specific to processing requirements that are being modeled, can be specified and used to predict performance and guide design decisions. Cognitive architectures are generally implemented in software.

Cognitive tasks: Tasks that predominantly consist of mental components and, in ERM terms, require mental performance and skill resources to perform.

Task: A goal-directed, procedural activity that is defined with regard to the resources (i.e., capabilities) that performing agents (i.e., humans or machines) must possess to accomplish the goal.

Task analysis: The process of (1) decomposing high-level tasks into their constituent, mutually exclusive, and lower-level tasks; (2) describing intertask relationships and dependencies; and (3) defining each task's goals, procedures, performance, and skill requirements.

References

Anderson, J. R. 2007. *How Can the Human Mind Occur in the Physical Universe?* New York, NY: Oxford University Press.

Barnard, P. J. and May, J. 1999. Representing cognitive activity in complex tasks. *Human-Computer Interaction* 14:1,2.

Boose, J. H. 1985. A knowledge acquisition program for expert systems based on personal construct psychology. *International Journal of Man-Machine Studies* 23:495.

Boy, G. and Nuss, N. 1988. Knowledge acquisition by observation: Application to intelligent tutoring systems. In *Proceedings of the Second European Knowledge Acquisition Workshop (EKAW-88)*, 11.1:14, Bonn, Germany.

Card, S. K., Moran, T. P., and Newell, A. 1983. *The Psychology of Human-Computer Interaction*. Hillsdale, NJ, Erlbaum.

Card, S. K., Moran, T. P., and Newell, A. 1986. The model human processor: An engineering model of human performance. *Handbook of Perception and Human Performance. Vol. 2: Cognitive Processes and Performance*, ed. K. R. Boff, L. Kaufman, and J. P. Thomas, 1–35. New York: Wiley.

Cooke, N. J. 1994. Varieties of knowledge elicitation techniques. *International Journal of Human-Computer Studies* 41:801.

Cooke, N. J. and Gorman, J. C. 2009. Interaction-based measures of cognitive systems. *Journal of Cognitive Engineering and Decision Making* 3:1.

Cooke, N. M. and McDonald, J. E. 1988. The application of psychological scaling techniques to knowledge elicitation for knowledge-based systems. *Knowledge-Based Systems, Vol 1: Knowledge Acquisition for Knowledge-Based Systems*, ed. J. H. Boose and B. R. Gaines, 65–82. New York: Academic Press.

Endsley, M. R. 1995. Measurement of situation awareness in dynamic systems. *Human Factors* 37:1.

Endsley, M. R. and Hoffman, R. R. 2002. The Sacagawea principle. *IEEE Intelligent Systems* 17:6.

Ericsson, K. A. and Simon, H. A. 1984. *Protocol Analysis*. Cambridge, MS: MIT Press.

Fleishman, E. A. and Quaintance, M. K. 1984. *Taxonomies of Human Performance: The Description of Human Tasks*. Orlando, FL: Academic Press.

Forlizzi, J., DiSalvo, C., and Gemperle, F. 2004. Assistive robots and an ecology of elders living independently in their homes. *Human-Computer Interaction* 19:1,2.

Fowlkes, J. E., Salas, E., Baker, D. P. et al. 2000. The utility of event-based knowledge elicitation. *Human Factors* 42:1.

Fu, W. and Pirolli, P. 2007. SNIF-ACT: A cognitive model of user navigation on the World Wide Web. *Human-Computer Interaction* 22:355–412.

Gettman, M. T., Kondraske, G. V., Traxer, O. et al. 2003. Assessment of basic human performance resources predicts operative performance of laparoscopic surgery. *Journal of the American College of Surgeons* 197:489.

Gray, W. D. 2008. Cognitive architectures: Choreographing the dance of mental operations with the task environment. *Human Factors* 50:497–505.

Helie, S. and Sun, R. 2010. Incubation, insight and creative problem solving: A unified theory and a connectionist model. *Psychological Review*, 117: 3.

Hoffman, R. R. and Militello, L. G. 2009. *Perspectives on Cognitive Task Analysis*. New York, NY: Psychology Press.

Hornoff, A. J. 2004. Cognitive strategies for the visual search of hierarchical computer displays. *Human-Computer Interaction* 19:3.

Kaptelinin, V. and Nardi, B. A. 2006. *Acting with Technology*. Cambridge, MA: MIT Press.

Kieras, D. E. 1988. Towards a practical GOMS model methodology for user interface design. *Handbook of Human-Computer Interaction*, ed. M. Helander, 135–157. New York: Elsevier Science Publishers.

Kieras, D. E. and Meyer, D. E. 1997. An overview of the EPIC architecture for cognition and performance with application to human–computer interaction. *Human-Computer Interaction* 12:4.

Kondraske, G. V. 2006. The elemental resource model for human performance. *The Biomedical Engineering Handbook*. Ed. J. D. Bronzino, Boca Raton, FL: CRC Press.

Laird, J. E. 2008. Extending the soar cognitive architecture. In *Proceedings of the First Conference on Artificial General Intelligence* (AGI-08). Memphis, TN.

Laird, J. E. and Rosenbloom, P. S. 1996. The evolution of the soar cognitive architecture. In: T. Mitchell (ed.) *Mind Matters*, 1–50.

Lehto, M. R., Boose, J., Sharit, J. et al. 1992. Knowledge acquisition. In: *Handbook of Industrial Engineering*, second ed. ed., G. Salvendy, New York: Wiley.

Lintern, G. 2009. *The Foundations and Pragmatics of Cognitive Work Analysis*. Edition 1.0, Cognitive Systems Design, CognitiveSystemsDesign.net.

Liu, Y., Feyen, R., and Tsimhoni, O. 2006. Queuing network–model human processor (QN–MHP): A computational architecture for multitask performance in human–machine systems. *ACM Transactions on Computer-Human Interaction* 13:1.

Miller, A. 2004. A work domain analysis framework for modelling intensive care unit patients. *Cognition Technology and Work* 6:207–222.

Newell, A. 1990. *Unified Theories of Cognition*. Cambridge, MA: Harvard University Press.

Newell, A. and Simon, H. 1972. *Human Problem Solving*. Englewood Cliffs, NJ: Prentice-Hall.

Payne, S. J. and Green, T. 1986. Task-action grammars: A model of mental representation of task languages. *Human-Computer Interaction* 2:93.

Rasmussen, J. 1983. Skills, rules, and knowledge: Signals, signs, and symbols and other distinctions in human performance models. *IEEE Transactions on Systems, Man and Cybernetics* SMC-13:257.

Rasmussen, J. 1986. *Information Processing and Human–Machine Interaction*. New York: North-Holland.

Rasmussen, J. and Goodstein, L. P. 1988. Information technology and work. *Handbook of Human-Computer Interaction*, ed. M. Helander, 175–201, New York: Elsevier Science Publishers.

Rehling, J., Lovett, M., Lebiere, C. et al. 2004. Modeling complex tasks: An individual difference approach. In *Proceedings of the 26th Annual Conference of the Cognitive Science Society*, 1137–1142. August 4–7, Chicago, USA.

Rogers, W. A., Mykityshyn, A. L., Cambell, R. H. et al. 2001. Analysis of a "simple" medical device. *Ergonomics in Design* 9:1.

Schiele, F. and Green, T. 1990. HCI formalisms and cognitive psychology: The case of task-action grammar. *Formal Methods in Human-Computer Interaction*, eds. M. Harrison and H. Thimbleby, 9–62. Cambridge, UK: Cambridge University Press.

Sun, R. 2009. Motivational representations with a computational cognitive architecture. *Cognitive Computation* 1:1.

Suri, J. F. 2000. Saving lives through design. *Ergonomics in Design* 8:3.

Vicente, K. H. 1999. *Cognitive Work Analysis: Towards Safe, Productive, and Healthy Computer-Based Work*. Mahwah, NJ: Lawrence Erlbaum Associates.

Weiss, D. J. and Shanteau, J. 2003. Empirical assessment of expertise. *Human Factors* 45:104–114.

Wickens, C. D. 1984. *Engineering Psychology and Human Performance*. Columbus, OH: Charles E Merrill.

Further Information

Durso, F. R. ed. 2007. *Handbook of Applied Cognition*. Second ed., New York, NY, Wiley.

The journals *Human Factors and Journal of Cognitive Engineering and Decision-Making*, published by the Human Factors and Ergonomics Society, are sources for new cognitive task-analytic techniques and application studies.

34

Task Analysis and Decomposition: Physical Components

Sheik N. Imrhan
University of Texas,
Arlington

A task can be viewed as a sequence of actions performed to accomplish one or more desired objectives. Task analysis and decomposition involve breaking down a task into identifiable elements or steps and analyzing them to determine the resources (human, equipment, and environmental) necessary for the accomplishment of the task. As indicated in earlier chapters, all human tasks require the interaction of mental and physical resources, but it is often convenient, for analytical purposes, to make a distinction between tasks that require predominantly physical resources of the person performing the tasks and tasks that require predominantly mental resources. These different types of tasks are often analyzed separately. Usually, in physical tasks, the mental requirements are described but are not analyzed as meticulously as the physical requirements. For example, a heavy-lifting task in industry requires musculoskeletal strength and *endurance*, decision making, and other resources, but the successful completion of such a task is limited by musculoskeletal strength. Decision-making and cognitive resources may be lightly tapped, and so the heavy-lifting task analysis will tend to focus only on those factors that modify the expression of musculoskeletal strength while keeping the other kinds of requirements at a descriptive level. The descriptions and analyses of manual materials handling tasks in Chaffin and Andersson (1991) and Ayoub and Mital (1991) exemplify this kind of focus. The degree with which a resource may be stressed depends on a number of factors, among which are the resource availabilities (capacities) of the person performing the task compared with the task demands.

This chapter deals with the analysis and decomposition of only the physical aspects of tasks. It is assumed that nonphysical resources are either available in nonlimiting quantities or are not crucial to task accomplishment. While the compartmentalization of task characteristics tends to blur the natural connections among the various human performance resources, it is still the most pragmatic method available for task analysis.

Physical task analysis first achieved scientific respectability in the early part of this century from the work of the industrial engineer Frederick Winslow Taylor (1911) and, shortly afterward, by Frank and Lillian Gilbreth (Gilbreth and Gilbreth, 1917). Taylor and the Gilbreths showed how a task can be broken down into a number of identifiable, discrete steps that can be characterized by type of physical motions, energy expenditure, and time required to accomplish the task. By this method, they argued that many task steps, normally taken for granted, may contribute little or nothing to the accomplishment of the task and can therefore be eliminated. As a result of these kinds of analyses, Taylor and the Gilbreths were able to enhance productivity of individual workers on a scale that was considered unrealistic at that time. The basic approach to the highest level of physical task analysis today has evolved from the motion and time studies of Taylor and the Gilbreths (known as Taylorism), both in the industrial and nonindustrial environments. The exact methods have become more sophisticated and refined, incorporating new technologies and knowledge accumulated about human–task interaction.

From its roots in time and motion studies, task analysis has become a very complex exercise. No longer is a single task considered in isolation, as shoveling was by Taylor and bricklaying by the Gilbreths. Today, different ideas in management and advanced data analytical methods have established the need for cohesion between physical tasks and (1) the more global processes, such as jobs and occupations encompassing them, and (2) the more detailed processes contained within them (the different types of subtasks and basic elements of performance). Campion and Medsker (1992) give examples of the first, and Kondraske (1995) gives examples of the second. This chapter describes physical task analysis, showing the approach for proceeding from higher-level tasks to lower-level ones. Figure 34.1 shows a summary of the overall approach.

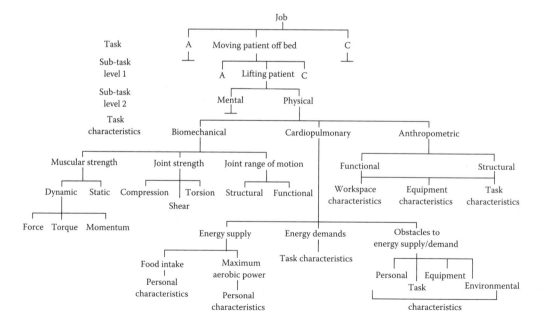

FIGURE 34.1 Diagram showing the concept of a hierarchical task analysis for physical tasks.

34.1 Fundamental Principles

The fundamental principle of physical task analysis is the establishment of the work relationships between the person performing the task and the elements of the task under specified environmental and social conditions. The main driving forces are performance enhancement, protection from injuries and illnesses, and decision making. The order of importance depends on the particular context in which the task analysis is performed. Performance enhancement is a concern in all disciplines that deal with human performance, though the approaches and objectives may differ. In physical rehabilitation, for example, performance enhancement focuses on improving the performance of basic physical functions of the human body, such as handgrip, elbow flexion, etc., that have deteriorated from injury or illness. In athletics, it focuses on improving performance to the highest possible levels, such as the highest jump or the fastest 100-m run. In exercise and fitness, it aims at improving body functions to enhance health and quality of life. Finally, in the discipline of ergonomics, it aims at enhancing task performance as well as the health and safety of people at work.

34.1.1 Speed–Accuracy Principle

Performance enhancement and protection from injuries and illnesses are not necessarily mutually exclusive. In performance enhancement, the aim is to complete a task as accurately and quickly as possible. Both accuracy and speed are important in the work environment, especially in manufacturing, and are influenced by other factors. When lack of accuracy or precision leads to dire consequences, as in air traffic control jobs, then a decision to sacrifice speed is usually made. The basic concept of Fitt's law (1954) is relevant to these situations. It is difficult to find examples of cases where gross inaccuracy is tolerable, but in many cases more speed is required and less accuracy is tolerable, and a different point on the speed–accuracy continuum is selected. In the manufacturing environment, speed translates into productivity and accuracy into quality, and both determine profitability of the production enterprise. Speed and accuracy are rarely attainable at the highest levels simultaneously. In practice, a certain amount of one may be sacrificed for the other. Thus, industrial engineers who set these tolerable limits talk of "optimum" speed instead of "fastest" speed and "optimum" quality instead of "perfect" quality. These facts must be borne in mind when analyzing physical tasks. A task analysis indicating that a person can increase his or her speed of performance should not necessarily imply that the task is being done inefficiently, because quality of performance may deteriorate with increased speed. This kind of flawed reasoning can occur when a variable is dealt with in isolation, without regard to its interaction with other variables.

34.1.2 Stress–Strain Concept

In task analysis, it is common practice to distinguish between stress and strain. However, these terms are sometimes used interchangeably and confusedly. In this chapter, stress refers to a condition that may lead to an adverse effect on the body, whereas strain refers to the effect of stress on the body. For example, working at a computer job in dim lighting often leads to headaches. The dim lighting is considered the stress, and the headache is the strain. The term stressor is also widely used as a synonym for stress. Strain has often been wrongly called stress. These terms must be clearly defined to determine which factors are causative ones (stresses) and which are consequences (strains). Stress is determined by task demands, while strain is determined by the amount of physical resources expended beyond some tolerable level, defined by the person's resource capacities. The stress–strain principle is pivotal to task analysis when one is concerned with errors, *cumulative traumas*, and injuries in the workplace and is applicable to task situations where task demands are likely to exceed human resource capacities.

Ayoub et al. (1987) developed a quantitative stress–strain index, called the *job severity index* (JSI), from empirical task analysis and epidemiologic data for manual materials handling tasks. This index computes the ratio of "job task physical demands to person physical capacities" from several interacting variables. The application of the JSI is also detailed in Ayoub and Mital (1991). Also, Kondraske (1995) defines a quantitative measure of stress that can be applied to individual performance resources. In this measure, defined as the "ratio of resource utilization to resource availability," an adverse effect may be noted when the stress level exceeds a threshold, which may be different for different types of performance resources (e.g., strength, range of motion, etc.).

34.1.3 Cumulative Strains

The elimination of motions and other physical actions that do not contribute directly to task performance (tayloristic practice) has led to a concentration of work at specific localities in the body and to consequent overwork at those localities, but this concentration often leads to rapid consumption of the limited resources of the working systems. For example, VDT data entry is a highly repetitive task with very little variation; work is concentrated heavily on the hands (rapid finger motions for operating the keyboard) and in the neck and trunk (prolonged static muscular contraction), and this often leads to cumulative trauma disorders of the hands, wrists, neck, and shoulders. By comparison, traditional typists performed a variety of tasks in addition to using the keyboard—changing paper on the typewriter, filing documents, using the phone, etc.—and this helped to stem the depletion of physiologic resources caused by rapid finger work or sustained static muscular contractions in the neck and shoulder. Also, it is now recognized that some functions of the body that have not been considered "productive" under Taylorism are highly stressed and may even be the limiting factors in task performance. In data processing, the muscles of the neck and back maintain prolonged static contractions that often result in muscular strains in the neck and back and limit work time. Traditional task analysis does not always consider this static muscular work as productive, even though it is absolutely necessary for steadying the arms (for keyboard and mouse use) and the head (for viewing the screen and documents). Likewise, *work pauses*, which have been considered wasteful, are now valued for their recuperative effects on the physical (and mental) working systems of the body. The increasing awareness of the causes of work-related cumulative trauma disorders will continue to influence the interpretation of data derived from task analyses.

34.2 Early Task-Analysis Methods

The history of physical task analysis does not show a trend toward the development of a single generalized model. The direction of physical task analysis has been influenced by Taylorism and by specific efforts in the military that were later adapted to the industrial and other nonmilitary environments. A list of influential methods, to which readers are referred, is given below:

1. Time studies of Fredrick Winslow Taylor (1911)
2. Time and motion studies of Frank and Lillian Gilbreth (Gilbreth and Gilbreth, 1917)
3. *Job analysis* developed by the U.S. Department of Labor in the 1930s (Drury et al., 1987)
4. The U.S. Air Force "method for man–machine task analysis" developed by R. Miller (1953)
5. Singleton's methods (Singleton, 1974)
6. *Hierarchical task analysis* (HTA) developed by Annette and Duncan (1974)
7. Checklist of worker activities developed by E.J. McCormick and others for the U.S. Office of Naval Research (Drury et al., 1987)
8. Position analysis questionnaire (McCormick et al., 1969)
9. The AET method (Arbeitswissenchaftliches Erhenbungsverfahen zur Tatigkeitsanalyse, or ergonomic job analysis) developed by Rohmert and Landau (Drury et al., 1987)

34.3 Methods of Physical Task Analysis

Methods of physical task analysis vary widely. Drury and colleagues (1987) point out that "the variation of task analysis format is the result of different requirements placed on the task analysis." While this is a pragmatic method for short-term results, a more general approach for long-term solutions is needed. Such an approach should aim to proceed from higher- to lower-level tasks, as discussed in other chapters (Kondraske, 1995). The following general sequence of analysis is recommended:

1. Statement of the objectives of the task analysis
2. Description of the system within which the tasks reside
3. Identification of jobs (if relevant) within the system
4. Identification of the tasks
5. Identification of subtasks that can stand independently enough to be analyzed as separate entities
6. Determination of the specific starting point of each task
7. Determination of the specific stopping point of each task
8. Characterization of the task as discrete, continuous, or branching (Drury et al., 1987)
9. Determination of task resources (human, equipment, and environmental) required to perform the task (this step is the essence of task description)
10. Determination of other support systems (e.g., in work situations, managerial and supervisory help may be needed)
11. Determination of possible areas of *person–task conflicts*
12. Determination of possible consequences of conflict, for example, errors, slowing down of work rate, deterioration of quality of end product, decline in comfort, harm to health, and decline in safety

After the task analysis is performed and the resulting data analyzed, solutions for solving the associated problems are formulated then implemented; for example, repositioning of the mechanical hoist used for lifting and moving a patient at the beginning of the lift to minimize human muscular input. This is then followed by an evaluation period in which enough data is gathered to compare the task states before or after the changes. The evaluation criteria must be compatible with the stated objectives of the task analysis.

34.3.1 General Methods for Background Information

Many different techniques for gathering information in physical task analysis have evolved over the years, especially in the industrial and biomedical engineering environments. The quality and quantity of information that the techniques provide are limited by available equipment, and it seems that the quality and quantity of available equipment lag far behind the state of the art in technology. General data-gathering techniques, which are somewhat self-descriptive, include:

- Direct observation (predominantly visual)
- Indirect observation (e.g., replay of videotape)
- Document review
- Questionnaire survey
- Personal interview

34.3.2 Specific Techniques

Specialized data-gathering techniques (Winter, 1990; Chaffin and Andersson, 1991; Niebel, 1993) that have evolved into powerful tools in the industrial environment and which can be used for task analysis in other situations include:

- *Motion study*—details the motions made by the various segments of the body while performing the task
- *Time study*—details the time taken to perform each motion element
- *Micromotion study*—detailed description of motion using mainly videotapes
- *Kinematic analysis*—measures or estimates various motion parameters for specified body segments, for example, displacement, velocity, acceleration. (It involves micromotion studies.) The

data are used for subsequent biomechanical analyses, for example, to determine mechanical strain in the musculoskeletal system (Chaffin and Andersson, 1991)

- *Kinetic analysis*—measures or estimates forces produced by body segments and other biomechanical parameters (e.g., center of mass, moment of inertia, etc.) and physical parameters of objects (e.g., mass, dimension, etc.) (the data are used for subsequent biomechanical analyses)

In the assessment of jobs in the occupational environment, two of the most useful motion-study methods are Rapid Upper Limb Assessment (RULA) and the Ovako Working Posture Analysis System (OWAS). These methods are used for assessing the risk to musculoskeletal cumulative strains from work postures. In RULA (McAtamney and Corlett, 1993), the geometric configurations of the upper arms, lower arms, wrists, neck, and trunk are estimated by visual observation and an overall score is calculated for posture. This score is then modified by incorporating data on the muscular forces exerted by the upper limbs and the frequency of exertion. Stressful postures and their contributing factors can therefore be identified and risk to injuries assessed. The OWAS method (Kahru et al., 1977) is similar to RULA but does not incorporate frequency of muscular force exertions.

Specialized data-analytic techniques include:

- Methods analysis—determines the overall relationships among various operations, the work force, and the equipment
- Operations analysis—determines the details of specific operations
- Worker–equipment relationship study—determines the interactions between people and their equipment

Examples of the above techniques that are frequently used for analyzing industrial jobs, but may also be used for other tasks involving people, are discussed in Gramopadhye and Thaker (1999). Among the most useful are flow charts such as sequence diagrams, functional flow analysis, and decision diagrams, which depict the links among tasks and subtasks. These charts may also be used in conjunction with summary tables of the number of activities, duration of activities, and distance traveled by the human worker. They therefore facilitate improvements in system efficiency and identification of sources of possible operation errors. Examples of their applications are shown in Barnes (1980) for baking soda crackers and by Lock and Strutt (1985, in Gramopadhye and Thacker, 1999) for inspection in transport aircraft structures. Other techniques such as link analysis (Chapanis, 1962), critical incident technique (Meister, 1985), fault tree analysis (Green, 1983), and failure modes and effects analysis are not specific to physical task analysis but may be used in systems analysis involving physical tasks.

34.3.3 Decomposition of Physical Tasks

Physical tasks can be viewed as exchanges of energy within a system consisting of the human, the task, the equipment, and the environment. In task analysis and decomposition, we look at the human on one side and the other system components on the other side and then determine the nature of the exchange. The energy is transmitted by muscular action. Tasks are hierarchical, however, and for systematic decomposition, it is useful to identify the various levels and proceed in a top-down sequence (see Figure 34.1). The items in the various levels given here are self-explanatory, but there is considerable content within each. Detailed descriptions of each is beyond the scope of this chapter, and readers should consult the references (Singleton, 1974; Corlett et al., 1979; Meister, 1985; Winter, 1990; Niebel, 1993; Chaffin and Andersson, 1994) for standard measurement procedures and analyses.

Level I: Identifying general types of tasks according to levels of energy requirements:

- Tasks requiring great muscular forces
- Tasks requiring medium to low levels of muscular forces

Tasks requiring very low levels of muscular forces are not predominantly physical. Their successful accomplishment is strongly dependent on cognitive resources. The application of strong and weak muscular forces is not necessarily mutually exclusive. Such forces may be exerted simultaneously by different muscular systems or may even alternate within the same system. For example, a typing task may require strong back extensor forces while sitting bent forward (if the workstation is poorly designed) and weak finger flexion forces for activating the keyboard keys, and a weak index finger flexion may be required to activate a trigger on a hand drill while strong handgrip forces stabilize the drill.

Level II: Identifying the crucial subsystems involved in the generation and transference of forces of varying intensities involved in tasks:

- Musculoskeletal—for great forces
- Cardiopulmonary—for medium to low forces
- General body posture
- Body motion
- Local segmental motion
- Local segmental configuration
- Anthropometry
- Workplace and equipment dimensions
- The last three subsystems modify directly the expression of muscular force

Level III: Identifying environmental requirements and constraints. Environmental conditions influence performance and functional capacities in humans. They should therefore be measured or estimated in task analyses. Table 34.1 describes common environmental constraints.

Level IV: Identifying body actions in relation to tasks. These actions can be decomposed into two major types:

1. Those which involve body motions. They are used for either changing body positions or moving objects
2. Those which do not involve body motions. They are used primarily for balancing and stabilizing the body for performing some task. Body posture is especially important here, especially when great muscular forces must be exerted

These actions are not mutually exclusive during task performance. One part of the body may move, while another part, involved in the task, may be still. For example, the fingers move rapidly when using a keyboard, but the rest of the hand is kept motionless while the fingers are moving. Tables 34.2 through 34.5 depict practical decompositions of these actions as well as those requiring muscular forces.

Level V: Identifying anthropometric variables. Human anthropometry interacts with workplace and equipment dimensions. Tasks are performed better when the interaction defines a close "match" between human body size and task-related physical dimensions. Therefore, physical task analysis may be inadequate without measurements of the dimensions of people performing the task and the corresponding dimensions of other aspects of the system of which the task is a part. This kind of matching is one of

TABLE 34.1 Environmental Factors in Task Analysis

Environmental Factor	Constraint	Examples of Effects
Illumination	Insufficient intensity	Errors
Heat	Excessive heat and humidity	Lowering of physiologic endurance
Cold	Excessive cold	Numbness of hands—inability to grasp hand tool properly
Vibration	Excessive amplitude	Loss of grip and control of vibrating tool
Noise	Excessive intensity	Inability to coordinate job with coworkers
Body supporting surface	Slipperiness	Difficulty in balancing body
Space	Insufficient workspace	Inability to position body properly

TABLE 34.2   Representative Actions with Motions

Class of Action	Subclass	Purpose of Action	Examples
Whole body		Positioning body	Walking, crawling, running, jumping, climbing
		Transporting object	Lifting, lowering, carrying horizontally, pushing, pulling, rotating
Gross segmental	Arm movement	Applying forces to object	Reaching for object, twisting, turning, lifting, lowering, transporting horizontally, positioning, pressing down, pushing, pulling, rotating
	Leg movement	Applying forces	Rotating (e.g., foot pedal), pushing
	Trunk movement	Generating momentum	Sitting and bending forward, backward, and sideways to retrieve items on a table
Fine segmental	Finger movement	Applying forces	Turning, pushing, pulling, lifting

TABLE 34.3   Representative Actions with Motions

Class of Action	Subclass	Purpose of Action	Examples
Whole body		Balancing body	Standing while preparing meal in kitchen
		Supporting or stabilizing object	Bracing ladder while coworker climbs on it
Segmental	Arm		Holding food item with one hand while cutting it with other hand
	Leg	Supporting body	Forcing foot on ground while sitting in constrained posture

TABLE 34.4   Representative Actions Requiring Forces, for Different Types of Forces

Class of Action	Subclass	Sub-subclass	Body–Object Contact	Purpose of Action	Examples
Whole body	Whole body	Dynamic	One hand, two hands, or other contact	Generate great forces that must be transmitted over small localized area or large area. The effort produces motion of whole body	Lift, push, pull
		Static	One hand, two hands, or other contact	Generate great forces that must be transmitted over small localized area or large area. The effort does not produce motion	Lift, push, pull
Segmental		Static	One hand, two hands, one foot, or two feet	Generate forces (over a wide range of magnitude) that must be transmitted over a relatively small localized area. The effort does not produce motion of the body segment	Gripping with whole hand, pinching, pressing down, twisting, turning, pushing, pulling, or combinations
		Dynamic	One hand, two hands, one foot, or two feet	Generate great forces that must be transmitted over small localized area or large area. The effort produces motion of the body segment	Pushing, pulling, pressing down

TABLE 34.5 Posture While Performing Tasks

Class	Subclass	Purpose	Examples
Whole body	Standing, sitting, kneeing, lying down, other	Optimize body leverage; position body for making proper contact with object; other	Squatting at beginning of a heavy lift to prevent excessive strain in the lower back
Segmental	Arms, legs, trunk, hands, other	Optimize segment leverage; position segment for making proper contact with object	Placing elbow at about right angles while using wrench to prevent excessive shoulder and muscle efforts

TABLE 34.6 Human Anthropometry and System Dimensions

Body Dimensions	System Dimensions
Height, arm length, shoulder width	Workspace—height of shelf, depth of space under work table, circumference of escape hatch
Leg length, knee height	Equipment size—distance from seat reference point to foot pedal of machine, height from floor to dashboard of vehicle
Hand length, grip circumference	Hand tool size—trigger length, handle circumference
Crotch height, arm length	Apparel size—leg length of pants, arm length of shirt
Face height, hand width	Personal protective equipment—height of respirator, width of glove

the basic thrusts in the discipline of ergonomics. Grandjean (1988) and Konz (1990) discuss these issues in many types of human–task environments, and Pheasant (1986) gives numerous body dimensions related to task design. Some important examples of human–system dimensions that must be considered during task analysis are shown in Table 34.6.

34.4 Factors Influencing the Conduct of Task Analysis

While task analysis traditionally focuses on what a person does and how he or she does it, other factors must be considered to complete the picture. In general, the characteristics of the task, the equipment used, and environmental conditions must all be accounted for. Human functional performance cannot be viewed in isolation because the person, the task, the equipment, and the environment form a system in which a change in one factor is likely to affect the way the person reacts to the others. For example, in dim lighting, a VDT operator may read from a document with marked flexion of the neck but with only slight flexion (which is optimal) when reading from the screen. Brighter ambient lighting may prevent sharp flexion when reading from documents but is likely to decrease contrast of characters on the screen. Screen character brightness must therefore be changed to maintain adequate reading performance to prevent sharp flexion of the neck again.

34.4.1 Knowing the Objectives of Task Analysis

Motion, speed, force, environment, and object (equipment) characteristics are common factors for consideration in task analysis. However, the reasons for performing a task are an equally important factor. Tasks that may involve the same equipment and which may seem identical may differ in their execution because of their objectives. Thus, a person opening a jar in the battlefield in the midst of enemy fire to retrieve medicines will not perform that task in exactly the same way as a person at home opening a similar jar to retrieve sugar for sweetening coffee. In the former case, speed is more important, and both the type of grasp used and the manual forces exerted are likely to be markedly different from the latter case. Napier (1980) recognized this principle, in relation to gripping tasks, when he wrote that the "nature of the intended activity influences the pattern of grip used on an object." These kinds of considerations in task analysis can influence the design of objects and other aids and the nature of education and training programs.

34.4.2 Levels of Effort

The level of required effort when performing similar tasks in different environments is not necessarily the same, and the interpretation of task-analysis data is influenced by these differences. Tasks in the workplace are designed so that human physical effort is minimized, whereas tasks in the competitive athletics environment are designed to tap the limits of human performance resources. There are other differences. An athlete paces himself or herself according to his or her own progress. He or she has greater freedom to stop performing a task should physical efforts become painful or uncomfortable. In the workplace, however, there is often little freedom to stop. Many workers often push themselves to the limits of their endurance in order to maintain (flawed) performance goals set by their employers. This is why cumulative strains are more prevalent in the workplace than in many other environments. These differences in performance levels may influence the way task analyses are performed among the different disciplines and the application of the data derived therefrom.

34.4.3 Criticality of Tasks

An inventory of task elements is necessary for describing the requirements of the task. It can tell us about the person, equipment, and environmental requirements for performing a job, but we must also be able to identify specific elements or factors that can prevent the successful completion of the task or that can lead to accidents and injuries. These critical elements are usually measured in detail or estimated and used for developing quantitative models for predicting success or failure in performance. One such widely researched element is the compression force on the L5/S1 disk in the human spine while performing heavy-lifting tasks (Chaffin and Andersson, 1984). This force is being used by the National Institute of Occupational Safety and Health as a criterion for determining how safe a lifting activity is. If analysis of task-analysis data indicates that the *safety limit* (3400 N of compression) is exceeded then work redesign, based on task-analysis information, must be implemented (National Technical Information Service, 1991; NIOSH, 1981).

34.5 Measurement of Task Variables

During task analysis, variables must be measured for subsequent data summary and analysis. It is important to know not only what the inventory of task-related variables is but also to what degree the variables are related to or affect overall performance. The measurement of task-related variables allows for quantification of the overall system. For example, the NIOSH lifting equation (National Technical Information Service, 1991) shows how task variables such as the horizontal distance of the load from the body, the initial height of the load, the vertical height of lift, the frequency of lifting, the angular displacement of the load from the saggital plane during lifting, and the type of hand–handle coupling affect the maximal weight of the load that can be lifted safely by most people in a manual materials-handling task. The number of task-related variables measured should be adequate for describing the task and for representing it quantitatively. However, there are often constraints. These include:

1. The number of variables that can be identified
2. The number of variables that can be measured at an acceptable level of reliability and accuracy
3. The availability of measurement instruments

Merely summarizing individual measurements seldom yields the desired information. Task performance is essentially a multivariable operation, and variables often must be combined by some quantitative method that can yield models representative of the performance of the task. Sometimes a variable cannot be measured directly but can be estimated from other measured variables. The estimated variable may then be used in a subsequent modeling process. A good example of this is the intraabdominal pressure achieved during heavy lifting. Though it can be predicted by a cumbersome process of swallowing a pressure-sensitive pill, it also can be estimated from the weights of the upper body and load lifted and other variables related to lifting posture. Its estimate can then be used to estimate the compressive force in the L5/S1 disk and the tension in the erector spinae muscles during lifting. Imrhan and Ayoub (1988) also show how estimated velocity and acceleration of elbow flexion and shoulder extension can be used, with other variables, to predict linear pulling strength.

34.5.1 Task-Related Variables

Variables that are usually measured during physical task analysis include:

1. Those related to the physical characteristics of task objects or equipment:
   a. Weight of load lifted, pushed, carried, etc.
   b. Dimensions of load
   c. Location of center of mass of load
2. Those related to the nature of the task:
   a. The frequency of performance of a cycle of the task
   b. The range of heights over which a load must be lifted
   c. The speed of performance
   d. The level of accuracy of performance
3. Those related to the capacities of various physical resources of the person:
   a. Muscular strength
   b. Joint range of motion
   c. Joint motion (velocity and acceleration)
   d. *Maximal aerobic power*
   e. Anthropometry
4. Those related to the environment:
   a. Temperature
   b. Illumination
   c. Vibration
5. Those related to workplace design:
   a. Amount of space available for the task
   b. Geometric and spatial relationships among equipment
   c. Furniture dimensions
6. Those related to anthropometry:
   a. Length, breadth, depth, or circumference of a body segment
   b. Mass and mass distribution of a body segment
   c. Range of motion of a skeletal joint

34.5.2 Instruments for Gathering Task-Analysis Data

A great number of instruments are available for measuring variables derived from task analyses. The choice of instruments depends on the type of variables to be measured and the particular circumstances. In general, there should be instruments for recording the sequence of actions during task, for example, videotape with playback feature, and instruments for measuring kinematic, kinetic, and anthropometric variables (Winter, 1990; Chaffin and Andersson, 1994). The main kinematic variables include displacement (of a body part), velocity, and acceleration. Kinetic variables include force and torque. Anthropometric variables include body segment length, depth, width, girth, segment center of mass, segment radius of gyration, segment moment of inertia, joint axis of rotation, and joint angle. Some variables are measured directly, for example, acceleration (with accelerometers), force applied at a point of contact between the body and an object (with load cells), and body lengths (with anthropometers); some may be measured indirectly, for example, joint angle (from a videotape image) and intraabdominal pressure (using swallowed pressure pill); and others may be estimated by mathematic computations from other measured variables, for example, compressive force on the lumbosacral (L5/S1) disk in the lower back. Posture targeting, a method for recording and analyzing stressful postures in work sampling (Corlett et al., 1979), is becoming popular.

The measurements of performance capacities associated with human functions should conform to certain criteria. Details can be found in Brand and Crownshield (1981) and Chaffin (1982). A general set of psychometric criteria is also discussed by Sanders and McCormick (1993). It includes measurement accuracy, reliability, validity, sensitivity, and freedom from contamination. Meeting these criteria depends not only on the instruments used but also on the methods of analysis and the expertise of the analyst. It is almost impossible to satisfy these criteria perfectly, especially when the task is being performed in its natural environment (as opposed to a laboratory simulation). However, the analyst must always be aware of them and must be pragmatic in measuring task variables. Meister (1985) lists the following practical requirements for measurements: (1) objective, (2) quantitative, (3) unobtrusive, (4) easy to collect, (5) requiring no special data-collection techniques or instrumentation, and (6) of relatively low cost in terms of money and effort by the experimenter. However, these are not necessarily mutually exclusive.

34.6 Uses and Applications of Task Analysis

The uses of task-analysis information depend on the objectives of performing the task, which, in turn, depend on the environment in which the task is performed. Table 34.7 gives the different situations.

TABLE 34.7   Uses and Applications of Task Analysis

Uses and Applications	Examples of Relevant Situations
Modeling human performance and determining decision-making strategies	A model showing the sequence of the various steps required to perform a task and the type of equipment needed at each step
Predicting human performance	Using a quantitative model to predict whether an elderly person has enough arm strength to lift a pot full of water from a cupboard onto a stove
Redesigning of the existing tasks or designing of new tasks	Eliminating an unnecessary step in the packaging of production items into cartons; designing a different package for a new item based on task-analytic data gathered for a related item
Determining whether to use task-performance aids	The analysis may show that most elderly persons do not possess enough strength to open many food jars and may, therefore, need a mechanical torqueing aid
Personnel selection or placement	Matching personnel physical characteristics with task requirements can reveal which person may be able to perform a task and, hence, be assigned to it
Determining whether to use aids that enhance health or safety	Task analysis may show that too much dust always gets into the atmosphere when opening packages of a powered material and that workers should wear a respirator
Determining educational and training procedures	Identification of difficult task steps or the need for using mechanical aids, together with knowledge of workers' skills, may indicate the level of education and training needed
Allocating humans to machines and machines to humans	Matching people skills and capacities with the resource demands of machines
Determining emergency procedures	Task-analysis information may indicate which steps are likely to result in dangerous situations, and therefore, require contingency plans

34.7 Future Developments

To date, there is no reliable quantitative model that can combine mental and physical resources. A general-purpose task-analysis method that uses active links between the various compartments of human functions would be an ideal method, but our lack of knowledge about the way in which many of these "compartments" communicate precludes the development of such a method. The present approach to compartmentalization seems to be the most pragmatic approach. It offers the analyst access to paths from a gross task or job to the myriad of basic task elements of performance. Unfortunately, actual systems and subsystems used in practice seem to be loosely defined and inconsistent, often with confusing metrics and terminologies for important variables. Moreover, available task-analysis models deal only with specific classes of application (Drury, 1987). A general-purpose model is badly needed for handling different mental and physical resources at the same time, dealing with wide ranges in a variable, and bridging the gaps across disciplines. Such a model should help us to perform task analyses and manipulate the resulting data from environments ranging from the workplace, the home (activities of daily living), athletics, exercise and fitness, and rehabilitation. Such a model can also help to eliminate the present trend of performing task analyses that are either too specific to apply to different situations or not specific enough to answer focused questions. Fleishman (1982) deals with the issue. At least one recent effort is active (Kondraske, 1995). However, as Landau et al. (1998) points out, such generalizability has a cost in that the associated data is produced at a higher level of abstraction, which is likely to be difficult for a practitioner to apply to specific problems.

There is also a need for better quantification of performance. We need to know not only what kind of shifting in resources a person resorts to when one route to successful task accomplishment is blocked (e.g., insufficient strength for pressing down in a certain sitting posture) but also the quantity and direction of that shift. For example, we need to know not merely that a change in posture can increase manual strength for torqueing but also what the various postures can yield and what quantity of specific mental resources are involved in the change. The models today that answer the quantitative questions are mainly ones of statistical regression, and they are limited by the number of variables and the number of levels of each variable that they can deal with.

Defining Terms

Anthropometry: The science that deals with the measure of body size, mass, shape, and inertial properties.

Cumulative trauma: The accumulation of repeated insults to body structures over a period of time (usually months or years) often leading to "cumulative trauma disorders."

Endurance: The maximum time for which a person can perform a task at a certain level under specified conditions without adverse effects on the body.

Fitts' law: The equation, derived by P. Fitts, showing the quantitative relationship between the time for a human (body segment) to move from one specific point to another (the target) as a function of distance of movement and width of the target.

Hierarchical task analysis: The analysis of a task by breaking it down to its basic components, starting from an overall or gross description (e.g., lifting a load manually) and moving down in a series of steps in sequence.

Job analysis: Any of a number of techniques for determining the characteristics of a job and the interactions among workers, equipment, and methods of performing the job.

Job severity index: An index indicating the injury potential of a lifting or lowering job. It is computed as the ratio of the physical demands of the job to the physical capacities of the worker.

Local segment: A specific body segment, usually the one in contact with an object required for performing a task or the one most active in the task.

Maximal aerobic power: The maximal rate at which a person's body can consume oxygen while breathing air at sea level.

Motion study: The analysis of a task or job by studying the motions of humans and equipment related to its component activities.

Person–task conflict: The situation in which task demands are beyond a person's capacities and the task is unlikely to be performed according to specifications by that person.

Position analysis questionnaire: A checklist for job analysis, developed by the Office of Naval Research in 1969, requiring the analyst to rate or assess a job from a list of 187 job elements.

Safety limit: The maximum stress (e.g., load to be lifted) that most workers can sustain under specified job conditions without adverse effects (injuries or cumulative strains) on their bodies.

Time study: The study of a task by timing its component activities.

Work pause: A short stoppage from work.

References

Ayoub M.M. and Mital A. 1991. *Manual Materials Handling*. London, Taylor & Francis.

Ayoub M.M., Bethea N.J., Deivanayagam S. et al. 1979. Determination and Modeling of Lifting Capacity. Final report, HEW (NIOSH), grant no. 5R01–OH–00545–02.

Barnes R. 1980. *Motion and Time Study Design and Measurement of Work*. New York, John Wiley and Sons.

Campion M.A. and Medsker G.J. 1992. *Handbook of Industrial Engineering*. New York, Wiley.

Chaffin D.B. and Andersson G.D. 1991. *Occupational Biomechanics*. New York, Wiley.

Chapanis A. 1962. *Research Techniques in Human Engineering*. Baltimore, Johns Hopkins University Press.

Corlett E.N., Madeley S.J., and Manenica I. 1979. Postural targeting: A technique for recording work postures. *Ergonomics* 22: 357.

Drury G.D., Paramore B., Van Cott H.P. et al. 1987. Task analysis. In: J. Salvendy (Ed.), *Handbook of Human Factors*, pp. 371–399. New York, Wiley.

Fitts P. 1954. The information capacity of the human motor system in controlling the amplitude of movement. *J. Exp. Psychol.* 47: 381.

Fleishman E.A. 1982. Systems for describing human tasks. *Am. Psychol.* 37: 821.

Gilbreth F.B. and Gilbreth F.M. 1917. *Applied Motion Study*. New York, Sturgis and Walton.

Gramopadhye A. and Thacker J. 1999. Task analysis. In W. Karwowski and W.S. Marras (Eds.), *The Occupational Ergonomics Handbook*, pp. 297–329. Boca Raton, FL, CRC Press.

Grandjean E. 1988. *Fitting the Task to the Man*, 4th ed. New York, Taylor & Francis.

Imrhan S.N. and Ayoub M.M. 1988. Predictive models of upper extremity rotary and linear pull strength. *Hum. Factors* 30: 83.

Kahru O., Kansi P., and Kuorinka I. 1977. Correcting working postures in industry. A practical method for analysis. *Appl. Ergon.* 8: 199–201.

Kondraske G.V. 1995. A working model for human system task interfaces. In J.D. Bronzino (Ed.), *Handbook of Biomedical Engineering*. Boca Raton, FL, CRC Press.

Konz S. 1990. *Work Design: Industrial Ergonomics*. Worthington, Ohio, Publishing Horizon.

Landau K.L., Rohmert W., and Brauchler R. 1998. Task analysis: Part I— guidelines for the practitioner. *Int. J. Indust. Ergon.* 22: 3–11.

McAtamney L. and Corlett E.N. 1993. RULA: A survey method for the investigation of work-related upper limb disorders. *Appl. Ergon.* 24: 91–99.

Meister D. 1985. *Behavioral Analysis and Measurement Methods*. New York, Wiley.

Napier J.R. 1980. *Hands*. New York, Pantheon.

National Technical Information Service. 1991. Scientific Support Documentation for the Revised 1991 NIOSH Lifting Equation. PB91-226274. U.S. Department of Commerce, Springfield, VA.

Niebel B.W. 1993. *Motion and Time Study*, 9th ed. Homewood, IL, Richard D. Irwin.

NIOSH, 1981. Work Practices Guide for Manual Lifting. NIOSH technical report no 81–122, US Department of Health and Human Services, National Institute of Occupational Safety and Health, Cincinnati, OH.

Pheasant S. 1986. *Bodyspace*. London, Taylor & Francis.

Singleton. 1974. *Man–Machine Systems*. London, Penguin.

Taylor F.W. 1911. *The Principles of Scientific Management*. New York, Harper.

Winter D.A. 1990. *Biomechanics and Motor Control of Human Movement*, 2nd ed. New York, Wiley.

Further Information

For the design of equipment in human work environments where task analysis is employed, see *Human Factors Design Handbook*, by W.E. Woodson [McGraw-Hill, New York, 1981]. For human anthropometric data that are useful to task analysis, see NASA Reference Publication 1024: Anthropometric Source Book, vol. 1: *Anthropometry for Designers* [Webb Associates, Yellow Springs, Ohio, 1978].

35

Human–Computer Interaction Design: Usability and User Experience Design

Ken Maxwell
IBM
MaxwellX

35.1 Introduction

The field of human–computer interaction (HCI) is about helping people realize their goals and fulfill their needs with the aid of information technology (IT) by making that technology useful, accessible, effective, and safe. Since the third edition of this handbook, the purposes for and means by which computing technology is used have expanded. Computing technologies are ubiquitous and capable of supporting a highly social, mobile, connected, and information-rich daily life.

IT systems, generally, and biomedical systems, particularly, now leverage social, mobile, embedded, and intelligent computing technologies to satisfy the interconnected needs of medical providers, consumers, and organizations. In doing so, biomedical systems are making the manner in which medical information is managed and medical care is provided highly collaborative, contextual, personalized, and intelligent. With biomedical systems (e.g., instruments, devices, robots, and bioinformatics systems) becoming highly reliant on new computing technologies, usability and user experience are now principal determinants of their adoption, effectiveness, and safe use.

Furthermore, biomedical technology is increasingly advantageous to expanding the user interaction capabilities of products and systems in general, helping to make them more accessible, usable, and useful. Consideration of biomedical factors affecting accessibility, usability, and overall user experience is increasingly needed as user interaction technology extends to incorporate alternative modalities for use in expanding mobile and real-world contexts.

This chapter provides the reader with fundamentals for addressing HCI in the design of interactive systems in general, and biomedical systems, in particular. To achieve their greatest benefit in today's highly interconnected information-based world, these systems need to be conceived from a holistic perspective that provides people with different abilities, motivations, lifestyles, and needs the capabilities to perform purposeful activities. Today's biomedical systems need to support data acquisition, analysis, and sharing in expanded social and environmental contexts to support medical purposes. Beyond this, biomedical systems are moving toward becoming a seamless component of broader everyday social and mobile activity, that is, toward becoming as much a part of everyday life as personal and social media and entertainment systems (and the content they generate, manage, and deliver) are today.

Work in HCI is abundant in academic, government, and commercial sectors. This chapter selects from this work essential and practical information needed to incorporate human experience into the engineering of biomedical systems. References to broaden the reader's knowledge of HCI are provided in the Further Information section.

35.2 HCI Directions and Design Challenges

Computing technology is increasingly used to support human purposes that require collaborative, contextual, analytic, personalized, and secure interaction in an expanding variety of real-world environments. To meet these requirements, computing and interaction technologies have broadened to support contexts of use that are social, mobile, embedded, and intelligent.

35.2.1 Supporting the Social Experience

Computing is currently a primary means to support and augment social activity among people and organizations. People increasingly embrace social networking technologies as a means to communicate and build community. Online social communities that provide support and resources for meeting medical needs abound. Medicine 2.0 is a term used to describe the use of Web 2.0 technologies to implement and support advanced medical systems. Medicine 2.0 uses social networking, user-generated content, crowd-sourcing techniques, multimedia, and personalization to enable web-based collaborative and personalized health-related services, education, information management, and awareness. The technologies being adopted by Medicine 2.0 foster collaboration, distribution of expertise, data sharing, and data analytics among medical professionals, consumers, and organizations.

Although the Medicine 2.0 technologies discussed above hold great promise for transforming the way medical information is used and medicine itself is practiced, there are still necessary advances to be made in the fit between existing medical systems and the technologies that can realize the future vision for delivering transformed health services. Technology is available today to support a medical information and practice landscape that leverages social media and advanced IT. However, obtaining this leveraged benefit is dependent on both (1) adapting to users' (i.e., consumers, providers, and organizations) varying interaction experiences and expectations, and (2) moving the existing health-related information into forms that are compatible and usable by the new technologies.

Overcoming the former requires systems that can cope with the varied needs of users with different levels of experience, usage patterns, abilities, motivations, and trust of and reliance on computing technologies. In addition, users expect services to be available and accessible seamlessly as they move through various contexts of use.

Overcoming the latter has proved difficult, for example, Google Health, an online service that enables people to upload, store, analyze, and share data shut down service in January 2012. In launching this online application, Google did not adequately anticipate the difficulties and barriers for consumers who are presented by the current differences in provider-systems and record-keeping methods (both electronic and nonelectronic).

35.2.2 Supporting the Mobile Experience

Computing is now mobile, being performed in all environments, situations, and contexts. Data services, including web browsing, email, and text messaging, are common on mobile phones and other personal devices. The Pew Internet and American Life Project, a project of the Pew Research Center, reports that of all smartphone owners, 25% say they go online mostly using their smartphones rather than their computers (Smith 2011).

Mobile applications for a myriad of general uses benefit from new modalities of interaction. Biomedical-oriented applications for personal mobile devices are now prolific and include a growing number of mobile applications intended for use by medical professionals to assist with patient care management and collaboration. In July 2011, the U.S. Federal Drug Administration issued draft guidelines for comment on mobile medical applications. In particular, applications that are used as an accessory to a regulated medical device or transform the mobile device into a regulated medical device are of interest (US Dept. of Health and Human Services 2011). Mobile medical applications have demonstrated that they can be of great help in acute as well as routine situations. For example, "Medical encyclopedia for home use" became the leading downloaded application in the Japan iTunes store in the aftermath of the March 2011 earthquake and tsunami. It provides basic first aid advice.

The number and nature of information and communication-based personal devices is increasing such that in the near future individuals will carry and wear several connected devices for the purposes of gathering and sharing information and assisting with both personal and social activities. For biomedical applications, mobile and wearable devices that monitor, analyze, and transmit data from a patient are becoming commonplace. These devices can be used to monitor vital signs, sleep patterns, motor activity, and even social interaction. All applications, whether biomedical or not, will increasingly make use of biomedical information to facilitate interaction with people and services. Mobile medical devices and applications expand contexts of use and in so doing promote more rapid collaboration, increase the opportunities for data sharing and collaboration, and extend possibilities for remote care through telepresence.

From the perspective of physical interaction, mobile form factors present interaction design challenges, including restricted display space and input mechanisms, function integration, management of multiple communication channels, and reduced computing power. When viewed from a broader user experience perspective, mobile devices are cultural accessories and must fit with the user's aesthetics and personality. Wearable devices must be comfortable emotionally as well as physically for the wearer, similar to the impact of an accessory to clothing.

35.2.3 Supporting the Blended Virtual–Physical World (Embedded) Experience

Computing is now embedded and ubiquitous in devices, instruments, and other products for both general and biomedical uses (Norman 1998). Computing technology has evolved to become part of the fabric of acting in the physical world. HCI design is increasingly addressing the integration of the physical with the virtual world (Streitz et al. 2002).

Because they may be of relatively specific use with narrow functionality, the interfaces to products that embed computing technology may have reduced complexity, and the HCI design task may appear to not require much consideration. Although the scale of the HCI design effort may be smaller for devices than for large information systems, attention to HCI factors should remain prominent. Rogers et al. (2001) in an analysis of a commonly used blood glucose meter found that although the instructions listed three general steps, these actually required a total of 52 substeps, many of which were sources of error in operating the device for the participants in the study. Many problems can sabotage the usability of simple products (Darnell, http://www.baddesigns.com/). These are unnecessary and can be avoided when proper methods are applied to understand users, identify potential problems, and design a quality user experience. Satisfying user needs represents value to customers and can present a competitive advantage.

Also, products with embedded computing technology are likely to be connected and be in communication with other devices or large systems. An understanding of the broader activities being performed with such products and the underlying human purposes they serve is paramount to realizing the benefits they can provide.

35.2.4 Supporting the Intelligent Interactive Experience

Computing technology now enables analytic and interactive capabilities that display a new horizon for biomedical systems in analysis of medical data, distribution of medical expertise, collaboration assisted by analytic insight, and improved evidence-based diagnosis. IBM's Watson is capable of analyzing very large volumes of medical data and identifying connections and patterns within that data. In the coming years, IBM plans to apply Watson to data-analytic needs in the healthcare industry as well as other industries.

In addition to its analytic capabilities, Watson also possesses an impressive capability to understand natural language. This capability will enable robust collaboration among providers and communication of information with all users. Bental and Cawsey (2002) use text analysis and natural language generation of medical record information, along with other techniques, to provide personalized and adaptive information to consumers. Text and data mining techniques are also described by Leroy et al. (2003).

35.2.5 Supporting Accessibility

Section 508, an amendment of the Rehabilitation Act, legislates requirements for U.S. Federal agencies to make electronic and information systems accessible to people with disabilities. The legislation covers the accessibility of a wide array of hardware and software products and systems by people with sensory-motor and cognitive disabilities.

International mandates and initiatives for e-accessibility and e-inclusion in the European Union highlight the growing need for accessibility for all users and for expanding the concept of accessibility universally. That is, accessibility is moving beyond the idea of providing access for people with injuries, illnesses, and ailments that are characterized by traditional disability labels and toward a greater holistic concept that includes age, social, and economic factors, experience with technology and emotion as factors affecting an individuals' capability for using products and systems effectively and safely.

35.3 Interaction Design Paradigms

Today's computing and interaction technology supports networked human activity being performed in a broad variety of environments with an array of interconnected information-based objects and systems. To meet the challenges presented by the expanding purposes supported by HCI, designers are exploring alternative design approaches that solve interaction problems from different perspectives and are moving beyond a singular human-centered design (HCD) focus. Taken as a whole, system designs are becoming more holistic in the combination of factors considered and the perspectives from which the designs are generated. Major paradigms that guide system design are discussed below.

35.3.1 Human-Centered Design

HCD (also referred to as *user-centered design*) is a modern design philosophy and methodology for deriving and allocating functional requirements, driving design concepts, and setting evaluation criteria from the perspectives of the person or persons who will use the products being developed. This philosophy was promoted as an alternative to design approaches that emphasized technology and market factors over user experience, resulting in designs that frequently and unnecessarily compromised the user's motivations, performance, safety, and emotional responses. HCD does not and should not exclude technology and market factors, but is meant to ensure that along with these factors the realized products or systems satisfy human needs and desires (Norman 1998). HCD is ubiquitous and is an enduring tradition toward achieving highly usable products. As testament to HCD's importance, an international standard (ISO 13407 1999) provides a guide to its application.

Usability refers to the capacity of a machine or system to be used by intended persons for accomplishing set purposes. It is a multifaceted concept that can include effectiveness, efficiency, time to learn, safety, and emotional satisfaction. International standard ISO 9241-11 (1998) defines usability as "the *effectiveness*, *efficiency*, and *satisfaction* with which specified users achieve specified goals in particular environments." Effectiveness is "the accuracy and completeness with which specified users can achieve specified goals in particular environments." Efficiency is "the resources expended in relation to the accuracy and completeness of goals achieved." Satisfaction relates specifically to the user and is "the comfort and acceptability of the work system to its users and other people affected by its use." A human-centered methodology is the widely accepted path toward realizing a design that embodies usability qualities. Usability is a major factor affecting the adoption, operational performance, availability, maintainability, and reliability of a human-product system.

The following are some characteristics of HCD:

- The purposes of all users involved are identified.
- The product is viewed as a tool that users employ to accomplish their purpose.
- The user is always performing a higher level task than the product.
- Tasks are allocated away from the users rather than to the users. This is not simply a matter of perspective but rather is fundamental to a human-centered approach. That is, the user is assumed to be performing a high-level task. Lower level tasks that are better performed by the computer are allocated from the user to the computer. This approach is opposed to one that considers the computer as the high-level task performer and allocates to the user lower-level tasks that the machine cannot do well.
- Tasks performed by users are meaningful.
- The user's responsibilities provide satisfaction and make use of the user's talents and skills.
- Intended users of the product participate in the design process.
- The user's skills and performance capabilities are explicitly considered in and accounted for in design decisions.

35.3.2 Activity-Centered Design

A different approach to the design of human interaction with products and systems focuses on the activity being performed. In activity theory, the foundation of activity-centered design (ACD), activity is considered as a fundamental construct that involves social and organizational factors, tools, agency, and context of use (Kaptelinin and Nardi 2006). In ACD, activities and the contexts in which they are performed are studied, modeled, and designed. People and organizations are agents that perform purposeful activities using tools within an environmental context. In ACD, activities comprise tasks that in turn comprise lower level actions and operations performed by agents in contexts.

For activities with a biomedical purpose, biomedical products and systems constitute part of the broader activity-performing system that includes agents, organizations, other tools, and the contexts of use.

The following are some characteristics of ACD:

- The purposes of the activity being performed and the agents having those purposes are identified.
- The contexts in which the activity is performed are identified.
- Activities are decomposed by the tasks and actions they comprise.
- Accomplishment of activities is modeled in terms of human, machine, and organizational agents doing tasks with tools in context.
- The user's responsibilities provide satisfaction and make use of the user's talents and skills.
- The user's skills and performance capabilities are explicitly considered in and accounted for in design decisions.

35.3.3 Embodied Interaction

Similar to ACD, embodied interaction is about activity and an agent acting in the world. That agent is embodied, that is, mediated and governed by the sensory-motor capabilities the agent possesses to act in the world. The philosophical basis of embodied interaction derives from phenomenology, especially as described by Hiedegger. Dourish (2001) translated these ideas into an approach to interaction design that uses embodied action with technology as a basis for product design. Adoption of the embodied approach has been catalyzed by the increase in social and mobile computing and embedding computational capabilities in various products that force interaction with tangible objects for performing activities.

In the embodied interaction view, the agency is manifested in real-world action and purpose is achieved through action. Agency can act only in ways it is equipped to act. Tools and social organizations extend the capability of an agent to act.

Biomedical products and systems are inherently amenable to a design approach that incorporates ideas of embodied interaction. For example, biomedical products and systems by design monitor, compensate for, augment, and utilize the embodiment of agency either by people or by robots. In this sense, embodied agency provides a congruent model for assistive biomedical systems.

35.3.4 Holistic Interaction Design

Today, computing technology is deeply embedded and broadly interconnected with real-world activities and social structures, and is used to fulfill a wide, and growing, spectrum of human needs and wants. To specify designs that effectively support these needs and wants, the design of interaction between people and today's computing technology and among people doing interrelated activities supported by technology is becoming increasingly holistic, expanding the factors that need to be considered to achieve successful products and systems. Many of these factors are biomedical in character and many of the systems are biomedical in purpose.

Interaction is becoming more multimodal. Alternative modes of interaction, such as speech, gesture, haptics, gaze, and the use of bioelectric signals, can provide the means for managing interaction across a variety of user needs, device form factors, and computing contexts. Interacting with computing technology is an expected part of everyday activity. Interfaces have become visually richer. Greater computing power has enabled the support of visualization and visual simulation techniques that enable a myriad of biomedical applications that were impractical not long ago. Interaction and interfaces are supporting more personalization and adapt to the needs of individuals. The design of interaction has moved beyond what Maxwell (2002) called basic usability concerns toward concern with broader elements of human experience, including social interaction and collaboration, motivations (Fogg 2003, Shneiderman 2002), emotions (Norman 2004, Cavazza and Simo 2003), context (Abowd and Mynatt 2002), and integration with real-world interactions (Streitz et al. 2002).

Holistic models, for example, Ruhala's Holistic Concept of Man (HCM), have been applied to the design of electronic health systems (Hakula 2009). Vanharanta and Salminen (2007) apply the HCM to the design of decision support systems. Young et al. (2011) point out that because social and emotional factors are particularly acute in human–robot interaction (HRI), HCI methods should be applied differently than they would be with other technologies and artifacts. They propose a *holistic interaction experience* view of social interaction with robots composed of three interaction perspectives. The first, visceral factors of interaction, such as smiling, are instinctual. The second, social mechanics, includes means of communicating between people and robots. The third, social structure, involves the social relationship between people and robots (e.g., domestic service, ambulatory assistance, and surgical team member). With regard to the third perspective, Forlizzi and DiSalvo (2006) demonstrate that the use of robots can change social structures and workflows. The use of a domestic robot, Roomba, can shift responsibilities for performing activities between generations and genders.

In the holistic view, embodied agents are all on different points in a multidimensional space that defines their capability to purposefully act in real-world environments. These dimensions include, among others, motivations, goals, mental and physical abilities, social needs and responsibilities, vocation, and lifestyles. The holistic approach draws from HCD, ACD, and embodied interaction to connect product and system design with the purposeful real-world and social needs of people, thereby creating augmented agency capable of acting to satisfy those needs. In making this connection, however, the holistic approach is not centered by the human or activity or nature of the embodied agent acting in the environment. These are all subsumed by attention to how they interrelate to form a unified system.

Holistic design attends to obtaining coordination across functional and interchangeable components toward realizing purposes greater than those of each component individually. Holistic design emphasizes that the individual components should not be designed and built in the absence of an understanding of how each might coordinate with other components toward achieving greater benefits through collective performance. Even a seemingly isolated wearable health monitor should be designed with a notion of how it could fit into the health information management and healthcare delivery systems for the users of the monitor, their care providers, and their health organizations.

Although holistic design provides a means to understand problems and their causes from both deeper and broader perspectives and to facilitate more reliable, robust, and resilient solutions, it is often not adopted because of barriers that are both structural—design processes are not generally set up to address solutions that encompass larger systems, and perceptual—the benefits and return on investment are not appreciated (Rohrer 2011).

35.4 User Interaction Design Processes

The design paradigms discussed above are frameworks that steer and orient the creation of products and systems for human use. The holistic approach is viewed here as the most applicable for applying advanced technology to creating products and systems that meet the health-related needs of consumers, providers, and organizations. These needs are increasingly met by a coordinated set of products and systems collecting, sharing, and analyzing data together with systems that assist or augment human agency in expanding real-world contexts. The design of any biomedical product or system will benefit by adopting a holistic design approach that not only considers the multidimensional needs of the users discussed above but also how the product or system can use social media, mobility, machine intelligence, and other means to interconnect with broader systems that are both biomedical and general in nature.

Creating a biomedical product or system for use by people involves performing and applying a set of techniques, methods, and tools for understanding users and the activities they perform; deriving a design that meets the purposeful, functional, and interaction needs of those users; and validating the design through test and evaluation. These means and processes are described below.

35.4.1 Purpose, User, and Activity Modeling Methods

Many techniques, methods, and tools have been developed for designers to acquire information about users, their activities, and their purposes very early in the product and system development process. These means are employed to inform the specification of function and design requirements and the synthesis of design concepts, as well as forming a basis for test and evaluation criteria.

Of foremost concern to designers is human purpose. As computing technology and HCI have progressed, there has been a transition from focusing on what computers can do to what humans can do (Shneiderman 2002). This transition is manifest in the evolution of human needs and wants that IT systems are intended to satisfy (Maxwell 2002). The human purpose for a product or system may be broad or specific. Purpose can translate directly into the function of a product or system but not necessarily so. For example, the function of a consumer blood pressure monitor is to measure a user's blood pressure, but its purpose is broader. It is to enable a convenient, frequent, and private monitoring of blood pressure, to inform the user, and toward the goal of keeping the user's blood pressure at a healthy level. In this broader sense, the purpose fulfills not only the needs of the user of the monitor (the medical consumer) but also purposes of the user's doctor and more broadly of the user's health insurer. From a very different human perspective, the monitor also needs to serve the purposes of the people who make and sell it. To satisfy this array of users and their purposes, design methods must consider user, market, technology, and context-of-use factors together.

A first step is to identify the needs and wants of intended users and to characterize those users with attributes relevant to satisfying their identified needs and wants. This involves characterizing users along any number of relevant dimensions, such as age, skill level, geographic location, and context of use (e.g., home or work). The purpose of such an analysis is to determine the range of these characteristics and the extent to which users are similar and different. Similarities can be used to categorize users and to direct design decisions to address the needs of these categories. Design requirements can be very different across user groups. Differences within groups can be used to inform the degree of flexibility, personalization, and adaptability needed.

As part of a project to improve the usability of bioinformatics websites, Javahery et al. (2004) report a user analysis of the biomedical research community. Their analysis described users with regard to seven characteristics: user's language, familiarity with the Internet, bioinformatics background, education level, profession, experience with specific websites, and the tasks performed on websites. Of course, the specific characteristics that are relevant will vary with the product or system being developed or evaluated.

Several methods for identifying, analyzing, and modeling purpose, people, and activities are described below. The various methods discussed in this section are not meant to be exclusive of one another and the use of more than one approach is encouraged. Carroll and Rosson (2007) provide a particularly good example of this, by combining participatory methods with a scenario-based design approach and ethnographic design techniques.

35.4.1.1 Ethnographic Research

Ethnographic research uses in-the-field studies that have been adopted from anthropology research. The researchers are embedded with the users and garner data on how they interact in real life with the products or systems under study or similar products or systems or to identify the need for such products. In an ethnographic study of independent elders, Forlizzi et al. (2004) identified two groups of elders, well and declining using characteristics of mobility, cognitive function, and household maintenance.

User groups can be defined along many different dimensions. Two typical and general grouping criteria are function based and resource needs based. For biomedical applications, functional user groups commonly include those identified below.

- Practitioners and service providers: This group includes doctors, nurses, psychologists, social workers, paramedics, and other providers of medical care.
- Biomedical science researchers: This group uses biomedical instruments, simulation tools, data analysis software, and data mining software to conduct research and development in laboratories or in the field.
- Administrators: This group represents hospital administration, doctor's office, and insurance personnel who use biomedical records and data as part of their daily work.
- Legal: This group includes lawyers, paralegals, court and government representatives, expert witnesses, and insurance industry representatives who employ biomedical products for legal purposes.
- Analysts: This group includes persons who perform data mining and other analyses of biomedical data using computer systems.
- Patients: This is a specific subset of the general public user group who uses biomedical products or systems under the advice of a doctor or during a period of care.
- General public: This group is maximally diverse and uses a variety of consumer instruments and products as well as accessing a variety of online medical information and belonging to online support networks.
- IT support personnel: This group includes persons who install, manage, configure, diagnose, and repair biomedical IT systems.
- Biomedical engineers: This group includes persons who use computer-based tools to design and build biomedical products.

Resource-needs-based groups typically are differentiated along the dimensions identified below. Users belonging to different groups along these dimensions will typically need different levels of assistance and training.

- *Age*: Elders and children comprise especially important broad groups.
- *Disabilities*: These typically are further grouped by type such as vision, hearing, motor skills, and cognition.
- *Current medical condition*: Groups can be defined by any condition needing current care.
- *Current lifestyle*: Any number of cultural variables can be used to identify groups.
- *History*: Any number of medical, lifestyle, or family variables can be used to specify the relevant groups.
- *Expertise*: This dimension differentiates the level of knowledge and skill users have with a particular product or system, or the functions they perform.

In addition to differences in the level of interactive assistance or training needs derived from the dimensions above are variables that affect the acceptance of computing technology. For example, Park et al. (2006) report that psychological factors, such as self-efficacy (a judgment of one's ability to use the technology effectively), are better predictors of acceptance than demographic factors such as age. Thus, older users with high self-efficacy are more likely to accept computing technology than low self-efficacy users even when the latter are younger. This same study reports several social and organizational factors that influence acceptance. These findings emphasize the need for holistic analysis and consideration of factors in the design of technological products and systems.

Another step in employing a human-centered approach is to describe what and how users will do interacting with the product or system. The methods discussed below can be employed to generate this needed information.

35.4.1.2 Contextual Inquiry

Contextual inquiry is a situated field interview (real-world use environment) method, related to ethnographic research, in which a researcher observes a user's interaction with and use of systems in real-world contexts. The researcher watches and periodically interviews the user and colleagues about the activities while they are being performed. The technique is less burdensome on the user because much of the time is devoted to direct observation of the user's actions. The combination of direct observation of users working in context together with probing users to articulate important aspects of their work leads the researcher to a deep understanding of the work.

35.4.1.3 Personas

The development of personas is a means to understand a group of users by personifying that group and their characteristics with a single user identity. The set of personas (usually just a few but sometimes dozens) represent not only the needs of users that a product must satisfy but also the workflows, lifestyles, preferences, and user experiences within which the product's use must fit. Personas can and are specified to various depths and breadths of analysis that may include social interactions, cultural practices, personality, and motivational variables. Because personas can capture many characteristics and dimensions about a user group, they represent a vehicle for addressing biomedical factors in concert with other human factors as a whole. In this respect, they are a basis for a holistic approach to design that goes beyond the usability of the product toward addressing a broader desired experience of use including the use of biomedical products and systems. Alan Cooper introduced the use of personas (Cooper 2004).

35.4.1.4 Use-Case Analysis

Use-case analysis is a part of the unified modeling language (UML) development process (Booch et al. 1999). This analysis is meant to specifically identify and characterize each use of a product or system by each user. UML calls these users "actors." Use-cases are valuable for identifying each functional type of user and the functions that they perform.

35.4.1.5 Scenario-Based Analysis and Design

In this analysis, a set of representative scenarios are defined and used to examine how a product or system will be used in the contexts of its use. Scenarios are especially useful for revealing and addressing highly critical, low-probability situations. Rosson (1999) develops a form of user interaction scenarios that are an expansion of use-case scenarios. These are particularly useful for modeling a user's goals, expectations, and reactions and provide a means of tracing these user factors through to design. See Carroll (2000) for more scenario-based designs.

35.4.1.6 User Journeys

User journeys are a way to understand the user's needs for the system by understanding broader patterns, habits, motivations, and needs. Describing the user journey combines personas with scenarios and ethnographic data to ensure that the system is fulfilling the user's needs. Constructing user journeys is a way of connecting the system being designed with real-world contexts of use in a deep and holistic way.

35.4.1.7 Participatory Design and Knowledge Acquisition

Participatory design is a cooperative approach that includes some users on the design team as active participants in the design process. This approach ensures that the design team includes domain expertise and as such represents the expectation that this expertise will translate into successful designs. Participatory design is very applicable to biomedical products because in many cases expert medical knowledge will need to be incorporated into the system and an understanding of the medical knowledge of the various user groups will be needed to inform the design.

35.4.1.8 Task Analysis, Allocation, and Modeling

Task analysis is a process of decomposing the activities and functions that need to be performed into their constituents. When humans interact with products or systems, two types of tasks are performed: an interaction task and an application task. The interaction task consists of the actions and operations that the user performs to manipulate the product or system. These activities include moving input devices, pressing virtual or physical buttons, gesturing, changing eye direction, changing the orientation of devices, viewing displays, reading instructions, setting preferences, and attaching wearable devices among many others.

The application task refers to the user's functional objectives that will in turn satisfy the user's purpose. These objectives vary widely and include planning a surgery, performing a statistical analysis, diagnosing a patient's condition, finding information in a database, monitoring blood pressure, and living independently. The application task is a higher level task than the interaction task, meaning that the interaction tasks are subtasks that contribute to accomplishing the application task. Figure 35.1 illustrates the relationships between these two task levels and the greater purpose being satisfied for a healthcare consumer employing a blood glucose monitor. The broader system and context of use that includes the healthcare provider and support groups is also depicted (Figure 35.1).

Tasks can be analyzed qualitatively and quantitatively. There are several methods for quantifying various aspects of HCI tasks. The GOMS (for goals, operators, methods, and selection rules) and keystroke-level models (Card et al. 1983, 1986), when used in combination with human performance models, such as the model human processor, provide task performance estimates and knowledge requirements. The NGOMSL (for natural GOMS language) (Kieras 1998) and TAG (task action grammar) (Payne and Green 1986, Schiele and Green 1990) models provide quantitative metrics for interaction task complexity and consistency.

Kondraske (1995) has developed an elemental resource model (ERM) of human performance that can be applied to quantify tasks in terms of the requirements for and availability of performance and skill resources. Each performance resource is defined in terms of a quantitative unidimensional capability to perform an elemental function. Skill resources are defined in terms of knowledge and experience.

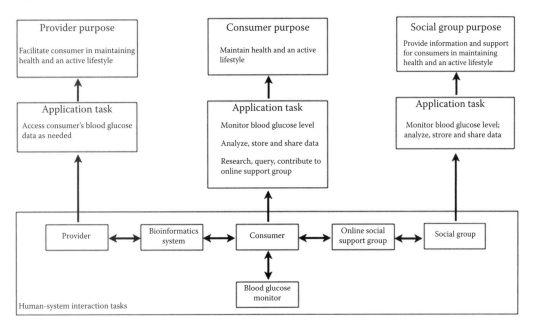

FIGURE 35.1 Each user group's purpose is satisfied by one or more application tasks that are accomplished through the interaction tasks performed among the users and systems.

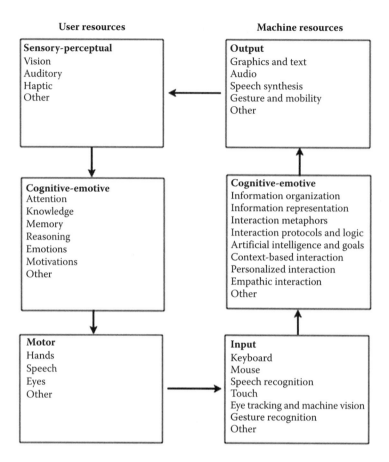

FIGURE 35.2   Resource correspondence between user resources and machine resources.

Adopting this model allows usability trade-offs in design decisions to be stated in terms of the relationships between (1) available resources and the sources that possess them and (2) required resources and the sinks that expend them. The capabilities of users and machine systems are sources of resources. The demands of performing interaction and application tasks are resource sinks.

Because, as in the example in Figure 35.1, humans and biomedical systems work together to satisfy the application tasks, the resources needed to accomplish the tasks are distributed between the humans and the machine systems. The designer has partial control over the resources required of the user to perform the interaction and application tasks by optimally off-loading (i.e., allocating) required resources to the machine systems. Figure 35.2 illustrates the resource correspondence between the users and machines. The arrows indicate the flow of information across the interface (Figure 35.2).

The designer has much control over the design of the interaction task. Although tempting, it is not necessarily optimal to let interaction tasks be defined in terms of existing ways of doing the task because existing means do not account for advanced machine systems that are being introduced to ease the task and augment user capabilities. Meaning, do not rely solely on existing task flows. Kramer et al. (2000) calls the process of creating innovative task flows for new environments "exploring the blue sky."

35.4.2 Design Generation

The methods described above generate the information needed by designers to develop conceptual and detailed designs. Early design concepts need not and should not be overly detailed. HCI design is an iterative process and the benefits of iteration are lost if too much detail is specified in early iterations. Generating quality designs requires imagination; unnecessary detail included too early will tend to block innovations at more abstract levels of the design. Iteration guides a graceful narrowing that matches design solutions to the level of understanding of the users and the tasks available. Each cycle either corrects design problems or refines the detail of design areas that work.

35.4.2.1 Information Architecture

Information architecture (IA) has its origins in library science and is concerned with the modeling of information and the application of that model to the structure of user interfaces. The IA establishes a structure for accomplishing tasks with the interface. As such, it is not just applicable to human interaction with bioinformatics or information management systems but for any interaction needed to perform an activity.

Card sorting is a popular technique in formulating an IA whereby a group of users is guided to generate taxonomies of information related to a product or system. Such taxonomies are also often evolved from a folksonomy that emerges from user tagging (i.e., associating characteristics and descriptors to) information and content items. The IA of an interface is integrally tied to navigation, and therefore task, complexity (Miller and Remington 2004).

35.4.2.2 Concept Modeling

A concept model describes the information entities being processed and activities being performed by the human–machine system. Concept models provide a means of exploring and examining the ways humans and machines can and need to interact to accomplish the purposes of the system as a whole.

35.4.2.3 Prototyping

After design concepts have been developed, they need to be prototyped and evaluated.

Prototypes are representations of the system and system design. These are early forms of a product or system that incorporate partially or fully the functions and features of a system. Prototypes can be developed at any of a range of fidelities and are an essential tool in evaluating usability as well as engineering feasibility and marketability. Early prototypes will generally be of low fidelity and may only model part of the functionality of the product. As with the design, prototypes will evolve to greater fidelity and functionality.

35.4.2.4 Design Standards and Guidelines

Following design standards and guidelines is an essential design practice. Standards and guidelines provide conformity and structure that promotes consistency and reuse of design patterns and components, grows and leverages user familiarity, and incorporates best practices. Standards and guidelines exist at many levels from international (like ISO 13407 and 9241-11 discussed earlier) to company specific.

35.4.3 Design Evaluation and Iteration

Evaluation is a matter of testing, measuring, and validating the usability of the design and the user experience in using the product or system. Evaluations are performed throughout the design, development, and deployment process. Because the designs and their prototypes will be at evolving levels of specification, their evaluations at different points will be performed in fundamentally different ways. Relatively inexpensive and expedient evaluations include cognitive walkthroughs and expert heuristic inspections (Nielsen and Mack 1994). More elaborate evaluations include formal empirical studies that can collect objective task performance data as well as subjective data. Recently, remote evaluation techniques, unmoderated testing software, and passive data collection and analysis (e.g., web analytics) have been increasingly adopted.

The goodness of a system's design and implementation with regard to satisfying user needs can be assessed with regard to several measurements. These include both subjective and objective measures of the utility, ease, effectiveness, efficiency, accessibility, safety, and satisfaction of use. In-depth coverage about collecting, analyzing, and presenting usability metrics is provided by Tullis and Albert (2008).

Evaluation results lead to reexamination of requirements, narrowing of the range of design concepts under consideration, and refinement of superior concepts in subsequent design iterations.

35.4.3.1 Heuristic Review

Usability can be improved by applying resource-demand-reducing HCI heuristics. Five major design heuristics that act to reduce task demands on performance and skill resources are described.

35.4.3.1.1 Naturalness and Familiarity of Interaction

Usability will be improved to the degree that the interaction is natural and familiar. Naturalness and familiarity reduce training requirements and increase available resources (e.g., available knowledge and sensory-motor performance). For physical components at a task level, this means that the user's sensory and effector modalities are properly matched to the required interactions, for example, keyboards used for typing, keypads for data entry, and mouse, pen, or touch-screen devices for pointing. For physical components at a feature level, this means that (1) user anthropometrics are employed in defining workstation and component configurations and dimensions and (2) the physical characteristics of controls and displays (e.g., operating force, sensitivity, brightness, intensity, and size of displayed information) are congruous with the users and physical capabilities. For mental components at a task level, natural interaction means that the HCI models the user's tasks in accordance with the user's knowledge and experience. For mental components at a feature level, natural interaction means that the user's perceptual and cognitive capabilities and limitations are employed in defining HCI features (e.g., icons, names, screen layouts, and the behavior of window controls such as scroll bars). Direct manipulation interaction techniques (e.g., drag and drop) are a form of natural interaction in that they create a software mechanism with a physical analogy.

35.4.3.1.2 Simplicity of Interaction

Simplicity applies across a wide variety of design issues and must be incorporated in every architectural category. Applying this principle reduces training requirements, memory demands, perceptual demands, and the cognitive demands for inference. For the physical interface component, applying this principle reduces the number of physical steps needed to select and invoke actions and reduces movement precision requirements.

35.4.3.1.3 Consistency

Consistency reduces training and memory requirements and promotes skill development. Consistency applies across a wide variety of design issues and must be incorporated in every architectural category. Examples include object, action, and information organizations, task flows, representations for objects and actions, and procedures. TAG (Payne and Green 1986, Schiele and Green 1990) provides a formal technique for analyzing consistency.

35.4.3.1.4 Robustness

Robustness refers to the ability of the design to tolerate user error and to span the functional requirements of the user. Error tolerance reduces resources needed to recover from errors and reduces initial accuracy requirements, allowing the user to increase operating speed. Users may commit errors because of a lack of knowledge. In this case, the user may be exploring the system to learn it. These are not errors. But this type of behavior should be expected, and the design should allow the user to do this exploration and to recover from anything he or she may do. Users may commit errors because of a misunderstanding or negative transfer from other systems. Thus, a user may infer that a menu item will elicit a given behavior because it does so on another system that he or she has used. Or the user may feel that he or she understands what a given menu item or icon means and be wrong. Users may commit errors through unintentional commands. For example, a user may inadvertently click a wrong button, hit a wrong key, or select a wrong item from a menu. Ensuring adequate functional coverage reduces the functional demands on the user.

35.4.3.1.5 *Accommodation of User Capabilities*

In resource terms, applying this design principle increases the fit between an individual user's available mental and physical resources and those required by the interaction and application tasks. There are two major dimensions on which users vary: experience and capability.

Along the experience dimension, users vary between experts and novices on either the interaction or the application task. Thus, a user could be very experienced with the applied task but not with doing that task on a computer. Similarly, a user may be very used to using computers but not skilled in the applied task. Novice users will (1) need more guidance and feedback, (2) require more structure to the task, (3) rely more on memory-aiding design features (e.g., menus), and (4) benefit more from online help facilities than expert users. Expert users will (1) want more flexibility in task control, (2) want shortcut methods to do high-level actions, (3) rely more on recall rather than memory aids, and (4) benefit more from the use of preferences and tailored configurations than novice users (Brown 1988, Galitz 1993).

Along the capacity dimension users vary between healthy and impaired. In the ERM, impairments are not defined differently from any other performance or skill differences among users. All differences are defined in terms of the amount of specific performance resources available to an individual. Impaired users will vary greatly in capacity and experience. Only through an analysis of resources demanded by the task and resources available to the user can an adequate design for an impaired user be accomplished successfully.

35.4.3.2 Cognitive Walkthrough

Cognitive walkthrough is a technique for evaluating the usability of a system early in the design process. The walkthrough consists of identifying a set of activities or tasks that are to be performed and specifying the steps required for performing them using one or more designs. A group of users or designers is selected or recruited for participation.

35.4.3.3 Usability Testing

Usability testing is a method to objectively assess the ability of a product or system to be effectively used by intended users to achieve their purposes and goals. The methods generally tend toward controlled formal studies of various activities and tasks performed with medium to high fidelity prototypes or mockups of the user interface. Usability testing is conducted before user acceptance testing, meaning also before the product or system is deployed.

35.4.3.4 Remote Usability Testing

Usability testing can be expensive and it is often difficult to recruit participants. In remote testing, the test environment is made available to participants using their own connections. Two types of remote testing are moderated and unmoderated. In moderated testing, the tester is in synchronous communication with the test participant and controls the test session. In unmoderated testing, participants autonomously perform a set of tasks or activities and the system collects and stores the data for use later by the tester. Both types of testing vastly increase the participant pool. Unmoderated testing enables more flexible scheduling by the tester and participant.

35.4.3.5 Web Analytics

Web analytics refers to the collection and analysis of data on system usage passively and automatically by capturing the user's interactions as the system is being used. The data can inform business as well as design decisions. The data typically provide behavioral data from actual use and are collected across the entire population of users not a sample. Patterns from the data can be used to better organize information or structure activities on a website.

35.4.4 Agile Development Process

Traditional software development processes (e.g., Waterfall) have increasingly given way to more flexible and responsive processes. "Agile" is a development process in which system requirements are not firmly fixed but can change and evolve as the system is developed. Requirements are incorporated over time and design and development occur iteratively. Frequent meetings among all stakeholders ensure that everyone is kept informed and that dependencies among requirements and needs from business, development, test, and user communities are addressed.

The iterative structure of agile development fits well with the iteration needed for usability and user experience design. However, the piecemeal manner in which functionality is introduced into the overall system necessitates developing a concept model early to guide consistent design and define reusable interaction patterns.

35.5 HCI in Biomedical Application Areas

35.5.1 Instruments and Devices

Biomedical instruments increasingly embed computing power, and to the extent they do, the instrument's interface involves HCI. These products include simple consumer devices for home use by the general public up through complex instruments used by researchers, physicians, and other professionals (Table 35.1).

35.5.2 Robotics

Robots are becoming a part of our everyday lives (UNECE and IFR 2004). Biomedical robotics promises an exciting future in which robots will augment people's bodies with active assistive limbs and exoskeletons. Physicians will increasingly perform remote and precise surgical procedures with robots. Robots will enable professionals to deliver care through mobile telepresence and the automation of routine medical tasks. Robots will assist people in their daily lives, providing cognitive, sensory, and physical aides. Robots will give comfort and emotional support. Professionals, as well as the general public, will receive training and education from robots. In recent years, the area of *human–robot interaction* has emerged as a separate area of focus, addressing many issues that go beyond usability (Yanco et al. 2004).

35.5.3 Medical Information Systems and Bioinformatics

Advanced computing power and computational tools have made possible the collection and complex analysis of very large amount of biomedical data, contributing to improvements in healthcare and understanding of biological processes. However, in many cases, these improvements can only be realized if researchers, practitioners, and patients themselves can effectively, satisfactorily, and safely operate equipment and systems. Medicine 2.0, discussed above, promises to provide many of these improvements by the application of advanced web-based, cloud, analytic, and visualization technologies to medical informatics. Intelligent technology such as IBM's Watson will capture and distribute state-of-the-art medical expertise and knowledge, playing an integral part in medical care. Raghupathi and Tan (2002) describe the rapid growth of strategic large-scale healthcare systems that address complex organizational management and decision-making activities rather than lower level routine administrative tasks.

TABLE 35.1 Biomedical Products and Systems

System Type	Examples	Major HCI Considerations
	Instruments and Devices	
Assistive	Hearing aids	Lifestyle
Cognitive and physical augmentation	Prosthetics	Personalization
	Cognitive aids	Mobility
Monitoring, analytic, storing	Blood pressure monitors	Security, trust, accuracy,
	Blood glucose monitors	intrusiveness, personalization,
	Vital sign monitors	connectivity, information display, mobility
	Robotics	
Surgical	Precision surgery	Precise real-time feedback
	Targeted radiation therapy	Precision control, information display
Assistive and routine tasks	Dispensing medication	Workflow, reporting
	Visit scheduling	
Emotional support		Social interaction
		Empathic interaction
	Bioinformatic Systems	
Medical advice systems	Diagnostic systems	Security, trust, accuracy,
	Crowd-sourcing systems	persuasiveness, search
Medical informatics	IT systems that store analyze,	Search
	retrieve, and otherwise manage	Social network
	health-related information	Mobility
		Information architecture
		Personalization
		Information display
Hospital management information systems	Systems for managing a hospital's administrative, financial, and clinical information in an integrated manner	Information architecture Information display Search
Visualization	Imaging	Information display
	Graphics	Visual sensation and perception
	Virtual reality	Provision for different views of data
	Visual data analysis	Sharing and collaboration of visual
	Computer vision	data

35.5.4 Interaction Technologies

The applications discussed above address the interaction between humans and biomedical products and systems that use embedded and connected information technologies. However, as HCI technology develops to address new paradigms, new modes of interaction (e.g., haptics, gestures, speech, bioelectric signals, and behaviometrics) will increasingly involve biomedical factors.

For example, early results from Keates et al. (2004) suggest that haptic force feedback is very promising for providing significant interaction performance improvements for motion-impaired users. Han et al. (2002) report that a 2D force feedback device could be used to present 3D shapes using a force-shading technique, a haptic analog to bump-mapping in computer graphics. Bach-y-Rita et al. (2003) found that a system in which electrotactile stimuli were delivered to the tongue via flexible electrode arrays placed in the mouth provided a feasible means for tactile vision substitution (Table 35.2).

TABLE 35.2   Emerging Interaction Technologies

Interaction Technology	Examples	Enablement
Haptics	Touch screens Joysticks Data gloves	Enables users to communicate with touch and obtain information in the form of felt sensations
Biosignal–ocular–gaze	EOG	Enables users to communicate and control with eye direction
Biosignal–muscular–gesture	EMG	Enables users to communicate and control with muscle movements and gestures
Biosignal–brain	EEG	Enables communication and control with brain signal patterns. Used in the expanding field of brain–computer interfaces
Biometric–physiological	Fingerprint, voice identification, corneal topography	Enables user identification via physiological signatures
Biometric–behavioral (behaviometric)	Behavioral patterns of interaction, such as key sequences, mouse movements, gestures, and microexpressions (facial muscle movement patterns)	Enables user identification via behavioral signatures. Can also be used to infer mood

Defining Terms

Activity-centered design (ACD): Activity-centered design refers to a philosophy of human–machine system design that places the focus of the design process on the activities being performed, the purposes of those activities, and the context in which they are performed.

Application task: Refers to the objectives the user is employing the product to accomplish. In this regard, it is akin to the activity that is the focus in ACD.

Holistic design: A nonisolationist approach to design that considers the impact and influences of the social and organizational contexts, high-level purposes, and other seemingly external factors on the product or system being designed.

Human-centered design (HCD): Human-centered design refers to a philosophy of human–machine system design that places the focus of the design process on the needs of the human who uses the system to accomplish a task.

Interaction task: Refers to the activities that the user performs to use the product (e.g., moving a mouse device, typing keyboard inputs, viewing displays, searching for and managing files, managing displays, setting preferences, and executing programs).

Usability: Usability is a multidimensional quality that affords the user practical and convenient interaction with the product for achieving applied objectives. The concept of usability is fundamental to the design of any human system.

User experience: A broad concept that encompasses the impressions, observations, and emotional responses as well as the perceptual-motor and cognitive demands and delights that a user undergoes and encounters while using a product or system in a real-world context of use.

References

Abowd G. D. and Mynatt E. D. 2002 Charting past, present, and future research in ubiquitous computing, In: *Human-Computer Interaction in the New Millennium*, ed. J. M. Carroll, 513–535. New York: ACM Press.

Bach-y-Rita, P., Tyler, M. E., and Kaczmarek, K. A. 2003. Seeing with the brain. *International Journal of Human-Computer Interaction*, 15: 287–297.

Bental, D. and Cawsey, A. 2002. Personalized and adaptive systems for medical consumer applications. *Communications of the ACM* 45: 5.

Booch, G., Rumbaughand, J., and Jacobson, I. 1999. *The Unified Modeling Language User Guide*. Reading, MA: Addison-Wesley.

Brown, C. M. 1988. *Human-Computer Interface Design Guidelines*. Norwood, NJ: Ablex Publishing.

Card, S. K., Moran, T. P., and Newell, A. 1983. *The Psychology of Human-Computer Interaction*. Hillsdale, NJ: Erlbaum.

Card, S. K., Moran, T. P., and Newell, A. 1986. The model human processor: An engineering model of human performance. *Handbook of Perception and Human Performance. Vol. 2: Cognitive Processes and Performance*, ed. K. R. Boff, L. Kaufman and J. P. Thomas, 1–35. New York: Wiley.

Carroll, J. M. 2000. *Making Use: Scenario-Based Design of Human-Computer Interactions*. Cambridge, MA: MIT Press.

Carroll, J. M. and Rosson, M.B. 2007. Participatory design in community infomatics. *Design Studies*, Special Issue on Participatory Design, 28, 243–261.

Cavazza, M. and Simo, A. 2003. *A Virtual Patient Based on Qualitative Simulation*. IUI'03, January 12–15, Miami, FL.

Cooper, A. 2004. *The Inmates Are Running the Asylum. Why High-Tech Products Drive Us Crazy* (second edition). Indianapolis, IN: Sams Publishing.

Darnell, M. J. Bad human factors designs. http://www.baddesigns.com/.

Dourish, P. 2001. *Where the Action Is: The Foundations of Embodied Interaction*. Cambridge, MA: MIT Press.

Fogg, B. J. 2003. *Persuasive Technology*. San Francisco, CA: Morgan Kaufmann.

Forlizzi, J. and DiSalvo, C. 2006. Service robots in the domestic environment: A study of the Roomba vacuum in the home. In *Proceedings of the 1st ACM SIGCHI/SIGART Conference on Human-Robot Interaction*, HRI'06, Salt Lake City, 2–4 March, 258–256. New York: ACM.

Forlizzi, J., DiSalvo, C., and Gemperle, F. 2004. Assistive robots and an ecology of elders living independently in their homes. *Human-Computer Interaction* 19:1,2.

Galitz, W. O. 1993. *User-Interface Screen Design*. Boston: QED Publishing Group.

Hakula, J. 2009. The Purola model and the holistic concept of man metaphor as bases for the networked view of decision-making in eHealth and eWelfare. *Finnish Journal of eHealth and eWelfare*, 1: 2.

Han, H., Yamashita, J., and Fujishiro, I. 2002. 3D haptic shape perception using a 2D device. *ACM SIGGRAPH*, 135.

ISO 9241-11. 1998. *Ergonomic Requirements for Office Work with Visual Display Terminals (VDTs) Part 11: Guidance on Usability*. International Organization for Standardization. Washington D.C.: Distributed by the American National Standards Institute.

ISO 13407. 1999. *Human-Entered Design Processes for Interactive Systems*. International Organization for Standardization. Washington D.C.: Distributed by the American National Standards Institute.

Javahery, H., Seffah, A., and Radhakrishnan, T. 2004. Beyond power: Making bioinformatics tools user-centered. *Communications of the ACM* 47:11.

Kaptelinin, V. and Nardi, B. A. 2006. *Acting with Technology*. Cambridge MA: MIT Press.

Keates, S., Clarkson, P. J., and Robinson, P. 2004. *Computer Assistance for Motion-Impaired Users*. Cambridge Engineering Design Centre. http://wwwedc.eng.cam.ac.uk/inclusivedesign/computeraccess/

Kieras, D. E. 1988. Towards a practical GOMS model methodology for user interface design. In: *Handbook of Human-Computer Interaction*, ed. M. Helander, 135–157. New York: Elsevier Science Publishers.

Kondraske, G. V. 1995. A working model for human-system-task interfaces. *The Biomedical Engineering Handbook*, ed. J. D. Bronzino, 2157–2174. Boca Raton, FL: CRC Press.

Kramer, J., Noronha, S., and Vergo, J. 2000. A user-centered design approach to personalization. *Communications of the ACM* 43: 8.

Leroy, G., Chen, H., Martinez J. D. et al. 2003. Genescene: Biomedical text and data mining. Information retrieval and data mining. *JCDL'03: Proceedings of the 3rd ACM/IEEE-CS Joint Conference on Digital Libraries.* 116–118.

Maxwell, K. 2002. The maturation of HCI: Moving beyond usability toward holistic interaction. In: *Human-Computer Interaction in the New Millennium,* ed. J. M. Carroll 191–209. New York: ACM Press.

Miller, C. S. and Remington, R. W. 2004. Modeling information navigation: Implications for information architecture. *Human-Computer Interaction.* 19: 3.

Nielsen, J. and Mack, R. L. eds. 1994. *Usability Inspection Methods.* New York, NY: John Wiley & Sons.

Norman, D. A. 1998. *The Invisible Computer.* Cambridge, MA: MIT Press.

Norman, D. A. 2004. *Emotional Design.* Cambridge, MA: Basic Books, Dept. of Perseus Book Group.

Park, S., O'Brien, M. A., Caine, K. E. et al. 2006. Acceptance of computer technology: Understanding the user and the organizational characteristics, *Proceedings of the Human Factors and Ergonomics Society 50th Annual Meeting.*

Payne, S. J. and Green, T. 1986. Task-action grammars: A model of mental representation of task languages. *Human-Computer Interaction* 2: 93.

Raghupathi, W. and Tan, J. 2002. Strategic IT applications in health care. *Communications of the ACM* 45: 12.

Rogers, W. A., Mykityshyn, A., Cambell, R. H. et al. 2001. Analysis of a "simple" medical device. *Ergonomics in Design* 9:1.

Rohrer, C. 2011. Barriers to holistic design solutions, UXmatters. http://uxmatters.com/mt/archives/2011/01/barriers-to-holistic-design-solutions.php.

Rosson, M. B. 1999. Integrating development of task and object models. *Communications of the ACM* 42: 1.

Schiele, F. and Green, T. 1990. HCI formalisms and cognitive psychology: The case of task-action grammar. *Formal Methods in Human-Computer Interaction,* eds. M. Harrison and H. Thimbleby, 9–62. Cambridge, UK: Cambridge University Press.

Shneiderman, B. 2002. *Leonardo's Laptop.* Cambridge, MA: MIT Press.

Smith, A. 2011. *Smartphone Adoption and Usage.* Pew Internet & American Life Project, Pew Research Center. http://www.pewinternet.org/Reports/2011/Smartphones.aspx.

Streitz, N. A., Tandler, P., Muller-Tomfelde, C. et al. 2002. Roomware: Toward the next generation of human-computer interaction based on an integrated design of real and virtual worlds. *Human-Computer Interaction in the New Millennium,* ed. J. M. Carroll, 553–578. ACM Press, New York.

Tullis, T. and Albert, B. 2008. *Measuring the User Experience.* Amsterdam: Elsevier.

UNECE and IFR. 2004. *United Nations Economic Commission for Europe and the International Federation of Robotics: World Robotics.* New York and Geneva: United Nations.

US Dept. of Health and Human Services. *Federal Drug Administration. Draft Guidance for Industry and Food and Drug Administration Staff—Mobile Medical Applications,* July 21, 2011. http://www.fda.gov/MedicalDevices/DeviceRegulationandGuidance/GuidanceDocuments/ucm263280.htm.

Vanharanta, H. and Salminen, T. 2007. Holistic interaction between the computer and the active human being. In: *Human-Computer Interaction: Interaction Design and Usability,* 12th International Conference, HCI International, Beijing, China, ed. J. A. Jacko, 252–261. New York: Springer.

Yanco, H. A., Drury, J. L., and Sholtz, J. 2004. Beyond usability evaluation: Analysis of human-robot interaction at a major robotics competition. *Human-Computer Interaction* 19: 1,2.

Young, J. E., Sung, J., Voida, A. et al. 2011. Evaluating human-robot interaction: Focusing on the holistic interaction experience. *International Journal of Social Robotics* 3: 53–67.

Further Information

Human-centered design: http://www.upassoc.org/usability_resources/about_usability/what_is_ucd.html

Usability standards: http://www.upassoc.org/usability_resources/guidelines_and_methods/standards.html
Usability methods: http://www.usability.gov/; http://usabilitynet.org/tools/methods.htm

General Information

Association for Computing Machinery, Special Interest Group in Computer-Human Interaction
    (ACM SIGCHI): http://www.acm.org/sigchi/
HCI Bibliography, suggested readings: http://www.hcibib.org/readings.html
Human Factors and Ergonomics Society: http://www.hfes.org/
Industrial Design Society of America: http://www.idsa.org/
Usability Net: http://usabilitynet.org
Usability Professionals' Association: http://www.upassoc.org/

36

Applications of Human Performance Measurements to Clinical Trials to Determine Therapy Effectiveness and Safety

Pamela J. Hoyes Beehler
University of Texas, Arlington

Karl Syndulko
UCLA School of Medicine

A *clinical trial* is a research study involving human subjects and an intervention (i.e., device, drug, surgical procedure, or other procedure) that is ultimately intended to either enhance the professional capabilities of physicians (i.e., improve the service delivered), improve the quality of life of patients, or contribute to the field of knowledge in those sciences which are traditionally in the medical field setting—for example, physiology, anatomy, pharmacology, epidemiology, neurology, cognitive psychology, etc. (Levin, 1986). Clinical trials research is in the business of evaluating therapeutic interventions intended to benefit humans. Its value is directly related to the relevance of the questions "Do our treatments work?" "How well do our treatments work?" and "Are our treatments safe?" For example, drug *A* is designed and anticipated to relieve sinus congestion. Is there a drug interaction when drug *A* is taken with drug *B* and/or moderate levels of alcohol consumption such that while congestion is relieved (i.e., drug *A* is effective), human information processing capacities are reduced (i.e., is drug *A* safe?). And what is the time course of effects with regard to positive and negative (or adverse) effects? Thus it is clear that not only steady-state issues buy also dynamic questions are on interest in clinical trials research.

While clinical trials research incorporates many different components, the focus of this chapter is limited to study questions associated with human *performance capacity* variables and their measurement as they contribute to the determination of therapy effectiveness and safety. Such variables have been incorporated into trials since the use of controlled studies in the medical field began. However, the methodology employed to address human performance variables has been slowly but steadily shifting from mostly subjective to more objective instrumented methods (e.g., Tourtellotte et al., 1965) as both the understanding of the phenomena at play and the demand for improved quality of studies have increased. This chapter begins by briefly examining a classification of typical clinical trials study models, presents a summary of methods employed and key methodologic issues in both the design and conduct of studies (with special emphasis on issues related to the selection of measures and interpretation of results), and ends with a walk-through of a typical example that demonstrates the methods described. Brief discussion of the benefits that can be attributed to the use of objective, instrumented measures of human performance capacities as well as their current limitations in clinical trials research is also presented. While it is emphasized that most methods and issues addressed are applicable to any intervention, the use of human performance variables in pharmaceutical clinical trials has been most prevalent, and special attention has been given here to this application.

36.1 Basic Principles: Types of Studies

Depending on the set of primary and secondary questions to be addressed, considerable variety can exist with respect to the structure of a given trial and the analysis that is performed. Within the focus and scope of this chapter, clinical trials are classified into two categories for discussion: (1) safety-oriented and (2) efficacy-oriented. According to the Food and Drug Administration (FDA) (1977), four phases of research studies are required before a drug can be marketed in the United States. Phase I is known as *clinical pharmacology* and is intended to include the initial introduction of a drug into humans. These studies are safety-oriented; one issue often addressed is determination of the maximum tolerable dose. Phases II and III are known as *clinical investigation* and *clinical trials*, respectively, consisting of controlled and uncontrolled clinical trials research. Phase IV is the *postmarketing of clinical trials* to supplement premarketing data. Both safety and efficacy are addressed in phases II to IV investigations. As specified earlier, not all interventions studied are drugs. However, a similar phased approach is also characteristic of the investigation of therapeutic devices and treatments.

Safety-oriented trials usually involve vital sign measures (e.g., heart rate, blood pressure, respiration rate), clinical laboratory tests (e.g., blood chemistries, urinalysis, ECG), and adverse reaction tests (both mental and physical performance capacities) to evaluate the risk of the intervention. In this chapter we focus on the adverse reaction components, most of which historically have been addressed with subjective reporting methods. In the case of drug interventions, different doses (e.g., small to large) are administered within the trial, and the dose-related effects are examined. Thus the rate at which a drug is metabolized (*pharmacokinetics*), as evidenced by changes in drug concentrations in blood, cerebral spinal fluid, urine, etc., is usually addressed in safety-oriented drug studies, as well as the maximum dosage which subjects can tolerate (Baker et al., 1985; Fleiss, 1986; Tudiver et al., 1992; Jennison and Turnbull, 1993).

Efficacy-oriented trials are usually conducted after initial safety-oriented trials have established that the intervention has met safety criteria, but they will always have safety questions and elements as well. In this type of study, the goal is to objectively determine the therapeutic effect. Whatever the type of intervention, these studies are designed around the bottom-line question "Is the intervention effective?" In many cases (e.g., drugs for neurologic disorders, exercise programs for musculoskeletal injuries, etc.), *effectiveness* implies improvement or retarding the rate of deterioration in one or more aspects of mental and/or physical performance. With regard to disease contexts, it is necessary to distinguish performance changes that merely reflect treatment of systems as opposed to those which reflect the slowing or reversal of the basic disease process. Studies typically include pre- and postintervention measurement points and, whenever feasible, a control group that is administered a placebo intervention (Fleiss, 1986; Weissman, 1991; Tang and Geller, 1993). The situation is complicated because there are many performance capacities that could be affected. In response to the intervention, some capacities may improve, some may remain unchanged, and some may be adversely affected. Thus efficacy-oriented studies typically include a number of secondary questions that address specificity of effects. When the intervention is a drug, both the pharmacokinetics and *pharmacodynamics* are often addressed. Pharmacodynamic studies attempt to relate physiologic and/or metabolic changes in the concentration of the agent over time to corresponding changes in the therapeutic effect. Thus repeated measurement of selected performance capacities are required over relatively short periods of time as part of these *protocols*.

Clinical trials involving human performance metrics generally use the *randomized clinical trial* (RCT) design. The RCT is a way to compare the efficacy and safety of two or more therapies or regimens. It was originally designed to test new drugs (Hill, 1963); however, over the last 25 years, it has been applied to the study of vaccinations, surgical interventions, and even social innovations such as multiphasic screening (Levin, 1986). Levin (1986) describes four key elements of RCTs: (1) the trials are "controlled," that is, part of the group of subjects receive a therapy that is tested while the other subjects receive either no therapy or another therapy; (2) the significance of its results must be established through statistical analysis; (3) a double-blind experimental design should be used whenever possible; and (4) the therapies being compared should be allocated among the subjects randomly. Levin (1986) further noted that "the RCT is the gold standard for evaluating therapeutic efficacy."

36.2 Methods

Studies are defined and guided by *protocols*, a detailed statement of all procedures and methods to be employed. Figure 36.1 summarizes the major steps in clinical trials in which human performance

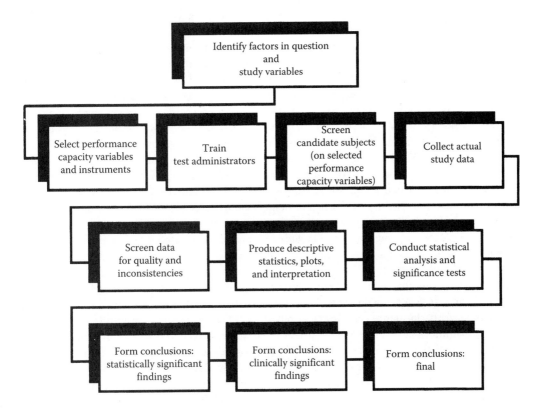

FIGURE 36.1 Summary of major steps in the conduct of a clinical trial involving human performance capacities.

variables represent those of primary interest, although the general process is similar for most trial involving human subjects.

36.2.1 Selecting Study Variables

In many clinical trials, performance measurements must be focused on the specific disease or set of symptoms against which a medication or intervention is directed. The critical element is selection of an outcome assessment that will indicate directly whether the intervention can eliminate key signs or symptoms of the disease, improve function affected by the disease, or even simply delay further disease progression and loss of function. Economic and statistical constraints of such trials often indicate that a minimal set of measures must be used to provide valid, reliable, and sensitive indicators of changes in underlying disease activity related to the treatments. In many instances, there is considerable controversy about what constitutes a valid and reliable assessment of the underlying disease process, or there may be de facto standards adopted by clinicians, pharmaceutical companies, and the FDA as to the choice of outcome assessments. In many diseases, these standards may be physician rating scales of disease severity. Thus objective studies may be required in the case of specific diseases and disorders to delineate the most sensitive set of performance measures for clinical trial evaluations (Mohr and Prouwers, 1991). Further, it often must be demonstrated to clinicians, drug companies, and the FDA that the objective performance measures selected as outcome assessments actually do provide equal or more sensitive indicators of disease progression (and improvement) than do existing rating scale measures traditionally utilized in clinical trials. Experience with human performance testing in multiple sclerosis clinical trials, discussed below, illustrates these issues.

When objective measurement of performance capacities has been incorporated into many clinical trials, concepts and tools from human performance engineering can facilitate the selection of variables and shed some light on issues noted above. In either safety- or efficacy-oriented studies, study variable selection can be characterized as a two-step process: (1) identification of the factors in question (Table 36.1) and (2) selection of the relevant *performance capacities* to be measured and associated measurement instruments. This link between these two steps often represents a challenge to researchers for a number of reasons. First, duality in terminology must be overcome. Concerns about an intervention are typically initially identified with "negative" terms such as "dizziness" and not in terms of performance capacities such as "postural stability." Human performance models based on systems engineering concepts (Kondraske, 1995) can be used to facilitate the translation of both formal and lay terms used to identify adverse effects to relevant performance capacities to be measured, as shown in Table 36.1.

In Kondraske's (1995) model, performance capacities are modeled as resources that a given system possesses and draws up to perform tasks. It also provides a basis for delineation of *hierarchical* human systems and their performance capacities as well as a basis to quantitatively explain the interaction of available performance capacities with demands of higher-level tasks (e.g., such as those encountered in daily living). The hierarchical aspect is particularly important in selecting performance capacities to be measured. It is generally good practice to include a combination of carefully selected lower-level and higher-level capacity measures. This combination allows careful tradeoffs between information content (i.e., specificity) and simplicity of the protocol (e.g., number of variables, time for test administration, etc.). Higher-level capacities (characterizing systems responsible for gait, postural stability, complex mental task, etc.) are dependent on the performance capacities of multiple lower-level subsystems. Thus a few higher-level performance capacities can reflect multiple lower-level capacities (e.g., knee flexor strength, visual information processing speed, etc.). However, lower-level capacity measures are typically less variable than higher-level capacities within individuals (i.e., on retest) and within populations. Therefore, small changes in performance can be more readily discriminated statistically if they exist and are attributable primarily to localized lower-level capacities (e.g., see data in Potvin et al. (1985)). Also, more specific information can provide valuable insights into physiologic effects if they are present. By combining both types, broad coverage can be achieved (so that aspects of human performance

TABLE 36.1 Representative Examples of Linking Factors in Question to Specific Measurable Performance Capacities

Factor in Question[a]	Selected Relevant Performance Capacities[b]
General central nervous system effects (of drug)	Selected activity of daily living execution speed
	Postural stability
	Upper extremity neuromotor channel capacity
	Manual manipulation speed
	Visual-upper extremity information processing speed
	Visual attention span
	Visual-spatial memory capacity
	Visual-numerical memory capacity
Alcohol interaction (of drug)	Selected activity of daily living execution speed
	Postural stability
	Visual information processing speed
	Visual–spatial memory capacity
Dizziness	Postural stability
Drowsiness	Selected activity of daily living execution speed
	Visual attention span
	Visual-upper extremity information procession speed
	Bond–Lader visual analog scale
Slowness of movement, psychomotor retardation	Visual-upper extremity information processing speed
	Upper extremity random reach movement speed
	Index finger (proximal intercarpal phalangeal joint), flexion–extension speed
Mood	Emotional stability (e.g., with Hamilton anxiety scale, Bond–Lader analog scale and other similar tools)
Speed	Reaction time
Coordination	Finger tapping
Tremors, abnormal movements	Limb steadiness
	Postural stability
	Vocal amplitude and pitch steadiness
Joint stiffness or pain	Extremes and range of motion
	Isomeric strength (selected joins)
Weakness, strength	Postural stability (one leg, eyes open)
	Isometric grip strength
	Isometric strength (representative set of upper and lower extremity, proximal and distal muscle groups)
Sensation	Vibration sensitivity
	Thermal sensitivity

[a] Terms used include those often used by pharmaceutical companies to communicate adverse effects to general public.

[b] Lists are illustrative and not exhaustive. More or fewer items can be included depending on time available or willingness to expend for data collection, with commensurate tradeoffs between specificity and protocol simplicity.

in which the expectation of an effect is less remain included), as well as a degree of specificity, while keeping the total number of study variables to a reasonable size. In addition, if an effect is found in both a higher-level capacity and a related lower-level capacity, an internal cross-validation of finding is obtained. Many earlier studies incorporated variables representing looks across different hierarchical levels but did not distinguish them by level during analysis and interpretation. While such logic begins to remove the guesswork, much work remains to refine variable-selection methodology.

To address the broad, bottom-line questions regarding safety and efficacy, the formation of *composite scores* (i.e., some combination of scores from two or more performance capacity challenges or "tests") is necessary. A resource model and the concept of hierarchical human systems also can be used to develop composite variables for practical use in clinical trials. Component capacities can be selected that are theoretically or empirically most sensitive to the disease or condition under study. The composite variable is then created by calculating a more traditional weighted arithmetic sum (Potvin et al., 1985) or product (Kondraske, 1989) of the component scores. In both cases, the definition of component scores is important (i.e., whether a smaller or larger number represents better performance). Treatments are not approved if only a small subset of individuals is helped. Composite measures provide the only objective means of integrating multidimensional information about an intervention's effects. The primary advantages of the composite variable are the creation of a single, global, succinct measure of the disease, condition, or intervention, which is often essential as the primary outcome assessment for efficacy. The major disadvantage is loss of detailed information about the unique profile of performance changes that each subject of a group as a whole may show. Such tradeoffs are to be expected. Thus both composite and component measures play important but different roles in clinical trials.

It is imperative that the selection of the study measures also consider a test's objectivity (nonbiased), reliability (consistency), and validity (measures what is intends to measure) to add to the quality of the measurements. Many complex issues, which are beyond the present scope, are associated with measuring and interpreting the quality of a measurement. (See Safrit (1990), Baumgartner and Jackson (1993), and Hastad and Lacy (1994) for more information.)

36.2.2 Formation of the Subject Pool

Clinical research investigations usually involve a *sample* group of subjects from a defined population. Selection of the study population so that generalizations from that sample accurately reflect the defined population is a dilemma that must be adequately addressed. If *probability sampling* is chosen, each subject in the defined population theoretically has an equal chance of being included in the sample. The advantage of this kind of sampling is that differences between treatment groups can be detected and the probability that these differences actually exist may be estimated. If *nonprobability sampling* is chosen, there is no way to ensure that each subject had an equal chance of being included in the sample. Conclusions of nonprobability sampling therefore have less merit (not as generalizable) than those based on probability sampling.

Studies with healthy subjects are believed to be necessary before exposing sick persons to some interventions because persons with disease or injuries commonly have impaired function of various organs that metabolize drugs and may take medications that can alter the absorption, metabolism, and/or excretion rates of the intervention. Gender issues also should be a concern in clinical trials because of new FDA regulations (Cotton, 1993; Merkatz et al., 1993; Stone, 1993).

All subjects selected as study candidates should be informed of the procedures that will be utilized in the clinical trials investigation by signing an informed consent document, as required by the Department of Health and Human Services *Code of Federal Regulations* (1985) and other federal regulations applicable to research involving human subjects. Using all or a subset of study measurement variables (in addition to medical history and examinations as necessary), a screening procedure is recommended to determine if each subject meets the minimum performance criteria established for subject inclusion. When patients are part of the sample group, this performance screening also can be used to establish that the sample includes the desired balance of subjects with different amounts of "room for improvement" on relevant variables. An added benefit of this screening process is that subjects and test administrators obtain experience with test protocols, equipment, an procedures that will add to the validity of the study.

Unless available from a previous similar study, it is typical for pilot data to be collected to estimate the expected size of outcome effects. With this information, the power of the statistical analysis (i.e., the likelihood that a significant difference will be detected) can be estimated so that sample size can be determined (Cochran and Cox, 1957; Kepple, 1982; Fleiss, 1986). Another concern is that some of the original subject pool will not complete the study or will have incomplete data. High attrition rates may damage the credibility of the study, and every effort should be made to not lose subjects. DeAngelis (1990) estimates that attrition rates higher than 50% make the interpretation of clinical trial research very difficult. Some researchers believe that no attempt should be made to replace these subjects because even random selection of new subjects will not ensure bias caused by differential participation of all the subjects.

36.2.3 Data Collection

Investigators should seek to minimize sources of variability by careful control of the test conditions and procedures. Proper control can be attained by (1) using rooms that are reasonably soundproof or sound-deadened, well lighted, and of a comfortable temperature; (2) selecting chairs and other accessories carefully (e.g., no wheels for tests in which the subject is seated); (3) testing subjects one at a time without other subjects in the test room; (4) using standardized written instructions for each test to eliminate variability in what is stated; (5) allowing for familiarization with the test instruments and procedures; (6) not commenting about subject performance to avoid biased raising or lowering of expectations; (7) arranging a test order to offset fatigue (mental and physical) or boredom and to include rest periods; and (8) training test administrators and evaluating their training using healthy subjects, especially in multicenter studies, so that consistent results can be obtained.

36.2.4 Data Integrity Screening

Despite all good efforts and features incorporated to ensure high-quality data, opportunities exist for error. It is therefore beneficial to subject data obtained during formal test sessions to quality screenings. This is a step toward forming the official study data set (i.e., the set that will be subjected to statistical and other analyses). Several independent analyses used to screen data, which are typically computer-automated, are described below.

Screening of baseline measures against inclusionary criteria: If human performance study variables with specific performance criteria are used as part of the subject selection process as recommended above, each subject's baseline score can be compared with the score obtained during inclusionary testing. For most variables, baseline scores should not differ from inclusionary testing by more than 20% (Potvin et al., 1985). Greater deviations point to examiner training, test procedure, or subject compliance problems.

Screening against established norms: For variables that are not included in inclusionary screenings or in studies where performance variables are not used as part of the subjects inclusionary criteria, baseline data can be screened against established reference data (e.g., human performance means and standard deviations). Data are considered acceptable if they fall within an established range (e.g., two standard deviation units of the reference population mean). From the perspective of risk associated with not identifying a data point that could be a potential problem, this is a fairly liberal standard that can still identify problems in data collection and management. Standards that lessen risk can, or course, be employed at the discretion of the investigator, but at the expense of the possible identification of a larger number of data points that require follow-up.

Screening against anticipated effects: It is more difficult to screen nonbaseline data for quality because of the possible influences of the intervention. However, criteria can be established based on (1) absolute level of variables (both maximums and minimums) and (2) rates and direction of change from one measurement period to the next. Even criteria that allow a rather wide range of data (or changes across repeated measures) can be useful in detecting gross anomalies and is recommended.

If anomalies are discovered using the screening methods described above, several outcomes are possible: (1) the anomaly can be traced and rectified (e.g., it may be attributable to a human or computer error with backup available); (2) the anomaly may be explainable as a procedural error, but it may not be possible to rectify; and (3) the anomaly may be unexplainable. Data anomalies that are explainable with supporting documentation could justify classification of the given data items as "missing data" or replacement of all data for the corresponding subject in the data set (i.e., the subject could be dropped from the study and replaced with another). There is no justification for eliminating or replacing data anomalies for which a documentable explanation does not exist.

36.2.5 Analysis and Interpretation of Results

Traditional inferential statistical analysis should be performed according to the statistical model and significance levels agreed on by the clinical research team when the study is designed. However, data also should be analyzed and interpreted from a clinical perspective as well.

In experimental research, tests of *statistical significance* are the most commonly used tools for assessing possible associations between independent and dependent variables as well as differences among treatment groups. The purpose of significance (i.e., statistical) tests is to evaluate the research hypothesis at a specific level of probability, or p value. For example, if a p value of .05 was chosen, the researcher is asking if the levels of treatment (for example) differ significantly so that these differences are not attributable to a chance occurrence more than 5 times out of 100. By convention, a p value of .01 (1%) or .05 (5%) is usually selected as the cutoff for statistical significance. Significance tests cannot accept a research hypothesis; all that significance tests can do is reject or fail to reject the research hypothesis (Thomas and Nelson, 1990). Ultimately, significance tests can determine if treatment groups are different, but not why they are different. Good experimental design, appropriate theorizing, and sound reasoning are used to explain why treatment groups differ.

Exclusive reliance on tests of statistical significance in the present context can mislead the clinical researcher, and interpretation of *clinical significance* is required. The key issue here is the size of the observed effect; p values give little information on the actual magnitude of a finding (i.e., decrement or improvement in performance, etc.). Also, statistical findings are partially a function of sample size. Thus even an effect that is small in size can be detected with tests of statistical significance in a study with a large sample. For example, a mean difference in grip strength of 2 kg may be found in response to drug therapy. This difference is a quite small fraction of the variability in grip strength observed across normal individuals, however. Thus, although statistically significant, such a change would perhaps have a minimal impact on an individual's ability to function in daily activities which make demands on grip strength performance resources. Thus clinical significance addresses cause-and-effect relationships between study variables and performance in activities of daily life or other broad considerations such as the basic disease process. The danger of not defining clinical significance appropriately can be either that a good intervention is not used in practice (e.g., it may be rejected for a safety finding that is statistically significant but small) or that a poor intervention is allowed into practice (e.g., it may result in statistically significant improvements that are small).

Ideally, if empirical data existed that established what amount of a given performance capacity such as visual information processing speed (VIPS) was necessary to perform a task (e.g., driving safely on the highway), then it would be possible to interpret statistically significant findings (e.g., a decrement in VIPS of a known amount) to determine if the change would be a magnitude that would limit the individual from successfully accomplishing the given task. Unfortunately, while general cause–effect relationships between laboratory-measured capacities and performance in high-level tasks are evident, quantitative models do not yet exist, and completely objective interpretations of clinical significance are not yet possible. As such, the process by which clinical significance is determined is less well developed and structured. More recent concepts introduced by Kondraske (1988a,b, 1989) based on the use of *resource economic* principles (i.e., the idea of a threshold "cost" associated with lower-level variables typically employed in clinical trials for achieving a given level of human performance in any given high-level task) may be helpful in defining objective criteria for clinical significance. This approach directly addresses cause-and-effect relationships between performance capacities and high-level tasks with an approach much like that which an engineer would employ to design a system capable of performing a specified task.

Despite known limitations, interpretation of clinical significance is always incorporated into clinical trials in some fashion. Any change in human performance for a given variable should be first documented to be statistically significant before it is considered to be a candidate for clinical significance (i.e., a statistically significant difference is a necessary but not a sufficient condition for clinical significance). Objective determination of clinical significance can be based in part on previous methods introduced by Potvin et al. (1985) in clinical trials involving neuromotor and central processing performance tests. They advocate the use of an objective criteria whereby a decrease or increase in a human performance capacity (with healthy test subjects, for example) should be greater than 20% to be classified as "clinically significant." Kondraske (1989) uses a similar approach that uses z-scores (i.e., number of standard deviation units form a population mean) as the basis for determining criteria. This accounts for population variability which is different for different performance capacity variables. A recent approach is to assess effect size, a statistical metric that is independent of sample size and which takes into account data variability. This method provides an objective basis for comparison of the magnitude of treatment effects among studies (Cohen, 1988; Ottenbacher and Barrett, 1991).

36.3 Representative Application Examples

36.3.1 Safety-Oriented Example: Drug–Alcohol Interaction

In this section, selected elements of an actual clinical trial are presented to further illustrate methods and issues noted above. To maintain confidentialities, the drug under test is simple denoted as drug *A*.

Identify factors in question: Upper respiratory infections are among the most frequent infections encountered in clinical practice and affect all segments of the general population. The pharmacologic agent of choice for upper respiratory infections are the antihistamines (reference drug), which possess a wide margin of safety and almost no lethality when taken alone in an overdose attempt. Although quite effective, antihistamines can produce several troublesome side effects (i.e., general CNS impairment, sedation, and drowsiness) and have been incriminated in automobile accidents as well as public transportation disasters. New drugs (e.g., drug *A*) are being developed to have similar benefits but fewer side effects. From prior animal studies, drug *A* has been shown to have minimal effects on muscle relaxation and muscular coordination as well as less sedative and alcohol-potentiating effects than those associated with classical antihistamines. Based on drug *A*'s history and concerns, the following factors in question were identified in this clinical trial: general CNS impairment, alcohol interaction, dizziness, drowsiness, mood, and slowness of movement/speed. The purpose of this investigation was to examine the effect of drug *A* on human performance capacity relative to a reference drug and placebo as well as the drug–alcohol potentiating interaction effects after multiple dose treatment.

Select performance capacity variables and instruments: With the factors in question identified, the following performance capacity variables and their testing instruments were selected for the clinical trial: visual information processing speed (VIPS), finger tapping speed (TS), visual arm lateral reach coordination (VALRC), visual spatial memory capacity (VSMC), postural performance (PP), digit symbol substitution task (DSST), and Bond-Lader Visual Analog Scale (BLS). These variables were collectively called the *human performance capacity test battery* (HPCTB) (Table 36.2). Due to space limitations, only one performance capacity variable (VMRS—visual information processing speed, i.e., VIPS) is discussed in this section.

Experimental design: The first primary objective of this investigation was to examine after 8 days of oral dosing the relative effects of drug *A*, reference drug, and placebo on the human performance capacity of healthy male and female adult volunteers (see Table 36.2). This effect was determined by examining the greatest decrease in human performance capacity from day 1 of testing (i.e., baseline at −0.5 h drug ingestion time) to day 8 of testing at drug ingestion times of 0.0, 1.0, 2.0, 4.0, and 6.0 h.

TABLE 36.2 Experimental Schedule for Human Performance Capacity Test Battery (HPCTB)

	Drug Ingestion Times (h)					
Test day	−0.5	0.0	1.0	2.0	4.0	6.0
1[a]	HPCTB					
8[b]		HPCTB	HPCTB	HPCTB	HPCTB	HPCTB
9[b,c]		HPCTB	HPCTB	HPCTB	HPCTB	HPCTB

Note: The human performance capacity test battery (HPCTB) was administered in the following order: VIPS, TS, VALRC, VSMC, PP, DSST, and BLS.

[a] On day 1 of testing only, the −0.5 HPCTB was performed and utilized as the baseline value for test days 8 and 9.

[b] The peak effect was determined by comparing baseline values (day 1) against the greatest detriment in performance for the eighth and ninth testing days at drug ingestion times of 0.0, 1.0, 2.0, 4.0, and 6.0 h.

[c] On day 9 of testing, an alcohol drink was served immediately after drug administration and was ingested over a 15-min period.

The second primary objective was to examine after 9 days of oral dosing the relative effects of drug A, reference drug, and placebo in combination with a single dose of alcohol served immediately after drug administration (male alcohol dose 0.85 g/kg body weight, female alcohol dose 0.75 g/kg body weight) on the human performance capacity of healthy male and female adult volunteers (see Table 36.2). This effect was determined by comparing the greatest decrease in performance on the ninth day of study drug treatment (at drug ingestion times of 0.0, 1.0, 2.0, 4.0, and 6.0 h) to baseline on day one of testing (−0.5 h drug ingestion time) for the HPCTB (see Table 36.2). Independent variables were treatment group (1 = drug A, 2 = reference drug, and 3 = placebo) and gender (male/female). The dependent variable was maximum decrease in performance (peak effect) for each human performance capacity study variable and was determined by comparing the baseline value (day 1) against the greatest decrease in performance at drug ingestion times of 0.0, 1.0, 2.0, 4.0, and 6.0 h for day 8 and day 9 of testing. Inferential statistical analysis of the data was performed using a 3 (treatment group: reference drug, drug A, and placebo) by 5 (hour; 0, 1, 2, 4, and 6) mixed factorial ANOVA with repeated measures on hour for each dependent variable. Statistical tests of significance of all ANOVAs were conducted at the 0.05 level.

Data screening: For each dependent variable, baseline treatment data were compared against the criteria established for subject inclusion using each subject's performance score from the HPCTB to identify data anomalies. Then the expected increases/decreases in human performance capacity from baseline treatment data were compared against the drug therapy-influenced data to determine if these changes were within "reasonable" limits. Potential anomalies were detected in less than 5% of the data, with most occurring within records for only a few subjects. These cases were investigated, and in consultation with the principal investigator, decisions were made and documented to arrive at the official data set.

Descriptive statistical analysis: Figure 36.2 illustrates the visual information processing speed (VIPS) for treatment groups reference drug, drug A, and placebo. On day 1 of testing (baseline), all treatment groups had similar VIPSs, with means between 5.7 and 5.8 stimuli per second. On day 8 of testing and at drug ingestion time of 2 h, VIPS decreased to 4.9 stimuli per second for drug A, to 5.1 stimuli per second for reference drug and to 5.65 stimuli per second for the placebo. On day 8, the greatest group impairment of VIPS occurred at drug ingestion time of 4 h. Drug A appeared to have the greatest impairment of VIPS (4.6 stimuli per second), followed by the reference drug group (4.9 stimuli per second). This decrease in performance was not present with the placebo group (5.61 stimuli per second). By the sixth hour after drug ingestion on day 8, VIPS improved toward baseline for treatment groups reference drug (5.1 stimuli per second) and drug A (5.3 stimuli per second), while the placebo group remained unchanged (5.58 stimuli per second). One day 9 of testing, all treatment groups received their assigned drug and alcohol. By 1 h after drug ingestion, all treatment groups' VIPSs were impaired from baseline, with drug A showing the greatest impairment (4.3 stimuli per second), followed by reference drug (4.6 stimuli per second) and placebo (4.9 stimuli per second). All treatment groups' VIPSs improved toward baseline values by the second hour after drug ingestion (5.0–5.1 stimuli per second) and the fourth hour

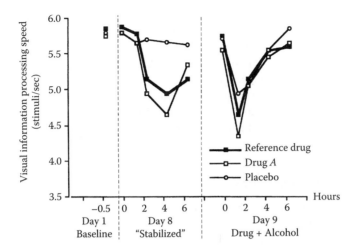

FIGURE 36.2 One performance capacity variable (visual information processing speed) for three treatment groups (drug *A*—the drug under test—reference drug, and placebo) taken from any actual efficacy-oriented study. Note changes from baseline to drug stabilization (day 8) and interaction with alcohol (day 9). See text for further explanation.

after drug ingestion (5.4–5.5 stimuli per second), respectively. By the sixth hour after drug ingestion, reference drug and drug *A* plateaued between 5.55 and 5.6 stimuli per second, respectively, while the placebo group improved slightly above the baseline value (5.8 stimuli per second). The basic pattern observed (i.e., decrease from baseline, return to baseline, impairment of all groups, including placebo, with alcohol) lend validity to the overall study.

Statistical analysis and significance test results: On day 8 of testing, significant differences in VIPS for main effects treatment group and hour were observed. There was a significant interaction, however, between treatment group and hour of drug ingestion. Post hoc analysis demonstrated that treatment groups drug *A* and reference drug were significantly slower in VIPS than the placebo group at drug ingestion times of 2, 4, and 6 h, but there was no difference in VIPS between treatment groups drug *A* and reference drug. (Simple main effects and simple, simple main effects showed that the placebo group had faster VIPSs than both reference drug and drug *A* treatment groups at drug ingestion times of 2, 4, and 6 h.)

On day 9 of testing when the drug–alcohol potentiating interaction effect was of primary interest, significant differences in VIPS occurred for main effects treatment group and hour, but there were no interactions between treatment group and hour of drug ingestion. Post hoc analysis demonstrated that treatment groups drug *A* and reference group were significantly slower in VIPS than the placebo group at 1 h after drug ingestion only, but there was no statistically significant difference in VIPS between treatment groups drug *A* and reference group at any hour after drug–alcohol ingestion. Also, the drug–alcohol interaction was significant 1 h after drug–alcohol ingestion for all treatment groups.

Conclusions from statistically significant findings: After 8 days of oral dosing, while a significant difference was found for both drug treatment groups compared with the placebo group, there was no significant difference in VIPS between drug *A* and reference drug treatment groups. The effect was apparent at approximately the same drug ingestion time of 4 h. It was concluded that drug *A* had the same effect on safety as the reference drug in terms of CNS impairment as measured by VIPS.

After 9 days of oral dosing in combination with alcohol consumption, drug *A* and reference drug caused a greater decrease in VIPS compared with the placebo group. This effect was most apparent at 1 h after drug ingestion. The placebo group also decreased its VIPS at 1 h after drug ingestion at a statistically significant level. It was concluded after 9 days of oral dosing that drug *A* in combination with alcohol produced the same effect as the reference drug in combination with alcohol in terms of CNS impairment as measured by VIPS.

Conclusions from clinically significant findings. Since there was no statistically significant difference between drug *A* and the reference drug on either day 8 or day 9, the only findings requiring an interpretation of clinical significance are the statistically significant findings for both drug *A* and reference drug relative to the placebo group. On both day 8 and day 9, these findings are clinically significant using either the Potvin et al. (1985) percentage change or Kondraske (1989) *z*-score approach. Using the resource economic model for human performance (Kondraske, 1988a,b, 1989), it can be argued that, for example, during critical events during tasks such as driving, all of an individual's available VIPS resource is drawn on. Clearly, the substantial decrease in VIPS observed can compromise safety during such events.

36.3.2 Efficacy-Oriented Study: Experiences in Neurology

Performance testing in clinical trials in neurology has grown tremendously within the last decade (Mohr and Prouwers, 1991), but within specific disease areas there remains reluctance to accept the replacement of traditional rating-scale evaluations of disease presence and progression by objective performance testing (Syndulko et al., 1993). The evolution of clinical evaluations in multiple sclerosis clinical trials illustrates this point.

Evaluation of disability change or deterioration in multiple sclerosis (MS) historically has been limited to physician rating scales that attempt to globally summarize some or most of the salient clinical features of the disease. General consensus in the use of rating scales for MS has been achieved in the specification of a minimal record of disability (MRD) for MS that incorporates several physician- and paramedical-administered rating scales for evaluating MS disease status and its effects on the patient's life (International Federation of Multiple Sclerosis Societies, 1984). However, there has been general dissatisfaction with the use of rating scales in MS clinical trials because of issues of lack or sensitivity to disease change, lack of interrater reliability, and simply the inherent reliance on subjective ratings of signs, symptoms, and unmeasured performance changes (Paty et al., 1992).

As an alternative to MS rating scales, comprehensive, quantitative evaluation of human performance was originally proposed and developed over 25 years ago for use in MS clinical trials (Tourtellotte et al., 1965). The first application of performance testing in a major MS clinical trial was the multicenter cooperative ACTH study (Rose et al., 1968). The study proved that human performance testing could be incorporated into a multicenter MS clinical trial and that examiners at multiple centers could be trained to administer the tests in a standardized, repeatable fashion. The results generally supported fairly comparable levels of sensitivity among the outcome measures, including performance testing (Dixon and Kuzma, 1974). Subsequent analyses showed that a priori composites that provided succinct summary measures of disease change in key functional areas could be formed from the data and that these composite measures were sensitive to treatment effects in relapsing/remitting MS patients (Henderson et al., 1978). Despite the favorable results of the ACTH study, performance testing did not achieve general acceptance in MS clinical studies. Comprehensive performance testing as conducted in the ACTH trial was considered time-consuming, the instrumentation was not generally available, and despite the use of composites, the number of outcome measures remained too large. In a recent double-blind, placebo-controlled collaborative study in 12 medical centers, the study design included both rating-scale and performance measures as outcome assessments in the largest sample of chronic progressive MS patients studied to date (The Multiple Sclerosis Study Group, 1990). Analyses of the change in performance composite scores from baseline over the 2-year course of the clinical trial showed that the drug-treated patients worsened significantly less than the placebo-treated patients. In contrast, the EDSS and other clinical rating scores did not show significant treatment effects for the subset of MS patients at the same center (Syndulko et al., 1993). This indicated that the performance composites were more sensitive than the clinical disability measures to disease progression and treatment effects. A more recent comparative analysis of the full data set also supports the greater sensitivity of composites based on performance testing compared with rating scales to both MS disease progression and to a treatment effect (Syndulko et al., 1994a,b). Although the biomedical community remains divided regarding the best outcome assessment in MS clinical trials, the accumulating evidence favors performance testing over clinical measures.

Another type of efficacy-oriented study of particular note in the context of this chapter involves the combination of pharmacodynamic models with instrumented, objective, and sensitive performance capacity measurements to optimize therapeutic effectiveness by fine-tuning dose prescription for individual subjects. For example, the results from a Parkinson's disease study by Hacisalihzade et al. (1989) suggest that performance capacity measurements, which would play a key role in a strategy to determine pharmacodynamics of a drug for the individual (i.e., not a population), could become a component in the management of some patients receiving long-term drug therapy.

36.4 Future Needs and Anticipated Developments

The field of clinical trials in which human performance variables are of interest has expanded at such a rapid rate in recent years that it has been difficult for researchers to keep up with all the new technologies, instrumentations, and methodologies. The type of evaluation employed has steadily shifted from mostly subjective to more objective, which can be argued to provide improved measurement quality. Increased standardization of human performance measurements has led to greater cost-effectiveness due to computer-based test batteries (Woollacott, 1983; Kennedy et al., 1993). Thus, even if the quality of measurement were the same with methodologies that used less sophisticated methods, the initial investment would frequently be saved with newer data management techniques. This sentiment has not yet been accepted by all segments of the relevant communities. Also, the speed at which data can now be collected (which is especially important when changes over short time periods are of interest, as in pharmacodynamic studies) has led to greater cost-effectiveness. Furthermore, since instrumented devices are becoming commercially available and more widely used, it is neither necessary nor desirable for researchers whose primary interest is the intervention of disease process to "reinvent" measurements (possibly with subtle but significant changes that ultimately inhibit standardization) for use in studies. Also, new measurements that may be different—but not necessarily better—must undergo long and expensive studies prior to their use in clinical trials. Although certain human performance measures are becoming standard in selected situations, more experience is needed before a substantial degree of standardization in human performance measurement is achieved in such situations.

The perfect research strategy in clinical trials involving human performance capacities to determine therapy effectiveness and safety may not be possible due to financial and/or ethical considerations. Thus the challenge of clinical trials research in the future is to maintain scientific integrity while conforming to legal mandates and staying within economic feasibility; that is, an optimization is almost always necessary. Multidisciplinary research efforts can be useful in these circumstances.

Defining Terms

Clinical significance: An additional level of interpretation of a statistically significant finding that addresses the size of the effect found.

Clinical trial: A research study involving human subjects and an intervention (i.e., device, drug, surgical procedure, or other procedure) that is ultimately intended to either enhance the professional capabilities of physicians, improve the quality of life of patients, or contribute to the field of knowledge in those sciences which are traditionally in the medical field setting.

Composite score: A score derived by combining two or more measured performance capacities.

Efficacy-oriented clinical trial: A study that is conducted to objectively determine an intervention's effectiveness along with any pharmacokinetic or pharmacodynamic interactions.

Nonprobability sampling: A method of sampling whereby no subject in a defined population has an equal chance of being included in the sample.

Performance capacities: Dimensional capabilities or resources (e.g., speed, accuracy, strength, etc.) that a given human subsystem (e.g., visual, central processing, gait production, posture maintenance, etc.) possesses to perform a given task.

Pharmacodynamics: The physiologic and/or metabolic changes in the concentration of a drug over time to corresponding measurable performance capacity changes in the therapeutic effect.

Pharmacokinetics: The rate at which a drug is metabolized, as evidenced by changes in drug concentrations in blood, cerebral spinal fluid, urine, etc.

Probability sampling: A method of sampling whereby each subject in a defined population theoretically has an equal chance of being included in the sample.

Protocol: A detailed statement of all procedures and methods to be employed in a research investigation.

Randomized clinical trial (RCT): A study that uses controlled trials whereby part of the group of subjects receives a therapy that is tested, while the other subjects receive either no therapy or another therapy.

Resource economics: A cause–effect type of relationship between available performance resources (i.e., capacities) and demands of higher-level tasks in which the relevant subsystems are used.

Safety-oriented clinical trial: A study that usually involves vital sign measures (e.g., heart rate, blood pressure, respiration rate), clinical laboratory tests (e.g., blood chemistries, urinalysis, ECG), and adverse reaction tests (both mental and physical performance capacities) to evaluate the risk of an intervention.

Sample: A proportion of the defined population that is studied. When used as a verb (sampling), it refers to the process of subject selection.

Significance (statistical) test: A tool used for assessing possible associations between independent and dependent variables as well as differences among treatment groups.

Statistical significance: An evaluation of the research hypothesis at a specific level of probability so that any differences observed are not attributable to a chance occurrence.

References

Baker, S.J., Chrzan, G.J., Park, C.N., and Saunders, J.H. 1985. Validation of human behavioral tests using ethanol as a CNS depressant model. *Neurobehav. Toxicol. Teratol.* 7:257.

Baumgartner, T.A. and Jackson, A.S. 1993. *Measurement for Evaluation*, 4th ed. Dubuque, Iowa, Wm. C. Brown.

Cochran, W.G. and Cox, G.M. 1957. *Experimental Designs*, 2nd ed. New York, John Wiley & Sons.

Cohen, J. 1988. *Statistical Power Analysis for the Behavioral Sciences*. Hillsdale, NJ, Lawrence Erlbaum Associates.

Cotton, P. 1993. FDA lifts ban on women in early drug tests, will require companies to look for gender differences. *JAMA* 269:2067.

DeAngelis, C. 1990. *An Introduction to Clinical Research*. New York, Oxford University Press.

Department of Health and Human Services. 1985. *Code of Federal Regulation of the Department of Health and Human Services*, title 45, part 46.

Dixon, W.J. and Kuzma, J.W. 1974. Data reduction in large clinical trials. *Commun. Stat.* 3:301.

Fleiss, J.L. 1986. *The Design and Analysis of Clinical Experiments*. New York, John Wiley & Sons.

Food and Drug Administration. 1977. *General Considerations for the Clinical Evaluation of Drugs*. DHEW Publication No. (FDA) 77–3040. Washington.

Hacisalihzade, S.S., Mansour, M., and Albani, C. 1989. Optimization of symptomatic therapy in Parkinson's disease. *IEEE Trans. Biomed. Eng.* 36:363.

Hastad, D.N. and Lacy, A.C. 1994. *Measurement and Evaluation*, 2nd ed. Scottsdale, Ariz, Gorsuch Scarisbrick.

Henderson, W.G., Tourtellotte, W.W., Potvin, A.R., and Rose, A.S. Methodology for analyzing clinical neurological data: ACTH in multiple sclerosis. *Clin. Pharmacol. Ther.* 24:146.

Hill, A.B. 1963. Medical ethics and controlled trials. *Br. Med. J.* 1: 1043.

Horne, J.A. and Gibbons, H. 1991. Effects of vigilance performance and sleepiness of alcohol given in the early afternoon (post lunch) vs early evening. *Ergonomics* 34: 67.

International Federation of Multiple Sclerosis Societies. 1984. Symposium on a minimal record of disability for multiple sclerosis. *Acta Neurol. Scand.* 70(Suppl): 101–217.

Jennison, C. and Turnbull, B.W. 1993. Group sequential tests for bivariate response: Interim analyses of clinical trials with both efficacy and safety endpoints. *Biometrics* 49:741.

Jones, B. and Kenward, M.G. 1989. *Design and Analysis of Crossover Trials*. New York, Chapman & Hall.

Kennedy, R.S., Turnage, J.J., and Wilkes, R.L. 1993. Effects of graded doses of alcohol on nine computerized repeated-measures tests. *Ergonomics* 36:1195.

Kepple, G. 1982. *Design and Analysis a Researcher's Handbook*, 2nd ed. Englewood Cliffs, NJ, Prentice-Hall.

Kondraske, G.V. 1988a. Workplace design: An elemental resource approach to task analysis and human performance measurements. *International Conference for the Advancement of Rehabilitation Technology, Montreal, Proceedings*, pp. 608–611.

Kondraske, G.V. 1988b. Experimental evaluation of an elemental resource model for human performance. *Tenth Annual IEEE Engineering in Medicine and Biology Society Conference, New Orleans, Proceedings*, pp. 1612–1613.

Kondraske, G.V. 1989. Measurement science concepts and computerized methodology in the assessment of human performance. In: T. Munsat (Ed.), *Quantification of Neurologic Deficit*. Stoneham, MA, Butterworth.

Kondraske, G.V. 1995. A working model for human system-task interfaces. In: J.D. Bronzino (Ed.), *Handbook of Biomedical Engineering*. Boca Raton, FL, CRC Press.

Levin, R.J. 1986. *Ethics and Regulation of Clinical Research*, 2nd ed. Baltimore, Urban & Schwarzenberg.

Merkatz, R.B., Temple, R., and Sobel, S. 1993. Women in clinical trials of new drugs: A change in Food and Drug Administration policy. *N. Engl. J. Med.* 329:292.

Mohr, E. and Prouwers, P. 1991. *Handbook of Clinical Trials: The Neurobehavioral Approach*. Berwyn, PA, Swets and Zeitlinger.

The Multiple Sclerosis Study Group. 1990. Efficacy and toxicity of cyclosporine in chronic progressive multiple sclerosis: A randomized, double-blind, placebo-controlled clinical trial. *Ann. Neurol.* 27:591.

Ottenbacher, K.J. and Barrett, K.A. 1991. Measures of effect size in the reporting of rehabilitation research. *Am. J. Phys. Med. Rehabil.* 70(suppl 1):S131.

Paty, D.E., Willoughby, E., and Whitakek, J. 1992. Assessing the outcome of experimental therapies in multiple sclerosis. In *Treatment of Multiple Sclerosis: Trial Design, Results, and Future Perspectives*, pp. 47–90. London, Springer-Verlag.

Potvin, A.R., Tourtellotte, W.W.T., Potvin, J.H. et al. 1985. *Quantitative Examination of Neurologic Function*, vols I and II. Boca Raton, FL, CRC Press.

Rose, A.S., Kuzma, J.W., Kurtzke, J.F. et al. 1968. Cooperative study in the evaluation of therapy in multiple sclerosis: ACTH vs placebo in acute exacerbations. Preliminary report. *Neurology* 18:1.

Safrit, M.J. 1990. *Evaluation in Exercise Science*. Englewood Cliffs, NJ, Prentice-Hall.

Salame, P. 1991. The effects of alcohol in learning as a function of drinking habits. *Ergonomics* 34:1231.

Stone, R. 1993. FDA to ask for data on gender differences. *Science* 260:743.

Syndulko, K., Ke, D., Ellison, G.W. et al. 1994a. Neuroperformance assessment of treatment efficacy and MS disease progression in the Cyclosporine Multicenter Clinical Trial. *Brain* (submitted).

Syndulko, K., Ke, D., Ellison, G.W. et al. 1994b. A comparative analysis of assessments for disease progression in multiple sclerosis: I. Signal to noise ratios and relationship among performance measures and rating scales. *Brain* (submitted).

Syndulko, K., Tourellotte, W.W., Baumhefner, R.W. et al. 1993. Neuroperformance evaluation of multiple sclerosis disease progression in a clinical trial. 7:69.

Tang, D. and Geller, N.L. 1993. On the design and analysis of randomized clinical trials with multiple endpoints. *Biometrics* 49:23.

Thomas, J.R. and Nelson, J.K. 1990. *Research Methods in Physical Activity*, 2nd ed. Champaign, IL, Human Kinetics Publishers.

Tourtellotte, W.W., Haerer, A.F., Simpson, J.F. et al. 1965. Quantitative clinical neurological testing: I. A study of a battery of tests designed to evaluate in part the neurologic function of patients with multiple sclerosis and its use in a therapeutic trial. *Ann. NY Acad. Sci.* 122:480.

Tudiver, F., Bass, M.J., Dunn, E.V. et al. 1992. *Assessing Interventions Traditional and Innovative Methods.* London, Sage Publications.

Weissman, A. 1991. On the concept "study day zero." *Perspect. Biol. Med.* 34:579.

Willoughby, P.D. and Whitaker, J.E. 1992. Assessing the outcome of experimental therapies in multiple sclerosis. In: R.A. Rudick and D.E. Goodkin (Eds.), *Treatment of Multiple Sclerosis: Trial Design, Results, and Future Perspectives*, pp. 47–90. London, Springer-Verlag.

Woollacott, M.H. 1983. Effects of ethanol on postural adjustments in humans. *Exp. Neurol.* 80:55.

Further Information

The original monograph, *Experimental and Quasi-Experimental Designs for Research*, by D.T. Campbell and J.C. Stanley (Boston: Houghton Mifflin, 1964), is a classic experimental design text. The book *Statistics in Medicine*, by T. Colton (Boston: Little, Brown, 1982), examines statistical principles in medical research and identifies common perils when drawing conclusions from medical research. The book *Clinical Epidemiology: The Essentials*, R.H. Fletcher, S.W. Fletcher, and E.H. Wagner (2nd ed., Baltimore: Williams and Wilkins, 1982), is a readable text with concise descriptions of various types of studies. *Clinical Trials: Design, Conduct, and Analysis*, by C.L. Meinert (New York: Oxford University Press, 1986), is a comprehensive text covering most details and provides many helpful suggestions about clinical trials research. R.J. Porter and B.S. Schoenberg, *Controlled Clinical Trials in Neurological Disease* (Boston: Kluwer Academic Publishers, 1990), is also a comprehensive text covering clinical trials with a special emphasis on neurologic diseases.

Applications of Quantitative Assessment of Human Performance in Occupational Medicine

Mohamad
Parnianpour
*Sharif University of
Technology*

37.1 Introduction

As early as 1700, Bernardino Ramazzini, one of the founders of occupational medicine, had associated certain physical activities with musculoskeletal disorders (MSD). He postulated that certain violent and irregular motions and unnatural postures of the body impair the internal structure (Snook et al., 1988). Currently, much effort is directed toward a better understanding of work-related MSD involving the back, cervical spine, and upper extremities (Mousavi et al. 2011). The World Health Organization (WHO) has defined occupational diseases as those work-related diseases where the relationship to specific causative factors at work has been fully established (WHO, 1985). Other work-related diseases may have a weaker or unclear association to working conditions. They may be aggravated, accelerated, or exacerbated by workplace factors and may lead to impairment of workers' performance. Hence, obtaining the occupational history is crucial for proper diagnosis and appropriate treatment of work-related disorders. The occupational physician must consider the conditions of both the workplace and the worker in evaluating injured workers. Biomechanical and ergonomic evaluators have developed a series of techniques for quantification of the task demands and evaluation of the stresses in the workplace. Functional capacity evaluation has also been advanced to quantify the maximum performance capability of workers. The motto of ergonomics is to avoid the mismatch between the task demand and functional capacity of individuals. A multidisciplinary group of physicians and engineers constitutes the rehabilitation team that work together to implement the prevention measures. Through proper workplace design, workplace stressors could be minimized. It is expected that one-third of the compensable low back pain (LBP) in industry could be prevented by proper ergonomic workplace or task design. In addition to reducing the probability of both the initial and recurring episodes, proper ergonomic design allows earlier return to work of injured workers by keeping the task demands at a lower level. Unfortunately, ergonomists are often asked to redesign the task or the workplace after a high incidence of injuries has already been experienced. The next preventive measure that has been suggested is preplacement of workers based on the medical history, strength, and physical examinations (Snook et al., 1988). Training and education have been the third prevention strategy in the reduction of MSD. Some components of these educational packages such as "back schools" and the teaching of "proper body mechanics" have been used in the rehabilitation phase of injured workers as well.

Title I of the Americans with Disability Act (ADA, 1990) prohibits discrimination with regard to any aspect of the employment process. Thus, the development of preplacement tests has been impeded by the possibility of discrimination against individuals based on gender, age, or medical condition. The ADA requires physical tests to simulate the "essential functions" of the task. In addition, one must be aware of "reasonable accommodations," such as lifting aids, that may make an otherwise infeasible task possible for a disabled applicant to perform. Healthcare providers who perform physical examinations and provide recommendations for job applicants must consider the rights of disabled applicants. It is extremely crucial to quantify the specific physical requirements of the job to be performed and to examine an applicant's capabilities to perform those specific tasks, taking into account any reasonable accommodations that may be provided. Hence, task analysis and functional capacity assessment are truly intertwined.

Work-related disorders of the upper extremities, unlike low back disorders, can better be related to specific anatomic sites such as a tendon or compressed nerve. Examples of the growing number of cumulative trauma disorders of the upper extremities and the neck are carpal tunnel syndrome (CTS), DeQuervain's disease, trigger finger, lateral epicondylitis (tennis elbow), rotator cuff tendinitis, thoracic outlet syndrome, and tension neck syndrome. The prevalence of these disorders is higher among some specific jobs, such as meat cutters, welders, sewer workers, grinders, meat packers, and keyboard operators. Some of the common risk factors leading to pain, impairment, and physical damage in the neck and upper extremities are forceful motion, repetitive motion, vibration, prolonged awkward posture, and mechanical stress (Kroemer et al., 1994).

This chapter illustrates the application of some principles and practices of human performance engineering, especially quantification of human performance in the field of occupational medicine. I have selected the problem of LBP to illustrate a series of concepts that are essential to evaluation of both the worker and the workplace, while realizing the importance of the disorders of the neck and upper extremities. By inference and generalization, most of these concepts can be extended to these situations.

37.2 Principles

The assessment of function across various dimensions of performance (i.e., strength, speed, endurance, and coordination) has provided the basis for a rational approach to clinical assessment, rehabilitation strategies, and determination of return-to-work potential for injured employees (Kondraske, 1990). To understand the complex problem of trunk performance evaluation of LBP patients, the terminology of muscle exertion must first be defined. However, it should be noted that several excellent reviews on trunk muscle function have been carried out (Andersson, 1991; Beimborn and Morrissey, 1988; Newton and Waddell, 1993; Pope, 1992). I do not intend to reproduce this extensive literature here because my motive is to provide a critical analysis that will lead the reader toward an understanding of the future of functional assessment techniques. A more extensive clinical application is provided elsewhere (Szpalski and Parnianpour, 1996; Parnianpour and Shirazi-adl, 1999).

37.2.1 Impairment, Disability, and Handicap

The tremendous human suffering and economic costs of disability present a formidable medical, social, and political challenge in the midst of growing healthcare costs and scarcity of resources. WHO (1980) distinguishes among impairment, disability, and handicap. Impairment is any loss or abnormality of psychological, physiological, or anatomical structure or function—impairment reflects disturbances at the organ level. Disability is any restriction or lack of ability (resulting from impairment) to perform an activity in the manner or within the range considered normal for a human being—disability reflects disturbances at the level of person. Handicap is a disadvantage for a given individual, resulting from an impairment or a disability, that limits or prevents the fulfillment of a role that is normal (depending on age, sex, and social and cultural factors) for that individual. Because disability is the objectification of an impairment, handicap represents the socialization of an impairment or disability. Despite the immense improvement presented by the International Classification of Impairments, Disabilities, and Handicaps (ICIDH), the classification is limited from an industrial medicine or rehabilitation perspective. The hierarchical organization lacks the specificity required for evaluating the functional state of an individual with respect to task demands.

Kondraske (1990) has suggested an alternative approach using the principles of resource economics. The resource economics paradigm is reflective of the principal goal of ergonomics: fitting the demands of the task to the functional capability of the worker. The elemental resource model (ERM) is based on the application of general performance theory that presents a unified theory for measurement, analysis, and modeling of human performance across different aspects of performance, across all human subsystems, and at any hierarchical level. This approach uses the same bases to describe both the fundamental dimensions of performance capacity and task demand (available and utilized resources) of each functional unit involved in performance of the high-level tasks. The elegance of the ERM is due to its hierarchical organization, allowing causal models to be generated based on assessment of the task demands and performance capabilities across the same dimensions of performance (Kondraske, 1990)).

37.2.2 Muscle Action and Performance Quantification

The details of the complex processes of muscle contraction in terms of the bioelectrical, biochemical, and biophysical interactions are under intense research. Muscle tensions are a function of the muscle length and its rate of change and can be scaled by the level of neural excitation. These relationships are called the length–tension and velocity–tension relationships. From a physiological point of view, the measured force or torque applied at the interface is a function of (1) the individual's motivation (magnitude of the neural drive for excitation and activation processes), (2) environmental conditions (muscle length, rate of change of muscle length, nature of the external load, metabolic conditions, pH level, temperature, and so forth), (3) history of activation (fatigue), (4) instructions and descriptions of the tasks given to the subject, (5) the control strategies and motor programs employed to satisfy the demands of the task, and (6) the biophysical state of the muscles and fitness (fiber composition, physiological cross-sectional area of the muscle, cardiovascular capability). It cannot be overemphasized that these processes are complex and interrelated (Kroemer et al., 1994). Other factors that may affect the performance of patients are misunderstanding of the degree of effort needed in maximal testing, test anxiety, depression, nociception, fear of pain and reinjury, as well as unconscious and conscious symptom magnification.

The following sections review some methods to quantify performance and lifting capability of isolated trunk muscles during a multilink coordinated manual materials-handling task. Relevant factors that influence the static and dynamic strength and endurance measures of trunk muscles will be addressed, and the clinical applications of these assessment techniques will be illustrated.

The central nervous system (CNS) appropriately excites the muscle, and the generated tension is transferred to the skeletal system by the tendon to cause motion, stabilize the joint, and resist the effect of external forces on the body. Hence, the functional evaluation of muscles cannot be performed without the characterization of the interfaced mechanical environment.

The four fundamental types of muscle exertion or action are isometric, isokinetic, isotonic, and isoinertial. In isometric exertion, the muscle length is kept constant, and there is no movement. Although mechanical work is not achieved, physiological work, that is, static work, is performed, and energy is consumed. When the internal force exerted by the muscle is greater than the external force offered by the resistance, then concentric, that is, shortening, muscle action occurs, whereas if the muscle is already activated and the external force exceeds the internal force of the muscle, then eccentric, that is, lengthening, muscle action occurs. When the muscle moves, either concentrically or eccentrically, dynamic work is performed. If the rate of shortening or lengthening of the muscle is constant, the exertion is called isokinetic. When the muscle acts on a constant inertial mass, the exertion is called isoinertial. Isotonic action occurs when the muscle tension is constant throughout the range of motion.

These definitions are very clear when dealing with isolated muscles during physiological investigations. However, terminology employed in the literature of strength evaluation is imprecise. The terms are intended to refer to the state of muscles, but they actually refer to the state of the mechanical interface, that is, the dynamometer. Isotonic exertion, as defined, is not as realizable physiologically because muscular tensions change as its lever arm changes despite the constancy of external loads. Special designs may vary the resistance level to account for changes in mechanical efficiency of the muscles. In addition, the rate of muscle length change may not remain constant even when the joint angular velocity is regulated by the dynamometer during isokinetic exertions. During isoinertial action, the net external resistance is not only a function of the mass (inertia) but also a function of the acceleration. The acceleration, however, is a function of the input energy to the mass. Hence, to fully characterize the net external resistance, we need to have both the acceleration and the inertial parameters (mass and moment of inertia) of the load and body parts. Future research should better quantify the inertial effects of the dynamometers, particularly during nonisometric and nonisokinetic exertions.

For any joint or joint complex, muscle performance can be quantified in terms of the basic dimensions of performance: strength, speed, endurance, steadiness, and coordination. Muscle strength is the capacity to produce torque or work by voluntary activation of the muscles, whereas muscle endurance is the ability to maintain a predetermined level of motor output—for example, torque, velocity, range of motion, work, or energy—over a period of time. Fatigue is considered to be a process under which the capability of muscles diminish. However, neuromuscular adjustments take place to meet the task demands (i.e., increase in neural excitation) until there is final performance breakdown—endurance time. Coordination, in this context, is the temporal and spatial organizations of movement and the recruitment patterns of the muscle synergies.

Despite the proliferation of various technologies for measurement, basic questions such as "What needs to be measured and how can it best be measured?" are still being investigated. However, there is a consensus on the need to measure objectively the performance capability along the following dimensions: range of motion, strength, endurance, coordination, speed, acceleration, and so on. Strength is one of the most fundamental dimensions of human performance and has been the focus of many investigations. Despite the general consensus about the abstract definition of strength, there is no direct method for measurement of muscle tension *in vivo*. Strength has often been measured at the interface of a joint (or joints) with the mechanical environment. A dynamometer, which is an external apparatus on which the body exerts force, is used to measure strength indirectly.

Different modes of strength testing have evolved based on different levels of technological sophistication. The practical implication of contextual dependencies on the provided mechanical environment of the strength measures must be considered during selection of the appropriate mode of measurement. In this regard, equipment that can measure strength in different modes is more efficient in terms of both initial capital investment, required floor space in the clinics or laboratories, and the amount of time it takes to get the person in and out of the dynamometer.

37.3 LBP and Trunk Performance

The problem of LBP is selected to present important models that could be used by the entire multi-disciplinary rehabilitation team for the measurement, modeling, and analysis of human performance (Kondraske, 1990). The inability to relate LBP to anatomic findings and the difficulties in quantifying pain have directed much effort toward quantification of spinal performance. The problem is made even more complex by the increasing demand of the healthcare system to quantify the level of impairment of patients reporting back pain without objective findings.

There are three basic impairment evaluation systems, each having its own merits and shortcomings: (1) anatomic, based on physical examination findings, (2) diagnostic, based on pathology, and (3) functional, based on performance or work capacity (Luck and Florence, 1988). The earlier systems were anatomic, based on amputation and ankylosis. Although this approach may be more applicable to the hand, it is very inappropriate for the spine. The diagnostic-based systems suffer from lack of correspondence between the degree of impairment for a given diagnosis and the resulting disability and even more from the lack of a clear diagnosis. A large percentage of symptom-free individuals have anatomic findings detectable by the imaging technologies, whereas some LBP patients have no structural anomalies.

The function-based systems are more desirable from an occupational medicine perspective for the following reasons: they allow the rehabilitation team to rationally evaluate the prospect for return to light-duty work and the type of "reasonable accommodations" needed (such as assistive devices) that could reduce the task demand below the functional capability of the individual. By focusing on remaining ability and transferable skills rather than the disability or structural impairment of the injured worker, the set of feasible jobs can be identified. These points are extremely important, given the natural history of work disability after a single LBP episode causing loss of work time: 40–50% of workers return to work by 2 weeks, 60–80% return by 4 weeks, and 85–90% return by 12 weeks. The small number of disabled workers who become chronic are responsible for the majority of the economic cost of LBP. It is, therefore, the primary goal of the rehabilitation team to prevent the LBP, which is self-correcting in most cases, no matter what kind of therapy is used, from becoming a chronic disabling predicament. Injured workers should neither be returned to work too early nor too late because both could complicate the prognosis. The results of functional capacity evaluation and task demand quantification should guide the timing for returning to work. It is clear that psychosocioeconomic factors become increasingly more important than physical factors as the disability progresses into "chronicity syndrome" and play a major role in defining the evolution of a low back disability claim. Future research should further establish the reliability and reproducibility of performance assessment tools to expedite their widespread use (Luck and Florence, 1988; Newton and Waddell, 1993).

37.3.1 Maximal and Submaximal Protocols

Biomechanical strength models of the trunk are usually based on static maximal strength measurement. In real-life work situations, individuals rarely exert lengthy or maximum static effort. In most clinical situations, submaximal protocols are recommended, especially in patients with pain or with cardio-vascular problems. Also, submaximal testing is less susceptible to fatigue and injury. The activities of daily living also have a great deal of submaximal efforts at the self-selected pace. Hence, it has been argued that testing at the preferred rate may be complementary to the maximal effort protocols. The preferred motion can be solicited by instructing the subject to perform repetitive movement at a pace and through the range of motion which he or she feels is the most comfortable. It has been shown that LBP patients and normal individuals have different resisted preferred flexion/extension motion characteristics. Having the subject perform against resistance is based on the hypothesis that, at higher resistance levels, the separation between the performance levels of patients and normal subjects becomes more evident. It has been shown, for example, that functional impairment of trunk extensors in LBP patients with respect to the normal population is larger at higher velocities during isokinetic trunk extension. However, the proponents of unconstrained testing have argued that separation of these groups can be performed based on the position, velocity, and acceleration profiles of the trunk during self-selected flexion/extension tasks. They have noted that pain and fear of reinjury may become the limiting factors. The sudden surge in acquiring performance measures of LBP patients during the initial rehabilitation process also underscores the validity of this concept.

37.3.2 Static and Dynamic Strength Measurements of Isolated Trunk Muscles

Weakness of the trunk extensor and abdominal muscles in patients with LBP was demonstrated using the cable tensiometer to measure isometric strength. The disadvantage of the cable tensiometer (which records applied force) is that it neglects to measure the lever arm distance from the center of trunk motion. It is also recommended that cable tensiometer be used to determine peak isometric torques rather than the stable average torque exerted over a 3-s period. Dynamometers used for testing dynamic muscle performances contain either hydraulic or servo motor systems to provide constant velocity, for example, isokinetic devices, or constant resistance, for example, isoinertial devices. The isokinetic devices can be further categorized into passive and active types. The robotics-based dynamometers can actively apply force on the body and hence allow eccentric muscle performance assessments, while only concentric exertions can be measured by the passive devices. Eccentric muscle action can stimulate the lowering phase of a manual materials handling task. On the basis of sports medicine literature, eccentric action has been implicated for its significant role in the muscle injury mechanism. Using isokinetic dynamometers, the isometric and isokinetic strengths of trunk extensor and abdominal muscles were shown to be weaker in LBP patients compared with healthy individuals. Dedicated trunk testing systems have become the cornerstone of objective functional evaluation and have been incorporated in the rehabilitation programs in many centers.

Two issues of importance for future research are the role of pelvic restraints and the significance of using newly developed triaxial dynamometers as opposed to more traditional uniaxial dynamometers. Studies on healthy volunteers have shown that trunk motions occur in more than one plane—lateral bending accompanies the primary motion of axial rotation. Numerous attempts have been made to measure the segmental range of motion three-dimensionally in the lumbar spine with the purpose of quantifying abnormal coupling and diagnosing instabilities.

The effect of posture on the maximum strength capability can be described based on the length–tension relationship of muscle action. Marras and Mirka (1989) studied the effect of trunk postural asymmetry, flexion angle, and trunk velocity (eccentric, isometric, and concentric) on maximal trunk torque production. It was shown that trunk torque decreased by about 8.5% of the maximum for every 15° of asymmetric trunk angle. At higher trunk flexion angles, extensor strength increased. Complex, significant interaction effects of velocity, asymmetry, and sagittal posture were detected. The ranges of velocity studies were more limited (±30°/s) than those used customarily in spinal evaluation. Tan et al. (1993) tested 31 healthy males for the effects of standing trunk-flexion positions (0°, 15°, and 35°) on triaxial torques and did *electromyograms* (EMGs) of 10 trunk muscles during isometric trunk extension at 30%, 50%, 70%, and 100% of maximum voluntary exertions (MVE). Trunk muscle strength was significantly increased at a more flexed position. However, the accessory torques in the transverse and coronal planes were not affected by trunk postures. The recorded lateral bending and rotation accessory torques were less than 5% and 16% of the primary extension torque, respectively. The rectus abdominis muscles were inactive during all the tests. The EMGs of the erector spinae varied linearly with higher values of MVE, whereas the latissimus dorsi had a nonlinear behavior. The obliques were coactivated only during 100% MVE. The neuromuscular efficiency ratio (NMER) was constructed as the ratio of the extension torque over the processed (RMS) EMG of the extensor muscles. It was hoped that NMER could be used in clinical settings where generation of the maximum exertion are not indicated. However, the NMER proved to have a limited clinical utility because it was significantly affected by both exertion level and posture. The NMER of the extensor muscles increased at more flexed position. Studies that have combined the EMG activities and dynamometric evaluations have the potential of discovering the neuromuscular adaptation during different phases of injury and rehabilitation processes.

37.3.3 Static and Dynamic Trunk Muscle Endurance

The high percentage of type I fibers in the back muscles, in addition to the better vascularization of these muscle groups, contributes to their superior endurance. Physiological studies indicate that at higher muscle utilization ratios (relative muscle loads), fatigue is detected earlier. Isometric endurance tests have been used to compute the median frequency (MF) of the myoelectrical activities of trunk muscles in both normal and LBP populations. The expected decline of the median frequency with fatigue is parameterized by the intercept (initial MF) and the slope of the fall. It has been shown that trunk range of motion (ROM) and isometric strength suffered from lower specificity and sensitivity than spectral parameters. Trunk muscle endurance does differ between healthy subjects and those reporting LBP. During isometric endurance testing, trunk flexors develop fatigue faster than extensors in symptom-free subjects. The flexor fatigability appeared significantly higher in patients with LBF as compared with controls. Chronicity also influences trunk muscle endurance. Chronic LBP patients showed reduced abdominal as well as back muscle endurance as compared with the healthy controls and lower back muscle endurance as compared with the intermittent LBP group. Individuals with a history of debilitating LBP demonstrated less isometric trunk extensor endurance than either normal individuals or patients with history of lesser LBP.

Soft tissues subjected to repetitive loading, because of their viscoelastic properties, demonstrate creep and load relaxation. The loss of precision, speed, and control of the neuromuscular system induced by fatigue reduces the ability of muscles to protect the weakened passive structure, which may explain many industrial, clinical, and recreational injury mechanisms. These results further indicate the necessity of relating clinical protocols to the job and show how short-duration maximal isometric testing alone cannot provide the complex functional interaction of strength, endurance, control, and coordination.

Parnianpour et al. (1988) studied the effect of isoinertial fatiguing of flexion and extension trunk movements on the movement pattern (angular position and velocity profile) and the motor output (torque) of the trunk. They showed that, with fatigue, there is a reduction of the functional capacity in the main sagittal plane. There is also a loss of motor control enabling a greater range of motion in the transverse and coronal planes while performing the primary sagittal task. Association of sagittal with coronal and transverse movements is considered more likely to induce back injuries; thus the effect of fatigue and reduction of motor control and coordination may be an important risk factor leading to injury-prone working postures. The endurance limit is a more useful predictor of incidence and recurrence of low back disorders than the absolute strength values. Although physiological criteria used in the National Institute for Occupational Safety and Health Lifting Guide (NIOSH, 1981) considered cardiovascular demands of dynamic repetitive lifting tasks, the limits of muscular endurance were not explicitly addressed. Future research should fill this gap because the maximum strength measures should not guide the design decisions. Maximum level of performance can only be maintained for short periods of time, and muscular fatigue should be avoided to prevent the development of MSD. This caveat should be applied to all dimensions of performance capability (Kondraske, 1990).

A prospective, randomized study among employees in a geriatric hospital showed that exercising during work hours to improve back muscle strength, endurance, and coordination proved cost-effective in preventing back symptoms and absence from work (Gundewall et al., 1993). Every hour spent by the physiotherapist on the exercise group reduced the work absence by 1.3 days. In this study, both training and testing equipment were very modest. Endurance training is based on exercises with high repetition and low resistance, whereas strength training requires exercise with high resistance and low repetition.

37.3.4 Lifting Strength Testing

NIOSH (1981) recommended static, that is, isometric, strength measurements as its standard for lifting tasks. This was based on the evidence that associated LBP with inadequate isometric strength. The incidence of an individual's sustaining an on-the-job back injury increases threefold when the task-lifting requirements approached or exceed the individual's strength capacity. However, lifting strength is not a true measure of trunk function but is a global measure taking into account arm, shoulder, and leg strength as well as the individual's lifting technique and overall fitness. It has been shown that strength tests were more valid and predictive of risk of low back disorders if they simulated the demands of the job. The clinicians must be aided with easy-to-use and validated instruments or questionnaires to gather information about the task demands to decide what testing protocol best simulates the applicant's spinal loading conditions.

Static strength measurements have been reported to underestimate significantly the loads on the spine during dynamic lifts. Comparing static and dynamic biomechanical models of the trunk, the predicted spinal loads under static conditions were 33–60% less than those under dynamic conditions, depending on the lifting technique. The recruitment patterns of trunk muscles (and thus the internal loading of the spine) are significantly different under isometric and dynamic conditions. General manual materials handling tasks require a coordinated multilink activity that can be simulated using classic psychophysical techniques or the robotics-based lift task simulators. Various lifting tests, including static, dynamic, maximal, and submaximal, are currently available. The experimental results of correlational studies have confirmed the theoretical prediction that strength will be dependent on the measurement technique. Because muscle action requires external resistance, the effect of muscle action will depend on the nature of the resistance. These results refute the implicit assumption that a generic strength test exists that can be used for preplacing workers (preemployment) and predicting the risk of injury or future occurrence of LBP. The psychometric properties of isokinetic and isoresistive modes of strength testing were recently addressed. The quantification of the surface response of strength as a function of joint angle and velocity was only possible for isokinetic testing, whereas isoresistive tests yielded a very sparse data set (Figures 37.1 and 37.2).

The wide conflicting results found in the literature regarding the relationship of an individual's strength to the risk of developing LBP may be because of inappropriate modes of strength measurements, that is, lack of job specificity. Isometric strength testing of the trunk is still widely used, especially in large-scale industrial or epidemiological studies, because it has been standardized and studied prospectively in industry. Compared with trunk dynamic strength testing protocols, the trunk isometric strength testing protocols are simpler and less expensive.

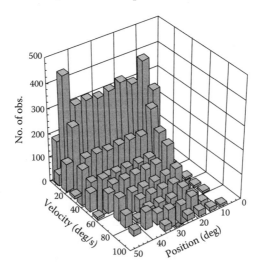

FIGURE 37.1 Bivariate distribution histogram of isokinetic trunk extension for 10 subjects.

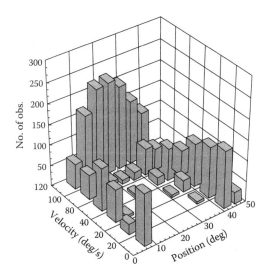

FIGURE 37.2 Bivariate distribution histogram of isotonic trunk extension for 10 subjects.

One outstanding issue during dynamic testing is the unresolved problem of how the wealth of information can be presented in a succinct and informative fashion. One approach has been to compare the statistical features of the data with the existing normal databases. This is particularly crucial because one does not have the option of comparing the results to the "contralateral asymptomatic joint," as one has with lower or upper extremity joints. Given the large differences between individuals, I recommend comparison be made to job-specific databases. For example, it is more appropriate for the trunk strength of an injured construction worker to be compared with age- and gender-controlled healthy construction workers than with data from healthy college graduate students or office workers. However, given the scarcity of such data, I argue for comparison of performance capacity with job demand based on task analysis. The performance capacity evaluation is once again linked to task demand quantification.

37.3.5 Inverse and Direct Dynamics

A major task of biomechanics has been to estimate the internal loading of musculoskeletal structure and establish the physiological loading during various daily activities. Kinematic studies deal with joint movement, with no emphasis on the forces involved. However, kinetic studies address the effect of forces that generate such movements. Using sophisticated experimental and theoretical stress/strain analyses, hazardous/failure levels of loads have been determined. The estimated forces and stresses are used to estimate the level of deformation in the tissues. This technique allows one to assess the risk of overexertion injury associated with any physical activity. Given repetitive motions and exertion levels much lower than the ultimate strength of the tissues, an alternative injury mechanism, the cumulative trauma model, has been used to describe much of the MSD of the upper extremities.

The experimental data on the joint trajectories are differentiated to obtain the angular velocity and acceleration. Appropriate inertial properties of the limb segments are used to compute the net external moments about each joint. This mapping from joint kinematics to net moments is called inverse dynamics. Direct dynamics refers to studies that simulate the motion based on known actuator torques at each joint. The key issue in these investigations is understanding the control strategies underlying the trajectory planning and performance of purposeful motion. A highly multidisciplinary field has emerged to address these unsolved questions (see Berme and Cappozzo (1990) for a comprehensive treatment of these issues).

It should be pointed out that determination of the external moments about different joints during manual materials-handling tasks is based on the well-established laws of physics (Figure 37.3). However, the

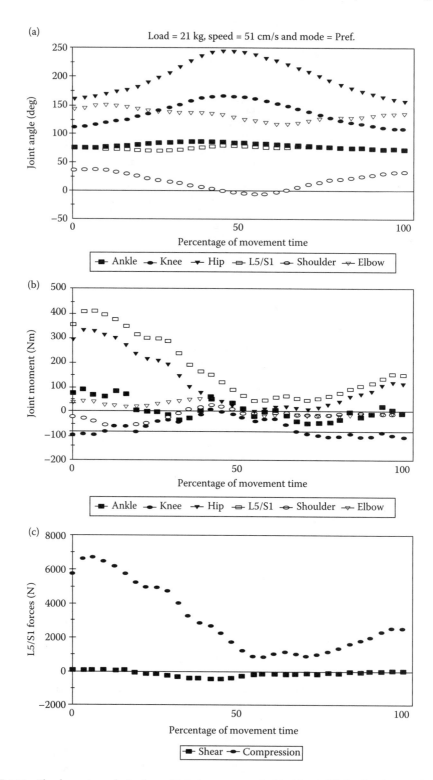

FIGURE 37.3 The dynamic analysis of a sagittal plane symmetrical isokinetic lift (load 21 kg, speed = 51 cm/s, mode = preferred method of lifting): (a) joint angle; (b) net muscular joint moment; and (c) the joint reaction forces at L5/S1.

determination of human performance and assessment of functional capacity are based on other disciplines, for example, psychophysics, that are not as exact or well developed. One can describe easily the job demand, in terms of the required moments about each joint, by analyzing the workers performing the tasks. However, one is unable to predict the ability to perform an arbitrary task based on the incomplete knowledge of functional capacities at the joint levels. A task is easily decomposed to its demands at the joint level; however, one cannot compose (construct) the set of feasible tasks based on one's functional capacity knowledge. The mapping from high-level task demands to the joint-level functional capacity for a given performance trial is unique. However, the mapping from joint-level functional capacity to the high-level task demand is one to many (not unique). The challenge to the human performance research community is to establish this missing link. Much of the integration of ergonomics and functional analysis depends on removal of this obstacle. The question of whether a subject can perform a task based on knowledge of his or her functional capacity at the joint level remains an area of open research. When ergonomists or occupational physicians evaluate the fitness of task demands and worker capability, the following clinical questions will be presented; (1) Which space should be explored for determining normalcy, fit, or equivalence? (2) Should we consider the performance of the multilink system in the joint space or end-effector (cartesian workspace)? These issues have profound effects on both the development of new technologies and the evaluation of trunk or lifting performance.

The enormous degrees of freedom existing in the neuromusculoskeletal system provide the control centers for both the kinematic and actuator redundancies. The redundancies provide optimization possibility. Because one can lift an object from point A to point B with infinite postural possibilities, it can be suggested that certain physical parameters maybe optimized for the learned movements. The possible candidates for objective function to be optimized are movement time, energy, smoothness, muscular activities, and so on. This approach, although still in its early stage, may be very important for spine functional assessment. One could compare the given performance with the optimal performance that is predicted by the model. This approach provides specific goals and gives biofeedback with respect to the individual's performance.

37.3.6 Comparison of Task Demands and Performance Capacity

The regression analysis was used to model the dynamic torque, velocity, and power output as a function of resistance level during flexion and extension using the B-200 Isostation (Parnianpour et al., 1990). Results indicated that the measured torque was not a good discriminator of the 10th, 50th, and 90th percentile population. However, velocity and power were shown to effectively discriminate the three populations (Figure 37.4). Based on these data, it was suggested that during clinical testing, sagittal plane resistance should not be set at higher than about 80 N m to minimize the internal loading of spine while taxing trunk functional capacity. This presentation of data may be useful to the physician or ergonomist in evaluating the functional capacity requirements of workplace manual materials-handling tasks. For example, a manual material-handling task that requires about 80 N m (61 ft lb) of trunk extensor strength could be performed by 90% of the population in the normal database if the required average trunk velocity does not exceed 40 deg/s, while only 50% could perform the task if the velocity requirement exceeds 70 deg/s. More importantly, only the top 10th percentile population could perform the task if the velocity requirement approaches 105 deg/s. A few versions of lumbar motion monitors that can record the triaxial motion in the workplace have been used to provide the trunk movement requirements. The preceding example also illustrates the importance of having the same bases for evaluation of both task and the functional capability of the worker.

37.4 Clinical Applications

37.4.1 Low Back Patient Evaluation and Identification

Clinical studies have utilized quantitative human performance, that is, strength and endurance measures, to predict the first incidence or recurrence of LBP and disability outcome and also as a prognosis

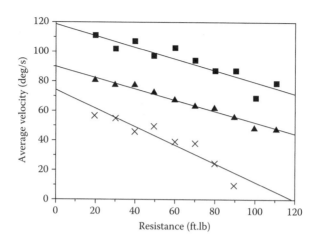

FIGURE 37.4 The average extension velocity measured during maximum trunk extension against a set resistance for 10th (×), 50th (▲), and 90th (■) percentile distribution.

measure during the rehabilitation process. Training programs to enhance the endurance and strength of workers have been implemented in some industries. More studies on the effectiveness of these programs are needed. It can be hypothesized that these programs complement the stress-management programs to enhance both worker satisfaction and coping strategies with regard to physical and nonphysical stressors at the workplace.

Functional-based impairment evaluation schemes traditionally have used spinal mobility. Given the poor reliability of range of motion (ROM), its large variability among individuals, and the static psychometric nature of ROM, the use of continuous dynamic profiles of motion with the higher order derivatives has been suggested. Dynamic performances of 281 consecutive patients from the Impairment Evaluation Center at the Mayo Clinic were used. As part of the comprehensive physical and psychological evaluation, 281 consecutive LBP patients underwent isometric and dynamic trunk testing using the B200 Isostation. *Feature extraction* and *cluster analysis* techniques were used to identify the main profiles in dynamic patient performances. The middle three cycles of movements were interpolated and averaged into 128 data points; thus, the data were normalized with respect to cycle time. This allowed for comparison between individuals. The number of patients in each group is also noted on the graph (Figure 37.5). Patients in the first (*n* = 48) and second (*n* = 55) groups had similar flexion mobility; however, those in the first group had more limited extension mobility. The time-to-peak sagittal position also varied among the five groups. Forty-seven patients in the fifth group showed extreme impairment in both flexion and extension. The third group (26 patients) showed differential impairments with respect to direction of motion. A marked improvement over the use of ROM has been achieved by preserving information in the continuous profiles. The LBP patients in this study are heterogeneous with respect to their movement profile. Uniform treatment of these patients is questionable, and rehabilitation programs should consider their specific impairments. Future research should incorporate the clinical profiles with these movement profiles to further delineate the heterogeneity of LBP patients. Marras et al. (1993) used similar feature-extraction techniques to characterize the movement profiles of 510 subjects belonging to normal (*n* = 339) and 10 LBP patient groups (*n* = 171). Subjects were asked to perform flexion/extension trunk movement at five levels of asymmetry, while the three-dimensional movement of the spine was monitored by the Lumbar Motion Monitor (an exoskeleton goniometer developed at the Biodynamics Lab of The Ohio State University). Trunk motions were performed against no resistance, and no pelvic stabilization was required (Ferguson et al. 2009). The quadratic discriminant analysis was able to correctly classify more than 80% of the subjects. The same technology was used to develop logistic regression

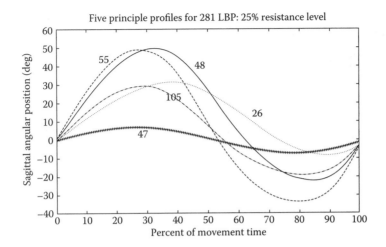

FIGURE 37.5   The five principle profiles of trunk sagittal movement for 281 low back pain patients.

models to identify the high-risk jobs in industrial workplaces. Hence, principles of human performance can be applied successfully to the worker and the task to avoid the mismatch between performance capability and task demand.

The key limitations in the development of the discriminate functions for classification purposes, are the data-driven nature of the algorithms and the lack of theoretical orientation in the process of development and validation of these models. It is suggested that the mathematical simulation of flexion or extension trunk movement may identify an objective basis for the evaluation and assessment of trunk kinematic performance. A catalog of movement patterns that are optimal with respect to physical and biomechanical quantities may contribute to the emergence of a more theoretically based computational paradigm for the evaluation of kinematic performance of normal subjects and patients. It must be emphasized that in this paradigm one has no intention to claim that the CNS actually optimizes any single or composite cost function.

To provide clinical insight for interpretation of the distinctive features in the movement profiles, Parnianpour et al. (1999) have suggested an optimization-based approach for simulation of dynamic point-to-point sagittal trunk movement (Zeinali-Davarani et al. 2011). The effect of strength impairment on movement patterns was simulated based on minimizing different physical cost functions: energy, jerk, peak torque, impulse, and work. During unconstrained simulations, the velocity patterns of all models are predicted, while time-to-peak velocity is distinct for each cost function (Figure 37.6). Imposing an 80% reduction in extensor muscle strength diminished the significant differences between unimpaired optimal movement profiles (Figure 37.7). The results indicate that the search for finding the objective function being used by the CNS is an ill-posed problem because we are sure if we have included all the active constraints in the simulation. The four application areas of these results are (1) providing optimized trajectories for biofeedback to patients during the rehabilitation process; (2) training workers to lift safely; (3) estimating the task demand based on the global description of the job; and (4) aiding the engineering evaluation to develop ergonomic and workplace interventions which are needed to accommodate individuals with prior disability.

37.4.2 LBP and Postural Sway during Quiet Standing

Postural balance is a fundamental activity of daily living that must be considered in the frail elderly and patients with various neurological or MSD. Byl and Sinnott (1991) were the first to investigate balance control in patients with LBP, by measuring postural sway. A recent review of published studies

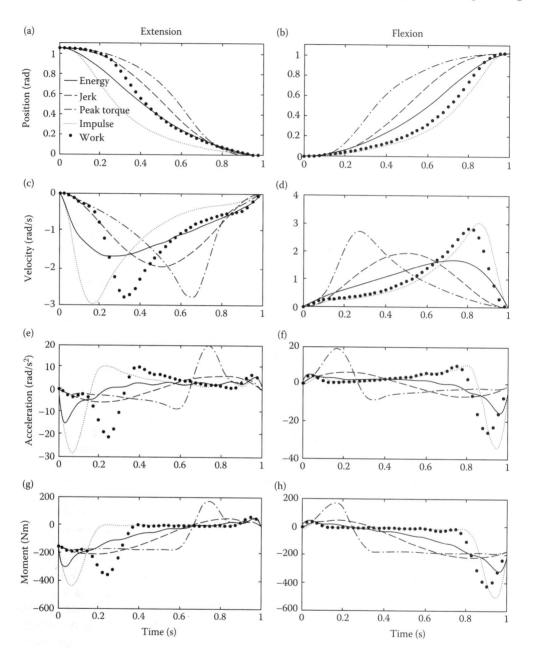

FIGURE 37.6 The optimized unconstrained trunk flexion and extension trajectories for the five cost functions: Energy, Jerk, Peak Torque, Impulse, and Work. The optimized unconstrained trunk flexion and extension trajectories are shown for the five cost functions. The magnitude and timing of velocity and acceleration are significantly different based on the different cost functions. The anthropometric data for an individual with height and weight of 1.7 m and 80 kg were used in these simulations.

concluded that there is consistent evidence that LBP coincides with increased sway amplitude and/ or sway velocity (Ruhe et al. 2011). However, a more detailed analysis of the original studies indicates that significant effects on postural sway are found in some experimental conditions and not in others (Mazaheri et al. 2011). Mientjes and Frank (1999) tested subjects under different conditions: comprising standing on firm and unstable surfaces, with eyes open and closed, standing upright and leaning

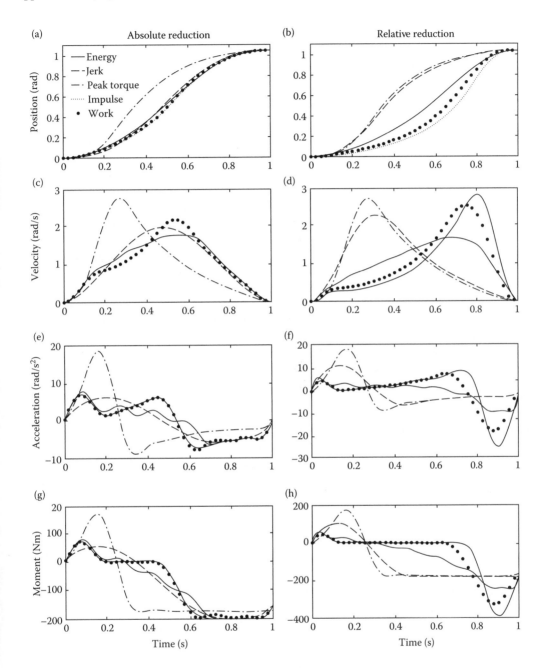

FIGURE 37.7 The optimized trunk flexion trajectories for the five cost functions with the relative and absolute peak extensor strength impairments. The relative strength reduction meant that the extensor strength was reduced to 80% of the peak extension moment required during unconstrained simulations. The absolute strength reduction meant that the extensor strength was set to 200 Nm.

forward, with head upright and tilted backward. Differences between groups were found only when visual information was removed (eyes closed) and/or when vestibular information was manipulated (head tilt). This suggests that impairments of balance control may not be present in LBP consistently and the nature of such contextual dependence on experimental conditions should be scrutinized to gain insight into the mechanisms underlying poor balance control in LBP (Mazaheri et al. 2011).

Impairments of lumbar proprioception is another factor associated with LBP that is likely to affect postural control as well (Gill and Callaghan, 1998; Leinonen et al. 2003; Brumagne et al. 2004). Increased postural sway when visual or vestibular input is removed or manipulated in subjects with LBP compared with healthy subjects has been observed in keeping with the above assertion. In addition, impaired motor control of the trunk as a result of LBP has been suggested to determine increased postural sway (Brumagne et al. 2004; Leinonen et al. 2003; Radebold et al. 2001). Radebold et al. (2001) found a correlation between poor balance control in an unstable sitting position and delayed trunk muscle responses after a sudden release perturbation in patients with idiopathic LBP, and Leinonen et al. (2003) reported a similar relationship in sciatica patients. Note that delayed muscle responses could actually be the result of sensory impairments. Furthermore, type of LBP (i.e., severity, disability, and origin), fear of pain or pain itself may affect results of postural sway. Interpretation of pain as catastrophic element may give rise to pain-related fear and avoidance of activities that have an impact on posture. Fear of pain may lead to more rigid control, as reflected by decreased sway in a subset of patients, while the effect of pain or proprioceptive deficits may dominate and lead to increased sensory and/or motor noise, which increase postural sway (Mazaheri et al. 2011). The studies of Mok et al. (2004) and Salavati et al. (2009) showed reduced sway in a group of LBP that had low levels of pain or even no pain at the time of testing. van Dieën et al. (2010) also reported that patients with a recent history of LBP showed a lower sway amplitude in unstable sitting than individuals with current and without LBP.

Information about the relationship between posture and cognition in LBP is scarce (van Daele et al. 2010). Influence of a secondary attention demanding task on sway has been investigated in LBP compared to healthy individuals under different sensory conditions. Therefore, dual tasking can be used in future studies on balance performance between in LBP. Furthermore, postural sway of LBP patients has been assessed mostly by linear measures of COP variability. Few studies have investigated the nonlinear dynamical pattern of sway in LBP. Further analysis of postural sway by nonlinear methods might reveal differential responses of LBP and healthy people to sensory and cognitive manipulations more consistently (Mazaheri et al. 2010; Van Daele et al. 2010; Bruijn et al. 2011).

Recurrence quantification analysis (RQA), a nonlinear method of postural analysis, was used to explore the effects of dual tasking on postural performance in people with nonspecific LBP compared with healthy participants (Mazaheri et al. 2010). Postural performance was quantified by RQA% recurrence% determinism, entropy, and trend. People with nonspecific LBP ($n = 22$) and unimpaired individuals ($n = 22$) randomly performed quiet standing tasks with three levels of difficulty (rigid-surface eyes open, rigid-surface eyes closed, and foam-surface eyes closed). These tasks were performed in isolation or concurrently with an easy or difficult cognitive task. Increasing postural difficulty was associated with higher% determinism, higher entropy, and lower trend in anteroposterior (AP) and mediolateral (ML) directions in people with LBP and healthy participants. All RQA variables in the ML direction decreased as cognitive conditions became more difficult. Significant interactions between group and cognitive difficulty were shown for % recurrence, % determinism, and trend in the AP direction. While healthy participants decreased % recurrence and trend by increasing the level of cognitive difficulty, the LBP patients did not.

37.4.3 Identification of Frequent Fallers and Variability and Stability Assessment of Gait

Much effort has been invested to find ways to identify frequent fallers to target them with prevention methods. The frequency of fall leading to injury and activity limitation increases among the elderly. These are significant concepts as a growing number of older workers may delay their retirements in the Western nations and because of unfavorable economic conditions and much longer life expectancy that is achieved by the improved medications and health conditions. Nonlinear and linear analyses of postural balance during gait and batteries of validated clinical tests have been developed to identify frequent fallers (Najafi et al. 2002; Ganea et al. 2011). Najafi et al. (2002) developed a method for evaluating

the characteristics of postural transition (PT) and their correlation with falling risk in elderly people using wearable inertial sensors. The time of sit-to-stand and stand-to-sit transitions and their duration were evaluated using a miniature gyroscope. On the basis of the discrete wavelet transform, the average and standard deviation of transition duration and the occurrence of abnormal successive transitions (number of attempts to have a successful transition) were significantly correlated with the falling risk during the previous year, balance and gait disorders (Tinetti score), visual disorders, and cognitive and depressive disorders ($p < 0.01$).

van Schooten et al. (2011) tested the sensitivity of measures of variability, local stability, and orbital stability of trunk kinematics to balance impairments during gait, using galvanic vestibular stimulation (GVS) to impair balance in 12 young adults while walking on a treadmill at different speeds. Variability in the medio-lateral direction and local and orbital stability were calculated for the trunk acceleration based on the measurements of inertial sensors. The short-term Lyapunov exponent and variability reflected the destabilizing effect of GVS, whereas the long-term Lyapunov exponent and Floquet multipliers suggested increased stability. They concluded that only short-term Lyapunov exponents and variability can be used to asses stability of gait. The feasibility of using these measures in screening for fall risk was investigated by prediction of the presence or absence of GVS with variability and the short-term Lyapunov exponent. Predictions were best at preferred walking speed, with a correct classification in 83.3% of the cases.

37.5 Conclusions

The outcome of trunk performance is affected by the many neural, mechanical, and environmental factors that must be considered during quantitative assessment. The objective evaluation of the critical dimensions of functional capacity and its comparison with the task demands is crucial to the decision-making processes in the different stages of the ergonomic prevention and rehabilitation process. Knowing the tissue tolerance limits from biomechanical studies, task demands from ergonomic analysis, and function capacities from performance evaluation, the rehabilitation team will optimize the changes to the workplace or the task that will maximize the functional reserves (unutilized resources) to reduce the occurrence of fatigue and overexertion. This will enhance worker satisfaction and productivity while reducing the risk of the MSD. On the basis of ergonomic and motor control literature, the testing protocols that best simulate the loading conditions of the task will yield more valid results and better predictive ability. Ergonomic principles indicate that the ratio of the functional capacity to the task demand (utilization ratio) is critical to the development of muscular fatigue, which may lead to more injurious muscle recruitment patterns and movement profiles due to loss of motor control and coordination. However, large prospective studies are still needed to verify this. The most promising application for these quantitative measures is to be used as a benchmark for the safe return to work of injured workers, given the enormous variations within the normal population. With the advent of technologies to monitor trunk performance in the workplace, one can obtain estimates of the injurious levels of task demands (kinematic and kinetic parameters), which can be used to guide preplacement and rehabilitation strategies. The more functional the clinical tests become, the more clinicians need a complex interpretation scheme. An increasingly complex interpretation scheme opens the possibility of using mathematical modeling with intelligent computer interfaces. The ability to identify subgroups of patients or high-risk individuals based on their functional performance will remain an open area of research to interested biomedical engineers within the multidisciplinary group of experts addressing neuromusculoskeletal occupational disorders.

Acknowledgments

The author would like to thank Drs. George V. Kondraske, Margareta Nordin, Victor H. Frankel, Elen Ross, Jackson Tan, Robert Gabriel, Robert R. Crowell, William Marras, Sheldon R. Simon, Heinz Hoffer,

Ali Sheikhzadeh, Jung Yong Kim, Sue Ferguson, Patrick Sparto, and Kinda Khalaf, Masood Mazaheri, Japp van Dieën, Aboulfazl Shirazi-adl, Hooshang Hemami, and Seyyed Javad Mousavi for their invaluable comments and contributions.

Defining Terms

Carpal tunnel syndrome (CTS): The result of compression of the median nerve in the carpal tunnel of the wrist.

Cluster analysis: A statistical technique to identify natural groupings in data.

DeQuervain's disease: A special case of tendosynovitis (swelling and irritation of the tendon sheath) which occurs in the abductor and extensor tendons of the thumb, where they share a common sheath.

Electromyogram: Recordings of the electric potentials produced by muscle action.

Feature extraction: A statistical technique to allow efficient representation of variability in the original signals while reducing the dimensions of the data.

Lateral epicondylitis (tennis elbow): Tendons attaching to the epicondyle of the humerus bone become irritated.

Rotator cuff tendinitis: The irritation and swelling of the tendon or the bursae of the shoulder that is caused by continuous muscle or tendon effort to keep the arm elevated.

Tension neck syndrome: An irritation of the levator scapulae and trapezius group of muscles of the neck commonly occurring after repeated or sustained overhead work.

Thoracic outlet syndrome: A disorder resulting from compression of nerves and blood vessels between the clavicle and the first and second ribs at the brachial plexus.

Trigger finger: A special case of tendosynovitis where the tendon becomes nearly locked so that forced movement is not smooth.

References

Andersson, G.B.J. 1991. Evaluation of muscle function. In: J.W. Frymoyer (Ed.), *The Adult Spine: Principles and Practice*, p. 241. New York, Raven Press.

Beimborn, D.S. and Morrissey, M.C. 1988. A review of literature related to trunk muscle performance. *Spine* 13:655.

Berme, N. and Cappozzo, A. 1990. *Biomechanics of Human Movement: Applications in Rehabilitation, Sports and Ergonomics.* Worthington, Ohio, Bertec Corporation.

Bruijn, S.M., Bregman, D.J., Meijer, O.G., Beek P.J., and van Dieën, J.H. 2011. The validity of stability measures: A modelling approach. *J Biomech* 44:2401.

Brumagne, S., Cordo, P., and Verschueren, S. 2004. Proprioceptive weighting changes in persons with low back pain and elderly persons during upright standing. *Neurosci Lett* 366:63.

Byl, N. and Sinnott, P. 1991. Variations in balance and body sway in middle-aged adults: Subjects with healthy backs compared with subjects with low-back dysfunction. *Spine* 16:325.

Ferguson, S.A., Marras, W.S., Burr, D.L., Woods, S., Mendel, E., and Gupta, P. 2009 Quantification of a meaningful change in low back functional impairment. *Spine* 34:2060.

Ganea, R., Paraschiv-Ionescu, A., Büla, C., Rochat, S., and Aminian, K. 2011. Multi-parametric evaluation of sit-to-stand and stand-to-sit transitions in elderly people. *Med Eng Phys* 33:1086.

Gill, K. and Callaghan, M. 1998. The measurement of lumbar proprioception in individuals with and without low back pain. *Spine* 23:371.

Gundewall, B., Liljeqvist, M., and Hansson, T. 1993. Primary prevention in back symptoms and absence from work. *Spine* 18:587.

Kondraske, G.V. 1990. Quantitative measurement and assessment of performance. In: R.V. Smith and J.H. Leslie (Eds.), *Rehabilitation Engineering*, Boca Raton, FL, CRC Press.

Kroemer, K.E., Kroemer, H., and Kroemer-Elbert, K. 1994. *Ergonomics: How to Design for the Ease & Efficiency*. Englewood Cliffs, NJ, Prentice-Hall.

Leinonen, V., Kankaanpaa, M., Luukkonen, M, Kansanen, M., Hanninen, O., Airaksinen, O., and Taimela, S. 2003. Lumbar paraspinal muscle function, perception of lumbar position, and postural control in disc herniation-related back pain. *Spine* 28:842–848.

Luck, J.V. and Florence, D.W. 1988. A brief history and comparative analysis of disability systems and impairment evaluation guides. *Office Practice* 19:839.

Marras, W.S. and Mirka, G.A. 1989. Trunk strength during asymmetric trunk motion. *Human Factors* 31:667.

Marras, W.S., Parnianpour, M., Ferguson, S.A. et al. 1993. Quantification and classification of low back disorders based on trunk motion. *Eur J Med Rehabil* 3:218.

Mazaheri, M., Coenen, P., Parnianpour, M., Kiers, H., and van Dieën, J. 2013. Low back pain and postural sway during quiet standing with and without sensory manipulation: A systematic review. *Gait Posture* 2011 Submitted.

Mazaheri, M., Salavati, M., Negahban, H., Sanjari, M.A., and Parnianpour, M. 2010. Postural sway in low back pain: Effects of dual tasks. *Gait Posture*, 31:116.

Mientjes, M. and Frank, J. 1999. Balance in chronic low back pain patients compared to healthy people under various conditions in upright standing. *Clin Biomech.* 14:710.

Mok, N., Brauer, S., and Hodges, P. 2004. Hip strategy for balance control in quiet standing is reduced in people with low back pain. *Spine*, 29:E107.

Mousavi, S.J., Akbari. M.E., Mehdian. H., Mobini. B., Montazeri. A., Akbarnia. B., and Parnianpour. M. 2011. Low back pain in Iran: A growing need to adapt and implement evidence-based practice in developing countries. *Spine* 36:E638.

Najafi, B., Aminian, K., Loew, F., Blanc, Y., and Robert, P.A. 2002. Measurement of stand-sit and sit-stand transitions using a miniature gyroscope and its application in fall risk evaluation in the elderly. *IEEE Trans Biomed Eng* 49:843.

National Institute for Occupational Safety and Health (NIOSH). 1981. *Work Practice Guide for Manual Lifting* (DHHS Publication No. 81122). Washington, DC: U.S. Government Printing Office.

Newton, M. and Waddell, G. 1993. Trunk strength testing with Iso-Machines, Part 1: Review of a decade of scientific evidence. *Spine* 18:801.

Parnianpour, M. and Shirazi-Adl, A. 1999. Quantitative assessment of trunk performance. In W. Karwowski and W.S. Marras (Eds.), *Handbook of Occupational Ergonomics*, pp. 985–1006, Boca Raton, FL, CRC Press.

Parnianpour, M., Nordin, M., Kahanovitz, N. et al. 1988. The triaxial coupling of torque generation of trunk muscles during isometric exertions and the effect of fatiguing isoinertial movements on the motor output and movement patterns. *Spine* 13:982.

Parnianpour, M., Nordin, M., and Sheikhzadeh, A. 1990. The relationship of torque, velocity and power with constant resistive load during sagittal trunk movement. *Spine* 15:639.

Parnianpour, M., Wang, J.L., Shirazi-Adl, A. et al. 1999. A computational method for simulation of trunk motion: Towards a theoretical based quantitative assessment of trunk performance. *Biomed Eng Appl Basis Commun* 11:1.

Pope, M.H. 1992. A critical evaluation of functional muscle testing. In J.N. Weinstein (Ed.), *Clinical Efficacy and Outcome in the Diagnosis and Treatment of Low Back Pain*, p. 101, Ltd., New York, Raven Press.

Radebold, A., Cholewicki, J., Polzhofer, G., and Greene, H. 2001. Impaired postural control of the lumbar spine is associated with delayed muscle response times in patients with chronic idiopathic low back pain. *Spine* 26:724.

Ruhe, A., Fejer, R., and Walker, B. 2011. Center of pressure excursion as a measure of balance performance in patients with non-specific low back pain compared to healthy controls: A systematic review of the literature. *Eur Spine J.* 20:358.

Salavati, M., Mazaheri, M., Negahban, H., Ebrahimi, I., Jafari, A., Kazemnejad, A., and Parnianpour, M. 2009. Effect of dual-tasking on postural control in subjects with nonspecific low back pain. *Spine* 34:1415.

Snook, S.H., Fine, L.J., and Silverstein, B.A. 1988. Musculoskeletal disorders. In B.S. Levy and D.H. Wegman (Eds.), *Occupational Health: Recognizing and Preventing Work-Related Disease*, pp. 345–370, Little, Brown and Co., Boston/Toronto.

Szpalski, M. and Parnianpour, M. 1996. Trunk performance, strength and endurance: Measurement techniques and application. In: S. Weisel and J. Weinstein (Eds.), *The Lumbar Spine*, 2nd ed., pp. 1074–1105, Philadelphia, W.B. Saunders.

Tan, J.C., Parnianpour, M., Nordin, M. et al. 1993. Isometric maximal and submaximal trunk exertion at different flexed positions in standing: Triaxial torque output and EMG. *Spine* 18:2480.

Van Daele, U., Hagman, F., Truijen, S., Vorlat, P., Van Gheluwe, B., and Vaes, P. 2010. Decrease in postural sway and trunk stiffness during cognitive dual-task in nonspecific chronic low back pain patients, performance compared to healthy control subjects. *Spine* 35:583.

van Dieën, J.H., Koppes, L.L., Twisk, J.W. 2010. Low back pain history and postural sway in unstable sitting. *Spine* 35:812.

van Schooten, K.S., Sloot, L.H., Bruijn, S.M., Kingma, H., Meijer, O.G., Pijnappels, M., and van Dieën, J.H. 2011. Sensitivity of trunk variability and stability measures to balance impairments induced by galvanic vestibular stimulation during gait. *Gait Posture*, 33:656.

World Health Organization. 1980. *International Classification of Impairments, Disabilities, and Handicaps.* Geneva, WHO.

World Health Organization. 1985. Identification and Control of Work-Related Diseases. Technical report no. 174. Geneva, WHO.

Zeinali-Davarani, S., Shirazi-Adl, A., Dariush, B., Hemami, H., and Parnianpour, M. 2011. The effect of resistance level and stability demands on recruitment patterns and internal loading of spine in dynamic flexion and extension using a simple trunk model. *Comput Methods Biomech Biomed Eng.* 14:645.

38

Human Performance Engineering Design and Analysis Tools

Paul J. Vasta
University of Texas,
Arlington

George V. Kondraske
University of Texas,
Arlington

38.1 Introduction

Computer software applications have been implemented in virtually every aspect of our lives and the field of human performance has not proven to be an exception. Due to the growing recognition of the role of human performance engineering in many different areas (e.g., clinical medicine, industrial design, etc.) and the resulting increase in requirements of the methods involved, having the "right tool for the job" is becoming of vital importance. Software developers bear the brunt of the responsibility of determining the qualities of a software application that define it as being "the right tool" for a specific job. In contrast, users of this class of tools must determine when their application extends a given tool beyond its intended scope. These abilities require a knowledge base spanning a number of different fundamental concepts and methods encompassing not only the obvious aspects of human performance and computer programming, but also many other less obvious issues related to database requirements, parameter standards, systems engineering principles, and software architecture. In addition, foresight of how specific components can best be integrated to fit the needs of a particular usage is also necessary.

    This chapter addresses selected aspects of computer software tools specifically directed toward human performance design and analysis. The majority of tools currently available emphasize biomechanical models, and as such, this emphasis is reflected here. However, a much broader scope in terms of the body systems incorporated is anticipated, and an effort is made to consider the evolution of more versatile and integrated packages. Selected key functional components of tools are described and a representative sample of currently emerging state-of-the-art packages is used to illustrate not only a snapshot of the capabilities now available, but also those which are needed and options that exist in terms of the fundamental approach taken to address similar problems.

In general, the development of computer software applications, especially in maturing fields such as human performance engineering, serves multiple purposes. The most apparent is the relative speed and accuracy that can be achieved in computationally intensive tasks (e.g., dynamic analysis) compared to performing the processes by hand. In addition, computers can handle large amounts of data and help keep track of the multitude of parameters associated with the human architecture. This allows otherwise impossible procedures, such as the detailed analysis of a complex *human–task interface*, visualization of a human figure in a *virtual workspace*, or the computation of time-series multibody joint torques, to be realized. Perhaps more important, though, are the indirect benefits provided. For example, relatively complex analytic methods utilized in research facilities can be directly implemented in the field by practitioners, with the need for only a complete knowledge of how to effectively *use* the capability available (which is substantially different than the knowledge required to *create* that ability). Moreover, because the software environment demands rigor (e.g., coding structure requirements, data handling and storage, etc.) and since the potential scope of end-user needs in terms of functional and parametric components encompassed is broad, decisions are forced and rules must be clearly delineated. These characteristics thus serve as a motivation to develop standards for (or at least decide upon the use of) many items including methods, parameters, parameter definition conventions, and units of measure. Such efforts can expose and correct inadequacies inherent in current standards while successful software tools (i.e., those which make their way into everyday use) facilitate dissemination of key knowledge and standards to both researchers and practitioners alike.

It can be anticipated that most analysis or decision-making tasks required of practitioners will be made available in computer-based form, including some that are not currently feasible to perform at all except, perhaps, by using intuitive methods that are inconsistently applied and produce results of questionable validity. Given the extent of the possible list of tools within a given package, and considering the substantial overlap of various support functions, classification of packages is difficult. This has been seen already in the relatively modest number of those currently available.

38.2 Selected Fundamentals

It is typical to think of a software capability in terms of a high-level process, for example "gait analysis," where the end result is of primary interest since the underlying processes are performed "invisibly." Yet these supportive processes, many of which have common mathematical methodologies and modeling approaches, determine the ultimate usability and applicability of the software to a given problem and, therefore, deserve closer examination. It makes sense to consider these methods generically not only because they are common to several existing packages, but also because they will undoubtedly be important in others.

38.2.1 Physics-Based Models and Methods

Physics-based methods are implemented when direct analysis of the system or its resources is feasible. With regard to the human system, such methods are commonly applied in biomechanical analysis where unknown parameters, such as joint torque, are derived from known characteristics, such as segment lengths and reaction forces, based on established physical laws and relationships. Given that relatively simple biomechanical analyses typically include multiple segments and degrees of freedom, the feasibility of employing such methods depends not only on the availability of the required input data, but on the capability to process large amounts of information as well. As the analytical complexity of the task increases, for example, with the inclusion of motion, the significance of implementing such processes within a computer software application becomes readily apparent.

Physical motion is common to most situations in which the human functions and is therefore fundamental to the analysis of performance. Parameters such as segment position, orientation, velocity, and acceleration are derived using kinematic or dynamic analysis or both. This approach is equally appropriate for operations on a single joint system or *linked multibody systems*, such as is typically required for human analysis. Depending on the desired output, foreword (direct) or inverse analysis may be employed to obtain the parameters of interest. For example, inverse dynamic analysis can provide joint torque, given motion and force data while foreword (direct) dynamic analysis uses joint torque to derive motion. Especially for three-dimensional analyses of multijoint systems, the methods are quite complex and are presently a focal point for computer implementation (Allard et al., 1994).

Physics models used to address biomechanical aspects of human performance are relatively well established and utilized in both research and applied domains. In contrast, concepts and methods directed toward other aspects of human performance, such as information processing (in purely perceptual contexts as well as in neuromotor control contexts), are based on strong science and have been incorporated into one-of-a-kind computer models, but to our knowledge have not been engineered into any general-purpose computer tools. It can be argued that Shannon's information theory provides the basis for a similar set of "physics-based" cause-and-effect models to support the incorporation of this aspect of human performance into computer-based modeling and analysis tools. Considerable work has gone into the application of information theory to human information processing (Lachman et al., 1979) within research domains. The definition of neuromotor *channel capacity* (Fitts, 1954) and metrics for the information content of a visual stimulus measured in bits (Hick, 1952; Hyman, 1953) are some examples of the influence of information theory that have become well established. Given the considerable science that now exists, useful computer-based analytic tools that use these ideas as basic modeling constructs are likely to emerge.

38.2.2 Inference-Based Models

Often, direct measurement of a *performance resource* or structural element is not feasible or practical and estimates must be inferred from models based on representative populations. Inferential-based methods, therefore, utilize derived relationships between parameters to provide an estimation (or prediction) of an unknown quantity based on other available measures. One type of modeling approach in such a situation is through statistical regression. This process utilizes data measured from a population of subjects with characteristics similar to the subject or population of interest, to derive a function which represents a "typical" relationship between the independent (measured) variable and the dependent (desired) variable. Specifically, this is achieved through the determination of the function that minimizes the error between the actual and the predicted value across all observations of the independent variable. This process results in an approximation of the desired parameter with a quantified standard error (Remington and Schork, 1985). Applications of this method require that the dependent variable is distributed normally and with constant variance, and correspondingly, that an estimation of its typical value (for a given population) is desired. Applied to the human system, regression is often implemented to develop *data models*, which are then used to estimate unknown structural parameter values from known parameters, such as the estimation of body segment moments of inertia from stature and weight (McConville et al. 1980). Regression has also been used to predict task performance from a wide variety of other variables (e.g., height, weight, age, other performance variables, etc.). A specific example is the determination of the maximum acceptable load during lifting tasks as a function of variables such as body weight and arm strength (Jiang and Ayoub, 1987).

A conceptually different and relatively new example of an inferential model, motivated by human performance problems specifically, is nonlinear causal resource analysis (NCRA) (Vasta and Kondraske, 1994; Kondraske, 1988). Quantitative task demands, in terms of performance variables that characterize the involved subsystems, are inferred from a population data set that includes measures of subsystem performance resource availabilities (e.g., speed, accuracy, etc.) and overall performance on the task in question. This method is based on the following simple concept: Consider a sample of 100 people, each with a known amount of cash (e.g., a fairly even distribution from $0 to $10,000). Each person is asked to try to purchase a specific computer, the "cost" of which is unknown. In the subgroup that was able to make the purchase (some would not have enough cash), the individual who had the least amount of cash provides the key clue. That "amount of cash availability" provides an estimate of the computer's cost (i.e., the unknown value). Thus, in human performance, demand is inferred from resource availabilities.

38.2.3 Fidelity

An important principle that has not often received the scrutiny it deserves is that of the level of fidelity desired, or perhaps more critically, necessary for a particular application. This includes anything that affects the range of applicability or quality of the results provided in a given application. Fidelity can be characterized in terms of three distinctly different components: (1) model scope, (2) computational quality (e.g., resolution limits, compounding of errors, convergence limits of numerical methods, etc.), and (3) data quality (e.g., noise, intrinsic resolution limits, etc.). Model scope considers the extent to which major systems are incorporated (e.g., neuromuscular, sensory, cognitive, etc.) and, as a separate issue, the extent to which these major subsystems are represented (e.g., peak torque and angle limits vs. a three-dimensional torque-angle-speed envelope for neuromuscular systems of rotational joints).

38.2.4 Parameter Conventions

Often, the exact definition of parameters across (and even within) scientific disciplines varies, limiting communication of findings and inhibiting dissemination of knowledge. Careful selection and clear documentation of *parameter conventions* is an important principle in producing analytic software that can be understood, accepted, and used.

Within the broad scope of parameters that could possibly be incorporated in analytic and other software tools, there are many parameter convention challenges that arise. Due to the fact that of the reported analyses in which various parameters that appear have been of restricted scope and largely special purpose, more generalized situations where convention is important have escaped standardization in terms broad enough to support all application needs. As one example, consider the description of relative orientation between two object-attached coordinate systems in three dimensions (in the context of the human system, this specifies joint angle). There are two basic forms of angle set representations, each derived in terms of the method of rotation of one coordinate system (attached to a moving object) about a specific axis: (1) Fixed angle representation, which involves referencing each rotation of the moving system to some fixed reference frame and, (2) Euler angle representation, indicating that each consecutive rotation of the moving system is referenced to the coordinate axes of its present orientation. Given multiple degrees of freedom, multiple angles result representing the amount of rotation about a specific axis and at a defined position in the order of rotations. The specification of these parameters defines the associated angle set convention (i.e., fixed or Euler). Utilization of the terms "roll, pitch, and yaw" (Chao, 1980) in communicating this convention, originally used to describe ship and aircraft orientation, can also lead to confusion. This is not only due to the lack of similarity between the defined reference frame of an aircraft and that of a human segment, but also due to its altered definition within other disciplines (e.g., fixed angle representation (Spong and Vidyasagar, 1989). Thus, depending on the "type" of Euler angle used and the sequence of axes about which the rotations occur, two entirely different orientations are likely to result. This discussion does not even consider the clinical perspective on joint angles, where only angles measured in three orthogonal planes (Panjabi et al., 1974) are considered. Despite the fact that the human architecture has remained constant (unlike many artificial systems), to our knowledge there is no standard convention that defines all angles in a total human link model for three-dimensional motion.

38.2.5 Data Formats

The utilization of data, especially within a software environment, involves both communication and manipulation not only within a single stand-alone application, but often across facilities, databases, and platforms. Data formats, in this light, can be considered among the most important of the components fundamental to analytic software. Problematic effects may result from aspects including inconsistent adoption of terminology (e.g., endurance vs. fatigue), units of measure specifications, file structures, parameter coding, and database structure. Computer-aided design (CAD) environments in traditional engineering disciplines (e.g., drafting, mechanical design, etc.) have confronted such issues with standardization such as the DXF file formats (used for two- and three-dimensional geometric drawings; even accepted by some numerical machining systems) and the Gerber format (used to communicate a printed circuit board specification to board manufacturers). Within the realm of human performance engineering, standards for data formats remain at the forefront of developmental needs. Some limited standards are emerging, such as the relatively consistent use of ASCII text files with either labeled or position-dependent parameters. However, there are currently no known, agreed upon, or de facto standards for positions, labels, units of measure, and so on.

38.3 Scope, Functionality, and Performance

As summarized in Figure 38.1, CAD-like human performance software depends on conceptual issues as well as decisions regarding fidelity, functionality, and implementation. There is also a great deal of interaction among these categories. Topics within each category were derived in part from a review of current packages (e.g., those described below) and an assessment of other issues and needs. These

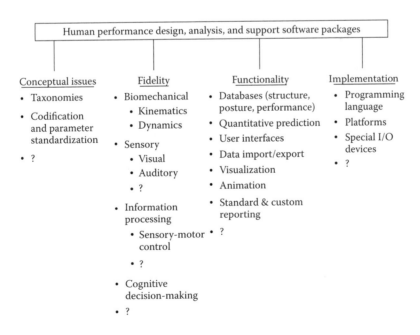

FIGURE 38.1 Related aspects of human design and performance software describe the diversity and scope of underlying issues.

lists are intended to be illustrative and not exhaustive. While *every* major category applies to *any* given software tool, not all topics listed within a category will always be relevant.

Conceptual issues include taxonomies on which a given package is based (e.g., basic approaches to motor control, system performance, task categorizations and analysis, data estimation, etc.), parameter choices and codification (e.g., hierarchical level of representation, identification in structured input/output file formats), and compliance with or deviation from accepted standards with the varied communities that deal with human performance. They may well deserve special recognition given the impressionable developmental stage of the class of software tools addressed. Perhaps because developers are so familiar with a given perspective or body of knowledge, key conceptual issues are often overlooked or incorporated de facto from previous work (e.g., research studies) that is similar (but perhaps not identical) to the intended purpose of a given package, which is frequently broader and more general than the research efforts or projects that inspired it. Software packages impose on users the constructs on which they are based and this may result in conflicts within an already structured environment. Conceptual foundations and approaches are not yet as clearly defined in human performance as they are in disciplines such as electrical and mechanical engineering. This is further complicated by the wide variety of disciplines (and therefore educational backgrounds) represented by those with interest in participating in software development. Clear and complete disclosure of the conceptual foundation used by developers is thus helpful to both users (potential and actual) and developers.

The concept and scope of fidelity in the present context has been delineated in Section 38.2.3 and is further represented by the subtopics in Figure 38.1. We have chosen to apply it here in its broadest sense. In a fairly recent National Research Council panel on human performance modeling (Baron et al., 1990), recommendations were made toward problems regarding design and implementation issues. Though not specifically addressing computer software, the extension of the discussion is natural given present technology and implementation methods. While it was concluded that an all-inclusive model (i.e., high fidelity, in the sense that biomechanical, information processing, sensory, and perceptual aspects, etc. are represented) might be desirable, it is highly unlikely that it could be achieved or would be useful, as the inherent complexity would impede effective usage. The basic recommendation made was to pursue more limited scope submodels. The implication is that two or more computer-based versions of such submodels could be integrated to achieve a wide range of fidelity, with the combination selected to meet the needs of particular situations. However, there is neither a general framework nor set of guidelines for developers of submodels (i.e., an *open-architecture concept*) that would facilitate integration of relatively independent software development efforts. Thus, integration is left to the end user and typically only cumbersome methods are available.

Fidelity should be considered in combination with productivity and both must be carefully assessed against needs. For example, a package that provides the user with control over a large number of parameters (e.g., joint stiffness, balance control, etc.) that define the human system under analysis, typically allows for greater intrinsic fidelity and can be valuable if the ability to specify parameters at that level of detail is an absolute user requirement. If not, this level of specificity only increases the number of prerequisite steps to achieve a given analysis and leads to a more complex program in terms of operation and function (which is perhaps most evident in the user interface). Furthermore, more accurate results are not necessarily obtained. Programs that are structured to automatically rely on default parameter values that can be inspected or changed when desired serve both types of needs. However, concern is typically raised that "lazy" users will forego the entry of values more appropriate to the situation at hand. Thus, while software developers can provide features that greatly simplify procedures and recommendations regarding their proper use, users bear the responsibility of choosing when to invoke such features. Fidelity issues are often viewed as "either" or "or" choices, when many times a "both" or "all" approach is quite feasible. This gives the user the decision-making power and responsibility for decisions that may affect quality of results. Such approaches also typically result in a greater user pool for a given package. The manner in how such flexibility is implemented, however, is critical. For example, if fidelity decisions are likely to be made once in a given installation, schemes that require decision making with each analysis can prove to be cumbersome and ineffective.

Functionality can be considered in terms of basic and special subcategories. Far too often, attention is given to special features while those that are more basic (such as import/export capabilities) are ignored. Most items listed in Figure 38.1 under the "functionality" category are self-explanatory, although it should be noted that features such as importing and exporting are more complex in the present context than one might anticipate due in part to the lack of standards for parameters representation (see above). Developers must carefully select functionality and potential users must carefully evaluate the impact of those choices against their specific needs. For example, the processing power required to display and animate contoured multisegment human figures in real time and in three dimensions is substantial. Programs with this ability typically require high-end platforms and also require that a large fraction of the programming effort and user interface be used for this functionality. The addition of processes such as a dynamic analysis places even a greater stress on processing power and complexity. Visualization of human figures in three dimensions along with some environmental components is essential for some applications. For many applications, such as those in which numerical results are required and conveyed to others with simple printed reports, such visualization are not required, or contribute little, to achieving the desired end purpose (although they are almost always viewed as "attractive" by potential users). Functionality options are further developed and exemplified in the discussion of actual software packages below (Section 38.4).

The last of these four categories describes the support structure upon which the software packages are built. Software implementation in today's ever-changing computer market requires careful thought. In addition to host platform and standard accessories, special input/output interfaces are often necessary (e.g., to allow direct access to laboratory-acquired kinematic data). Support software for such special hardware is not always available on all platforms, preventing operation with analytic software in the same environment. Choice of programming language (supporting modules and libraries, platform diversity) and the operating system (Macintosh®, Windows™, Unix, etc.) are also critical. As exemplified in Section 38.4, no existing packages run on all platforms and under all operating systems users who wish to employ multiple packages are left with cumbersome and often costly solutions.

As computing power at the single-user level (i.e., personal computer) increases, there is little doubt that a full set of state-of-the-art features covering a broad scope of human performance and data needs *could* be integrated into a single package. At present, though, limitations are real and necessary. These are the result of specific trade-offs that must be considered during development when determining target users. Operational costs include software acquisition, maintenance, basic platform acquisition and outfitting, and training costs. A large feature set and high performance are not always indicative of a software tool's value. Value is lost if a user's requirements are either unfulfilled or greatly exceed by the functionality and performance of a program. Unfortunately, general trade-offs that are acceptable within different groups of users have not yet become evident.

38.4 Functional Overview of Representative Packages

In this section, a selected set of different types of software packages intended specifically for human design and performance analysis applications are described. At least one example of each type exists and is noted for reference and to illustrate the types of functionality developers are addressing in response to perceived needs. No endorsement of any example cited is implied. The packages included vary widely in function and performance and should not be considered to be directly comparable. Operational costs reflect this diversity, ranging from relatively inexpensive (e.g., approximately $100.00 plus the price of a moderately equipped PC™) to the level defined by high-end workstations (e.g., thousands of dollars for software licenses plus the cost of a Unix-based workstation). As with desktop computer applications, such as word processors and spreadsheets, the packages used to illustrate functionality are under constant development, and changing feature-sets, performance, and cost are to be anticipated.

The types of packages included illustrate fundamental options with regard to general or dedicated analysis (e.g., user-defined tasks vs. gait), different levels of analysis (e.g., "muscle" vs. "joint" levels in biomechanical analyses), body-function-specific or general-purpose analysis (e.g., gait vs. user-defined function), fidelity in terms of scope (e.g., biomechanical, sensory, neuromotor control, etc.), and target user orientation (medical vs. nonmedical design; although overlap is possible). It should be noted that while particular packages are highlighted under certain categories, underlying features and functions are common across many applications.

38.4.1 Human Parameter Databases

The need for data is evident in all aspects of human-related CAD and the analysis of human performance. In certain situations, requirements may be for a specific individual or a representative population. In the former case, there are certain parameters that are not readily attainable (e.g., location of center of mass for a segment, inertia, etc.) and therefore must be estimated, as in the latter case, from normative values derived from studies. For a number of years, these estimates have been available in book form primarily as lookup tables. This format, however, does not take advantage of current technology and is not sufficient for use with software-based analytic tools. Some currently available packages, in addressing this need, have included data tables that are utilized exclusively within the program. Programs such as *MannequinPro* and *SafeWork* (detailed below) for example, each include a significant database of anthropometric measures for various populations. The user specifies design parameter values by choosing characteristics such as gender, ethnic origin, and morphology representative of the desired population. Various other stand-alone database software packages, for example, *PeopleSize* (targeted initially for clothing design), allow data to be exported, thereby providing at least an indirect support for external applications.

In addition to measures such as segment lengths, parameters including reach and range of motion for selected postures are frequently provided in databases (e.g., horizontal sitting reach, etc.). Because it is prohibitive (if not impossible) to measure and report all possible situations, this issue may be more adequately addressed through the use of parametric data models. Data derived from such models would provide estimates for all possible conditions as well as having the additional advantage of requiring lesser storage and management requirements. Caution is warranted with regard to issues such as model validity, statistical sample sizes and variations, combinatory effects of merging databases or data models, and traceability of data to original sources.

38.4.2 Biomechanical, Muscle-Level Modeling and Analysis

Software for interactive musculoskeletal modeling *SIMM* is a graphics-based tool for modeling and visualization of any human or animal musculoskeletal system and is directed at lower-level structures, that is, individual muscles. The program allows users to model any type of musculoskeletal system using files, which specify (1) the skeletal structure through polygonal surface objects, (2) the joint kinematics, and (3) the muscle architecture through specifications of a line of action for each muscle and isometric force data. *SIMM* contains various tools for observing and editing the model (see Figure 38.2). The user can visualize and animate the model, display or hide the individual muscles (shown as line segments), manipulate joint angles, muscle forces, and moment arms. Joint torques (static) can be analyzed via plots and graphs and all of the muscle parameters may be edited including visual alteration of muscle lines of action. Finally, the user also has control over joint kinematics by altering the cubic splines used to control the animated joint movements. Developers claim that *SIMM* is aimed at biomechanics researchers, kinesiologists, workspace designers, and students who can benefit from visual feedback showing muscle locations and actions.

Musculographics, the developers of *SIMM*, also produce a component as part of the SIMM suite specifically directed toward gait analysis that provides ground reaction force vectors and color-highlighted

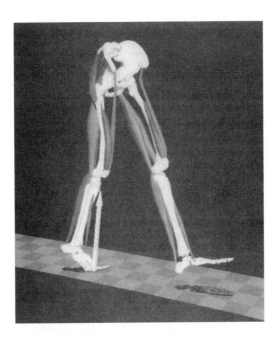

FIGURE 38.2 Muscle attachments and utilization (indicated by shading) for the lower extremities during gait, created and displayed using SIMM software.

muscle activity through animation of the model. The software is designed to input data files written by movement analysis systems and can display plots of data such as muscle lengths and ground reaction forces. Another application, the *Dynamics Pipeline*, is a general-purpose package that provides forward and inverse dynamics to calculate motions resulting from forces or torques required to generate a given motion, respectively. *SIMM* was also made available for Microsoft Windows. However, the original Unix-based version is still available.

38.4.3 Body Function–Specific Tools

GaitLab is a Windows™-based software package that allows fundamental parameters of human gait to be derived, analyzed, and inspected. At this time it is available inexpensively ($49.95) as part of a larger package from Kiboho Publishers. The program is divided into two main sections (i.e., subprograms that run under the "shell" of the main application): (1) a mathematics section, which provides processes for generating text files representing various gait parameters throughout a gait cycle; and (2) a graphics section that creates plots of the parameters as well as a representation of gait through an animated stick figure. Documentation covers the gait parameters and equations associated with the software package as well as the underlying principles for their use in gait analysis. Software accepts different, custom-formatted data files (ASCII text) based on direct measurements of a human subject. These include anthropometric, kinematic (i.e., three-dimensional positions of anatomic landmarks), force plate, and electromyographic (EMG) measures. Sample files are included for a healthy adult male, female, and an adult male with cerebral palsy. From these data, text files are created for lower-extremity body segment parameters (mass, center of gravity position, and moment of inertia), linear kinematics (joint center, heel, and toe locations, segment reference frames), center of gravity (position, velocity, and acceleration), angular kinematics (joint angles, angular velocity, and acceleration), and dynamics (joint forces and torques). The package can also display up to three simultaneous plots of these parameters in any combination. Time, percent of gait cycle, and marker position scales are also available for plotting against any of the variables.

GaitLab provides a useful function in its ability to generate the above mentioned parameters and is effective with its simplistic stick figure animation, allowing minimal processing power/speed requirements while providing the nuances of lower limb movement pertinent to gait analysis. It is just one of many examples of function-specific packages.

38.4.4 Biomechanical, Joint-Level, Total Human Analysis

ADAMS is a software package designed for mechanical design and system simulation in general. It is an extensive package incorporating specific components for both modeling and kinematic/dynamic analysis. What sets *ADAMS* apart from other nonperformance-based simulation/dynamics packages is the availability of a module, LifeMOD, specifically designed to allow the user to create a human model. The human model may be edited as needed but is provided in a default configuration of a 19 joint-body architecture with five anthropometric body size databases. Because the package focuses on mechanical systems in general, a great deal of control is provided to the user over the parameters of the model including contact forces, joint friction, damping, and nonlinear stiffness as well as control parameters. Having this capability, the human model is able to affect control over objects in its environment as well as responding biomechanically to contact. Supplemental toolsets may be (custom) developed to provide proper control over model parameters such as motion resistance relationships, joint strength and range of motion limits, and delays in neuromuscular response. For a given model, kinematic or dynamic simulations may be run and values for any parameter can be plotted on screen. Both forward and inverse dynamic analyses are available and graphics-based facilities such as the specification of trajectories via mouse input are available. The simulations may be used to generate detailed animation movie (.avi) files.

Because *ADAMS'* capabilities are so extensive, it has become one of the most widely used mechanical system simulation packages. Outside of the realm of human performance analysis, the package is targeted at engineers and scientists who require complete observation and control of the model parameters across many hierarchical levels. While this format affords great fidelity and specificity in the analysis, there is also a great deal of complexity and detail that must be addressed in every new simulation run. Though *performance assessment* is not an inherent or recognized feature in the package, custom modules may be incorporated, which would allow for direct comparison of system resource utilization and stress against the demands of the task.

38.4.5 Visualization for Low-End Computer Platforms

MannequinPro, while having inherent database functionality, is essentially a visualization tool that allows users to quickly create three-dimensional humanoid figures, which may be represented in stick-figure form, as a wireframe "robot" with polygonal segments, or as its name implies, a mannequin with higher-resolution segments. These figures may be postured within preset (i.e., noneditable) range-of-motion limits, as well as viewed from many different perspectives. They are created automatically by the program according to user-defined structural aspects chosen from a list of specifications for gender, population percentile, body type, age, and nationality. The package also provides a modest drawing (CAD-type) tool for creating various objects to be placed in the scene with the figure. Two additional features extend *MannequinPro* beyond the domain of a "simple" object rendering tool. The first is provided through animation effects, allowing the mannequin to walk via an internally generated gait sequence (a specific path may be defined through a virtual workspace), reach to a specific location, or move through any sequence of positions created on a frame-by-frame basis by the user. The second feature allows the user to specify forces acting on the mannequins hands or feet from which static torques are calculated for both left and right wrists, elbows, shoulders, neck, back, hips, knees, and ankles.

As a visualization tool, *MannequinPro* provides a needed capability for a modest price and requires only a personal computer to run. Figures are easily produced to the anthropometric specifications available and posing, reaching, and walking functions, though limited, are simple to control. The package is primarily operated from mouse input with standard point, click, and drag operations that should be familiar to most users of current commercial software. Once the scene is created with humans and objects in their workspace, it is up to the user to extract any information regarding function and performance from the visual images presented by the package. These features, as well as others, are also contained within the software package *Jack* and *SafeWork* (described below), which provide greater functionality but are targeted toward workstation environments. In sum, *MannequinPro*, with a good price-to-performance ratio, is an effective tool when human visualization with moderate graphics is required at the single-user platform level.

38.4.6 Extended Visualization for the High-End Workstations

Jack, developed within the University of Pennsylvania Center for Human Modeling and Simulation (Badler et al., 1993), and *SafeWork* are a high-end CAD-oriented design and visualization packages. Similar in function to *MannequinPro* (above), but with considerably more flexibility and detail, they are designed to allow human factors engineers to place a human in a virtual workstation environment while still in the design phase. Both extend far beyond the capabilities of *MannequinPro*, trading simplicity for specificity in that they provide users with control over a large range of variables regarding many aspects of the human figure and its virtual environment. Human models are fully articulated and preset or user-definable anthropometric parameters that include segment dimensions, joint limits, moments of inertia, and strength allow highly specific representation. The total functionality of these packages are far too great to list the individual aspects here, but examples include reach, hand gripping, balance (including reorientation behavior), collision detection, light and camera (view) manipulation, animation, and kinematic/dynamic analysis. *Jack* also allows for real-time posture tracking of a human operator through position and orientation sensors (see Figure 38.3).

Similar to the functionality of *ADAMS*, these packages provide a great deal of control over the design and manipulation of the human figure. Because of the large number of controllable parameters and the difficulty involved in providing an interface allowing three-dimensional manipulation of high-end graphics in a two-dimensional environment, the majority of users will require training. *Jack* and *SafeWork* require a Silicon Graphics workstation to run.

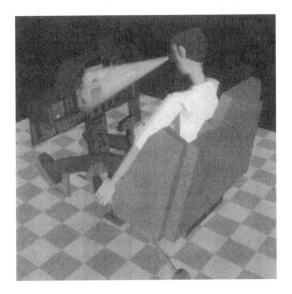

FIGURE 38.3 A human/workspace figure created and displayed using Jack software.

38.4.7 Total Human, Performance-Based, Human–Task Interface Analysis

While now under development, *HMT–CAD* represents yet a different perspective in that it is based primarily on performance modeling constructs (e.g., Kondraske, 2005) and is aimed at producing bottom-line assessments regarding human-to-task, human-to-machine, and eventually machine-to-task interfaces using a logic similar to that used by systems-level designers. In a joint effort between Photon Research Associates, Inc. and the University of Texas at Arlington Human Performance Institute, performance models and decision-making strategies are combined with advanced multibody dynamic analysis.

HMT-CAD's initial development emphasized a top-down approach that set out with the goal of realizing a shell that would allow systematic incorporation of increasingly higher fidelity in a modular, stepwise fashion. The initial modules encompass biomechanical and neuromuscular aspects of performance that bases analyses on knowledge of range/extremes of motion, torque, and speed capacities. Gross total human (23 links and 41 degrees of freedom) and hand link models (16 links and 22 degrees of freedom each) are included. The Windows™-based tool provides a predefined framework for specifying human structure and performance parameters (e.g., anthropometry, strength, etc.) for individuals or populations. A task library is included based on an object-oriented approach to task analysis. HMT–CAD attempts to help communicate information about many parameters via a custom graphical–button interface. For example, one analysis result screen shows a human figure surrounded by buttons connected to body joints. Button color (e.g., red or green) communicates whether an analysis found limiting factors for the specified person in the specified task associated with that joint system. Using computer mouse input, clicking on red buttons produces a new window showing a list of performance capacities and stress levels associated with systems of that joint. Maximally stressed performance resources are tagged. *HMT–CAD* uses the same systems of level modeling constructs for human and artificial systems. A novel technique that transparently draws upon a large set of data models as needed is used to provide "the best analysis possible" with the data provided by the user. This allows users to directly specify values for all parameters if desired, but does not require this for each analysis (see Figure 38.4).

In the present prototype, analysis scope is very limited (upper extremity, object moving tasks). Databases are being populated to allow a similar fidelity of analysis for trunk and lower-extremity analyses. Development of an optimization engine based on minimizing stress across performance resources (Kondraske and Khoury, 1992) to solve problems in which redundant approaches are possible is underway. No capability is currently provided for animation of human movement, as binary assessments (e.g., red and green buttons) and numerical results (stress levels on performance capacities) are emphasized. However, an interface to emerging general-purpose animation tools is planned. Long-term development will proceed to increase fidelity in a stepwise fashion by the inclusion of performance capacities for other major systems (e.g., information processing associated with motor control) as well as additional performance capacities for major systems represented at any given time (e.g., the inclusion of neuromuscular endurance limits).

The inferential NCRA methodology discussed earlier has recently been used to create a companion NCRA software package by the University of Texas at Arlington's Human Performance Institute. It is based on General System Performance Theory concepts and the Elemental Resource Model (Kondraske, 2005) and performs the following functions:

- *Perform Task Analyses (Build NCRA models):* Models consist of a set of Resource Demand Functions, each of which relates the amount of a given performance resource required to achieve a specific level of High Level Task (HLT) performance.
- *Predict HLT Performance:* Using an NCRA model and a set of measures representing basic performance resource availability (i.e., performance capacities) for a set of "n" subjects as "inputs" to the model (i.e., independent variables), individualized predictions of performance in the HLT are computed.

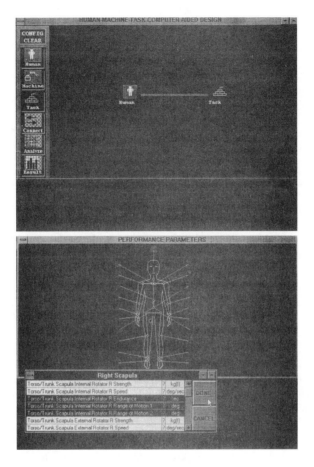

FIGURE 38.4 A desktop environment of the HMT-CAD performance assessment package including system model development and analysis result reporting.

- *Identify Limiting Performance Resources:* In addition to a prediction of HLT performance, for each subject in a Prediction Source Data set, the performance resource that prevents that subject from "performing better" is identified.
- *Obtain Other Useful Performance-Related Measures:* Various options are available to explore the stress on the performance resources of individuals associated with a given level of HLT performance.

Importantly, NCRA allows models to be formulated that mix neuromuscular, information processing, sensory, and life-sustaining performance resources. It is anticipated that many existing data sets, which have been previously used to develop regression-based models, can be used with NCRA (see Figure 38.5).

38.5 Anticipated Development

While it is relatively easy to outline the functionality and unique aspects of the software discussed above, it is a great deal harder to describe the level of difficulty required to achieve a desired end result and to characterize how well functions are performed. Online "help" systems, multimedia components, associated software development tools, improved parameter measurement tools, and higher-fidelity models will no doubt impact these aspects.

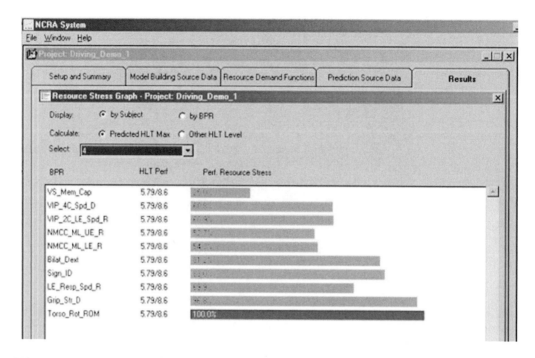

FIGURE 38.5 Screen capture from NCRA software illustrating results for one individual applied to a model of driving performance. Overall driving performance level (HLT performance) and limiting performance resources (in this case "torso rotation range of motion") are predicted based on a set of more basic performance resource measures (BPRs). BPR measures are lower-level performance capacities relative to the higher-level task modeled.

As mundane as it may seem, perhaps nothing is more important to the overall advancement of this class of software tools than the development of standards for parameters used, parameter conventions, and data formats. It is likely that de facto standards will emerge from individual commercial endeavors. Due to the diversity of professionals involved, it is difficult to envision the evolution of "standards by committee." Observation of success stories in analogous efforts also supports this opinion. This, in turn, will enable progress to be made in database and data model development, which is vital to the many of the more routine functions such software will perform. Combined with modular object-oriented programming techniques, the emergence of true multitasking operating systems on desktop computers, and the support for interprocess communication (such as dynamic data exchange) will encourage developers. Many new tools, both similar to and completely different than those described here, can be anticipated.

Defining Terms

Channel capacity: The maximum rate of information flow through a specific pathway from source to receiver. In the context of the human, a sensorimotor pathway (e.g., afferent sensory nerves, processors, descending cerebrospinal nerve and α-motoneuron) is an example of a channel through which motor control information flows from sensors to actuators (muscle).

Data model: A mathematical equation derived as a representation of the relationship between a dependent variable and one or more independent variables. Similar in function to a database, data models provide parameter values across conditions of other related parameters.

Human–task interface: The common boundary between the human and a task specified by the demands of a task on the respective resources of the human and the capacities of the human's resources involved in performing the task.

Linked multibody system: A system of three or more individual segments joined (as an open or closed chain) in some manner with the degree of freedom between any two segments defined by the characteristics of the corresponding hinge.

Open-architecture concept: A general methodology for the development of functional modules that may be readily integrated to form a higher-level system through well-defined design and interface constructs.

Parameter conventions: Aspects and usage of a parameter that are specifically defined with respect to general implementation.

Performance assessment: The process of determining the level or degree in which a system can perform a specific task given the demands required and the availabilities of the resources of the system which are involved in performing the task.

Performance resource: Defined as a functional unit and an associated dimension of performance (e.g., knee extensor strength) that is available to a system.

Virtual workspace: A representation of a three-dimensional physical workspace generated by computer software and displayed on a video monitor or similar device. This enables, for example, the inclusion and manipulation of computer-generated objects within the virtual workspace such that designs can be tested and modified prior to manufacturing.

References

Allard, P., Stokes, I.A.F., and Blanchi, J.P. (Eds.) 1994. *Three-Dimensional Analysis of Human Movement*, Human Kinetics, Champaign, IL.

Badler, N.I. 1989. Task-oriented animation of human figures. In *Applications of Human Performance Models to System Design*, G.R. McMillan, D. Beevis, and E. Salas, (Eds.), Plenum Press, New York.

Badler, N.I., Phillips, C.B., and Webber, B.L. 1993. *Simulating Humans: Computer Graphics Animation and Control*, Oxford University Press, New York.

Baron, S., Kruser, D.S., and Huey, B.M. (Eds.) 1990. *Quantitative Modeling of Human Performance in Complex, Dynamic Systems*, National Academy Press, Washington, DC.

Chao, E.Y.S. 1980. Justification of triaxial goniometer for the measurement of joint rotation. *Biomechanics*, 13: 989–1006.

Craig, J.J. 1989. *Introduction to Robotics Mechanics and Control*, 2nd ed., Addison-Wesley, New York.

Delp, S.L., Loan, J.P., Hoy, M.G., Zajac, F.E., Topp, E.L., and Rosen, J.M. 1990. An interactive graphics-based model of the lower extremity to study orthopaedic surgical procedures. *IEEE Trans. Biomed. Eng.*, 37: 757–767.

Fitts, P. 1954. The information capacity of the human motor system in controlling the amplitude of movement, *J. Exp. Psychol.*, 47: 381–391.

Hick, W. 1952. On the rate of gain of information, *Quart. J. Exp. Psychol.*, 4: 11–26.

Hyman, R. 1953. Stimulus information as a determinant of reaction time, *J. Exp. Psychol.*, 45: 423–432.

Jiang, B.C. and Ayoub, M.M. 1987. Modelling of maximum acceptable load of lifting by physical factors. *Ergonomics*, 30: 529–538.

Khan, C. 1991. Humanizing AutoCAD. *Cadence*, June.

Kondraske, G.V. 1988. Experimental evaluation of an elemental resource model for human performance. In *Proceedings, Tenth Annual IEEE Engineering in Medicine and Biology Society Conference*, New Orleans, pp. 1612–1613.

Kondraske, G.V. 2005. The elemental resource model for human performance. In *Handbook of Biomedical Engineering*. J.D. Bronzino (Ed.) CRC Press Inc., Boca Raton, FL.

Kondraske, G.V. and Khoury, G.J. 1992. Telerobotic system performance measurement: Motivation and methods. In *Cooperative Intelligent Robotics in Space III* (*Proceedings of the SPIE 1829*), J.D. Erickson (Ed.), pp. 161–172, SPIE.

Lachman, R., Lachman, J.L., and Butterfield, E.C. 1979. *Cognitive Psychology and Information Processing: An Introduction*, Lawrence Erlbaum Assoc., Hillsdale, NJ.

McConville, J.T., Churchill, T.D., Kaleps, I., Clauser, C.E., and Cuzzi, J. 1980. *Anthropometric Relationships of Body and Body Segment Moments of Inertia*, Air Force Aerospace Medical Research Laboratory, AFAMRL-TR-80-119, Wright-Patterson Air Force Base, Ohio.

Panjabi, M.M, White III, A.A., and Brand, R.A. 1974. A note on defining body parts configurations. *J. Biomech.*, 7: 385–387.

Pheasant, S.T. 1986. *Bodyspace: Anthropometry, Ergonomics and Design*, Taylor & Francis, Philadelphia, PA.

Remington, R.D. and Schork, M.A. 1985. *Statistics with Applications to the Biological and Health Sciences*, Prentice-Hall, NJ.

Spong, M.W. and Vidyasagar, M. 1989. *Robot Dynamics and Control*, John Wiley & Sons, New York.

Vasta, P.J. and Kondraske, G.V. 1994. Performance prediction of an upper extremity reciprocal task using non-linear causal resource analysis. In *Proceedings, Sixteenth Annual IEEE Engineering in Medicine and Biology Society Conference*, Baltimore, MD, pp. 305–306.

Vaughan, C.L., Davis, B.L., and O'Connor, J.C. 1992. *Dynamics of Human Gait*, Human Kinetics, Champaign, IL.

Winter, D.A. 1990. *Biomechanics and Motor Control of Human Movement*, 2nd ed. John Wiley & Sons, New York.

Further Information

For explicit information regarding the software packages included in this chapter, the developers may be directly contacted as follows:

ADAMS: Mechanical Dynamics, 2301 Commonwealth Blvd., Ann Arbor, MI 48105, USA, 800-88-ADAMS, http://www.adams.com.

GaitLab: originally published by Human Kinetics,1607 N. Market St., Box 5076, Champaign, IL 61825, (217) 351-5076, Now available from Kiboho Publishers, http://www.kiboho.co.za/GaitCD/.

HMT-CAD: Human Performance Institute, The University of Texas at Arlington, PO Box 19180, Arlington, TX 76019, (817) 272-2335.

Jack: Center for Human Modeling and Simulation, The University of Pennsylvania, 200 South 33rd St., Philadelphia, PA 19104-6389, (215) 573-9463, http://www.cis.upenn.edu/~ hms/jack.html.

MannequinPro: HumanCAD, a division of Biomechanics Corporation of America, 1800 Walt Whitman Road, Melville, NY, 11747, (516) 752-3568, http://www.humancad.com.

Nonlinear Causal Resource Analysis (NCRA): Human Performance Institute, The University of Texas at Arlington, PO Box 19180, Arlington, TX 76019, (817) 272-2335.

PeopleSize: Open Ergonomics Ltd., Loughborough Technology Centre, Epinal Way, Loughborough, LE11 3GE, UK, + 44 (0) 1509 218 333, http://www.openerg.com/psz.htm.

SafeWork: Genicom Consultants Inc., 3400 de Maisonneuve Blvd. West, 1 Place Alexis Nihon, Suite 1430, Montreal, Quebec, CANADA, H3Z 3B8, (514) 931-3000, http://www.safework.com.

SIMM: Musculographics, Inc. c/o Motion Analysis. Corp., 3617 Westwind Blvd., Santa Rosa, CA 95403, (707) 579-6500, ww.musculographics.com.

Readers are also encouraged to simply perform web searches on the relevant package keywords or acronyms to discover a wide range of application examples, use issues, and discussions relevant to specific packages.

A broad perspective of issues related to those presented here may be found in: Matilla, M. and Karwowski, W., eds. 1992. Computer applications in ergonomics, occupational safety, and health, In: *Proceedings of the International Conference on Computer-Aided Ergonomics and Safety '92*, Tampere, Finland, North-Holland Publishers, Amsterdam.

Additionally, periodic discussions of related topics may be found in the following publications: CSERIAC Gateway, published by the Crew System Ergonomics Information Analysis Center. For subscription information contact AL/CFH/CSERIAC, Bldg. 248, 2255 H St., Wright-Patterson Air Force Base, Ohio, 45433; IEEE Transactions on Biomedical Engineering or IEEE Engineering in Medicine & Biology Magazine. For further information contact: IEEE Service Center, 445 Hoes Lane, PO Box 1331, Piscataway, NJ, 08855-1331.

Numerous other related sites can be found on the Internet. Among those of interest are:

Biomechanics World Wide: includes a very thorough listing of various topics related to biomechanics including links to educational, corporate, and related sites of interest. http://www. per.ualberta.ca/biomechanics/bwwframe.htm.

Biomch-L: an Internet list-server supporting discussions regarding topics relating to biomechanics. http://isb.ri.ccf.org/isb/biomch-l/.

Motion Lab Systems, Inc.: a collection of information and links to a variety of Internet sites focused on electromyography, biomechanics, gait analysis, and motion capture. Includes both commercial and non-commercial sites. http://www.emgsrus.com/links.htm.

39

Human Performance Engineering: Challenges and Prospects for the Future

George V. Kondraske
University of Texas,
Arlington

39.1 Introduction

Human Performance Engineering is a dynamic area with rapid changes in many facets and constantly emerging developments that affect application possibilities. Materials presented in other chapters of this section of the text illustrate the breadth and depth of effort required as well as the variety of applications in this field. At the same time, the field is relatively young and as is often the case in such instances, some "old" issues remain unresolved and new issues emerge with new developments. With the other material in this section as background, this chapter focuses on selected issues of a general nature (i.e., cutting across various human subsystem types and applications) in three major areas vital to the future of the field: (1) human performance modeling; (2) measurement; and (3) data-related topics. In addition to the identification of some key issues, some speculation is presented with regard to the lines along which future work may develop. Awareness of the specific issues raised is anticipated to be helpful to practitioners who must operate within the constraints of the current state of the art. Moreover, the issues selected represent scientific and engineering challenges for the future that will require not only awareness but also the collaboration of researchers and practitioners from the varied segments of the community to resolve.

39.2 Models

It is important to distinguish various types of models encountered in human performance. They include conceptual, statistically based predictive models, predictive models based on cause and effect

(Kondraske et al., 1997), and data models (Vasta and Kondraske, 1995). Issues related to data models are described in Section 39.4 of this chapter, while those related to the remaining types are discussed in this section.

Traditionally, a tremendous amount of activity in various segments of the human performance community has been directed toward development of statistically based predictive models (e.g., regression models). This remains the most popular approach. By their very nature, each of these is very application specific. Even within the intended application, success of these models has mostly ranged from poor to marginal, with a few reports of models that look "very good" in the populations in which they were tested. However, the criteria for "good" has been skewed by the early performance achieved with these methods and statistically significant "r" values of 0.6 have come to be considered "good." Even if predictive performance was excellent, the long-term merit of statistically based prediction methods can be questioned on the basis that this approach is intrinsically inefficient. A unique and time-consuming modeling effort, requiring new data collection with human subjects, is required for every situation. At the same time, powerful computer-based tools are commonly available that facilitate the generation of what is estimated to be hundreds and perhaps thousands of these regression models on an annual basis. It appears that many researchers and practitioners have forgotten that one purpose of such statistical methods is to provide insight into the cause-and-effect principles at play and into generalizations that might be more broadly applied. Statistically-based regression models will continue to serve useful purposes within the specific application contexts for which they are developed. However, the future of predictive modeling in human performance engineering must be based on cause-and-effect principles. The sentiment for the need to shift from statistical to more physically based models is present and growing in several of the related application disciplines as evidenced by a sampling of quotations from the literature presented in Table 39.1.

A National Research Council panel on human performance modeling (Baron et al., 1990) conducted one of the more broad-looking investigations regarding complex human performance models; that is, those that consider one or more major attributes (e.g., biomechanical, sensory, cognitive, structural details, etc.) of a total or near-total human. The convening of this panel itself underscored the interest in and need for human performance models. As an interesting aside, while the panel's focus was on modeling, a large fraction of the efforts cited as background represented major software packages, most of which were developed to support defense industry needs. A major application for such models is in computer simulation of humans in various circumstances, which could be used to support prediction and other analysis needs. A series of useful recommendations were included in panel's report regarding the direction that should be taken in future work. However, recommendations were quite general in nature and no specific plans were outlined regarding how some of these objectives might actually be achieved. Nonetheless, it was clear from the choice of the previous works cited and from the

TABLE 39.1 Representative Quotations Illustrating the Need for a Shift toward the Development of Causal Models

Quote	Field	References
… there has been little advancement of the science of ergonomics … the degree of advancement is so low that, in my opinion, ergonomics does not yet qualify as a science … There has been no progress in the accumulation of general knowledge … because nearly all studies have not been general studies.	Human factors	Smith (1987)
… experiments are performed year after year to answer the same questions, those questions—often fundamental ones—remain unanswered … the methodology employed today is a hodgepodge of quick fixes that evolved over the years into a paradigm that is taught and employed as sacrosanct, when in fact it is woefully inadequate and frequently incompetent …	Human factors	Simmon (1987)
…authors and users of these instruments lacked a conceptual model … lack of a well-developed conceptual model is unfortunately characteristic of the entire history of the field…	Rehabilitation	Frey (1987)

recommendations that development of cause and effect, general-purpose models should receive priority. The elemental resource model presented at the beginning of this section of the text (Kondraske, 2005) is one example of a causal, integrative model that reflects an initial attempt to incorporate many of this panel's recommendations.

Whether primarily statistical or causal in nature, frustration with what has been characterized or perceived as "limited success" achieved to date in efforts to unlock and formalize the underpinnings of complex human functions such as speech, gait, lifting, and memory have led to attacks in recent years on the basic reductionistic approach that has been pursued most aggressively. In fact, reductionism has been characterized as a "dead end" methodology—one that has been tried and has failed (Gardner, 1985; Bunge, 1977), as further evidenced by the following somewhat representative quote (Weismer and Liss, 1991):

> [T]his view held the scientific community spellbound until people started looking past the technological issues, and asking how well the reductionist observations were doing at explaining behavior, and the answer was, miserably. Many microscopic facts had been accumulated, and incredible technological advances had been made, but the sum of all of these reductionist observations could not make good sense of macroscopic levels of movement behavior.

Prior to total abandonment, it is perhaps wise not only to characterize the performance of reductionism, but also to question why it might have failed *thus far*. For example, it may be prudent to entertain the proposition that reductionism may be "a correct approach" that has failed to date because of a problem with one or more components associated with its implementation. Are we certain that this is not the case?

One potential explanation for an apparent failure of reductionism is simply the manner in which manpower has been organized (i.e., the research infrastructure) to attack problems of the magnitude of those considered, for example, by the National Research Council panel noted earlier. With some exceptions, the majority of funded research efforts is short term and involve very small teams. Is it possible that the amount of information "to reduce" is too much to produce results that would be characterized as "success" (i.e., does the equivalent of an undercapitalized business venture exist?)? It is further observed that the value of *reduction* is often only demonstrable by the ability to *assemble*. As noted, the prime tool of assembly thus far has been statistical in nature and relatively few causal models have been seriously entertained. With regard to human systems, it is clear that there are many such "items" to assemble and many details to consider if "assembly"—with high fidelity—is to result. Furthermore, it is clear that tools (i.e., special computer software) are needed to make such assembly efforts efficient enough to consider undertaking. Has the data management and analytic power of computers, which have only been readily available in convenient-to-use forms and with required capacities for less than a decade, been fully exploited in a "fair test" of reductionism?

Reductionism is clearly a methodology for understanding "that which is." Drawing by inference from engineering design in general, a close relationship can be observed to systems engineering synthesis methods used to define "that which will be." In artificial systems (as opposed to those which naturally occur, like humans), reverse engineering (basically, a reductionistic method) has been used quite successfully to create functionally equivalent replicas of products. The methodology employed is guided by knowledge of the synthesis process. The implementation of reductionism in human performance modeling can possibly benefit from the reverse mental exercise of "building a human," which may not be so abstract given current efforts and achievements in rehabilitation engineering. In looking toward the future, it is fair to ask, "To what extent have those who have attempted to apply reductionism, or who have dismissed it, attempted to bring to bear methods of synthesis?" The real support for reductionism is success obtained with methods based on this concept; new findings of an extremely encouraging nature are beginning to come forth (Kondraske et al., 1997).

The issue of biological variability is also frequently raised in the context of the desire to develop predictive models of human performance. It is perhaps noteworthy that variability is an issue with which one must deal in the manufacture of man-made products (i.e., particularly with regard to quality assurance in manufacturing), which are designed almost exclusively using causal principles. Taguchi methods (Bendell et al., 1988), a collection of mathematics and concepts, have been used in widespread fashion with remarkable success in modeling and controlling variability in the characteristics of a final product, which is based on the combination of many components, each of which has multiple characteristics, which also range within tolerance bands. Similarity of these circumstances suggests that Taguchi methods may also be valuable in human performance engineering. Investigations of this nature are likely to be a part of future work.

39.3 Measurements

39.3.1 Standardization of Variables and Conditions

Human performance literature is replete with different measures that characterize human performance. Despite the number and magnitude of efforts where human performance is of interest, a standard set of measurement variables has yet to emerge. Relatively loose, descriptive naming conventions are used to identify variables reported leading to the perception of differences when, upon careful inspection, the variables used in two different studies or modeling efforts are the same. In other cases, the names of variables are the same, but conditions under which measures are acquired are different or not reported with enough detail to evaluate if numerical data are comparable (across the reports in question) or not.

The needs of science and engineering are considerably different. Although standardization is generally considered to be desirable in both arenas, the former stresses that only those methods used must be accurately reported so that they may be replicated. There has been, unfortunately, little motivation to achieve standardization in any broad sense in the human performance research world. In traditional areas of engineering, it is the marketplace that has forced the development of standards for naming of variables such as performance characteristics of various components (e.g., sensors, actuators, etc.) and for conditions under which these variables are measured. In more recent years, product databases (e.g., for electronic, mechanical, and electromechanical components) and systems level modeling software (i.e., computer-aided design and computer-aided manufacturing), along with the desire to reduce concept-to-production cycle times, have further increased the levels of standardization in these areas.

Despite the somewhat gloomy circumstance at present, there are some signs of potential improvement. An increasing number of research groups are beginning to attack problems of larger scale and interest is growing with regard to the ability to exchange data and models. Several small standards development efforts have surfaced recently in specific areas such as biomechanics to develop, for example, standards for kinematic representation of various body joints. The advent of an increasing number of commercially available measurement tools has also driven a trend to similarity in conventions used in some specific subareas. However, the quest for standardization in measurement that is often heard or voiced is still a distant vision. A willingness to suffer the inconvenience of "standardizing" in the short run in exchange for a greater convenience and "power" over the long run must be recognized by a critical mass of researchers, instrument manufacturers, and practitioners before a significant breakthrough can occur. The large number of different professional bodies and societies that may potentially become involved in promulgating an official set of standards will most likely contribute to slow progress in this area.

39.3.2 New Instruments

Instruments to acquire measures of both human structure and performance have been improving at a rapid pace, commensurate with the improvement of base technologies (e.g., sensors, signal conditioning, microprocessors, and desktop computer systems, etc.). Compared to one decade ago, a practitioner or researcher can today assemble a relatively sophisticated and broad-based measurement laboratory with commercially available devices instead of facing the burden of fabricating his or her own instruments. However, a considerable imbalance still exists across the profile of human performance with regard to commercial availability of necessary tools. This imbalance extends to the profile of tools seen in use in contexts such as rehabilitation and sports training. In particular, devices that measure sensory performance capacities are not nearly as commonplace or well developed as those which measure, for example, strength and range of motion. Likewise, there are few commercially available instruments that measure aspects of neuromotor control in any general sense other than, for example, in a selected task such as maintaining stable posture. The complexity and diversity of higher-level human cognitive processes has also hindered development of measurement instruments in this domain that possess any true degree of commonality in content across products. A wide variety of computer-based test batteries have been proliferating that are more or less implementations of the great number of tests formerly administered in paper–pencil format.

From a practitioner's perspective, prospects for the future are both good and bad. There is some evidence that suppliers of instruments that cover areas of the performance where there has been vigorous competition (e.g., dynamic strength) are experiencing market saturation and uncertainty on the part of consumers regarding what is "the best way" to acquire necessary information. This may force some groups to drop product lines, while others are expressing subtle interests in expanding measurement instrument product lines to fill empty niches. This latter behavior is good in that it will likely increase the scope of measurement tools that are commercially available. However, problems associated with standardization often confuse potential users and this, in general, has slowed progress in the adoption of more objective measurement instruments (compared to subjective methods) in some application areas. This, in turn, has inhibited product providers from taking the risk associated with the introduction of new products.

Compared to the commercial availability of tools that characterize the performance of various human subsystems, instruments that quantify task attributes are much less prevalent. However, the perception that increased emphasis on this area will increase the utility of measures that characterize the human will likely motivate a substantial increase in the number and variety of products available for task characterization. In addition, factors such as the Americans with Disabilities Act (ADA), which encourages worksite evaluations and modifications to facilitate employment of individuals with disabilities and the increase in work-site-related injuries such as carpal tunnel syndrome have led to an increased demand for such tools.

There has been a subtle but noticeable developing sense of awareness in the various communities that there is room for more than one kind of instrument to measure a given variable. Thus, debates regarding "the correct approach," which were commonplace, are beginning to be replaced with debates concerned with determining "the best approach for a given situation." A prime example is in the area of strength measurement. Devices range from relatively inexpensive handheld dynamometers that provide rapid measurements and meaningful results with neurologic patients to expensive devices with electric or hydraulic servomotor systems that are more suited, for example, for use in sports-medicine contexts. This trend is quite healthy and is likely to spread too though it has been driven by different constraints in different circumstances.

39.3.3 Measuring the Measurements

Reliability and validity have been the keywords associated with characterizing the quality of measures of human structure and performance (Potvin et al., 1985). Often, these terms are used in a manner that implies that a given test "has it" or "does not have it" (i.e., reliability or validity) when in fact both should be recognized as continuums.

There are traditional, well-known methods used in academic circles to quantify reliability. The result produced implies an interpretation of "how much" reliability a given test has, but there is no corresponding way to determine how much is needed (in the same terms that reliability of a test is measured) so that one could determine if one has "enough." Other aspects of the academic treatment of human performance measurement quality are similarly troublesome with regard to the implications for widespread, general use of measurements. For example, there is an inherent desire (and need) to generalize the results of a given reliability study for a given instrument and, at the same time, a reluctance on the part of those who conduct such studies to do so in writing. The strictly academic position is that one can *never* generalize a reliability study; that is, it applies only to a situation which is identical to that reported (i.e., that instrument, those subjects, that examiner, that room, that time of day, etc.). So, one may ask, what is the value of reporting any such study? The purely academic view may be the most correct, but strict interpretation is completely useless to a practitioner who needs to reach a conclusion regarding the applicability of a given instrument in given application. The mere fact that reliability studies are reported implies that there is an expectation of generalization to *some* degree. The question is, "How much generalization can one make? This issue has not been adequately addressed from a general methodological standpoint. However, awareness of this issue and the need for improved methods are growing.

What is the general "quality" of measurement available today? The following is offered as a reasonably "healthy" perspective on this complex issue:

1. Technology has advanced to the point where it is now possible to measure many of the basic physical variables employed on measurement such as time, force, torque, angles, linear distance, etc. very accurately, with high repeatability and with high resolution without significant difficulty.
2. Most of the difference on test–retest is due to limitations in how well one can reasonably control procedures and actual variability of the parameter measured—even in the most ideal test subjects.
3. Many studies have been conducted on the reliability of a wide variety of human performance capacities. Some true generalization can be achieved by looking at this body of work as a whole and not from attempts to generalize from only single studies.
4. Across the many types of variables investigated, results of such studies are amazingly quite similar. Basically, they say that if your instrumentation is good, and if you carefully follow established, optimal test administration procedures, then it should be possible to obtain results on repeated testing that are within a range of 5–20% of each other. The exact location achieved in this range depends in large part on the particular variable in question (e.g., repeated measures associated with complex tasks with many degrees of freedom such as lifting or gait will differ more than repeated measures of hinge joint range of motions). In addition, the magnitude of the given metric will influence such percentage characterizations since errors are often fixed amounts and independent of the size of the quantity measured. Thus, when measuring quantities with small magnitudes, a larger variability (i.e., more like 20%) should be anticipated. One can usually determine an applicable working value in these straightforward, usable terms (e.g., 5% or 20%) that allow direct comparison to an evaluation of needs by careful review of the relevant reliability studies.

A major point of this discussion is to illustrate that traditional methods used to "measure the measurements" do not adequately communicate the information that current and potential users of measurements often need to know. Traditional methods were valuable to some degree in providing relative indicators within the context of academic group studies. However, methods that are more similar to those used to characterize measurement system performance in physics and other traditional engineering areas (e.g., accuracy, signal–noise ratio concepts, etc.) are needed. This will help practitioners who must make single measurements on individual subjects (i.e., not populations) to support clinical decision making (Mayer et al., 1997). As the manner in which measurements are used continues to change to include more of the latter, new interest and methods for quantifying the quality of measurements can be anticipated.

39.4 Databases and Data Modeling

Much research has been conducted to define measurements of human structure and performance and to collect and characterize data as basis to increase understanding and make inferences in different contexts. A wide variety of problems of major medical and other societal significance require the use of such data

1. For diagnostic purposes (i.e., when assessing measures obtained from a subject-under-test, such as to determine the efficacy of an intervention or treatment in a medical context).
2. For modeling and simulation (e.g., analyses for return-to-work decisions of injured employees, to support job-site modifications for individuals with disabilities, and design specifications for virtual reality systems).
3. Status/capacity evaluations (e.g., disability determinations for insurance settlements, worker's compensation claims, etc.).
4. To obtain a better understanding of disease and aging processes (e.g., associated with problems such as falls in elderly populations, etc.).
5. To gain insight into the impact of environmental and occupational factors (e.g., as in epidemiologic studies, such as in lead toxicity or carpal tunnel syndrome).
6. To support ergonomic design of consumer products and living environments for use by the public in general. Despite such a diverse range in needs for basically the same information, there has been little—if any—attempt to organize, integrate, and represent available data in a compact, accessible form that can serve the cited needs.

Figure 39.1 illustrates the scope of the general problem and infers a potential approach to integration. At the most basic level, individual measurements for a given variable must be collected and databased. In addition, databases of data from published studies are required to identify specific gaps that limit either analytic functionality or fidelity in the types of tasks, which data must support. Data from the literature are typically available only in summary form, that is, in terms of means and standard deviations for defined populations. Future research is required to define and validate methods for integrating data, for example, from multiple studies to form a single, more robust data model for a given performance

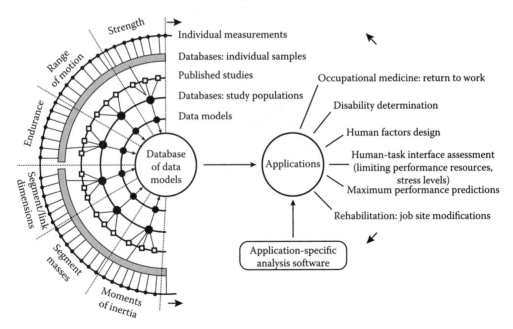

FIGURE 39.1 Schematic summary of proposed integration of human structural and performance data to realize compact representations (i.e., parametric data models) to support analyses in multiple application areas. Only several types of performance resources and aspects of structure are represented. The problem of realizing a complete array of such models in a form generally useable by multiple analysis tools is complex.

or structure parameter. This will involve testing data models developed from databases of individual measures and databases of studies against each other. Development of data warping methods (e.g., to adapt predictions of expected performance levels to subjects of different body sizes and ages) is required to provide models that would be transparent operationally and would allow analyses to proceed in data-limited situations with predictable tradeoffs in fidelity. In many areas, especially with regard to practitioners such as occupational and physical therapists, performance characterization has been viewed only unidimensionally. More multidimensional perspectives are needed for an adequate representation of fidelity (e.g., Kondraske, 2000). Another major aspect of data modeling therefore involves the development of multivariate models of performance envelopes (Vasta and Kondraske, 1997) for individual human subsystems (e.g., knee flexors, visual information processors, etc.). Such models would support, for example, prediction of available torque production capacity under different specified conditions (e.g., joint angle, speed, etc.). In summary, a basic strategy is required for harvesting the vast amount of previously collected data to obtain compact, accessible representations. Means must be incorporated in this strategy to allow for integration of data from multiple sources and continuous update as new data are collected to enhance fidelity and range of applicability of composite models.

As previously noted, individuals within the human performance community typically adopt a variety of terms or identification schemes for structures and parameters employed in both the execution and communication of their work. The sheer number of parameters and variety of combinations in which they may be required to meet analysis needs may be sufficient to justify a more formal approach (e.g., Kondraske, 1993), thereby facilitating the development of common data structures. The engineering contexts in which data models can be envisioned to be used require more rigor and stability. Computer-based models and analyses beg for codification of terms and parameters (i.e., for databases, etc.). In this regard, these emerging applications bring to light the lack of precision in terminology and confusion in definitions. Moreover, the ability to integrate models and analysis modules developed independently within more narrow subsets of the field to address more complex problems requires standardized notation if for no other reason than for efficiency. Development of a standardized systematic notation is compelling; it is postulated that without such a notation, progress to the next level of sophistication cannot occur.

39.5 Measure or Predict?

The large number of different human performance parameters discussed in this section of the text motivates an often-heard question from practitioners: "What is the most important thing to measure?" Clearly, the interest behind such questions is efficiency; it takes time to measure and practitioners are generally under many pressures to be efficient. Figure 39.2 casts the issue in a way that reflects a hierarchical organization of parameters, where each box can represent many different parameters. It can generally be argued that in many situations the "need to know" exists at multiple levels in this hierarchy. Thus, this presents a somewhat bleak outlook for practitioners that generally results in the use of only the most gross level of measurement (e.g., subjective rating scales) because it is "quick." Significant advancement in applications beyond the research lab demands that this problem be addressed.

One possibility that could contribute to solving this dilemma is to utilize models to estimate performance at a given hierarchical level using measurements obtained at lower hierarchical levels. It is argued that this may be an optimal long-term strategy (see Figure 39.3). Methods such as Nonlinear Causal Resource Analysis and others discussed in Chapter 156 (Vasta and Kondraske, 2005), and promising results that have been obtained thus far in limited contexts, provide a basis for believing in the promise of this strategy. In the ideal situation, many different laboratories could contribute to building and evaluating high-quality models for many different "higher-level tasks" (emphasizing that "higher level" is a relative concept). Independently developed models could be integrated into computer-based tools available to practitioners. A reasonable set of measurements made at selected levels could then be used with such tools to obtain a huge "added value" by having performance in a number of different

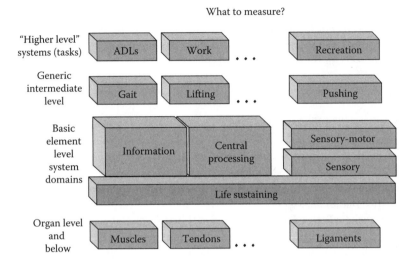

FIGURE 39.2 Performance capacity and related parameters are of interest at many hierarchical levels, posing the problem of deciding what to measure in any given application and presenting a problem of complexity for which solutions must be defined.

higher-level tasks estimated through use of the models. In essence, one would obtain the equivalent of measurements that would otherwise require hours of measurement time in an instant.

39.6 Summary

A relatively high degree of sophistication currently exists with regard to the science, engineering, and technology of human performance. The field is, nonetheless, relatively young and undergoing natural maturation processes. Remaining needs in terms of both conceptual underpinnings and tools (which

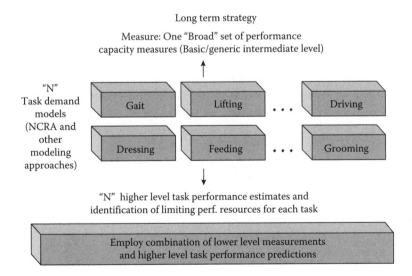

FIGURE 39.3 Summary of a long-term strategy in which models are used to predict performance capacities at higher levels using measurements obtained at lower levels to provide the required scope of information that is generally of interest.

are not independent) are enormous. Future progress, however, is likely to be more dependent on collaborative efforts of different types. The magnitude and nature of problems that are at the forefront demand the achievement of agreement among a critical mass of researchers and practitioners. Both the challenges and prospects for the future are significant.

References

Bendell, A., Disney, J., and Pridmore, W.A. 1988. *Taguchi Methods: Applications in World Industry*, IFS Publishing, London.

Bunge, M. 1977. Levels and reduction. *Am. J. Physiol.*, 233: R75–R82.

Frey, W.D. 1987. Functional assessment in the '80s: A conceptual enigma, a technical challenge. In: Halpern, A.S. and Fuhrer, M.J. (eds.), *Functional Assessment in Rehabilitation*, Paul H. Brookes Publishing Co., Baltimore, MD.

Gardner, H. 1985. *The Mind's New Science: A History of Cognitive Revolution.* Basic Books, Inc., New York, NY.

Kondraske, G.V. 1993. *The HPI Shorthand Notation System for Human System Parameters, (Technical Report 92-001R V1.5)*, The University of Texas at Arlington, Human Performance Institute, Arlington, TX.

Kondraske, G.V. 1995. A working model for human system–task interfaces. In: Bronzino, J.D. (ed.), *Handbook of Biomedical Engineering.* CRC Press, Boca Raton, FL.

Potvin, A.R., Tourtellotte, W.W., Potvin, J.H., Kondraske, G.V., and Syndulko, K. 1985. *The Quantitative Examination of Neurologic Function.* CRC Press, Boca Raton, FL.

Simmon, C.W. Will egg-sucking ever become a science? *Hum. Factors Soc. Bull.*, 30: 1.

Smith, L.L. 1987. Whyfore human factors. *Hum. Factors Soc. Bull.*, 30: 1.

Vasta, P.J. and Kondraske, G.V. 1992. *Standard Conventions for Kinematic and Structural Parameters for the "Gross Total Human" Link Model*, Technical Report 92-003R V1.0, The University of Texas at Arlington, Human Performance Institute.

Vasta, P.J. and Kondraske, G.V. 2005. Human performance engineering: Design and analysis tools. In: Bronzino, J.D. (ed.), *Handbook of Biomedical Engineering.* CRC Press, Boca Raton, FL.

Weismer, G. and Liss, J.M. 1991. Reductionism is a dead-end in speech research, In: Moore, C.A., Yorkston, K.M., and Beukelman, D.R. (eds.), *Dysarthria and Apraxia of Speech.* Paul H. Brookes Publishing Co., Baltimore, MD.

Further Information

The section of this handbook titled *"Human Performance Engineering"* contains chapters that address human performance modeling and measurement in considerably more detail.

Manufacturers of instruments used to characterize different aspects of human performance often provide technical literature and bibliographies of studies related to measurement quality, technical specifications of instruments, and application examples.

Future articles of relevance can be expected on a continuing basis in the following journals:

American Journal of Occupational Therapy; *Archives of Physical Medicine and Rehabilitation*; *Human Factors*; *IEEE Transactions on Rehabilitation Engineering* and *IEEE Transactions on Biomedical Engineering*; *Journal of Biomechanics*; *Journal of Occupational Rehabilitation*; *Physical Therapy*; *Rehabilitation Management*; and *Rehabilitation Research and Development*.

IV

Rehabilitation Engineering

Charles Robinson
Clarkson University

Preface

Engineering advances have resulted in enormous strides in the field of rehabilitation. Individuals with reduced or no vision can be given "sight"; those with severe or complete hearing loss can "hear" by being provided with a sense of their surroundings; those unable to talk can be aided to "speak" again; and those without full control of a limb (or with the limb missing) can by artificial means "walk" or regain other movement functions. But the current level of available functional restoration for seeing, hearing, speaking, and moving still pales in comparison to the capabilities of individuals without disability. As is readily apparent from the content of many of the chapters in this handbook, the human sensory and motor (movement) systems are marvelously engineered, both within a given system and integrated across systems. The rehabilitation engineer thus faces a daunting task in trying to design augmentative or replacement systems when one or more of these systems is impaired.

Rehabilitation engineering had its origins in the need to provide assistance to individuals who were injured in World War II. Rehabilitation engineering can be defined in a number of ways. Perhaps the most encompassing (and the one adopted here) is that proposed by Reswick (1982): rehabilitation engineering is the application of science and technology to ameliorate the handicaps of individuals with disabilities. With this definition, any device, technique, or concept used in rehabilitation that has a technological basis falls under the purview of rehabilitation engineering. This contrasts with the much narrower view that is held by some that rehabilitation engineering is only the design and production phase of a broader field called assistive technology. Lest one consider this distinction trivial, consider that the US Congress has mandated that rehabilitation engineering and technology services be provided by all states; an argument has ensued among various groups of practitioners about who can legally provide such services because of the various interpretations of what rehabilitation engineering is.

There is a core body of knowledge that defines each of the traditional engineering disciplines. Biomedical engineering is less precisely defined, but in general, a biomedical engineer must be proficient in a traditional engineering discipline and have a working knowledge of things biological or medical. The rehabilitation engineer is a biomedical engineer who must not only be technically proficient as an engineer and know biology and medicine but also integrate artistic, social, financial, psychological, and physiological considerations to develop or analyze a device, technique, or concept that meets the needs of the population that the engineer is serving. In general, rehabilitation engineers deal with musculoskeletal or sensory disabilities. They often have a strong background in biomechanics. Most work in a multidisciplinary team setting.

Rehabilitation engineering deals with many aspects of rehabilitation, including applied, scientific, clinical, technical, and theoretical. Various topics include but are not limited to assistive devices and other aids for those with disability, sensory augmentation and substitution systems, functional electrical stimulation (for motor control and sensory–neural prostheses), orthotics and prosthetics, myoelectric devices and techniques, transducers (including electrodes), signal processing, hardware, software, robotics, systems approaches, technology assessment, postural stability, wheelchair seating systems, gait analysis, biomechanics, biomaterials, control systems (both biological and external), ergonomics, human performance, and functional assessment (Robinson, 1993).

In this section of the handbook we focus only on applications of rehabilitation engineering. The basic concepts of rehabilitation engineering, rehabilitation science, and rehabilitation technology are outlined in Robinson's Chapter 43. Two chapters in this section cover sensory input, and two cover movement or communication output. Gill (Chapter 41) and Remus (Chapter 40) cover sensory rehabilitation or remediation (blindness and low vision, deafness, and hearing loss). Fite's Chapter 42 looks at orthopedic rehabilitation in terms of prosthetics. Hill, Romich, and Vanderheiden (Chapter 47) look at the output side as they explore augmentative and alternative communication systems and their scientific bases. Treffler's Chapter 49 covers concepts involved in the day-to-day provision of rehabilitation technology.

For the purposes of this handbook, many topics that partially fall under the rubric of rehabilitation engineering are covered elsewhere. These include chapters on electrical stimulation, hard tissue replacement—long bone repair and joints, biomechanics, musculoskeletal soft-tissue mechanics, analysis of gait, sports biomechanics/kinesiology, biodynamics, cochlear mechanics, measurement of neuromuscular performance capabilities, human factors applications in rehabilitation engineering, electrical stimulators, prostheses and artificial organs, nerve guidance channels, bioactive brain implants, and tracheal, laryngeal, and esophageal replacement devices.

Rehabilitation engineering can be described as an engineering systems discipline. Imagine being the design engineer on a project that has an unknown, highly nonlinear plant, with coefficients whose variations in time appear to follow no known or solvable model, where time (yours and your client's) and funding are severely limited, where no known solution has been developed (or if it has, will need modification for nearly every client, so no economy of scale exists). Further, there will be severe impedance mismatches between available appliances and your client's needs. Or the low residual channel capacity of one of your client's senses will require enormous signal compression to get a signal with any appreciable information content through it. Welcome to the world of the rehabilitation engineer!

Bibliography

Reswick, J. 1982. What is a rehabilitation engineer? In *Annual Review of Rehabilitation*, Vol. 2 (eds. E.L. Pan, T.E. Backer, C.L. Vash), Springer-Verlag, New York.

Robinson, C.J., 1993. Rehabilitation engineering: An editorial. *IEEE Transactions on Rehabilitation Engineering*, 1(1):1–2.

40

Hearing Loss and Deafness: Augmentation and Substitution

Jeremiah J. Remus
Clarkson University

40.1 Introduction

This chapter presents rehabilitative technologies that have been developed to provide clinical solutions to sufferers of hearing loss and deafness. According to the National Institute on Deafness and Other Communication Disorders (NIDCD), 36 million American adults (17% of the adult population) report some degree of hearing loss. These self-reported hearing losses affect an individual's ability to communicate and can be detrimental to the quality of life. However, many years of interdisciplinary collaboration by speech scientists, neurobiologists, audiologists, and engineers has resulted in the development of successful devices that the medical community can use to help patients with hearing loss and deafness.

40.2 Typical Disorders and Causes of Hearing-Related Impairments

This section will begin with a brief background on the components and functioning of the human auditory system. The auditory system can be divided into three areas: the outer ear which consists of the pinna and ear canal, the middle ear which includes the ossicles (malleus, incus, and stapes), and the inner ear which includes the cochlea and the auditory nerve (VIIIth cranial nerve). The process of hearing is a sequence of energy transfers that starts with the acoustic waveform impinging on the tympanic membrane (i.e., eardrum) at the end of the ear canal. The tympanic membrane converts the acoustic energy to mechanical energy which is relayed through the three bones of the middle ear to the oval window of the inner ear. The middle ear ossicles also provide critical impedance matching that enables the transfer of energy into the fluid-filled cochlea. The motion of the ossicles is transferred into the cochlea and produces compression waves in the fluid-filled ducts of the cochlea, resulting in a displacement of the basilar membrane at a location that is dependent on the frequency of the acoustic source waveform. Thus, the cochlea performs a frequency-dependent spatial mapping of the incoming waveform. Located on the basilar membrane within the cochlea is the organ of Corti, containing cilia-lined hair cells that are stimulated by the displacement of the basilar membrane. The inner hair cells generate an action potential that is transmitted via the auditory nerve to the auditory centers of the brain, producing a sound percept.

In a clinical setting, the loss of normal hearing function can most easily be described by two metrics: hearing thresholds and masking level. Hearing loss produces increased threshold levels, and the increases in threshold level that result from hearing loss can be frequency specific. Audiologists often view a patient's thresholds in the form of an audiogram, which plots frequency-specific hearing thresholds that are measured using pure-tone sinusoids at a range of frequencies. Often, audiometric testing focuses on the range of frequencies most critical for speech understanding (250 Hz–8 kHz). The second metric that is useful for describing hearing loss is the masking level. Masking is a perceptual effect in which one stimulus "masks" a subsequent lower amplitude probe stimulus that is temporally or spectrally similar to the first stimulus. Although masking levels are informative, the time required to measure them prevents their frequent use by audiologists, and they are more commonly used in research settings for device development. Often, individuals suffering from hearing impairments can be measured to have abnormal values of both threshold and masking level.

Hearing losses can be localized to a specific range of frequencies (e.g., higher frequencies) or can affect the entire range of hearing. Hearing losses are often categorized according to the degree of impairment: slight, mild, moderate, severe, and profound. The various degrees of hearing loss as defined by the American Speech-Language-Hearing Association are as follows [1]:

Degree of Hearing Loss	Hearing Threshold Range (dB)
Normal	−10–15
Slight	16–25
Mild	26–40
Moderate	41–55
Moderately severe	56–70
Severe	71–90
Profound	91+

Hearing losses can typically be classified as conductive hearing loss or sensorineural hearing loss, although some patients do simultaneously suffer from both conditions. Conductive hearing loss is the result of an obstruction of the mechanical pathways in the middle ear. This can be caused, for example, by otosclerosis, an abnormal growth of bone in the ear that mitigates normal transfer of energy from the eardrum to the inner ear, or otitis media, an infection of the middle and inner ear. In most circumstances it is possible to treat conductive hearing loss using medication or a medical procedure; for example, stapedotomy to correct an immobilized stapes due to otosclerosis. The second category of hearing loss is sensorineural hearing loss. Sensorineural hearing loss refers to hearing loss that occurs in the inner ear and VIIIth cranial (auditory) nerve. In this case, the cause of hearing loss is deterioration of the neural transmission pathway that includes the cochlea, the inner hair cells along the organ of Corti, and the auditory nerve. Because sensorineural hearing affects the underlying neural transmission path, it is considered a permanent disability that requires rehabilitative devices.

There are a variety of potential causes of sensorineural hearing loss. Prolonged exposure to high levels of noise can damage the cilia of the inner hair cells [2]. Exposure to certain ototoxic chemicals and medications can have side effects that include hearing loss and deafness [3]. Certain illnesses, such as Meniere's disease or Usher syndrome, are also capable of producing severe to profound hearing loss. In sensorineural hearing loss, the inner hair cells in the organ of Corti are the most likely source of the disruption in normal operation of the auditory system. As mentioned previously, the inner hair cells are responsible for producing an action potential in response to displacement of the basilar membrane in the cochlea. Thus, the inner hair cells serve as the link between the cochlea and the auditory nerve.

40.3 Methods of Remediation

The two most widely used technologies for remediation of hearing impairments are the hearing aid and the cochlear implant. The hearing aid is most appropriate for individuals with mild-to-moderate hearing loss. More severe hearing impairments affecting both ears might require cochlear implants to restore some percept of hearing. A combination of hearing aids and cochlear implants is common in individuals with varying levels of impairment affecting each ear [4,5]. Hearing loss does not necessarily affect both ears equally; it is possible to have a higher degree of hearing impairment in one of the ears, or for the impairment to have been present for a longer time in one ear. This can often become a consideration during treatment because there is still debate on whether assistive technologies are more effective when applied to the "better" or "worse" ear, and how to utilize the remaining ear. The additional cost of bilateral cochlear implantation is also weighed against the potential benefits in terms of improved speech recognition [6,7]. These rehabilitation technologies have been commercially available for many years and are the focus of this chapter. We will briefly address advanced efforts, such as hair cell regeneration, at the end of the chapter.

The electronic hearing aid operates essentially as a sound amplifier, and consists of a microphone, amplifier electronics, and a speaker. Hearing aids are available in three basic structures: behind the ear (BTE), in the ear (ITE), and in the canal (ITC) devices. The various structures differ most significantly in their cost of fitting, cost of the hardware, and levels of potential hearing loss compensation. In general, hearing aids have benefited from advances in technology that have allowed for miniaturization of the components and improved power management, which has also driven a shift from analog-to-digital technology as costs decrease and additional features are enabled through digital signal processing.

As digital hearing aids become more common, the development of more advanced digital signal processing should add greater capabilities to hearing aids. One of the significant challenges in hearing aids is performance in situations with high background noise and multiple talkers. To address these challenges, hearing aid manufacturers are focusing on digital signal processing techniques to provide advanced noise suppression [8], as well as taking advantage of multiple microphones and using algorithms to perform beamforming [9], which tunes the directional sensitivity of the hearing and attenuates signals (i.e., noise sources) arriving at angles away of the targeted direction. Digital hearing aids are also able to provide higher levels of gain, and actively work to reduce feedback using adaptive signal processing. Another capability of digital hearing aids is the potential for binaural hearing. Binaural hearing strategies utilize a wireless RF link between the hearing aids in each ear to synchronize the devices, providing natural binaural cues that normal-hearing individuals use for sound localization. Further development of this technology will lead to additional improvements in hearing aid performance in noisy and multitalker environments.

The second hearing rehabilitation device is the cochlear implant. Cochlear implants are neural prosthetic devices intended to restore some degree of hearing to severely hearing-impaired individuals. As thresholds rise far above the level of normal hearing, hearing aids are no longer capable of providing a sufficient level of remediation. In these situations, a cochlear implant is necessary to bypass the middle and inner ear, including the inner hair cells that are often responsible for sensorineural hearing loss, and directly stimulate the spiral ganglion of the auditory nerve.

Cochlear implants can be divided into two components: the external speech processor and the implanted electrode array and electronics. A diagram of a cochlear implant is shown in Figure 40.1. Sounds recorded by the microphone are sent to the speech processor, which decomposes the incoming waveform and extracts certain cues that allow the speech signal to be represented as a pulse sequence. The information about the pulse sequence is then transmitted transcutaneously to the implanted electronics through a radio-frequency link, where it is decoded and used to specify stimuli that are delivered via the implanted electrode array.

The electrode array, depending on the specific device, consists of 16–28 contacts spread over a 12–30 mm distance. Cochlear implants take advantage of the tonotopic arrangement of the cochlea;

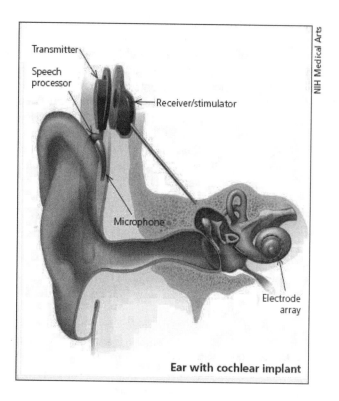

FIGURE 40.1 Diagram of cochlear implant showing external speech processor and transmitter and internal receiver/stimulator and electrode array. (From Medical illustrations by NIH, Medical Arts & Photography Branch.)

different locations in the cochlea correspond to different perceived frequencies. The multiple frequency-specific channels provide greater spectral resolution by allowing the division of the speech spectrum into several channels that are allocated to a corresponding region of the cochlea. Several studies, most notably that of Greenwood [10], have mapped the distance from the round window of the cochlea to a corresponding frequency percept. Each contact in the electrode array stimulates a different site in the cochlea; based on the cochlear physiology, each site in the cochlea corresponds to a unique presentation frequency. Early cochlear implants had a single electrode and a separate ground electrode typically placed in the tissue outside the cochlea. Current cochlear implant devices use a multielectrode array to create more focused stimuli by constraining the stimulus to a local population of nerve fibers. This allows different sections of the cochlea to be stimulated independently. Recent developments in cochlear implants are investigating the use of current steering, which includes simultaneous stimulation of neighboring electrodes to produce a percept at a "virtual electrode" located between the two physical electrodes [11]. In the speech processor of the multielectrode cochlear implant, the incoming sound is filtered with a bank of nonoverlapping bandpass filters, creating a set of channels containing different regions of the frequency spectrum. Each of these speech processor channels is presented to one of the electrodes, thereby improving the frequency resolution over the single electrode cochlear implant.

Current cochlear implant technology allows many device recipients to perform very well in tests of speech recognition and to function normally in daily life. However, cochlear implantees have displayed a wide range of scores in tests evaluating speech perception abilities [12,13]. One potential source of variation in speech perception abilities is deviation from the assumptions about how cochlear implants transmit speech information under ideal conditions. In any particular cochlear implant patient, researchers and clinicians cannot be certain about the number of surviving spiral ganglion or how the surviving population of nerve fibers in the vicinity of the electrode will respond to electrical stimulation. With the multichannel cochlear implant, the possibility of interaction between channels interfering with the transmission of speech information must also be considered. Current research is seeking to determine methods for patient-specific tuning of the speech processor and to identify early predictors of the level of speech perception improvement that a patient will receive from a cochlear implant. There is also a significant effort to determine the best strategies for utilizing bilateral implants as a growing number of patients are receiving a cochlear implant in their second ear, especially prelingual deaf individuals who will see the greatest benefits from bilateral implantation while learning to communicate.

While still in the basic research stage, a potentially transformative development in the treatment of sensorineural hearing loss would be the ability to regenerate hair cells. Researchers have been actively pursuing this line of research for more than 20 years, and some studies have shown successful regeneration in avian species [14]. However, the technology is still many years from use as a treatment option for human patients. Despite the amount of work that remains to transfer this technology from the laboratory to the clinic, it is a promising avenue of investigation that will hopefully provide significant capabilities for restoring hearing in many instances of sensorineural hearing loss.

References

1. Clark, J.G., Uses and abuses of hearing loss classification, *ASHA,* 23(7), 1981, 493–500.
2. Rabinowitz, P.M., Noise-induced hearing loss, *American Family Physician,* 61(9), 2000, 2759–2760.
3. Seligmann, H., Podoshin, L., and Ben-David, J., Drug-induced tinnitus and other hearing disorders, *Drug Safety: An International Journal of Medical Toxicology and Drug Experience,* 14(3), 1996, 198–212.
4. Ching, T.Y.C., Incerti, P., and Hill, M., Binaural benefits for adults who use hearing aids and cochlear implants in opposite ears, *Ear and Hearing,* 25(1), 2004, 9.
5. Tyler, R.S., Parkinson, A.J., and Wilson, B.S., Patients utilizing a hearing aid and a cochlear implant: Speech perception and localization, *Ear and Hearing,* 23(2), 2002, 98.
6. Litovsky, R.Y., Johnstone, P.M., and Godar, S.P., Benefits of bilateral cochlear implants and/or hearing aids in children, *International Journal of Audiology,* 45, 2006, 78–91.
7. Summerfield, A.Q., Marshall, D.H., and Barton, G.R., A cost-utility scenario analysis of bilateral cochlear implantation, *Archives of Otolaryngology-Head and Neck Surgery,* 128(11), 2002, 1255–1262.
8. Plomp, R., Noise, amplification, and compression: Considerations of three main issues in hearing aid design, *Ear and Hearing,* 15(1), 1994, 2.
9 Berghe, J.V. and Wouters, J., An adaptive noise canceller for hearing aids using two nearby microphones, *The Journal of the Acoustical Society of America,* 103, 1998, 3621.
10. Greenwood, D.D., A cochlear frequency-position function for several species—29 years later, *Journal of the Acoustical Society of America,* 87(6), 1990, pp. 2592–2605.
11. Firszt, J.B., Koch, D.B., and Downing, M., Current steering creates additional pitch percepts in adult cochlear implant recipients, *Otology & Neurotology,* 28(5), 2007, 629.
12. Shannon, R.V., Multichannel electrical stimulation of the auditory nerve in man. II. Channel interaction, *Hearing Research,* 12, 1983, 1–16.
13. Shannon, R.V., Temporal modulation transfer functions in patients with cochlear implants, *Journal of the Acoustical Society of America,* 91(4), 1992, 2156–2164.
14. Ryals, B.M. and Rubel, E.W., Hair cell regeneration after acoustic trauma in adult Coturnix quail, *Science,* 240(4860), 1988, 1774.

41

Low Vision and Blindness: Augmentation and Substitution

John Gill
John Gill Technology Ltd

The number of people with disabilities is gradually increasing since more people are living to an older age and many disabilities are correlated with age. About 1.5% of the population in the United Kingdom have such vision that they could be registered as "blind" or "partially sighted." However, the effect depends on a number of factors including medical condition (e.g., macular degeneration), environment (e.g., illumination), and contrast.

The more common conditions are

1. Macular degeneration
   Age-related macular degeneration accounts for about half of all registerable visual impairments in the United Kingdom. It typically results in the loss of central vision (see Figure 41.1). Since most of the color receptors are in the macula (the central area of the retina), those with macular degeneration see colors less vividly.

   Frequently enlarging text will improve legibility and readability, but it is important that there is high contrast between the text and the background.
2. Diabetic retinopathy
   This is the single most common cause of registerable visual impairment among those of the working age group in the United Kingdom. It is more likely to occur if the control of diabetes is poor. Typically it results in hemorrhages in the back of the eye (see Figure 41.2); laser treatment can reduce the spread of the hemorrhages by sealing the edges.

   Individuals with diabetes often have poor circulation which can result in problems with their feet. However, it frequently adversely affects their sense of touch, so the ability to read braille is rare.
3. Cataracts
   A cataract is an opaqueness of the lens at the front of the eye. The effect is not dissimilar to driving a car with a dirty windscreen; if the sun is behind you, visibility is reasonably good, but if the sun is in front of you, visibility may be severely impaired (Figure 41.3).

   Surgically it is possible to remove the cataract and replace it with a plastic lens. However it is not uncommon to then find macular degeneration which has not been diagnosed because it was obscured by the cataract.
4. Tunnel vision
   Tunnel vision (Figure 41.4) is associated with a late stage of glaucoma and some forms of retinitis pigmentosa. Glaucoma is caused by an increase in pressure in the fluid in the eye; at an early stage

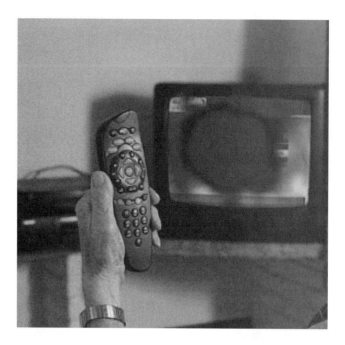

FIGURE 41.1   How someone with macular degeneration might see their television screen.

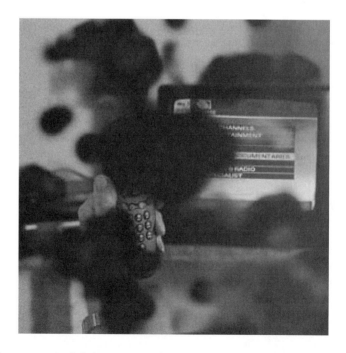

FIGURE 41.2   How someone with diabetic retinopathy might see their television screen.

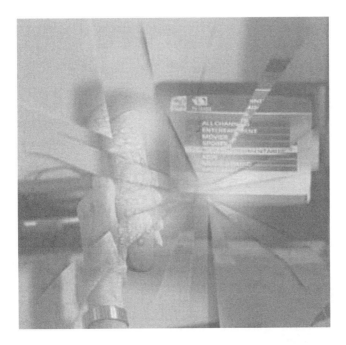

FIGURE 41.3 How someone with cataracts might see their television screen.

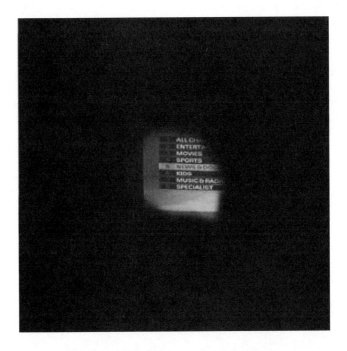

FIGURE 41.4 How someone with tunnel vision might see their television screen.

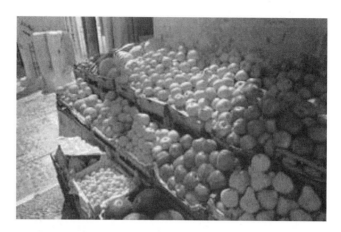

FIGURE 41.5   Normal color vision.

it can be treated with tablets, but surgical intervention may be necessary if it has not been treated at a sufficiently early stage.

Retinitis pigmentosa (RP) represents a group of conditions whose common factors are that they are genetic and result in night blindness. In the classic form, the onset is typically between the age of 30 and 40 and results in reduced peripheral vision.

Individuals with tunnel vision may have difficulties in not walking into objects on a sidewalk even though they can read road signs. Often they will find it easier to read in print which is smaller so that a whole word fits into their visual field.

5. Dyslexia

This is a cognitive impairment which can result in difficulty in reading or writing textual characters. It can also result in problems in remembering a series of digits (e.g., a PIN at a cash dispenser) in the correct order. The design of the typeface can make a significant difference to the readability of text which is also affected by foreground and background colors.

6. Color blindness

Total color blindness is rare, but difficulty in distinguishing between red and green is common (see Figures 41.5 and 41.6). About 8% of the male population in the United Kingdom have red/green color blindness, but only 0.5% of the female population are affected. About 2% of the population can have difficulties with blue/yellow differentiation.

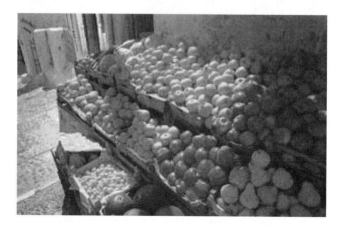

FIGURE 41.6   How someone with red/green color vision might view the same scene.

7. Aging

There are a number of effects of the aging process including:

a. Lessening in the ability of the eye to focus at different distances (visual accommodation).
b. The need for higher levels of illumination since less light reaches the retina. Typically in a 60-year old, only a third as much light reaches their retina compared to when they were aged 20.
c. The need for greater contrast to be able to accurately read text.
d. Multitasking becomes less easy.

In addition the individual may not have a current correct optical prescription for their spectacles (or may have left the appropriate spectacles at home).

41.1 Electronic Vision Systems

For many years scientists have addressed the problem of how to use electronic systems to replace some of the functions of the human eye. Up to recently these were just interesting laboratory experiments, but new developments in electronics and wearable computers could turn these prototypes into devices of practical benefit at affordable prices.

The three main approaches are

- Vision enhancement
- Vision substitution
- Vision replacement

Vision enhancement involves input from a camera, processing of the information, and output on a visual display. In its simplest form it may be a miniature head-mounted camera with the output on a head-mounted visual display (as used in some virtual reality systems). However, modern fast wearable computers make feasible sophisticated processing of the information in real time, and it is this factor which could transform interesting research projects into products of practical benefit to the blind and partially sighted people.

For instance, a more sophisticated system might incorporate a combination of visual and ultrasonic cameras. The ultrasonic camera can provide information about the distance of an object from the camera. The user could then instruct that he or she is only interested in viewing items less than 2 m away. The processor would then delete all data at a distance of more than 2 m; this would significantly reduce the clutter on the visual display.

Another possibility could be that the user is looking for a post box which he knows is painted bright red; he could request that anything which is not red is shown with lower brightness. Yet another possibility is for the user to instruct that only the edges of objects should be displayed. There are many other possibilities for processing the information to meet the specific needs of an individual at that moment.

Research is needed to determine what facilities are required and how to optimally design the user interface. This is a nontrivial research task since users will have little understanding of what facilities could be offered and the types of user interface that could be utilized. However, without the research being done systematically, progress on electronic vision systems will be slow and fragmentary.

Vision substitution is similar to vision enhancement but with the output being nonvisual—typically tactual or auditory or some combination of the two. Since the senses of touch and hearing have a much lower information capacity than vision, it is essential to process the information to a level that can be handled by the user.

Vision replacement involves displaying the information directly to the visual cortex of the human brain or via the optic nerve. Considerable research has been done on how to interface to the brain but problems have been experienced in obtaining a reliable link of sufficient bandwidth, as well as the human brain interpreting the data it is receiving.

Vision enhancement systems have already appeared on the market, but are often limited to providing image enhancement. It is anticipated that they will gradually incorporate more options for the image processing. Vision substitution systems already exist, mainly as developments of electronic mobility devices, but it is likely to be some years before they come into widespread use. They will need to be accompanied by appropriate training.

Affordable vision replacement systems are farther into the future since much more needs to be known about how to optimally connect to the visual cortex. Since this will involve a surgical procedure, there will need to be stringent testing to ensure that there are no adverse effects.

Over the next few years it will be important to differentiate advertising hype from the real benefits to some people from the appropriate use of these systems. There is a tendency to dismiss developments if they do not live up to the stories in the newspapers, but it would be unwise to dismiss these systems even if claims are made that they "solve the problems of blind people."

42

Orthopedic Prosthetics in Rehabilitation

Kevin Fite
Clarkson University

42.1 Fundamentals

A prosthetic limb is an external device that replaces musculoskeletal function lost because of limb amputation. Such limb loss may be attributed to trauma-related injury, cancer, or complications of the vascular system. The ultimate goal of prostheses is the restoration of full limb control and functionality using an engineered artificial limb. As evidenced by the current state of the art in upper and lower extremity prostheses, there continues to be significant gaps between artificial limbs and the intact appendages for which they are designed as replacements. Historically, the major limitations in prosthetic limb development have been twofold: (1) the lack of a power/actuation system with human-scale size, weight, and power outputs, and (2) the lack of a multi-degree-of-freedom neural interface to the amputee user for purposes of command and control. Because of these constraints, typical commercial prostheses have limited degrees of freedom capable of only a subset of an intact limb's full suite of output capability.

With regard to external power sources, prosthetic limb development benefits from continuing advances in robotic system technologies. In the field of robotics, researchers have demonstrated the ability to build robotic arms capable of dexterous manipulations and power outputs comparable to an intact human limb. However, many of these robotic systems achieve such performance specifications with little regard to the size/weight of the required actuators or the source used to power them. Achieving the same output capabilities with a self-contained artificial limb proves to be a continuing challenge for prosthetic limb design. The common approach to external power and actuation in self-contained limbs is to use battery-powered, motor-driven designs. State-of-the-art commercial motors provide power densities inferior to that of natural muscle and in a form factor that complicates their integration within the envelope boundaries of a limb replacement. These issues, combined with the limited energy densities of lithium battery technology, serve to significantly constrain both the performance and the operation duration of current state-of-the-art prosthetic limbs.

In addition to the mechanical performance limitations of prosthetic limbs, the other major impediment to full restoration of limb capability with an artificial device is the command and control interface between the prosthesis and amputee user. The typical approach for direct amputee control of a prosthetic limb is to use myoelectric potentials from muscles in the amputee's residual limb as user commands to the limb controller. One benefit of this method is that residual-limb muscles can be targeted for the control of limb functions that they would have previously controlled before amputation, thereby easing the learning curve for the amputee user. One of the major issues is the ability to obtain a large number of independent efferent control channels from the amputee's residual musculature, much of which may no longer be available because of the amputation procedure. In the absence of multiple independent control sites, the ability to control a multi-degree-of-freedom limb in a manner comparable to that of an intact limb is compromised. The other major constraint lies in the limitations of afferent neural integration. Haptic and proprioceptive feedback constitutes sensory information critical to many limb functions of the upper and lower extremity. Without such afferent feedback, the amputee user is left to control the artificial limb behavior using visual information coupled with indirect haptic cues transmitted through the load-bearing interface of the socket. An amputee's ability to accurately control limb–environment interaction using visual cues as the primary component of feedback renders the simplest of manipulation tasks quite difficult.

In light of the aforementioned constraints, many of the advances in prosthetic limb technology have been achieved with innovative designs that optimize function for specific task sets rather than develop artificial limbs that yield suboptimal performance for all applications. Only with continued evolution in state-of-the-art technology for both power/actuation and neural integration will the gap in performance between an intact human limb and its artificial counterpart narrow to the degree necessary for complete restoration of functionality lost because of amputation.

42.2 General Design Factors

42.2.1 Cosmesis

The choice of prosthesis for a particular amputee is driven by various factors, some of which include the activity level of the amputee, the desired mechanical functionality of the prosthesis, and its cosmetic appearance. Some amputees choose to be fitted with a prosthesis designed primarily for naturalness of appearance. Such cosmetic designs, an example of which is shown in Figure 42.1, generally sacrifice mechanical functionality in favor of a device that visually looks as close as possible to the limb it is intended to replace. Conversely, other persons may prefer to use a highly functional limb that achieves its level of performance at the expense of cosmetic appearance. This type of limb, an example of which is shown in Figure 42.2, may use a cable-actuated hook as the terminal device. Although not cosmetic in appearance, the hook provides a functional design for effective amputee–environment interaction. A prosthetist

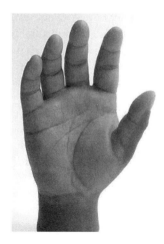

FIGURE 42.1   A living skin hand. (Touch Bionics Inc., Hilliard, OH, USA.)

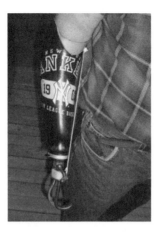

FIGURE 42.2 Cable-driven body-powered arm prosthesis. (Courtesy of Mountain Orthotic and Prosthetic Services, Lake Placid, NY, USA.)

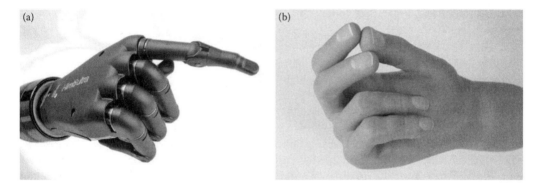

FIGURE 42.3 (a) The i-limb ultra myoelectric hand and (b) i-limb skin natural cosmetic covering. (Touch Bionics Inc., Hilliard, OH, USA.)

or rehabilitation technologist will often fabricate multiple prosthetic limbs, each with their own proportions of functionality and cosmetic appearance, to bracket the range of intended uses for a given amputee. Advances in state-of-the-art prosthesis componentry continue to decrease the disparity between function and cosmesis. The i-limb ultra hand (Touch Bionics Inc., Hilliard, OH, USA) of Figure 42.3 is one example of an upper-extremity terminal device that combines anthropomorphic function with cosmetically natural appearance, holding the promise of both looking and functioning like an intact human hand.

42.2.2 Weight and Amputee Attachment

The overall weight of the prosthesis imposes a significant constraint on artificial limb design. Most artificial limbs attach to the user through a body harness or with a socket interface designed to achieve intimate contact with the tissue of the user's residual limb. Different means of socket suspension are used depending on the intended use and function of the prosthetic limb and the comfort of the user. Sockets may leverage the structural anatomy of the user's residual limb and suspend the limb from bony protrusions. Other sockets incorporate two layers comprising a flexible silicone inner sleeve that adheres to the residual limb and a hard thermoplastic or composite outer socket. The inner sleeve can be custom molded to fit a particular residual limb or selected from a set of stock sizes. The sleeves connect to the outer socket via a direct mechanical connection or by suction acting between themselves and the

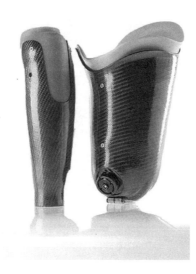

FIGURE 42.4   Otto Bock SiOCX socket system (Otto Bock Healthcare, GmbH, Duderstadt, Germany). The socket consists of an inner made of HTV silicone that connects to the outer composite socket using a mechanical screw interface.

outer socket. Figure 42.4 shows one such socket from Otto Bock Healthcare for use with lower extremity prosthetic limbs. The inner socket uses high temperature vulcanization (HTV) silicone of varying durometers combined with integrated gel pads, providing enhanced comfort, hygiene, and adhesion.

Because prostheses are not directly attached to the user's skeletal structure, the amputee perceives the device as an external load. The overall weight of a prosthetic limb is thus constrained to be less than that of the limb for which it is intended to replace. Otherwise, the likelihood for broad user acceptance of the device may be limited. Osseointegration is an emerging technology that offers the possibility for eliminating the need for a prosthetic socket (Hagberg and Branemark, 2009). The method of osseointegration comprises the surgical implantation of a titanium anchor directly into living bone tissue. The titanium implant consists of a fixture that is inserted into the amputee's residual bone (e.g., the femur in the case of a transfemoral amputation) connected to an abutment that protrudes from the skin at the distal end of the residual limb. Following the implant procedure and subsequent soft-tissue surgery, the patient progresses through a graded rehabilitation protocol until full osseointegration is achieved. The patient is then left with an abutment anchored to the residual skeleton that can then be attached directly to an artificial limb. Figure 42.5 shows an example of a transfemoral prosthesis attached to the user via osseointegration. Such an interface provides for improved fit without the discomforts associated with a socket. Despite these advantages, serious complications do exist with osseointegration. Patients face risks including superficial infections around the area of skin penetration, deep tissue infections, mechanical complications, and the potential for loosening of the implant. As its surgical and rehabilitative aspects continue to advance, osseointegration should offer a clinically feasible alternative to conventional prosthetic sockets.

42.2.3 Source of Power

The final major consideration in prosthetic limb design is the choice of power source. For all but the completely passive cosmetic prostheses, power source selection plays a significant role in the resulting weight and functionality of the artificial limb. The states of the art in upper and lower extremity prosthetics are anthropomorphic designs with motor-actuated joints that offer the possibility of near-human-like output behavior. That said, energetically passive and body-powered limbs offer significant functionality, albeit in a less anthropomorphic package, which should not be overlooked. Given the differences in the functional requirements of upper and lower extremity devices, the discussion below is segregated accordingly.

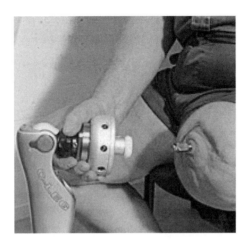

FIGURE 42.5 Osseointegration of a transfemoral prosthesis. (Courtesy of Dr. Rickard Branemark, MD, MSc, PhD.)

42.2.3.1 Upper Extremity Prostheses

Articulating artificial arms can be divided into body-powered and externally powered devices. In the case of a body-powered limb, the user's own musculature is used to control the prosthetic limb. Body-powered actuation is typically achieved using intact muscle power to apply tension to Bowden cables (consisting of a cable sliding within a fixed outer housing). A transhumeral prosthesis such as that shown in Figure 42.2 may include an articulating elbow and a single-degree-of-freedom terminal device. The user actuates Bowden cables to perform functions such as locking/unlocking of the elbow, flexion/extension of the elbow, and opening/closing of the terminal device. Owing, in part, to their technological simplicity, cable-actuated devices offer the benefits of intuitive, reliable, and robust output behavior. Furthermore, Bowden cables provide a degree of kinesthetic feedback because of mechanical interaction between the user and cable. Such feedback gives the user a sense of the interaction between the artificial limb and environment during manipulation tasks, providing an effective interface for command and control of prosthesis behavior.

Alternatively, an external power and actuation system may be incorporated to control each degree of freedom of the limb. Early work in powered arms focused on the use of pneumatic actuators powered by CO_2 cartridges (Marquardt, 1965; Burrows et al., 1972). The relatively low energy-storage density of CO_2 was a major constraint on the operation longevity of these gas-actuated devices. The common approach to external power in current prosthetic arms is the use of electrochemical batteries combined with direct current (DC) motors (Mann and Reimers, 1970; Jacobsen et al., 1982). Improvements in the energy and power densities of battery-powered DC motors have led to the development of advanced externally powered artificial limbs that exhibit near-human-like mechanical output capabilities. Commercially available options include the Boston Elbow III (Liberating Technologies, Inc.), the Utah Arm (Motion Control, Inc.) and the Dynamic Arm (Otto Bock Healthcare, GmbH). These devices use myoelectric commands from the user's residual biceps and triceps muscles to control the motion of the elbow joint. When combined with an electric terminal device, the resulting transhumeral prosthesis can provide the user with sequential, but not simultaneous, myoelectric control of each powered degree of freedom.

Highly articulating prosthetic hands, such as the Otto Bock Michelangelo Bionic Hand of Figure 42.6 and the Touch Bionics iLIMB Hand of Figure 42.3, offer the potential of significantly improved biomimicry. These multi-degree-of-freedom designs enable enhanced dexterous manipulation capacity but require an increased number of independent commands from the user. The residual limb of

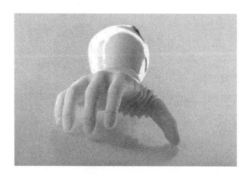

FIGURE 42.6   The Michelangelo Bionic Hand. (Otto Bock Healthcare, GmbH, Duderstadt, Germany.)

a transradial amputee may have a sufficient number of independent myoelectric sites because of the potentially large number of muscle groups available for myoelectric targeting. For a user with a trans-humeral amputation or shoulder disarticulation, the decreased number of myoelectric control sites imposes major constraints on the individual's ability to control advanced anthropomorphic arms. Targeted muscle reinnervation (TMR) is one emerging technology that offers the potential for obtaining an increased number of independent myoelectric control channels (Kuiken et al., 2004; Huang et al., 2008). TMR is a surgical intervention that transfers residual peripheral nerves to intact muscles that, because of the amputation, no longer have biomechanical functionality. After this surgical intervention, the patient gains the ability to activate the reinnervated muscles using neural commands that previously would have activated muscles in the amputated limb. TMR-based control provides a more intuitive amputee–limb control interface and allows the user to exploit the enhanced capabilities of an advanced anthropomorphic prosthesis in a biomechanically natural way.

42.2.3.2 Lower Extremity Prostheses

Artificial limbs for lower extremity amputees have been limited to passive devices, in large part because of the lack of appropriately sized power and actuation systems capable of human-scale power outputs. Despite the absence of power production in lower extremity artificial limbs, several important advances have been achieved for improved functionality of a passive artificial leg in restoring locomotive function. The least-complex prosthetic knee joint, appropriate for amputees with low activity levels, incorporates single-axis rotation with a manually actuated locking joint. Such designs can also incorporate internal extension-assist mechanisms and joint friction for swing-phase control. Advances to this design include a polycentric linkage structure in which the instantaneous center of rotation changes as a function of the knee angle, thereby providing knee stabilization during stance and increased ground clearance during swing. Improvements in knee performance during swing have been achieved with the integration of pneumatic or hydraulic fluid components to provide tunable damping characteristics. The most recent advances incorporate microprocessor-controlled damping characteristics for improved performance in both stance and swing, examples of which are the Otto Bock Genium (Figure 42.7a) and the Össur RHEO KNEE® (Figure 42.7b). The microprocessor uses measured knee position in conjunction with flexion movements measured from heel strike to toe-off to adjust the flexor and extensor resistance of the knee during both stance and swing. Such a system provides real-time adaptation to changes in cadence, allowing effective operation over a large range of walking speeds.

With regard to prosthetic feet and ankles, commercially available designs typically incorporate compliant components for shock absorption or energy-storage elements that can store and return mechanical energy during ground interaction. Energy-storage designs enable energy to be stored during impact

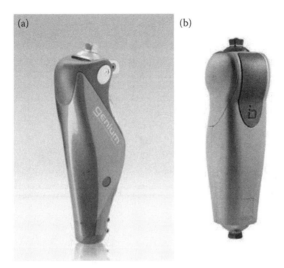

FIGURE 42.7 Microprocessor-controlled knee joints: (a) Genium (Otto Bock Healthcare, GmbH, Duderstadt Germany) and (b) RHEO KNEE®. (Image courtesy Össur, Inc.)

with the ground at the beginning of support and released during the transition to swing. In contrast to prosthetic knee joints, prosthetic ankles and feet typically do not incorporate the large ranges of motion exhibited by their intact counterparts. Instead, these devices often use composite structures that store and return energy over relatively small-magnitude deflections. The current state-of-the-art feet, such as the Össur PROPRIO FOOT® and Endolite élan foot, incorporate active dorsiflexion and plantarflexion. Although incapable of significant power output, the active articulate provides improved toe clearance during swing and adaptation to varied terrains. Figure 42.8 shows a representative sample of commercially available prosthetic feet.

Despite significant improvements that have been achieved with the development of the microprocessor-controlled knees and energy-storage ankles and feet, the fundamentally passive nature of the devices has not been altered. Although capable of damping modulation and energy storage, these devices remain unable to provide net-positive power outputs. As such, the current passive transtibial and transfemoral prostheses can restore normal limb function only over the extent to which normal limb function remains energetically conservative or dissipative. Passive artificial legs perform adequately for walking on level ground, ascent/descent of low-grade slopes, and descent of stairs. Owing to the largely passive nature of

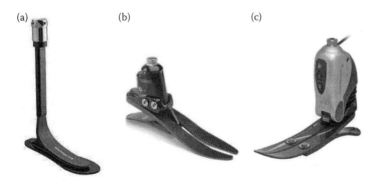

FIGURE 42.8 Prosthetic feet: (a) 1E50/1E51 Advantage DP2 foot (Otto Bock Healthcare, Duderstadt, Germany), (b) Endolite echelon foot (Image courtesy Endolite, USA), and (c) PROPRIO FOOT® (Image courtesy Össur, Inc.).

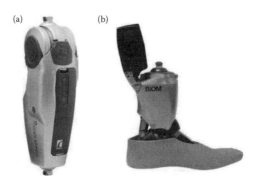

FIGURE 42.9 (a) The Össur POWER KNEE™ (Image courtesy Össur, Inc., Ossur, Reykjavik, Iceland) and (b) the BiOM Ankle System (Image courtesy of BiOM).

intact-limb biomechanics during these functions, a passive prosthetic leg provides much of the required functionality. However, the absence of net-positive power output prevents their use, in a biomechanically natural way, for limb functions that require significant mechanical output power (e.g., ascent of moderate grade slopes, ascent of stairs, and standing from a sitting position).

The emergence of prosthetic legs with externally powered ankle and/or knee joints offers the potential for expanding artificial leg functionality to realize these net-positive power outputs and more fully restore a user's locomotive capacity. A number of transtibial prostheses (Au et al., 2009; Hitt et al., 2010) and transfemoral prostheses (Popovic et al., 1991; Sup et al., 2009) that incorporate battery-powered, motor-actuated joints are in advanced stages of development. Additionally, there are two powered prosthetic legs with limited commercial availability: the Össur POWER KNEE™ of Figure 42.9a and the BiOM Ankle System of Figure 42.9b. In contrast to the difficulties faced in the command and control interface of anthropomorphic arms, the decreased number of degrees of freedom in prosthetic legs and the reciprocal nature of leg function during locomotion enable biomechanically natural gaits to be obtained without needing a direct interface to the user's neuromuscular system. Instead of using myoelectric commands from the user's residual limb, many of the externally powered lower extremity devices are controlled based on the intent of the user as inferred from contralateral limb dynamics, mechanical interaction at the socket interface, and/or mechanical interaction between the limb and ground. Although myoelectric control in lower extremity prosthetics is a research area of current interest, much of a powered limb's functional capability can be exploited without such a direct interface between the limb and amputee.

42.3 Summary

The field of prosthetics continues to be an area of active research and development, combining clinical and engineering technologies to address the restoration of limb function lost because of amputation. As is evident from the preceding discussion, effective solutions span the technological spectrum from relatively low-level to advanced technologies. Although the state of the art in prosthetic limbs is evolving toward anthropomorphic designs with outputs commensurate with the natural biomechanics of intact limbs, there continues to be various technical challenges that limit the practical ability of such anthropomorphic designs in fully restoring the lost functionality of the amputated limb. Limb functionality, the resulting weight, and its ease of use are the important design considerations when choosing among the variety of prosthetic components. The clinical skills of the prosthetist continue to be critical to the selection and implementation of a prosthetic solution that addresses the functional requirements of the user under a control architecture that the user can effectively exploit.

References

Au, S. K., Weber, J., and Herr, H. 2009. Powered ankle–foot prosthesis improves walking metabolic economy. *IEEE Transactions on Robotics*, 25(1), 51–66.

Burrows, C. R., Martin, D. J., and Ring, N. D. 1972. Investigation into the dynamics and control of a pneumatically powered artificial elbow. *International Journal of Control*, 15(2), 337–352.

Hagberg, K. and Branemark, R. 2009. One hundred patients treated with osseointegrated transfemoral amputation prostheses—Rehabilitation perspective. *Journal of Rehabilitation Research and Development*, 46(3), 331–344.

Hitt, J. K., Sugar, T. G., Holgate, M. H., and Bellman, R. 2010. An active foot–ankle prosthesis with biomechanical energy regeneration. *ASME Journal of Medical Devices*, 4(1), 011003.

Huang, H., Zhou, P., Li, G., and Kuiken, T. A. 2008. An analysis of EMG electrode configuration for targeted muscle reinnervation based neural machine interface. *IEEE Transactions on Neural Systems and Rehabilitation Engineering*, 16(1), 37–45.

Jacobsen, S. C., Knutti, D. F., Johnson, R. T., and Sears, H. H. 1982. Development of the Utah arm. *IEEE Transactions on Biomedical Engineering*, 29(3), 249–269.

Kuiken, T. A., Dumanian, G. A., Lipschutz, R. D., Miller, L. A., and Stubblefield, K. A. 2004. The use of targeted muscle reinnervation for improved myoelectric prosthesis control in a bilateral shoulder disarticulation amputee. *Prosthetics Orthotics International*, 28, 245–253.

Mann, R. W. and Reimers, S. D. 1970. Kinesthetic sensing for the EMG controlled "Boston Arm." *IEEE Transactions on Man-Machine Systems*, 11(1), 110–115.

Marquardt, E. 1965. The Heidelberg pneumatic arm prosthesis. *Journal of Bone and Joint Surgery*, 47 B(3), 425–434.

Popovic, D. B., Tomovic, R., Schwirtlich, L., and Tepavac, D. 1991. Control aspects of an active above-knee prosthesis. *International Journal of Man-Machine Studies*, 35, 751–767.

Sup, F., Varol, H. A., Mitchell, J., Withrow, T. J., and Goldfarb, M. 2009. Preliminary evaluations of a self-contained anthropomorphic transfemoral prosthesis. *IEEE/ASME Transactions on Mechatronics*, 14(6), 667–676.

Further Information

International Society for Prosthetics and Orthotics (ISPO), 22–24 Rue du Luxembourg, B-1000 Brussels, Belgium [http://ispoint.org/].

American Academy of Orthotists & Prosthetists, 1331 H Street NW, Suite 501, Washington, DC 20005 [http://www.oandp.org/].

U.S. Department of Veterans Affairs, Rehabilitation Research and Development Service, 810 Vermont Avenue NW, Washington, DC 20420 [http://www.rehab.research.va.gov/].

The Open Prosthetics Project, 107 N. Church Street, Durham, NC 27701 [http://openprosthetics.org/].

43

Rehabilitation Engineering, Science, and Technology

Charles J. Robinson
Clarkson University

43.1 Introduction

Rehabilitation engineering requires a multidisciplinary effort. To put rehabilitation engineering into its proper context, we need to review some of the other disciplines with which rehabilitation engineers must be familiar. Robinson (1993) has reviewed or put forth the following working definitions and discussions:

Rehabilitation is the (re)integration of an individual with a disability into society. This can be done either by enhancing existing capabilities or by providing alternative means to perform various functions or to substitute for specific sensations.

Rehabilitation engineering is the "application of science and technology to ameliorate the handicaps of individuals with disabilities" (Reswick, 1982). In actual practice, many individuals who say that they practice "rehabilitation engineering" are not engineers by training. While this leads to controversies from practitioners with traditional engineering degrees, it also has the de facto benefit of greatly widening the scope of what is encompassed by the term "rehabilitation engineering."

Rehabilitation medicine is a clinical practice that focuses on the physical aspects of functional recovery, but that also considers medical, neurological, and psychological factors. Physical therapy, occupational therapy, and rehabilitation counseling are professions in their own right. On the sensory–motor side, other medical and therapeutical specialties practice rehabilitation in vision, audition, and speech.

Rehabilitation technology (or assistive technology) narrowly defined is the selection, design, or manufacture of augmentative or assistive devices that are appropriate for the individual with a disability. Such devices are selected based on the specific disability, the function to be augmented or restored, the user's wishes, the clinician's preferences, cost, and the environment in which the device will be used.

Rehabilitation science is the development of a body of knowledge, gleaned from rigorous basic and clinical research, which describes how a disability alters specific physiological functions or anatomical structures, and that details the underlying principles by which residual function or capacity can be measured and used to restore function of individuals with disabilities.

43.2 Rehabilitation Concepts

Effective rehabilitation engineers must be well versed in all the areas described above since they generally work in a team setting, in collaboration with physical and occupational therapists, orthopedic surgeons, physical medicine specialists, and/or neurologists. Some rehabilitation engineers are interested in certain activities that we do in the course of a normal day that could be summarized as *activities of daily living* (ADL). These include eating, toileting, combing hair, brushing teeth, reading, and so on. Other engineers focus on *mobility* and the limitations to mobility. Mobility can be personal (e.g., within a home or office) or public (automobile, public transportation, and accessibility questions in buildings). Mobility also includes the ability to move functionally through the environment. Thus, the question of mobility is not limited to that of getting from place to place, but also includes such questions as whether one can reach an object in a particular setting or whether a paralyzed urinary bladder can be made functional again. Barriers that limit mobility are also studied. For instance, an ill-fitted wheelchair cushion or support system will most assuredly limit mobility by reducing the time that an individual can spend on a wheelchair before he or she must vacate it to avoid serious and difficult-to-heal pressure sores. Other groups of rehabilitation engineers deal with *sensory disabilities*, such as sight or hearing, or with *communications disorders*, both in the production side (e.g., the nonvocal) or in the comprehension side. For any given client, a rehabilitation engineer might have all these concerns to consider (i.e., ADLs, mobility, sensory, and communication dysfunctions).

A key concept in physical or sensory rehabilitation is that of *residual function or residual capacity*. Such a concept implies that the function or sense can be quantified, that the performance range of that function or sense is known in a nonimpaired population, and that the use of residual capacity by a disabled individual should be encouraged. These measures of human performance can be made subjectively by clinicians or objectively by some rather clever computerized test devices.

A rehabilitation engineer asks three key questions: Can a diminished function or sense be successfully augmented? Is there a substitute way to return the function or to restore a sense? And is the solution appropriate and cost-effective? These questions give rise to two important rehabilitation concepts: orthotics and prosthetics. An *orthosis* is an appliance that aids an existing function. A *prosthesis* provides a substitute.

An artificial limb is a *prosthesis*, as is a wheelchair. An ankle brace is an *orthosis*. So are eyeglasses. In fact, eyeglasses might well be the penultimate rehabilitation device. They are inexpensive, have little social stigma, and are almost completely unobtrusive to the user. They have let many millions of individuals with correctable vision problems who lead productive lives. But in essence, a pair of eyeglasses is an optical device, governed by traditional equations of physical optics. Eyeglasses can be made out of simple glass (from a raw material as abundant as the sands of the earth!) or complex plastics such as those that are ultraviolet sensitive. They can be ground by hand or by sophisticated computer-controlled optical grinders. Thus, crude technology can restore functional vision. Increasing the technical content of the eyeglasses (either by material or manufacturing method) in most cases will not increase the amount of function restored, but it might make the glasses cheaper, lighter, and more prone to be used.

43.2.1 Engineering Concepts in Sensory Rehabilitation

Of the five traditional senses, vision and hearing mostly define the interactions that permit us to be human. These two senses are the main input channel through which data with high information content can flow. We read, listen to speech or music, and view art. A loss of one or the other of these senses (or both) can have a devastating impact on the individual affected. Rehabilitation engineers attempt to restore the functions of these senses either through augmentation or via sensory substitution systems. Eyeglasses and hearing aids are examples of augmentative devices that can be used if some residual capacity remains. A major area of rehabilitation engineering research deals with *sensory substitution systems*.

The visual system has the capability to detect a single photon of light, yet also has a dynamic range that can respond to intensities many orders of magnitude greater. It can work with high contrast items and with those of almost no contrast, and across the visible spectrum of colors. Millions of parallel data channels form the optic nerve that comes from an eye; each channel transmits an asynchronous and quasi-random (in time) stream of binary pulses. While the temporal coding on any one of these channels is not fast (on the order of 200 bits/s or less), the capacity of the human brain to parallel process the entire image is faster than any supercomputer yet built.

If sight is lost, how can it be replaced? A simple pair of eyeglasses will not work, since the sensor (the retina), the communication channel (the optic nerve and all its relays to the brain), or one or more essential central processors (the occipital part of the cerebral cortex for initial processing; the parietal and other cortical areas for information extraction) have been damaged. For replacement within the system, one must determine where the visual system has failed and whether a stage of the system can be artificially bypassed. If one uses another sensory modality (e.g., touch or hearing) as an alternate input channel, one must determine whether the there is sufficient bandwidth in that channel and whether the higher-order processing hierarchy is plastic enough to process information coming via a different route.

While the above discussion might seem just philosophical, it is more than that. We normally read printed text with our eyes. We recognize words from their (visual) letter combinations. We comprehend what we read via a mysterious processing in the parietal and temporal parts of the cerebral cortex. Could we perhaps read and comprehend this chapter or other forms of writing through our fingertips with an appropriate interface? The answer surprisingly is yes! And, the adaptation actually goes back to one of the earliest applications of coding theory—that of the development of Braille. Braille condenses all text characters to a raised matrix of 2×3 dots (26 combinations), with certain combinations reserved as indicators for the next character (such as a number indicator) or for special contractions. Trained readers of Braille can read over 250 words per minute of grade 2 Braille (as fast as most sighted readers can read printed text!). Thus, the Braille code is in essence a rehabilitation engineering concept where an alternate sensory channel is used as a substitute and where a recoding scheme has been employed.

Rehabilitation engineers and their colleagues have designed other ways to read the text. To replace the retina as a sensor element, a modern high-resolution, high-sensitivity, fast imaging sensor (CCD, etc.) is employed to capture a visual image of the text. One method, used by various page-scanning devices, converts the scanned image to text by using optical character-recognition schemes and then outputs the text as speech via text-to-speech algorithms. This machine essentially recites the text, much as a sighted helper might do when reading aloud to the blind individual. The user of the device is thus freed of the absolute need for a helper. Such *independence* is often the goal of rehabilitation.

Perhaps, the most interesting method presents an image of the scanned data directly to the visual cortex or retina via an array of implantable electrodes that are used to electrically activate nearby cortical or retinal structures. The visual cortex and retina are laid out in a topographic fashion such that there is an orderly mapping of the signal from different parts of the visual field to the retina, and from the retina to corresponding parts of the occipital cortex. The goal of stimulation is to mimic the neural activity that would have been evoked had the signal come through normal channels. And, such stimulation does produce the sensation of light. Since the "image" stays within the visual system, the rehabilitation solution is said to be *modality specific*. However, substantial problems dealing with biocompatibility, image processing, and reduction remain in the design of the electrode arrays and processors that serve to interface the electronics and neurological tissue.

Deafness is another manifestation of a loss of a communication channel, this time for the sense of hearing. Totally deaf individuals use vision as a substitute input channel when communicating via sign language (also a substitute code) and can sign at information rates that match or exceed that of verbal communication. Hearing aids are now commercially available that can adaptively filter out background noise (a predictable signal) while amplifying speech (unpredictable) using autoregressive, moving average (ARMA) signal processing. With the recent advent of powerful digital signal processing chips, true digital hearing aids are now available. The previous analog aids or digitally programmable analog aids provided a set of tunable filters and amplifiers to cover the low-, mid-, and high-frequency ranges of the hearing spectrum. But the digital aids can be specifically and easily tailored (i.e., programmed) to compensate for the specific losses of each individual client across the frequency continuum of hearing, and still provide automatic gain control and one or more user-selectable settings that have been adjusted to perform optimally in differing noise environments.

An exciting development is occurring outside the field of rehabilitation that will have a profound impact on the ability of the deaf to comprehend speech. Electronics companies are now marketing universal translation aids for travelers, where a phrase spoken in one language is captured, parsed, translated, and restated (either spoken or displayed) in another language. The deaf would simply require that the visual display must be in the language that they use for writing.

Deafness is often brought on (or occurs congenitally) by damage to the cochlea. The cochlea normally transduces variations in sound pressure intensity at a given frequency into patterns of neural discharge. This neural code is then carried by the auditory (eighth cranial) nerve to the brain stem where it is preprocessed and relayed to the auditory cortex for initial processing and onto the parietal and other cortical areas for information extraction. Similar to the case for the visual system, the cochlea, auditory nerve, auditory cortex, and all relays in between maintain a topological map, this time based on tone frequency (tonotopic). If deafness is solely due to cochlear damage (as is often the case) and if the auditory nerve is still intact, a cochlear implant can often be substituted for the regular transducer array (the cochlea) while still sending the signal through the normal auditory channel (to maintain modality–specificity).

At first glance, the design of a cochlear prosthesis to restore hearing appears daunting. The hearing range of a healthy young individual is 20–16,000 Hz. The transducing structure, the cochlea, has 3500 inner and 12,000 outer hair cells, each best activated by a specific frequency that causes a localized mechanical resonance in the basilar membrane of the cochlea. Deflection of a hair cell causes the cell to fire an all-or-none (i.e., pulsatile) neuronal discharge, whose rate of repetition depends to a first approximation on the amplitude of the stimulus. The outputs of these hair cells have an orderly convergence on the 30,000–40,000 fibers that make up the auditory portion of the eighth cranial nerve. These afferent fibers in turn go to brain stem neurons that process and relay the signals onto higher brain centers (Klinke, 1983). For many causes of deafness, the hair cells are destroyed, but the eighth nerve remains intact. Thus, if one could elicit activity in a specific output fiber by means other than the hair cell motion, perhaps some sense of hearing could be restored. The geometry of the cochlea helps in this regard as different portions of the nerve are closer to different parts of the cochlea.

Electrical stimulation is now used in the cochlear implant to bypass hair cell transduction mechanisms (Loeb, 1985; Clark et al., 1990). These sophisticated devices have required that complex signal processing, electronic, and packaging problems must be solved. One current cochlear implant has 22 stimulus sites along the scala tympani of the cochlea. Those sites provide excitation to the peripheral processes of the cells of the eighth cranial nerve, which are splayed out along the length of the scala. The electrode assembly itself has 22 ring electrodes spaced along its length and some additional guard rings between the active electrodes and the receiver to aid in securing the very flexible electrode assembly after it is snaked into the cochlea's very small (a few mm) round window (a surgeon related to me that positioning the electrode was akin to pushing a piece of cooked spaghetti through a small hole at the end of a long tunnel). The electrode is attached to a receiver that is inlaid into a slot milled out of the temporal bone. The receiver contains circuitry that can select any electrode ring to be a source and any other electrode to be a sink for the stimulating current, and that can rapidly sequence between various pairs of electrodes. The receiver is powered and controlled by a radio-frequency link with an external transmitter, whose alignment is maintained by means of a permanent magnet imbedded in the receiver.

A digital signal processor stores information about a specific user and his or her optimal electrode locations for specific frequency bands. The objective is to determine what pair of electrodes best produces the subjective perception of a certain pitch *in the implanted individual himself or herself,* and then to associate a particular filter with that pair via the controller. An enormous amount of compression occurs in taking the frequency range necessary for speech comprehension and reducing it to a few discrete channels. Much fundamental research is being carried out in speech processing, compression, and recognition. But, what is amazing is that a number of totally deaf individuals can relearn to comprehend speech exceptionally well without speech–reading through the use of these implants. Other individuals find that the implant aids in speech–reading. For some, only an awareness of environmental sounds is apparent; and for another group, the implant appears to have had little effect. But, if you could (as I have been able to) finally converse in unaided speech with an individual who had been rendered totally blind and deaf by a traumatic brain injury, you begin to appreciate the power of rehabilitation engineering.

43.2.2 Engineering Concepts in Motor Rehabilitation

Limitations in mobility can severely restrict the quality of life of an individual so affected. A wheelchair is a prime example of a prosthesis that can restore personal mobility to those who cannot walk. Given the proper environment (fairly level floors, roads, etc.), modern wheelchairs can be highly efficient. In fact, the fastest times in one of man's greatest tests of endurance, the Boston Marathon, are achieved by the wheelchair racers. Although they do gain the advantage of being able to roll, they still must climb the same hills and do so with only one-fifth of the muscle power available to an able-bodied marathoner.

While a wheelchair user could certainly go down a set of steps (not recommended), climbing steps in a normal, manual, or electric wheelchair is a virtual impossibility. Ramps or lifts are engineered to provide accessibility in these cases or special climbing wheelchairs can be purchased. Wheelchairs also do not work well on surfaces with high rolling resistance or viscous coefficients (e.g., mud, rough terrain, etc.); so, alternate mobility aids must be found if access to these areas is to be provided to the physically disabled. Hand-controlled cars, vans, tractors, and even airplanes are now driven by wheelchair users. The design of appropriate control modifications falls to the rehabilitation engineer.

Loss of a limb can greatly impair functional activity. The engineering aspects of artificial limb design increase in complexity as the amount of residual limb decreases, especially if one or more joints are lost. As an example, a person with a mid-calf amputation could use a simple wooden stump to extend the leg and could ambulate reasonably well. But such a leg is not cosmetically appealing and completely ignores any substitution for ankle function.

Immediately following World War II, the United States government began the first concerted effort to foster better engineering design for artificial limbs. Dynamically lockable knee joints were designed for artificial limbs for above-knee amputees. In the ensuing years, energy-storing artificial ankles have been designed, some with prosthetic feet so realistic that beach thongs could be worn with them! Artificial hands, wrists, and elbows were designed for upper-limb amputees. Careful design of the actuating cable system also provided for a sense of hand-grip force, so that the user had some feedback and did not need to rely on vision alone for guidance.

Perhaps, the most transparent (to the user) artificial arms are the ones that use electrical activity generated by the muscles remaining in the stump to control the actions of the elbow, wrist, and hand (Stein et al., 1988). This electrical activity is known as myoelectricity and is produced as the muscle contraction spreads through the muscle. Note that these muscles, if intact, would have controlled at least one of these joints (e.g., the biceps and triceps for the elbow). Thus, a high level of modality–specificity is maintained since the functional element is substituted only at the last stage. All the batteries, sensor electrodes, amplifiers, motor actuators, and controllers (generally analog) reside entirely within these myoelectric arms. An individual trained in the use of a myoelectric arm can perform some impressive tasks with this arm. Current engineering research efforts involve the control of simultaneous multijoint movements (rather than the single joint movement now available) and the provision for sensory feedback from the end effector of the artificial arm to the skin of the stump via electrical means. A recent Defense Advanced Research Projects Agency Research and Development (DARPA R&D) project is working on developing a true bionic arm, with human-like sensors and actuators for disabled soldiers.

43.2.3　Engineering Concepts in Communications Disorders

Speech is a uniquely human means of interpersonal communication. Problems that affect speech can occur at the initial transducer (the larynx) or at other areas of the vocal tract. They can be of neurological (due to cortical, brain stem, or peripheral nerve damage), structural, and/or cognitive origin. A person might only be able to make a halting attempt by talking or might not have sufficient control of other motor skills to type or write.

If only the larynx is involved, an externally applied artificial larynx can be used to generate a resonant column of air that can be modulated by other elements in the vocal tract. If other motor skills are intact, typing can be used to generate text, which in turn can be spoken via text-to-speech devices described above. And the rate of typing (either whole words or via coding) might be fast enough so that reasonable speech rates could be achieved.

The rehabilitation engineer often becomes involved in the design or specification of *augmentative communication aids* for individuals who do not have good muscle control, either for speech or for limb movement. A whole industry has developed around the design of symbol or letter boards, where the user can point out (often painstakingly) letters, words, or concepts. Some of these boards now have speech output. Linguistics and information theory have been combined in the invention of acceleration techniques intended to speedup the communication process. These include alternative language representation systems based on semantic (iconic), alphanumeric, or other codes; and prediction systems, which provide choices based on previously selected letters or words. A general review of these aids can be found in Hill, Romich, and Vanderheiden's chapter in this section, whereas Goodenough-Trepagnier (1994) edited a good publication dealing with human factors and cognitive requirements.

Some individuals can produce speech, but it is dysarthric and very hard to understand. Yet, the utterance does contain information. Can this limited information be used to figure out what the individual wanted to say, and then voice it by artificial means? Research labs are now employing neural-network theory to determine which pauses in an utterance are due to content (i.e., between a word or sentence) and those due to unwanted halts in speech production.

43.3　Appropriate Technology

Rehabilitation engineering lies at the interface of a wide variety of technical, biological, and other concerns. A user might (and often does) put aside a technically sophisticated rehabilitation device in favor of a simpler device that is cheaper and easier to use and maintain. The cosmetic appearance of the device (or cosmesis) sometimes becomes the overriding factor in acceptance or rejection of a device. A key design factor often lies in the use of the *appropriate technology* to accomplish the task adequately given the extent of the resources available to solve the problem and the residual capacity of the client. Adequacy can be verified by determining that increasing the technical content of the solution results in disproportionately diminishing gains or escalating costs. Thus, a rehabilitation engineer must be able to distinguish applications where high technology is required from those where such technology results in an incremental gain in cost, durability, acceptance, and other factors. Further, appropriateness very much depends on location. What is appropriate to a client near a major medical center in a highly developed country might not be appropriate to one in a rural setting or in a developing country.

This is not to say that rehabilitation engineers should shun advances in technology. In fact, a fair proportion of rehabilitation engineers work in a research setting where state-of-the-art technology is being applied to the needs of the disabled. However, it is often difficult to transfer complex technology from a laboratory to disabled consumers not directly associated with that laboratory. Such devices are often designed for use only in a structured environment, are difficult to repair properly in the field, and often require a high level of user interaction or sophistication.

Technology transfer in the rehabilitation arena is difficult due to the limited and fragmented market. Advances in rehabilitation engineering are often piggybacked onto advances in commercial electronics. For instance, the exciting developments in text-to-speech and speech-to-text devices mentioned above are being driven by the commercial marketplace and not by the rehabilitation arena. But such developments will be welcomed by rehabilitation engineers no less.

43.4 The Future of Engineering in Rehabilitation

The traditional engineering disciplines permeate many aspects of rehabilitation. Signal processing, control and information theory, materials design, and computers are all in widespread use from an electrical engineering perspective. Neural networks, microfabrication, fuzzy logic, virtual reality, image processing, and other emerging electrical and computer engineering tools are increasingly being applied. Mechanical engineering principles are used in biomechanical studies, gait and motion analysis, prosthetic fitting, seat cushion and back-support design, and the design of artificial joints. Materials and metallurgical engineers provide input on newer biocompatible materials. Chemical engineers are developing implantable sensors. Industrial engineers are increasingly studying rehabilitative ergonomics.

The challenge to rehabilitation engineers is to find advances in *any* field, engineering, or otherwise, which will aid their clients who have a disability.

Defining Terms

Activities of daily living (ADL): Personal activities that are done by almost everyone in the course of a normal day including eating, toileting, combing hair, brushing teeth, reading, and so on. ADLs are distinguished from hobbies and from work-related activities (e.g., typing).

Appropriate technology: The technology that will accomplish a task adequately given the resources available. Adequacy can be verified by determining that increasing the technological content of the solution results in diminishing gains or increasing costs.

Disability*: Inability or limitation in performing tasks, activities, and roles to levels expected within physical and social contexts.

Functional limitation*: Restriction or lack of ability to perform an action in the manner or within the range consistent with the purpose of an organ or organ system.

Impairment*: Loss or abnormality of cognitive, emotional, physiological, or anatomical structure or function, including all losses or abnormalities, not just those attributed to the initial pathophysiology.

Modality specific: A task that is specific to a single sense or movement pattern.

Orthosis: A modality-specific appliance that aids the performance of a function or movement by augmenting or assisting the residual capabilities of that function or movement. An orthopedic brace is an orthosis.

Pathophysiology*: Interruption or interference with normal physiological and developmental processes or structures.

Prosthesis: An appliance that substitutes for the loss of a particular function, generally by involving a different modality as an input and/or output channel. An artificial limb, a sensory substitution system, and an augmentative communication aid are prosthetic devices.

---

* This term has been proposed by the National Center for Medical Rehabilitation and Research (NCMRR) of the U.S. National Institutes of Health (NIH).

Residual function or residual capacity: Residual function is a measure of the ability to carry out one of more general tasks using the methods normally used. Residual capacity is a measure of the ability to carry out these tasks using any means of performance. These residual measures are generally more subjective than other more quantifiable measures such as residual strength.

Societal limitation*: Restriction, attributable to social policy or barriers (structural or attitudinal), which limits fulfillment of roles, or denies access to services or opportunities that are associated with full participation in society.

References

Clark, G.M., Y.C. Tong, and J.F. Patrick, 1990. *Cochlear Prostheses,* Churchill Livingstone, Edinburgh.

Goodenough-Trepagnier, C., 1994. Guest editor of a special issue of *Assistive Technology* 6(1) dealing with mental loads in augmentative communication.

Klinke, R., 1983. Physiology of the sense of equilibrium, hearing and speech. Chapter 12 in: *Human Physiology* (eds. R.F. Schmidt and G. Thews), Springer-Verlag, Berlin.

Loeb, G.E., 1985. The functional replacement of the ear, *Scientific American* 252:104–111.

Reswick, J. 1982. What is a rehabilitation engineer? in *Annual Review of Rehabilitation,* Vol. 2 (eds. E.L. Pan, T.E. Backer and C.L. Vash), Springer-Verlag, New York.

Robinson, C.J. 1993. Rehabilitation engineering—An editorial, *IEEE Transactions on Rehabilitation Engineering* 1(1):1–2.

Stein, R.B., D. Charles, and K.B. James, 1988. Providing motor control for the handicapped: A fusion of modern neuroscience, bioengineering, and rehabilitation, in *Advances in Neurology, vol. 47: Functional Recovery in Neurological Disease* (ed. S.G. Waxman), Raven Press, New York.

Further Information

The readers interested in rehabilitation engineering can contact RESNA—an interdisciplinary association for the advancement of rehabilitation and assistive technologies, 1101 Connecticut Ave., N.W., Suite 700, Washington, DC 20036. RESNA publishes a quarterly journal called *"Assistive Technology."*

The United States Department of Veterans Affairs puts out a quarterly *"Journal of Rehabilitation R&D."* The January issue of each year contains an overview of most of the rehabilitation engineering efforts occurring in the United States and Canada, with over 500 listings.

The IEEE Engineering in Medicine and Biology Society publishes the *"IEEE Transactions on Neural Systems and Rehabilitation Engineering,"* a quarterly journal. The reader should contact the IEEE at PO Box 1331, 445 Hoes Lane, Piscataway, NJ 08855-1331, USA for further details.

44

Orthopedic Prosthetics and Orthotics in Rehabilitation

Marilyn Lord
King's College Hospital,
London

Alan Turner-Smith
King's College Hospital,
London

An *orthopedic prosthesis* is an internal or external device that *replaces* lost parts or functions of the *neuroskeletomotor system*. In contrast, an *orthopedic orthosis* is a device that *augments* a function of the skeletomotor system by controlling motion or altering the shape of body tissue. For example, an artificial leg or hand is a prosthesis, whereas a caliper (or brace) is an orthosis. This chapter addresses only orthoses and external orthopedic prostheses; internal orthopedic prostheses, such as artificial joints, are a subject on their own.

When a human limb is lost through disease or trauma, the integrity of the body is compromised in so many ways that an engineer may well feel daunted by the design requirements for a prosthetic replacement. Consider the losses from a lower limb amputation. Gone is the structural support for the upper body in standing, along with the complex joint articulations and muscular motor system involved in walking. Also lost is the multimode sensory feedback, from *inter alia* pressure sensors on the sole of the foot, length and force sensors in the muscles, and position sensors in the joints, which closed the control loop around the skeletomotor system. The body also has lost a significant percentage of its weight and is now asymmetrical and unbalanced.

We must first ask if it is desirable to attempt to replace all these losses with like-for-like components. If so, we need to strive to make a bionic limb of similar weight embodying anthropomorphic articulations with equally powerful motors and distributed sensors connected back into the wearer's residual neuromuscular system. Or, is it better to accept the losses and redefine the optimal functioning of the new unit of person-plus-technology? In many cases, it may be concluded that a wheelchair is the optimal solution for lower limb loss. Even if engineering could provide the bionic solution, which it certainly cannot at present despite huge inroads made into aspects of these demands, there remain additional problems inherent to prosthetic replacements to consider. Of these, the unnatural mechanical interface between the external environment and the human body is one of the most difficult. Notably, in place of weight bearing through the structures of the foot that are well adapted for this purpose, load must now be transferred to the skeletal structures via intimate contact between the surface of residual limb and prosthesis; the exact distribution of load becomes critical. To circumvent these problems, an alternative direct **transcutaneous** fixation to the bone has been attempted in limited experimental trials, but this brings its own problems of materials **biocompatability** and prevention of infection ingress around the opening through the skin. Orthotic devices are classified by acronyms that describe the joint which they cross. Thus an AFO is an ankle–foot orthosis, a CO is a cervical orthosis (neck brace or collar), and a TLSO is a thoracolumbosacral orthosis (spinal brace or jacket). The main categories are braces for the cervix (neck), upper limb, trunk, lower limb, and foot. Orthoses are generally simpler devices than prostheses, but because orthoses are constrained by the existing body shape and function, they can present an equally demanding design challenge. Certainly the interaction with body function is more critical, and successful application demands an in-depth appreciation of both residual function and the probable reaction to external interference. External orthotics are often classified as structural or functional, the former implying a static nature to hold an unstable joint and the latter a flexible or articulated system to promote the correct alignment of the joints during dynamic functioning. An alternative orthotic approach utilizes functional electrical stimulation (FES) of the patient's own muscles to generate appropriate forces for joint motion; this is dealt with in Chapter 45.

44.1 Fundamentals

Designers of orthotic and prosthetic devices are aware of the three cardinal considerations—function, structure, and *cosmesis*.

For requirements of function, we must be very clear about the objectives of treatment. This requires first an understanding of the clinical condition. *Functional prescription* is now a preferred route for the medical practitioner to specify the requirements, leaving the implementation of this instruction to the prosthetist, orthotist, or rehabilitation technologist. The benefits of this distinction between client specification and final hardware will be obvious to design engineers. Indeed, the influence of design procedures on the supply process is a contribution from engineering that is being appreciated more and more.

The second requirement for function is the knowledge of the biomechanics that underlies both the dysfunction in the patient and the function of proposed device to be coupled to the patient. Kinematics, dynamics, energy considerations, and control all enter into this understanding of function. Structure is the means of carrying the function, and finally both need to be embodied into a design that is cosmetically acceptable. Some of the fundamental issues in these concepts are discussed here.

To function well, the device needs an effective coupling to the human body. To this end, there is often some part that is molded to the contours of the wearer. Achieving a satisfactory mechanical interface of a molded component depends primarily on the shape. The internal dimensions of such components are not made by an exact match to the external dimensions of the limb segment, but by a process of *rectification*, the shape is adjusted to relieve areas of skin with low load tolerance. The shapes are also evolved to achieve appropriate load distribution for stability of coupling between prosthetic socket and limb or, in orthotic design, a system of usually three forces that generates a moment to stabilize a collapsing joint (Figure 44.1). Alignment is a second factor influencing the interface loading. For lower limb prostheses particularly, the alignment of the molded socket to the remainder of the structural components also will be critical in determining the moments and forces transmitted to the interface when the foot is flat on the ground. The same is true for lower limb orthoses, where the net action of the ground reaction forces and consequent moments around the natural joints are highly dependent on the alignment taken up by the combination of orthosis and shoe. Adjustability may be important, particularly for children or progressive medical conditions. Functional components that enable desirable motions are largely straightforward engineering mechanisms such as hinges or dampers, although the specific

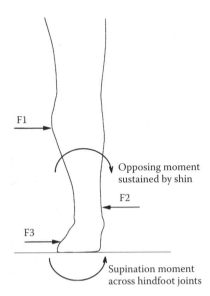

F1

Opposing moment
sustained by shin

F2

F3

Supination moment
across hindfoot joints

FIGURE 44.1 Three-force system required in an orthosis to control a valgus hindfoot due to weakness in the hindfoot supinators.

design requirements for their dynamic performance may be quite complex because of the biomechanics of the body. An example of the design of knee joints is expanded below. These motions may be driven from external power sources but more often are passive or body-powered mechanisms. In orthoses where relatively small angular motions are needed, these may be provided by material flexibility rather than mechanisms.

The structural requirements for lower limb prosthetics have been laid down at a consensus meeting (1978) bases on biomechanical measurement of forces in a gait laboratory, referred to as the *Philadelphia standards* and soon to be incorporated into an ISO standard (ISO 13404,5; ISO 10328). Not only are the load level and life critical, but also is the mode of failure. Sudden failure of an ankle bolt resulting in disengagement of an artificial foot is not only potentially life threatening to an elderly amputee who falls and breaks a hip but also can be quite traumatic to unsuspecting witnesses of the apparent event of autoamputation. Design and choice of materials should ensure a controlled slow yielding, not brittle fracture. A further consideration is the ability of the complete structure to absorb shock loading, either the repeated small shocks of walking at the heel strike or rather more major shocks during sports activities or falls. This minimizes the shock transmitted through the skin to the skeleton, known to cause both skin lesions and joint degeneration. Finally, the consideration of hygiene must not be overlooked; the user must be able to clean the orthosis or prosthesis adequately without compromising its structure or function.

Added to the two elements of structure and function, the third element of *cosmesis* completes the trilogy. Appearance can be of great psychological importance to the user, and technology has its contribution here, too. As examples, special effects familiar in science fiction films also can be harnessed to provide realistic cosmetic covers for hand or foot prostheses. Borrowing from advanced manufacturing technology, optical shape scanning linked to three-dimensional (3D) computer-aided design, and *CNC machining* can be pressed into service to generate customized shapes to match a contralateral remaining limb. Up-to-date materials and component design each contribute to minimize the "orthopedic appliance" image of the devices (Figure 44.2). In providing cosmesis, the views of the user must remain paramount. The wearer will often choose an attractive functional design in preference to a life-like design that is not felt to be part of his or her body.

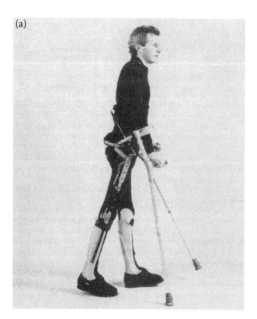
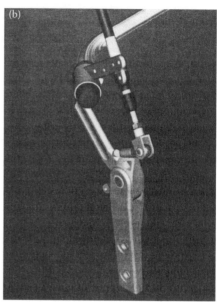

FIGURE 44.2   The ARGO reciprocating-gait orthosis, normally worn under the clothing, with structural components produced from 3D CAD. (Courtesy of Hugh Steeper, Ltd., UK.)

Upper limb prostheses are often seen as a more interesting engineering challenge than lower limb, offering the possibilities for active motor/control systems and complex articulations. However, the market is an order of magnitude smaller and cost/benefit less easy to prove—after all, it is possible to function fairly well with one arm, but try walking with one leg. At the simplest end, an arm for a below-elbow amputee might comprise a socket with a terminal device offering a pincer grip (hand or hook) that can be operated through a Bowden cable by shrugging the shoulders. Such body-powered prostheses may appear crude, but they are often favored by the wearer because of a sense of position and force feedback from the cable, and they do not need a power supply. Another, more elegant method of harnessing body power is to take a muscle-made redundant by an amputation and tether its tendon through an artificially fashioned loop of skin: the cable can then be hooked through the loop (Childress, 1989).

Externally powered devices have been attempted using various power sources with degrees of success. Pneumatic power in the form of a gas cylinder is cheap and light, but recharging is a problem that exercised the ingenuity of early suppliers: where supplies were not readily available, even schemes to involve the local fire services with recharging were costed. Also, contemplate the prospect of bringing a loaded table fork toward your face carried on the end of a position-controlled arm powered with spongy, low-pressure pneumatic actuators, and you will appreciate another aspect of difficulties with this source. Nevertheless, gas-powered grip on a hand can be a good solution. Early skirmishes with stiffer hydraulic servos were largely unsuccessful because of power supply and actuator weight and oil leakage. Electric actuation, heavy and slow at first, has gradually improved to establish its premier position. Input control to these powered devices can be from surface electromyography or by mechanical movement of, for example, the shoulder or an ectromelic limb. Feedback can be presented as skin pressure, movement of a sensor over the skin, or electric stimulation. Control strategies range from position control around a single joint or group of related joints through combined position and force control for hand grip to computer-assisted coordination of entire activities such as feeding.

The physical designs in prosthetic and orthotic devices have changed substantially over the past decade. One could propose that this is solely the introduction of new materials. The sockets of artificial limbs have always been fashioned to suit the individual patient, historically by carving wood, shaping

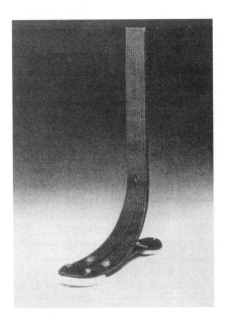

FIGURE 44.3   Flex foot.

leather, or beating sheet metal. Following the introduction of thermosetting fiber-reinforced plastics hand shaped over a plaster cast of the limb residuum, substitution of thermoforming plastics that could be automatically vacuum formed made a leap forward to give light, rapidly made, and cosmetically improved solutions. Polypropylene is the favored material in this application. The same materials permitted the new concept of custom-molded orthoses. Carbon fiber composites substituted for metal have certainly improved the performance of structural components such as limb shanks. But some of the progress owes much to innovative thinking. The flex foot is a fine example, where a traditional anthropomorphic design with imitation of ankle joint and metatarsal break is completely abandoned and a functional design is adopted to optimize energy storage and return. This is based on two leaf springs made from Kevlar, joined together at the ankle with one splaying down toward the toes to form the forefoot spring and the other rearward to form the heel spring (Figure 44.3). Apart from the gains for the disabled athletes for whom the foot was designed—and these are so remarkable that there is little point in competing now without this foot—clients across all age groups have benefited from the adaptability to rough ground and shock-absorption capability.

44.2 Applications

44.2.1 Computer-Aided Engineering in Customized Component Design

Computer-aided engineering has found a fertile ground for exploitation in the process of design of customized components to match to body shape. A good example is in sockets for artificial limbs. What prosthetists particularly seek is the ability to produce a well-fitting socket during the course of a single-patient consultation. Traditional craft methods of casting the residual limb in plaster of Paris, pouring a positive mold, manual rectification, and then socket fabrication over the *rectified* cast takes too long.

By using advanced technology, residual limb shapes can be captured in a computer, rectified by computer algorithms, and CNC machined to produce the rectified cast within an hour so that with the addition of vacuum-formed machinery to pull a socket rapidly over the cast, the socket can be ready for trial fitting in one session. There are added advantages too, in that the shape is now stored in digital form in the computer and can be reproduced or adjusted whenever and wherever desired. Although such systems are still in an early stage of introduction, many practicing prosthetists in the United States have now had hands-on experience of this technology, and a major evaluation by the Veterans Administration has been undertaken (Houston et al., 1992).

Initially, much of the engineering development work went into the hardware components, a difficult brief in view of the low-cost target for a custom product. Requirements are considerably different from those of standard engineering, for example, relaxation in the accuracies required (millimeters, not microns); a need to measure limb or trunk parts that are encumbered by the attached body, which may resist being oriented conveniently in a machine and which will certainly distort with the lightest pressure; and a need to reproduce fairly bulky items with strength to be used as a sacrificial mold. Instrumentation for body shape scanning has been developed using methods of silhouettes, Moiré fringes, contact probes measuring contours of plaster casts, and light triangulation. Almost universally the molds are turned by "milling on a spit" (Duncan and Mair, 1983), using an adapted lathe with a milling head to spiral down a large cylindrical plug of material such as plaster of paris mix. Rehabilitation engineers watch with great interest, some with envy, the developments in rapid prototyping manufacture, which is so successful in reducing the cycle time for one-off developments elsewhere in industry, but alas the costs of techniques such as stereolithography are as yet beyond economic feasibility for our area.

Much emphasis also has been placed on the graphics and algorithms needed to achieve rectification. Opinions vary as to what extent the computer should simply provide a more elegant tool for the prosthetist to exercise his or her traditional skills using 3D modeling and on-screen sculpting as a direct replacement for manual plaster rectification or to what extent the computer system should take over the bulk of the process by an expert systems approach. Systems currently available tend to do a little of each. A series of rectification maps can be held as templates, each storing the appropriate relief or buildup to be applied over a particular anatomic area of the limb. Thus the map might provide for a ridge to be added down the front of the shin of a lower limb model so that the eventual socket will not press against the vulnerable bony prominence of the tibia (Figure 44.4). Positioning of the discrete regions to match individual anatomy might typically be anchored to one or more anatomic features indicated by the prosthetist. The prosthetist is also able to free-form sculpt a particular region by pulling the surface interactively with reference to graphic representation (Figure 44.5); this is particularly useful where the patient has some unusual feature not provided for in the templates.

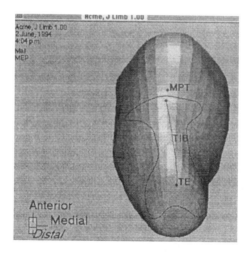

FIGURE 44.4   Rectification requirement defined over the tibia of lower limb stump using the Shapemaker application for computer-aided socket design.

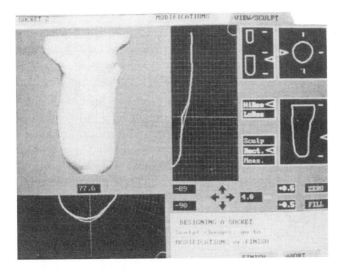

FIGURE 44.5 Adjusting a socket contour with reference to 3D graphics and cross-sectional profiles in the UCL CASD system. (Reproduced from Reynolds, D.P. and Lord, M. 1992. *Med. Biol. Eng. Comput.* 30: 419. With permission.)

As part of this general development, finite-element analysis has been employed to model the soft-tissue distortion occurring during limb loading and to look at the influence of severity of rectification in the resultant distribution of interface stress (Reynolds and Lord, 1992) (Figure 44.6). In engineering terms, this modeling is somewhat unusual and decidedly nonlinear. For a start, the tissues are highly deformable but nearly incompressible, which raises problems of a suitable Poisson ratio to apply in the modeling. Values of $n = 0.3$–$n = 0.49$ have been proposed, based on experimental matching of stress–strain curves from indentation of limb tissue *in vivo*. In reality, though, compression (defined as a loss of volume) may be noted in a limb segment under localized external pressure due to loss of mass as first the

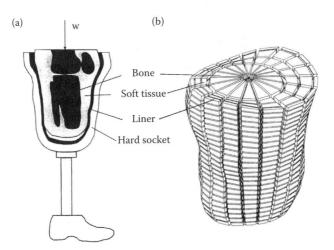

FIGURE 44.6 Finite-element analysis employed to determine the sensitivity of interface pressure to socket-shaped rectification: (a) limb and socket; (b) elements in layers representing idealized geometry of bone, soft tissue, and socket liner; (c) rectification map of radial differences between the external free shape of the limb and the internal dimensions of socket; and (d) FE predictions of direct pressure. (Courtesy of Zhang Ming, King's College, London.)

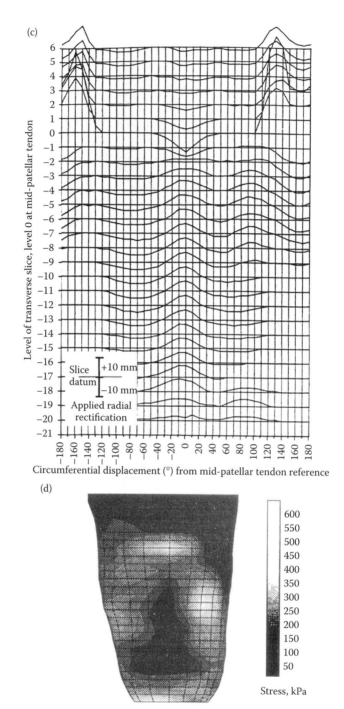

FIGURE 44.6 (continued) Finite-element analysis employed to determine the sensitivity of interface pressure to socket-shaped rectification: (a) limb and socket; (b) elements in layers representing idealized geometry of bone, soft tissue, and socket liner; (c) rectification map of radial differences between the external free shape of the limb and the internal dimensions of socket; and (d) FE predictions of direct pressure. (Courtesy of Zhang Ming, King's College, London.)

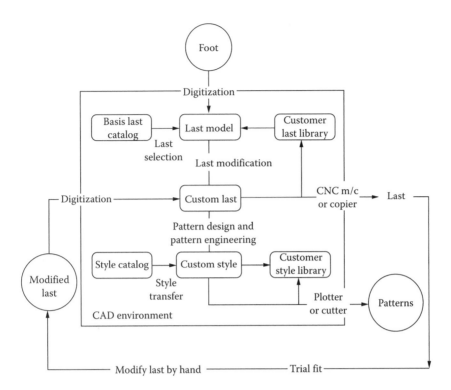

FIGURE 44.7   Schematic of operation of the Shoemaster shoe design system based on selection of a basis last from a database of model lasts. A database of styles is also employed to generate the upper patterns.

blood is rapidly evacuated and then interstitial fluids are more slowly squeezed out. Also, it is difficult to define the boundaries of the limb segment at the proximal end, still attached to the body, where soft tissues can easily bulge up and out. This makes accurate experimental determination of the stress–strain curves for the tissue matrix difficult. A nonlinear model with interface elements allowing slip to occur between skin and socket at the limit of static friction may need to be considered, since the frictional conditions at the interface will determine the balance between shear and direct stresses in supporting body weight against the sloping sidewalls. Although excessive shear at the skin surface is considered particularly damaging, higher pressures would be required in its complete absence.

In a similar vein, computer-aided design (CAD) techniques are also finding application in the design of bespoke orthopedic footwear, using CAD techniques from the volume fashion trade modified to suit the one-off nature of bespoke work. This again requires the generation of a customized mold, or shoe last, for each foot, in addition to the design of patterns for the shoe uppers (Lord et al., 1991). The philosophy of design of shoe lasts is quite different from that of sockets, because last shapes have considerable and fundamental differences from foot shapes. In this instance, a library of reference last shapes is held, and a suitable one is selected both to match the client's foot shape and to fulfill the shoemaking needs for the particular style and type of shoe. The schematic of the process followed in development of the Shoemaster system is shown in Figure 44.7.

Design of shoe inserts is another related application, with systems to capture, manipulate, and reproduce underfoot contours now in commercial use. An example is the Ampfit system, where the foot is placed on a platform to which preshaped arch supports or other wedges or domes may first be attached. A matrix of round-ended cylinders is then forced up by gas pressure through both platform and supports, supporting the foot over most of the area with an even-load distribution. The shape is captured from the cylinder locations and fed into a computer, where rectification can be made similar to that described for prosthetic sockets. A benchtop CNC machine then routs the shoe inserts from specially provided blanks while the client waits.

44.2.2 Examples of Innovative Component Design

44.2.2.1 Intelligent Prosthetic Knee

The control of an artificial lower limb turns out to be most problematic during the swing phase, during which the foot is lifted off the ground to be guided into contact ahead of the walker. A prosthetic lower limb needs to be significantly lighter than its normal counterpart because the muscular power is not present to control it. Two technological advances have helped. First, carbon fiber construction has reduced the mass of the lower limb, and second, pneumatic or hydraulically controlled damping mechanisms for the knee joint have enabled adjustment of the swing phase to suit an individual's pattern of walking.

Swing-phase control of the knee should operate in three areas:

1. Resistance to flexion at late stance during toe-off controls any tendency to excessive heel rise at early swing.
2. Assistance to extension after midswing ensures that the limb is fully extended and ready for heel strike.
3. Resistance before a terminal impact at the end of the extension swing dampens out the inertial forces to allow a smooth transition from flexed to extended knee position.

In conventional limbs, parameters of these controls are determined by fixed components (springs, bleed valves) that are set to optimum for an individual's normal gait at one particular speed, for example, the pneumatic controller in Figure 44.8. If the amputee subsequently walks more slowly, the limb will tend to lead, while if the amputee walks more quickly, the limb will tend to fall behind; the usual compensatory actions are, respectively, an unnatural tilting of the pelvis to delay heel contact or abnormal kicking through the leg.

In a recent advance, intelligence is built into the swing-phase controller to adjust automatically for cadence variations (Figure 44.9). A 4-bit microprocessor is used to adjust a needle valve, via a linear stepper motor, according to duration of the preceding swing phase (Zahedi, 1995). The unit is programmed by the prosthetist to provide optimal damping for the particular amputee's swing phase at slow, normal, and fast walking paces. Thereafter, the appropriate damping is automatically selected for any intermediate speed.

44.2.3 Hierarchically Controlled Prosthetic Hand

Control of the intact hand is hierarchical. It starts with the owner's intention, and an action plan is formulated based on knowledge of the environment and the object to be manipulated. For gross movements, the numerous articulations rely on "preprogrammed" coordination from the central nervous system. Fine control leans heavily on local feedback from force and position sensors in the joints and tactile information about loading and slip at the skin. In contrast, conventional prostheses depend on the conscious command of all levels of control and so can be slow and tiring to use.

Current technology is able to provide both the computing power and transducers required to recreate some of a normal hand's sophisticated proprioceptive control. A concept of extended physiologic proprioception (EPP) was introduced for control of gross arm movement (Simpson and Kenworthy, 1973) whereby the central nervous system is retrained through residual proprioception to coordinate gross actions applying to the geometry of the new extended limb. This idea can be applied to initiate gross hand movements while delegating fine control to an intelligent controller.

Developments by Chappell and Kyberd (1991) and others provide a fine example of the possibilities. A suitable mechanical configuration is shown in Figure 44.10. Four 12-V dc electric motors with gearboxes

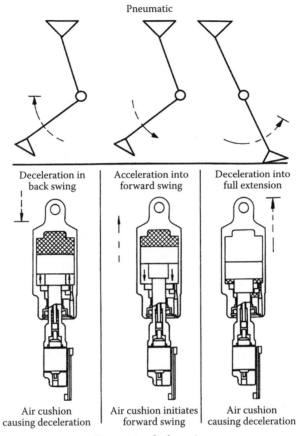

FIGURE 44.8 Pneumatic cylinder action in a swing-phase controller. (Reprinted with permission from S. Zahedi, *The Results of the Field Trial of the Endolite Intelligent Prosthesis, Internal Publication*, Chas. A. Blatchford & Sons, UK.)

control, respectively, thumb adduction, thumb flexion, forefinger flexion, and flexion of digits 3, 4, and 5. Digits 3, 4, and 5 are linked together by a double-swingletree mechanism that allows all three to be driven together. When one digit touches an object the other two can continue to close until they also touch or reach their limit of travel. The movement of the digits allows one of several basic postures:

- *Three-point chuck*: Precision grip with digits 1, 2, and 3 (thumb set to oppose the midline between digits 2 and 3); digits 4 and 5 give additional support.
- *Two-point grip*: Precision grip with digits 1 and 2 (thumb set to oppose forefinger); digits 3, 4, and 5 are fully flexed and not used or fully extended.
- *Fist*: As two-point grip but with thumb fully extended to allow large objects to be grasped.
- *Small fist*: As fist but with thumb flexed and abducted to oppose side of digit 2.
- *Side or key*: Digits 2–5 half or fully flexed with thumb opposing side of second digit.
- *Flat hand*: Digits 2–5 fully extended with thumb abducted and flexed, parked beside digit 2.

The controller coordinates the transition between these positions and ensures that trajectories do not tangle. Feedback to the controller is provided by several devices. Potentiometers detect the angles of flexion of the digits; touch sensors detect pressure on the palmer surfaces of the digits; and a combined contact force (Hall effect) and slip sensor (from acoustic frequency output of force sensor) is mounted at

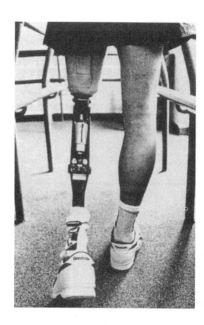

FIGURE 44.9   Endolite intelligent prosthesis in use, minus its cosmetic covers.

the fingertips. The latter detects movement of an object and so controls grip strength appropriate to the task—whether holding a hammer or an egg (Kyberd and Chappell, 1993).

The whole hand may be operated by electromyographic signals from two antagonistic muscles in the supporting forearm stump, picked up at the skin surface. In response to tension in one muscle, the hand opens progressively and then closes to grip with an automatic reflex. The second muscle controls the mode of operation as the hand moves between the states of touch, hold, squeeze, and release.

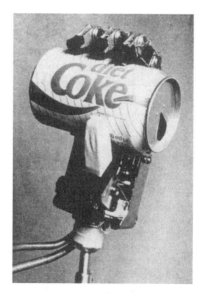

FIGURE 44.10   Southampton hand prosthesis with four degrees of freedom in a power grip. An optical/acoustic sensor is mounted on the thumb. (Reprinted from Chappell, P.H. and Kyberd, P.J. 1991. *J. Biomed. Eng.* 13: 363.)

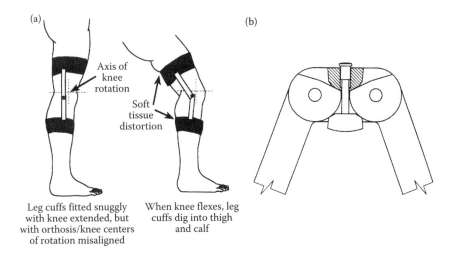

FIGURE 44.11 Problem caused by misplacement of a single-axis orthotic joint (a) is overcome by an orthosis (b) with a self-aligning axis. (From The Laser System, courtesy of Hugh Steeper, Ltd., UK.)

44.2.4 Self-Aligning Orthotic Knee Joint

Knee orthosis is often supplied to resist knee flexion during standing and gait at an otherwise collapsing joint. The rigid locking mechanisms on these devices are manually released to allow knee flexion during sitting. Fitting is complicated by the difficulty of attaching the orthosis with its joint accurately aligned to that of the knee. The simple diagram in Figure 44.11 shows how misplacement of a simple hinged orthosis with a notional fixed knee axis would cause the cuffs on the thigh and calf to press into the soft tissues of the limb (known as pistoning).

The human knee does not have a fixed axis, though, but is better represented as a polycentric joint. In a sagittal (side) view, it is easy to conceptualize the origin of these kinematics from the anatomy of the cruciate ligaments running crisscross across the joint, which together with the base of the femur and the head of the tibia form a classic four-bar linkage. The polycentric nature of the motion can therefore be mimicked by a similar geometry of linkage on the orthosis.

The problem of alignment still remains, however, and precision location of attachment points is not possible when gripping through soft tissues. In one attempt to overcome this specific problem, the knee mechanism has been designed with not one but two axes (Figure 44.11). The center of rotation is then free to self-align. This complexity of the joint while still maintaining the ability to fixate the knee and meeting low-weight requirements is only achieved by meticulous design in composite materials.

44.3 Summary

The field of prosthetics and orthotics is one where at present traditional craft methods sit alongside the application of high technology. Gradually, advanced technology is creeping into most areas, bringing vast improvements in hardware performance specifications and aesthetics. This is, however, an area where the clinical skills of the prosthetist and orthotist will always be required in specification and fitting and where many of the products have customized components. The successful applications of technology are those which assist the professional to exercise his or her judgment, providing him or her with good tools and means to realize a functional specification.

Since the demand for these devices is thankfully low, their design and manufacture are small scale in terms of volume. This taxes the skills of most engineers, both to design the product at reasonable up-front costs and to manufacture it economically in low volume. For bespoke components, we are moving from a base of craft manufacture through an era when modularization was exploited to allow small-batch production toward the use of CAD. In the latter, the engineering design effort is then embodied in the CAD system, leaving the prosthetist or orthotist to incorporate clinical design for each individual component.

Specific examples of current applications have been described. These can only represent a small part of the design effort that is put into prosthetics and orthotics on a continuing basis, making advances in materials and electronics in particular available.

We are also aware that in the space available, it has not been possible to include a discussion of the very innovative work that is being done in intermediate technology for the third world, for which the International Society of Prosthetics and Orthotics (address below) currently has a special working group.

Defining Terms

Biocompatability: Compatibility with living tissue, for example, in consideration of toxicity, degradability, and mechanical interfacing.

CNC machining: Use of a computer numerically controlled machine.

Cosmesis: Aesthetics of appearance.

Ectromelia: Congenital gross shortening of the long bones of a limb.

Functional prescription: A doctor's prescription for supply of a device written in terms of its function as opposed to embodiment.

Neuroskeletomotor system: The skeletal frame of the body with the muscles, peripheral nerves, and central nervous system of the spine and brain, which together participate in movement and stabilization of the body.

Rectified, rectification: Adjustment of a model of body shape to achieve a desirable load distribution in a custom-molded prosthesis or orthosis.

Soft tissues: Skin, fat, connective tissues, and muscles which, along with the hard tissues of bone, teeth, etc. and the fluids, make up the human body.

Transcutaneous: Passing through the skin.

References

Chappell, P.H. and Kyberd, P.J. 1991. Prehensile control of a hand prosthesis by a microcontroller. *J. Biomed. Eng.* 13: 363.

Childress, D.S. 1989. Control philosophies for limb prostheses. In: J. Paul et al. (eds.), *Progress in Bioengineering*, pp. 210–215. New York, Adam Hilger.

Duncan, J.P. and Mair, S.G. 1983. *Sculptured Surfaces in Engineering and Medicine*. Cambridge, England, Cambridge University Press.

Houston, V.L., Burgess, E.M., Childress, D.S. et al. 1992. Automated fabrication of mobility aids (AFMA): Below-knee CASD/CAM testing and evaluation. *J. Rehabil. Res. Dev.* 29: 78.

Kyberd, P.J. and Chappell, P.H. 1993. A force sensor for automatic manipulation based on the Hall effect. *Meas. Sci. Technol.* 4: 281.

Lord, M., Foulston, J., and Smith, P.J. 1991. Technical evaluation of a CAD system for orthopaedic shoe-upper design. *Eng. Med. Proc. Instrum. Mech. Eng.* 205: 109.

Reynolds, D.P. and Lord, M. 1992. Interface load analysis for computer-aided design of below-knee prosthetic sockets. *Med. Biol. Eng. Comput.* 30: 419.

Simpson, D.C. and Kenworthy, G. 1973. The design of a complete arm prosthesis. *Biomed. Eng.* 8: 56.

Zahedi, S. 1995. Evaluation and biomechanics of the intelligent prosthesis: A two-year study. *Orthop. Tech.* 46: 32–40.

Further Information

Bowker, P., Condie, D.N., Bader, D.L., and Pratt, D.J. (eds.). 1993. *Biomechanical Basis of Orthotic Management*. Oxford, Butterworth-Heinemann.

Murdoch, G. and Donovan, R.G. (eds.). 1988. *Amputation Surgery and Lower Limb Prosthetics*. Boston, Blackwell Scientific Publications.

Nordin, M. and Frankel, V. 1980. *Basic Mechanics of the Musculoskeletal System*, 2nd ed. Philadelphia, Lea & Febiger.

Smidt, G.L. (ed). 1990. *Gait in Rehabilitation*. New York, Churchill-Livingstone.

Organizations

International Society of Prosthetics and Orthotics (ISPO), Borgervaenget 5, 2100 Copenhagen Ø, Denmark [tel (31) 20 72 60].

Department of Veterans Affairs, VA Rehabilitation Research and Development Service, 103 Gay Street, Baltimore, MD 21202-4051.

Rehabilitation Engineering Society of North America (RESNA), Suite 1540, 1700 North Moore Street, Arlington, VA 22209-1903.

Externally Powered and Controlled Orthoses and Prostheses

Dejan B. Popović
University of Belgrade and
Aalborg University

Rehabilitation of humans with sensory-motor disability requires effective assistive systems that would allow their fast and maximal reintegration into the normal life. The cost-benefit functions that humans with disability likely appreciate and optimize comprise elements, such as (1) the quality of life measured by reintegration into the social and work environments; (2) reliability of the assistive system; (3) energy rate and cost with respect to the one used for accomplishing the same task with alternative methods; (4) disruption of normal activities when employing the assistive system; (5) cosmetics; (6) maintenance; and (7) cost. The same elements are considered, but, in a different order by the developers of the rehabilitation technology, practitioners of physical medicine, and rehabilitation and healthcare providers.

Here, we present technical aspects of the available externally powered orthoses and prostheses that interface directly or indirectly with the human neuro-musculo-skeletal system. We elaborate here two methods for the restoration of movements in humans with paralysis: functional activation of paralyzed muscles termed functional electrical stimulation (FES) or functional neuromuscular stimulation (FNS or NMS), and parallel application of FES and a mechanical orthosis called hybrid assistive system (HAS). We also describe externally controlled and powered leg and arm/hand prostheses.

45.1 Neural Prostheses Based on FES

Assistive systems that apply FES to restore sensory or motor function are called neural prostheses. A *neural prosthesis* (NP) could improve sensory or motor function in subjects after cerebro-vascular accident (CVA), spinal cord injury (SCI), and some other diseases of the central nervous system (CNS) [1]. A motor NP applies electrical stimulation to artificially generate muscle contractions required for executing of a functional task in subjects who have lost voluntary control because of a disease or injury. The basic phenomena of the FES are the contraction of a muscle due to the direct stimulation of motorneurons, and reflexive responses due to the activation of sensory pathways and CNS. An NP sends a burst of short electric pulses (pulse duration: $0-250$ μs, pulse amplitude: $10-150$ mA) to generate a function. The key element for achieving functional movement is the appropriate sequencing of bursts of electrical pulses. To achieve a smooth contraction of the extremity, the burst of pulses has to have a frequency of about 20 pulses/s. If less than 20 pulses/s are induced into the motor nerve the muscle generates a series of twitches, instead of a fused smooth contraction of the muscle. In order to generate stronger force (tetanic contraction) higher frequencies (e.g., $30-50$ pulses/s) need to be applied. The higher the stimulation, the more the fatigue that will be developed in the stimulated muscle. Other types of stimulation (e.g., intermittent stimulation, use of doublets, or n-plets) could improve the force vs. fatigue ratio. If the motor nerve is missing, then the muscle becomes denervated and it cannot generate functional force by means of NP. Recently, new methods were suggested that claim to be applicable for stimulation of denervated muscles [2,3]. The motor nerves can be stimulated using monophasic and biphasic current or voltage pulses. The monophasic pulses are used only with the surface electrodes because they lead to unbalanced charge delivery to the tissues, potentially causing the damage. Most NPs implement monophasic compensated current or voltage pulses.

The motor nerves can be stimulated using either surface (transcutaneous), percutaneous, or implanted electrodes. The transcutaneous stimulation is performed with self-adhesive or nonadhesive electrodes that are placed on the subject's skin in the vicinity of the motor point of the muscle that needs to be stimulated. Recently, new technology that uses electrode arrays positioned on the skin instead of single-filed electrodes was suggested [4]. This electrode array allows variation of the stimulation effects without moving of the electrode (e.g., simultaneous control of agonist and antagonistic muscles resulting with the variable stiffness of the joint, in parallel with the strong activation of the prime movers needed for the desired movement, and dynamic adaptation to the change of the position of the muscle vs. electrode during the movement) [5].

The alternative to surface electrodes is the implantable electrodes. One type of electrodes is wire electrodes that are applied percutaneously, that is, the electrode connects to the stimulator outside of the body, while the stimulation point is close to the motor point (inside the body). Another option is fully implantable electrodes that are sutured to the fascia placed close to the entry point of the motor nerve (epimysial electrodes). More recently, cuff electrodes have been introduced as the NP interface to the tissues. The cuff electrode allows selective stimulation of specific nerve fascicles. Implanted electrodes compared to surface electrodes guarantee higher stimulation selectivity with much less electrical charge applied, both being desired characteristics of NPs. The technology that was introduced few years ago uses miniature implantable stimulator that communicates with the external unit via radio-frequency electromagnetic field. The current version of the small implants called Bion comprises the rechargeable battery that is charged when not used and is discharged during operation [6–8].

45.1.1 Restoration of Hand Functions

During the last 50 years several NPs for grasping have been designed and tested; yet, only few were brought to the market [9–11]. An important recent finding is that NPs have therapeutic effects if applied appropriately and timely [12]. The proof of the long-term therapeutic effect of NPs could be the milestone for the healthcare providers to change their attitude and start paying for this important rehabilitation modality.

The neural prosthesis for grasping is most frequently used to help tetraplegic subjects to restore or hemiplegic patients to promote the recovery of the grasping function. Among tetraplegic subjects, the patients who benefit the most have a complete C5/C6 spinal lesion. Typically, these patients have preserved proximal upper-limb muscles allowing them to perform limited reaching and manipulation, while their wrist and finger movements are greatly compromised. In hemiplegic subjects one arm is often fully functional, while the other arm is paretic or paralyzed because of the CVA. Hemiplegic subjects feel unpleasant stimulation because the sensory mechanisms are intact. One can decrease the unpleasant sensation by applying stimulation at higher frequency (e.g., 50 pulses/s). The unpleasant sensation can also be decreased by using the pulses with the exponential rising edge.

The NP for grasping restores the two most frequently used grasp types: the palmar and the lateral grasp. The palmar grasp provides the opposition of the palm and the thumb; hence, allows holding bigger and heavier objects such as cans and bottles. The lateral grasp provides the opposition of the flexed index finger and the thumb and it is used to hold thinner objects such as keys, paper, etc. Finger flexion is performed by stimulating the *Flexor Digitorum Superficialis m.* and the *Flexor Digitorum Profundus m.* Finger extension is obtained by stimulating the *Extensor Communis Digitorum m.* Stimulation of the thumb's Thenar muscle or the median nerve produces thumb flexion. The FES can also be applied to generate elbow extension by stimulating the *Triceps Brachii m.* Such elbow extension in combination with the voluntary *Biceps Brachii m.* contraction can be used to augment the reaching. The FES could be used to stimulate elbow flexion (*Biceps Brachii m.*) or even the shoulder muscles to provide upper-arm movements; yet, these systems have not been developed into practical devices.

The NPs for grasping can be classified upon the source of control signals that trigger or regulate the stimulation pattern to the following groups: shoulder control [13], voice control [14,15], respiratory control [16], joystick control [13], position transducers [18,19], and trigger [11,20]. The classification can also be made upon the interface between the stimulator and the tissues to the following groups: one- or two-channel surface-electrode systems [17–20], multichannel surface stimulation system [11,15,17], multichannel percutaneous systems with intramuscular electrodes [10,13,14,16], and fully implanted systems [10].

The first grasping system used to provide prehension and release [21] used a splint with a spring for closure and electrical stimulation of the thumb extensor for release. Rudel et al. [22] suggested the use of a simple two-channel stimulation system and a position transducer (sliding potentiometer). The shift of the potentiometer generated by the user controlled the opening and closing of the hand. This technique was used for the therapy of hemiplegic patients and as an orthosis for tetraplegic patients.

The approach taken at Ben Gurion University, Israel [15] used a voice-controlled multichannel surface-electrode system. Up to 12 bipolar stimulation channels and a splint were used to control elbow, wrist, and hand functions. Daily mounting and fitting of the system were complex, but the experience leads to the commercial device called Handmaster NMS1 [23]. The Handmaster is an NP for grasping with three surface stimulation channels. One stimulation channel is used to stimulate the finger extensors, the second for finger flexors, and the third generates the thumb opposition. The Handmaster is controlled with a push-button switch that triggers the hand opening and closing functions. One of the major advantages of the Handmaster in comparison with other surface stimulation systems is that it is easy to do on and off. The second feature is that Handmaster stabilizes the wrist being important for effective grasping, yet also limiting from some movements (e.g., supination and pronation).

Prochazka et al. [18] introduced an assistive system that enhances tenodesis grasp that was controlled by a wrist flexion and extension. This, so-called Bionic glove comprised three channels of stimulation to interface the paralyzed sensory-motor systems. The self-adhering surface electrodes, with the metal pin contacting the flexible garment, were positioned over the prime movers contributing to finger flexors, finger extensors, and thumb opposition/flexion. The wrist-joint angle sensor triggered the "close the hand" pattern once the wrist extension was bigger than the selected threshold and vice versa, that is, the "open the hand" stimulation pattern was triggered once the sensor measured the wrist flexion bigger than the preset threshold. Clinical evaluation of the Bionic glove [24] indicated that the 6 months of use of the Bionic glove was beneficial for tetraplegic patients both therapeutically and as an orthosis; yet, the overall acceptance rate remained insufficient.

Recently, an assistive system called Actigrip CS® (Figure 45.1b) was brought to the market by the company Neurodan A/S, Denmark [11]. This device follows the development of the system introduced as the Belgrade Grasping-Reaching System (BGS®) [17]. The BGS had four stimulation channels, three of which were used to control the hand, while the fourth channel was used to control the elbow extension (stimulation of the *Triceps Brachii m.*) allowing a tetraplegic subject to reach objects that he/she was not

(a)   (b)

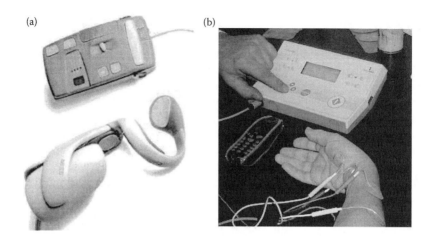

FIGURE 45.1 Handmaster NMS1 (NESS, Israel) grasping device for tetraplegic and hemiplegic patients (a). Actigrip CS (Neurodan A/S, Denmark) is the surface functional electrical therapy system (b). (See text for details.)

able to do without the NP. The grasping function was controlled by a push-button switch that triggered the hand opening and closing. The grasping was separated into three phases: prehension that forms the correct aperture; relaxation that allows the hand to get in good contact with the object; and closing the hand by opposing either the palm and the thumb, or the side of the index finger and the thumb. The releasing function included two stages, opening of the hand and resting. The reaching function was controlled by implementing the synergy typical for able-bodied humans between the shoulder flexion/extension and elbow flexion/extension.

The Actigrip CS uses four channels of stimulation to control the hand functions. The novelty is the use of the life-like control: the use of triphasic pattern of agonist and antagonistic muscles and use of parallel stimulation of agonist and antagonistic muscles to control the joint stiffness [5]. Clinical studies with the Actigrip CS in poststroke humans suggested excellent recovery compared with the recovery following the conventional therapy.

The ETHZ-ParaCare NP was designed to improve grasping and walking functions in SCI and stroke patients [25]. This surface NP is fully programmable. The system has four stimulation channels, and can be interfaced with many sensors or sensory systems. The ETHZ-ParaCare neural prosthesis for grasping provides both palmar and lateral grasps. The system can be controlled with proportional EMG (electromyography), discrete EMG, push button, and sliding resistor-control strategies [25–27].

The group at the Institute for Biokybernetik, Karlsruhe, Germany, suggested the use of EMG recordings from the muscle that is stimulated [28]. The aim of this device was to enhance grasping using weak muscles. It was possible to use retained recordings from the volar side of the forearm to trigger on and off the stimulation of the same muscle groups. In this case, it was essential to eliminate the stimulation artifact and the evoked potential caused by the stimulus in order to eliminate positive feedback effects, which could generate a tetanic contraction that could not be turned off. Sennels et al. (1997) [29] have further developed this approach. In order to implement EMG control the NP has to include electrodes positioned over the muscle that can be voluntarily controlled [30]. The electrodes should be connected to low noise, high impedance, and high common-mode rejection ratio preamplifier. The output from the preamplifier should be fed to a blanking device in order to eliminate the stimulation artifact. The obtained integrated signal can be used as a trigger (switch) or as an input to a state machine. If the EMG recordings are to be used only as a trigger, a comparator that is connected to the reference voltage at the second input can achieve effective operation [30]. A state control relying on a multithreshold detection could be used to allow the user to vary the strength of the grasp or select other modalities of grasping.

The alternatives to surface electrodes are implantable electrodes or fully implantable systems. In the early 1980s the FES group in Sendai developed a microcomputer-controlled NP for grasping by means of implanted electrodes [31]. The system comprised several intramuscular electrodes that were positioned by the hypodermal needles. These external parts comprised the NEC PC-98LT personal computer and an external microcontroller-based stimulator. The stimulation patterns were "cloned" from the muscle activities recorded during voluntary grasping movements of able-bodied subjects. The stimulation sequences were triggered with a push button or a pneumatic pressure sensor. The subsequent version of the same system had 30 stimulation channels. This system demonstrated that post-SCI subjects with complete C4–C6 spinal cord lesion could achieve both reaching and grasping functions. Since 1994, in collaboration with NEC Inc., the Sendai FES team has developed a fully implantable 16-channel electric stimulator NEC FESMate. Two hundred of these stimulators were manufactured [32]. The operation of the NEC FESMate system is similar to the earlier Sendai stimulator.

The Freehand system (NeuroControl Co, Cleveland, OH, USA) (Figure 45.2) has eight implanted epimysial stimulation electrodes and an implanted stimulator [33]. The stimulation electrodes are used to generate flexion and extension of the fingers and the thumb in C5 and C6 SCI subjects in order to provide them with lateral (key pinch) or palmar grasp. The stimulation sequences that are used to generate both palmar and lateral grasps are individually tuned and are preprogrammed in the form of a "muscle contraction map." The hand closure and the hand opening are commanded using a position sensor that is placed on the shoulder of the subject's opposite arm. The position sensor monitors two axes of shoulder motion, protraction/retraction, and elevation/depression. Typically, the protraction/retraction motion of the shoulder is used as a proportional signal for hand opening and closing. The shoulder elevation/depression motion is used to generate logic commands that are used to establish a zero level for the protraction/retraction command and to "freeze" the stimulation levels until the next logic command is issued. An additional switch is also provided to allow a user to choose between palmar

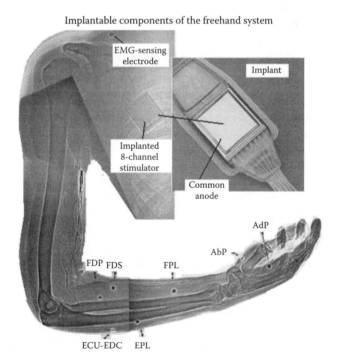

FIGURE 45.2 Freehand fully implantable grasping system (Neurocontrol, Cleveland, OH). The system comprises eight epimysial electrodes for interfacing the muscles. The device is driven and controlled by an external unit that transmits energy and control signals to the implantable unit.

and lateral grasp strategies. The shoulder position sensor and the controller are not implanted. Besides this sensor configuration, the Freehand system also allows one to use either external or implanted transducer mounted on ipsilateral wrist. This transducer measures the dorsal/volar flexion of the wrist and uses this motion to control hand opening and closing in a way similar to the shoulder position sensor [34,35]. The output of the shoulder or the wrist sensor is sent to an external control unit that generates an appropriate stimulation sequence for each stimulation electrode. This sequence is then sent via an inductive link to an implanted stimulator that generates the stimulation trains for each implanted stimulation electrode. More than 250 tetraplegic subjects have received the Freehand neural prosthesis at more than a dozen sites around the world. The subjects have demonstrated the ability to grasp and release objects and performing of typical daily activities more independently when using the neural prosthesis compared with no NP.

The idea of controlling the whole arm and assisting manipulation in humans lacking shoulder and elbow control is getting more attention recently by the research team at the Case Western Reserve University (CWRU) in Cleveland, OH [36–39]. The system was designed to combine a fully implantable grasping system with some additional channels to control elbow extension, flexion, and shoulder movements. The control of reaching, unlike the control in the BGS NP, measures the position of the arm in space and for certain arm positions automatically triggers stimulation of the *Triceps Brachii m.*

Scott et al. [40] suggested the use of EMG recordings from sternocleidomastoid (SCM) muscles to control an FES system for hand control of tetraplegic individuals. Surface electrodes were applied over the SCM muscles to record the EMG. The control could be described as a three-state machine (1) Strong flexion of the ipsilateral SCM opens the hand, (2) weaker flexion closes the hand, and (3) no flexion (below a selected threshold) locks the grasp. This is to say that three levels of EMG recordings trigger the controller to activate the following programs: (1) increase the stimulation of the muscles that are contributing to the opening of the hand, (2) increase the stimulation of the muscles that are contributing to the closing of the hand, and (3) keep the activation of the muscles at the selected level. The control has been implemented using a fully implantable Freehand® grasping system. The use of SCM muscles could be of specific importance for bilateral application of commercial open-loop FES systems to improve hand grasp since the contralateral shoulder could be used for the control of the respective hand.

The development of implantable cuff electrodes to be used for sensing contact, slippage, and pressure [41–43] opened a new prospective in controlling grasping devices; and the Center for Sensory Motor Interactions in Aalborg, Denmark was pursuing a series of experiments combining their sensing technique with the fully implantable CWRU system.

45.1.2 Restoration of Standing and Walking

The application of NP to the restoration of gait was first investigated systematically in Ljubljana, Slovenia [44]. Currently, NP for gait rehabilitation is used in a clinical setting in several rehabilitation centers [45–51], and there is a growing trend for the design of devices for home use (see Figure 45.3).

Current surface NP systems use various numbers of stimulation channels. The simplest one, from a technical point, is a single-channel stimulation system. This system is only suitable for hemiplegic patients, and a limited group of incomplete paraplegic patients. These individuals can perform limited ambulation with assistance of the upper extremities without NP. The NP in these humans is used to activate a single muscle group. The first demonstrated application of this technique was in hemiplegic patients [52] following the patent and research of Liberson et al. [53]. The stimulation was applied to ankle dorsiflexors so that the "foot-drop" can be eliminated. Several versions of foot-drop stimulators with the shoe trigger switch were developed and tested with various levels of success [54–56]. A commercial system was designed by Stein and coworkers [57] integrating a single-channel stimulator and a tilt sensor that replaced the foot trigger switch. Single- and dual-channel correcting foot drop is now a regular clinical treatment in some rehabilitation institution [58].

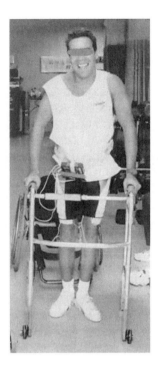

FIGURE 45.3 Complete paraplegic subject walking assisted with the Parastep I (Sigmedics, Chicago, IL). The walking assist comprises six channels that stimulate hip and knee extensors and withdrawal reflex bilaterally. The patient is wearing an ankle-foot orthosis and uses the rolling walker instrumented with the switches for control of stepping.

A version of the foot-drop stimulator that is being introduced is called Actigait, and it was brought to the market by the company Neurodan A/S, DK. The Actigait uses a cuff electrode to selectively stimulate peroneal nerve, thereby, effectively controlling the foot drop and assisting the paretic limb during the swing. The heel switch or, potentially, the implantable sensor that records activity from a sensory nerve innervating the lateral side of the foot [59] triggers the dorsiflexion by means of a multichannel cuff electrode (see Figure 45.4).

A multichannel NP with a minimum of four stimulation channels is required for ambulation of a patient with a complete motor lesion of lower extremities and preserved balance and upper-body motor control [44]. Appropriate bilateral stimulation of the quadriceps muscles locks the knees during standing. Stimulating the common peroneal nerve on the ipsilateral side, while switching off the quadriceps stimulation on that side, produces a withdrawal of that leg. This withdrawal (flexion) combined with an adequate movement of the upper body and use of the upper extremities for propulsion and support allow ground clearance. This withdrawal is considered as the swinging of the leg. Hand or foot switches can provide the flexion-extension alternation needed for a slow forward or backward progression. Sufficient arm strength must be available to provide balance in parallel bars, rolling walker, or crutches. These systems evolved into a commercial six-channel assistive system called Parastep-1R (Sigmedics, Chicago, IL) approved for home usage by the Food and Drugs Administration (FAD) in 1994.

Multichannel percutaneous systems for gait restoration, with many channels, were suggested [60–62]. The main advantage of these systems is the plausibility to selectively activate many muscle groups. The implantable system also activates deep muscles that are not accessible by surface stimulation. A preprogrammed stimulation pattern that is a replica of the EMG pattern typical for humans with no motor disorders is delivered to muscles controlling the ankle, knee, and hip joints as well as to some trunk muscles. The experience of the Cleveland research team suggested that 48 channels are required

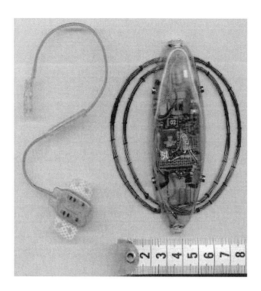

FIGURE 45.4 Components of the prototype of the Actigait system. The Actigait is an implantable foot-drop preventer for poststroke hemiplegic patients. The picture shows the cuff electrode that selectively stimulates the peroneal nerve connected to the implantable two-channel stimulator (left side of the image). The right side of the image shows the external unit with the cooper winding (transmitting antenna).

for a complete paraplegic patient to achieve an acceptable and effective walking pattern. More recently, the Cleveland group changed its stimulation strategy and is suggesting limited external bracing to operate in parallel to the electrical stimulation. Fine-wire intramuscular electrodes are cathodes positioned close to the motor point within selected muscles. Knee extensors (rectus femoris, vastus medialis, vastus lateralis, and vastus intermedius), hip flexors (sartorius, tensor fasciae latae, gracilis, and iliopsoas), hip extensors (semimembranosus, gluteus maximus), hip abductors (gluteus medius), ankle dorsiflexors (tibialis anterior, peroneus longus), ankle plantar flexors (gastrocnemius lateralis and medialis, plantaris and soleus), and paraspinal muscles are selected for activation. A surface electrode is used as a common anode. Interleaved pulses are delivered with a multichannel, battery-operated, portable stimulator. The hand controller allows the selection of gait activity. These systems were limited to the clinical environment. The application was investigated in complete spinal cord lesions and in stroke patients. The same strategy and selection criteria for implantation were used for both stroke and SCI patients. Recent developments use the CWRU system with eight channels per leg to be activated and improved control.

A multichannel totally implanted FES system [51] was proposed and tested in few subjects. This system uses a 16-channel implantable stimulator and was attached to the epineurium electrodes. Femoral and gluteal nerves were stimulated for hip and knee extension. The so-called round-about stimulation was applied in which four electrodes were located around the nerve and stimulated intermittently. This stimulation method reduces muscle fatigue.

The development of the stimulation technology is giving new hopes. Two new techniques are especially important (1) application of remotely controlled wireless microstimulators [63,64], and (2) so-called stimulator for all seasons [65]. There are several attempts to design effective wireless stimulator that is believed to be capable of selectively stimulating fascicles [66,67]. Using the technology of cochlear implants is finding its way for standing and walking restoration [68].

Some essentials limit effectiveness of FES-based NPs: muscle fatigue caused by nonphysiological activation of sensory-motor systems, reduced muscle forces compared with the forces in naturally controlled muscles, modified reflex activities, spasticity, etc. From the engineering point of view the further development of NPs has to address the following issues: the interface between an FES system and neuromuscular structures in the organism, biocompatibility of the FES system, and overall practicality. The least-resolved solution in FES-based motor NPs is automatic control (see Chapter 15 of this book).

45.1.3 Hybrid Assistive Systems for Walking

The combination of FES and external skeleton for restoring motor functions in humans with sensory-motor disability is called hybrid assistive system (HAS) [69–71]. Several HAS designs have been proposed that combine relatively simple rigid mechanical structures for passive stabilization of lower limbs during stance phase and FES systems. These systems combine use of a *reciprocating-gait orthosis* with multichannel stimulation, the use of an ankle-foot orthosis or an extended ankle-foot orthosis with a knee cage, or the use of a *self-fitting modular orthosis* [72–78]. Each trend in the design of HAS implies different applications as well as specific hardware and control problems. On the basis of accumulated experience, the following features can serve as criteria for a closer description of various HAS designs: (1) partial mechanical support, (2) parallel operation of the biological and mechanical system, (3) sequential operation of the biological and the mechanical system. The partial mechanical support refers to the use of braces to assist FES only at specific events within a walking cycle [75]. The advanced version of powered orthoses to be used with FES is being developed by Goldfarb and colleagues [76]. Control of joints in mechanical orthosis is becoming again a target of research and development mainly because of new technological tools [77,78].

45.2 Active Prostheses

The role of active prosthesis is to extend the function provided by a "nonexternally" powered and controlled artificial organ (see Chapter 137 of previous edition), hence to improve the overall performance of motor function, ultimately providing better quality of life.

45.2.1 Externally Controlled Transfemoral Prostheses

Effective restoration of walking and standing of handicapped humans is an important element to improve the quality of life. Artificial legs of different kinds have been in use for a long time, but in many cases they are inadequate for the needs of amputees, specifically for high transfemoral (above the knee) amputees (e.g., hip disarticulation), bilateral amputees, and highly active patients (e.g., subjects involved in sport).

Modern technology has led to greatly improved design of transtibial (below the knee) prostheses (TTP). Below-knee amputees perform many normal locomotor activities, and participate in many sports requiring running, jumping, and other jerky movements [79]. The biggest progress was made using readily available and easy-to-work-with plastic and graphite alloys for building the artificial skeletal portion of the shank and foot [80]. TTP are light, easy to assemble, and overall very reliable. TTP provide good support and excellent energy absorption leading to reduced impacts and jerks; yet, allowing storing of the energy helps in the push-off phase in the gait cycle. Existing TTP, although without ankle joints, duplicate closely the dynamics of the normal foot-ankle complex during swing and stance phases of the step cycle.

The same technology has been introduced into the design of transfemoral prostheses (TFP). The requirements for a TFP were stated by Wagner and Catranis [81]. The prosthesis must support the body weight of the amputee like the normal limb during the stance phase of level walking, on slopes, and on soft or rough terrain. This implies that the prosthesis provides "stability" during weight bearing: that is, it prevents sudden or uncontrolled flexion of the knee during weight bearing. The second requirement is that the body is supported such that undesirable socket/stump interface pressures and gait abnormalities due to painful socket/stump contact are prevented. The analysis of biomechanical factors that influence the shaping, fitting, and alignment of the socket is a problem in itself. If the fitting has been accomplished, allowing the amputee to manipulate and control the prosthesis in an active and comfortable manner, the socket and stump can be treated as one single body. The third requirement, which is somewhat controversial, is that the prosthesis should duplicate as nearly as possible the kinematics and dynamics of normal gait. The amputee should walk with a normal-looking gait over a useful range of speeds associated with typical activities for normal persons of similar age. The latter requirement has received attention in recent years and fully integrated systems, so-called self-contained active TFPs are being incorporated into modern rehabilitation. The self-contained principle implies that the artificial leg contains the energy source, actuator, controller, and sensors.

The externally controlled knee is a recent development that provides some solutions that fulfill the said requirements. Two microprocessor-controlled pneumatic knee prosthesis using the Kobe technology [82] is available: the Endolite Intelligent Prosthesis (Blatchford and Sons, London, UK) and the Seattle Limb Systems Power Knee (Seattle Limb Systems, Seattle, WA). Intelligent Prosthesis was first developed in 1993 and an improved version was further introduced in 1995 (Intelligent Prosthesis Plus) and 1998 (Adaptive Prosthesis) [83].

The Adaptive Prosthesis uses two microprocessor-controlled motor valves to control a hybrid hydraulic and pneumatic system. The hydraulic system controls stance, flexion, and terminal impact. The pneumatic portion of the system controls both swing phase and knee extension. The Adaptive Prosthesis also offers a voluntary locking mechanism for extended standing and a stumble control that responds to prevent knee buckling. The Adaptive Prosthesis has batteries that power the system for several months and a software design that prevents memory loss during battery replacement [83–85].

The C-leg® produced by Otto Bock was introduced in 1997. The C-leg comprises the microprocessor-controlled knee with both hydraulic stance and swing-phase control [86]. It has force sensors in the shin that use heel, toe, and axial loading data to determine stance-phase stability. A knee-angle sensor provides data for control of swing phase, angle, velocity, and direction of the movement created by the knee. Sensor technology adapts to movement by measuring angles and moments 50 times/s. The unit transfers information to the hydraulic valve allowing reaction to changing conditions. This mechanism results in an individual's gait that resembles natural walking on many different types of terrain. The C-leg uses a rechargeable battery that lasts 25–30 h. When the battery drains off power, the knee goes into safety mode [86]. The company claims that C-leg immediately adapts to different walking speeds and provides knee stability (see Figure 45.5).

The application of prostheses starts to be more complex when subjects are to walk stairs, slope, and uneven terrain. Walking downstairs and down the slope requires the controlled flexion of the knee joint, and the flexion is totally dependent on the environmental conditions. James et al. [87] introduced a microcomputer control of the hydraulic system affecting stiffness in both flexion and extension from free to lock states. C-leg from Otto Bock, Germany is the first microprocessor-controlled knee joint which incorporates some of these features. Electronic sensors supply basic data for stance-phase stability and stance-phase control. This is the closest approximation to natural gait where subjects no longer have to think about walking. Walking upstairs and up slopes requires a powered knee joint, which is still not commercially available and has not been developed even for experimental purposes to the satisfaction of researchers, clinical, and over all potential users. Powered transfemoral prostheses have been suggested [88,89] but the technology and control have not been adequate.

There are two groups of patients who will benefit greatly from the powered leg: patients with hip disarticulation and bilateral amputees. In both cases, amputees are not able to generate movement of the thigh that is required to drive the underpowered system; hence, the externally powered knee joint will compensate for lack of power by the user.

45.2.2 Powered Hand and Arm Prostheses

The power for active hand and arm prostheses can come from the body (body-powered prosthesis) or from external sources (externally powered prosthesis) [90–97]. Gross body movement controls a body-powered prosthesis. The movement of the shoulder, upper arm, or chest is captured by a harness system,

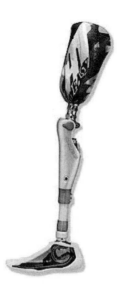

FIGURE 45.5   C-leg. The C-leg is a transfemoral prosthesis that incorporates intelligent knee mechanism allowing controlled swing and stance phases of the gait cycle.

which is attached to a cable that is connected to a terminal device (hook or hand). For some levels of amputation or deficiency, an elbow system can be added to provide the amputee additional function. An amputee must possess at least one or more of the following gross body movements: glenohumeral flexion, scapular abduction or adduction, shoulder depression and elevation, and chest expansion in order to control body-powered prosthesis. In addition, sufficient residual limb length and sufficient musculature must exist.

There are two types of controls for body-powered hands and hooks, voluntary opening and voluntary closing: voluntary opening gives the subject grasping control even when he/she is relaxed. The trade-off for this is limited grip force, often less than 30 N. Voluntary closing allows the subject to have substantially greater grip force, often over 150 N, but does not allow the subject to relax without losing grasp.

Many amputees who wear a body-powered prosthesis develop increased control due to a phenomenon called extended proprioception [90]. Extended proprioception gives the wearer feedback as to the position of the terminal device. The subject will know whether the hook is open or closed by the extent of pressure the harness is exerting on his or her shoulder area without having to visually inspect the operation. Many amputees do not like the cosmetic appearance of the hook and control cables and they request a "natural-like" part of the body replacement.

Externally powered prostheses use electrical power to provide function. The electrical power is applied via motors located in the terminal device (hand or hook), wrist, and elbow. The grip force of the hand can be in excess of 100 N. Command signals are generated either by voluntary contraction of muscles, so-called *myoelectric control*, or by using switches of different kinds. For applications that are more complex, both the command signals are used for different operations (e.g., control of several degrees of freedom).

Myoelectric control is a very popular command method [95]. It relies on the ability of the amputee to generate voluntary contraction of a muscle that he or she would normally use for the same function before the disability, or some other synergistic muscle at his/her subconscious level. Muscle contraction can be registered by recording of the electrical activity of muscles (electromyogram—EMG). Electrodes that contact the skin capture EMG signal. The EMG can be recorded accurately if the appropriate technology is used. EMG has to be carefully extracted from "electrical noise." Many individuals prefer this type of control because it only requires the wearer to contract his muscles. This eliminates the need for a tight, often-uncomfortable control harness. Another advantage of a myoelectric prosthesis is that because it does not require a control cable or harness, a cosmetic skin can be applied in either latex or silicone, greatly enhancing the cosmetic restoration.

An example of the profound designs is the Utah Arm 2 for the transhumeral amputees (see Figure 45.6) [92]. The Utah Arm and hand system for transhumeral amputees allows sensitive control of elbow, hand, and wrist (optional) using only EMG signals from two muscles. The exclusive myoelectric system eliminates cables, letting the amputee move the arm and hand slowly or quickly in any position, ultimately leading to a more natural response with less effort. The Utah Arm, combined with its high-performance hand control, supplies the wearer with superior cosmetic appearance. Smooth exterior hand covers provide natural look. For rugged tasks, the hand can be changed to another hand or terminal device. The optional electrically driven wrist joint allows hand pronation and supination. Proportional or on-off myoelectric controls are both available based on the subject's request and abilities.

The ServoPro, an exclusive feature of the Utah Arm, is designed for amputees with shoulder disarticulation, interscapulothoracic, or brachial plexus injuries. The ServoPro eliminates the electrodes normally required to operate the Utah Arm. The system may be the only option, which can provide functional control of both elbow and hand. The ServoPro is based on a harness, but instead of cables, electronic components are pushed and pulled to generate command signals that will control the electrically powered prosthesis. The ServoPro requires much smaller excursion of movement and less effort compared with body-powered cables in equivalent mechanical systems. The servo control is accurate and it uses feedback from sensors in the elbow and hand.

Hybrid prosthesis utilizes a body-powered elbow and a myoelectrically controlled terminal device—hook or hand. Most important ability provided to the patient is to simultaneously control elbow flexion and extension while opening or closing the electric hand/hook or while rotating the wrist. The other prosthetic options generally require the wearer to control one function at a time (flex the elbow, lock the elbow, open, or close the terminal device). The hybrid prosthesis weighs less and is less expensive than a similar prosthesis with an electrically powered elbow and hand. An example is the Ergo arm from Otto Bock that uses the new elbow system that can be unlocked or locked in any position, even under loads up to 250 N. A slight pull on the cable lowers the forearm gradually. Releasing the cable immediately locks the elbow in that position. For normal locking or unlocking, the cable has to be pulled stronger. The elbow is designed to support myoelectric hand. When the prosthetic arm is extended, the system stores the energy to facilitate flexion. The arm swings smoothly while walking. Subject-adjustable counterbalance makes the arm feel lighter, even with an electric wrist and terminal device.

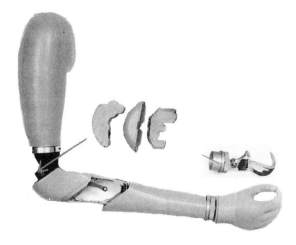

FIGURE 45.6 Utah Arm is a self-contained battery-powered artificial arm-hand complex. The system comprises myoelectric control of the elbow, wrist, and grasping movements.

Otto Bock Sensor Hand provides secure grasps of various objects. The system frees the user from constant watch on the objects in the hand since the automatic grasping feature senses when an object is about to slip and makes necessary adjustments. The Flexi-Grip function gives the amputee a natural look and flexible grip. The hand is controlled by volitional contraction of muscles that are touching the socket. The electrodes are built into the socket. This hand is used with the passive wrist rotation with ratchet mechanism or optional friction wrist. The Sensor Hand senses the change in the center of gravity and readjusts its grip automatically. The hand closes at maximum speed and grips an object with the least amount of force. When the contact of fingers and the object are sensed, the control changes to grip-force control and increases the force to its maximum. Two programs can be executed, namely, (1) controlling the opening speed by the strength of the muscle signal (contraction) in addition to controlling the closing speed based on a decrease in muscle tension and (2) controlling both speeds by the strength of the muscle contraction.

The current commercial hand prostheses have extremely limited performance compared with the able-bodied arm and hand. The Southampton Artificial Hand has been in existence for several decades and is based on the original hypothesis for the development of a hierarchically controlled myoelectric prosthesis. The mechanics of the Southampton hand has undergone several stages; however, the main hypothesis remains the same. Vast quantities of information are utilized to form a stable and comfortable grip in able-bodied humans. The grip is constantly adjusted to prevent the slip, deforming or crushing of the object, and incorrect orientation (e.g., spilling the content of a container). In all systems described above the grasping force is preselected based on experience, and rarely voluntarily adjusted based on visual feedback. The philosophy behind the development of the Southampton hand is to come with the adaptive, mechanical structure that uses sensors and intelligent control to generate optimum grip. The basis of the control is a finite state of modeling and use of synergistic model of movement of fingers and the thumb. The hand has five functioning digits and four degrees of freedom. The index finger acts independently from the other three fingers, which move in tandem. The other two degrees of freedom are in the thumb. Slip transducers are built in the pads of the fingers.

Defining Terms

Artificial reflex control: A sensory-driven control algorithm based on knowledge representation (production rule-based system).

Externally controlled assistive system: Assistive system for restoration of motor functions with automatic control.

Externally powered assistive system: Assistive system for restoration of motor functions that uses external power to control muscles of driven actuators.

Hybrid assistive systems: Combination of a functional electrical stimulation and a mechanical orthosis.

Myoelectric (EMG) control: Use of voluntary-generated myoelectric activity as control signals for an externally controlled and powered assistive system.

Neural prosthesis—Assistive systems for replacing or augmenting sensory-motor function, functional electrical stimulation, or functional neuromuscular stimulation: Patterned electrical stimulation of neuromuscular structures dedicated to restore motor functions.

Reciprocating-gait orthosis: A walking and standing assistive system with a reciprocating mechanism for hip joints, which extends the contralateral hip when the ipsilateral hip is flexed.

Self-fitting modular orthosis: A modular, self-fitting, and mechanical orthosis with a soft interface between human body and the orthosis.

Transfemoral prosthesis: Artificial leg for amputees with the amputation between the knee and hip joint (transfemur).

Transtibial prosthesis: Artificial leg for amputees with the amputation between the ankle and the knee joints (transtibia).

References

1. Popović, D.B. and Sinkjær, T., *Control of Movement for the Physically Disabled*. Springer, London, 2000.

2. Salmons, S., Ashley, H. et al., FES of denervated muscles: Basic issues. In Bijak, M., Mayr, W., and Pichler, M. (eds.) *Proceedings of 8th International Workshop on FES*, Vienna, Austria, Sept. 10–13, pp. 52–57, 2004.

3. Kern, H., Mödlin, M., and Fostner, C., The RISE patient study: FES in the treatment of flaccid paraplegia. In: Bijak, M., Mayr, W., and Pichler, M. (eds.) *Proceedings of 8th International Workshop on FES*, Vienna, Austria, Sept. 10–13, pp. 27–31, 2004.

4. Popović-Bijelić, A., Bijelić, G. et al., Multi-field surface electrode for selective electrical stimulation. In: Bijak, M., Mayr, W., and Pichler, M. (eds.) *Proceedings of 8th International Workshop on FES*, Vienna, Austria, Sept. 10–13, pp. 195–198, 2004.

5. Popović, M.B. and Popović, D.B., Hierarchical hybrid control for therapeutic electrical stimulation of upper extremities. In: Bijak, M., Mayr, W., and Pichler, M. (eds.) *Proceedings of 8th International Workshop on FES*, Vienna, Austria, Sept. 10–13, pp. 142–145, 2004.

6. Loeb, G., Implantable device having an electrolytic storage electrode, United States Patent 5,312,439, www.uspto.gov/patfv/index.html, 1994.

7. Schulman, J. et al., Implantable microstimulator, United States Patent 5,324,316, www.uspto.gov/patfv/index.html, 1995.

8. Cameron, T., Loeb, G.E., Peck, R. et al., Micromodular implants to provide electrical stimulation of paralyzed muscles and limbs, *IEEE Trans. Biomed. Eng.* BME-44: 781–790, 1997.

9. Nathan, R., Device for generating hand function, Patent application 5,330,516, www.uspto.gov/patfv/index.html, 1994.

10. Peckham, P.H. et al., Functional neuromuscular stimulation system, United States Patent 5,167,229. www.uspto.gov/patfv/index.html, 1992.

11. Sinkjær, T. and Popović, D.B., Functional electrical therapy systems (FETS). United States Patent Application US2004147975, www.uspto.gov/patfv/index.html, 2004.

12. Popović, D.B., Popović, M.B., Sinkjær, T., Stefanović, A., and Schwirtlich, L., Therapy of paretic arm in hemiplegic subjects augmented with a neural prosthesis: A cross-over study, *Can. J. Physio. Pharmacol.* 82: 749–756, 2004.

13. Buckett, J.R., Peckham, H.P. et al., A flexible, portable system for neuro-muscular stimulation in the paralyzed upper extremities, *IEEE Trans. Biomed. Eng.* BME-35: 897–904, 1988.

14. Handa, Y., Handa, T. et al., Functional electrical stimulation (FES) systems for restoration of motor function of paralyzed muscles—Versatile systems and a portable system, *Front. Med. Biol. Eng.* 4: 241–255, 1992.

15. Nathan, R.H., Control strategies in FNS systems for the upper extremities, *Crit. Rev. Biomed. Eng.* 21: 485–568, 1993.

16. Hoshimiya, N., Naito, N., Yajima, M., and Handa, Y., A multichannel FES system for the restoration of motor functions in high spinal cord injury patients: A respiration-controlled system for multijoint upper extremity, *IEEE Trans. Biomed. Eng.* BME-36: 754–760, 1989.

17. Popović, D., Popović, M. et al., Clinical evaluation of the Belgrade grasping system. *Proceedings of 5th Vienna International Workshop on Functional Electrical Stimulation*, Vienna, 1998.

18. Prochazka, A., Gauthier, M., Wieler, M., and Kenwell, Z., The Bionic glove: An electrical stimulator garment that provides controlled grasp and hand opening in quadriplegia, *Arch. Phys. Med. Rehabil.* 78: 608–614, 1997.

19. Reberšek, S. and Vodovnik, L., Proportionally controlled functional electrical stimulation of hand, *Arch. Phys. Med. Rehabil.* 54: 378–382, 1973.

20. Nathan, R., Handmaster NMS—Present technology and the next generation. In: Popović, D. (ed.) *Proceedings of 2nd International Symposium on FES*, Burnaby, pp. 139–140, 1997.

21. Long, C. II and Masciarelli, C.V., An electrophysiologic splint for the hand, *Arch. Phys. Med. Rehabil.* 44: 499–503, 1963.
22. Rudel, D., Bajd, T., Reberšek, S., and Vodovnik, L., FES assisted manipulation in quadriplegic patients. In: Popović, D. (ed.) *Advances in External Control of Human Extremities VIII*, pp. 273–282, ETAN, Belgrade, 1984.
23. Ijzerman, M., Stoffers, T. et al., The NESS Handmaster orthosis: Restoration of hand function in C5 and stroke patients by means of electrical stimulation, *J. Rehab. Sci.* 9: 86–89, 1996.
24. Popović, D., Stojanović, A. et al., Clinical evaluation of the Bionic glove, *Arch. Phys. Med. Rehabil.* 80: 299–304, 1999.
25. Keller, T., Curt, A. et al., Grasping in high lesioned tetraplegic subjects using the EMG controlled neural prosthesis, *J. NeuroRehab.* 10: 251–255, 1998.
26. Popović, M.R., Keller, T. et al., Surface stimulation technology for grasping and walking neural prosthesis, *IEEE Eng. Med. Biol. Mag.* 20: 82–93, 2001.
27. Keller, T. and Popović, M.R., Real-time stimulation artifact removal in EMG signals for neural prosthesis control applications. *Proceedings of 6th Annual IFESS Conference*, Cleveland, OH, June 10–13, pp. 208–210, 2001.
28. Holländer, H.J., Huber, M., and Vossius, G., An EMG controlled multichannel stimulator. In: Popović, D. (ed.) *Advances in External Control of Human Extremities IX*, pp. 291–295, Published by ETAN, Belgrade, 1987.
29. Sennels, S., Biering-Soerensen, F., Anderson, O.T., and Hansen, S.D., Functional neuromuscular stimulation control by surface electromyographic signals produced by volitional activation of the same muscle: Adaptive removal of the muscle response from the recorded EMG-signal, *IEEE Trans. Rehab. Eng.* TRE-5:195: 206, 1997.
30. Saxena, S., Nikolić, S., and Popović, D., An EMG controlled FES system for grasping in tetraplegics, *J. Rehabil. Res. Dev.* 32: 17–23, 1995.
31. Hoshimiya, N. and Handa, Y., A master-slave type multichannel functional electrical stimulation (FES) system for the control of the paralyzed upper extremities, *Automedica* 11: 209–220, 1989.
32. Takahashi, K., Hoshimiya, N., Matsuki, H., and Handa, Y., Externally powered implantable FES system, *Jap. J. Med. Electron. Biol. Eng.* 37: 43–51, 1999.
33. *The Neurocontrol Freehand System, Manual, NeuroControl*, Cleveland, OH, USA, 1998.
34. Hart, R.L., Kilgore, K.L., and Peckham, P.H., A comparison between control methods for implanted FES hand-grasp systems, *IEEE Trans. Rehab. Eng.* 6: 208–218, 1998.
35. Kilgore, K.L., Peckham, P.H. et al., An implanted upper-extremity neural prosthesis: Follow-up of five patients, *J. Bone Joint Surg. Am.* 79: 533–541, 1997.
36. Grill, J.H. and Peckham, P.H., Functional neuromuscular stimulation for combined control of elbow extension and hand grasp in C5 and C6 quadriplegics, *IEEE Trans. Rehab. Eng.* TRE-6: 190–199, 1998.
37. Crago, P.E., Memberg, W.D., Usey, M.K. et al., An elbow extension neuroprosthesis for individuals with tetraplegia, *IEEE Trans. Rehab. Eng.* TRE-6: 1–6, 1998.
38. Johnson, M.W. and Peckham, P.H., Evaluation of shoulder movement as a command control source, *IEEE Trans. Biomed. Eng.* BME-37: 876–885, 1990.
39. Smith, B.T., Mulcahey, M.J., and Betz, R.R., Development of an upper extremity FES system for individuals with C4 tetraplegia, *IEEE Trans. Rehab. Eng.* TRE-4: 264–270, 1996.
40. Scott, T.R.D., Peckham, P.H., and Kilgore, K.L., Tri-state myoelectric control of bilateral upper extremity neuroprosthesis for tetraplegic individuals, *IEEE Trans. Rehab. Eng.* TRE-4: 251–263, 1996.
41. Haugland, M., Lickel, A., Haase, J., and Sinkjær, T., Control of FES thumb force using slip information obtained from the cutaneous electroneurogram in quadriplegic man, *IEEE Trans. Rehab. Eng.* TRE-7: 215–227, 1999.
42. Haugland, M.K. and Hoffer, J.A., Slip information provided by nerve cuff signals: Application in closed-loop control of functional electrical stimulation, *IEEE Trans. Rehab. Eng.* TRE-2: 29–37, 1994.

43. Haugland, M.K., Hoffer, J.A., and Sinkjaer, T., Skin contact force information in sensory nerve signals recorded by implanted cuff electrodes, *IEEE Trans. Rehab. Eng.* TRE-2: 18–27, 1994.

44. Kralj, A. and Bajd, T., *Functional Electrical Stimulation, Standing and Walking after Spinal Cord Injury*, CRC Press, Boca Raton, FL, 1989.

45. Andrews, B.J., Baxendale, R.H. et al., Hybrid FES orthosis incorporating closed loop control and sensory feedback, *J. Biomed. Eng.* 10: 189–195, 1988.

46. Brindley, G.S., Polkey, C.E., and Rushton, D.N., Electrical splinting of the knee in paraplegia, *Paraplegia* 16: 428–435, 1978.

47. Jaeger, R., Yarkony, G.Y., and Smith, R., Standing the spinal cord injured patient by electrical stimulation: Refinement of a protocol for clinical use, *IEEE Trans. Biomed. Eng.* BME-36: 720–728, 1989.

48. Mizrahi, J., Braun, Z., Najenson, T., and Graupe, D., Quantitative weight bearing and gait evaluation of paraplegics using functional electrical stimulation, *Med. Biol. Eng. Comput.* 23: 101–107, 1985.

49. Petrofsky, J.S. and Phillips, C.A., Computer controlled walking in the paralyzed individual, *J. Neurol. Orthop. Surg.* 4: 153–164, 1983.

50. Solomonow, M., Biomechanics and physiology of a practical powered walking orthosis for paraplegics. In: Stein, R.B., Peckham, H.P., and Popović, D. (eds.) *Neural Prostheses: Replacing Motor Function after Disease or Disability*, Oxford University Press, New York, pp. 202–230, 1992.

51. Thoma, H., Frey, M. et al., Functional neurostimulation to substitute locomotion in paraplegia patients, In: Andrade, D. et al. (eds.), *Artificial Organs*, VCH Publishers, pp. 515–529, 1987.

52. Gračanin, F., Prevec, T., and Trontelj, J., Evaluation of use of functional electronic peroneal brace in hemiparetic patients. In *Advances in External Control of Human Extremities III*, ETAN, Belgrade, pp. 198–210, 1967.

53. Liberson, W.T., Holmquest, H.J., Scott, D., and Dow, A., Functional electrotherapy. Stimulation of the peroneal nerve synchronized with the swing phase of the gait of hemiplegic patients, *Arch. Phys. Med. Rehab.* 42: 101–105, 1961.

54. Burridge, J.H., Taylor, P.N. et al., The effect of common peroneal stimulation on the effort and speed of walking. A randomised controlled trial of chronic hemiplegic patients, *Clin. Rehab.* 11: 201–210, 1997.

55. Taylor, P.N., Burridge, J.H. et al., Clinical use of the Odstock dropped foot stimulator: Its effect on the speed and effort of walking, *Arch. Phys. Med. Rehab.* 80: 1577–1583, 1999.

56. Waters, R.L., McNeal, D.R., Fallon, W., and Clifford, B., Functional electrical stimulation of the peroneal nerve for hemiplegia, *J. Bone Joint Surg.* 67: 792–793, 1985.

57. Dai, R., Stein, R.B. et al., Application of tilt sensors in functional electrical stimulation, *IEEE Trans. Rehab. Eng.* TRE-4: 63–72, 1996.

58. Taylor, P., Burridge, J.H. et al., Clinical audit of 5 years provision of the Odstock dropped foot stimulator, *Artif. Organs* 23: 440–442, 1999.

59. Childs, C., *Application of Selective Stimulation in Human Peripheral Nerves*, PhD thesis, Aalborg University, Denmark, 2004.

60. Marsolais, E.B. and Kobetic, R., Implantation techniques and experience with percutaneous intramuscular electrode in the lower extremities, *J. Rehab. Res.* 23: 1–8, 1987.

61. Kobetic, R. and Marsolais, E.B., Synthesis of paraplegic gait with multichannel functional electrical stimulation, *IEEE Trans. Rehab. Eng.* TRE-2: 66–79, 1994.

62. Abbas, J.J. and Triolo, R.J., Experimental evaluation of an adaptive feedforward controller for use in functional neuromuscular stimulation systems, *IEEE Trans. Rehab. Eng.* TRE-5: 12–22, 1997.

63. Cameron, T., Liinama, T., Loeb, G.E., and Richmond, F.J.R., Long term biocompatibility of a miniature stimulator implanted in feline hind limb muscles, *IEEE Trans. Biomed. Eng.* BME-45: 1024–1035, 1998.

64. Cameron, T., Richmond, F.J.R., and Loeb, G.E., Effects of regional stimulation using a miniature stimulator implanted in feline posterior biceps femoris, *IEEE Trans. Biomed. Eng.* BME-45: 1036–1045, 1998.

65. Strojnik, P., Whitmoyer, D., and Schulman, J., An implantable stimulator for all season, In: Popović, D. (ed.) *Advances in External Control of Human Extremities X*, Nauka, Belgrade, pp. 335–344, 1990.
66. Ziaie, B., Nardin, M.D., Coghlan, A.R., and Najafi, K., A single channel implantable microstimulator for functional neuromuscular stimulation, *IEEE Trans. Biomed. Eng.* BME-44: 909–920, 1997.
67. Haugland, M.K., A miniature implantable nerve stimulator. In: Popović, D. (ed.) *Proceedings of 2nd International Symposium on FES*, Burnaby, pp. 221–222, 1997.
68. Houdayer, T., Davis, R. et al., Prolonged closed-loop standing in paraplegia with implanted cochlear FES-22 stimulator and Andrews ankle-foot orthosis. In: Popović, D. (ed.) *Proceedings of 2nd International Symposium on FES*, Burnaby, pp. 168–169, 1997.
69. Andrews, B.J., Baxendale, R.M. et al., A hybrid orthosis for paraplegics incorporating feedback control. In *Advances in External Control of Human Extremities IX*, ETAN, Belgrade, pp. 297–310, 1987.
70. Popović, D., Tomović, R., and Schwirtlich, L., Hybrid assistive system—Neuroprosthesis for motion, *IEEE Trans. Biomed. Eng.* BME-37: 729–738, 1989.
71. Solomonow, M., Baratta, R. et al., Evaluation of 70 paraplegics fitted with the LSU RGO/FES. In Popović, D. (ed.) *Proceedings of 2nd International Symposium on FES*, Burnaby, p. 159, 1997.
72. Andrews, B.J., Barnett, R.W. et al., Rule-based control of a hybrid FES orthosis for assisting paraplegic locomotion, *Automedica* 11: 175–199, 1989.
73. Schwirtlich, L. and Popović, D., Hybrid orthoses for deficient locomotion. In: Popović, D. (ed.) *Advances in External Control of Human Extremities VIII*, ETAN, Belgrade, pp. 23–32, 1984.
74. Phillips, C.A., An interactive system of electronic stimulators and gait orthosis for walking in the spinal cord injured, *Automedica* 11: 247–261, 1989.
75. Popović, D., Schwirtlich, L., and Radosavljević, S., Powered hybrid assistive system. In Popović, D. (ed.) *Advances in External Control of Human Extremities X*, Nauka, Belgrade, pp. 191–200, 1990.
76. Goldfarb, M. and Durfee, W.K., Design of a controlled-brake orthosis for FES-aided gait, *IEEE Trans. Rehab. Eng.* TRE-4: 13–24, 1996.
77. Irby, S.E., Kaufman, K.R., and Sutherland, D.H., A digital logic controlled electromechanical long leg brace. In *Proceedings of 15th Southern Biomedical Engineering Conference*, Dayton, OH, p. 28, 1996.
78. Kaufman, K.R., Irby, S.E., Mathewson, J.W. et al., Energy efficient knee-ankle-foot orthosis, *J. Prosthet. Orthot.* 8: 79–85, 1996.
79. Inman, V.T., Ralston, J.J., and Todd, F., *Human Walking*. Williams & Wilkins, Baltimore, London, 1981.
80. Doane, N.E. and Holt, L.E., A comparison of the SACH foot and single axis foot in the gait of the unilateral below-knee amputee, *Prosthet. Orthot. Int.* 7: 33–36, 1983.
81. Wagner, E.M. and Catranis, J.G., New developments in lower-extremity prostheses. In: Klopsteg, P.E., Wilson, P.D. et al. (eds.) *Human Limbs and Their Substitutes*, McGraw-Hill Book Company, New York, (Reprinted 1968), 1954.
82. Michael, J.W., Modern prosthetic knee mechanisms, *Clin. Orthop. Relat. Res.* 361: 39–47, 1999.
83. The adaptive prosthesis: For transfemoral amputees. From http://www. blatchford.co.uk/products/products.
84. Pike, A., The new high tech prostheses. From www.amputee-coalition.orq/inmotion/mav iun 99/hitech.html
85. Schuch, C.M., A guide to lower limb prosthetics. Part I— Prosthetic design: Basic concepts. From www.amputeecoalition.orq/inmotion/mar apr 98/pros primer/paqe2.html
86. 3C100 C-leg system. New generation leg system revolutionizes lower limb prosthesis. From www. ottobockus.com/products/op lower cleg.asp
87. James, K., Stein, R.B., Rolf, R., and Tepavac, D., Active suspension above-knee prosthesis. In: Goh, D. and Nathan, A. (eds.) *Proceedings of 6th International Conference on Biomedical Engineering*, pp. 317–320, 1991.

88. Tomović, R., Popović, D., Turajlić S., and McGhee, R.B., Bioengineering actuator with non-numerical control. In *Proceedings of IFAC Conference Orthotics and Prosthetics*, Columbus, OH, Pergamon Press, pp. 145–151, 1982.

89. Popović, D. and Schwirtlich, L., Belgrade active *A/K* prosthesis. In: deVries J. (ed.) *Electrophysiological Kinesiology*, Excerpta Medica, Amsterdam, *Intern. Cong. Ser*, 804: 337–343, 1988.

90. Simpson, D.C., The choice of control system for the multi-movement prosthesis: Extended physiological proprioception (EPP). In *The Control of Upper-Extremity Prostheses and Orthoses,* Chapter 15, pp. 146–150, 1973.

91. Sheridan, T.B. and Mann, R.W., Design of control devices for people with severe motor impairment, *Hum. Factors* 20: 312–338, 1978.

92. Jacobsen, S.C., Knutti, F.F., Johnson, R.T., and Sears, H.H., Development of the Utah artificial arm, *IEEE Trans. Biomed. Eng.* BME-29: 249–269, 1982.

93. Gibbons, D.T., O'Riain, M.D., and Philippe-Auguste, J.S., An above-elbow prosthesis employing programmed linkages, *IEEE Trans. Biomed. Eng.* BME-34: 251–258, 1987.

94. Kyberd, P.J., Holland, O.E., Chappel, P.H. et al., MARCUS: A two degree of freedom hand prosthesis with hierarchical grip control, *IEEE Trans. Rehab. Eng.* TRE-3: 70–76, 1995.

95. Park, E. and Meek, S.G., Adaptive filtering of the electromyographic signal for prosthetic and force estimation, *IEEE Trans. Biomed. Eng.* BME-42: 1044–1052, 1995.

96. Kurtz, I., Programmable prosthetic controller. In *Proceedings of MEC '97*, Frederciton, NB, p. 33, 1997.

97. Bertos, Y.A., Hechathorne, C.H., Weir, R.F., and Childress, D.S., Microprocessor based EPP position controller for electric powered upper limb prostheses. In *Proceedings of IEEE International Conference on EMBS*, Chicago, 1997.

Further Reading

Agnew, W.V. and McCreery, D.B., *Neural Prostheses: Fundamental Studies*, Prentice-Hall, Englewood Cliffs, NJ, 1990.

Dhilon, G. and Horch, K. (eds.). *Neuroprosthetics: Theory and Practice*, World Science Publications, 2004.

Popović, D. (ed.). *Advances in External Control of Human Extremities I-X*, Aalborg University, 2002, ISSN (Electronic version of the 10 Proceedings from Dubrovnik meetings, 1963–1990).

Popović, D. and Sinkjær, T., *Control of Movement for the Physically Disabled*, Springer, 2000.

Stein, R.B., Peckham, H.P., and Popović, D., *Neural Prostheses: Replacing Motor Function after Disease or Disability*, Oxford University Press, New York, 1992.

46

Sensory Augmentation and Substitution

Kurt A. Kaczmarek
*University of Wisconsin,
Madison*

This chapter will consider methods and devices used to present visual, auditory, and tactual (touch) information to persons with sensory deficits. *Sensory augmentation systems* such as eyeglasses and hearing aids enhance the existing capabilities of a functional human sensory system. *Sensory substitution* is the use of one human sense to receive information normally received by another sense. Braille and speech synthesizers are examples of systems that substitute touch and hearing, respectively, for information that is normally visual (printed or displayed text).

The following three sections will provide theory and examples for aiding the visual, auditory, and tactual systems. Because capitalizing on an *existing* sensory capability is usually superior to substitution, each section will consider first augmentation and then substitution, as shown below:

Human Sensory Systems

Visual	Auditory	Tactual
Visual augmentation	Auditory augmentation	Tactual augmentation
Tactual vision substitution	Visual auditory substitution	Tactual substitution
Auditory vision substitution	Tactual auditory substitution	

46.1 Visual System

With a large number of receptive channels, the human visual system processes information in a parallel fashion. A single glimpse acquires a wealth of information; the field of view for two eyes is 180° horizontally and 120° vertically (Mehr and Shindell, 1990). The spatial resolution in the central (foveal) part of the visual field is approximately 0.5–1.0 min of arc (Shlaer, 1937), although Vernier acuity, the specialized task of detecting a misalignment of two lines placed end to end, is much finer, approximately 2 s of arc (Stigmar, 1970). Low-contrast presentations substantially reduce visual acuity.

The former resolution figure is the basis for the standard method of testing visual acuity, the Snellen chart. Letters are considered to be "readable" if they subtend approximately 5 min of arc and have details one-fifth this size. Snellen's 1862 method of reporting visual performance is still used today. The ratio 20/40, for instance, indicates that a test was conducted at 20 ft and that the letters that were recognizable at that distance would subtend 5 min of arc of 40 ft (the distance at which a normally sighted, or "20/20," subject could read them). Although the standard testing distance is 20, 10 and even 5 ft may be used, under certain conditions, for more severe visual impairments (Fonda, 1981).

Of the approximately 6–11.4 million people in the United States who have visual impairments, 90% have some useful vision (NIDRR, 1993). In the United States, *severe visual impairment* is defined to be 20/70 vision in the better eye with best refractive correction (see below). Legal blindness means that the best corrected acuity is 20/200 or that the field of view is very narrow (<20°). People over 65 years of age account for 46% of the legally blind and 68% of the severely visually impaired. For those with some useful vision, a number of useful techniques and devices for visual augmentation can allow performance of many everyday activities.

46.1.1 Visual Augmentation

People with certain eye disorders see better with higher- or lower-than-normal light levels; an **illuminance** from 100 to 4000 lx may promote comfortable reading (Fonda, 1981). Ideal illumination is diffuse and directed from the side at a 45-degree angle to prevent glare. The surrounding room is preferably 20–50% darker than the object of interest.

Refractive errors cause difficulties in focusing on an object at a given distance from the eye (Mountcastle, 1980). Myopia (near-sightedness), hyperopia (far-sightedness), astigmatism (focus depth that varies with radial orientation), and presbyopia (loss of ability to adjust focus, manifested as far-sightedness) are the most common vision defects. These normally can be corrected with appropriate eyeglasses or contact lenses and are rarely the cause of a disability.

Magnification is the most useful form of image processing for vision defects that do not respond to refractive correction. The simplest form of image magnification is getting closer; halving the distance to an object doubles its size. Magnifications up to 20 times are possible with minimal loss of field of view. At very close range, eyeglasses or a loupe may be required to maintain focus (Fonda, 1981). Hand or stand magnifiers held 18–40 cm (not critical) from the eye create a virtual image that increases rapidly in size as the object-to-lens distance approaches the focal length of the lens. Lenses are rated in diopters ($D = 1/f$, where f is the focal length of the lens in centimeters). The useful range is approximately 4–20 D; more powerful lenses are generally held close to the eye as a loupe, as just mentioned, to enhance field of view. For distance viewing, magnification of 2–10 times can be achieved with hand-held telescopes at the expense of a reduced field of view.

Closed-circuit television (CCTV) systems magnify print and small objects up to 60 times, with higher effective magnifications possible by close viewing. Users with vision as poor as 1/400 (20/8000) may be able to read ordinary print with CCTV (Fonda, 1981). Some recent units are portable and contain black/white image reversal and contrast enhancement features.

Electrical (or, more recently, magnetic) stimulation of the visual cortex produces perceived spots of light called *phosphenes*. Some attempts, summarized in Webster et al. (1985), have been made to map these sensations and display identifiable patterns, but the phosphenes often do not correspond spatially with the specific location on the visual cortex. Although the risk and cost of this technique do not yet justify the minimal "vision" obtained, future use cannot be ruled out.

46.1.2 Tactual Vision Substitution

With sufficient training, people without useful vision can acquire sufficient information via the tactile sense for many activities of daily living, such as walking independently and reading. The traditional long cane, for example, allows navigation by transmitting surface profile, roughness, and elasticity to the hand. Interestingly, these features are *perceived* to originate at the tip of the cane, not the hand where they are transduced; this is a simple example of *distal attribution* (Loomis, 1992). Simple electronic aids such as the hand-held Mowat sonar sensor provide a tactile indication of range to the nearest object.

Braille reading material substitutes raised-dot patterns on 2.3-mm centers for visual letters, enabling reading rates up to 30–40 words per minute (wpm). Contracted Braille uses symbols for common words and affixes, enabling reading at up to 200 wpm (125 wpm is more typical).

More sophisticated instrumentation also capitalizes on the spatial capabilities of the tactile sense. The Optacon (optical-to-tactile converter) by TeleSensory, Inc. (Mountain View, Calif.) converts the outline of printed letters recorded by a small, hand-held camera to enlarged *vibrotactile* letter outlines on the user's fingerpad. The camera's field of view is divided into 100 or 144 pixels (depending on the model), and the reflected light intensity at each pixel determines whether a corresponding vibrating pin on the fingertip is active or not. Ordinary printed text can be read at 28 (typical) or 90 (exceptional) wpm.

Spatial orientation and recognition of objects beyond the reach of a hand or long cane are the objective of experimental systems that convert an image from a television-type camera to a matrix of *electrotactile* or vibrotactile stimulators on the abdomen, forehead, or fingertip. With training, the user can interpret the patterns of tingling or buzzing pints to identify simple, high-contrast objects in front of the camera, as well as experience visual phenomena such as looming, perspective, parallax, and distal attribution (Bach-y-Rita, 1972; Collins, 1985).

Access to graphic or spatial information that cannot be converted into text is virtually impossible for blind computer users. Several prototype devices have been built to display computer graphics to the fingers via vibrating or stationary pins. A fingertip-scanned display tablet with embedded electrodes, under development in our laboratory (Kaczmarek et al., 1997), eliminates all moving parts; ongoing tests will determine if the spatial performance and reliability are adequate.

46.1.3 Auditory Vision Substitution

Electronic speech synthesizers allow access to electronic forms of text storage and manipulation. Until the arrival of graphic user interfaces such as those in the Apple Macintosh® and Microsoft Windows® computer-operating systems, information displayed on computer screens was largely text based. A number of products appeared that converted the screen information to speech at rates of up to 500 wpm, thereby giving blind computer users rapid access to the information revolution. Fortunately, much of the displayed information in graphic-operating systems is not essentially pictorial; the dozen or so common graphic features (e.g., icons, scroll bars, and buttons) can be converted to a limited set of words, which can then be spoken. Because of the way information is stored in these systems, however, the screen-to-text conversion process is much more complex, and the use of essentially spatial control features such as the mouse await true spatial display methods (Boyd et al., 1990).

Automated optical character recognition (OCR) combined with speech synthesis grants access to the most common printed materials (letters, office memorandums, and bills), which are seldom available in Braille or narrated-tape format. First popularized in the Kurzweil reading machine, this marriage of technologies is combined with a complex set of lexical, phonetic, and syntactic rules to produce understandable speech from a wide variety of, but not all, print styles.

Mobility of blind individuals is complicated, especially in unfamiliar territory, by hazards that cannot be easily sensed with a long cane, such as overhanging tree limbs. A few devices have appeared that convert the output of sonar-like ultrasonic ranging sensors to discriminable audio displays. For example, the Wormald Sonicguide uses interaural intensity differences to indicate the azimuth of an object and frequency to indicate distance (Cook, 1982); subtle information such as texture can sometimes also be discriminated.

46.2 Auditory System

The human auditory system processes information primarily serially; having at best two receptive channels, spatial information must be built up by integration over time. This latter capability, however, is profound. Out of a full orchestra, a seasoned conductor can pinpoint an errant violinist by sound alone.

Human hearing is sensitive to sound frequencies from approximately 16 to 20,000 Hz and is most sensitive at 1000 Hz. At this frequency, a threshold root-mean-square pressure of 20 Pa (200 µbar) can be perceived by normally hearing young adults under laboratory conditions. Sound pressure level (SPL) is measured in decibels relative to this threshold. Some approximate benchmarks for sound intensity are a whisper at 1 m (30 dB), normal conversion at 1 m (60 dB), and a subway train at 6 m (90 dB). Sounds increasing from 100 to 140 dB become uncomfortable and painful, and short exposures to a 160-dB level can cause permanent hearing impairment, while continuous exposure to sound levels over 90 dB can cause slow, cumulative damage (Sataloff et al., 1980).

Because hearing sensitivity falls off drastically at lower frequencies, clinical audiometric testing uses somewhat different scales. With the DIN/ANSI reference threshold of 6.5 dB SPL at 1 kHz, the threshold rises to 24.5 dB at 250 Hz and 45.5 dB at 125 Hz (Sataloff et al., 1980). Hearing loss is then specified in decibels relative to the reference threshold, rather than the SPL directly, so that a normal audiogram would have a flat threshold curve at approximately 0 dB.

46.2.1 Auditory Augmentation

Loss of speech comprehension, and hence interpersonal communication, bears the greatest effect on daily life and is the main reason people seek medical attention for hearing impairment. Functional impairment begins with 21- to 35-dB loss in average sensitivity, causing difficulty in understanding faint speech (Smeltzer, 1993). Losses of 36–50 dB and 51–70 dB cause problems with normal and loud speech. Losses greater than 90 dB are termed *profound* or *extreme* and cannot be remedied with any kind of hearing aid; these individuals require auditory substitution rather than augmentation.

Hearing loss can be caused by conduction defects in the middle ear (tympanic membrane and ossicles) or by sensorineural defects in the inner ear (cochlear transduction mechanisms and auditory nerve). Conduction problems often can be corrected medically or surgically. If not, hearing aids are often of benefit because the hearing threshold is elevated uniformly over all frequencies, causing little distortion of the signal. Sensorineural impairments differentially affect different frequencies and also cause other forms of distortion that cannot be helped by amplification or filtering. The dynamic range is also reduced, because while loud sounds (>100 dB) are often still perceived as loud, slightly softer sounds are lost. Looked at from this perspective, it is easy to understand why the amplification and automatic gain control of conventional hearing aids do not succeed in presenting the 30 dB or so dynamic range of speech to persons with 70 + dB of sensorineural impairment.

Most hearing aids perform three basic functions. (1) Amplification compensates for the reduced sensitivity of the damaged ear. (2) Frequency-domain filtering compensates for hearing loss that is not spectrally uniform. For example, most sensorineural loss disproportionately affects frequencies over 1 kHz or so; so, high-frequency preemphasis may be indicated. (3) Automatic gain control (ACG) compresses the amplitude range of desired sounds to the dynamic range of the damaged ear. Typical AGC systems respond to loud transients in 2–5 ms (attack time) and reduce their effect in 100–300 ms (recovery time).

Sophisticated multiband AGC systems have attempted to normalize the ear's amplitude/frequency response, with the goal of preserving intact the usual intensity relationships among speech elements. However, recent research has shown that only certain speech features are important for intelligibility (Moore, 1990). The fundamental frequency (due to vocal cord vibration), the first and second formants (the spectral peaks of speech that characterize different vowels), and place of articulation are crucial to speech recognition. In contrast, the overall speech envelope (the contour connecting the individual peaks in the pressure wave) is not very important; articulation information is carried in second-formant and high-frequency spectral information and is not well represented in the envelope (Van Tasell, 1993). Therefore, the primary design goal for hearing aids should be to preserve and make audible the individual spectral components of speech (formants and high-frequency consonant information).

The cochlear implant could properly be termed an auditory augmentation device because it utilizes the higher neural centers normally used for audition. Simply stated, the implant replaces the function of the (damaged) inner ear by electrically stimulating the auditory nerve in response to sound collected by an external microphone. Although the auditory percepts produced are extremely distorted and noise-like due to the inadequate coding strategy, many users gain sufficient information to improve their lipreading and speech-production skills. The introductory chapter in this section provides a detailed discussion of this technology.

46.2.2 Visual Auditory Substitution

Lipreading is the most natural form of auditory substitution, requiring no instrumentation and no training on the part of the speaker. However, only about one-third to one-half of the 36 or so phonemes (primary sounds of human speech) can be reliably discriminated by this method. The result is that 30–50% of the words used in conversational English look just like, or very similar to, other words (homophones) (Becker, 1972). Therefore, word pairs such as buried/married must be discriminated by grammar, syntax, and context.

Lipreading does not provide information on voice, fundamental frequency, or formants. With an appropriate hearing aid, any residual hearing (<90-dB loss) often can supply some of this missing information, improving lipreading accuracy. For the profoundly deaf, technological devices are available to supply some or all of the information. For example, the Upton eyeglasses, an example of a cued-speech device, provide discrete visual signals for certain speech sounds such as fricatives (letters like *f* of *s*, containing primarily high-frequency information) that cannot be readily identified by sight.

Fingerspelling, a transliteration of English alphabet into hand symbols, can convey everyday words at up to 2 syllables per second, limited by the rate of manual symbol production (Reed et al., 1990). American sign language uses a variety of upper-body movements to convey words and concepts rather than just individual letters, at the same effective rate as ordinary speech, 4–5 syllables per second.

Closed captioning encodes the full text of spoken words on television shows and transmits these data in a nonvisible part of the video signal (the vertical blanking interval). Since July of 1993, all new television sets sold in the United States with screens larger than 33 cm diagonal have been required to have built-in decoders that can optionally display the encoded text on the screen. Over 1000 h per week of programming is closed captioned (National Captioning Institute, Falls Church, VA, 1994, personal communication.).

Automatic speech-recognition technology may soon be capable of translating ordinary spoken discourse accurately into visually displayed text, at least in quiet environments; this may eventually be a major boon for the profoundly hearing impaired. Presently, such systems must be carefully trained on individual speakers and/or must have a limited vocabulary (Ramesh et al., 1992). Because there is much commercial interest in speech command of computers and vehicle subsystems, this field is advancing rapidly.

46.2.3 Tactual Auditory Substitution

Tadoma is a method of communication used by a few people in the deaf–blind community and is of theoretical importance for the development of tactual auditory substitution devices. While sign language requires training by both sender and receiver, in Tadoma, the sender speaks normally. The trained receiver places his or her hands on the face and neck of the sender to monitor lip and jaw movements, airflow at the lips, and vibration of the neck (Reed et al., 1992). Experienced users achieve 80% keyword recognition of everyday speech at a rate of 3 syllables per second. Using no instrumentation, this is the highest speech communication rate recorded for any tactual-only communication system.

Alternatively, tactile vocoders perform a frequency analysis of incoming sounds, similar to the ear's cochlea (Békésy, 1955), and adjust the stimulation intensity of typically 8–32 tactile stimulators (vibrotactile or electrotactile) to present a linear spectral display to the user's abdominal or forehead skin. Several investigators (Blamey and Clark, 1985; Boothroyd and Hnath-Chisolm, 1988, Brooks and Frost, 1986; Saunders et al., 1981) have developed laboratory and commercial vocoders. Although vocoder users cannot recognize speech as well as Tadoma users, research has shown that vocoders can provide enough "auditory" feedback to improve the speech clarity of deaf children and to improve auditory discrimination and comprehension in some older patients (Szeto and Riso, 1990) and aid in discrimination of phonemes by lipreading (Hughes, 1989; Rakowski et al., 1989). An excellent review of earlier vocoders appears in Reed et al. (1982). The most useful information provided by vocoders appears to be the second-formant frequency (important for distinguishing vowels) and position of the high-frequency plosive and fricative sounds that often delineate syllables (Bernstein et al., 1991).

46.3 Tactual System

Humans receive and combine two types of perceptual information when touching and manipulating objects. *Kinesthetic* information describes the relative positions and movements of body parts as well as muscular effort. Muscle and skin receptors are primarily responsible for kinesthesis; joint receptors serve primarily as protective limit switches (Rabischong, 1981). Tactile information describes spatial pressure patterns on the skin given a fixed body position. Everyday touch perception combines tactile and kinesthetic information; this combination is called *tactual* or *haptic perception*. Loomis and Lederman (1986) provide an excellent review of these perceptual mechanisms.

Geldard (1960) and Sherrick (1973) lamented that as a communication channel, the tactile sense is often considered inferior to sight and hearing. However, the tactile system possesses some of the same spatial and temporal attributes as both of the "primary" senses (Bach-y-Rita, 1972). With over 10,000 parallel channels (receptors) (Collins and Saunders, 1970), the tactile system is capable of processing a great deal of information if it is properly presented.

The human kinesthetic and tactile senses are very robust and, in the case of tactile, very redundant. This is fortunate, considering their necessity for the simplest of tasks. Control of movement depends on kinesthetic information; tremors and involuntary movements can result from disruption of this feedback control system. Surgically repaired fingers may not have tactile sensation for a long period or at all, depending on the severity of nerve injuries; it is known that insensate digits are rarely used by patients (Tubiana, 1988). Insensate fingers and toes (due to advanced Hansen's disease or diabetes) are often injured inadvertently, sometimes requiring amputation. Anyone who has had a finger numbed by cold realizes that it can be next to useless, even if the range of motion is normal.

The normal sensitivity to touch varies markedly over the body surface. The threshold forces in dynes for men (women) are lips, 9 (5); fingertips, 62 (25); belly 62 (7); and sole of foot, 343 (79) (Weinstein, 1968). The fingertip threshold corresponds to 10-μm indentation. Sensitivity to vibration is much higher and is frequency- and area dependent (Verillo, 1985). A 5-cm² patch of skin on the palm vibrating at 250 Hz can be felt at 0.16-μm amplitude; smaller areas and lower frequencies require more displacement. The minimal separation for two nonvibrating points to be distinguished is 2–3 mm on the fingertips, 17 mm on the forehead, and 30–50 mm on many other locations. However, size and localization judgments are considerably better than these standard figures might suggest (Vierck and Jones, 1969).

46.3.1 Tactual Augmentation

Although we do not often think about it, kinesthetic information is reflected to the user in many types of human-controlled tools and machines, and lack of this feedback can make control difficult. For example, an automobile with power steering always includes some degree of "road feel" to allow the driver to respond reflexively to minor bumps and irregularities without relying on vision. Remote-control robots (telerobots) used underwater or in chemical- or radiation-contaminated environments are slow and cumbersome to operate, partly because most do not provide force feedback to the operator; such feedback enhances task performance (Hannaford and Wood, 1992).

Tactile display of spatial patterns on the skin uses three main types of transducers (Kaczmarek et al., 1991; Kaczmarek and Bach-y-Rita, 1995). *Static tactile* displays use solenoids, shape–memory alloy actuators, and scanned air or water jets to indent the skin. Vibrotactile displays encode stimulation intensity as the amplitude of a vibrating skin displacement (10–500 Hz); both solenoids and piezoelectric transducers have been used. *Electrotactile* stimulation uses 1–100 mm^2-area surface electrodes and careful waveform control to electrically stimulate the afferent nerves responsible for touch, producing a vibrating or tingling sensation.

Tactile rehabilitation has received minimal attention in the literature or medical community. One research device sensed pressure information normally received by the fingertips and displayed it on the forehead using electrotactile stimulation (Collins and Madey, 1974). Subjects were able to estimate surface roughness and hardness and detect edges and corners with only one sensor per fingertip. Phillips (1988) reviews prototype tactile feedback systems that use the intact tactile sense to convey hand and foot pressure and elbow angle to users of powered prosthetic limbs, often with the result of more precise control of these devices.

Slightly more attention has been given to tactile augmentation in special environments. Astronauts, for example, wear pressurized gloves that greatly diminish tactile sensation, complicating extravehicular repair and maintenance tasks. Efforts to improve the situation range from mobile tactile pins on the fingertips to electrotactile stimulation on the abdomen of the information gathered from fingertip sensors (Bach-y-Rita et al., 1987).

46.3.2 Tactual Substitution

Because of a paucity of adequate tactual display technology, spatial pressure information from a robot or remote manipulator is usually displayed to the operator visually. A three-dimensional bar graph, for example, could show the two-dimensional pressure pattern on the gripper. While easy to implement, this method suffers from two disadvantages (1) the visual channel is required to process more information (it is often already heavily burdened), and (2) reaction time is lengthened, because the normal human tactual reflex systems are inhibited. An advantage of visual display is that accurate measurements of force and pressure may be displayed numerically or graphically.

Auditory display of tactual information is largely limited to warning systems, such as excessive force on a machine. Sometimes such feedback is even inadvertent. The engine of a bulldozer will audibly slow down when a heavy load is lifted; by the auditory and vibratory feedback, the operator can literally "feel" the strain.

The ubiquity of such tactual feedback systems suggests that the human–machine interface on many devices could benefit from intentionally placed tactual feedback systems. Of much current interest is the **virtual environment**, a means by which someone can interact with a mathematical model of a place that may or may not physically exist. The user normally controls the environment by hand, head, and body movements; these are sensed by the system, which correspondingly adjusts the information presented on a wide-angle visual display and sometimes also on a spatially localized sound display. The user often describes the experience as "being there," a phenomenon known as *telepresence* (Loomis, 1992). One can only imagine how much the experience could be enhanced by adding kinesthetic and tactile feedback (Shimoga, 1993), quite literally putting the user in touch with the virtual world.

Defining Terms

Distal attribution: The phenomenon whereby events are normally perceived as occurring external to our sense organs—but also see Loomis' (1992) engaging article on this topic. The environment or transduction mechanism need not be artificial; for example, we visually perceive objects as distant from our eyes.

Electrotactile: Stimulation that evokes tactile (touch) sensations within the skin at the location of the electrode by passing a pulsatile, localized electric current through the skin. Information is delivered by varying the amplitude, frequency, etc. of the stimulation waveform. Also called *electrocutaneous stimulation.*

Illuminance: The density of light falling on a surface, measured in lux. One lux is equivalent to 0.0929 ft-candles, an earlier measure. Illuminance is inversely proportional to the square of the distance from a point of light source. A 100-W incandescent lamp provides approximately 1280 lx at a distance of 1 ft (30.5 cm). Brightness is a different measure, depending also on the reflectance of the surrounding area.

Kinesthetic perception: Information about the relative positions of and forces on body parts, possibly including efference copy (internal knowledge of muscular effort).

Sensory augmentation: The use of devices that assist a functional human sense; eyeglasses are one example.

Sensory substitution: The use of one human sense to receive information normally received by another sense. For example, Braille substitutes touch for vision.

Sound pressure level (SPL): The root-mean-square pressure difference from atmospheric pressure ($\approx$ 100 kPa) that characterizes the intensity of sound. The conversion SPL = 20 log(P/P_0) expresses SPL in decibels, where P_0 is the threshold pressure of approximately 20 Pa at 1 kHz.

Static tactile: Stimulation that is a slow local mechanical deformation of the skin. It varies the deformation amplitude directly rather than the amplitude of vibration. This is "normal touch" for grasping objects, etc.

Tactile perception: Information about spatial pressure patterns on the skin with a fixed kinesthetic position.

Tactual (haptic) perception: The seamless, usually unconscious combination of tactile and kinesthetic information; this is "normal touch."

Vibrotactile: Stimulation that evokes tactile sensations using mechanical vibration of the skin, typically at frequencies of 10–500 Hz. Information is delivered by varying the amplitude, frequency, etc. of the vibration.

Virtual environment: A real-time interactive computer model that attempts to display visual, auditory, and tactual information to a human user as if he or she was present at the simulated location. The user controls the environment with head, hand, and body motions. An airplane cockpit simulator is one example.

References

Bach-y-Rita, P. 1972. *Brain Mechanisms in Sensory Substitution.* New York, Academic Press.

Bach-y-Rita, P., Kaczmarek, K.A., Tyler, M., and Garcia-Lara, M. 1998. Form perception with a 49-point electrotactile stimulus array on the tongue. *J. Rehab. Res. Dev.* 35:427–430.

Bach-y-Rita, P., Webster, J.G., Tompkins, W.J., and Crabb, T. 1987. Sensory substitution for space gloves and for space robots. In: *Proceedings of the Workshop on Space Telerobotics, Jet Propulsion Laboratory, Publication 87-13,* pp. 51–57.

Barfield, W., Hendrix, C., Bjorneseth, O., Kaczmarek, K.A., and Lotens, W. 1996. Comparison of human sensory capabilities with technical specifications of virtual environment equipment. *Presence* 4: 329–356.

Becker, K.W. 1972. *Speechreading: Principles and Methods.* Baltimore, MD, National Educational Press.

Békésy, G.V. 1955. Human skin perception of traveling waves similar to those of the cochlea. *J. Acoust. Soc. Am.* 27:830.

Bernstein, L.E., Demorest, M.E., Coulter, D.C., and O'Connell, M.P. 1991. Lipreading sentences with vibrotactile vocoders: Performance of normal-hearing and hearing-impaired subjects. *J. Acoust. Soc. Am.* 90:2971.

Blamey, P.J. and Clark, G.M. 1985. A wearable multiple-electrode electrotactile speech processor for the profoundly deaf. *J. Acoust. Soc. Am.* 77:1619.

Boothroyd, A. and Hnath-Chisolm, T. 1988. Spatial, tactile presentation of voice fundamental frequency as a supplement to lipreading: Results of extended training with a single subject. *J. Rehab. Res. Dev.* 25(3):51.

Boyd, L.H., Boyd, W.L., and Vanderheiden, G.C. 1990. *The Graphical User Interface Crisis: Danger and Opportunity.* September, Trace R&D Center, University of Wisconsin–Madison.

Brooks, P.L. and Frost, B.J. 1986. The development and evaluation of a tactile vocoder for the profoundly deaf. *Can. J. Public Health* 77:108.

Collins, C.C. 1985. On mobility aids for the blind. In D.H. Warren and E.R. Strelow (eds.), *Electronic Spatial Sensing for the Blind.* pp. 35–64. Dordrecht, the Netherlands, Martinus Nijhoff.

Collins, C.C. and Madey, J.M.J. 1974. Tactile sensory replacement. In *Proceedings of the San Diego Biomedical Symposium,* pp. 15–26.

Collins, C.C. and Saunders, F.A. 1970. Pictorial display by direct electrical stimulation of the skin. *J. Biomed. Syst.* 1:3–16.

Cook, A.M. 1982. Sensory and communication aids. In: A.M. Cook and J.G. Webster (eds.), *Therapeutic Medical Devices: Application and Design,* pp. 152–201. Englewood Cliffs, NJ, Prentice-Hall.

Fonda, G.E. 1981. *Management of Low Vision.* New York, Thieme-Stratton.

Geldard, F.A. 1960. Some neglected possibilities of communication. *Science* 131:1583.

Hannaford, B. and Wood L. 1992. Evaluation of performance of a telerobot. *NASA Tech. Briefs* 16(2): 62.

Hughes, B.G. 1989. A new electrotactile system for the hearing impaired. National Science Foundation final project report, ISI-8860727, Sevrain-Tech, Inc.

Kaczmarek, K.A. and Bach-y-Rita, P. 1995. Tactile displays. In: W. Barfield and T. Furness (eds.), *Virtual Environments and Advanced Interface Design.* New York, Oxford University Press.

Kaczmarek, K.A., Tyler, M.E., and Bach-y-Rita, P. 1997. Pattern identification on a fingertip-scanned electrotactile display. *Proceedings of the 19th Annual International Conference on IEEE Engineering Medical Biological Society,* pp. 1694–1697.

Kaczmarek, K.A., Webster, J.G., Bach-y-Rita, P., and Tompkins, W.J. 1991. Electrotactile and vibrotactile displays for sensory substitution systems. *IEEE Trans. Biomed. Eng.* 38:1.

Loomis, J.M. 1992. Distal attribution and presence. *Presence: Teleoper. Virtual Environ.* 1(1):113.

Loomis, J.M. and Lederman, S.J. 1986. Tactual perception. In K.R. Boff et al. (eds.), *Handbook of Perception and Human Performance, Vol II: Cognitive Processes and Performance,* pp. 31.1–31.41. New York, Wiley.

Mehr, E. and Shindell, S. 1990. Advances in low vision and blind rehabilitation. In: M.G. Eisenberg and R.C. Grzesiak (eds.), *Advances in Clinical Rehabilitation,* Vol. 3, pp. 121–147. New York, Springer.

Moore, B.C.J. 1990. How much do we gain by gain control in hearing aids? *Acta Otolaryngol. (Stockh)* Suppl. 469:250.

Mountcastle, V.B. (ed.). 1980. *Medical Physiology.* St. Louis, Mosby.

NIDRR. 1993. Protocols for choosing low vision devices. US Department of Education. Consensus Statement 1(1–28).

Phillips, C.A. 1988. Sensory feedback control of upper- and lower-extremity motor prostheses. *CRC Crit. Rev. Biomed. Eng.* 16:105.

Rabischong, P. 1981. Physiology of sensation. In R. Tubiana (ed.), *The Hand,* pp. 441–467. Philadelphia, PA, Saunders.

Rakowski, K., Brenner, C., and Weisenberger, J.M. 1989. Evaluation of a 32-channel electrotactile vocoder (abstract). *J. Acoust. Soc. Am.* 86 (Suppl.1):S83.

Ramesh, P., Wilpon, J.G., McGee, M.A. et al. 1992. Speaker independent recognition of spontaneously spoken connected digits. *Speech Commun.* 11:229.

Reed, C.M., Delhorne, L.A., Durlach, N.I., and Fischer, S.D. 1990. A study of the tactual and visual reception of fingerspelling. *J. Speech Hear. Res.* 33:786.

Reed, C.M., Durlach, N.I., and Bradia, L.D. 1982. Research on tactile communication of speech: A review. *AHSA Monogr.* 20:1.

Reed, C.M., Rabinowitz, W.M., Durlach, N.I. et al. 1992. Analytic study of the Tadoma method: Improving performance through the use of supplementary tactile displays. *J. Speech Hear. Res.* 35:450.

Sataloff, J., Sataloff, R.T., and Vassallo, L.A. 1980. *Hearing Loss*, 2nd ed. Philadelphia, PA, Lippincott.

Saunders, F.A., Hill, W.A., and Franklin, B. 1981. A wearable tactile sensory aid for profoundly deaf children. *J. Med. Syst.* 5:265.

Sherrick, C.E. 1973. Current prospects for cutaneous communication. In *Proceedings of the Conference on Cutaneous Communication System Development*, pp. 106–109.

Shimoga, K.B. 1993. A survey of perceptual feedback issues in dextrous telemanipulation: II. Finger touch feedback. In *IEEE Virtual Reality Annual International Symposium*, pp. 271–279.

Shlaer, S. 1937. The relation between visual acuity and illumination. *J. Gen. Physiol.* 21:165.

Smeltzer, C.D. 1993. Primary care screening and evaluation of hearing loss. *Nurse Pract.* 18:50.

Stigmar, G. 1970. Observation on vernier and stereo acuity with special reference to their relationship. *Acta Ophthalmol.* 48:979.

Szeto, A.Y.J. and Riso, R.R. 1990. Sensory feedback using electrical stimulation of the tactile sense. In R.V. Smith and J.H. Leslie, Jr. (eds.), *Rehabilitation Engineering*, pp. 29–78. Boca Raton, FL, CRC Press.

Tubiana, R. 1988. Fingertip injuries. In R. Tubiana (ed.), *The Hand*, pp. 1034–1054. Philadelphia, PA Saunders.

Van Tasell, D.J. 1993. Hearing loss, speech, and hearing aids. *J. Speech Hear. Res.* 36:228.

Verrillo, R.T. 1985. Psychophysics of vibrotactile stimulation. *J. Acoust. Soc. Am.* 77:225.

Vierck, C.J. and Jones, M.B. 1969. Size discrimination on the skin. *Science* 163:488.

Webster, J.G., Cook, A.M., Tompkins, W.J., and Vanderheiden, G.C. (eds.). 1985. *Electronic Devices for Rehabilitation*. New York, Wiley.

Weinstein, S. 1968. Intensive and extensive aspects of tactile sensitivity as a function of body part, sex and laterality. In D.R. Kenshalo (ed.), *The Skin Senses*, pp. 195–218. Springfield, IL, Charles C. Thomas.

Further Information

Presence: Teleoperators and Virtual Environments is a bimonthly journal focusing on advanced human–machine interface issues. In an effort to develop tactile displays without moving parts, our laboratory has demonstrated simple pattern recognition on the fingertip (Kaczmarek et al., 1997) and tongue (Bach-y-Rita et al., 1998) using electrotactile stimulation.

The Trace Research and Development Center, Madison, Wisconsin, publishes a comprehensive resource book on commercially available assistive devices, organizations, etc. for communication, control, and computer access for individuals with physical and sensory impairments.

Electronic Devices for Rehabilitation, edited by J.G. Webster (Wiley, 1985), summarizes the technological principles of electronic assistive devices for people with physical and sensory impairments.

47

Augmentative and Alternative Communication

Katya Hill
University of Pittsburgh
AAC Institute

Barry Romich
Prentke Romich Company
AAC Institute

Gregg Vanderheiden
University of Wisconsin,
Madison

47.1 Introduction

The inability to express oneself through either speech or writing is perhaps the most limiting of physical disabilities. Meaningful participation in life requires the communication of information, desires, needs, feelings, and aspirations. The lack of full interpersonal communication results from a variety of congenital and acquired disabilities, including but not limited to amyotrophic lateral sclerosis, aphasia, autism, brain injury, cerebral palsy, and Parkinson's disease. Also, the use of natural speech to communicate may be interrupted due to hospitalization. The complex communication disorders associated with these conditions substantially reduce an individual's quality of life and potential for education, employment, and independence.

Today, through multidisciplinary contributions, individuals who cannot speak or write have access to a wide variety of therapies, techniques, and systems designed to ameliorate challenges to effective communication. The field of augmentative and alternative communication (AAC) has the goal to optimize the communication of individuals with significant communication disorders (ASHA, 2004). Biomedical and rehabilitation engineering play a significant role in the research and development of AAC and related assistive technology. Engineering contributions range from relatively independent work on product definition and design to the collaborative development and evaluation of tools to support the contributions of other professions, such as linguistics, speech-language pathology, special education, and occupational therapy.

Augmentative communication can be classified in a variety of ways ranging from techniques that require no technology or apparatuses, that is, gestures, signs, and eye pointing, to sophisticated electronic devices (Lloyd et al., 1980; Beukelman and Mirenda, 2013). This chapter focuses on the review of

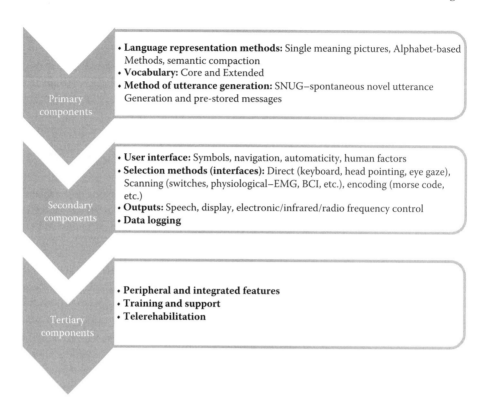

FIGURE 47.1 Primary, secondary, and tertiary components of an augmentative and alternative communication (AAC) system.

high technology-based techniques and related issues, because of the importance engineering principles play in the effectiveness of the achieved communication performance of an AAC system.

Technology-based AAC systems are designed and evaluated based on primary, secondary, and tertiary components (Cooper et al., 2006; Hill, 2010). See Figure 47.1 identifying the AAC components that are considered when designing systems and during an assessment. The primary components involve how language is represented and generated. The secondary components consist of the user and control interfaces and various output features. Tertiary features include various peripherals to improve performance and additional considerations such as training and technical support. Generally, a multidisciplinary team evaluates the current and projected skills and needs of the individual, determines the most effective language representation method(s) (LRMs) and physical access technique(s), and then selects a system, including training and other supports, with characteristics that will lead to the best communication performance.

47.2 Primary Factors: Language Considerations

To achieve communication competence, the person using an AAC system must have access to language components capable of handling the various vocabulary and message construction demands of the environment. Professionals rely on the theoretical models of language development and linguistics to evaluate the effectiveness of how language is represented and generated using an AAC system. Three critical features are considered: (1) the method of utterance generation; (2) the selection and organization of vocabulary; and (3) the availability of the three AAC LRMs.

Individuals using AAC systems have two options or methods to generate utterances. Preprogrammed or prestored messages can be added to most AAC systems that allow a person to select a key or button to speak or write a sentence or series of sentences (Todman, 2000). Prestored messages, the first option, are typically used for highly predictable or frequently needed information, such as providing personal contact information, requesting daily medications, and social scripts. However, the nature of daily communication is such that specific messages related to topics of conversation are highly unpredictable. Spontaneous novel utterance generation (SNUG), the second option, is the method most frequently used for interactive communication (Hill, 2006). SNUG is real-time construction of utterances and is the preferred method for individuals to say what they want to say and not what the programmer presumed was appropriate. Vocabulary organization and access to the various LRMs influence the efficiency of generating real-time conversation by the AAC user.

AAC research on vocabulary use has documented the phenomenon of core and fringe vocabulary and the reliance on a relatively limited core vocabulary to express a majority of communication utterances (Vanderheiden and Kelso, 1987; Yorkston et al., 1988). Core or high-frequency vocabulary is the relatively small number of words that constitute the vast majority of what is said or written, ~80% of the words used in conversations. Detail, fringe, or extended vocabulary is a large number of words that are used for the remaining small part of communication. It is only around 20% of what is said or written but it is the meat of the communication. Whereas fringe vocabulary is specific to topic, activity, and situations, core vocabulary is used across different types of conversation and is needed for fluent communication. Engineering AAC systems to provide the most efficient methods to access core vocabulary is critical to effective word-by-word communication performance (Anderson and Baker, 2003) because they are the words used most often. But communication with core words only needs to be taught to be efficient and functional. For example, in technical writing, core words constitute a much smaller percentage of the vocabulary than in daily conversation (see paragraph below: core words are bolded). However, AAC intervention can maximize the use of core vocabulary to improve the functional communication of individuals who rely on AAC. For example, the following sentences can be generated to meet a person's communication needs using only core vocabulary. *Examples:* "This is the one I want." "I need your help." "What are we doing next?"

The ways in which symbols **or** letters **are used to** generate communication **are** referred **to as** LRMs. **The three** AAC LRMs **are**: (1) alphabet-based methods; (2) single meaning pictures; and (3) Semantic Compaction™ (Baker, 1986). **In addition, various** keystroke savings techniques **can be** applied **with the** LRMs **on a** system **in an** attempt to improve **the** efficiency **for** generating real-time conversation. Communication **by users of** AAC systems **is far slower than that of the** general population. Yet **the** speed **of** communication **is a** significant factor influencing **the** perceptions **by the** user's communication partner, **and the** potential **for** personal achievement **for the** person relying **on** AAC. **The** development **and** application **of** techniques **to** reduce keystrokes **and/or** accelerate communication rates **is** critical. Further, **these** techniques **are most** effective **when** developers pay attention **to** human factors design principles (Demasco, 1994; Goodenough-Trepagnier, 1994).

Alphabet-based language representation methods involve the use of traditional orthography and keystroke savings techniques that require spelling and reading skills. AAC systems using orthography require the user to spell each word using a standard keyboard or alphabet overlay on a static or touch screen display. A standard or customized alphabet overlay provides use for successful conversations; however, spelling letter by letter can be a slow and inefficient AAC strategy if a person's individual selection rate is slow and keystroke savings techniques are not used.

Abbreviation systems represent language elements using a number of keystrokes typically smaller than that required by spelling. For example, words or sentences are abbreviated using principled approaches based on vowel elimination or the first letters of salient words. Abbreviation systems can be fast but require not only spelling and reading skills but also memorization of abbreviation codes. Typically, people with spelling and reading skills have large vocabulary needs and increased demands on the production of text. Principled approaches soon experience abbreviation code conflicts or memory overload.

Word prediction is another technique available to consider. Based on previously selected letters and words, the system presents the user with best guess choices for completing the spelling of a word. The user then chooses one of the predictions or continues spelling, resulting in yet another set of predictions.

Prediction systems have demonstrated a reduction in the number of keystrokes, but decades of research show that the actual communication rate does not represent a statistical improvement over spelling (Koester and Levine, 1994, 1996). The reason for word predication's failure to improve the actual communication rate is that increased time is needed to read and select the word table choices. The cost of discontinuity and increased cognitive load in the task seems to match or exceed the benefits of reduced keystrokes (Koester and Levine, 1996).

Single meaning picture symbols involve the use of graphic or line-drawn symbols to represent single word vocabulary or messages (phrases, sentences, and paragraphs). A variety of AAC symbol sets are available on devices or software to depict the linguistic elements available through the system. Universal considerations regarding the selection of a symbol set include research on symbol characteristics such as size, transparency, complexity, and iconicity (Fuller et al., 1992, 1997; Romski and Sevcik, 1988). The use of a goal-driven graphic symbol selection process (Schlosser et al., 1997) and understanding the strategies to teach a symbol are necessary to make clinical decisions about system selection and vocabulary organization (VanTatenhove, 2009).

Vocabulary size and representation of linguistic rules (grammar) are concerns for users relying on graphic symbol sets. Users of static display systems have a limited number of symbols available on any one overlay; however, they have ready access to that vocabulary. Touch screen display users have an almost unlimited number of symbols available as vocabulary for message generation; however, they must navigate through pages or displays to locate a word. Figure 47.3 represents this organizational challenge to word selection. Frequently, morphology and syntax are not graphically represented. Since research has strongly supported the need for users to construct spontaneous, novel utterances (Beukelman et al., 1984), neither method is efficient for interactive communication.

Semantic Compaction is perhaps the most efficient AAC LRM (Baker, 1986, 1994). With this method, language is represented by a relatively small set of multimeaning icons. The specific meaning of each icon is a function of the context in which it is used. Semantic Compaction makes use of a meaningful relationship between the icon and the information it represents; it does not require spelling and reading skills, and yet is powerful even for people with these skills. The performance of Semantic Compaction stems from its ability to handle both vocabulary and linguistic structures as found in the Semantic Compaction Application Programs (MAPS) of Words Strategy and Unity in languages such as English, German, French, Spanish, and Mandarin. These MAPS support the concept of a core and fringe vocabulary. They provide the architecture for handling rules of grammar and morphology. The number of required keystrokes is significantly reduced relative to spelling. Semantic Compaction however does require more extensive training. As a result it may not be as applicable in temporary disability. The picture nature of the technique may also be an undesirable format for some adults.

47.3 Secondary Factors: User Interfaces, Control Interfaces, and Outputs

The AAC software and hardware components can be classified in terms of how the user interfaces and control interfaces organize and provide access to the language components. AAC systems employ a user interface based on the selection of items that will produce the desired output (Vanderheiden and Lloyd, 1996). Engineering decisions include the use of symbols, navigation methods, possibility of automaticity, and related human factors influencing learning and long-term use (Romich, 1994). Each engineered consideration may influence communication performance or user preference and satisfaction.

Items being selected from the user interface may be individual letters, as used in spelling, whole words, or picture symbols to represent single word vocabulary or phrases and sentences. Basic user interface design considerations include the type of display, for example, keyboard, static overlay, or touch screen display; number of buttons or locations on the display, for example, 8, 32, or 144; the color scheme, for example, primary or muted colors and color coding; and the symbol type, for example, photos, icons, letters, and words.

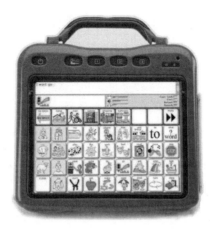

FIGURE 47.2 Example of a touch screen AAC user interface with a language software application with 45 locations that provides all three language representation methods.

The size of the desired stored vocabulary influences navigation needs for the AAC system. For example, a display with 30 locations can provide access to all the letters of the alphabet for spelling to use this LRM. However, providing access to numbers, punctuation, and function keys would require an additional display. Using a single meaning picture LRM approach, a stored vocabulary of 300 words would require at least 10 pages using 30 location displays to access all the items, thus requiring navigation among the screens or pages. Figure 47.2 shows a user interface designed using 45 locations organized based on four core or high-frequency vocabulary row and one activity row to access extended vocabulary. Such engineering avoids frequent navigation to generate a word-by-word message.

Figure 47.3 illustrates the engineering considerations in juggling the number of items required for effective communication with the number of locations the person can access accurately. As the number of items increases, so does the number of pages. As the number of pages increases, the navigational and memory demands increase too. Navigation prevents individuals from becoming automatic with their

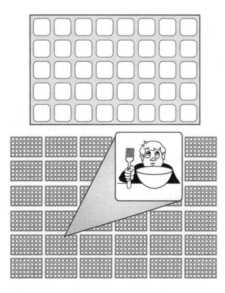

FIGURE 47.3 Navigation to a page is required for a single meaning picture approach to select a word from one of the many pages on the system. (AAC Institute©.)

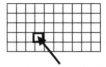

FIGURE 47.4   Direct selection.

language software and more dependent on visual references to locate items and slows real-time communication. Finally, for many AAC users with multiple disabilities, literacy skills are delayed and reading symbol labels to assist with vocabulary selection adds additional demands to the navigation process.

The control interface provides the various selection methods available on the AAC system. High-technology AAC systems frequently offer several selection techniques with various features that can be manipulated to improve selection performance. The numerous techniques for making selections are based on either direct selection or scanning.

Direct selection refers to techniques by which a single selection from a set of choices indicates the desired item (Vanderheiden and Grilley 1976, Beukelman and Mirenda, 2013). A common example of this method is the use of a computer keyboard. Each key is directly selected by finger. Expanded keyboards accommodate more gross motor actions, such as using the fist or foot. In some cases, pointing can be enhanced through the use of technology. Sticks are held in the mouth or attached to the head using a headband or helmet. Light pointers are used to direct a light beam at a target. Light pen-type techniques can also direct a visual pointer. Indirect pointing systems might include the common computer mouse, trackball, or joystick. Alternatives to these for people with disabilities are based on the movement of the head or other body part. Figure 47.4 depicts direct selection in that the desired location is pointed to directly.

Remote eye gaze and brain–computer interface (BCI) technologies are two direct selection technique advances with growing clinical uses. Remote eye gaze is a vision-controlled direct selection technique that uses a camera to detect the eye movement to select a target based on the held gaze. A BCI creates a nonmuscular output channel for the brain. Instead of being executed through peripheral nerves and muscles, the user's selections are conveyed by brain signals (such as EEG), not dependent on neuromuscular activity (Wolpaw et al., 2002).

Scanning refers to techniques in which the individual is presented with a time sequence of choices and indicates when the desired choice appears (Vanderheiden and Grilley 1976; Romich et al., 2000). A simple linear scanning system might be a clock face-type display with a rotating pointer to indicate a letter, word, or picture. Additional dimensions of scanning can be added to reduce the selection time when the number of possible choices is larger. A common technique involves the arrangement of choices in a matrix of rows and columns. The selection process has two steps. First, rows are scanned to select the row containing the desired element. The selected row is then scanned to select the desired element. This method is called row–column scanning. See Figure 47.5. Either by convention or by the grouping of the elements, the order might be reversed. For example, in the United Kingdom, column–row scanning is preferred over row–column scanning. Other scanning techniques also exist and additional dimensions can be employed.

47.4 Acceleration Techniques

Both direct selection and scanning are used to select elements that might not of themselves define an output. In these cases, the output may be defined by a code or sequence of selected elements (Vanderheiden and Grilley, 1976). A common example is Morse code by which dots and dashes are directly selected but must be combined to define letters and numbers. Another example, more common to AAC, has an output defined by a sequence of two or more pictures or icons, such as Semantic Compaction.

Scanning, and to some degree direct selection, can be faster when the choices are arranged such that those most frequently used are easiest to access. For example, in a row–column scanning spelling system

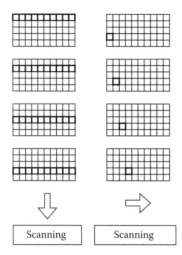

FIGURE 47.5 Illustration representing row-column scanning as a selection method.

that scans top to bottom and left to right, the most frequently used letters are usually grouped toward the upper left corner.

Predictive selection is an acceleration technique used with Semantic Compaction. When this feature is enabled, only those choices that complete a meaningful sequence can be selected. With scanning, for example, the selection process can be significantly faster because the number of possible choices is automatically reduced and the scanning process skips over the nonselectable icons.

Generally, the selection technique of choice should be that which results in the fastest communication possible. (Selection rate can be measured in bits per second.) Consideration of factors such as cognitive load, environmental changes, fatigue, aesthetics, and stability of physical skill often influence the choice of the best selection technique (Cress and French, 1994).

47.5 Other Outputs

AAC system outputs in common use are speech, displays, printers, beeps, data, infrared, Bluetooth, and other formats. Outputs are used to facilitate the interactive nature of "real-time" communication. Users may rely on auditory and visual feedback to enhance vocabulary selection and the construction of messages. The speech and display outputs may be directed toward the communication partner to support the exchange of information. Auditory feedback such as beeps and key clicks, while useful to the individual using the system, also provide the communication partner with information that a user is in the process of generating a message. Finally, outputs may be used to control other items or devices such as printers.

AAC speech output normally consists of two types: synthetic and digitized.

Synthetic speech usually is generated from text input following a set of rules. Synthetic speech is usually associated with AAC systems that are able to generate text. These systems have unlimited vocabulary and are capable of speaking any word or expression that can be spelled. With some systems it is actually possible to sing songs, another feature that enhances social interaction. Most synthetic speech systems are limited to a single language, although bilingual systems are available. Further limitations relate to the expression of accent and emotion. Research and development in artificial speech technology is attacking these limitations.

Digitized speech is essentially speech that has been recorded into digital memory. Relatively simple AAC systems typically use digitized speech. The vocabulary is entered by speaking into the system through a microphone. People who use these systems can say only what someone else said in programming them. They are independent of language and can replicate the song, accent, and emotion of the original speaker.

USB and infrared output are used to achieve a variety of functional outcomes. These outputs permit the AAC system to replace the keyboard and mouse for computer access, known as emulation. The advantage of emulation is that the LRM and physical access method used for speaking is used for writing and other computer tasks (Buning and Hill, 1999). Another application for these outputs is environmental control. Users are able to operate electrical and electronic items in their daily-living surroundings. Particular sequences of characters, symbols, or icons are used to represent commands such as answering the telephone, turning off the stereo, and even setting a thermostat. In addition, the serial output may also be used to monitor the language activity for purposes of clinical intervention, progress reporting, and research (Hill and Romich, 2001).

47.6 Tertiary Factors: Outcomes and Other Issues

The selection an AAC system is not complete without considering several factors that will influence ongoing use and overall communication performance. Tertiary factors include considerations such as mounting options, safe transportation of systems, training, and technical support and maintenance. Intervention and training should extend beyond the initial application of the system. People who rely on AAC frequently live unstable lives. Consequently, they have a need for ongoing, changing services across the life span. Monitoring and evaluation of changing needs and physical skill levels is needed to ensure that AAC systems are upgraded when appropriate and not abandoned due to lack of support.

The choice of an AAC system should rely primarily on the best interests of the person who will be using the system. Since outcomes and personal achievement will be related directly to the ability to communicate, the choice of a system will have lifelong implications. The process of choosing the most appropriate system is not trivial and can be accomplished best with a multidisciplinary team focusing on quantitative performance and outcomes. Team members should realize that the interests of the individual served professionally are not necessarily aligned with those of the providers and/or payers of AAC devices and services. The temptation to select a system that is easy to apply or inexpensive to purchase frequently exists, especially with untrained and novice teams. Teams that identify outcomes and have the goal of achieving interactive communication make informed decisions.

47.7 Future

Technological development in and of itself will not solve the problems of people with disabilities (Romich, 1993). Technology advancements, however, will continue to provide more powerful tools allowing the exploration of new and innovative approaches to support users and professionals. As access to lower cost, more powerful computer systems increases, the availability of alternative sources of information, technical support and training is possible either through software or the Internet. Users and professionals will have increased opportunities to learn and exchange ideas and outcomes.

References

American Speech Language Hearing Association 2004. *Preferred Practice Patterns for the Profession of Speech-Language Pathology.* Rockville, MD: Author, 2004.

Anderson, A. and Baker, B.R. 2003. Navigating AAC devices for early communicators. *Presented at the Assistive Technology Industry Association (ATIA)*, Orlando, FL.

Baker, B.R. 1986. Semantic compaction lets speech-impaired people quickly and effectively communicate in a variety of environments. *Byte*, 11, 160–168.

Baker, B.R. 1994. Semantic compaction: An approach to a formal definition. *Proceedings of the Sixth Annual European Minspeak Conference*, Swinstead, Lincs, UK: Prentke Romich Europe.

Beukelman, D.R. and Mirenda, P. 2013. *Augmentative and Alternative Communication: Management of Severe Communication Disorders in Children and Adults.* Baltimore, MD: Paul H. Brookes Publishing Co.

Beukelman, D.R., Yorkson, K., Poblete, M., and Naranjo, C. 1984. Frequency of word occurrence in communication samples produced by adult communication aid users. *Journal of Speech and Hearing Disorders,* 49, 360–367.

Buning, M.E. and Hill, K. 1999. An AAC device as a computer keyboard: More bang for the buck. *AOTA Annual Conference,* Indianapolis.

Cooper, R.A., Ohnabe, H., and D. Hobson, 2006. *An Introduction to Rehabilitation Engineering.* London: Institute of Physics Publishing.

Cress, C.J. and French, C.J. 1994. The relationship between cognitive load measurements and estimates of computer input control skills. *Assistive Technology,* 6.1, 54–66.

Demasco, P. 1994. Human factors considerations in the design of language interfaces in AAC. *Assistive Technology,* 6.1, 10–25.

Fuller, D., Lloyd, L., and Schlosser, R., 1992. Further development of an augmentative and alternative communication symbol taxonomy. *Augmentative and Alternative Communication,* 8, 67–74.

Fuller, D., Lloyd, L., and Stratton, M., 1997. Aided AAC symbols. In: L. Lloyd, D. Fuller, and H. Arvidson (Eds.), *Augmentative and Alternative Communication: Principles and Practice* (pp. 48–79), Needham Heights, MA: Allyn & Bacon.

Goodenough-Trepagnier, C., 1994. Design goals for augmentative communication. *Assistive Technology,* 6.1, 3–9.

Hill, K., 2006. Augmentative and alternative communication (AAC) research and development: The challenge of evidence-based practice. *International Journal of Computer Processing of Oriental Languages,* 19(4), 249–262.

Hill, K., 2010. Advances in augmentative and alternative communication as quality-of-life technology. *Physical Medicine and Rehabilitation Clinics of North America,* 21(1), 43–58.

Hill, K. and Romich, B., 2001. A language activity monitor for supporting AAC evidence-based clinical practice. *Assistive Technology,* 13, 12–22.

Horstmann Koester, H. and Levine, S.P., 1994. Learning and performance of able-bodied individuals using scanning systems with and without word prediction. *Assistive Technology,* 6.1, 42–53.

Horstmann Koester, H. and Levine, S.P., 1996. Effect of a word prediction feature on user performance. *Augmentative and Alternative Communication,* 12, 155–168.

Lloyd, L., Fuller, D.R., and Arvidson, H.A., 1980. *Augmentative and Alternative Communication: A Handbook of Principles and Practices.* Boston: Allyn and Bacon.

Norman, D.A. *The Psychology of Everyday Things.* New York: Basic Books, Inc.

Romich, B., 1993. Assistive technology and AAC: An industry perspective. *Assistive Technology,* 5.2, 74–77.

Romich, B., 1994. Knowledge in the world vs. knowledge in the head: The psychology of AAC systems. *Communication Outlook,* 14(4), 1–2.

Romich, B., Vanderheiden, G., and Hill, K., 2000. Augmentative communication. In J.D. Bronzine (Ed.), *Biomedical Engineering Handbook, 2nd ed.,* (pp. 101–122), Boca Raton, FL: CRC Press.

Romski, M. and Sevcik, R., 1988. Augmentative and alternative communication systems: Considerations for individuals with severe intellectual disabilities. *Augmentative and Alternative Communication,* 4, 83–93.

Schlosser, R.W., Lloyd, L.L., and McNaughton, S. 1997. Graphic symbol selection in research and practice: Making the case for a goal-driven process, Communication… Naturally: Theoretical and methodological issues in augmentative and alternative communication. Edited by E. Bjorck-Akesson and P. Lindsay, *Proceedings of the Fourth ISAAC Research Symposium,* (pp. 126–139), Vancouver, Canada.

Todman, J., 2000. Rate and quality of conversations using a text-storage AAC system: A training study. *Augmentative and Alternative Communication,* 16, 164–179.

Vanderheiden, G. and Grilley, K. (Eds.) 1976. *Non-Vocal Communication Techniques and Aids for the Severely Physically Handicapped.* Baltimore, MD: University Park Press.

Vanderheiden, G.C. and Kelso, D. 1987. Comparative analysis of fixed-vocabulary communication acceleration techniques. *Augmentative and Alternative Communication,* 3, 196–206.

Vanderheiden, G.C. and Lloyd, L.L. 1996. Communication systems and their components. In S. Blackstone (Ed.), *Augmentative Communication: An Introduction* (pp. 49–161). Rockville, MD: American Speech-Language Hearing Association.

VanTatenhove, G.M. 2009. The pixon project kit: A language development curriculum. *Semantic Compaction Systems.* Pittsburgh, PA: Semantic Compaction Systems, Inc.

Wolpaw, J., Birbaumer, N., McFarland, D., Pfurtscheller, G., and Vaughan, T., 2002. Brain-computer interfaces for communication and control. *Clinical Neurophysiology,* 113(6), 767–791.

Yorkston, K.M., Dowden, P.A., Honsinger, M.J., Marriner, N., and Smith, K., 1988. A comparison of standard and user vocabulary list. *Augmentative and Alternative Communication,* 4, 189–210.

Further Information

There are a number of organizations and publications that relate to AAC and accessibility:

AAC (*Augmentative and Alternative Communication*) is the quarterly refereed journal of ISAAC. It is published by Decker Periodicals Inc., PO Box 620, L.C.D. 1, Hamilton, Ontario, L8N 3K7 Canada, Tel. 905-522-7017, Fax. 905-522-7839. http://www.isaac-online.org.

AAC Institute is a not-for-profit, charitable organization dedicated to the most effective communication for people who rely on AAC. AAC Institute 1401 Forbes Ave., Suite 206, Pittsburgh, PA 15219, Tel. 412-523-6424. http://www.aacinstitute.org.

American Speech-Language-Hearing Association (ASHA) is the professional organization of speech-language pathologists. ASHA has a Special Interest Division on augmentative communication. ASHA, 10801 Rockville Pike, Rockville, MD, 20852, Tel. 301-897-5700, Fax. 301-571-0457. http://www.asha.org.

ISAAC is the International Society for Augmentative and Alternative Communication). USSAAC is the United States chapter. Both can be contacted at PO Box 1762 Station R, Toronto, Ontario, M4G 4A3, Canada, Tel. 905-737-9308, Fax. 905-737-0624. http://www.isaac-online.org.

National Public Inclusive Infrastructure (NPII) is a coalition of academic, industry, and nongovernmental organizations and individuals coming together to promote the creation of a National Public Inclusive Infrastructure (NPII). The purpose is to ensure that everyone who faces accessibility can access and use the Internet and all its information, communities, and services for education, employment, daily living, civic participation, health, and safety. http://npii.org.

Raising the Floor (RtF) is an international coalition of individuals and organizations working to ensure that the Internet is accessible to people experiencing accessibility or literacy problems, even if they have very limited or no financial resources. http://raisingthefloor.net.

RESNA is an interdisciplinary association for the advancement of rehabilitation and assistive technologies. RESNA has many Special Interest Groups including those on Augmentative and Alternative Communication and Computer Applications. RESNA, 1700 North Moore Street, Suite 1540, Arlington, VA, 22209-1903, Tel. 703-524-6686, Fax. 703-524-6630. http://resna.org.

Trace Research & Development Center is a part of the College of Engineering at the University of Wisconsin-Madison. Trace has been a pioneer in the field of technology and disability with a mission to create a world that is as accessible and usable as possible for as many people as possible. Trace, University of Wisconsin-Madison, 2107 Engineering Centers Bldg. Madison, WI 53706, Tel. 608-262-6966, Fax. 608-262-8848, http://www.trace.wisc.edu.

48

Measurement Tools and Processes in Rehabilitation Engineering

George V. Kondraske
University of Texas,
Arlington

In every engineering discipline, measurement facilitates the use of structured *procedures* and decision-making processes. In rehabilitation engineering, the presence of "a human," the only or major component of *the system of interest*, has presented a number of unique challenges with regard to measurement. This is especially true with regard to the routine processes of rehabilitation that either do or could incorporate and rely on measurements. This, in part, is due to the complexity of the human system's architecture, the variety of ways in which it can be adversely affected by disease or injury, and the versatility in the way it can be used to accomplish various *tasks* of interest to an individual.

Measurement supports a wide variety of assistive device design and prescription activities undertaken within rehabilitation engineering (e.g., Webster et al. 1985, Smith and Leslie 1990, and other chapters within this section). In addition, rehabilitation engineers contribute to the specification and design of measurement instruments that are used primarily by other service providers (such as physical and occupational therapists). As measurements of human *structure, performance*, and *behavior* become more rigorous and instruments used have taken advantage of advanced technology, there is also a growing role for rehabilitation engineers to assist these other medical professionals with the proper application of measurement instruments (e.g., for determining areas that are most deficient in an individual's performance profile, objectively documenting progress during rehabilitation, etc.). This is in keeping with the team approach to rehabilitation that has become popular in clinical settings. In short, the role of measurement in rehabilitation engineering is dynamic and growing.

In this chapter, a top-down overview of measurement tools and processes in rehabilitation engineering is presented. Many of the measurement concepts, processes, and devices of relevance are common to applications outside the rehabilitation engineering context. However, the nature of the human population with which rehabilitation engineers must deal is arguably different in that each individual must be assumed to be unique with respect to at least a subset of his or her performance capacities and/or structural parameters; that is, population reference data cannot be assumed to be generally applicable. While there are some exceptions, population labels frequently used such as "head-injured" or "spinal cord-injured" represent only a gross classification that should not be taken to imply homogeneity with regard to parameters such as range of motion, strength, movement speed, information-processing speed, and other performance capacities. This is merely a direct realization that many different ways exist in which the human system can be adversely affected by disease or injury and recognition of the continuum that exists with regard to the degree of any given effect. The result is that in rehabilitation engineering, compared with standard human factors design tasks aimed at the average healthy population, many measurement values must be acquired directly for the specific client.

Measurement in the present context encompasses actions that focus on (1) the human (e.g., structural aspects and performance capacities of subsystems at different hierarchical levels ranging from specific neuromuscular subsystems to the total person and his or her activities in daily living, including work), (2) assistive devices (e.g., structural aspects and demands placed on the human), (3) tasks (e.g., distances between critical points, masses of objects involved, etc.), and (4) overall systems (e.g., performance achieved by a human-assistive device–task combination, patterns of electrical signals representing the timing of muscle activity while performing a complex maneuver, behavior of an individual before and after being fitted with a new prosthetic device, etc.). Clearly, an exhaustive treatment is beyond the scope of this chapter. Measurements are embedded in every specialized subarea of rehabilitation engineering. However, there are also special roles served by measurement in a broader and more generic sense, as well as principles that are common across the many special applications. Emphasis here is placed on these.

There is no lack of other literature regarding the types of measurement outlined to be of interest here and their use. However, it is diffusely distributed, and gaps exist with regard to how such tools can be integrated to accomplish *goals* beyond simply the acquisition of numeric data for a given parameter. With rapidly changing developments over the last decade, there is currently no comprehensive source that describes the majority of instruments available, their latest implementations, procedures for their use, evaluation of effectiveness, etc. While topics other than measurement are discussed, Leslie and coworkers (1990) produced what is perhaps the single most directly applicable source with respect to rehabilitation engineering specifically, although it too is not comprehensive with regard to measurement, nor does it attempt to be.

48.1 Fundamental Principles

Naturally, the fundamental principles of human physiology manifest themselves in the respective sensory, neuromuscular, information-processing, and life-sustaining systems and impact approaches to measurement. In addition, psychological considerations are vital. Familiarization with this material is essential to measurement in rehabilitation; however, treatment here is far beyond the scope of this chapter. The numerous reference works available may be most readily found by consulting relevant chapters in this *Handbook* and the works that they reference. In this section, key principles that are more specific to measurement and of general applicability are presented.

48.1.1 Structure, Function, Performance, and Behavior

It is necessary to distinguish between structure, *function*, performance, and behavior and measurements thereof for both human and artificial systems. In addition, hierarchical systems concepts are necessary both to help organize the complexity of the systems involved and to help understand the various needs that exist.

Structural measures include dimensions, masses (of objects, limb segments), moments of inertia, circumferences, contours, compliances, and any other aspects of the physical system. These may be considered hierarchically as being pertinent to the total human (e.g., height, weight, etc.), specific body segments (e.g., forearm, thigh, etc.), or components of basic systems such as tendons, ligaments, and muscles.

Function is the *purpose* of the system of interest (e.g., to move a limb segment, to communicate, to feed, and care for oneself). Within the human, there are many single-purpose systems (e.g., those that function to move specific limb segments, process specific types of information, etc.). As one proceeds to higher levels, such as the total human, systems that are increasingly more multifunctional emerge. These can be recognized as higher-level configurations of more basic systems that operate to feed oneself, to conduct personal hygiene, to carry out task of a job, etc. This multilevel view of just functions begins to help place into perspective the scope over which measurement can be applied.

In rehabilitation in general, a good deal of what constitutes measurement involves the application of structured subjective observation techniques (see also the next subsection) in the form of a wide range of rating scales (e.g., Granger and Greshorn, 1984; Potvin et al., 1985; Fuhrer, 1987). These are often termed *functional assessment scales* and are typically aimed at obtaining a global index of an individual's ability to function independently in the world. The global index is typically based on a number of items within a given scale, each of which addresses selected, relatively high-level functions (e.g., personal hygiene, mobility, etc.). The focus of measurement for a given item is often in estimate of the *level* of independence or dependence that the subject exhibits or needs to carry out the respective function. In addition, inventories of functions that an individual is able or not able to carry out (with and without assistance) are often included. The large number of such scales that have been proposed and debated is a consequence of the many possible functions and combinations thereof that exist on which to base a given scale. Functional assessment scales are relatively quick and inexpensive to administer and have a demonstrated role in rehabilitation. However, the nature and levels of measurements obtained are not sufficient for many rehabilitation engineering purposes. This latter class of applications generally begins with a function at the level and of the type used as a constituent component of functional assessment scales, considers the level of performance at which that function is executed more quantitatively, and incorporates one or more lower levels in the hierarchy (i.e., the human subsystems involved in achieving the specific functions of daily life that are of interest and their capacities for performance).

Where functions can be described and inventoried, *performance* measures directly characterize *how well* a physical system of interest executes its intended function. Performance is multidimensional (e.g., strength, range, speed, accuracy, steadiness, endurance, etc.). Of special interest are the concepts of *performance capacity* and *performance capacity measurement*. Performance capacity represents the *limits* of a given system's ability to operate in its corresponding multidimensional performance space. In this chapter, a resource-based model for both human and artificial system performance and measurement of their performance capacities is adopted (e.g., Kondraske, 1990, 1995). Thus the *maximum* knee flexor strength available (i.e., the resource availability) under a stated set of conditions represents one unique performance capacity of the knee flexor system. In rehabilitation, the terms *impairment, disability*, and *handicap* (World Health Organization, 1980) have been prominently applied and are relevant to the concept of performance. While these terms place an emphasis on what is missing or what a person cannot do and imply not only a measurement but also the incorporation of an assessment or judgment based on one or more observations, the resource-based performance perspective focuses on "what is present" or "what is right" (i.e., performance resource availability). From this perspective, an impairment can be determined to exist if a given performance capacity is found to be less than a specified level (e.g., less than 5th percentile value of a health reference population). A disability exists when performance resource insufficiency exists in a specified task.

While performance relates more to what a system can do (i.e., a challenge or maximal stress is implied), *behavior* measurements are used to characterize what a system does naturally. Thus a given variable such as movement speed can relate to both performance and behavior depending on whether the system (e.g., human subsystem) was maximally challenged to respond "as fast as possible" (performance) or simply observed in the course of operation (behavior). It is also possible to observe a system that it is behaving at one or more of its performance capacities (e.g., at the maximum speed possible, etc.) (see Table 48.1).

48.1.2 Subjective and Objective Measurement Methods

Subjective measurements are made by humans without the aid of instruments and objective measurements result from the use of instruments. However, it should be noted that the mere presence of an instrument does not guarantee complete objectivity. For example, the use of a ruler requires a human judgment in reading the scale and thus contains a subjective element. A length-measurement system with an integral data-acquisition system would be more objective. However, it is likely that even this system would involve human intervention in its use, for example, the alignment of the device and making the decision as to exactly what is to be measured with it by selection of reference points. Measures with more objectivity (less subjectivity) are preferred to minimize questions of bias. However, measurements that are intrinsically more objective are frequently more costly and time consuming to obtain. Well-reasoned trade-offs must be made to take advantage of the ability of a human (typically a skilled professional) to quickly "measure" many different items subjectively (and often without recording the results but using them internally to arrive at some decision).

It is important to observe that identification of the variable of interest is not influenced by whether it is measured subjectively or objectively. This concept extends to the choice of instrument used for objective measurements. This is an especially important concept in dealing with human performance and behavior, since variables of interest can be much more abstract than simple lengths and widths (e.g., coordination, postural stability, etc.). In fact, many measurement variables in rehabilitation historically have tended to be treated as if they were inextricably coupled with the measurement method, confounding debate regarding *what should be measured with what should be used to measure it* in a given context.

48.1.3 Measurements and Assessments

The basic representation of a measurement itself in terms of the actual units of measure is often referred to as the *raw form*. For measures of performance, the term *raw score* is frequently applied. Generally, some form of *assessment* (i.e., judgment or interpretation) is typically required. Assessments may be applied to (or, viewed from a different perspective, may require) either a single measure of groups of them. Subjective assessments are frequently made that are based on the practitioner's familiarity with values for a given parameter in a particular context. However, due to the large number of parameters and the amount of experience that would be required to gain a sufficient level of familiarity, a more formal and objective realization of the process that takes place in subjective assessments is often employed. This process combines the measured value with objectively determined reference values to obtain new metrics or scores, that facilitate one or more steps in the assessment process.

For aspects of performance, *percent normal scores* are computed by expressing subject Y's availability of performance resource $k[R_{A_k}(Y)]$ as a fraction of the mean availability of that resource in a specified reference population $[R_{A_k}(pop)]$. Ideally, the reference population is selected to match the characteristics of the individual as closely as possible (e.g., age range, gender, handedness, etc.).

$$\text{Percent normal} = \frac{R_{A_k}(Y)}{R_{A_k}(pop)} \times 100 \qquad (48.1)$$

TABLE 48.1 The Scope of Measurement in Rehabilitation Is Broad

Hierarchical Level	Structure	Function	Performance	Behavior
Global/composite • Total human • Human with artificial systems	• Height • Weight • Postures • Subjective and instrumented methods	• Multifunction, reconfigurable system • High-level functions: tasks of daily life (working, grooming, recreation, etc.) • Functional assessment scales • Single-number global index • Level of independent estimates	• No single-number direct measurement is possible • Possible models to integrate lower-level measures • Direct measurement (subjective and instrumented) of selected performance attribute for selected functions	• Subjective self- and family reports • Instrumented ambulatory activity monitors (selected attributes) • See notes under "function"
Complex body systems • Cognitive • Speech • Lifting, gait • Upper extremity • Cardiovascular/ respiratory • Etc.	• Dimensions • Shape • Etc. • Instrumented methods	• Multifunction, reconfigurable systems • System-specific functions	• Function-specific subjective rating scales • Often based on impairment/ disability concepts • Relative metrics • Some instrumented performance capacity measures also known as "functional capacity" (misnomer)	• Subjective and automated (objective) videotape evaluation • Instrumented measures of physical quantities versus time (e.g., forces, angles, and motions) • Electromyography (e.g., muscle-timing patterns, coordination)
Basic systems • Visual information processors • Flexors, extensors • Visual sensors • Auditory sensors • Lungs • Etc.	• Dimensions • Shape • Masses • Moments of inertia • Instrumented methods	• Single function • System-specific functions	• Subjective estimates by clinician for diagnostic and routine monitoring purposes • Instrumented measures of performance capacities (e.g., strength, extremes/range of motion, speed, accuracy, endurance, etc.)	• Instrumented systems • Measure and log electrophysiological, biomechanical, and other variables versus time • Post hoc parameterization
Components of basic systems • Muscle • Tendon • Nerve • Etc.	• Mechanical properties • Instrumented methods/imaging	• Generally single function • Component-specific functions	• Difficult to assess for individual subjects • Infer from measures at "basic system level" • Direct measurement methods with lab samples, research applications	• Difficult to assess for individual subject • Direct measurement methods with lab samples, research applications

Note: Structure, function, performance, and behavior are encompassed at multiple hierarchical levels. Both subjective and objective, instrumented methods of measurement are employed.

Aside from the benefit of placing all measurements on a common scale, a percent normal representation of a performance capacity score can be loosely interpreted as a probability. Consider grip strength as the performance resource. Assume that there is a uniform distribution of demands placed on grip strength across a representative sample of tasks of daily living, with requirements ranging from zero to the value representing mean grip strength availability in the reference population. Further assuming that grip strength was the only performance resource that was in question for subject Y (i.e., all others were available in nonlimiting amounts), the percent normal score would represent the probability that a task involving grip strength, randomly selected from those which average individuals in the reference population could execute (i.e., those for which available grip strength would be adequate), could be successfully executed by subject Y. While the assumptions stated here are unlikely to be perfectly true, this type of interpretation helps place measurements that are most commonly made in the laboratory into daily-life contexts.

In contrast to percent normal metrics, *z-scores* take into account variability within the selected reference population. Subject Y's performance is expressed in terms of the difference between it and the reference population mean, normalized by a value corresponding to one standard-deviation unit (σ) of the reference population distribution:

$$z = \frac{R_{A_k}(Y) - R_{A_k}(\text{pop})}{\sigma} \tag{48.2}$$

It is important to note that valid *z*-scores assume that the parameter in question exhibits a normal distribution in the reference population. Moreover, *z*-scores are useful in assessing measures of structure, performance, and behavior. With regard to performance (and assuming that measures are based on a resource construct, that is, a larger numeric value represents better performance), a *z*-score of zero is produced when the subject's performance equals that of the mean performance in the reference population. Positive *z*-scores reflect performance that is better than the population mean. In a normal distribution, 68.3% of the samples fall between *z*-scores of −1.0 and +1.0, while 95.4% of these samples fall between *z*-scores of −2.0 and +2.0. Due to variability of a given performance capacity within a healthy population (e.g., some individuals are stronger, faster, and more mobile than others), a subject with a raw performance capacity score that produces a percent normal score of 70% could easily produce a *z*-score of −1.0. Whereas this percent normal score might raise concern regarding the variable of interest, the *z*-score of −1.0 indicates that a good fraction of healthy individuals exhibits lower level of performance capacity.

Both percent normal and *z*-scores require reference population data to compute. The best reference (i.e., most sensitive) is data for that specific individual (e.g., preinjury or predisease onset). In most cases, these data do not exist. However, practices such as preemployment screenings and regular checkups are beginning to provide individualized reference data in some rehabilitation contexts.

In yet another alternative, it is frequently desirable to use values representing demands imposed by tasks $[R_{D_k}(\text{task A})]$ as the reference for assessment of performance capacity measures. Demands on performance resources can be envisioned to vary over the time course of a task. In practice, an estimate of the worst-case value (i.e., highest demand) would be used in assessments that incorporate task demands as reference values. In one form, such assessments can produce binary results. For example, availability can be equal to or exceed demand (resource sufficiency), or it can be less than demand (resource insufficiency). These rule-based assessments are useful in identifying limiting factors, that is, those performance resources that inhibit a specified type of task from being performed successfully or that prevent achievement of a higher level of performance in a given type of task.

If R_{A_k} (subject Y) $\geq R_{D_k}$ (task A), then R_{A_k} (subject Y) is sufficient,

else R_{A_k} (subject Y) is insufficient $\tag{48.3}$

These rule-based assessments represent the basic process often applied (sometimes subliminally) by experienced clinicians in making routine decisions, as evidenced by statements such as "not enough strength," "not enough stability," etc. It is natural to extend and build on these strategies for use with objective measures. Extreme care must be employed. It is often possible, for example, for an individual to substitute another performance resource that is not insufficient for one that is. Clinicians take into account many such factors, and objective components should be combined with subjective assessments that provide the required breadth that enhances validity of objective components of a given assessment.

Using the same numeric values employed in rule-based binary assessments, a *preference capacity stress* metric can be computed:

$$\text{Performance capacity stress}(\%) = \frac{R_{D_k}(\text{task A})}{R_{A_k}(\text{subject Y})} \times 100 \tag{48.4}$$

Binary assessments also can be made using this metric and a threshold of 100%. However, the stress value provides additional information regarding how far (or close) a given performance capacity value is from the sufficiency threshold.

48.2 Measurement Objectives and Approaches

48.2.1 Characterizing the Human System and Its Subsystems

Figure 48.1 illustrates various points at which measurements are made over the course of a disease or injury, as well as some of the purposes for which they are made. The majority of measurements made in rehabilitation are aimed at characterizing the human system.

Measurements of human structure (Pheasant, 1986) play a critical role in the design and prescription of components such as seating, wheelchairs, workstations, artificial limbs, etc. Just like clothing,

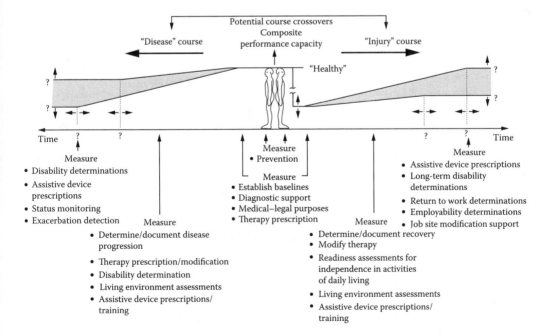

FIGURE 48.1 Measurements of structure, performance, and behavior serve many different purposes at different points over the course of a disease or injury that results in the need for rehabilitation services.

these items must "fit" the specific individual. Basic tools such as measuring tapes and rulers are becoming supplemented with three-dimensional digitizers and devices found in computer-aided manufacturing. Measurements of structure (e.g., limb segment lengths, moments of inertia, etc.) are also used with computer models (Vasta and Knodraske, 1994) in the process of analyzing tasks to determine demands in terms of performance capacity variables associated with basic systems such as flexors and extensors.

After nearly 50 years, during which a plethora of mostly disease- and injury-specific functional assessment scales were developed, the *functional independence measure* (FIM) (Hamilton et al., 1987; Keith et al., 1987) is of particular note. It is the partial result of a task-force effort to produce a systematic methodology (Uniform Data System for Medical Rehabilitation) with the specific intent of achieving standardization throughout the clinical service-delivery system. This broad methodology uses subjective judgments exclusively, based on rigorous written guidelines, to categorize demographic, diagnostic, functional, and cost information for patients within rehabilitation settings. Its simplicity to use once learned and its relatively low cost of implementation have helped in gaining a rather widespread utilization for tracking progress of individuals from admission to discharge in rehabilitation programs and evaluating effectiveness of specific therapies within and across institutions.

In contrast, many objective measurement tools of varying degrees of technological sophistication exist (Potvin et al., 1985; Smith and Leslie, 1990; Jones, 1995; Kondraske, 1995; Smith, 1995) (also see Further Information below). A good fraction of these has been designed to accomplish the same purposes as corresponding subjective methods, but with increased resolution, sensitivity, and repeatability. The intent is not always to replace subjective methods completely but to make available alternatives with the advantages noted for situations that demand superior performance in the aspects noted. There are certain measurement needs, however, that cannot be accomplished via subjective means (e.g., measurement of a human's visual information-processing speed, which involves the measurement of times of <1 s with millisecond resolution). These needs draw on the latest technology in a wide variety of ways, as demonstrated in the cited material.

With regard to instrumented measurements that pertain to a specific individual, performance capacity measures at both complex body system and basic system levels (Figure 48.1) constitute a major area of activity. A prime example is methodology associated with the implementation of industrial lifting standards (NIOSH, 1981). Performance capacity measures reflect the limits of availability of one or more selected resources and require test strategies in which the subject is commanded to perform at or near a maximum level under controlled conditions. Performance tests typically last only a short time (seconds or minutes). To improve estimates of capacities, multiple trials are usually included in a given "test" from which a final measure is computed according to some established reduction criterion (e.g., average across five trials, best of three trials). This strategy also tends to improve test–retest repeatability. Performance capacities associated with basic and intermediate-level systems are important because they are "targets of therapy" (W.W. Tourtellotte, 1993, personal communication), that is, the entities that patients and service providers want to increase to enhance the chance that enough will be available to accomplish the tasks of daily life. Thus measurements of baseline levels and changes during the course of a rehabilitation program provide important documentation (for medical, legal, insurance, and other purposes) as well as feedback to both the rehabilitation team and the patient.

Parameters of human behavior are also frequently acquired, often to help understand an individual's response to a therapy or new circumstance (e.g., obtaining a new wheelchair or prosthetic device). Behavioral parameters reflect what the subject does normally and are typically recorded over longer time periods (e.g., hours or days) compared with that required for a performance capacity measurement under conditions that are more representative of the subject's natural habitat (i.e., less laboratory like). The general approach involves identifying the behavior (i.e., an event such as "head flexion," "keystrokes," "steps," "repositionings," etc.) and at least one parametric attribute of it. Frequency, with units of "events per unit time," and time spent in a given behavioral or activity state (Ganapathy and Kondraske, 1990) are the most commonly employed behavioral metrics. States may be detected with electromyographic means or electronic sensors that respond to force, motion, position, or orientation. Behavioral measures can be used as feedback to a subject as a means to encourage desired behaviors or discourage undesirable behaviors.

48.2.2 Characterizing Tasks

Task characterization or *task analysis*, like the organization of human system parameters, is facilitated with a hierarchical perspective. A highly objective, algorithmic approach could be delineated for task analysis in any given situation (Imrhan, 2000; Maxwell, 2000). The basic objective is to obtain both descriptive and quantitative information for making decisions about the interface of a system (typically a human) to a given task. Specifically, function, procedures, and goals are of special interest. *Function* represents the purpose of a task (e.g., to flex the elbow, to lift an object, and to communicate). In contrast, task goals relate to performance, or how well the function is to be executed, and are quantifiable (e.g., the mass of an object to be lifted, the distance over which the lift must occur, the speed at which the lift must be performed, etc.). In situations with human and artificial systems, the term *overall task goals* is used to distinguish between goals of the combined human–artificial system and goals associated with the task of operating the artificial system. Procedures represent the process by which goals are achieved. Characterization of procedures can include descriptive and quantitative components (e.g., location of a person's hands at beginning and end points of a task, path in three-dimensional space between beginning and end points). Partial or completely unspecified procedures allow for variations in *style*. Goals and *procedures* are used to obtain numeric estimates of task demands in terms of the performance resources associated with the systems anticipated to be used to execute the task. Task demands are time dependent. Worst-case demands, which may occur only at specific instants in time, are of primary interest in task analysis.

Estimates of task demand can be obtained as (1) direct measurement (i.e., of goals and procedures), (2) the use of physics-based models to map direct measurements into parameters that relate more readily to measurable performance capacities of human subsystems, or (3) inference. Examples of direct measurement include key dimensions and mass of objects, three-dimensional spatial locations between "beginning" and "end points" of objects in tasks involving the movement of objects, etc. Instrumentation-supporting task analysis is available (e.g., load cells, video and other systems for measuring human position, and orientation in real time during dynamic activities), but it is not often integrated into systems for task analysis per se. Direct measurements of forces based on masses of objects and gravity often must be translated (to torques about a given body joint): this requires the use of static and dynamic models and analysis (Winter, 1990; Vasta and Kondraske, 1994).

An example of an inferential task-analysis approach that is relatively new is nonlinear causal resource analysis (NCRA) (Kondraske, 1988, 1999; Kondraske et al., 1997). This method was motivated by human performance analysis situations where direct analysis is not possible (e.g., determination of the amount of visual information-processing speed required to drive safely on a highway). Quantitative task demands, in terms of performance variables that characterize the involved subsystems, are inferred from a population data set that includes measures of subsystem performance, resource availabilities (e.g., speed, accuracy, etc.), and overall performance on the task in question. This method is based on the simple observation that the individual with the *least amount* of the given resource (i.e., the lowest performance capacity) who is still able to accomplish a given goal (i.e., achieve a given level of performance in the specified high-level task) provides the key clue. That amount of availability is used to infer the amount of demand imposed by the task.

The ultimate goal to which task characterization contributes is to identify limiting factors or unsafe conditions when a specific subject undertakes the task in question; this goal must not be lost while carrying out the basic objectives of task analysis. While rigorous algorithmic approaches are useful to make evident the true detail of the process, they are generally not performed in this manner in practice at present. Rather, the skill and experience of individuals performing the analysis are used to simplify the process, resulting in a judicious mixture of subjective estimates and objective measurements. For example, some limiting factors (e.g., grip strength) may be immediately identified without measurement of the human or the task requirements because the margin between availability and demand is so great that quick subjective "measurements" followed by an equally quick "assessment" can be used to arrive at the proper conclusion (e.g., "grip strength is a limiting factor in this task").

48.2.3 Characterizing Assistive Devices

Assistive devices can be viewed as artificial systems that either completely or partially bridge a gap between a given human (with his or her unique profile of performance capacities, i.e., available performance resources) and a particular task or class of tasks (e.g., communication, mobility, etc.). It is thus possible to consider the aspects of the device that constitute the user–device interface and those aspects which constitute, more generally, the device–task interface. In general, measurements supporting assessment of the user–device interface can be viewed to consist of (1) those which characterize the human and (2) those which characterize tasks (i.e., "operating" the assistive device). Each of these was described earlier. Measurements that characterize the device–task interface are often carried out in the context of the complete system, that is, the human-assistive device–task combination (see next subsection).

48.2.4 Characterizing Overall Systems in High-Level Task Situations

This situation generally applies to a human–artificial system–task combination. Examples include an individual using a communication aid to communicate, an individual using a wheelchair to achieve mobility, etc. Here, concern is aimed at documenting how well the task (e.g., communication, mobility, etc.) is achieved by the composite or overall system. Specific aspects or *dimensions of performance* associated with the relevant function should first be identified. Examples include speech, accuracy, stability, efficiency, etc. The total system is then maximally challenged (tempered by safety considerations) to operate along one or more of these dimensions of performance (usually not more than two dimensions are maximally challenged at the same time). For example, a subject with a communication device may be challenged to generate a single selected symbol "as fast as possible" (stressing speed without concern for accuracy). Speed is measured (e.g., with units of symbols per second) over the course of short trial (so as not to be influenced by fatigue). Then the "total system" may be challenged to generate a subset of specific symbols (chosen at random from the set of those available with a given device) one at a time, "as accurately as possible" (stressing accuracy while minimizing stress on speed capacities). Accuracy is then measured after a representative number of such trials are administered (in terms of "percent correct," for example). To further delineate the speed–accuracy performance envelope, "the system" may be challenged to select symbols at a fixed rate while accuracy is measured. Additional dimensions can be evaluated similarly. For example, endurance (measured in units of time) can be determined by selecting an operating point (e.g., by reference to the speed–accuracy performance envelope) and challenging the total system "to communicate" for "as long as possible" under the selected speed–accuracy condition.

In general, it is more useful if these types of characterizations consider all relevant dimensions with some level of measurements (i.e., subjective or objective) than it would be to apply a high-resolution, objective measurement in a process that considers only one aspect of performance.

48.3 Decision-Making Processes

Measurements that characterize the human, task, assistive device, or combination thereof are themselves only means to an end; the end is typically a decision. As noted previously, decisions are often the result of assessment processes involving one or more measurements. Although not exhaustive, many of the different types of assessments encountered are related to the following questions: (1) Is a particular aspect of performance normal (or impaired)? (2) Is a particular aspect of performance improving, stable, or getting worse? How should therapy be modified? (3) Can a given subject utilize (and benefit from) a particular assistive device? (4) Does a subject possess the required capacity to accomplish a given higher-level task (e.g., driving, a particular job after a work-related injury, etc.)?

In Figure 48.2, several of the basic concepts associated with measurement are used to illustrate how they enter into and facilitate systematic decision-making processes. The upper section shows raw score values as well as statistics for a healthy normal reference population in tabular form (left). It is difficult to reach any decision by simple inspection of just the raw performance capacity values. Tabular data are used to obtain percent normal (middle) and z-score (right) assessments. Both provide a more directly interpretable result regarding subject A's impairments. By examining the "right shoulder flexion extreme of motion" item in the figure, it can be seen that a raw score value corresponding to 51.2% normal yields a very large-magnitude, negative z-score (-10.4). This z-score indicates that virtually no one in the reference population would have a score this low. In contrast, consider similar scores for the "grip strength" item (56.2% normal, z-score = -1.99). On the basis of percent normal scores, it would appear that both these resources are similarly affected, whereas the z-score basis provides a considerably different perspective due to the fact that grip strength is *much more variable* in healthy populations than the extreme angle obtained by a given limb segment about a joint, relatively speaking. As noted, z-scores account for this variability.

The lower section of Figure 48.2 considers a situation in which the issue is a specific individual (subject A) considered in a specific task. Tabular data now include raw score values (which are the same as in upper section of the figure) and quantitative demands (typically worst case) imposed on the respective performance resources by task X. The lower-middle plot illustrates the process of individually assessing sufficiency of each performance resource in this task context using a rule-based assessment that incorporates the idea of a threshold (i.e., availability must exceed demand for sufficiency). The lower-right plot illustrates an analogous assessment process that is executed after computation of a stress metric for each of the performance capacities. Here, any demand that corresponds to more than a 100% stress level is obviously problematic. In addition to binary conclusions regarding whether a given capacity is or is not a limiting factor, it is possible to observe that of the two *limiting resources* (e.g., grip strength and right shoulder flexion extreme of motion), the former is more substantial. This might suggest, for example, that the task must be modified so as to decrease the grip strength demand (i.e., gains in performance capacity required would be substantial to achieve sufficiency) and the use of focused exercise therapy to increase shoulder flexion mobility (i.e., gains in mobility required are relatively small).

48.4 Current Limitations

48.4.1 Quality of Measurements

Key issues are measurement validity, reliability (or repeatability), accuracy, and discriminating power. An issue in terms of current limitations is not necessarily the quality of measurements but limitations with regard to methods employed to determine the quality of measurements and their interpretability.

A complete treatment of these complex topics is beyond the present scope. However, it can be said that standards are such (Potvin et al., 1985) that most published works regarding measurement instruments do address quality of measurements to some extent. Validity (i.e., how well does the measurement reflect the intended quantity) and reliability are most often addressed. However, one could easily be left with the impression that these are binary conditions (i.e., measurement is or is not reliable or valid), when in fact a continuum is required to represent these constructs. Of all attributes that relate to measurement quality, reliability is most commonly expressed in quantitative terms. This is perhaps because statistical methods have been defined and promulgated for the computation of so-called reliability coefficients (Winer, 1971). Reliability coefficients range from 0.0 to 1.0, and the implication is that 1.0 indicates a perfectly reliable or repeatable measurement process. Current methods are adequate, at best, for making

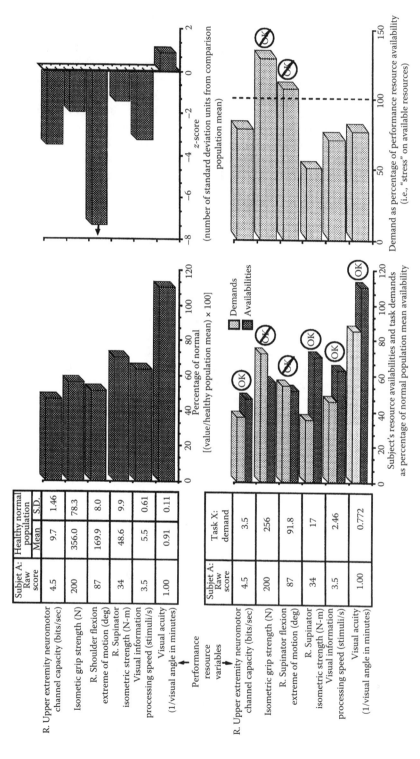

FIGURE 48.2 Examples of different types of assessments that can be performed by combining performance capacity measures and reference values of different types. The upper section shows raw score values as well as statistics for a healthy normal reference population in tabular form (*left*). It is difficult to reach any decision by simple inspection of just the raw performance capacity values. Tabular data are used to obtain a percent normal assessment (*middle*) and a z-score assessment (*right*). Both of these provide a more directly interpretable result regarding subject A's impairments. The lower section shows raw score values (same as in upper section) and quantitative demands (typically worst case) imposed on the respective performance resources by task X. The lower-middle plot illustrates the process of individually assessing sufficiency of each performance resource in this task context using a threshold rule (i.e., availability must exceed demand for sufficiency). The lower-right plot illustrates a similar assessment process after computation of a stress metric for each of the performance capacities. Here, any demand that corresponds to more than a 100% stress level is obviously problematic.

inferences regarding the relative quality of two or more methods of quantifying "the same thing." Even these comparisons require great care. For example, measurement instruments that have greater intrinsic resolving power have a great opportunity to yield smaller-reliability coefficients simply because they are capable of measuring the true variability (on repeated measurement) of the parameter in question within the system under test. While there has been widespread determination or reliability coefficients, there has been little or no effort directed toward determination of what value of a reliability coefficient is "good enough" for a particular application. In fact, reliability coefficients are relatively abstract to most practitioners.

Methods for determining the quality of a measurement process (including the instrument, procedures, examiner, and actual noise present in the variable of interest) that allow a practitioner to easily reach decisions regarding the use of a particular measurement instrument in a specific application and limitations thereof are currently lacking. As the use of different measurements increases and the number of options available for obtaining a given measurement grows, this topic will undoubtedly receive additional attention. Caution in interpreting literature, common sense, and the use of simple concepts such as "I need to measure range of motion to within 2 degrees in my application" are recommended in the meantime (Mayer et al., 1997).

48.4.1.1 Standards

Measurements and concepts with which they are associated, can contribute to a shift from experience-based knowledge acquisition to rule-based, engineering-like methods. This requires (1) a widely accepted conceptual framework (i.e., known to assistive device manufacturers, rehabilitation engineers, and other professionals within the rehabilitation community), (2) a more complete set of measurement tools that are at least standardized with regard to the definition of the quantity measured, (3) special analysis and assessment software (that removes the resistance to the application of more rigorous methods by enhancing the quality of decisions as well as the speed with which they can be reached), and (4) properly trained practitioners. Each is a necessary *but not sufficient* component. Thus balanced progress is required in each of these areas.

48.4.2 Rehabilitation Service Delivery and Rehabilitation Engineering

In a broad sense, it has been argued that all engineers can be considered rehabilitation engineers who merely work at different levels along a comprehensive spectrum of human performance, which itself can represent a common denominator among all humans. Thus an automobile is a mobility aid, a telephone is a communication aid, and so on. Just as in other engineering disciplines, measurement must be recognized not only as an important end in itself (in appropriate instances) but also as an integral component or means within the overall scope of rehabilitation and rehabilitation engineering processes. The service-delivery infrastructure must provide for such means. At present, one should anticipate and be prepared to overcome potential limitations associated with factors such as third-party reimbursement for measurement procedures, recognition of equipment and maintenance costs associated with obtaining engineering-quality measurements, and education of administrative staff and practitioners with regard to the value and proper use of measurements.

Defining Terms

Behavior: A general term that relates to what a human or artificial system does while carrying out its function(s) under given conditions. Often, behavior is characterized by measurement of selected parameters or identification of unique system states over time.

Function: The purpose of a system. Some systems map to a single primary function (e.g., process visual information). Others (e.g., the human arm) map to multiple functions, although at any given time multifunction systems are likely to be executing a single function (e.g., polishing a car).

Functions can be described and inventoried, whereas level of performance of a given function can be measured.

Functional assessment: The process of determining, from a relatively global perspective, an individual's ability to carry out tasks in daily life. Also, the result of such a process. Functional assessments typically cover a range of selected activity areas and include (at a minimum) a relatively gross indication (e.g., can or cannot do, with or without assistance) of status in each area.

Goal: A desired endpoint (i.e., result) typically characterized by multiple parameters, at least one of which is specified. Examples include specified task goals (e.g., move an object of specified mass from point A to point B in 3 s) or estimated task performance (maximum mass, range, speed of movement obtainable given a specified elemental performance resource availability profile), depending on whether a reverse or forward analysis problem is undertaken. Whereas function describes the general process of task, the goal directly relates to performance and is quantitative.

Limiting resource: A performance resource at any hierarchical level (e.g., vertical lift strength, knee flexor speed) that is available in an amount that is less than the worst-case demand imposed by a task. Thus a given resource can be "limiting" only when considered in the context of a specific task.

Overall task goals: Goals associated with a task to be executed by a human–artificial system combination (to be distinguished from goals associated with the task of operating the artificial system).

Performance: Unique qualities of a human or artificial system (e.g., strength, speed, accuracy, and endurance) that pertain to how well that system executes its function.

Performance capacity: A quantity in finite availability that is possessed by a system or subsystem, drawn on during tasks, and limits some aspect (e.g., speed, force, production, etc.) of a system's ability to execute tasks, or, the limit of that aspect itself.

Performance capacity measurement: A general class of measurements, performed at different hierarchical levels, intended to quantify one or more performance capacities.

Procedure: A set of constraints placed on a system in which flexibility exists regarding how a goal (or set of goals) associated with a given function can be achieved. Procedure specification requires specification of initial, intermediate, and/or final states or conditions dictating how the goal is to be accomplished. Such specification can be thought of in terms of removing some degrees of freedom.

Structure: Physical manifestation and attributes of a human or artificial system and the object of one type of measurements at multiple hierarchical levels.

Style: Allowance for variation within a procedure, resulting in the intentional incomplete specification of a procedure or resulting from either international or unintentional incomplete specification of procedure.

Task: That which results from (1) the combination of specified functions, goals, and procedures or (2) the specification of function and goals and the observation of procedures utilized to achieve the goals.

References

Fuhrer, M.J. 1987. *Rehabilitation Outcomes: Analysis and Measurement.* Baltimore, MD, Brookes.

Ganapathy, G. and Kondraske, G.V. 1990. Microprocessor-based instrumentation for ambulatory behavior monitoring. *J. Clin. Eng.* 15(16): 459.

Granger, C.V. and Greshorn, G.E. 1984. *Functional Assessment in Rehabilitation Medicine.* Baltimore, MD, Williams & Wilkins.

Hamilton, B.B., Granger, C.V., Sherwin, F.S. et al. 1987. A uniform national data system for medical rehabilitation. In: M.J. Fuhrer (ed.), *Rehabilitation Outcomes: Analysis and Measurement,* pp. 137–147. Baltimore, MD, Brookes.

Imrhan, S. 2000. Task analysis and decomposition: Physical components. In: J.D. Bronzino (ed.), *Handbook of Biomedical Engineering,* 2nd ed. Boca Raton, FL, CRC Press.

Jones, R.D. 1995. Measurement of neuromotor control performance capacities. In: J.D. Bronzino (ed.), *Handbook of Biomedical Engineering*. Boca Raton, FL, CRC Press.

Keith, R.A., Granger, C.V., Hamilton, B.B., and Sherwin, F.S. 1987. The functional independence measure: A new tool for rehabilitation. In: M.G. Eisenberg and R.C. Grzesiak (eds.), *Advances in Clinical Rehabilitation*, Vol. 1, pp. 6–18. New York, Springer-Verlag.

Kondraske, G.V. 1988. Experimental evaluation of an elemental resource model for human performance. In *Proceedings of the Tenth Annual IEEE Engineering in Medicine and Biology Society Conference*, pp. 1612–1613, New Orleans.

Kondraske, G.V. 1990. Quantitative measurement and assessment of performance. In: R.V. Smith and J.H. Leslie (eds.), *Rehabilitation Engineering*, pp. 101–125. Boca Raton, FL, CRC Press.

Kondraske, G.V. 2000. A working model for human system–task interfaces. In: J.D. Bronzino (ed.), *Handbook of Biomedical Engineering*, 2nd ed. Boca Raton, FL, CRC Press.

Kondraske, G.V., Johnston, C., Pearson, A., and Tarbox, L. 1997. Performance prediction and limiting resource identification with nonlinear causal resource analysis. In *Proceedings of the Nineteenth Annual Engineering in Medicine and Biology Society Conference*, pp. 1813–1816.

Kondraske, G.V. and Vasta, P.J. 2000. Measurement of information processing performance capacities. In: J.D. Bronzino (ed.), *Handbook of Biomedical Engineering*, 2nd ed. Boca Raton, FL, CRC Press.

Maxwell, K.J. 2000. High-level task analysis: Mental components. In: J.D. Bronzino (ed.), *Handbook of Biomedical Engineering*, 2nd ed. Boca Raton, FL, CRC Press.

Mayer, T., Kondraske, G.V., Brady, B.S., and Gatchel, R.J. 1997. Spinal range of motion: Accuracy and sources of error with inclinometric measurement. *Spine* 22(17): 1976–1984.

National Institute of Occupational Safety and Health (NIOSH). 1981. *Work Practices Guide for Manual Lifting (DHHS Publication No. 81122)*. Washington, US Government Printing Office.

Pheasant, S.T. 1986. *Bodyspace: Anthropometry, Ergonomics and Design*. Philadelphia, PA, Taylor & Francis.

Potvin, A.R., Tourtellotte, W.W., Potvin, J.H. et al. 1985. *The Quantitative Examination of Neurologic Function*. Boca Raton, FL, CRC Press.

Smith, R.V. and Leslie, J.H. 1990. *Rehabilitation Engineering*. Boca Raton, FL, CRC Press.

Smith, S.S. 2000. Measurement of neuromuscular performance capacities. In: J.D. Bronzino (ed.), *Handbook of Biomedical Engineering*, 2nd ed. Boca Raton, FL, CRC Press.

Vasta, P.J. and Kondraske, G.V. 1994. Performance prediction of an upper extremity reciprocal task using non-linear causal resource analysis. In *Proceedings of the Sixteenth Annual IEEE Engineering in Medicine and Biology Society Conference*, Baltimore, MD.

Vasta, P.J. and Kondraske, G.V. 2000. Human performance engineering: Computer based design and analysis tools. In: J.D. Bronzino (ed.), *Handbook of Biomedical Engineering*, 2nd ed. Boca Raton, FL, CRC Press.

Webster, J.G., Cook, A.M., Tompkin, W.J., and Vanderheiden, G.C. 1985. *Electronic Devices for Rehabilitation*. New York, Wiley.

Winer, B.J. 1971. *Statistical Principles in Experimental Design*, 2nd ed. New York, McGraw-Hill.

Winter, D.A. 1990. *Biomechanics and Motor Control of Human Movement*, 2nd ed. New York, Wiley.

World Health Organization. 1980. *International Classification of Impairments, Disabilities, and Handicaps*. Geneva, World Health Organization.

Further Information

The section of this *Handbook* entitled *"Human Performance Engineering"* contains chapters that address human performance modeling and measurement in considerably more detail.

Manufacturers of instruments used to characterize different aspects of human performance often provide technical literature and bibliographies with conceptual backgrounds, technical specifications, and application examples. A partial list of such sources is included below. (No endorsement of products is implied.)

Baltimore Therapeutic Equipment Co.
7455-L New Ridge Road
Hanover, MD 21076-3105
http://www.bteco.com/

Chattanooga Group
4717 Adams Road
Hixson, TN 37343
http://www.chattanoogagroup.com/

Henley Healthcare
120 Industrial Blvd.
Sugarland, TX 77478
http://www.henleyhealth.com/

Human Performance Measurement, Inc.
PO Box 1996
Arlington, TX 76004-1996
http://www.flash.net/~ hpm/

Lafayette Instrument
3700 Sagamore Parkway North
Lafayette, IN 47904-5729
http://www.lafayetteinstrument.com

The National Institute on Disability and Rehabilitation Research (NIDRR), part of the Department of Education, funds a set of Rehabilitation Engineering Research Centers (RERCs) and Research and Training Centers (RTCs). Each has a particular technical focus; most include measurements and measurement issues. Contact NIDRR for a current listing of these centers.

Measurement devices, issues, and application examples specific to rehabilitation are included in the following journals:

American Journal of Occupational Therapy
The American Occupational Therapy Association, Inc.
4720 Montgomery Ln.,
Bethesda, MD 20814-3425
http://www.aota.org/

Archives of Physical Medicine and Rehabilitation
Suite 1310
78 East Adams Street
Chicago, IL 60603-6103

IEEE Transactions on Rehabilitation Engineering
IEEE Service Center
445 Hoes Lane
PO Box 1331
Piscataway, NJ 08855-1331
http://www.ieee.org/index.html

Journal of Occupational Rehabilitation
Subscription Department
Plenum Publishing Corporation
233 Spring St.

New York, NY 10013
http://www.plenum.com/

Journal of Rehabilitation Research and Development
Scientific and Technical Publications Section
Rehabilitation Research and Development Service
103 South Gay St., 5th floor
Baltimore, MD 21202-4051
http://www.vard.org/jour/jourindx.htm

Physical Therapy
American Physical Therapy Association
1111 North Fairfax St.
Alexandria, VA 22314
http://www.apta.org/

49

Rehabilitation Engineering Technologies: Principles of Application

Douglas Hobson
University of Pittsburgh

Elaine Trefler
University of Pittsburgh

Rehabilitation engineering is the branch of *biomedical engineering* that is concerned with the application of science and technology to improve the quality of life of individuals with disabilities. Areas addressed within rehabilitation engineering include wheelchairs and seating systems, access to computers, sensory aids, prosthetics and orthotics, alternative and augmentative communication, home and worksite modifications, and universal design. Because many products of rehabilitation engineering require careful selection to match individual needs and often require custom fitting, rehabilitation engineers have necessarily become involved in service delivery and application as well as research, design, and development. Therefore, as we expand on later, it is not only engineers who practice within the field of rehabilitation engineering.

As suggested above, and as in many other disciplines, there are really two career tracks in the field of rehabilitation engineering. There are those who acquire qualifications and experience to advance the state of knowledge through conducting research, education, and product development, and there are others who are engaged in the application of technology as members of service delivery teams. At one time it was possible for a person to work in both arenas. However, with the explosion of technology and the growth of the field over the past decade, one must now specialize not only within research or service delivery but often within a specific area of technology.

One can further differentiate between rehabilitation and assistive technology. *Rehabilitation technology* is a term most often used to refer to technologies associated with the acute-care rehabilitation process. Therapy evaluation and treatment tools, clinical dysfunction measurement and recording instrumentation, and prosthetic and orthotic appliances are such examples. *Assistive technologies* are those devices and services that are used in the daily lives of people in the community to enhance their ability to function independently, examples being specialized seating, wheelchairs, environmental control devices, workstation access technologies, and services are now communication aids. Recognition and support of assistive technology devices and services are now embedded in all the major disability legislation that has been enacted over the last decade.

The primary focus of this chapter is on the role of the rehabilitation engineering practitioner as he or she carries out the responsibilities demanded by the application of assistive technology.

Before launching into the primary focus of this chapter, let us first set a conceptual framework for the *raison d'etre* for assistive technology and the role of the assistive technology professional.

49.1 The Conceptual Frameworks

The application of assistive technology can be conceptualized as minimizing the functional gap between the person and his or her environment. This reality is what technology does for all of us to varying degrees. For example, if you live in a suburban area that has been designed for access only by car and your car breaks down, you are handicapped. If your house has been designed to be cooled by air conditioning in the "dog days" of summer and you lose a compressor, your comfort is immediately compromised by your incompatibility with your environment. Similarly, if you live in a home that has only access by steps and you have an impairment requiring the use of a wheelchair, you are handicapped because you no longer have abilities that are compatible with your built environment. Because our environments, homes, workplaces, schools, and communities have been designed to be compatible with the abilities of the norm, young children, persons with disabilities, and many elderly people experience the consequences of their mismatch as a matter of course. The long-term utopian solution would be to design environments and their contents so that they can be used by all people of all ages, which is the essence of the universal design concept. However, given that today we do not have many products and environments that have been universally designed, rehabilitation engineers attempt to minimize the effects of the mismatch by designing, developing, and providing technologies that will allow persons with disabilities to pursue their life goals in a manner similar to any other person. Of course, the rehabilitation engineer cannot accomplish this working in isolation but rather must function as a part of a consumer-responsive team that can best deal with the multiplicity of factors that usually impact on the successful application of assistive technology.

Let us now move to another conceptual framework, one that conceptualizes how people actually interact with technology.

The following conceptualization has been adapted from the model proposed by Roger Smith (1992). In Figure 49.1, Smith suggests that there are three cyclic elements that come into play when humans interact with technology: the human and his or her innate sensory, cognitive, and functional abilities; the human factor's characteristics of the interface between the human and the technology; and the technical characteristics of the technology itself in terms of its output as a result of a specific input by the user. People with disabilities may have varying degrees of dysfunction in their sensory, cognitive, and functional abilities. The interface will have to be selected or adapted to these varying abilities in order to allow the person to effectively interact with the technology. The technology itself will need to possess specific electronic or mechanical capabilities in order to yield the desired outcome. The essence of assistive technology applications is to integrate all three of these elements into a functional outcome that meets the specific needs of a user. This is usually done by selecting commercially available devices and technologies at a cost that can be met by either the individual or his or her third-party payment source. When technologies are not available, then they must be modified from existing devices or designed and fabricated as unique custom solutions. It is particularly in these latter activities that a rehabilitation engineer can make his or her unique contribution to team process.

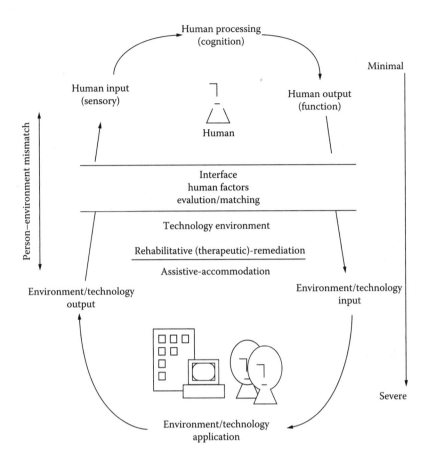

FIGURE 49.1 Conceptual framework of technology and disability. (Modified from Smith, R.O. 1992. Technology and disability. *AJOT* 1:22.)

Cook and Hussey (1995), published an excellent text, *Assistive Technologies—Principles and Practice*. As well as comprehensively addressing many of the assistive technologies briefly covered in this chapter, they also present a conceptual framework which builds on the one developed by Smith above. They introduce the additional concepts of activity and context. That is, understanding of a person's activity desires and the context (social, setting, and physical) in which they are to be carried out are essential components to successful assistive technology intervention.

It should be realized that there are several levels of assistive technology. The first level might be termed *fundamental technology* in contrast to advanced technology. Fundamental technologies, such as walkers, crutches, many wheelchairs, activities of daily living (ADL) equipment, etc., usually do not require the involvement of the rehabilitation engineer in their application. Others on the team can better assess the need, confirm the interface compatibility, and verify that the outcome is appropriate. The rehabilitation engineer is most often involved in the application of advanced technologies, such as powered wheelchairs, computerized workstation designs, etc., that require an understanding of the underlying technological principles in order to achieve the best match with the abilities and needs of the user, especially if custom modifications or integration of devices are required to the original equipment. The rehabilitation engineer is usually the key person if a unique solution is necessary.

Let's now discuss a few fundamental concepts related to the process by which assistive technology is typically provided in various service delivery programs.

49.2 The Provision Process

49.2.1 The Shifting Paradigm

In the traditional rehabilitation model of service delivery, a multidisciplinary team of professionals is already in place. Physicians, therapists, counselors, and social worker meet with the client and, based on the findings of a comprehensive evaluation, plan a course of action. In the field of assistive technology, the rules of the team are being charted anew. First, the decision making often takes place in a nonmedical environment and often without a physician as part of the team. Second, the final decision is rapidly moving into the hands of the consumer, not the professionals. The third major change is the addition of a rehabilitation engineer to the team. Traditional team members have experience working in groups and delegating coordination and decision making to colleagues depending on the particular situation. They are trained to be team players and are comfortable working in groups. Most engineers who enter the field of rehabilitation engineering come with a traditional engineering background. Although well versed in design and engineering principles, they often do not receive formal training in group dynamics and need to learn these skills if they are to function effectively. As well, engineers are trained to solve problems with technical solutions. The psychosocial aspects of assisting people with disabilities to make informed choices must be learned most often outside the traditional education stream. Therefore, for the engineer to be a contributing member of the team, not only must he or she bring engineering expertise, but it must be integrated in such a manner that it supports the overall objectives of the technology delivery process, which is to respond to the needs and desires of the consumer.

People with disabilities want to have control over the process and be informed enough to make good decisions. This is quite different from the traditional medical or rehabilitation model, in which well-meaning professionals often tell the individual what is best for him or her. Within this new paradigm, the role is to inform, advise, and educate, not to decide. The professional provides information as to the technical options, prices, etc. and then assists the person who will use the technology to acquire it and learn how to use it.

49.2.2 The Evaluation

An evaluation is meant to guide decision making for the person with a disability toward appropriate and cost-effective technology. Often, more than one functional need exists for which assistive technology could be prescribed. Costly, frustrating, and time-consuming mistakes often can be avoided if a thorough evaluation based on a person's total functional needs is performed before any technology is recommended. Following the evaluation, a long-range plan for acquisition and training in the chosen technology can be started.

For example, suppose a person needs a seating system, both a powered and manual wheelchair, an augmentative communication device, a computer workstation, and an environmental control unit (ECU). Where does one begin? Once a person's goals and priorities have been established, the process can begin. First, a decision would likely be made about the seating system that will provide appropriate support in the selected manual chair. However, the specifications of seating system should be such that the components also can be interfaced into the powered chair. The controls for the computer and augmentative communication device must be located so that they do not interfere with the display of the communication device and must in some way be compatible with the controls for the ECU. Only if all functional needs are addressed can the technology be acquired in a logical sequence and in such a manner that all components will be compatible. The more severely disabled the individual, the more technology he or she will need, and the more essential is the process of setting priorities and ensuring compatibility of technical components.

In summary, as suggested by the conceptual model, the process begins by gaining an understanding of the person's sensory, cognitive, and functional abilities, combined with clarification of his or her desires and needs. These are then filtered through the technology options, both in terms of how the interface will integrate with the abilities of the user and how the technology itself will be integrated to meet the defined needs. This information and the associated pros and cons are conveyed to the user, or in some cases, their caregiver, who then has the means to participate in the ultimate selection decisions.

49.2.3 Service Delivery Models

People with disabilities can access technology through a variety of different service delivery models. A team of professionals might be available in a university setting where faculty not only teaches but also delivers technical services to the community. More traditionally, the team of rehabilitation professionals, including a rehabilitation engineer, might be available at a hospital or rehabilitation facility. More recently, technology professionals might be in private practice either individually, as a team, or part of the university, hospital, or rehabilitation facility structure. Another option is the growing number of rehabilitation technology suppliers (RTSs) who offer commercial technology services within the community. They work in conjunction with an evaluation specialist and advise consumers as to the technical options available to meet their needs. They then sell and service the technology and train the consumer in its use. Local chapters of national disability organizations such as United Cerebral Palsy and Easter Seals also may have assistive technology services. In recent years, a growing number of centers for independent living (CILs) have been developed in each state with federal support. Some of these centers have opted to provide assistive technology services, in addition to their information and referral services, which are common to all CILs. And finally, there are volunteers, either in engineering schools or community colleges (student-supervised projects) or in industry (high-technology industries often have staff interested in doing community service), such as the Telephone Pioneers. Each model has its pros and cons for the consumer, and only after thoroughly researching the options will the person needing the service make the best choice as to where to go with his or her need in the community. A word of caution. Only if there is timely provision and follow-up available is a service delivery system considered appropriate, even if the cost of the service is less.

A more extensive description of service delivery options may be reviewed in a report that resulted from a RESNA-organized conference on service delivery (ANSI/RESNA, 1990).

49.3 Education and Quality Assurance

Professionals on the assistive technology team have a primary degree and credential in their individual professions. For example, the occupational or physical therapist will have a degree and most often state licensure in occupational or physical therapy. The engineer will have recognized degrees in mechanical, electrical, biomedical, or some other school of engineering. However, in order to practice effectively in the field of assistive technology, almost all will need advanced training. A number of occupational therapy curriculums provide training in assistive technology, but not all. The same is true of several of the others. Consumers and payers of assistive technology need to know that professionals practicing in the field of assistive technology have a certain level of competency. For this reason, all professionals, including rehabilitation engineers, are pursuing the ATP (assistive technology practitioner) credential through RESNA.

49.3.1 RESNA

RESNA, an interdisciplinary association of persons dedicated to the advancement of assistive technology for people with disabilities, has a credentialing program that credentials individuals on the assistive technology team. As part of the process, the minimum skills and knowledge base for practitioners is tested. Ties with professional organizations are being sought so that preservice programs will include at least some of the knowledge and skills base necessary. Continuing education efforts by RESNA and others also will assist in building the level of expertise of practitioners and consumers. At this time RESNA has a voluntary credentialling process to determine if a person meets a predetermined minimal standard of practice in the field of Assistive Technology. Persons who meet the prerequisite requirements, pass a written exam, and agree to abide by the RESNA Standards of Practice can declare themselves as RESNA certified. They can add the ATP if they are practitioners or ATS if they are suppliers of assistive technology.

Payment for technology and the services required for its application are complex and changing rapidly as healthcare reform evolves. It is beyond the scope of this discussion to detail the very convoluted and individual process required to ensure that people with disabilities receive what they need. However, there are some basic concepts to be kept in mind. Professionals need to be competent. The documentation of need and the justification of selection must be comprehensive. Time for a person to do this must be allocated if there is to be success. Persistence, creativity, education of the payers, and documentation of need and outcomes are the key issues.

49.4 Specific Impairments and Related Technologies

Current information related to specific technologies is best found in brochures, trade magazines (*Report Rehab*), exhibit halls of technology-related conferences, and databases such as ABLEDATA. Many suppliers and manufacturers are now maintaining Websites, which provide a quick means to locate information on current products. What follows is only a brief introduction to specific disabilities areas to which assistive technology applications are commonly used.

49.4.1 Mobility

Mobility technologies include wheelchairs, walkers, canes, orthotic devices, FES (functional electrical stimulation), laser canes, and any other assistive device that would assist a person with a mobility impairment, be it motor or sensory, to move about in his or her environment. There are very few people who have a working knowledge of all the possible commercial options. Therefore, people usually acquire expertise in certain areas, such as wheelchairs. There are hundreds of varieties of wheelchairs, each offering a different array of characteristics that need to be understood as part of the selection process. Fortunately, there are now several published ways that the practitioner and the consumer can obtain useful information. A classification system has been developed that sets a conceptual framework for understanding the different types of wheelchairs that are produced commercially (Hobson, 1990). *Paraplegic News and Sports and Spokes* annually publish the specifications on most of the manual and powered wheelchairs commonly found in the North American marketplace. These reviews are based on standardized testing that is carried out by manufacturers following the ANSI/RESNA wheelchair standards (ANSI/RESNA, 1990). Since the testing and measurements of wheelchairs are now done and reported in a standard way, it is possible to make accurate comparisons between products, a tremendous recent advancement for the wheelchair specialist and the users they serve (Axelson et al., 1994).

Possibly the most significant advancement in wheelchairs is the development and application of industry, on an international scale, for testing the safety and durability of their products. These standards also mandate what and how the test information should be made available in the manufacturer's presale literature. The Rehabilitation Engineering Research Center and University of Pittsburgh (RERC, 1999) maintains a large Website, where among its many resources is a listing of wheelchair research publications and a general reference site, termed Wheelchairnet (Wheelchairnet, 1999). The RERC site also tracks the current activities occurring in many of the wheelchair standards working groups. Finally, Cooper (1995, 1998) has published two excellent reference texts on rehabilitation engineering with emphasis on wheeled mobility.

49.4.2 Sitting

Many people cannot use the wheelchairs as they come from the manufacturer. Specialized seating is required to help persons to remain in a comfortable and functional seated posture for activities that enable them to access work and attend educational and recreational activities. Orthotic supports, seating systems in wheelchairs, chairs that promote dynamic posture in the workplace, and chairs for the elderly that fit properly, are safe and encourage movement all fit into the broad category of sitting technology.

49.4.3 Sensation

People with no sensation are prone to skin injury. Special seating technology can assist in the preventions of tissue breakdown. Specially designed cushions and backs for wheelchairs and mattresses that have pressure-distributing characteristics fall into this category. Technology also has been developed to measure the interface pressure. These tools are now used routinely to measure and record an individual's pressure profile, making cushion selection and problem solving more of a science than an art.

Again, a classification system of specialized seating has been developed that provides a conceptual framework for understanding the features of the various technologies and their potential applications. The same reference also discusses the selection process, evaluation tools, biomechanics of supported sitting, and materials properties of weight-relieving materials (Hobson, 1990).

49.4.4 Access (Person–Machine Interface)

In order to use assistive technology, people with disabilities need to be able to operate the technology. With limitations in motor and/or sensory systems, often a specially designed or configured interface system must be assembled. It could be as simple as several switches or a miniaturized keyboard or as complex as an integrated control system that allows a person to drive a wheelchair and operate a computer and a communication device using only one switch.

49.4.5 Communication

Because of motor or sensory limitations, some individuals cannot communicate with spoken or written word. There are communication systems that enable people to communicate using synthesized voice or printed output. Systems for people who are deaf allow them to communicate over the phone or through computer interfaces. Laptop computers with appropriate software can enable persons to communicate faster and with less effort than previously possible. Some basic guidelines for selecting an augmentative communication system, including strategies for securing funding, have been proposed in an overview chapter by James Jones and Winifred Jones (Jones and Jones, 1990).

49.4.6 Transportation

Modified vans and cars enable persons with disabilities to independently drive a vehicle. Wheelchair tie-downs and occupant restraints in personal vehicles and in public transportation vehicles are allowing people to be safely transported to their chosen destination. Fortunately, voluntary performance standards for restraint and tie-down technologies have been developed by a task group within the Society for Automotive Engineers (SAE). Standards for car hand controls, van body modifications, and wheelchair lifts are also available from SAE. These standards provide the rehabilitation engineer with a set of tools that can be used to confirm safety compliance of modified transportation equipment. Currently in process and still requiring several more years of work are transport wheelchair and vehicle power control standards.

49.4.7 Activities of Daily Living (ADL)

ADL technology enables a person to live independently as much as possible. Such devices as environmental control units, bathroom aids, dressing assists, automatic door openers, and alarms are all considered aids to daily living. Many are inexpensive and can be purchased through careful selection in stores or through catalogues. Others are quite expensive and must be ordered through vendors who specialize in technology for independent living.

Ron Mace, now deceased and creator of the Center for Universal Design at the North Carolina State University, is widely acknowledged as the father of the Universal Design concept. The concept of universal design simply means that if our everyday built environments and their contained products could be designed to meet the needs of a wider range of people, both young and old, then the needs of more persons with disabilities would be met without the need for special adaptations (Center for Universal Design, 1999). Others like Paul Grayson have also published extensively regarding the need to rethink how we design our living environments (Grayson, 1991). Vanderheiden and Denno have prepared human factors guidelines that provide design information to allow improved access by the elderly and persons with disabilities (Vanderheiden and Vanderheiden, 1991; Denno et al., 1992; Trace Center, 1999).

49.4.8 School and Work

Technology that supports people in the workplace or in an educational environment can include applications such as computer workstations, modified restrooms, and transportation to and from work or school. Students need the ability to take notes and do assignments, and people working have a myriad of special tasks that may need to be analyzed and modified to enable the employee with the disability to be independent and productive. Weisman has presented an extensive overview of rehabilitation engineering in the workplace, which includes a review of different types of workplaces, the process of accommodation, and many case examples (Weisman, 1990).

49.4.9 Recreation

A component of living that is often overlooked by the professional community is the desire and, in fact, need of people with disabilities to participate in recreational activities. Many of the adaptive recreational technologies have been developed by persons with disabilities themselves in their effort to participate and be competitive in sports. Competitive wheelchair racing, archery, skiing, bicycles, and technology that enables people to bowl, play pool, and fly their own airplanes are just a few areas in which equipment has been adapted for specific recreational purposes.

49.4.10 Community and Workplace Access

There is probably no other single legislation that is having a more profound impact on the lives of people with disabilities then the Americans with Disabilities Act (ADA), signed into law by President Bush in August of 1990. This civil rights legislation mandates that all people with disabilities have access to public facilities and that reasonable accommodations must be made by employers to allow persons with disabilities to access employment opportunities. The impact of this legislation is now sweeping America and leading to monumental changes in the way people view the rights of persons with disabilities.

49.5 Future Developments

The field of rehabilitation engineering, both in research and in service delivery, is at an important crossroad in its young history. Shifting paradigms of services, reduction in research funding, consumerism, credentialing, healthcare reform, and limited formal educational options all make speculating on what the future may bring rather hazy. Given all this, it is reasonable to say that one group of rehabilitation engineers will continue to advance the state of the art through research and development, while another group will be on the front lines as members of clinical teams working to ensure that individuals with disabilities receive devices and services that are most appropriate for their particular needs.

The demarcation between researchers and service providers will become clearer, since the latter will become credentialed. RESNA and its professional specialty group (PSG) on rehabilitation engineering are working out the final credentialing steps for the Rehabilitation Engineer (RE) and the Rehabilitation Engineering Technologist (RET). Both must also be an ATP. They will be recognized as valued members of the clinical team by all members of the rehabilitation community, including third-party payers, who will reimburse them for the rehabilitation engineering services that they provide. They will spend as much or more time working in the community as they will in clinical settings. They will work closely with consumer-managed organizations who will be the gatekeepers of increasing amounts of government-mandated service dollars.

If these predictions come to pass, the need for rehabilitation engineering will continue to grow. As medicine and medical technology continue to improve, more people will survive traumatic injury, disease, and premature birth, and many will acquire functional impairments that impede their involvement in personal, community, educational, vocational, and recreational activities. People continue to live longer lives, thereby increasing the likelihood of acquiring one or more disabling conditions during their lifetime. This presents an immense challenge for the field of rehabilitation engineering. As opportunities grow, more engineers will be attracted to the field. More and more rehabilitation engineering education programs will develop that will support the training of qualified engineers, engineers who are looking for exciting challenges, and opportunities to help people live more satisfying and productive lives.

References

ANSI/RESNA. 1990. *Wheelchair Standards*. RESNA Press, RESNA, 1700 Moore St., Arlington, VA 22209-1903.

Axelson, P., Minkel, J., and Chesney, D. 1994. *A Guide to Wheelchair Selection: How to Use the ANSI/RESNA Wheelchair Standards to Buy a Wheelchair*. Paralyzed Veterans of America (PVA).

Bain, B.K. and Leger, D. 1997. *Assistive Technology. An Interdisciplinary Approach*. Churchill Livingstone, New York.

Center for Universal Design, 1999. http://www.design.ncsu.edu/cud/

Cook, A.M. and Hussey, S.M. 1995. *Assistive Technologies: Principles and Practice*. Mosby, St. Louis, MO.

Cooper, R.A. 1995. *Rehabilitation Engineering Applied to Mobility and Manipulation*. Institute of Physics Publishing, Bristol, UK

Cooper, R.A. 1998. *Wheelchair Selection and Configuration*. Demos Medical Publishing, New York.

Deno, J.H. et al. 1992. *Human Factors Design Guidelines for the Elderly and People with Disabilities*. Honeywell, Inc., Minneapolis, MN 55418 (Brian Isle, MN65-2300).

Galvin, J.C. and Scherer, M.J. 1996. *Evaluating, Selecting, and Using Appropriate Assistive Technology*, Aspen Publishers, Gaithersburg, MD.

Hobson, D.A. 1990. Seating and mobility for the severely disabled. In: R. Smith and J. Leslie (eds.), *Rehabilitation Engineering*, pp. 193–252. CRC Press, Boca Raton, FL.

Jones, D. and Jones, W. 1990. Criteria for selection of an augmentative communication system. In: R. Smith and J. Leslie (eds.), *Rehabilitation Engineering*, pp. 181–189. CRC Press, Boca Raton, FL.

Medhat, M. and Hobson, D. 1992. *Standardization of Terminology and Descriptive Methods for Specialized Seating*. RESNA Press, RESNA, 1700 Moore St. , Arlington, VA 22209-1903.

Rehabilitation Technology Service Delivery—*A Practical Guide*. 1987. RESNA Press, RESNA, 1700 Moore St., Arlington, VA 22209-1903.

Smith, R.O. 1992. Technology and disability. *AJOT* 1: 22.

Society for Automotive Engineers. 1994. *Wheelchair Tie-Down and Occupant Restraint Standard (Committee Draft)*. SAE. Warrendale, PA.

Trace Center, 1999. http://trace.wisc.edu/

Vanderheiden, G. and Vanderheiden, K. 1991. *Accessibility Design Guidelines for the Design of Consumer Products to Increase their Accessibility to People with Disabilities or Who Are Aging*. Trace R&D Center, University of Wisconsin, Madison, WI.

Weisman, G. 1990. Rehabilitation engineering in the workplace. In: R. Smith and J. Leslie (eds.), *Rehabilitation Engineering*, pp. 253–297. CRC Press, Boca Raton, FL.

WheelchairNet, 1999. http://www.wheelchairnet.org

Further Information

AbleData, 8455 Colesville Rd., Suite 935, Silver Spring, MD 20910-3319.

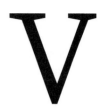

Clinical Engineering

Yadin David
Biomedical Engineering Consultants

Preface

During the past 100 years, the dependence of the healthcare system on medical technology for the delivery of its services has grown continuously. To some extent, all practitioners and clinical staff are dependent on technology, be it in the area of preventive medicine, diagnosis procedures, therapeutic care, rehabilitation, administration, or health-related education and training. Healthcare technology enables practitioners to integrate their interventions through connected decision-support systems and to manage their interactions with patients' condition in a cost-effective, efficient, and safe manner. As a result, the field of clinical engineering has continued to emerge as the discipline of biomedical engineering that fulfills the need to safely and efficiently manage the deployment of healthcare technology and to integrate it appropriately to support achieving desired clinical outcomes.

The healthcare delivery system presents a very complex environment in which human interventions taking place 365 days per year and 24 h per day in interacted environment of facilities, equipment, application software, materials, supplies, and a full range of patient population are involved. It is in this clinical environment that patients of various ages and conditions, trained staff, and the wide variety of medical technology converge. This complex mix of interactions may lead to unacceptable risk when programs for assessing, monitoring, controlling, improving, and educating all entities involved are not appropriately integrated or not managed by qualified professionals. Recent focus on the management of risk associated with networks that are connected to medical devices has magnified the need for new skills and for robust technology management program. New skills that support team approach and collaboration among various stakeholders include clinical engineering, information technology (IT), clinical, and administrative communities.

This section of clinical engineering focuses on the methodology for administering clinical engineering services that stretch from the facilitation of product innovation and technology transfer to the performance of technology assessment and operations verification support and onto the management tools with which today's clinical engineer needs to be familiar. With increased utilization of technological tools and of the awareness of the value obtained by these services, new career opportunities are created for clinical engineers.

In addition to highlighting the important roles that clinical engineers serve in many areas, this section focuses on those areas of the clinical engineering field that enhance the understanding of the "bigger picture." With such an understanding, the participation in and contribution by clinical engineers to improvements in their organization operation can be fully realized. The adoption of the tools described here will enable clinical engineers to fulfill their new role in the evolving objectives of today's healthcare delivery system.

All the authors in this section recognize this opportunity for volunteering their talent and time so that others can excel as well.

50

Clinical Engineering: Evolution of a Discipline

Joseph D. Bronzino
Trinity College

50.1 Who Is a Clinical Engineer?

As discussed in the introduction to this *Handbook*, biomedical engineers apply the concepts, knowledge, and techniques of virtually all engineering disciplines to solve specific problems in the biosphere, that is, the realm of biology and medicine. When biomedical engineers work within a hospital or clinic, they are more appropriately called *clinical engineers*. But what exactly is the definition of the term *clinical engineer*? For the purposes of this handbook, a *clinical engineer* is defined as an engineer who has graduated from an accredited academic program in engineering or who is licensed as a professional engineer or engineer-in-training and is engaged in the application of scientific and technological knowledge developed through engineering education and subsequent professional experience within the healthcare environment in support of clinical activities. Furthermore, clinical environment means that portion of the healthcare system in which patient care is delivered, and clinical activities include direct patient care, research, teaching, and public service activities intended to enhance patient care.

50.2 Evolution of Clinical Engineering

Engineers were first encouraged to enter the clinical scene during the late 1960s in response to concerns about patient safety as well as the rapid proliferation of clinical equipment, especially in academic medical centers. In the process, a new engineering discipline—clinical engineering—evolved to provide the technological support necessary to meet these new needs. During the 1970s, a major expansion of clinical engineering occurred, primarily due to the following events:

- The Veterans' Administration (VA), convinced that clinical engineers were vital to the overall operation of the VA hospital system, divided the country into biomedical engineering districts, with a chief biomedical engineer overseeing all engineering activities in the hospitals in that district.
- Throughout the United States, clinical engineering departments were established in most of the large medical centers and hospitals and in some smaller clinical facilities with at least 300 beds.

- Clinical engineers were hired in increasing numbers to help these facilities use existing technology and incorporate new technology.

Having entered the hospital environment, routine electrical safety inspections exposed the clinical engineer to all types of patient equipment that was not being maintained properly. It soon became obvious that electrical safety failures represented only a small part of the overall problem posed by the presence of medical equipment in the clinical environment. The equipment was neither totally understood nor properly maintained. Simple visual inspections often revealed broken knobs, frayed wires, and even evidence of liquid spills. Investigating further, it was found that many devices did not perform in accordance with manufacturers' specifications and were not maintained in accordance with manufacturers' recommendations. In short, electrical safety problems were only the tip of the iceberg. The entrance of clinical engineers into the hospital environment changed these conditions for the better. By the mid-1970s, complete performance inspections before and after use became the norm, and sensible inspection procedures were developed. In the process, clinical engineering departments became the logical support center for all medical technologies and became responsible for all the biomedical instruments and systems used in hospitals, the training of medical personnel in equipment use and safety, and the design, selection, and use of technology to deliver safe and effective healthcare.

With increased involvement in many facets of hospital/clinic activities, clinical engineers now play a multifaceted role (Figure 50.1). They must interface successfully with many "clients," including clinical staff, hospital administrators, regulatory agencies, etc., to ensure that the medical equipment within the hospital is used safely and effectively.

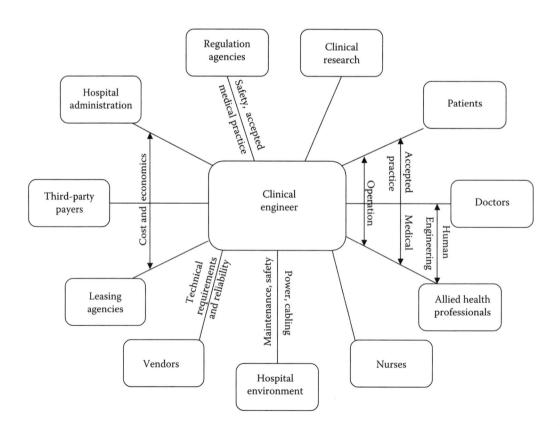

FIGURE 50.1   Diagram illustrating the range of interactions of a clinical engineer.

Today, hospitals that have established centralized clinical engineering departments to meet these responsibilities use clinical engineers to provide the hospital administration with an objective option of equipment function, purchase, application, overall system analysis, and preventive maintenance policies.

Some hospital administrators have learned that with the in-house availability of such talent and expertise, the hospital is in a far better position to make more effective use of its technological resources (Bronzino, 1992). By providing health professionals with needed assurance of safety, reliability, and efficiency in using new and innovative equipment, clinical engineers can readily identify poor-quality and ineffective equipment, thereby resulting in faster, more appropriate utilization of new medical equipment. Typical pursuits of clinical engineers, therefore, include:

- Supervision of a hospital clinical engineering department that includes clinical engineers and biomedical equipment technicians (BMETs)
- Prepurchase evaluation and planning for new medical technology
- Design, modification, or repair of sophisticated medical instruments or systems
- Cost-effective management of a medical equipment calibration and repair service
- Supervision of the safety and performance testing of medical equipment performed by BMETs
- Inspection of all incoming equipment (i.e., both new and returning repairs)
- Establishment of performance benchmarks for all equipment
- Medical equipment inventory control
- Coordination of outside engineering and technical services performed by vendors
- Training of medical personnel in the safe and effective use of medical devices and systems
- Clinical applications engineering, such as custom modification of medical devices for clinical research, evaluation of new noninvasive monitoring systems, etc.
- Biomedical computer support
- Input to the design of clinical facilities where medical technology is used, for example, operating rooms (ORs), intensive- care units, etc.
- Development and implementation of documentation protocols required by external accreditation and licensing agencies

Clinical engineers thus provide extensive engineering services for the clinical staff and, in recent years, have been increasingly accepted as valuable team members by physicians, nurses, and other clinical professionals. Furthermore, the acceptance of clinical engineers in the hospital setting has led to different types of engineering–medicine interactions, which in turn have improved healthcare delivery.

50.3 Hospital Organization and the Role of Clinical Engineering

In the hospital, management organization has evolved into a diffuse authority structure that is commonly referred to as the *triad model*. The three primary components are the governing board (trustees), hospital administration (CEO and administrative staff), and the medical staff organization. The role of the governing board and the chief executive officer are briefly discussed below to provide some insight regarding their individual responsibilities and their interrelationship.

50.3.1 Governing Board (Trustees)

The *Joint Commission on the Accreditation of Healthcare Organizations (JCAHO)* summarizes the major duties of the governing board as "adopting by-laws in accordance with its legal accountability and its responsibility to the patient." The governing body, therefore, requires both medical and paramedical departments to monitor and evaluate the quality of patient care, which is a critical success factor in hospitals today. To meet this goal, the governing board essentially is responsible for establishing the mission statement and defining the specific goals and objectives that the institution must satisfy. Therefore, the trustees are involved in the following functions:

- Establishing the policies of the institution
- Providing equipment and facilities to conduct patient care
- Ensuring that proper professional standards are defined and maintained (i.e., providing quality assurance)
- Coordinating professional interests with administrative, financial, and community needs
- Providing adequate financing by securing sufficient income and managing the control of expenditures
- Providing a safe environment
- Selecting qualified administrators, medical staff, and other professionals to manage the hospital

In practice, the trustees select a hospital chief administrator who develops a plan of action that is in concert with the overall goals of the institution.

50.3.2 Hospital Administration

The hospital administrator, the chief executive officer of the medical enterprise, has a function similar to that of the chief executive officer of any corporation. The administrator represents the governing board in carrying out the day-to-day operations to reflect the broad policy formulated by the trustees. The duties of the administrator are summarized as follows:

- Preparing a plan for accomplishing the institutional objectives, as approved by the board
- Selecting medical chiefs and department directors to set standards in their respective fields
- Submitting for board approval an annual budget reflecting both expenditures and income projections
- Maintaining all physical properties (plant and equipment) in safe operating condition
- Representing the hospital in its relationships with the community and health agencies
- Submitting to the board annual reports that describe the nature and volume of the services delivered during the past year, including appropriate financial data and any special reports that may be requested by the board

In addition to these administrative responsibilities, the chief administrator is charged with controlling cost, complying with a multitude of governmental regulations, and ensuring that the hospital conforms to professional norms, which include guidelines for the care and safety of patients.

50.4 Clinical Engineering Programs

In many hospitals, administrators have established clinical engineering departments to manage effectively all the technological resources, especially those relating to medical equipment, that are necessary for providing patient care. The primary objective of these departments is to provide a broad-based engineering program that addresses all aspects of medical instrumentation and systems support.

Figure 50.2 illustrates the organizational chart of the medical support services division of a typical major medical facility. Note that within this organizational structure, the director of clinical engineering reports directly to the vice president of medical support services. This administrative relationship is extremely important because it recognizes the important role clinical engineering departments play in delivering quality care. It should be noted, however, that in other common organizational structures, clinical engineering services may fall under the category of "facilities," "materials management," or even just "support services." Clinical engineers also can work directly with clinical departments, thereby bypassing much of the hospital hierarchy. In this situation, clinical departments can offer the clinical engineer both the chance for intense specialization and, at the same time, the opportunity to develop personal relationships with specific clinicians based on mutual concerns and interests.

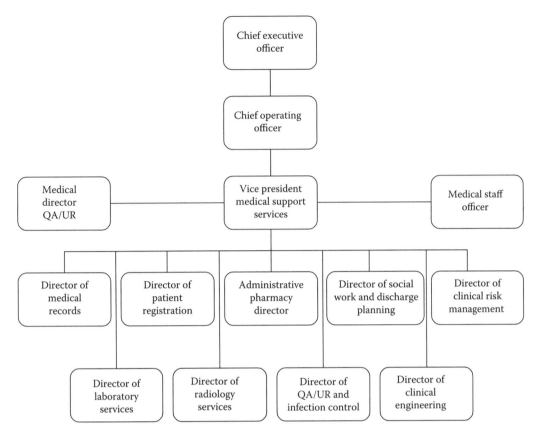

FIGURE 50.2 Organizational chart of medical support services division for a typical major medical facility. This organizational structure points out the critical interrelationship between the clinical engineering department and the other primary services provided by the medical facility.

Once the hospital administration appoints a qualified individual as director of clinical engineering, the person usually functions at the department-head level in the organizational structure of the institution and is provided with sufficient authority and resources to perform the duties efficiently and in accordance with professional norms. To understand the extent of these duties, consider the job title for "clinical engineering director" as defined by the World Health Organization (Issakov et al., 1990):

General Statement. The clinical engineering director, by his or her education and experience, acts as a manager and technical director of the clinical engineering department. The individual designs and directs the design of equipment modifications that may correct design deficiencies or enhance the clinical performance of medical equipment. The individual may also supervise the implementation of those design modifications. The education and experience that the director possesses enables him or her to analyze complex medical or laboratory equipment for purposes of defining corrective maintenance and developing appropriate preventive maintenance or performance assurance protocols. The clinical engineering director works with nursing and medical staff to analyze new medical equipment needs and participates in both the prepurchase planning process and the incoming testing process. The individual also participates in the equipment management process through involvement in the system development, implementation, maintenance, and modification processes.

Duties and Responsibilities. The director of clinical engineering has a wide range of duties and responsibilities. For example, this individual

- Works with medical and nursing staff in the development of technical and performance specifications for equipment requirements in the medical mission.
- Once equipment is specified and the purchase order developed, it generates appropriate testing of the new equipment.
- Does complete performance analysis on complex medical or laboratory equipment summarizes results in brief, concise, and easy-to-understand terms for the purposes of recommending corrective action or for developing appropriate preventive maintenance and performance assurance protocols.
- Designs and implements modifications that permit enhanced operational capability. May supervise the maintenance or modification as it is performed by others.
- Must know the relevant codes and standards related to the hospital environment and the performance assurance activities. (Examples in the United States are NFPA 99, UL 544, and JCAHO, and internationally, IEC-TC 62.)
- Is responsible for obtaining the engineering specifications (systems definitions) for systems that are considered unusual or one-of-a-kind and are not commercially available.
- Supervises in-service maintenance technicians as they work on codes and standards and on preventive maintenance, performance assurance, corrective maintenance, and modification of new and existing patient care and laboratory equipment.
- Supervises parts and supply purchase activities and develops program policies and procedures for the same.
- Sets departmental goals, develops budgets and policy, prepares and analyzes management reports to monitor department activity, and manages and organizes the department to implement them.
- Teaches measurement, calibration, and standardization techniques that promote optimal performance.
- In equipment-related duties, works closely with maintenance and medical personnel. Communicates orally and in writing with medical, maintenance, and administrative professionals. Develops written procedures and recommendations for administrative and technical personnel.

Minimum Qualifications. A bachelor's degree (4 years) in an electrical or electronics program or its equivalent is required (preferably with a clinical or biomedical adjunct). A master's degree is desirable. A minimum of 3 years' experience as a clinical engineer and 2 years in a progressively responsible supervisory capacity is needed. Additional qualifications are as follows:

- Must have some business knowledge and management skills that enable him or her to participate in budgeting, cost accounting, personnel management, behavioral counseling, job description development, and interviewing for hiring or firing purposes. Knowledge and experience in the use of microcomputers are desirable.
- Must be able to use conventional electronic troubleshooting instruments such as multimeters, function generators, oscillators, and oscilloscopes. Should be able to use conventional machine shop equipment such as drill presses, grinders, belt sanders, brakes, and standard hand tools.
- Must possess or be able to acquire knowledge of the techniques, theories, and characteristics of materials, drafting, and fabrication techniques in conjunction with chemistry, anatomy, physiology, optics, mechanics, and hospital procedures.
- Clinical engineering certification or professional engineering registration is required.

50.4.1 Major Functions of a Clinical Engineering Department

It should be clear by the preceding job description that clinical engineers are first and foremost engineering professionals. However, as a result of the wide-ranging scope of interrelationships within the medical setting, the duties and responsibilities of clinical engineering directors are extremely diversified. Yet a common thread is provided by the very nature of the technology they manage. Directors of clinical engineering departments are usually involved in the following core functions:

Technology Management: Developing, implementing, and directing equipment management programs. Specific tasks include accepting and installing new equipment, establishing preventive maintenance and repair programs, and managing the inventory of medical instrumentation. Issues such as cost-effective use and quality assurance are integral parts of any *technology management* program. The director advises the hospital administrator of the budgetary, personnel, space, and test equipment requirements necessary to support this equipment management program.

Risk management: Evaluating and taking appropriate action on incidents attributed to equipment malfunctions or misuse. For example, the clinical engineering director is responsible for summarizing the technological significance of each incident and documenting the findings of the investigation. He or she then submits a report to the appropriate hospital authority and, according to the Safe Medical Devices Act of 1990, to the device manufacturer, the Food and Drug Administration (FDA), or both.

Technology assessment: Evaluating and selecting new equipment. The director must be proactive in the evaluation of new requests for capital equipment expenditures, providing hospital administrators and clinical staff with an in-depth appraisal of the benefits/advantages of candidate equipment. Furthermore, the process of *technology assessment* for all equipment used in the hospital should be an ongoing activity.

Facilities design and project management: Assisting in the design of new or renovated clinical facilities that house specific medical technologies. This includes operating rooms, imaging facilities, and radiology treatment centers.

Training: Establish and deliver instructional modules for clinical engineering staff as well as clinical staff on the operation of medical equipment.

In the future, it is anticipated that clinical engineering departments will provide assistance in the application and management of many other technologies that support patient care, including computer support (which includes the development of virtual instrumentation), telecommunications, and facilities operations.

Defining Terms

JCAHO, Joint Commission on the Accreditation of Healthcare Organizations: The accrediting body responsible for checking compliance of a hospital with approved rules and regulations regarding the delivery of healthcare.

Technology assessment: Involves an evaluation of the safety, efficiency, and cost-effectiveness, as well as consideration of the social, legal, and ethical effects, of medical technology.

References

Bronzino J.D. 1992. *Management of Medical Technology: A Primer for Clinical Engineers*. Boston, Butterworth.

ICC. 1991. International Certification Commission's Definition of a Clinical Engineer, International Certification Commission Fact Sheet. Arlington, VA, ICC.

Issakov A., Mallouppas A., and McKie J. 1990. Manpower development for a healthcare technical service. Report of the World Health Organization, WHO/SHS/NHP/90.4.

Further Reading

1. Journals: *Journal of Clinical Engineering and Journal of Medical Engineering and Physics, Biomedical Instrumentation and Technology*.

51

Management and Assessment of Healthcare Technology

Yadin David
*Biomedical Engineering
Consultants*

Thomas M. Judd
Kaiser Permanente

As medical technology continues to evolve, so does its impact on patient outcome, hospital operations, and financial efficiency. The ability to optimally guide and integrated this evolution and its subsequent implications has become a major challenge in most decisions-making processes within healthcare delivery organizations and their related industries. Therefore, there is a need to adequately plan for and apply those management tools that optimize the deployment of medical technology and the facilities that house it and the integration with legacy systems. Successful management of the technology and facilities will ensure a good match between the needs and the capabilities of staff and technology, respectively. Although different types and sizes of hospitals will consider various strategies of action plans, they all share the need to efficiently manage utilization of their limited resources and their ability to integrate systems. Systems integration and systems performance assurance programs will be critical for successful and compliant hospital regardless of their size. Technology is one of these resources, and although it is frequently cited as the culprit behind cost increases, the well-managed technology program contributes to a significant containment of the cost of providing consistent quality patient care. The clinical engineer's skills and expertise are needed to facilitate the adoption of an objective methodology for implantation of an integrated program that will match the hospital's needs, operational conditions, and expected clinical outcomes. Whereas both the knowledge and practice patterns of management in general are well organized in today's literature, the management of the healthcare delivery systems and that of integrated medical technology in the clinical environment have not yet reached that same high level. Recent standards [1] and publications [2] highlighted the unique conditions that connected healthcare technology present, especially, with regard to the risk assessment and controlling of risks in networking and interconnecting of technology in the clinical environment. However, as we begin to understand the relationship between the methods and information that guide the decision-making processes regarding the management of medical technology that is being deployed in this highly complex environment, the role of the qualified clinical engineer becomes more valuable as a member of the team that manages systems. This is achieved by reformulating the technology management process, which starts with team approach to the strategic planning process, continues with the technology assessment process, leads to the equipment planning and procurement processes, and finally ends with the life cycle management of assets performance assurance program that combined together under the administration of comprehensive clinical engineering management. Definitions of terms used in this chapter are provided at the end of the chapter.

51.1 Healthcare Delivery System

Recent rethinking of how the U.S. healthcare system should be structured brought about significant changes. Healthcare reform was enacted nationally through two bills: the Patient Protection and Affordable Care Act that became law on March 23, 2010 [3] and was shortly amended thereafter by the Health Care and Education Reconciliation Act of 2010 (H.R. 4872). This response to societal demands on the healthcare delivery system revolve around extending coverage to the uninsured population, containment of financial burden, prediction for expected outcomes, and facilitate more consistent quality. In each of these parts, the technology plays a significant role. To respond effectively, the delivery system must identify its goals, select and define its priorities, and then wisely allocate its limited resources.

As healthcare systems and care providers become more mobile, more connected issues with systems integration, safety, and security will only become increasingly complex. For most organizations, this means that they will be limited to selecting access to only the most needed and appropriate technologies and manage their assets more effectively over their life cycle. To improve performance and reduce costs, the delivery system must recognize and respond to the key dynamics in which it operates, must shape and mold its planning efforts around several existing healthcare objectives and directions, and must respond proactively and positively to the pressures of environment within which it operates. These issues and the fact that technological advances provide critical ability to better manage patient conditions and to better restore patient functions mean for the technology manager the need for competencies and plan that meet them. These are outlined here as follows: (1) technology's positive impact on care quality and effectiveness will continue, (2) delivering services in stressful financial conditions brought about by limitation and reallocation of spending for healthcare services, (3) an increase in the volume of insured Americans and their access to healthcare, (4) increase in relating deployment of specific technology to expected achievement of clinical outcomes, (5) a changing mix of healthcare services and where these services are delivered, and (6) advancement of technological tools with growing pressures to further integrate information and biomedical technologies to facilitate continuum of care throughout the acute, chronic, outpatient, and home-care budgets.

51.1.1 Major Healthcare Trends and Directions

The major trends and directions in healthcare include (1) changing location and design of care and treatment areas, (2) evolving benefits, coverage, and choices, (3) continuing growth of intelligent support within the technology used at the point of care, (4) extreme pressures to manage costs, (5) treating of more acutely ill patients and at higher volume, (6) changing job competencies, structures, and demand for skilled labor, (7) need for visionary management to integrate the support of construction, equipment, and information technology system interoperability, (8) increased competition, (9) meeting compliance for reward associated with the use of information systems and electronic health record that effectively integrate clinical and decision-making issues, (10) changing reimbursement policies that reduce new purchases and lead to the expectation for extended equipment life cycles, (11) multidisciplinary technology planning and service management programs with joint decision-making process, (12) technology planning teams to coordinate absorption of new and replacement technologies while legacy systems are still in place, as well as to manage systems conversions, and (13) containment of service costs of systems and medical equipment that place demand for efficient collaborative technical leadership.

51.1.2 System Pressures

System pressures include (1) effect of healthcare reform; (2) society's expectations—highest quality care at the lowest risk and at reasonable price, where quality is a function of outcomes, personnel, facilities, technology, and clinical procedures offered; (3) economic conditions—driven often by reallocation and reimbursement criteria; (4) legal pressures—resulting primarily from careful identification of risk exposure and dealing with rule-intensive "government" clients; (5) regulatory–multistate delivery systems with increased management complexity or heavily regulated medical device industries facing free-market competition, and hospitals facing the deployment of consumer-based applications that are considered less regulated as compared with medical device, increase workforce mobility, and larger systems integration; (6) ethics—deciding who gets care and when; and (7) technology pressures—organizations not having sufficient capabilities to meet their community needs and to compete successfully in their marketplaces.

51.1.3 Technology Manager's Responsibility

Technology managers should (1) become deeply involved and committed to deliver technology planning and service management programs for their organization, often involving the need for greater personal responsibilities and expanded skills and credentials, (2) understand how the factors mentioned above impact their organization and how technology can be safely used to improve outcomes, reduce costs, and improve quality of life for patients, (3) educate other healthcare professionals about demonstrating the value of individual technology and that of system technologies through parameters, including financial, engineering, quality of care, and system's resiliency perspective, and (4) assemble a team of support staff and caregivers with sufficient broad clinical expertise and administrators with planning and financial expertise to monitor their assessment process and overall satisfaction with the technology management [4].

51.2 Strategic Technology Planning

51.2.1 Strategic Planning Process

Leading healthcare organizations combine strategic technology planning with other technology management activities in the program that effectively integrate new technologies with their legacy technology base. This has resulted in high-quality care at a reasonable cost. Among those who have been its leading catalysts are institutions such as the Kaiser-Permanente, Mass General Hospital, and ECRI Institute that are known for articulating this program [5] and encouraging its proliferation initially among regional healthcare systems and now for single- or multihospital systems as well [6]. The key components of the program include clinical strategic planning, technology strategic planning, technology assessment, interaction with capital budgeting, acquisition and deployment, resource (or equipment assets) management, and monitoring and evaluation. A proper technology strategic plan is derived from and supports as well-defined clinical strategic plan [7].

51.2.2 Clinical and Technology Strategic Plan

Usually considered long range and continually evolving, a clinical strategic plan is updated annually. For a given year, the program begins when key hospital stakeholders, through the strategic planning process, assess what changes in clinical services coverage the hospital will be considering and how it relates to its referral area and branch facilities. They usually will take into account healthcare trends, demographic and market share data, expertise needed, space, facilities, and technology plans. They analyze their facility's strengths and weaknesses, goals and objectives, competition, and impact on the existing technology base. The outcome of this process is a clinical strategic plan that establishes the organization's vision for the year, community coverage area needs, and the hospital's objectives in meeting them.

It is not possible to adequately complete a clinical strategic plan without engaging in the process of strategic technology planning. A key role for technology managers is to assist their organizations throughout the combined clinical and technology strategic planning processes by matching available technical capabilities, both existing and new ones, with the clinical objectives. To accomplish this, technology managers must understand why their institution's values and mission are set as they are, pursue their institution's strategic plans through that knowledge, and plan in a way that effectively allocates their limited resources. Although a technology manager may not be assigned to develop an institution's overall strategic plan, he or she must be part of it, understand, and be able to translate it into tools integration vision to offer good guidance for hospital leadership. In providing this input, a technology manager should determine a plan for evaluating the current state of the hospital's technological deployment, assist in providing a review of emerging technological innovations and their possible impact on the hospital, articulate justifications and provisions for adoption of new technologies or enhancement of existing ones, perform gap analysis, visit research and laboratories and exhibit areas at major medical and scientific meetings to view introduction of new technologies, and be familiar with the institution and its equipment users' abilities to assimilate the new technology. As interoperability between devices and between systems at times will be accomplished by collaboration among multivendor, it is also imperative that the technology manager will be familiar with current regulatory and compliance issues for both medical devices and nonmedical devices. Assessment of risk, mitigation, and management of risk residue are all part of technology management program. It must be performed by a team of stakeholders that includes internal and at times, when specific expertise is needed, external to the organization.

The past decade has shown a trend toward increased legislation in support of more federal regulations in healthcare. These and other pressures will require that additional or replacement medical technology be well anticipated and justified. As a rationale for technology adoption, a children's hospital in a large medical center focused on the issues of clinical necessity, management support, and market preference. Addressing the issue of clinical necessity, the hospital considers the technology's comparison against medical standard of care, its impact on the level of care and quality of life, its improvement on intervention's accuracy and safety, its impact on the rate of recovery, the needs or desires of the community, and the change in service volume or focus. On the issue of management support, the hospital estimates whether the technology will create a more effective care plan and decision-making process, improve operational efficiency in the current service programs, decrease liability exposure, increase compliance with regulations, reduce workload and dependence on user skill level, ameliorate departmental support, or enhance clinical proficiency. Weighting the issue of market preference, the hospital contemplates whether it will improve access to care, increase customer convenience and satisfaction, enhance the organization's image and market share, decrease the cost of adoption and ownership, or provide a return on its investment.

51.2.3 Technology Strategic Planning Process

When the annual clinical strategic planning process begins and hospital leaders begin to analyze or reaffirm the clinical services they want to offer to the community, the hospital can then conduct efficient technology strategic planning. Key elements of this planning involve (1) performing an initial audit of existing technologies, (2) conducting a technology assessment for new and emerging technologies for fitting with current or desired clinical services, (3) planning for replacement and selection of new technologies, (4) setting priorities for technology acquisition, and (5) developing processes to implement equipment acquisition and monitor ongoing utilization. "Increasingly, hospitals are designating a senior manager (e.g., an administrator, the director of planning, the director of clinical engineering) to take the responsibility for technology assessment and planning. That person should have the primary responsibility for developing the strategic technology plan with the help of key physicians, department managers, and senior executives" [5].

Hospitals can form a medical technology advisory committee (MTAC), overseen by the designated senior manager and consisting of the types of members mentioned above, to conduct the strategic technology planning process and to annually recommend technology priorities to the hospital strategic planning committee and capital budget committee. It is especially important to involve physicians and nurses in this process.

In the initial technology audit, each major clinical service or product line must be analyzed to determine how well the existing technology base supports it. The audit can be conducted along service lines (radiology, cardiology, and surgery) or technology function (e.g., imaging, therapeutic, and diagnostic) by a team of designated physicians, department heads, and technology managers. The team should begin by developing a complete hospital-wide assets inventory, including the quantity and quality of equipment. The team should compare the existing technology base against known and evolving standards-of-care information, patient outcome data, and known equipment problems. The team should then collect and examine information on technology utilization to assess its appropriate use, the opportunities for improvement, and the risk level. After reviewing the technology users' education needs as they relate to the application and servicing of medical equipment, the team should progress to credential users for competence in the application of new technologies. Also, the auditing team should keep up with published clinical protocols and practice guidelines using available healthcare *standards* directories and utilize clinical outcome data for quality-assurance and risk-management program feedback [8].

Although it is not expected that every hospital has all the required expertise in-house to conduct the initial technology audit or ongoing technology assessment, the execution of this planning process is sufficiently critical for a hospital's success that outside expertise should be obtained when necessary. The audit allows for the gathering of information about the status of the existing technology base and enhances the capability of the MTAC to assess the impact of new and emerging technologies on their major clinical services.

All the information collected from the technology audit results and technology assessments is used in developing budget strategies. Budgeting is part of strategic technology planning in that a 2- to 5-year long-range capital-spending plan should be created. This is in addition to the annual capital budget preparation that takes into account 1 year at a time. The MTAC, as able and appropriate, provides key information regarding capital budget requests and makes recommendations to the capital budget committee (CBC) each year. The MTAC recommends priorities for replacement as well as new and emerging technologies that during a period of several years guides that acquisition that provides the desired service developments or enhancements. Priorities are recommended on the basis of need, risk, cost (acquisition, operational, and maintenance), utilization, and fit with the clinical strategic plan.

51.3 Technology Assessment

As medical technology continues to evolve, so does its impact on patient outcome, hospital operations, and financial resources. The ability to manage this evolution and its subsequent implications has become a major challenge for all healthcare organizations. Successful management of technology will ensure a good match between needs and capabilities and between staff and technology. To be successful, an ongoing technology assessment process must be an integral part of an ongoing technology planning and management program at the hospital, addressing the needs of the patient, the user, and the support team. This facilitates better equipment planning and utilization of the hospital's resources. The manager who is knowledgeable about his or her organization's goals and culture, technology users' needs and capabilities, the environment within which the technology will be integrated and applied, risk management methodology [9], and emerging technological trends will be successful in proficiently implementing and managing technological changes [10].

It is in the technology assessment process that the clinical engineering/technology manager professional needs to wear two hats: that of project manager and of the engineer. This is a unique position, requiring expertise and detailed preparation, which allows one to be a team player and contributor to the decision-making process of a team such as the MTAC.

The MTAC uses an ad hoc team approach to conduct technology assessment of selected services and technologies throughout the year. The ad hoc teams may incorporate representatives of equipment users, equipment service providers, physicians, purchasing agents, reimbursement mangers, representatives of administration, and other members from the institution as applicable.

51.3.1 Prerequisites for Technology Assessment

Medical technology is a major strategic factor in positioning and creating a positive community perception of the hospital. Exciting new biomedical devices and systems are continually being introduced. And they are introduced at a time when the pressure on hospitals to contain expenditures is mounting. Therefore, forecasting the deployment of medical technology and the capacity to continually evaluate its impact on the hospital require that the hospital be willing to provide the support for such a program. (Note: Many organizations are aware of the principle that an in-house "champion" is needed to provide for the leadership that continually and objectively plans ahead. The champion and the program being "championed" may use additional in-house or independent expertise as needed. To get focused attention on the technology assessment function and this program in larger, academically affiliated, and government hospitals, the position of a chief technology officer is being created.) Traditionally, executives rely on their staff to produce objective analyses of the hospital's technological needs. Without such analyses, executives may approve purchasing decisions of sophisticated biomedical equipment only to discover later that some needs or expected features were not included with this installation, that those features are not yet approved for delivery, or that the installation has not been adequately planned.

Many hospitals perform technology assessment activities to project needs for new assets and to better manage existing assets. Because the task is complex, an interdisciplinary approach and a cooperative attitude among the assessment team leadership is required. The ability to integrate information from disciplines such as clinical, technical, financial, administrative, and facility in a timely and objective manner is critical to the success of the assessment. This chapter emphasizes how technology assessment fits within a technology planning and management program and recognizes the importance of corporate skills forecasting medical equipment changes and determining the impact of changes on the hospital's market position. Within the technology planning and management program, the focus on capital assets management of medical equipment should not lead to the exclusion of accessories, supplies, and the disposables also required.

Medical equipment has a life cycle that can be identified as (1) the innovation phase, which includes the concept, basic and applied research, and development, and (2) the adoption phase, which begins with the clinical studies, through diffusion and then widespread use. These phases are different from each other in the scope of professional skills involved, their impact on patient care, compliance with regulatory requirements, and the extent of the required operational support. In evaluating the applicability of a device or a system for use in the hospital, it is important to note in which phase of its life cycle the equipment currently resides.

51.3.2 Technology Assessment Process

More and more hospitals are faced with the difficult phenomenon of a capital equipment requests list that is much larger than the capital budget allocation. The most difficult decision, then, is the one that matches clinical needs with the financial capability. In doing so, the following questions are often raised:

How do we avoid costly technology mistakes? How do we wisely target capital dollars for technology? How do we avoid medical staff conflicts as they relate to technology? How do we control equipment-related risks? And how do we maximize the useful life of the equipment or systems while minimizing the cost ownership? A hospital's clinical engineering department can assist in providing the right answers to these questions.

Technology assessment is a component of technology planning that begins with the analysis of the hospital's existing technology base. It is then easy to perceive that technology assessment, rather than an equipment comparison, is a new major function for a clinical engineering department [11]. It is important that clinical engineers be well prepared for the challenge. They must have a complete understanding of the mission of their particular hospitals, a familiarity with the healthcare delivery system, and the cooperation of hospital administrators and the medical staff. To aid in the technology assessment process, clinical engineers need to utilize the following tools: (1) access to national database services, directories, and libraries, (2) visits to scientific and clinical exhibits, (3) a network with key industry contacts, and (4) a relationship with peers throughout the country [12].

The need for clinical engineering involvement in the technology assessment process becomes evident when recently purchased equipment or its functions are underutilized, users have ongoing problems with equipment, equipment maintenance costs become excessive, the hospital is unable to comply with standards or guidelines (i.e., Joint or requirements) for equipment management, a high percentage of equipment is awaiting repair, or training for equipment operators is inefficient because of shortage of allied health professionals. A deeper look at the symptoms behind these problems would likely reveal a lack of a central clearinghouse to collect, index, and monitor all technology-related information for future planning purposes, the absence of procedures for identifying emerging technologies for potential acquisition, the lack of a systematic plan for conducting technology assessment, resulting in an ability to maximize the benefits from deployment of available technology, the inability to benefit from the organization's own previous experience with a particular type of technology, the random replacement of medical technologies rather than a systematic plan based on a set of well-developed criteria, and the lack of integration of technology acquisition into the strategic and capital planning of the hospital.

To address these issues, efforts to develop a technology microassessment process were initiated at one leading private hospital with the following objectives: (1) accumulate information on medical equipment, (2) facilitate systematic planning, (3) create an administrative structure supporting the assessment process and its methodology, (4) monitor the replacement of outdated technology, and (5) improve the capital budget process by focusing on long-term needs relative to the acquisition of medical equipment [13].

The process, in general, and the collection of up-to-date pertinent information, in particular, requires the expenditure of certain resources and the active participation of designated hospital staff in networks providing technology assessment information. For example, corporate membership in organizations and societies that provide such information needs to be considered, as well as subscriptions to certain computerized database and printed sources [14].

At the example hospital, an MTAC was formed to conduct technology assessment. It was chaired by the director of clinical engineering. Other managers from equipment user departments usually serve as the MTAC's 12pt designated technical coordinators for specific task forces. Once the committee accepts a request from an individual user, it identifies other users who might have an interest in that equipment or system and authorized the technical coordinator to assemble a task force consisting of users identified by the MTAC. This task force then takes up responsibility for the establishment of performance criteria that would be used during this particular assessment. The task force also answers the questions of effectiveness, safety, and cost-effectiveness as they relate to the particular assessment. During any specific period, there may be multiple task forces, each focusing on a specific equipment investigation.

The task force technical coordinator cooperates with the material management department in conducting a market survey, obtaining the specified equipment for evaluation purposes, and in scheduling vendor-provided in-service training. The coordinator also confers with the clinical staff to determine whether they have experience with the equipment and the maturity level of the equipment under assessment. After the establishment of a task force, the MTACs technical coordinator is responsible for analyzing the clinical experiences associated with the use of this equipment, for setting evaluation objectives, and for devising appropriate technical tests in accordance with recommendations from the task force. The only equipment that successfully passes the technical tests will proceed to a clinical trial. During the clinical trial, a task force-appointed clinical coordinator collects and reports a summary of experiences gained. The technical coordinator then combines the results from both the technical tests and the clinical trial into a summary report for MTAC review and approval. In this role, the clinical engineer/technical coordinator serves as a multidisciplinary professional, bridging the gap between the clinical and technical needs of the hospital. To complete the process, financial staff representatives review the protocol.

The technology assessment process at this example hospital begins with a department or individual filling out two forms (1) a request for review (RR) form and (2) a capital asset request (CAR) form. These forms are submitted to the hospital's product standards committee, which determines whether an assessment process is to be initiated and the priority for its completion. It also determines whether a previously established standard for this equipment already exists (if the hospital is already using such a technology)—if so, an assessment is not needed.

On the RR, the originator delineates the rationale for acquiring the medical device. For example, the originator must tell how the item will improve the quality of patient care, who will be its primary user, and how it will improve the ease of use. On the CAR, the originator describes the item, estimates its cost, and provides purchase justification. The CAR is then routed to the capital budget office for review. During this process, the optimal financing method for acquisition is determined. If funding is secured, the CAR is routed to the material management department, where, together with the RR, it will be processed. The rationale for having the RR accompany the CAR is to ensure that financial information is included as part of the assessment process. The CAR is the tool by which the purchasing department initiates a market survey and later sends product requests for bid. Any request for evaluation that is received without a CAR or any CAR involving medical equipment that is received without a request for evaluation is returned to the originator without action. Both forms are then sent to the clinical engineering department, where a designated technical coordinator will analyze the requested technology maturity level and results of clinical experience with its use, review trends, and prioritize various manufactures' presentations for MTAC review.

Both forms must be sent to the MTAC if the item requested is not currently used by the hospital or if it does not conform to previously adopted hospital standards. The MTAC has the authority to recommend either acceptance or rejection of any RR, based on a consensus of its members. A task force consisting of potential equipment users will determine the "must have" equipment functions, review the impact of the various equipment configurations, and plan technical and clinical evaluations.

If the request is approved by the MTAC, the requested technology or equipment will be evaluated using technical and performance standards. On completion of the review, a recommendation is returned to the hospital's products standard committee, which reviews the results of the technology assessment, determines whether the particular product is suitable as a hospital standard, and decides if it should be purchased. If approved, the request to purchase will be reviewed by the CBC to determine whether the required expenditure meets with available financial resources and if or when it may be feasible to make the purchase. To ensure coordination of the technology assessment program, the chairman of the MTAC also serves as a permanent member of the hospital's CBC. In this way, there is a planned integration between technology assessment and budget decisions.

51.4 Equipment Assets Management

An accountable, systematic approach will ensure that cost-effective, efficacious, safe, and appropriate equipment is available to meet the demands of quality patient care. Such an approach requires that existing medical equipment resources be managed and the resulting management strategies have measurable outputs that are monitored and evaluated. Technology managers/clinical engineers are well positioned to organize and lead this function. It is assumed that cost accounting is managed and monitored by the healthcare organization's financial group.

51.4.1 Equipment Management Process

Through traditional assets management strategies, medical equipment can be comprehensively managed by clinical engineering personnel. First, the management should consider a full range of strategies for equipment technical support [15]. Plans may include the use of a combination of equipment service providers, such as manufacturers, third-party service groups, shared services, and hospital-based (in-house) engineers and biomedical equipment technicians (BMETs). All these service providers should be under the general responsibility of the technology manager to ensure optimal equipment performance through comprehensive and ongoing best-value equipment service. After obtaining a complete hospital medical equipment inventory (noting both original manufacturer and typical service provider), the management should conduct a thorough analysis of hospital accounts payable records for at least the past 2 years, compiling all service reports and preventative maintenance-related costs from all possible sources. The manager should then document in-house and external provider equipment service costs, extent of maintenance coverage for each inventory time, equipment-user-operating schedule, quality of maintenance coverage for each item, appropriateness of the service provider, and reasonable maintenance costs. Thereafter, he or she should establish an effective equipment technical support process. With an accurate inventory and best-value service providers identified, service agreements/contracts should be negotiated with external providers using prepared terms and conditions, including a log-in system. There should be an in-house clinical engineering staff ensuring ongoing external provider cost control utilizing several tools. By asking the right technical questions and establishing friendly relationships with the staff, the manager will be able to handle service purchase orders (POs) by determining whether the equipment is worth repairing and obtaining exchange prices for parts. The staff should handle service reports to review them for accuracy and proper use of the log-in system. They should also match invoices with the service reports to verify opportunities and review service histories to look for symptoms such as need for user training, repeated problems, run-on calls billed months apart, or evidence of defective or worn-out equipment. The manager should take responsibility for emergency equipment rentals. Finally, the manager should develop, implement, and monitor all the service performance criteria.

To optimize technology management programs, clinical engineers should be willing to assume responsibilities for technology planning and management in all related areas. They should develop policies and procedures for their hospital's management program. With life cycle costs determined for key high-risk or high-cost devices, they should evaluate methods to provide additional cost savings in equipment operation and maintenance. They should be involved with computer networking systems within the hospital. As computer technology applications increase, the requirements to review technology-related information in various hospital locations will increase. They should determine what environmental conditions and facility changes are required to accommodate new technologies or changes in standards and guidelines. Finally, they should use documentation of equipment performance and maintenance costs along with their knowledge of current clinical practices to assist other hospital personnel in determining the best time and process for planning equipment replacement [16].

51.4.2 Technology Management Activities

A clinical engineering department, through outstanding performance in traditional equipment management, will win its hospital's support and will be asked to be involved in a full range of technology management activities. The department should start an equipment control program that encompasses routine performance testing, inspection, periodic and preventive maintenance (PM), on-demand repair services, incidents investigation, and actions on recalls and hazards. The department should have multidisciplinary involvement in equipment acquisition and replacement decisions, development of new services, and planning of new construction and major renovations, including intensive participation by clinical engineering, materials management, and finance. The department should also initiate programs for training all users of patient care equipment, quality improvement (QI), as it relates to technology use, and technology-related risk management [17].

As convergence between devices and systems has taken powerful effect, hospitals are faced with the need for better and more effective life cycle technology support. As devices are becoming more intelligent, are able to process more information, and are connected, wired as well as wirelessly, the management of technology includes networks, access points, radio frequency (RF) spectrum, and other telecommunication tools working together. Service support for these systems is also converging, bringing clinical engineering and information technology (IT) program operation closer than ever before. However, these programs historically evolved from different points but are now searching for the business model that will help them succeed in the new reality. Visionary technical leadership will progress collaborative strategy toward convergence with anticipated accomplishment of both service success and staff on the job satisfaction.

51.4.3 Case Study: A Focus on Medical Imaging

In the mid-1980s, a large private multihospital system contemplated the start-up of a corporate clinical engineering program. The directors recognized that the involvement in a diagnostic imaging equipment service would be key to the economic success of the program. They further recognized that maintenance cost reductions would have to be balanced with achieving equal or increased quality of care in the utilization of that equipment.

Programs start-up was in the summer of 1987 in three hospitals that were geographically in close proximity. Within the first year, clinical engineering operations began in 11 hospitals in three regions over a two-state area. By the fall of 1990, the program included seven regions and 21 hospitals in a five-state area. The regions were organized, typically, into teams including a regional manager and 10 service providers, serving 3–4 hospitals, whose average size was 225 beds. Although the staffs were stationed at the hospitals, some specialists traveled between sites in the region to provide equipment service. Service providers included individuals specializing in the areas of diagnostic imaging (x-ray and computed tomography [CT]), clinical laboratory, general biomedical instrumentation, and respiratory therapy.

At the end of the first 18 months, the program documented more than $1 million in savings for the initial 11 hospitals, a 23% reduction from the previous annual service costs. More than 63% of these savings were attributable to "in-house" service, x-ray, and CT scanner equipment. The mix of equipment maintained by 11 imaging service providers—from a total staff of 30—included approximately 75% of the radiology systems of any kind found in the hospitals and five models of CT scanners from the three different manufacturers.

At the end of 3 years in 1990, program-wide savings had exceeded 30% of previous costs for participating hospitals. Within the imaging areas of the hospitals, savings approached and sometimes exceed 50% of initial service costs. The 30 imaging service providers—of a total staff of 62—had increased their coverage of radiology equipment to more than 95%, had increased involvement with CT to include nine models from five different manufacturers, and had begun in-house work in other key imaging modalities.

Tracking the financial performance of the initial 11 hospitals during the first 3 years of the program yields the following composite example: a hospital of 225 beds was found to have equipment service costs of $540,000 before program start-up. Sixty-three percent of these initial costs (or $340,000) was for the maintenance of the hospital's x-ray and CT scanner systems. Three years later, annual service costs for this equipment were cut in half, to approximately $170,000. That represents a 31% reduction in hospital-wide costs because of the imaging service alone.

This corporate clinical engineering operation is, in effect, a large in-house program serving many hospitals that all have common ownership. The multihospital corporation has significant purchasing power in the medical device marketplace and provides central oversight of the larger capital expenditures for its hospitals. The combination of the parent organization's leverage and the program's commitment to serve only hospitals in the corporation facilitated the development of positive relationships with medical device manufacturers. Most of the manufacturers did not see the program as competition but rather as a potentially helpful ally in the future marketing and sales of their equipment and systems. What staff provided these results? All service providers were either medical imaging industry or military trained. All were experienced at troubleshooting electronic subsystems to component level, as necessary. Typically, these individuals had prior experience on the manufacture's models of equipment under their coverage. Most regional managers had prior industry, third-party, or in-house imaging service management experience. Each service provider had the test equipment necessary for day-to-day duties. Each individual could expect at least 2 weeks of annual service training to keep appropriate skills current. Desired service training could be acquired in a timely manner from manufactures and third-party organizations. Spare or replacement parts inventory was minimal because of the program's ability to get parts from manufacturers and other sources either locally or shipped in overnight.

As quality indicators for the program, the management measured user satisfaction, equipment downtime, documentation of technical staff service training, types of user equipment errors and their effect on patient outcomes, and regular attention to hospital technology problems. User satisfaction surveys indicated a high degree of confidence in the program service providers by imaging department managers. Problems relating to technical, management, communication, and financial issues did occur regularly, but the regional manager ensured that they were resolved in a timely manner. Faster response to daily imaging equipment problems, typically by onsite service providers, coupled with regular PM according to established procedures led to reduced equipment downtime. PM and repair service histories were captured in a computer documentation system that also tracked service times, costs, and user errors and their effects. Assisting the safety committee became easier with the ability to draw a wide variety of information quickly from the program's documenting system.

Early success in imaging equipment led to the opportunity to do some additional value-added projects such as the moving and reinstallation of x-ray rooms that preserved exiting assets and opened up valuable space for installation of newer equipment and upgrades of CT scanner systems. The parent organization came to realize that these technology management activities could potentially have a greater financial and quality impact on the hospital's healthcare delivery than equipment management. In the example of one CT upgrade (which was completed over two weekends with no downtime), there was a positive financial impact on excess of $600,000 and improved quality of care by allowing faster off-line diagnosis of patient scans. However, the opportunity for this kind of contribution would never have occurred without the strong base of a successful equipment management program staffed with qualified individuals who receive ongoing training.

51.5 Equipment Acquisition and Deployment

51.5.1 Process of Acquiring Technology

Typically, medical device systems will emerge from the strategic technology planning and technology assessment processes as required and budgeted needs. At acquisition time, needs analysis should be conducted, reaffirming clinical needs and device-intended applications. The "request for review" documentation from the assessment process or capital budget request and incremental financial analysis from the planning process may provide appropriate justification information and a CAR form should be completed [18]. Materials management and clinical engineering personnel should ensure that this item is a candidate for centralized and coordinated acquisition of similar equipment with other hospital departments. Typical hospital prepurchase evaluation guidelines include an analysis of needs and development of a specification list, formation of a vendor list and requesting proposals, analyzing proposals and site planning, evaluating samples, selecting finalists, making the award, delivery and installation, and acceptance testing [19]. Formal request for proposals (RFPs) from potential equipment vendors are required for intended acquisitions whose initial or life-cycle cost exceeds a certain threshold, for example, $250,000. Finally, the purchase takes place, wherein final equipment negotiations are conducted and purchase documents are prepared, including a purchase order.

51.5.2 Acquisition Process Strategies

The cost-of-ownership concept can be used when considering what factors to include in cost comparisons of competing medical devices. Cost of ownership encompasses all the direct and indirect expenses associated with medical equipment over its lifetime [7]. It expresses the cost factors of medical equipment for both the initial price of the equipment (which typically includes the equipment, its installation, and initial training cost) and over the long term. Long-term costs include ongoing training, equipment service, supplies, connectivity, upgrades, and other costs. Healthcare organizations are just beginning to account for a full range of cost-of-ownership factors in their technology assessment and acquisition processes, such as acquisition costs, operating costs, and maintenance costs (installation, supplies, downtime, training, spare parts, test equipment and tools, and depreciation). It is estimated that the purchase price represents only 20% of the life cycle cost of ownership.

When conducting needs analysis, actual utilization information from the organization's existing same or similar devices can be very helpful. One leading private multihospital system has implemented the following approach to measuring and developing relevant management feedback concerning.equipment utilization. It is conducting equipment utilization review for replacement planning, for ongoing accountability of equipment use, and to provide input before more equipment is purchased. This private system attempts to match the product to its intended function and to measure daily (if necessary) the equipment's actual utilization. The tools they use include knowing their hospital's entire installed base of certain kinds of equipment, that is, imaging systems. Utilization assumptions for each hospital and its clinical procedural mix are made. Equipment functional requirements to meet the demands of the clinical procedures are also taken into account.

Life cycle cost analysis is a tool used during technology planning, assessment, or acquisition "either to compare high-cost, alternative means for providing a service or to determine whether a single project or technology has a positive or negative economic value. The strength of the life-cycle cost analysis is that it examines the cash flow impact of an alternative over its entire life, instead of focusing solely on initial capital investments" [7].

"Life-cycle cost analysis facilitates comparisons between projects or technologies with large initial cash outlays and those with level outlays and inflows over time. It is most applicable to complex, high-cost choices among alternative technologies, new service, and different means for providing a given service. Life-cycle cost analysis is particularly useful for decisions that are too complex and ambiguous for experience and subjective judgment alone. It also helps decision makers perceive and include costs that often are hidden or ignored, and that may otherwise invalidate results" [16].

"Perhaps the most powerful life-cycle cost technique is net present value (NPV) analysis, which explicitly accounts for inflation and foregone investment opportunities by expressing future cash flows in present dollars" [16].

Examples where LCC and NPV analysis proves very helpful are in deciding whether to replace/rebuild or buy/lease medical imaging equipment. The various costs captured in life cycle cost analysis include decision-making costs, planning agency/certificate of need costs (if applicable), financing, initial capital investment costs including facility changes, life cycle maintenance and repair costs, personnel costs, and others (reimbursement consequences, resale, etc.).

One of the best strategies to ensure that a desired technology is truly of value to the hospital is to conduct a careful analysis in preparation for its assimilation into hospital operations. The process of equipment prepurchase evaluation provides information that can be used to screen unacceptable performance by either the vendor or the equipment before it becomes a hospital problem.

Once the vendor has responded to informal requests or formal RFPs, the clinical engineering department should be responsible for evaluating the technical response, whereas the materials management department should devaluate the financial responses.

In translating clinical needs into a specification list, key features or "must have" attributes of the desired device are identified. In practice, clinical engineering and materials management should develop a "must have" list and an extras list. The extras list should contain features that may tip the decision in favor of one vendor, all other factors being even. These specification lists are sent to the vendor and are effective in a self-elimination process that results in a time savings for the hospital. Once the "must have" attributes have been satisfied, the remaining candidate devices are evaluated technically and the extras are considered. This is accomplished by assigning a weighting factor (i.e., 0–5) to denote the relative importance of each of the desired attributes. The relative ability of each device to meet the defined requirements is then rated [20].

One strategy that strengthens the acquisition process is the conditions-of-sale document. This multifaceted document integrates equipment specifications, performance, installation requirements, and follow-up services. The conditions-of-sale document ensures that negotiations are completed before a purchase order is delivered and each participant is in agreement about the product to be delivered. As a document of compliance, the conditions-of-sale document specifies the codes and standards having jurisdiction over that equipment. This may include provisions for future modification of the equipment, compliance with standards under development, compliance with national codes, and provision for software upgrades.

Standard POs that include the conditions of sale for medical equipment are usually used to initiate the order. At the time the order is placed, clinical engineering is notified of the order. In addition to current facility conditions, the management must address installation and approval requirements, responsibilities, and timetable; payment, assignment, and cancelation; software requirements and updates; documentation; clinical and technical training; acceptance testing (hospital facility and vendor); warranty, spare parts, and service; and price protection.

All medical equipment must be inspected and tested before it is placed into service regardless of whether it is purchased, leased, rented, or borrowed by the hospital. In any hospital, clinical engineering should receive immediate notification if a very large device or system is delivered directly into another department (e.g., imaging or cardiology) for installation. Clinical engineering should be required to sign-off on all POs for devices after installation and validation of satisfactory operation. Ideally, the warranty period on new equipment should not begin until installation and acceptance testing are completed. It is not uncommon for a hospital to lose several months of free parts and service by the manufacturer when new equipment is, for some reason, not installed immediately after delivery.

51.5.3 Clinical Team Requirements

During the technology assessment and acquisition processes, clinical decision makers analyze the following criteria concerning proposed technology acquisitions, specifically as they relate to clinical outcomes team requirements: ability of the staff to assimilate the technology, medical staff satisfaction (short term and long term), impact on staffing (numbers, functions), projected utilization, ongoing related supplies required, effect on delivery of care and outcomes (convenience, safety, or standard of care), result of what is written in the clinical practice guidelines, credentialing of staff required, clinical staff initial and ongoing training required, and the effect on existing technology in the department or on other services/departments. The critical role of technological tools that sense, process, collect, distribute, display, and archive health information has increased and is critical for meeting compliance with federal requirements such as the "meaningful use" parameters. This highlights the need for the clinical team to include technology managers and to collaborate especially throughout the planning and implementation phases of the technology life cycle.

Defining Terms

Appropriate technology [20]: A term used initially in developing countries, referring to selecting medical equipment that can "appropriately" satisfy the following constraints: funding shortages, insufficient numbers of trained personnel, lack of technical support, inadequate supplies of consumables/accessories, unreliable water and power utilities/supplies, and lack of operating and maintenance manuals. In the context of this chapter, appropriate technology selection must take into consideration local health needs and disease prevalence, the need for local capability of equipment maintenance, and availability of resources for ongoing operational and technical support.

Clinical engineers/biomedical engineers: As we began describing the issues with the management of medical technology, it became obvious that some of the terms are being used interchangeably in the literature. For example, the terms engineers, clinical engineers, BMETs, equipment managers, and healthcare engineers are frequently used. For clarification, in this chapter, we will refer to clinical engineers and the clinical engineering department as a representative group for all these terms.

Cost-effectiveness [20]: A mixture of quantitative and qualitative considerations. It includes the health priorities of the country or region at the macroassessment level and the community needs at the institution microassessment level. Product life cycle cost analysis (which, in turn, includes initial purchase price, shipping, renovations, installation, supplies, associated disposables, cost per use, and similar quantitative measures) is a critical analysis measure. Life cycle cost also takes into account staff training, ease of use, service, and many other cost factors. But experience and judgment about the relative importance of features and the ability to fulfill the intended purpose also contribute critical information to the cost-effectiveness equation.

Equipment acquisition and deployment: Medical device systems and products typically emerge from the strategic technology planning process as "required and budgeted" needs. The process that follows, which ends with equipment acceptance testing and placement into general use, is known as the equipment acquisition and deployment process.

Healthcare technology: Healthcare technology includes the devices, equipment, systems, software, supplies, pharmaceuticals, biotechnologies, and medical and surgical procedures used in the prevention, diagnosis, and treatment of disease in humans, for their rehabilitation, and for assistive purposes. In short, technology is broadly defined as encompassing virtually all the human interventions intended to cope with disease and disabilities, short of spiritual alternatives. This chapter focuses on medical equipment products (devices, systems, and software) rather than pharmaceuticals, biotechnologies, or procedures [20]. The concept of technology also encompasses the facilities that house both patients and products. Facilities cover a wide spectrum—from the modern hospital on one end to the mobile imaging trailer on the other.

Quality of care (QA) and quality of improvement (QI): Quality assurance (QA) and quality improvement (QI) are formal sets of activities to measure the quality of care provided; these usually include a process for selecting, monitoring, and applying corrective measures. The 1994 Joint Commission on the Accreditation of Healthcare Organizations (JCAHO) standards require hospital QA, programs to focus on patient outcomes as a primary reference. JCAHO standards for plant, technology, and safety management (PTSM), in turn, require certain equipment management practices and QA or QI activities. Identified QI deficiencies may influence equipment planning, and QI audits may increase awareness of technology overuse or under utilization.

Risk management: Risk management is a program that helps the hospital avoid the possibility of risks, minimize liability exposure, and stay compliant with regulatory reporting requirements. The Joint's standards require minimum technology-based risk-management activities. These include clinical engineering's determination of technology-related incidents with follow-up steps to prevent recurrences and evaluation and documentation of the effectiveness of these steps.

Safety: Safety is the condition of being safe from danger, injury, or damage. It is judgment about the acceptability of risk in a specified situation (e.g., for a given medical problem) by a provider with specified training at a specified type of facility equipment.

Standards [20]: A wide variety of formal standards and guidelines related to healthcare technology now exists. Some standards apply to design, development, and manufacturing practices for devices, software, and pharmaceuticals; some are related to the construction and operation of a healthcare facility; some are safety and performance requirements for certain classes of technologies, such as standards related to radiation or electrical safety; and others relate to performance or even construction specifications, for specific types of technologies. Other standards and guidelines deal with administrative, medical, and surgical procedures and the training of clinical personnel. Standards and guidelines are produced and adopted by government agencies, international organizations, and professional and specialty organizations and societies. ECRI Institute's Healthcare Standards Directory lists more than 20,000 individual standards and guidelines produced by more than 600 organizations and agencies from North America alone.

Strategic technology planning: Strategic technology planning encompasses both technologies new to the hospital and replacements for existing equipment that are to be acquired over several quarters. Acquisitions can be proposed for reasons related to safety, standard-of-care issues, and age or obsolescence of existing equipment. Acquisitions can also be proposed to consolidate several service areas, expand a service area to reduce cost of service, or add a new service area. Strategic technology planning optimizes the way the hospital's capital resources contribute to its mission. It encourages choosing new technologies that are cost-effective and it also allows the hospital to be competitive in offering state-of-the-art services. Strategic technology planning works for a single department, product line, or clinical service. It can be limited to one or several high-priority areas. It can also be used for an entire multihospital system or geographic region [5].

Technology assessment: Assessment of medical technology is any process used for examining and reporting properties of medical technology used in healthcare, such as safety, efficacy, feasibility, and indications for use, cost, and cost-effectiveness, as well as social, economic, and ethical consequences, whether intended or unintended [21]. A primary technology assessment is one that seeks new, previously nonexistent data through research, typically employing long-term clinical studies of the type described below. A secondary technology assessment is usually based on published data, interviews, questionnaires, and other information-gathering methods rather than original research that create new, basic data. In technology assessment, there are six basic objectives that the clinical engineering department should have in mind. First, there should be ongoing monitoring of developments concerning new and emerging technologies. For new technologies, there should be an assessment of the clinical efficacy, safety, and cost/benefit ratio, including their effects on established technologies. There should be an evaluation of the short- and long-term costs and benefits of alternate approaches to managing specific clinical conditions. The appropriateness of existing technologies and their clinical uses should be estimated, whereas outmoded technologies should be identified and eliminated from their duplicative uses. The department should rate specific technology-based interventions in terms of improved overall value (quality and outcomes) to patients, providers, and payers. Finally, the department should facilitate a continuous uniformity between needs, offerings, and capabilities [22]. The locally based (hospital or hospital group) technology assessment described in this chapter is a process of secondary assessment that attempts to judge whether a certain medical equipment/product can be assimilated into the local operational environment.

Technology diffusion [20]: This is the process by which a technology is spread over time in a social system. The progression of technology diffusion can be described in four stages. The emerging or applied research stage occurs around the time of initial clinical testing. In the new stage, the technology has passed the phase of clinical trials but is not yet in widespread use. During the established stage, technology is considered by providers to be a standard approach to a particular condition and diffuses into general use. Finally, in the obsolete/outmoded stage, the technology is superseded by another and is demonstrated to be ineffective or harmful.

Technology life cycle: Technology has a life cycle—a process by which technology is created, tested, applied, and replaced or abandoned. Because the life cycle varies from basic research and innovation to obsolescence and abatement, it is critical to know the maturity of a technology before making decisions regarding its adoption. Technology forecast assessment of pending technological changes are the investigative tools that support systematic and rational decisions about the utilization of a given institution's technological capabilities.

Technology planning and management [22]: Technology planning and management are an accountable, systematic approach to ensure that cost-effective, efficacious, appropriate, and safe equipment is available to meet the demands of quality patient care and allow an institution to remain competitive. Elements include in-house service management, management and analysis of equipment external service providers, involvement in the equipment acquisition process, involvement of appropriate hospital personnel in facility planning and design, involvement in reducing technology-related patient and staff incidents, training equipment users, reviewing equipment replacement needs, and ongoing assessment of emerging technologies [5].

References

1. Cooper T., David Y., and Eagles S., *Getting Started with IEC 80001, Association for the Advancement of Medical Instrumentation*, AAMI, 2011.
2. American National Standard, ANSI/AAMI/IEC 80001-1:2010, *Application of Risk Management for IT Networks Incorporating Medical Devices—Part 1: Roles, Responsibilities and Activities*. Association for the Advancement of Medical Instrumentation, Arlington, VA, USA, 2010, ISBN 1-57020-400-4.
3. Stolberg S.G. (March 23, 2010). Obama signs health care overhaul bill, with a flourish. *The New York Times*. http://www.nytimes.com/2010/03/24/health/policy/24health.html. Retrieved February 11, 2011.
4. ECRI. *Healthcare Technology Assessment Curriculum*. Philadelphia, August 1992.
5. Banata H.D. *Institute of Medicine. Assessing Medical Technologies*. Washington, National Academy Press, 1985.
6. Lumsdon K. Beyond technology assessment: Balancing strategy needs, strategy. *Hospitals* 15: 25, 1992.
7. ECRI. *Capital, Competition, and Constraints: Managing Healthcare in the 1990s. A Guide for Hospital Executives*, Philadelphia, 1992.
8. Berkowtiz D.A. and Solomon R.P. Providers may be missing opportunities to improve patient outcomes. *Costs, Outcomes Measure Manage* May–June: 7, 1991.
9. Eagles S. *An Introduction to IEC 80001: Aiming for Patient Safety in the Networked Healthcare Environment*, IT Horizon, 4th edition, AAMI, 2008. Arlington, VA, USA.
10. ECRI. *Regional Healthcare Technology Planning and Management Program*. Plymouth, PA, 1990.
11. Sprague G.R. Managing technology assessment and acquisition. *Health Executives* 6: 26, 1988.

12. David Y. Technology-related decision-making issues in hospitals. In *IEEE Engineering in Medicine and Biology Society. Proceedings of the 11th Annual International Conference*, Crain Communications, Inc., Washington, D.C., 1989.
13. Wagner M. Promoting hospitals high-tech equipment. *Modern Healthcare* 46, 1989.
14. David Y. Medical technology 2001. In *CPA Healthcare Conference*, Proceeding of the Health Care Conference, Texas Society of Certified Public Accountants, San Antonio, Texas, July 1992.
15. Bingseng W. *Strategic Health Technology Incorporation, Synthesis Lectures on Biomedical Engineering #32*. Morgan & Claypool Publishers, San Rafael, CA, 2009.
16. ECRI. Special report on technology management, health technology, Philadelphia, 1989.
17. ECRI. Special report on devices and dollars, Philadelphia, 1988.
18. Gullikson M.L., David Y., and Brady M.H. An automated risk management tool. *JCAHO, Plant, Technology and Safety Management Review, PTSM series*, no. 2, 1993.
19. David Y. and Jahnke E.G. Planning hospital medical technology management. *IEEE/Engineering in Medicine and Biology Magazine*, May/June 2004. ISBN 0739-5175/04.
20. David Y., Judd T., and ECRI. Special report on devices and dollars, Philadelphia, 1988. Medical Technology Management, SpaceLabs Medical, Inc., Redmond, WA, 1993.
21. Bronzino J.D. (ed). *Management of Medical Technology: A Primer for Clinical Engineers*. Stoneham, MA, Butterworth, 1992.
22. David Y. *Risk Measurement for Managing Medical Technology*. Conference Proceedings, PERM-IT 1997, Australia.

52

Managing Medical Equipment Risks

Larry Fennigkoh
*Milwaukee School of
Engineering*

The management and mitigation of medical equipment-related risk is complex and multidimensional in scope. There are also cultural, administrative, and procedural aspects unique to each healthcare organization that also influences how such risks are effectively identified and managed. In this regard, it then becomes the responsibility of each organization to develop their own internal methods and procedures for addressing medical equipment risks. While this is preferably done within the larger organizational context of risk management or patient safety, risk may also be effectively managed from a focused equipment perspective as long as the emphasis covers the entire institution. Despite the unique character of these organizational procedures, they can have a common paradigm from which such individual procedures are developed and maintained. The focus of this chapter is on the use of such a paradigm for the hospital-wide management and control of medical equipment-related risk.

James Reason's "Swiss cheese" model of accident causation and system failures has, indeed, become the dominate paradigm for incident investigation and accident reconstruction [1]. It not only provides a tremendously useful way of metaphorically looking at how accidents happen but also how the intrinsic hazards particularly within high-tech, high-risk enterprises, for example, hospitals, can be further identified, eliminated, or their effects minimized. Since this model is focused on systems and the organization rather than on blaming the individual, its appeal and acceptance has been further enhanced.

Reason's original model was first described in his 1990 book, *Human Error*, and included four primary barriers to accidents: organizational influences, unsafe supervision, preconditions for unsafe acts, and the unsafe acts themselves [2]. The imperfections or weaknesses within these barriers are further represented by the holes; hence the analogy of these barriers and their weaknesses to slices of Swiss cheese [3]. System failures occur when these constantly moving and/or size varying weaknesses (holes) align. Now, the threats intrinsic to the organization's primary mission have a free, unrestricted path toward doing patient harm.

An adaptation of Reason's original model specifically for the management of medical equipment-related risk is offered and shown in Figure 52.1. In this form, the model is particularly applicable to healthcare because it encourages a focus on three areas that lend themselves to a continued vigilance or

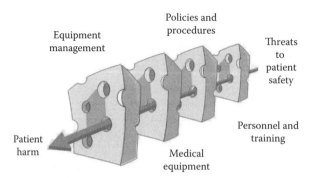

FIGURE 52.1 The use of Reason's Swiss cheese model of accident causation for the management of medical equipment risk. (Adapted from Reason, J. 2000. *British Medical Journal*, 320:768–770, 18 March.)

toward developing an organizational safety mindset or what Weick et al. termed *intelligent wariness* [4]. These areas include:

- Identifying, eliminating, or minimizing the nature of the intrinsic threats to patient safety themselves. Unfortunately, hospitals are loaded with such threats—from infections, falls, wrong-site surgeries, medication errors, equipment failures and use errors, caregiver communication problems, and so on. Once such threats are identified, the next best course is to determine which ones can actually be eliminated. For if a particular threat can truly be eliminated, there is no longer a need to develop a barrier against it. A prime example here is using only those infusion pumps that, by design, make fluid free flow simply impossible. Some pumps provide such assurance while others do not.

- Improving the effectiveness of the processes, procedures, people, equipment, or other things that constitute a particular barrier (i.e., the slices of cheese within the model). This effectively translates to making applicable policies meaningful and self-sustaining, hiring qualified people and then investing in keeping them competent, designing facilities that encourage the safe and efficient transport of patients, and purchasing and maintaining—in the best reasonable manner—those medical devices supplies needed to provide the best, safest care.

- Lastly, the model also forces the mindful organization to become more proactive in looking for and plugging the holes or weaknesses in its established barriers. Reason defines these "holes"—within his Swiss cheese model—as those due to *active failures* and *latent conditions*. Here, the former are those unsafe acts committed by people in direct contact with the patient or system [3]. These are the mistakes typically associated with human error, for example, lapses in judgment and procedural violations. The less obvious *latent conditions*, or as Reason also refers to as the "resident pathogens," are those weaknesses introduced during the design or decision making process that are unknown at the time and possibly laying dormant for years before their presence manifest themselves [3]. However, and unlike the fixed size and position of holes within slices of cheese, the real-life holes associated with these active failures and latent conditions are constantly changing their size and position. For example, the disastrous consequences of a free-flowing infusion pump containing a potent vasodilator such as sodium nitroprusside are reduced for the IV containing only normal saline. A crucial feature of Reason's model also recognizes the dynamic nature of these holes within any given slice of cheese (or institutional barrier).

The reader is encouraged to visualize these holes as both changing size as well as moving around within any slice of cheese. This feature of the model acknowledges the element of chance or random occurrences associated with many accidents.

However, and unlike that represented by the model, the holes—especially those due to the latent conditions—are invisible to the organization; typically not revealing themselves until some catastrophic event makes them now "obvious." As also illustrated in Figure 52.1, it is only when single holes in each of the available barriers align that the intrinsic threats to patient safety get a clear shot at doing the patient harm. These general concepts have made Reason's model readily adaptable to a variety of high-tech, high-risk enterprises—from aerospace, nuclear power plants, and aircraft carriers. As such, the model has established itself as a tremendously useful tool in the design of risk management systems. It also provides a useful template from which to conduct an accident reconstruction.

When applied to the delivery of healthcare, however, the model fails to acknowledge an additional complexity—one not typically encountered in other industries; namely, the highly variable nature of the patient themselves. A medication error, for example, that tunnels its way through all of the available barriers and reaches the patient may be life-threatening to one highly allergic patient but harmless to another. Further, some patients may simply be more physiologically tolerant of mistakes than others. A slip and fall may produce only a minor bruise to one patient, but result in a fractured hip in an osteoporotic elderly woman. Designing adequate barriers and plugging or minimizing likely "holes" is much more challenging and problematic given the highly variable nature of living things.

Nonetheless, hospital-based clinical engineering departments—if adequately staffed and prepared—are often the best suited to the task of managing the equipment-related risks. To do so, however, also requires a thorough, organizational-wide understanding and awareness of each of the model's major elements and—especially—their interactions. Even if the hospital's risk management department is not familiar with Reason's model, they may be a tremendous resource in the development and dissemination of the overall plan.

52.1 Threats to Patient Safety

The clinical engineering literature is replete with examples, case histories, and horror stories involving medical device-related patient injuries and deaths. Somewhat unfortunately, many of these examples have also been accompanied with blaming the caregiver for having made some type of mistake. While the end user of the device may have played a role in the resulting injury or death, they are rarely the only and primary cause. Many medical devices—especially those of a therapeutic nature—are intrinsically hazardous in ways that the nontechnical caregiver cannot even begin to imagine. Consider, for example:

- Electrosurgical units—generically often referred to as "Bovies" or "cautery machines"—that utilize high-frequency, high-voltage electrical waveforms to cut and cauterize tissue. These devices have been implicated in causing an untold number of unintentional and often full-thickness (third degree) burns at unwanted sites.
- The intentional sparks produced by these machines have also been blamed in a number of surgical drape fires. The high-frequency nature of these therapeutic electrical waveforms also makes it easier for them to become capacitively coupled to other tissue or conductive pathways. Burns due to such coupling and/or insulation failures during laparoscopic procedures are often the result. Since such burns are usually outside the surgeon's visual field, they often go untreated.
- Ventilators for the management of patient oxygenation (O_2 delivery) and ventilation (CO_2 removal) have been associated with a number of patient injuries and deaths through accidental tubing disconnects, inappropriate alarm level settings, infections, or lung damage due to excessive pressure (barotrauma) or volume (volutrauma).
- Surgical lasers have caused unwanted patient burns and retinal damage to physician users.
- Infusion pumps continue to accidentally deliver more or less medication than intended—at times with fatal consequences.
- External cardiac defibrillators are intentionally designed to deliver 200 J or more of electrical energy into a patient's chest. These devices have caused burns at the paddle sites as well as becoming the ignition sources within oxygen-enriched environments (see Figure 52.2).

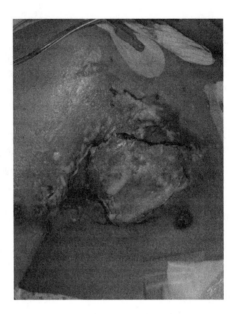

FIGURE 52.2   Patient burns from defibrillator-induced fire.

In short, any of the medical devices that apply some form of energy to patients—electrical, mechanical, or pneumatic—has the propensity to do harm. While continued improvement in device design can and has reduced the incidence of such injuries, these devices—by their very therapeutic nature—remain intrinsically dangerous. As such, users of such technology will now have to rely upon the development and use of appropriate and meaningful barriers to ensure patient safety.

52.2 Personnel and Training

While all organizations presumably seek to hire and retain the best employees possible, in reality not all people possess the same skills, abilities, or dedication to consistently performing their jobs at the best possible level. Nonetheless, hospital employees offer, perhaps, one of the most effective barriers against patient harm because they are potentially the most adaptable to changing threats and changes in patient vulnerability. Employees are also the only one within the organization capable of maintaining that level of *intelligent wariness*—an almost persistent expectation that things are going to go wrong. It is through such heightened awareness that employees become best prepared to appropriately react when things do go wrong. It is what also allows them to anticipate and identify the latent defects roaming throughout any given organization. Next to designing them out in the first place, simply identifying the existence of such latent conditions is the next best step in mitigating their effects. Developing and maintaining such staff wariness is also precisely how the equipment risk program becomes proactive rather than merely reactive.

52.3 Policies and Procedures

When appropriately developed, disseminated, and regularly reviewed, meaningful policies and procedures can offer a formidable barrier against equipment-related patient harm. The relatively common practice of requiring the presence of two nurses before administering patient blood transfusions is a prime example. When such a life-threatening procedure is checked and double checked by two different people, the likelihood of error drops considerably. The aviation industry and its crew resource management model offers considerable support and evidence for the value of checklists, repeating commands, and double checking all critical actions. John Nash, in his book *Why Hospitals Should*

Fly [5], makes an excellent case for the use and transfer of such aviation practices to healthcare. Even though the industries are very different, many of the concepts and practices within aviation are directly transferable to healthcare. The hospitals within the Veteran's Administration have already embraced and implemented many of these concepts through its National Center for Patient Safety (see http://www.patientsafety.gov).

52.4 Medical Equipment and Facilities

Fortunately, the intrinsic safety associated with a host of medical devices has continued to evolve and improve. Somewhat ironically, however, not until the safety weaknesses (i.e., latent conditions) have been exposed through patient injury, death, or costly lawsuits. The development of the return electrode monitor within electrosurgical units is a prime example. By continually interrogating the impedance within the return electrode–patient circuit, this feature disables the electrosurgical unit should the impedance become too high. Burns due to compromised or failed return electrodes are now largely prevented.

In addition to improvements in device design, there remain two additional equipment-related elements that offer tremendous potential for the further reduction in equipment-related risk.

- Continued acknowledgment and improvement in device human factors—especially as they apply to the device–user interface. As devices become increasingly human-friendly and their operation more intuitively obvious, the consequence of use errors is minimized, and patient injuries and deaths are also reduced. One of the best ways of assessing the human factors associated with device design is still done through prepurchase evaluations performed within the user's actual clinical environment. Here, the Agency for Healthcare Research and Quality also recommends:

  > Device purchasers should strongly consider institution-specific human factors testing. Usability testing at the institutional level establishes built-in redundancies to capture any design problems missed by manufacturers. Furthermore, the users and environments at individual institutions will differ, possibly in important ways, from the users and environments in which the device or program was initially designed and tested. It is important for an institution to be aware of who the intended users of the device or software will be, as well as where and when they plan to use the device. [6]

- Equipment standardization, while being at times difficult and costly to achieve, can be very helpful in minimizing use errors—especially in times of stress. At the very least, every effort should be made to standardize the life support devices, for example, defibrillators, ventilators, intra-aortic balloon pumps, and electrosurgical units.

52.4.1 Hospital Facilities Impact on Risk

There are also a variety of hospital facility-related or environmental factors that also become potential threats to patient safety. These include but are not limited to

- High ambient noise levels—which have repeatedly been cited as sources of psychological and physiological stress for both patients and clinicians [7]. While such noise levels may not result in permanent hearing loss, the greater concern are temporary threshold shifts that may interfere with hearing alarms and make communication difficult. Tijunelis et al. reported that time-weighted average sound levels measured in a large urban emergency department over both 12- and 8-h shifts exceeded 52 dB with measured peak noise levels of 94–117 dB occuring each minute during their measurement period [8]. It is in this context of hospital noise pollution that the many issues and problems surrounding medical device alarms need to be examined. Ironically, as the hospital ambient noise levels increase, so must the sound levels of medical device alarms in order that they be heard—which only increases ambient noise even more.

- Facilities design—including the physical layout and placement of devices relative to the patient. The often crammed and crowded critical care environment may contain a variety of tangled cables and lines, reach problems, and tripping hazards. Similarly, the often lengthy distances, multiple thresholds, and elevators that patients are often moved while being precariously tethered to multiple infusion pumps only adds to the potential risk of harm. The influence of such environmental factors on the patient–device interface is another compelling reason for hospitals to do extensive prepurchase usability testing.
- To a lesser extent, but no less important, are the intensity, position, and color temperature of available lighting. Such lighting factors may contribute to glare on monitors and instrument panels, artificially alter skin tones, and increase annoyance for both the patient and the clinician.

52.4.2 Equipment Management Program

As a highly regulated industry, hospitals also have obligations and requirements surrounding their management of medical devices. Of the many regulatory agencies involved, none have been more influential, perhaps, as the Joint Commission. Regardless of how the *letter* of their equipment-related codes and standards has changed over the years, the *intent* has remained fundamentally unchanged. Namely, that hospitals have a legal, moral, and ethical obligation of insuring that its medical technology is wisely purchased, performs properly, consistently, safely, and is routinely maintained. The well-designed and well-maintained equipment management program offers the best way of meeting these obligations and satisfying the intent of the Joint Commission requirements. While hospitals have been given considerable flexibility in how to design such programs, they all should include four, inextricably related components:

- An accurate, meaningful, and regularly maintained equipment inventory. While considerable debate continues on how best to develop and what to include in such an inventory, the essence being that the organization cannot begin to manage and maintain equipment if it does not know what it has, who manufactured it, where it is located, when it was purchased, and how much it cost. It is from such an inventory that preventive maintenance schedules are developed, staffing levels estimated, and device hazard alerts monitored. Without an accurate, meaningful equipment inventory, the equipment cannot be properly managed.
- An effective, meaningful, and practical preventive maintenance program. Unfortunately, and despite the age of the clinical engineering profession, considerable debate and disagreement continue as to what constitutes such a program. Nonetheless and fundamentally, such a program at the least should include: a meaningful inspection schedule based upon the needs of the device, its criticality to the hospital, and manufacturer-based recommendations; a practical set of inspection procedures; and documentation that the device was inspected according to these procedures and associated schedule.
- A well-educated and competently trained staff that also possesses the needed tools, test equipment, and access to the parts and supplies needed to properly repair, calibrate, and maintain the equipment. A well-functioning preventive maintenance program is also extremely dependent on such repair capabilities.
- The last essential link in the equipment management program "chain" is an involvement and input into the equipment acquisition process. The lack of such involvement can and often does introduce error into the equipment inventory if the clinical engineering department does not know when a new equipment is purchased. Further, if the staff is not adequately trained or has the needed access to repair parts, diagnostic software, and so on, the preventive maintenance and repair ability of the department will also be severely compromised.

52.5 Conclusions

The effective management of medical equipment-related risk requires a meaningful and practical framework or paradigm from which to start. As described here, Reason's modified Swiss cheese model provides one such paradigm. Metaphorically and conceptually, the model also tends to be readily understood, which further aids in its acceptance as a risk management tool.

References

1. Perneger, T.V. 2005. The Swiss cheese model of safety incidents: Are there holes in the metaphor? *BMC Health Services Research*. 5:71.
2. Reason, J. 1990. *Human Error*, Cambridge University Press, New York.
3. Reason, J. 2000. Human error: Models and management. *British Medical Journal*, 320:768–770, 18 March.
4. Weick, K., Sutcliffe, K., Obstfeld, D. 1991. Organizing for high reliability: Processes of collective mindfulness. *Research in Organizational Behavior*, 21:23–81.
5. Nance, J. 2008. *Why Hospitals Should Fly—The Ultimate Flight Plan to Patient Safety and Quality Care*. Montana: Second River Healthcare Press.
6. Making Health Care Safer: A critical analysis of patient safety practices. Evidence report/technology assessment no. 43, 2001, 461. Available at: http://archive.ahrq.gov/clinic/ptsafety/pdf/ptsafety.pdf. Accessed January 1, 2011.
7. McLaughlin, A. 1996. Noise levels in a cardiac surgical intensive care unit: A preliminary study conducted in secret. *Intensive and Critical Care Nursing*, 12:226–230.
8. Tijunelis, M. 2005. Noise in the ED. *American Journal of Emergency Medicine*, 23:332–335.

53

Clinical Engineering Program Indicators

Dennis D. Autio
Dybonics, Inc.

Robert L. Morris
Dybonics, Inc.

The role, organization, and structure of clinical engineering departments in the modern healthcare environment continue to evolve. During the past 10 years, the rate of change has increased considerably faster than mere evolution due to fundamental changes in the management and organization of healthcare. Rapid, significant changes in the healthcare sector are occurring in the United States and in nearly every country. The underlying drive is primarily economic, the recognition that resources are finite.

Indicators are essential for survival of organizations and are absolutely necessary for effective management of change. Clinical engineering departments are not exceptions to this rule. In the past, most clinical engineering departments were task driven and their existence was justified by the tasks performed. Perhaps the most significant change occurring in clinical engineering practice today is the philosophical shift to a more business-oriented, cost-justified, bottom-line-focused approach than has been generally the case in the past.

Changes in the healthcare delivery system will dictate that clinical engineering departments justify their performance and existence on the same basis as any business, the performance of specific functions at a high-quality level, and at a competitive cost. Clinical engineering management philosophy must change from a purely task-driven methodology to one that includes the economics of department performance. Indicators need to be developed to measure this performance. Indicator data will need to be collected and analyzed. The data and indicators must be objective and defensible. If it cannot be measured, it cannot be managed effectively.

Indicators are used to measure performance and function in three major areas. Indicators should be used as internal measurements and monitors of the performance provided by individuals, teams, and the department. These essentially measure what was done and how it was done. Indicators are essential during quality improvement and are used to monitor and improve a process. A third important type of program indicator is the benchmark. It is common knowledge that successful businesses will continue to use benchmarks, even though differing terminology will be used. A business cannot improve its competitive position unless it knows where it stands compared with similar organizations and businesses.

Different indicators may be necessary depending on the end purpose. Some indicators may be able to measure internal operations, quality improvement, and external benchmarks. Others will have a more restricted application.

It is important to realize that a single indicator is insufficient to provide the information on which to base significant decisions. Multiple indicators are necessary to provide cross-checks and verification. An example might be to look at the profit margin of a business. Even if the profit margin per sale is 100%, the business will not be successful if there are few sales. Looking at single indicators of gross or net profit will correct this deficiency but will not provide sufficient information to point the way to improvements in operations.

53.1 Department Philosophy

A successful clinical engineering department must define its mission, vision, and goals as related to the facility's mission. A mission statement should identify what the clinical engineering department does for the organization. A vision statement identifies the direction and future of the department and must incorporate the vision statement of the parent organization. Department goals are then identified and developed to meet the mission and vision statements for the department and organization. The goals must be specific and attainable. The identification of goals will be incomplete without at least implied indicators. Integrating the mission statement, vision statement, and goals together provides the clinical engineering department management with the direction and constraints necessary for effective planning.

Clinical engineering managers must carefully integrate mission, vision, and goal information to develop a strategic plan for the department. Since available means are always limited, the manager must carefully assess the needs of the organization and available resources, set appropriate priorities, and determine available options. The scope of specific clinical engineering services to be provided can include maintenance, equipment management, and technology management activities. Once the scope of services is defined, strategies can be developed for implementation. Appropriate program indicators must then be developed to document, monitor, and manage the services to be provided. Once effective indicators are implemented, they can be used to monitor internal operations and quality-improvement processes and complete comparisons with external organizations.

53.1.1 Monitoring Internal Operations

Indicators may be used to provide an objective, accurate measurement of the different services provided in the department. These can measure specific individual, team, and departmental performance parameters. Typical indicators might include simple tallies of the quantity or level of effort for each activity, productivity (quantity/effort), percentage of time spent performing each activity, percentage of scheduled IPMs (inspection and preventive maintenance procedures) completed within the scheduled period, mean time per job by activity, repair jobs not completed within 30 days, parts order for greater than 60 days, etc.

53.1.2 Process for Quality Improvement

When program indicators are used in a quality-improvement process, an additional step is required. Expectations must be quantified in terms of the indicators used. Quantified expectations result in the establishment of a threshold value for the indicator that will precipitate further analysis of the process. Indicators combined with expectations (threshold values of the indicators) identify the opportunities for program improvement. Periodic monitoring to determine if a program indicator is below (or above, depending on whether you are measuring successes or failures) the established threshold will provide a flag to whether the process or performance is within acceptable limits. If it is outside acceptable limits for the indicator, a problem has been identified. Further analysis may be required to define the problem better. Possible program indicators for quality improvement might include the number of repairs completed within 24 or 48 h, the number of callbacks for repairs, the number of repair problems caused by user error, the percentage of hazard notifications reviewed and acted on within a given time frame, meeting time targets for generating specification, evaluation or acceptance of new equipment, etc.

An example might be a weekly status update of the percentage of scheduled IPMs completed. Assume that the department has implemented a process in which a group of scheduled IPMs must be completed within 8 weeks. The expectation is that 12% of the scheduled IPMs will be completed each week. The indicator is the percentage of IPMs completed. The threshold value of the indicator is 12% per week increase in the percentage of IPMs completed. To monitor this, the number of IPMs that were completed must be tallied, divided by the total number scheduled, and multiplied by 100 to determine the percentage completed. If the number of completed IPMs is less than projected, then further analysis would be required to identify the source of the problem and determine solutions to correct it. If the percentage of completed IPMs was equal to or greater than the threshold or target, then no action would be required.

53.1.3 External Comparisons

Much important and useful information can be obtained by carefully comparing one clinical engineering program with others. This type of comparison is highly valued by most hospital administrators. It can be helpful in determining performance relative to competitors. External indicators or benchmarks can identify specific areas of activity in need of improvement. They offer insights when consideration is being given to expanding into new areas of support. Great care must be taken when comparing services provided by clinical engineering departments located in different facilities. There are number of factors that must be included in making such comparisons; otherwise, the results can be misleading or misinterpreted. It is important that the definition of the specific indicators used must be well understood, and great care must be taken to ensure that the comparison utilizes comparable information before interpreting the comparisons. Failure to understand the details and nature of the comparison and just using the numbers directly will likely result in inappropriate actions by managers and administrators. The process of analysis and explanation of differences in benchmark values between a clinical engineering department and a competitor (often referred to as gap analysis) can lead to increased insight into department operations and target areas for improvements.

Possible external indicators could be the labor cost per hour, the labor cost per repair, the total cost per repair, the cost per bed supported, the number of devices per bed supported, percentage of time devoted to repairs vs. IPMs vs. consultation, cost of support as a percentage of the acquisition value of capital inventory, etc.

53.2 Standard Database

In God we trust ... all others bring data!

—Florida Power and Light

Evaluation of indicators requires the collection, storage, and analysis of data from which the indicators can be derived. A standard set of data elements must be defined. Fortunately, one only has to look at commercially available equipment management systems to determine the most common data elements used. Indeed, most of the high-end software systems have more data elements than many clinical engineering departments are willing to collect. These standard data elements must be carefully defined and understood. This is especially important if the data will later be used for comparisons with other organizations. Different departments often have different definitions for the same data element. It is crucial that the data collected be accurate and complete. The members of the clinical engineering department must be trained to properly gather, document, and enter the data into the database. It makes no conceptual difference if the database is maintained on paper or using computers. Computers and their databases are ubiquitous and so much easier to use that usually more data elements are collected when computerized systems are used. The effort required for analysis is less and the level of sophistication of the analytical tools that can be used is higher with computerized systems.

The clinical engineering department must consistently gather and enter data into the database. The database becomes the practical definition of the services and work performed by the department. This standardized database allows rapid, retrospective analysis of the data to determine specific indicators identifying problems and assist in developing solutions for implementation. A minimum database should allow the gathering and storage of the following data:

In-House Labor. This consists of three elements: the number of hours spent providing a particular service, the associated labor rate, and the identity of the individual providing the service. The labor cost is not the hourly rate the technician is paid multiplied by the number of hours spent performing the service. It should include the associated indirect costs, such as benefits, space, utilities, test equipment, and tools, along with training, administrative overhead, and many other hidden costs. A simple, straightforward approach to determine an hourly labor rate for a department is to take the total budget of the department and subtract parts' costs, service contract costs, and amounts paid to outside vendors. Divide the resulting amount by the total hours spent providing services as determined from the database. This will provide an average hourly rate for the department.

Vendor Labor. This should include hours spent and rate, travel, and zone charges and any per-diem costs associated with the vendor-supplied service.

Parts. Complete information on parts is important for any retrospective study of services provided. This information is similar for both in-house and vendor-provided service. It should include the part number, a description of the part, and its cost, including any shipping.

Timeless. It is important to include a number of time stamps in these data. These should include the date the request was received, data assigned, and date completed.

Problem Identification. Both a code for rapid computer searching and classification and a free text comment identifying the nature of the problem and description of service provided are important. The number of codes should be kept to as few as possible. Detailed classification schemes usually end up with significant inaccuracies due to differing interpretations of the fine gradations in classifications.

Equipment Identification. Developing an accurate equipment history depends on reliable means of identifying the equipment. This usually includes a department- and/or facility-assigned unique identification number as well as the manufacturer, vendor, model, and serial number. Identification numbers provided by asset management are often inadequate to allow tracking of interchangeable modules or important items with a value less than a given amount. Acquisition cost is a useful data element.

Service Requester. The database should include elements allowing identification of the department, person, telephone number, cost center, and location of the service requester.

53.3 Measurement Indicators

Clinical engineering departments must gather objective, quantifiable data in order to assess ongoing performance, identify new quality-improvement opportunities, and monitor the effect of improvement action plans. Since resources are limited and everything cannot be measured, certain selection criteria must be implemented to identify the most significant opportunities for indicators. High-volume, high-risk, or problem-prone processes require frequent monitoring of indicators. A new indicator may be developed after analysis of ongoing measurements or feedback from other processes. Customer feedback and surveys often can provide information leading to the development of new indicators. Department management, in consultation with the quality-management department, typically determines what indicators will be monitored on an ongoing basis. The indicators and resulting analysis are fed back to individuals and work teams for review and improvement of their daily work activities. Teams may develop new indicators during their analysis and implementation of solutions to quality-improvement opportunities.

An indicator is an objective, quantitative measurement of an outcome or process that relates to performance quality. The event being assessed can be either desirable or undesirable. It is objective in that the same measurement can be obtained by different observers. This indicator represents quantitative, measured data that are gathered for further analysis. Indicators can assess many different aspects of quality, including accessibility, appropriateness, continuity, customer satisfaction, effectiveness, efficacy, efficiency, safety, and timeliness.

A program indicator has attributes that determine its utility as a performance measure. The reliability and variability of the indicator are distinct but related characteristics. An indicator is reliable if the same measurement can be obtained by different observers. A valid indicator is one that can identify opportunities for quality improvement. As indicators evolve, their reliability and validity should improve to the highest level possible.

An indicator can specify a part of a process to be measured or the outcome of that process. An outcome indicator assesses the results of a process. Examples include the percentage of uncompleted, scheduled IPMs, or the number of uncompleted equipment repairs not completed within 30 days. A process indicator assesses an important and discrete activity that is carried out during the process. An example would be the number of anesthesia machines in which the scheduled IPM failed or the number of equipment repairs awaiting parts that are uncompleted within 30 days.

Indicators can also be classified as sentinel-event indicators and aggregate data indicators. A performance measurement of an individual event that triggers further analysis is called a sentinel-event indicator. These are often undesirable events that do not occur often. These are often related to safety issues and do not lend themselves easily to quality-improvement opportunities. An example may include equipment failures that result in a patient injury.

An aggregate data indicator is a performance measurement based on collecting data involving many events. These events occur frequently and can be presented as a continuous variable indicator or as rate-based indicators. A continuous variable indicator is a measurement where the value can fall anywhere along a continuous scale. Examples could be the number of IPMs scheduled during a particular month or the number of repair requests received during a week. A rate-based variable indicator is the value of a measurement that is expressed as a proportion or a ratio. Examples could be the percentage of IPMs completed each month or the percentage of repairs completed within one workday.

General indicators should be developed to provide a baseline monitoring of the department's performance. They should also provide a cross-check for other indicators. These indicators can be developed to respond to a perceived need within a department or to solve a specific problem.

53.4 Indicator Management Process

The process to develop, monitor, analyze, and manage indicators is shown in Figure 53.1. The different steps in this process include defining the indicator, establishing the threshold, monitoring the indicator, evaluating the indicator, identifying quality-improvement opportunities, and implementing action plans.

> *Define Indicator.* The definition of the indicator to be monitored must be carefully developed. This process includes at least five steps. The event or outcome to be measured must be described. Define any specific terms that are used. Categorize the indicator (sentinel event or rate based, process or outcome, desirable, or undesirable). The purpose for this indicator must be defined, as well as how it is used in specifying and assessing the particular process or outcome.

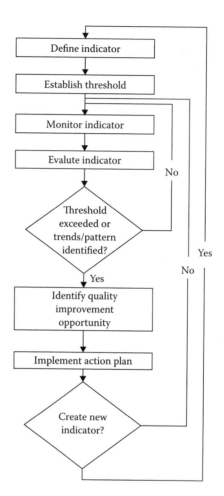

FIGURE 53.1 Indicator management process.

Establish Threshold. A threshold is a specific data point that identifies the need for the department to respond to the indicator to determine why the threshold was reached. Sentinel-event indicator thresholds are set at zero. Rate indicator thresholds are more complex to define because they may require expert consensus or definition of the department's objectives. Thresholds must be identified, including the process used to set the specific level.

Monitor Indicator. Once the indicator is defined, the data-acquisition process identifies the data sources and data elements. As these data are gathered, they must be validated for accuracy and completeness. Multiple indicators can be used for data validation and cross-checking. The use of a computerized database allows rapid access to these data. A database management tool allows quick sorting and organization of these data. Once gathered, these data must be presented in a format suitable for evaluation. Graphic presentation of data allows rapid visual analysis for thresholds, trends, and patterns.

Evaluate Indicator. The evaluation process analyzes and reports the information. This process includes comparing the information with established thresholds and analyzing for any trends or patterns. A trend is the general direction the indicator measurement takes over a period of time and may be desirable or undesirable. A pattern is a grouping or distribution of indicator measurements. A pattern analysis is often triggered when thresholds are crossed or trends are identified. Additional indicator information is often required. If an indicator threshold has not been reached, no further action may be necessary, other than continuing to monitor this indicator. The department may also decide to improve its performance level by changing the threshold.

Factors may be present leading to variation of the indicator data. These factors may include failure of the technology to perform properly, failure of the operators to use the technology properly, and failure of the organization to provide the necessary resources to implement this technology properly. Further analysis of these factors may lead to quality-improvement activities later.

Identify Quality-Improvement Opportunity. A quality-improvement opportunity may present itself if an indicator threshold is reached, a trend is identified, or a pattern is recognized. Additional information is then needed to further define the process and improvement opportunities. The first step in the process is to identify a team. This team must be given the necessary resources to complete this project, a timetable to be followed, and an opportunity to periodically update management on the status of the project. The initial phase of the project will analyze the process and establish the scope and definition of the problem. Once the problem is defined, possible solutions can be identified and analyzed for potential implementation. A specific solution to the problem is then selected. The solution may include modifying existing indicators or thresholds to more appropriate values, modifying steps to improve existing processes, or establishing new goals for the department.

Implement Action Plan. An action plan is necessary to identify how the quality-improvement solution will be implemented. This includes defining the different tasks to be performed, the order in which they will be addressed, who will perform each task, and how this improvement will be monitored. Appropriate resources must again be identified and a timetable must be developed prior to implementation. Once the action plan is implemented, the indicators are monitored and evaluated to verify appropriate changes in the process. New indicators and thresholds may need to be developed to monitor the solution.

53.5 Indicator Example 1: Productivity Monitors

Define Indicator. Monitor the productivity of technical personnel, teams, and the department. Productivity is defined as the total number of documented service support hours compared with the total number of hours available. This is a desirable rate-based outcome indicator. Provide feedback to technical staff and hospital administration regarding utilization of available time for department support activities.

Establish Threshold. At least 50% of available technician time will be spent providing equipment maintenance support services (revolving equipment problems and scheduled IPMs). At least 25% of available technician time will be spent providing equipment management support services (installations, acceptance testing, incoming inspections, equipment inventory database management, and hazard notification review).

Monitor Indicator. Data will be gathered every 4 weeks from the equipment work order history database. A trend analysis will be performed with data available from previously monitored 4-week intervals. These data will consist of hours worked on completed and uncompleted jobs during the past 4-week interval.

Technical staff available hours are calculated for the 4-week interval. The base time available is 160 h (40 h/week × 4 weeks) per individual. Add to this any overtime worked during the interval. Then subtract any holidays, sick days, and vacation days within the interval.

CJHOURS: Hours worked on completed jobs during the interval.
UJHOURS: Hours worked on uncompleted jobs during the interval.
AHOURS: Total hours available during the 4-week interval.

$$\text{Productivity} = (\text{CJHOURS} + \text{UJHOURS})/\text{AHOURS}$$

Evaluate Indicator. The indicator will be compared with the threshold, and the information will be provided to the individual. The individual team member data can be summed for team review. The data from multiple teams can be summed and reviewed by the department. Historical indicator information will be utilized to determine trends and patterns.

Quality-Improvement Process. If the threshold is not met, a trend is identified, or a pattern is observed, a quality-improvement opportunity exists. A team could be formed to review the indicator, examine the process that the indicator measured, define the problem encountered, identify ways to solve the problem, and select a solution. An action plan will then be developed to implement this solution.

Implement Action Plan. During implementation of the action plan, appropriate indicators will be used to monitor the effectiveness of the action plan.

53.6 Indicator Example 2: Patient Monitors IPM

53.6.1 Completion Time

Define Indicator. Compare the mean to complete an IPM for different models of patient monitors. Different manufacturers of patient monitors have different IPM requirements. Identify the most timely process to support this equipment.

Establish Threshold. The difference between the mean time to complete an IPM for different models of patient monitors will not be greater than 30% of the lesser time.

Monitor Indicator. Determine the mean time to complete an IPM for each model of patient monitor. Calculate the percentage difference between the mean time for each model and the model with the least mean time.

Evaluate Indicator. The mean time to complete IPMs was compared between the patient monitors, and the maximum difference noted was 46%. A pattern was also identified in which all IPMs for that one particular monitor averaged 15 min longer than those of other vendors.

Quality-Improvement Process. A team was formed to address this problem. Analysis of individual IPM procedures revealed that manufacturer X requires the case to be removed to access internal filters. Performing an IPM for each monitor required moving and replacing 15 screws for each of the 46 monitors. The team evaluated this process and identified that 5 min could be saved from each IPM if an electric screwdriver was utilized.

Implement Action Plan. Electric screwdrivers were purchased and provided for use by the technician. The completion of one IPM cycle for the 46 monitors would pay for two electric screwdrivers and provide 4 h of productive time for additional work. Actual savings were greater because this equipment could be used in the course of daily work.

53.7 Summary

In the ever-changing world of healthcare, clinical engineering departments are frequently being evaluated based on their contribution to the corporate bottom line. For many departments, this will require difficult and painful changes in management philosophy. Administrators are demanding quantitative measures of performance and value. To provide the appropriate quantitative documentation required by corporate managers, a clinical engineering a manager must collect available data that are reliable and accurate. Without such data, analysis is valueless. Indicators are the first step in reducing these data to meaningful information that can be easily monitored and analyzed. The indicators can then be used to determine department performance and identify opportunities for quality improvement.

Program indicators have been used for many years. What must change for clinical engineering departments is a conscious evaluation and systematic use of indicators. One traditional indicator of clinical engineering department success is whether the department's budget is approved or not. Unfortunately, approval of the budget as an indicator, while valuable, does not address the issue of predicting long-term survival, measuring program and quality improvements, or allowing frequent evaluation and changes.

There should be monitored indicators for every significant operational aspect of the department. Common areas where program indicators can be applied include monitoring interval department activities, quality-improvement processes, and benchmarking. Initially, simple indicators should be developed. The complexity and number of indicators should change as experience and needs demand.

The use of program indicators is absolutely essential if clinical engineering departments are to survive. Program and survival are now determined by the contribution of the department to the bottom line of the parent organization. Indicators must be developed and utilized to determine the current contribution of the clinical engineering department to the organization. Effective utilization and management of program indicators will ensure future department contributions.

References

AAMI. 1993. *Management Information Report MIR 1: Design of Clinical Engineering Quality Assurance Risk Management Programs*. Arlington, VA, Association for the Advancement of Medical Instrumentation.

AAMI. 1993. *Management Information Report MIR 2: Guideline for Establishing and Administering Medical Instrumentation Maintenance Programs*. Arlington, VA, Association for the Advancement of Medical Instrumentation.

AAMI. 1994. *Management Information Report MIR 3: Computerized Maintenance Management Systems for Clinical Engineering*. Arlington, VA, Association for the Advancement of Medical Instrumentation.

Bauld T.J. 1987. Productivity: Standard terminology and definitions. *J. Clin. Eng.* 12: 139.

Betts W.F. 1989. Using productivity measures in clinical engineering departments. *Biomed. Instrum. Technol.* 23: 120.

Bronzino J.D. 1992. *Management of Medical Technology: A Primer for Clinical Engineers*. Stoneham, MA, Butterworth-Heinemann.

Coopers and Lybrand International, AFSM. 1994. *Benchmarking Impacting the Boston Line*. Fort Myers, FL, Association for Services Management International.

David Y. and Judd T.M. 1993. Risk management and quality improvement. In: *Medical Technology Management*, pp. 72–75. Redmond, WA, SpaceLab Medical.

David Y. and Rohe D. 1986. Clinical engineering program productivity and measurement. *J. Clin. Eng.* 11: 435.

Downs K.J. and McKinney W.D. 1991. Clinical engineering workload analysis: A proposal for standardization. *Biomed. Instrum. Technol.* 25: 101.

Fennigkoh L. 1986. ASHE technical document no 055880: Medical equipment maintenance performance measures. Chicago, American Society for Hospital Engineers.

Furst E. 1986. Productivity and cost-effectiveness of clinical engineering. *J. Clin. Eng.* 11: 105.

Gordon G.J. 1995. *Breakthrough Management—A New Model for Hospital Technical Services*. Arlington, VA, Association for the Advancement of Medical Instrumentation.

Hertz E. 1990. Developing quality indicators for a clinical engineering department. In: *Plant, Technology and Safety Management Series: Measuring Quality in PTSM*. Chicago, Joint Commission on Accreditation of Healthcare Organizations.

JCAHO. 1990. *Primer on Indicator Development and Application, Measuring Quality in Health Care*. Oakbrook, IL, Joint Commission on Accreditation of Healthcare Organizations.

JCAHO. 1994. *Framework for Improving Performance*. Oakbrook, IL, Joint Commission on Accreditation of Healthcare Organizations.

Keil O.R. 1989. The challenge of building quality into clinical engineering programs. *Biomed. Instrum. Technol.* 23: 354.

Lodge D.A. 1991. Productivity, efficiency, and effectiveness in the management of healthcare technology: An incentive pay proposal. *J. Clin. Eng.* 16: 29.

Mahachek A.R. 1987. Management and control of clinical engineering productivity: A case study. *J. Clin. Eng.* 12: 127.

Mahachek A.R. 1989. Productivity measurement. Taking the first steps. *Biomed. Instrum. Technol.* 23: 16.

Selsky D.B. et al. 1991. Biomedical equipment information management for the next generation. *Biomed. Instrum. Technol.* 25: 24.

Sherwood M.K. 1991. Quality assurance in biomedical or clinical engineering. *J. Clin. Eng.* 16: 479.

Stiefel R.H. 1991. Creating a quality measurement system for clinical engineering. *Biomed. Instrum. Technol.* 25: 17.

Quality of Improvement and Team Building

Joseph P. McClain
*Walter Reed Army Medical
Center*

In today's complex healthcare environment, quality improvement and team building must go hand in hand. This is especially true for Clinical Engineers and Biomedical Equipment Technicians as the diversity of the field increases and technology moves so rapidly that no one can know all that needs to be known without the help of others. Therefore, it is important that we work together to ensure quality improvement. Ken Blachard, the author of the *One Minute Manager* series, has made the statement that "all of us are smarter than any one of us"—a synergy that evolves from working together.

Throughout this chapter we will look closely at defining quality and the methods for continuously improving quality, such as collecting data, interpreting indicators, and team building. All this will be put together, enabling us to make decisions based on scientific deciphering of indicators.

Quality is defined as conformance to customer or user requirements. If a product or service does what it is supposed to do, it is said to have high quality. If the product or service fails its mission, it is said to be low quality. Dr. W. Edward Demings, who is known to many as the "father of quality," defined it as surpassing customer needs and expectations throughout the life of the product or service.

Dr. Demings, a trained statistician by profession, formed his theories on quality during World War II while teaching industry how to use statistical methods to improve the quality of military production. After the war, he focused on meeting customer or consumer needs and acted as a consultant to Japanese organizations to change consumers' perceptions that "Made in Japan" meant junk. Dr. Demings predicted that people would be demanding Japanese products in just 5 years, if they used his methods. However, it only took 4 years, and the rest is history.

54.1 Deming's 14 Points

1. Create constancy of purpose toward improvement of product and service, with an aim to become competitive and to stay in business and provide jobs.
2. Adopt the new philosophy. We are in a new economic age. Western management must awaken and lead for change.
3. Cease dependence on inspection to achieve quality. Eliminate the needs for mass inspection by first building in quality.
4. Improve constantly and forever the system of production and service to improve quality and productivity and thus constantly decrease costs.
5. Institute training on the job.
6. Institute leadership: The goal is to help people, machines, and gadgets to do a better job.
7. Drive out fear so that everyone may work effectively for the organization.
8. Break down barriers between departments.
9. Eliminate slogans, exhortations, and targets for the workforce.
10. Eliminate work standards (quota) on the factory floor.
11. Substitute leadership: Eliminate management by objective, by numbers, and numerical goals.
12. Remove barriers that rob the hourly worker of the right to pride of workmanship.
13. Institute a vigorous program of education and self-improvement.
14. Encourage everyone in the company to work toward accomplishing transformation. Transformation is everyone's job.

54.2 Zero Defects

Another well-known quality theory, called zero defects (ZDs), was established by Philip Crosby. It got results for a variety of reasons. The main reasons are as follows:

1. *A strict and specific management standard.* Management, including the supervisory staff, does not use vague phrases to explain what it wants. It made the quality standard very clear: Do it the right way from the start. As Philip Crosby said, "What standard would you set on how many babies nurses are allowed to drop?"
2. *Complete commitment of everyone.* Interestingly, Crosby denies that ZD was a motivational program. But ZD worked because everyone got deeply into the act. Everyone was encouraged to spot problems, detect errors, and prescribe ways and means for their removal. This commitment is best illustrated by the ZD pledge: "I freely pledge myself to make a constant, conscious effort to do my job right the first time, recognizing that my individual contribution is a vital part of the overall effort."
3. *Removal of actions and conditions that cause errors.* Philip Crosby claimed that at ITT, where he was vice president for quality, 90% of all error causes could be acted on and fully removed by first-line supervision. In other words, top management must do its part to improve conditions, but supervisors and employees should handle problems directly. Errors, malfunctions, and/or variances can best be corrected where the rubber hits the road—at the source.

54.3 Total Quality Management

The most recent quality theory that has found fame is called TQM (Total Quality Management). It is a strategic, integrated management system for achieving customer satisfaction which involves all managers and employees and uses quantitative methods to continuously improve an organization's processes. Total Quality Management is a term coined in 1985 by the Naval Air Systems Command to describe its management approach to quality improvement. Simply put, TQM is a management approach to long-term success through customer satisfaction. TQM includes the following three principles: (1) achieving customer satisfaction, (2) making continuous improvement, and (3) giving everyone responsibility. TQM includes eight practices. These practices are (1) focus on the customer, (2) effective and renewed communications, (3) reliance on standards and measures, (4) commitment to training, (5) top management support and direction, (6) employee involvement, (7) rewards and recognition, and (8) long-term commitment.

54.4 Continuous Quality Improvement

Step 8 of the total quality management practices leads us to the quality concept coined by the Joint Commission on Accreditation of Healthcare Organizations and widely used by most healthcare agencies. It is called CQI (Continuous Quality Management). The principles of CQI are as follows:

Unity of Purpose

- Unity is established throughout the organization with a clear and widely understood vision.
- Environment nurtures total commitment from all employees.
- Rewards go beyond benefits and salaries to the belief that "We are family" and "We do excellent work."

Looking for Faults in the Systems

- Eighty percent of an organization's failures are the fault of management-controlled systems.
- Workers can control fewer than 20% of the problems.
- Focus on rigorous improvement of every system and cease blaming individuals for problems (the 80/20 rule of J.M. Juran and the nineteenth-century economist Vilfredo Pareto).

Customer Focus

- Start with the customer.
- The goal is to meet or exceed customer needs and give lasting value to the customer.
- Positive returns will follow as customers boast of the company's quality and service.

Obsession with Quality

- Everyone's job.
- Quality is relentlessly pursued through products and services that delight the customer.
- Efficient and effective methods of execution.

Recognizing the Structure in Work

- All work has structure.
- Structure may be hidden behind workflow inefficiency.
- Structure can be studied, measured, analyzed, and improved.

Freedom through Control

- There is control, yet freedom exists by eliminating micromanagement.
- Employees standardize processes and communicate the benefits of standardization.
- Employees reduce variation in the way work is done.
- Freedom comes as changes occur resulting in time to spend on developing improved processes, discovering new markets, and adding other methods to increase productivity.

Continued Education and Training

- Everyone is constantly learning.
- Educational opportunities are made available to employees.
- Greater job mastery is gained and capabilities are broadened.

Philosophical Issues on Training

- Training must stay tuned to current technology.
- Funding must be made available to ensure that proper training can be attained.
- Test, measurement, and diagnostic equipment germane to the mission must be procured and technicians trained on its proper use, calibration, and service.
- Creativity must be used to obtain training when funding is scarce.
- Include training in equipment procurement process.
- Contact manufacturer or education facility to bring training to the institution.
- Use local facilities to acquire training, thus eliminating travel cost.
- Allow employees to attend professional seminars where a multitude of training is available.

Teamwork

- Old rivalries and distrust are eliminated.
- Barriers are overcome.
- Teamwork, commitment to the team concept, and partnerships are the focus.
- Employee empowerment is critical in the CQI philosophy and means that employees have the authority to make well-reasoned, data-based decisions. In essence, they are entrusted with the legal power to change processes through a rational, scientific approach.

Continuous quality improvement is a means for tapping knowledge and creativity, applying participative problem solving, finding and eliminating problems that prevent quality, eliminating waste, instilling pride, and increasing teamwork. Further it is a means for creating an atmosphere of innovation for continued and permanent quality improvement. Continuous quality improvement as outlined by the Joint Commission on Accreditation of Healthcare Organizations is designed to improve the work processes within and across organizations.

54.5 Tools Used for Quality Improvement

The tools listed in the following sections will assist in developing quality programs, collecting data, and assessing performance indicators within the organization. These tools include several of the most frequently used and most of the seven tools of quality. The seven tools of quality are tools that help healthcare organizations understand their processes in order to improve them. The tools are the cause-and-effect diagram, check sheet, control chart, flowchart, histogram, Pareto chart, and scatter diagram. Additional tools shown are the Shewhart cycle (PDCA process) and the bar chart. The Clinical Engineering Manager must access the situation and determine which tool will work best for his/her situational needs.

Two of the seven tools of quality discussed above are not illustrated. These are the scatter diagram and the check sheet. The scatter diagram is a graphic technique to analyze the relationship between two variations and the check sheet is a simple data-recording device. The check sheet is custom designed by the user, which facilitates interpretation of the results. Most Biomedical Equipment Technicians use the check sheet on a daily basis when performing preventive maintenance, calibration, or electrical safety checks.

54.5.1 Cause and Effect or Ishikawa Chart

This is a tool for analyzing process dispersion (Figure 54.1). The process was developed by Dr. Karou Ishikawa and is also known as the fishbone diagram because the diagram resembles a fish skeleton. The

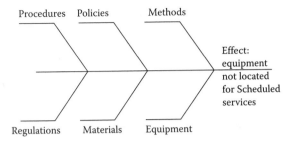

FIGURE 54.1   Cause and effect or Ishikawa chart.

diagram illustrates the main causes and subcauses leading to an effect. The cause-and-effect diagram is one of the seven tools of quality.

The following is an overview of the process:

1. Used in group problem solving as a brainstorming tool to explore and display the possible causes of a particular problem.
2. The effect (problem, concern, or opportunity) that is being investigated is stated on the right side, while the contributing causes are grouped in component categories through group brainstorming on the left side.
3. This is an extremely effective tool for focusing a group brainstorming session.
4. Basic components include environment, methods (measurement), people, money information, materials, supplies, capital equipment, and intangibles.

54.5.2 Control Chart

A control chart is a graphic representation of a characteristic of a process showing plotted values of some statistic gathered from that characteristic and one or two control limits (Figure 54.2). It has two basic uses:

1. As a judgment to determine if the process is in control.
2. As an aid in achieving and maintaining statistical control.

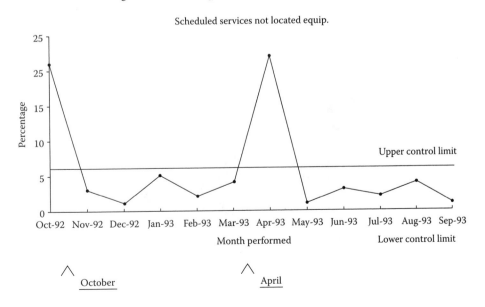

FIGURE 54.2   Control chart.

(This chart was used by Dr. W.A. Shewhart for a continuing test of statistical significance.) A control chart is a chart with a baseline, frequently in time order, on which measurement or counts are represented by points that are connected by a straight line with an upper and lower limit. The control chart is one of the seven tools of quality.

54.5.3 Flowchart

A flowchart is a pictorial representation showing all the steps of a process (Figure 54.3). Flowcharts provide excellent documentation of a program and can be a useful tool for examining how various steps in a process are related to each other. Flowcharting uses easily recognizable symbols to represent the type of processing performed. The flowchart is one of the seven tools of quality.

54.5.4 Histogram

A graphic summary of variation in a set of data is a histogram (Figure 54.4). The pictorial nature of the histogram lets people see patterns that are difficult to see in a simple table of numbers. The histogram is one of the seven tools of quality.

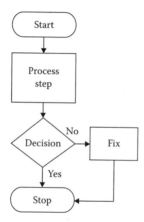

FIGURE 54.3   Flowchart.

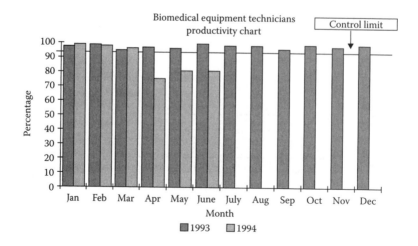

FIGURE 54.4   Histogram.

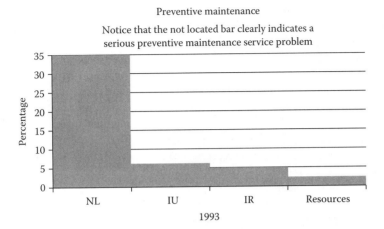

FIGURE 54.5   Pareto chart.

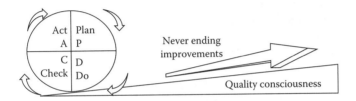

FIGURE 54.6   Shewhart cycle.

54.5.5 Pareto Chart

A Pareto chart is a special form of vertical bar graph that helps us to determine which problems to solve and in what order (Figure 54.5). It is based on the Pareto principle, which was first developed by J.M. Juran in 1950. The principle, named after the nineteenth-century economist Vilfredo Pareto, suggests that most effects come from relatively few causes; that is, 80% of the effects come from 20% of the possible causes.

Doing a Pareto chart, based on either check sheets or other forms of data collection, helps us direct our attention and efforts to truly important problems. We will generally gain more by working on the tallest bar than tackling the smaller bars. The Pareto chart is one of the seven tools of quality.

54.5.6 The Plan-Do-Check Act or Shewhart Cycle

This is a four-step process for quality improvement that is sometimes referred to as the Deming cycle (Figure 54.6). One of the consistent requirements of the cycle is the long-term commitment required. The Shewhart cycle or PDCA cycle is outlined here and has had overwhelming success when used properly. It is also a very handy tool to use in understanding the quality-cycle process. The results of the cycle are studied to determine what was learned, what can be predicted, and appropriate changes to be implemented.

54.6 Quality Performance Indicators

An indicator is something that suggests the existence of a fact, condition, or quality—an omen (a sign of future good or evil). It can be considered as evidence of a manifestation or symptom of an incipient failure or problem. Therefore, quality performance indicators (QPI) are measurements that can be used to ensure that quality performance is continuous and will allow us to know when incipient failures are starting so that we may take corrective and preventive actions.

QPI analysis is a five-step process:

Step 1: Decide what performance we need to track
Step 2: Decide the data that need to be collected to track this performance
Step 3: Collect the data
Step 4: Establish limits, a parameter, or control points
Step 5: Utilize BME (management by exception)—where a performance exceeds the established control limits, it is indicating a quality performance failure, and corrective action must be taken to correct the problem

In the preceding section, there were several examples of QPIs. In the Pareto chart, the NL = not located, IU = in use, and IR = in repair. The chart indicates that during the year 1994, 35% of the equipment could not be located to perform preventive maintenance services. This indicator tells us that we could eventually have a serious safety problem that could impact on patient care, and if not corrected, it could prevent the healthcare facility from meeting accreditation requirements. In the control chart example, an upper control limit of 6% "not located equipment" is established as acceptable in any one month. However, this upper control limit is exceeded during the months of April and October. This QPI could assist the clinical and Biomedical Equipment Manager in narrowing the problem down to a 2-month period. The histogram example established a lower control limit for productivity at 93%. However, productivity started to drop off in May, June, and July. This QPI tells the manager that something has happened that is jeopardizing the performance of his or her organization. Other performance indicators have been established graphically in Figures 54.7 and 54.8. See if you can determine what the indicators are and what the possible cause might be. You may wish to use these tools to establish QPI tracking germane to your own organization.

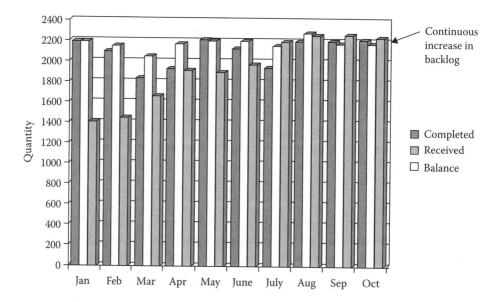

FIGURE 54.7 Sample repair service report.

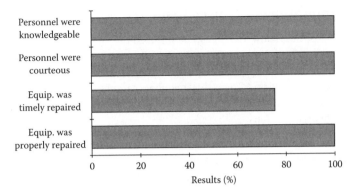

FIGURE 54.8 Customer satisfaction survey, August–September 1994.

54.7 Teams

A team is a formal group of persons organized by the company to work together to accomplish certain goals and objectives. Normally, when teams are used in quality improvement programs, they are designed to achieve the organization's vision. The organization's vision is a statement of the desired end state of the organization articulated and deployed by the executive leadership. Organizational visions are inspiring, clear, challenging, reasonable, and empowering. Effective visions honor the past, while they prepare for the future. The following are types of teams that are being used in healthcare facilities today. Some of the names may not be common, but their definitions are very similar if not commensurate.

54.7.1 Process Action Teams

Process action teams (PAT) are composed of those who are involved in the process being investigated. The members of a PAT are often chosen by their respective managers. The primary consideration for PAT membership is knowledge about the operations of the organization and consequently the process being studied. The main function of a PAT is the performance of an improvement project. Hence customers are often invited to participate on the team. PATs use basic statistical and other tools to analyze a process and identify potential areas for improvement. PATs report their findings to an Executive Steering Committee or some other type of quality management improving group. ("A problem well defined is half solved." John Dewey, American philosopher and educator; 1859–1952.)

54.7.2 Transition Management Team

The transition management team (TMT) (see *Harvard Business Review*, November–December 1993, pp. 109–118) is normally used for a major organizational change such as restructuring or reengineering. The TMT can be initiated due to the findings of a PAT, where it has been indicated that the process is severely broken and unsalvageable. The TMT is not a new layer of bureaucracy or a job for fading executives. The TMT oversees the large-scale corporate-change effort. It makes sure that all change initiatives fit together. It is made up of 8–12 highly talented leaders who commit all their time making the transition a reality. The team members and what they are trying to accomplish must be accepted by the power structure of the organization. For the duration of the change process, they are the CEO's version of the National Guard. The CEO should be able to say, "I can sleep well tonight, the TMT is managing this." In setting up a TMT, organizations should adopt a fail–safe approach: Create a position to oversee the emotional and behavioral issues unless you can prove with confidence that you do not need one.

54.7.3 Quality Improvement Project Team

A quality improvement project team (QIPT) can be initiated due to the findings of a PAT, where it has been indicated that the process is broken. The main agenda of the QIPT is to improve the work process that managers have identified as important to change. The team studies this process methodically to find permanent solutions to problems. To do this, members can use many of the tools described in this chapter and in many other publications on quality and quality improvement available from schools, bookstores, and private organizations.

54.7.4 Executive Steering Committee

This is an executive-level team composed of the Chief Executive Officer (CEO) of the organization and the executive staff that reports directly to the CEO. Whereas an organization may have numerous QMBs (Quality Management Board), PATs, and QIPTs, it has only one Executive Steering Committee (ESC). The ESC identifies strategic goals for organizational quality improvement efforts. It obtains information from customers to identify major product and service requirements. It is through the identification of these major requirements that quality goals for the organization are defined. Using this information, the ESC lists, prioritizes, and determines how to measure the organization's goals for quality improvement. The ESC develops the organization's improvement plan and manages the execution of that plan to ensure that improvement goals are achieved.

54.7.5 Quality Management Board

This is a permanent cross-functional team made up of top and midlevel managers who are jointly responsible for a specific product, service, or process. The structure of the board intended to improve communication and cooperation by providing vertical and horizontal "links" throughout the organization.

54.8 Process Improvement Model

This process is following the Joint Commission on the Accreditation of Healthcare Organizations' Quality Cube, a method of assessing the quality of the organization.

Plan:

1. Identify the process to be monitored
2. Select important functions and dimensions of performance applicable to the process identified
3. Design a tool for collection of data

Measure (Under this heading, you will document how, when, and where data were collected):

1. Collect data
2. Select the appropriate tool to deliver your data (charts, graphs, tables, etc.)

Assess (Document findings under this heading):

1. Interpret data collected
2. Design and implement change
   - Redesign the process or tool if necessary
   - If no changes are necessary, then you have successfully used the Process Improvement pathway

Improvement (Document details here):

1. Set in place the process to gain and continue the improvement

Outcome (Document all changes here):

1. Positive changes made to improve quality of care based on Performance Improvement Activity

54.8.1 Problem-Solving Model

The FOCUS-PDCA/PMAIO Process Improvement Model is a statistical-based quality-control method for improving processes. This approach to problem solving could be used by all process action teams to ensure uniformity within an organization. FOCUS-PDCA/PMAIO is as follows:

F—Find a process to improve.
O—Organize a team that knows the process.
C—Clarify current knowledge of the process.
U—Understand the cause or variations.
S—Select the process to improve.
P—Plan the improvement. P—Plan
D—Do the improvement (pilot test). M—Measure
C—Check the results of the improvement. A—Assess
A—Act to hold the gain. I—Improve
O—Outcome.

54.9 Summary

Although quality can be simply defined as conformity to customer or user requirements, it has many dimensions. Seven of them are described here (1) performance, (2) aesthetics, (3) reliability (how dependably it performs), (4) availability (there when you need it), (5) durability (how long it lasts), (6) extras or features (supplementary items), and (7) serviceability (how easy it is to get serviced). The word PARADES can help you remember this.

54.9.1 PARADES: Seven Dimensions of Quality

1. *Performance*: A product or service that performs its intended function well scores high on this dimension of quality.
2. *Aesthetics*: A product or service that has a favorable appearance, sound, taste, or smell is perceived to be of good quality.
3. *Reliability*: Reliability or dependability is such an important part of product quality that quality-control engineers are sometimes referred to as reliability engineers.
4. *Availability*: A product or service that is there when you need it.
5. *Durability*: Durability can be defined as the amount of use one gets from a product before it no longer functions properly and replacement seems more feasible than constant repair.
6. *Extras*: Feature or characteristics about a product or service that supplements its basic functioning (i.e., remote-control dialing on a television).
7. *Serviceability*: Speed, courtesy, competence, and ease of repair are all important quality factors.

54.9.2 Quality Has a Monetary Value!

Good quality often pays for itself, while poor quality is expensive in both measurable costs and hidden costs. The hidden costs include loss of goodwill, including loss of repeat business and badmouthing of the firm. High-quality goods and services often carry a higher selling price than do those of low quality. This information is evidenced by several reports in the *Wall Street Journal, Forbes Magazine, Money*

Magazine, Business Week Magazine, etc. A good example is the turnaround of Japanese product sales using quality methodologies outlined in *The Deming Guide to Quality and Competitive Position*, by Howard S. and Shelly J. Gitlow. As Dr. Demings has stated, quality improvement must be continuous!

Quality is never an accident; it has always the result of intelligent energy.

John Ruskin, 1819–1900, English art critic and historian
Seven Lamps of Architecture

References

Bittel L.R. 1985. *Every Supervisor Should Know*, 5th ed., pp. 455–456. New York, Gregg Division/ McGraw-Hill.

DuBrin A.J. 1994. *Essentials of Management*, 3rd ed. Cleveland, South-Western Publishing Co.

Duck J.D. 1993. Managing change—The art of balancing. *Harvard Business Review*, November–December 1993, pp. 109–118.

Gitlow H.S. and Gitlow S.J. 1987. *The Deming Guide to Quality and Competitive Position*. Englewood Cliffs, NJ, Prentice-Hall.

Goal/QPC. 1988. *The Memory Jogger. A Pocket Guide of Tools for Continuous Improvement*. Massachusetts, Goal/QPC.

Ishikawa K. 1991. *Guide to Quality Control*. New York, Quality Resources (Asian Productivity Organization, Tokyo, Japan).

Joint Commission on Accreditation of Healthcare Organizations—*Comprehensive Accreditation Manual for Hospitals—Official Handbook*, Library of Congress Number 96-076721, 1998, Oakbrook Terrace, IL 60181.

Juran J.M. 1979. *Quality Control Handbook*, 3rd ed. New York, McGraw-Hill.

Katzenbach J.R. and Smith D.K. 1994. *The Wisdom of Teams*. New York, Harper Business. A division of Harper Collins Publishers.

Mizuno S. 1988. *Management for Quality Improvement. The Seven New QC Tools*. Boston, Productivity Press.

Sholters P.R. 1993. *The Team Handbook. How to Use Teams to Improve Quality*. Madison, WI, Joiner Associates, Inc.

Walton M. 1986. *The Deming Management Method*. New York, Putnam Publishing Group.

55

A Standards Primer for Clinical Engineers

Alvin Wald
Columbia University

55.1 Introduction

The development, understanding, and use of standards is an important component of a clinical engineer's activities. Whether involved in industry, a healthcare facility, governmental affairs, or commercial enterprise, one way or another, the clinical engineer will find that standards are a significant aspect of professional activities. With the increasing emphasis on healthcare cost containment and efficiency, coupled with the continued emphasis on patient outcome, standards must be viewed both as a mechanism to reduce expenses and as another mechanism to provide quality patient care. In any case, standards must be addressed in their own right, in terms of technical, economic, and legal implications.

It is important for the clinical engineer to understand fully how standards are developed, how they are used, and most importantly, how they affect the entire spectrum of health-related matters. Standards exist that address systems (protection of the electrical power distribution system from faults), individuals (means to reduce potential electric shock hazards), and protection of the environment (disposal of deleterious waste substances).

From a larger perspective, standards have existed since biblical times. In the *Book of Genesis* (Chap. 6, ver. 14), Noah is given a construction standard by God, "Make thee an ark of gopher wood; rooms shalt thou make in the ark, and shalt pitch it within and without with pitch." Standards for weights and measures have played an important role in bringing together human societies through trade and commerce. The earliest record of a standard for length comes from ancient Egypt, in Dynasty IV (ca. 3000 BC). This length was the royal cubit, 20.620 in. (52.379 cm), as used in construction of the Great Pyramid.

The importance of standards to society is illustrated in the Magna Carta, presented by the English barons to King John in 1215 on the field at Runnymede. Article 35 states:

There shall be standard measures of wine, beer, and corn—the London quarter—throughout the whole of our kingdom, and a standard width of dyed, russet and halberject cloth—two ells within the selvedges; and there shall be standard weights also.

The principles of this article appear in the English Tower system for weight and capacity, set in 1266 by the assize of Bread and Ale Act:

An English penny called a sterling, round and without any clipping, shall weigh thirty-two wheat-corns in the midst of the ear; and twenty ounces a pound: and eight pounds do make a gallon of wine, and eight gallons of wine do make a bushell, which is the eighth part of a quarter.

In the United States, a noteworthy use of standards occurred after the Boston fire of 1689. With the aim of rapid rebuilding of the city, the town fathers specified that all bricks used in construction were to be $9 \times 4 \times 4$ in. An example of standardization to promote uniformity in manufacturing practices was the contract for 10,000 muskets awarded to Eli Whitney by President Thomas Jefferson in 1800. The apocryphal story is that Eli Whitney (better known to generations of grammar school children for his invention of the cotton gin) assembled a large number of each musket part, had one of each part randomly selected, and then assembled a complete working musket. This method of production, the complete interchangeability of assembly parts, came to be known as the "armory method," replacing hand crafting, which at that time had been the prevailing method of manufacturing throughout the world.

55.2 Definitions

A most general definition of a standard is given by Rowe (1983). "A standard is a multi-party agreement for establishing an arbitrary criterion for reference." Each word used in the definition by Rowe corresponds to a specific characteristic that helps to define the concept of a standard. Multi means more than one party, organization, group, government, agency, or individual. Agreement means that the concerned parties have come to some mutually agreed upon understanding of the issues involved and of ways to resolve them. This understanding has been confirmed via some mechanism such as unanimity, consensus, ballot, or other means that has been specified. Establishing defines the purpose of the agreement—to create the standard and carry forth its provisions.

Arbitrary emphasizes an understanding by the parties that there are no absolute criteria in creating the standard. Rather, the conditions and values chosen are based on the most appropriate knowledge and conditions available at the time the standard was established. Criterions are those features and conditions that the parties to the agreement have chosen as the basis for the standard. Not all issues may be addressed, but only those deemed, for whatever reasons, suitable for inclusion.

A different type of definition of a standard is given in The United States Office of Management and Budget Circular A-119:

… a prescribed set of rules, conditions, or requirements concerned with the definition of terms; classification of components; delineation of procedures; specifications of materials, performance, design, or operations; or measurement of quality and quantity in describing materials, products, systems, services, or practices.

A code is a compilation of standards relating to a particular area of concern, that is, a collection of standards. For example, local government health codes contain standards relating to providing of healthcare to members of the community. A regulation is an organization's way of specifying that some particular standard must be adhered to. Standards, codes, and regulations may or may not have legal implications, depending on whether the promulgating organization is governmental or private.

55.3 Standards for Clinical Engineering

There is a continually growing body of standards that affect healthcare facilities, and hence clinical engineering. The practitioner of healthcare technology must constantly search out, evaluate, and apply appropriate standards. The means to reconcile the conflicts of technology, cost considerations, the different jurisdictions involved, and the implementation of the various standards is not necessarily apparent. One technique that addresses these concerns and has proven to yield a consistent practical approach is a structured framework of the various levels of standards. This hierarchy of standards is a conceptual model that the clinical engineer can use to evaluate and apply to the various requirements that exist in the procurement and use of healthcare technology.

Standards have different purposes, depending on their particular applications. A hierarchy of standards can be used to delineate those conditions for which a particular standard applies. There are four basic categories, any one or all of which may be in simultaneous operation:

1. Local or proprietary standards (perhaps more properly called regulations) are developed to meet the internal needs of a particular organization.
2. Common interest standards serve to provide uniformity of product or service throughout an industry or profession.
3. Consensus standards are agreements amongst interested participants to address an area of mutual concern.
4. Regulatory standards are mandated by an authority having jurisdiction to define a particular aspect of concern.

In addition, there are two categories of standards adherence (1) voluntary standards, which carry no inherent power of enforcement, but provide a reference point of mutual understanding, and (2) mandatory standards, which are incumbent upon those to whom the standard is addressed, and enforceable by the authority having jurisdiction.

The hierarchy of standards model can aid the clinical engineer in the efficient and proper use of standards. More importantly, it can provide standards developers, users, and the authorities having jurisdiction in these matters with a structure by which standards can be effectively developed, recognized, and used to the mutual benefit of all.

55.4 A Hierarchy of Standards

Local, or proprietary standards, are developed for what might be called internal use. An organization that wishes to regulate and control certain of its own activities issues its own standards. Thus, the standard is local in the sense that it is applied in a specific venue, and it is proprietary in that it is the creation of a completely independent administration. For example, an organization may standardize on a single type of an electrocardiograph monitor. This standardization can refer to a specific brand or model, or to specific functional or operational features. In a more formal sense, a local standard may often be referred to as an institutional Policy and Procedure. The policy portion is the why of it; the procedure portion is the how. It must be kept in mind that standards of this type that are too restrictive will limit innovation and progress, in that they cannot readily adapt to novel conditions. On the other hand, good local standards contribute to lower costs, operational efficiency, and a sense of coherence within the organization.

Sometimes, local standards may originate from requirements of a higher level of regulation. For example, the Joint Commission for Accreditation of Healthcare Organizations (JCAHO) (formerly the Joint Commission for Hospital Accreditation (JCAH), a voluntary organization (but an organization that hospitals belong to for various reasons, for example, accreditation, reimbursement, approval of training programs), does not set standards for what or how equipment should be used. Rather, the JCAHO requires that each hospital set its own standards on how equipment is selected, used, and maintained. To monitor compliance with this requirement, the JCAHO inspects whether the hospital follows its own standards. In one sense, the most damaging evidence that can be adduced against an organization (or an individual) is that it (he) did not follow its (his) own standards.

Common interest standards are based on a need recognized by a group of interested parties, which will further their own interests, individually or collectively. Such standards are generally accepted by affected interests without being made mandatory by an authority; hence they are one type of voluntary standard. These standards are often developed by trade or professional organizations to promote uniformity in a product or process. This type of standard may have no inducement to adherence except for the benefits to the individual participants. For example, if you manufacture a kitchen cabinet that is not of standard size, it will not fit into the majority of kitchens and thus it will not sell. Uniformity of screw threads is another example of how a product can be manufactured and used by diverse parties, and yet be absolutely interchangeable. More recently, various information transfer standards allow the interchange of computer-based information among different types of instruments and computers.

Consensus standards are those that have been developed and accepted in accordance with certain well defined criteria so as to assure that all points of view have been considered. Sometimes, the adjective "consensus" is used as a modifier for a "voluntary standard." Used in this context, consensus implies that all interested parties have been consulted and have come to a general agreement on the provisions of the standard. The development of a consensus standard follows an almost ritualistic procedure to insure that fairness and due process are maintained. There are various independent voluntary and professional organizations that sponsor and develop standards on a consensus basis (see below). Each such organization has its own particular rules and procedures to make sure that there is a true consensus in developing a standard.

In the medical products field, standards are sometimes difficult to implement because of the independent nature of manufacturers and their high level of competition. A somewhat successful standards story is the adoption of the DIN configuration for ECG lead-cable connection by the Association for the Advancement of Medical Instrumentation (AAMI). The impetus for this standard was the accidental electrocution of several children brought about by use of the previous industry standard lead connection (a bare metal pin, as opposed to the new recessed socket). Most (but not all) manufacturers of ECG leads and cables now adhere to this standard. Agreement on this matter is in sharp contrast to the inability of the healthcare manufacturing industry to implement a standard for ECG cable connectors. Even though a standard was written, the physical configuration of the connector is not necessarily used by manufacturers in production, nor is it demanded by medical users in purchasing. Each manufacturer uses a different connector, leading to numerous problems in supply and incompatibility for users. This is an example of a voluntary standard, which for whatever reasons, is effectively ignored by all interested parties.

However, even though there have been some failures in standardization of product features, there has also been significant progress in generating performance and test standards for medical devices. A number of independent organizations sponsor development of standards for medical devices. For example, the American Society for Testing and Materials (ASTM) has developed, "Standard Specification for Minimum Performance and Safety Requirements for Components and Systems of Anesthesia Gas Machines (F1161-88)." Even though there is no statutory law that requires it, manufacturers no longer produce, and thus hospitals can no longer purchase anesthesia machines without the built-in safety features specified in this standard. AAMI has sponsored numerous standards that relate to performance of specific medical devices, such as defibrillators, electrosurgical instruments, and electronic sphygmomanometers. These standards are compiled in the AAMI publication, "Essential Standards for Biomedical Equipment Safety and Performance." The National Fire Protection Association (NFPA) publishes "Standard for Health Care Facilities (NFPA 99)," which covers a wide range of safety issues relating to facilities. Included are sections that deal with electricity and electrical systems, central gas and vacuum supplies, and environmental conditions. Special areas such as anesthetizing locations, laboratories, and hyperbaric facilities are addressed separately. Mandatory standards have the force of law or other authority having jurisdiction.

Mandatory standards imply that some authority has made them obligatory. Mandatory standards can be written by the authority having jurisdiction, or they can be adapted from documents prepared by others as proprietary or consensus standards. The authority having jurisdiction can be a local hospital or even a department within the hospital, a professional society, a municipal or state government, or an agency of the federal government that has regulatory powers.

In the United States, hospitals are generally regulated by a local city or county authority, and/or by the state. These authorities set standards in the form of health codes or regulations, which have the force of law. Often, these local bodies consider the requirements of a voluntary group, the Joint Commission for Accreditation of Healthcare Organizations, in their accreditation and regulatory processes.

American National Standards. The tradition in the United States is that of voluntary standards. However, once a standard is adopted by an organization, it can be taken one step further. The American National Standards Institute (ANSI) is a private, nongovernment, voluntary organization that acts as a coordinating body for standards development and recognition in the United States. If the development process for a standard meets the ANSI criteria of open deliberation of legitimate concerns, with all interested parties coming to a voluntary consensus, then the developers can apply (but are not required) to have their standard designated as an American National Standard. Such a designation does not make a standard any more legitimate, but it does offer some recognition as to the process by which it has been developed. ANSI also acts as a clearing house for standards development, so as to avoid duplication of effort by various groups that might be concerned with the same issues. ANSI is also involved as a U.S. coordinating body for many international standards activities.

An excellent source that lists existing standards and standards generating organizations, both nationally and internationally, along with some of the workings of the FDA (see below), is the "Medical Device Industry Fact Book" (Allen, 1996).

55.5 Medical Devices

On the national level, oversight is generally restricted to medical devices, and not on operational matters. Federal jurisdiction of medical devices falls under the purview of the Department of Health and Human Services, Public Health Service, Food and Drug Administration (FDA), Center for Devices and Radiological Health. Under federal law, medical devices are regulated under the "Medical Device Amendments of 1976" and the "Radiation Control for Health and Safety Act of 1968." Additional regulatory authorization is provided by the "Safe Medical Devices Act of 1990," the "Medical Device Amendments of 1992," the "FDA Reform and Enhancement Act of 1996," and the "Food and Drug Administration Modernization Act of 1997."

A medical device is defined by Section 201 of the Federal Food, Drug, and Cosmetic Act (as amended), as an:

Instrument, apparatus, implement, machine, contrivance, implant, *in vitro* reagent, or other similar or related article including any component, part, or accessory which is recognized in the official National Formulary, or the United States Pharmacopeia, or any supplement to them;
Intended for use in the diagnosis of disease or other conditions, or in the care, mitigation, treatment, or prevention of disease, in man or other animals, or

Intended to affect the structure of any function of the body of man or other animals; and which does not achieve its primary intended purposes through chemical action within or on the body of man ... and which is not dependent upon being metabolized for the achievement of its primary intended purposes.

The major thrust of the FDA has been in the oversight of the manufacture of medical devices, with specific requirements based on categories of perceived risks. The 1976 Act (Section 513) establishes three classes of medical devices intended for human use:

Class I. General controls regulate devices for which controls other than performance standards or premarket approvals are sufficient to assure safety and effectiveness. Such controls include regulations that (1) prohibit adulterated or misbranded devices; (2) require domestic device manufacturers and initial distributors to register their establishments and list their devices; (3) grant FDA authority to ban certain devices; (4) provide for notification of risks and of repair, replacement, or refund; (5) restrict the sale, distribution, or use of certain devices; and (6) govern Good Manufacturing Practices, records, and reports, and inspections. These minimum requirements apply also to Class II and Class III devices.

Class II. Performance Standards apply to devices for which general controls alone do not provide reasonable assurance of safety and efficacy, and for which existing information is sufficient to establish a performance standard that provides this assurance. Class II devices must comply not only with general controls, but also with an applicable standard developed under Section 514 of the Act. Until performance standards are developed by regulation, only general controls apply.

Class III. Premarket Approval applies to devices for which general controls do not suffice or for which insufficient information is available to write a performance standard to provide reasonable assurance of safety and effectiveness. Also, devices which are used to support or sustain human life or to prevent impairment of human health, devices implanted in the body, and devices which present a potentially unreasonable risk of illness or injury. New Class III devices, those not "substantially equivalent" to a device on the market prior to enactment (May 28, 1976), must have approved Premarket Approval Applications (Section 510 k).

Exact specifications for General Controls and Good Manufacturing Practices (GMP) are defined in various FDA documents. Aspects of General Controls include yearly manufacturer registration, device listing, and premarket approval. General Controls are also used to regulate adulteration, misbranding and labeling, banned devices, and restricted devices. Good Manufacturing Practices include concerns of organization and personnel; buildings and equipment; controls for components, processes, packaging, and labeling; device holding, distribution, and installation; manufacturing records; product evaluation; complaint handling; and a quality assurance program. Design controls for GMP were introduced in 1996. They were motivated by the FDA's desire to harmonize its requirements with those of a proposed international standard (ISO 13485). Factors that need to be addressed include planning, input and output requirements, review, verification and validation, transfer to production, and change procedures, all contained in a history file for each device. Device tracking is typically required for Class III life-sustaining and implant devices, as well as postmarket surveillance for products introduced starting in 1991.

Other categories of medical devices include combination devices, in which a device may incorporate drugs or biologicals. Combination devices are controlled via intercenter arrangements implemented by the FDA.

Transitional devices refer to devices that were regulated as drugs, prior to the enactment of the Medical Device Amendments Act of 1976. These devices were automatically placed into Class III, but may be transferred to Class I or II.

A custom device may be ordered by a physician for his/her own use or for a specific patient. These devices are not generally available, and cannot be labeled or advertised for commercial distribution.

An investigational device is one that is undergoing clinical trials prior to premarket clearance. If the device presents a significant risk to the patient, an Investigational Device Exemption must be approved by the FDA. Information must be provided regarding the device description and intended use, the origins of the device, the investigational protocol, and proof of oversight by an Institutional Review Board to insure informed patient consent. Special compassionate or emergency use for a nonapproved device or for a nonapproved use can be obtained from the FDA under special circumstances, such as when there is no other hope for the patient.

Adverse Events. The Safe Medical Devices Act of 1990 included a provision by which both users and manufacturers (and distributors) of medical devices are required to report adverse patient events that may be related to a medical device. Manufacturers must report to the FDA if a device (a) may have caused or contributed to a death or serious injury, or (b) malfunctioned in such a way as would be likely to cause or contribute to a death or serious injury if the malfunction were to reoccur. Device users are required to notify the device manufacturer of reportable incidents, and must also notify the FDA in case of a device-related death. In addition, the FDA established a voluntary program for reporting device problems that may not have caused an untoward patient event, but which may have the potential for such an occurrence under altered circumstances.

New devices. As part of the General Controls requirements, the FDA must be notified prior to marketing any new (or modifying an existing) device for patient use. This premarket notification, called the 510(k) process after the relevant section in the Medical Device Amendments Act, allows the FDA to review the device for safety and efficacy.

There are two broad categories that a device can fall into. A device that was marketed prior to May 28, 1976 (the date that the Medical Device Amendments became effective) can continue to be sold. Also, a product that is "substantially equivalent" to a preamendment device can likewise be marketed. However, the FDA may require a premarket approval application for any Class III device (see below). Thus, these preamendment devices and their equivalents are approved by "grandfathering." (Premarket notification to the FDA is still required to assure safety and efficacy.) Of course, the question of substantial equivalency is open to an infinite number of interpretations. From the manufacturer's perspective, such a designation allows marketing the device without a much more laborious and expensive premarket approval process.

A new device that the FDA finds is not substantially equivalent to a premarket device is automatically placed into Class III. This category includes devices that provide functions or work through principles not present in preamendment devices. Before marketing, this type of device requires a Premarket Approval Application by the manufacturer, followed by an extensive review by the FDA. (However, the FDA can reclassify such devices into Class I or II, obviating the need for premarket approval.) The review includes scientific and clinical evaluation of the application by the FDA and by a Medical Advisory Committee (composed of outside consultants). In addition, the FDA looks at the manufacturing and control processes to assure that all appropriate regulatory requirements are being adhered to. Clinical (use of real patients) trials are often required for Class III devices in order to provide evidence of safety and efficacy. To carry out such trials, an Investigational Device Exemption must be issued by the FDA.

The Food and Drug Administration Modernization Act of 1997, which amends section 514 of the Food, Drug, and Cosmetic Act, has made significant changes in the above regulations. These changes greatly simplify and accelerate the entire regulatory process. For example, the law exempts from premarket notification Class I devices that are not intended for a use that is of substantial importance in preventing impairment of human health, or that do not present a potential unreasonable risk of illness or injury. Almost 600 Class I generic devices have been so classified by the agency. In addition, the FDA will specify those Class II devices for which a 510(k) submission will also not be required.

Several other regulatory changes have been introduced by the FDA to simplify and speed up the approval process. So-called "third party" experts will be allowed to conduct the initial review of all

Class I and low-to-intermediate risk Class II devices. Previously, the FDA was authorized to create standards for medical devices. The new legislation allows the FDA to recognize and use all or parts of various appropriate domestic and internationally recognized consensus standards that address aspects of safety and effectiveness relevant to medical devices.

55.6 International Standards

Most sovereign nations have their own internal agencies to establish and enforce standards. However, in our present world of international cooperation and trade, standards are tending towards uniformity across national boundaries. This internationalization of standards is especially true since formation of the European Common Market. The aim here is to harmonize the standards of individual nations by promulgating directives for medical devices that address "Essential Requirements" (Freeman, 1993) (see below). Standards in other areas of the world (Asia, Eastern Europe) are much more fragmented, with each country specifying regulations for its own manufactured and imported medical devices.

There are two major international standards generating organizations, both based in Europe, the International Electrotechnical Commission (IEC) and the International Organization for Standardization (ISO). Nations throughout the world participate in the activities of these organizations.

The IEC, founded in 1906, oversees, on an international level, all matters relating to standards for electrical and electronic items. Membership in the IEC is held by a National Committee for each nation. The United States National Committee (USNC) for IEC was founded in 1907, and since 1931 has been affiliated with ANSI. USNC has its members representatives from professional societies, trade associations, testing laboratories, government entities, other organizations, and individual experts. The USNC appoints a technical advisor and a technical advisory group for each IEC Committee and Subcommittee to help develop a unified United States position. These advisory groups are drawn from groups that are involved in the development of related U.S. national standards.

Standards are developed by Technical Committees (TC), Subcommittees (SC), and Working Groups (WG). IEC TC 62, "Electrical Equipment in Medical Practice," is of particular interest here. One of the basic standards of this Technical Committee is document 601-1, "Safety of Medical Electrical Equipment, Part 1: General Requirements for Safety," 2nd Edition (1988) and its Amendment 1 (1991), along with Document 601-1-1, "Safety Requirements for Medical Electrical Systems" (1992).

The International Organization for Standardization (ISO) oversees aspects of device standards other than those related to electrotechnology. This organization was formed in 1946 with a membership comprised of the national standards organizations of 26 countries. There are currently some 90 nations as members. The purpose of the ISO is to "facilitate international exchange of goods and services and to develop mutual cooperation in intellectual, scientific, technological, and economic ability." ISO addresses all aspects of standards except for electrical and electronic issues, which are the purview of the International Electrotechnical Commission. ANSI has been the official United States representative to ISO since its inception. For each Committee or Subcommittee of the ISO in which ANSI participates, a U.S. Technical Advisory Group (TAG) is formed. The administrator of the TAG is, typically, that same U.S. organization that is developing the parallel U.S. standard.

Technical Committees (TC) of the ISO concentrate on specific areas of interest. There are Technical Committees, Subcommittees, Working Groups, and Study Groups. One of the member national standards organizations serves as the Secretariat for each of these technical bodies.

One standard of particular relevancy to manufacturers throughout the world is ISO 9000. This standard was specifically developed to assure a total quality management program that can be both universally recognized and applied to any manufacturing process. It does not address any particular product or process, but is concerned with structure and oversight of how processes are developed, implemented, monitored, and documented. An independent audit must be passed by any organization to obtain ISO 9000 registration. Many individual nations and manufacturers have adopted this standard and require that any product that they purchase be from a source that is ISO 9000 compliant.

The European Union was, in effect, created by the Single Europe Act (EC-92), as a region "without internal frontiers in which the free movement of goods, persons, and capital is ensured." For various products and classes of products, the European Commission issues directives with regard to safety and other requirements, along with the means for assessing conformity to these directives. Products that comply with the appropriate directives can then carry the CE mark. EU member states ratify these directives into national law.

Two directives related to medical devices are the Medical Devices Directive (MDD), enacted in 1993 (mandatory as of June 15, 1998), and the Active Implanted Medical Devices Directive (AIMDD), effective since 1995. Safety is the primary concern of this system, and as in the United States, there are three classes of risk. These risks are based on what and for how long the device touches, and its effects. Safety issues include electrical, mechanical, thermal, radiation, and labeling. Voluntary standards that address these issues are formulated by the European Committee for Standardization (CEN) and the European Committee for Electrotechnical Standardization (CENELEC).

55.7 Compliance with Standards

Standards that were originally developed on a voluntary basis may take on mandatory aspects. Standards that were developed to meet one particular need may be used to satisfy other needs as well. Standards will be enforced and adhered to if they meet the needs of those who are affected by them. For example, consider a standard for safety and performance for a defibrillator. For the manufacturer, acceptance and sales are a major consideration in both the domestic and international markets. People responsible for specifying, selecting, and purchasing equipment may insist on adherence to the standard so as to guarantee safety and performance. The user, physician, or other healthcare professional, will expect the instrument to have certain operational and performance characteristics to meet medical needs. Hospital personnel want a certain minimum degree of equipment uniformity for ease of training and maintenance. The hospital's insurance company and risk manager want equipment that meets or exceeds recognized safety standards. Third-party payers, that is, private insurance companies or government agencies, insist on equipment that is safe, efficacious, and cost effective. Accreditation agencies, such as local health agencies or professional societies, often require equipment to meet certain standards. More basically, patients, workers, and society as a whole have an inherent right to fundamental safety. Finally, in our litigatious society, there is always the threat of civil action in the case of an untoward event in which a "non-standard," albeit "safe," instrument was involved. Thus, even though no one has stated "this standard must be followed," it is highly unlikely that any person or organization will have the temerity to manufacture, specify, or buy an instrument that does not "meet the standard."

Another example of how standards become compulsory is via accreditation organizations. The Joint Commission for Accreditation of Healthcare Organizations has various standards (requirements). This organization is a private body that hospitals voluntarily accept as an accrediting agent. However, various health insurance organizations, governmental organizations, and physician specialty boards for resident education use accreditation by the JCAHO as a touchstone for quality of activities. Thus, an insurance company might not pay for care in a hospital that is not accredited, or a specialty board might not recognize resident training in such an institution. Thus, the requirements of the JCAHO, in effect, become mandatory standards for healthcare organizations.

A third means by which voluntary standards can become mandatory is by incorporation. Existing standards can be incorporated into a higher level of standards or codes. For example, various state and local governments incorporate standards developed by voluntary organizations, such as the National Fire Protection Association, into their own building and health codes. These standards then become, in effect, mandatory government regulations, and have the force of (civil) law. In addition, as discussed above, the FDA will now recognize voluntary standards developed by recognized organizations.

55.8 Limitations of Standards

Standards are generated to meet the expectations of society. They are developed by organizations and individuals to meet a variety of specific needs, with the general goals of promoting safety and efficiency. However, as with all human activities, problems with the interpretation and use of standards do occur. Engineering judgment is often required to help provide answers. Thus, the clinical engineer must consider the limits of standards, a boundary that is not clear and is constantly shifting. Yet clinical engineers must always employ the highest levels of engineering principles and practices. Some of the limitations and questions of standards and their use will be discussed below.

55.8.1 Noncompliance with a Standard

Sooner or later, it is likely that a clinical engineer will either be directly involved with or become aware of deviation from an accepted standard. The violation may be trivial, with no noticeable effect, or there may be serious consequences. In the former case, either the whole incident may be ignored, or nothing more may be necessary than a report that is filed away, or the incident can trigger some sort of corrective action. In the latter case, there may be major repercussions involving investigation, censure, tort issues, or legal actions. In any event, lack of knowledge about the standard is not a convincing defense. Anyone who is in a position that requires knowledge about a standard should be fully cognizant of all aspects of that standard. In particular, one should know the provisions of the standard, how they are to be enforced, and the potential risks of noncompliance. Nonetheless, noncompliance with a standard, in whole or in part, may be necessary to prevent a greater risk or to increase a potential benefit to the patient. For example, when no other recourse is available, it would be defensible to use an electromagnet condemned for irreparable excessive leakage current to locate a foreign body in the eye of an injured person, and thus save the patient's vision. Even if the use of this device resulted in a physical injury or equipment damage, the potential benefit to the patient is a compelling argument for use of the noncompliant device. In such a case, one should be aware of and prepared to act on the possible hazard (excessive electrical current, here). A general disclaimer making allowance for emergency situations is often included in policy statements relating to use of a standard. Drastic conditions require drastic methods.

55.8.2 Standards and the Law

Standards mandated by a government body are not what is called "black letter law," that is a law actually entered into a criminal or civil code. Standards are typically not adopted in the same manner as laws, that is, they are not approved by a legislative body, ratified by an elected executive, and sanctioned by the courts. The usual course for a mandated standard is via a legislative body enacting a law that establishes or assigns to an executive agency the authority to regulate the concerned activities. This agency, under the control of the executive branch of government, then issues standards that follow the mandate of its enabling legislation. If conflicts arise, in addition to purely legal considerations, the judiciary must interpret the intent of the legislation in comparison with its execution. This type of law falls under civil rather than criminal application.

The penalty for noncompliance with a standard may not be criminal or even civil prosecution. Instead, there are administrative methods of enforcement, as well as more subtle yet powerful methods of coercion. The state has the power (and the duty) to regulate matters of public interest. Thus, the state can withhold or withdraw permits for construction, occupancy, or use. Possibly more effective, the state can withhold means of finance or payments to violators of its regulations. Individuals injured by failure to abide by a standard may sue for damages in civil proceedings. However, it must be recognized that criminal prosecution is possible when the violations are most egregious, leading to human injury or large financial losses.

55.8.3 Incorporation and Revision

Because of advances in technology and increases in societal expectations, standards are typically revised periodically. For example, the National Fire Protection Association revises and reissues its "Standard for Health Care Facilities" (NFPA 99) every three years. Other organizations follow a five-year cycle of review, revision, and reissue of standards. These voluntary standards, developed in good faith, may be adapted by governmental agencies and made mandatory, as discussed above. When a standard is incorporated into a legislative code, it is generally referenced as to a particular version and date. It is not always the case that a newer version of the standard is more restrictive. For example, ever since 1984, the National Fire Protection Association "Standard for Health Care Facilities" (NFPA 99) does not require the installation of isolated power systems (isolation transformers and line isolation monitors) in anesthetizing locations that do not use flammable anesthetic agents, or in areas that are not classified as wet locations. A previous version of this standard, "Standard for the Use of Inhalation Anesthetics (Flammable and Nonflammable)," (NFPA 56A-1978) did require isolated power. However, many State Hospital Codes have incorporated, by name and date, the provisions of the older standard, NFPA 56A. Thus, isolated power may still be required, by code, in new construction of all anesthetizing locations, despite the absence of this requirement in the latest version of the standard that addresses this issue. In such a case, the organization having jurisdiction in the matter must be petitioned to remedy this conflict between new and old versions of the standard.

55.8.4 Safety

The primary purpose of standards in clinical practice is to assure the safety of patient, operator, and bystanders. However, it must be fully appreciated that there is no such thing as absolute safety. The more safety features and regulations attached to a device, the less useful and the more cumbersome and costly may be its actual use. In the development, interpretation, and use of a standard, there are questions that must be asked: What is possible? What is acceptable? What is reasonable? Who will benefit? What is the cost? Who will pay?

No one can deny that medical devices should be made as safe as possible, but some risk will always remain. In our practical world, absolute safety is a myth. Many medical procedures involve risk to the patient. The prudent physician or medical technologist will recognize the possible dangers of the equipment and take appropriate measures to reduce the risk to a minimum. Some instruments and procedures are inherently more dangerous than others. The physician must make a judgment, based on his/her own professional knowledge and experience, as well as on the expectations of society, whether using a particular device is less of a risk than using an alternative device or doing nothing. Standards will help—but they do not guarantee complete safety, a cure, or legal and societal approval.

55.8.5 Liability

Individuals who serve on committees that develop standards, as well as organizations involved in such activities, are justifiably concerned with their legal position in the event that a lawsuit is instituted as a result of a standard that they helped to bring forth. Issues involved in such a suit may include restraint of trade, in case of commercial matters, or to liability for injury due to acts of commission or of omission. Organizations that sponsor standards or that appoint representatives to standards developing groups often have insurance for such activities. Independent standards committees and individual members of any standards committees may or may not be covered by insurance for participation in these activities. Although in recent times only one organization and no individual has been found liable for damages caused by improper use of standards (see following paragraph), even the possibility of being named in a lawsuit can intimidate even the most self-confident "expert." Thus, it is not at all unusual for an individual who is asked to serve on a standards development committee first to inquire as to liability insurance coverage. Organizations that develop standards or appoint representatives also take pains to insure that all of their procedures are carefully followed and documented so as to demonstrate fairness and prudence.

The dark side of standards is the implication that individuals or groups may unduly influence a standard to meet a personal objective, for example, to dominate sales in a particular market. If standards are developed or interpreted unfairly, or if they give an unfair advantage to one segment, then restraint of trade charges can be made. This is why standards to be deemed consensus must be developed in a completely open and fair manner. Organizations that sponsor standards that violate this precept can be held responsible. In 1982, the United States Supreme Court, in the Hydrolevel Case (Perry, 1982), ruled that the American Society of Mechanical Engineers was guilty of antitrust activities because of the way some of its members, acting as a committee to interpret one of its standards, issued an opinion that limited competition in sales so as to unfairly benefit their own employers. This case remains a singular reminder that standards development and use must be inherently fair.

55.8.6 Inhibition

Another charge against standards is that they inhibit innovation and limit progress (Flink, 1984). Ideally, standards should be written to satisfy minimum, yet sufficient, requirements for safety, performance, and efficacy. Improvements or innovations would still be permitted so long as the basic standard is followed. From a device users point of view, a standard that is excessively restrictive may limit the scope of permissible professional activities. If it is necessary to abrogate a standard in order to accommodate a new idea or to extend an existing situation, then the choice is to try to have the standard changed, which may be very time consuming, or to act in violation of the standard and accept the accompanying risks and censure.

55.8.7 Ex Post Facto

A question continually arises as to what to do about old equipment (procedures, policies, facilities, etc.) when a new standard is issued or an old standard is revised so that existing items become obsolete. One approach, perhaps the simplest, is to do nothing. The philosophy here being that the old equipment was acquired in good faith and conformed to the then existing standards. As long as that equipment is usable and safe, there is no necessity to replace it. Another approach is to upgrade the existing equipment to meet the new standard. However, such modification may be technically impractical or financially prohibitive. Finally, one can simply throw out all of the existing equipment (or sell it to a second-hand dealer, or use the parts for maintenance) and buy everything new. This approach would bring a smile of delight from the manufacturer and a scream of outrage from the hospital administrator. Usually what is done is a compromise, incorporating various aspects of these different approaches.

55.8.8 Costs

Standards cost both time and money to propose, develop, promulgate, and maintain. Perhaps the greatest hindrance to more participation in standards activities by interested individuals is the lack of funds to attend meetings where the issues are discussed and decisions are made. Unfortunately, but nonetheless true, organizations that can afford to sponsor individuals to attend such meetings have considerable influence in the development of that standard. On the other hand, those organizations that do have a vital interest in a standard should have an appropriate say in its development. A consensus of all interested parties tempers the undue influence of any single participant. From another viewpoint, standards increase the costs of manufacturing devices, carrying out procedures, and administering policies. This incremental cost is, in turn, passed on to the purchaser of the goods or services. Whether or not the increased cost justifies the benefits of the standard is not always apparent. It is impossible to realistically quantify the costs of accidents that did not happen or the confusion that was avoided by adhering to a particular standard. However, it cannot be denied that standards have made a valuable contribution to progress, in the broadest sense of that word.

55.9 Conclusions

Standards are just like any other human activity, they can be well used or a burden. The danger of standards is that they will take on a life of their own; and rather than serve a genuine need will exist only as a justification of their own importance. This view is expressed in the provocative and iconoclastic book by Bruner and Leonard (1989), and in particular in their Chapter 9, *"Codes and Standards: Who Makes the Rules?"* However, the raison d'être of standards is to do good. It is incumbent upon clinical engineers, not only to understand how to apply standards properly, but also how to introduce, modify, and retire standards as conditions change. Furthermore, the limitations of standards must be recognized in order to realize their maximum benefit. No standard can replace diligence, knowledge, and a genuine concern for doing the right thing.

References

Allen, A. (ed.) 1996. *Medical Device Industry Fact Book*, 3rd ed. Canon Communications, Santa Monica, CA.

American Society for Testing and Materials (ASTM). 1916. *Race Street*, Philadelphia, PA 19103.

Association for the Advancement of Medical Instrumentation (AAMI) 3330 Washington Boulevard, Suite 400, Arlington, VA 22201.

Bruner, J.M.R. and Leonard, P.F. 1989. *Electricity, Safety and the Patient*, Year Book Medical Publishers, Chicago.

Flink, R. 1984. Standards: Resource or constraint? *IEEE Eng. Med. Biol. Mag.*, 3: 14–16.

Food and Drug Administration, Center for Devices and Radiological Health, 5600 Fishers Lane, Rockville, MD 20857. URL: http://www.fda.gov/

Freeman, M. 1993. The EC medical devices directives, *IEEE Eng. Med. Biol. Mag.*, 12: 79–80.

International Electrotechnical Commission (IEC), Central Office, 3 rue de Varembé, PO Box 131, CH-1211, Geneva 20, Switzerland. URL: http://www.iec.ch/

International Organization for Standardization (ISO), Central Secretariat, 1 rue de Varembe, Case postale 56, CH 1211, Geneva 20, Switzerland. URL: http://www.iso.ch/index.html.

Joint Commission for Accreditation of Healthcare organizations (JCAHO) 1 Renaissance Boulevard, Oakbrook, IL 60181.

National Fire Protection Association (NFPA) *Batterymarch Park*, Quincy, MA 02269.

Perry, T.S. 1982. Antirust ruling chills standards setting, *IEEE Spectrum*, 19: 52–54.

Rowe, W.D. 1983. Design and performance standards. In *Medical Devices: Measurements, Quality Assurance, and Standards*, C.A. Caceres, H.T. Yolken, R.J. Jones, and H.R. Piehler (eds.), pp. 29–40. American Society for Testing and Materials, Philadelphia, PA.

56

Regulatory and Assessment Agencies

Mark E. Bruley
ECRI Institute

Vivian H. Coates
ECRI Institute

Effective management and development of clinical and biomedical engineering departments (hereafter called clinical engineering departments) in hospitals requires a basic knowledge of relevant regulatory and technology assessment agencies. Regulatory agencies set standards of performance and record keeping for the departments and the technology for which they are responsible. Technology assessment agencies are information resources for what should be an ever expanding role of the clinical engineer in the technology decision-making processes of the hospital's administration.

This chapter presents an overview of regulatory and technology assessment agencies in the United States, Canada, Europe, and Australia that are germane to clinical engineering. Due to the extremely large number of such agencies and information resources, we have chosen to focus on those of greatest relevance and/or informational value. The reader is directed to the references and sources of further information presented at the end of the chapter.

56.1 Regulatory Agencies

Within the healthcare field, there are over 38,000 applicable standards, clinical practice guidelines, laws, and regulations (ECRI, 1999). Voluntary standards are promulgated by more than 800 organizations; mandatory standards by more than 300 state and federal agencies. Many of these organizations and agencies issue guidelines that are relevant to the vast range of healthcare technologies within the responsibility of clinical engineering departments. Although many of these agencies also regulate the manufacture and clinical use of healthcare technology, such regulations are not directly germane to the management of a clinical department and are not presented.

For the clinical engineer, many agencies promulgate regulations and standards in the areas of, for example, electrical safety, fire safety, technology management, occupational safety, radiology and nuclear medicine, clinical laboratories, infection control, anesthesia and respiratory equipment, power distribution, and medical gas systems. In the United States medical device problem reporting is also regulated by many state agencies and by the U.S. Food and Drug Administration (FDA) via its MEDWATCH program. It is important to note that, at present, the only direct regulatory authority that the FDA has over U.S. hospitals is in the reporting of medical device-related accidents that result in serious injury or death. Chapter 80 discusses in detail many of the specific agency citations. Presented below are the names and addresses of the primary agencies whose codes, standards, and regulations have the most direct bearing on clinical engineering and technology management:

American Hospital Association
1 North Franklin
Chicago, IL 60606
(312) 422-3000
Website: www.aha.org

American College of Radiology
1891 Preston White Drive
Reston, VA 22091
(703) 648-8900
Website: www.acr.org

American National Standards Institute
11 West 42nd Street
13th Floor, New York, NY 10036
(212) 642-4900
Website: www.ansi.org

American Society for Hospital Engineering
840 North Lake Shore Drive
Chicago, IL 60611
(312) 280 5223
Website: www.ashe.org

American Society for Testing and Materials
1916 Race Street
Philadelphia, PA 19103
(215) 299-5400
Website: www.astm.org

Association for the Advancement of Medical
  Instrumentation
3330 Washington Boulevard
Suite 400, Arlington, VA 22201
(703) 525-4890
Website: www.aami.org

Australian Institute of Health and Welfare
GPO Box 570
Canberra, ACT 2601
Australia, (61) 06-243-5092
Website: www.aihw.gov.au

British Standards Institution
2 Park Street
London, W1A 2BS
United Kingdom
(44) 071-629-9000
Website: www.bsi.org.uk

Canadian Healthcare Association
17 York Street
Ottawa, ON K1N 9J6
Canada, (613) 241-8005
Website: www.canadian-healthcare.org

CSA International
178 Rexdale Boulevard
Etobicoke, ON M9W 1R3

Canada, (416) 747-4000
Website: www.csa-international.org

Center for Devices and Radiological Health
Food and Drug Administration
9200 Corporate Boulevard
Rockville, MD 20850
(301) 443-4690
Website: www.fda.gov/cdrh

Compressed Gas Association, Inc.
1725 Jefferson Davis Highway
Suite 1004, Arlington, VA 22202
(703) 412-0900

ECRI
5200 Butler Pike
Plymouth Meeting, PA 19462
(610) 825-6000; (610) 834-1275 (fax)
Websites: www.ecri.org;
www.ecriy2 k.org
www.mdsr.ecri.org

Environmental Health Directorate
Health Protection Branch
Health Canada
Environmental Health Centre
19th Floor, Jeanne Mance Building
Tunney's Pasture
Ottawa, ON K1A 0L2 Canada
(613) 957-3143
Website: www.hc-sc.gc.ca/hpb/index_e.html

Food and Drug Administration MEDWATCH,
  FDA Medical Products
Reporting Program
5600 Fishers Lane
Rockville, MD 20857-9787
(800) 332-1088
Website: www.fda.gov/cdrh/mdr.html

Institute of Electrical and Electronics Engineers
445 Hoes Lane
P.O. Box 1331
Piscataway, NJ 08850-1331
(732) 562-3800
Website: www.standards.ieee.org

International Electrotechnical Commission
Box 131
3 rue de Varembe, CH 1211
Geneva 20, Switzerland
(41) 022-919-0211
Website: www.iec.ch

International Organization for Standardization
1 rue de Varembe
Case postale 56, CH 1211
Geneva 20
Switzerland

(41) 022-749-0111
Website: www.iso.ch

Joint Commission on Accreditation of Healthcare
 Organizations
1 Renaissance Boulevard
Oakbrook Terrace, IL 60181
(630) 792-5600
Website: www.jcaho.org

Medical Devices Agency Department of Health
Room 1209, Hannibal House
Elephant and Castle
London, SE1 6TQ
United Kingdom
(44) 171-972-8143
Website: www.medical-devices.gov.uk

National Council on Radiation Protection and
 Measurements
7910 Woodmont Avenue, Suite 800
Bethesda, MD 20814
(310) 657-2652
Website: www.ncrp.com

National Fire Protection Association
1 Batterymarch Park
PO Box 9101
Quincy, MA 02269-9101
(617) 770-3000
Website: www.nfpa.org

Nuclear Regulatory Commission
11555 Rockville Pike, Rockville
MD 20852, (301) 492-7000
Website: www.nrc.gov

Occupational Safety and Health Administration
US Department of Labor
Office of Information and Consumer Affairs
200 Constitution Avenue, NW
Room N3647, Washington, DC 20210
(202) 219-8151
Website: www.osha.gov

ORKI
National Institute for Hospital and Medical Engineering
Budapest dios arok 3, H-1125
Hungary, (33) 1-156-1522

Radiation Protection Branch
Environmental Health Directorate
Health Canada, 775 Brookfield Road
Ottawa, ON K1A 1C1
Website: www.hc-sc.gc.ca/ehp/ehd/rpb

Russian Scientific and Research Institute
Russian Public Health Ministry
EKRAN, 3 Kasatkina Street
Moscow, Russia 129301
(44) 071-405-3474

Society of Nuclear Medicine, Inc.
1850 Samuel Morse Drive
Reston, VA 20190-5316, (703) 708-9000
Website: www.snm.org

Standards Association of Australia
PO Box 1055, Strathfield
NSW 2135, Australia
(61) 02-9746-4700
Website: www.standards.org.au

Therapeutic Goods Administration
PO Box 100, Wooden, ACT 2606
Australia, (61) 2-6232-8610
Website: www.health.gov.au/tga

Therapeutic Products Programme
Health Canada
Holland Cross, Tower B
2nd Floor, 1600 Scott Street
Address Locator #3102D1
Ottawa, ON K1A 1B6
(613) 954-0288
Website: www.hc-sc.gc.ca/hpb-dgps/therapeut

Underwriters Laboratories, Inc.
333 Pfingsten Road
Northbrook, IL 60062-2096
(847) 272-8800
Website: www.ul.com

VTT, Technical Research Center of Finland
Postbox 316
SF-33101 Tampere 10
Finland, (358) 31-163300
Website: www.vti.fi

56.2 Technology Assessment Agencies

Technology assessment is the practical process of determining the value of a new or emerging technology in and of itself or against existing or competing technologies using safety, efficacy, effectiveness, outcome, risk management, strategic, financial, and competitive criteria. Technology assessment also considers ethics and law as well as health priorities and cost effectiveness compared to competing technologies. A "technology" is defined as devices, equipment, related software, drugs, biotechnologies, procedures, and therapies; and systems used to diagnose or treat patients. Processes of technology management are discussed in detail in Chapters 51 and 52.

Technology assessment is not the same as technology acquisition/procurement or technology planning. The latter two are processes for determining equipment vendors, soliciting bids, and systematically determining a hospital's technology-related needs based on strategic, financial, risk management, and clinical criteria. The informational needs differ greatly between technology assessment and the acquisition/procurement or planning processes. This section focuses on the resources applicable to technology assessment.

Worldwide, there are nearly 400 organizations (private, academic, and governmental), providing technology assessment information, databases, or consulting services. Some are strictly information clearing houses, some perform technology assessment, and some do both. For those that perform assessments, the quality of the information generated varies greatly from superficial studies to in-depth, well referenced analytical reports. In 1997, the U.S. Agency for Health Care Policy and Research (AHCPR) designated 12 "Evidence-Based Practice Centers" (EPC) to undertake major technology assessment studies on a contract basis. Each of these EPCs are noted in the list below and general descriptions of each center may be viewed on the Internet at the AHCPR website http://www.ahcpr.gov/clinic/epc/.

Language limitations are a significant issue. In the ultimate analysis, the ability to undertake technology assessment requires assimilating vast amounts of information, most of which exists only in the English language. Technology assessment studies published by the International Society for Technology Assessment in Health Care (ISTAHC), by the World Health Organization, and other umbrella organizations are generally in English. The new International Health Technology Assessment database being developed by ECRI in conjunction with the U.S. National Library of Medicine contains more than 30,000 citations to technology assessments and related documents.

Below are the names, mailing addresses, and Internet website addresses of some of the most prominent organizations undertaking technology assessment studies:

Agence Nationale pour le Develeppement
de l'Evaluation Medicale
159 Rue Nationale
Paris 75013
France
(33) 42-16-7272
Website: www.upml.fr/andem/andem.htm

Alberta Heritage Foundation for Medical Research
125 Manulife Place
10180-101 Street
Edmonton, AB T5J 345
(403) 423-5727
Website: www.ahfmr.ab.ca

leAgencia de Evaluacion de Technologias
  Sanitarias
Ministerio de Sanidad y Consumo
Instituto de Salud Carlos III, AETS
Sinesio Delgado 6, 28029 Madrid
Spain, (34) 1-323-4359
Website: www.isciii.es/aets

American Association of Preferred
Provider Organizations
601 13th Street, NW
Suite 370 South

Washington, DC 20005
(202) 347-7600

American Academy of Neurology
1080 Montreal Avenue
St. Paul, MN 55116-2791
(612) 695-2716
Website: www.aan.com

American College of Obstetricians and Gynecologists
409 12th Street, SW
Washington, DC 20024
(202) 863-2518
Website: www.acog.org

Australian Institute of Health and Welfare
GPO Box 570
Canberra, ACT 2601
Australia
(61) 06-243-5092
Website: www.aihw.gov.au

Battelle Medical Technology
Assessment and Policy
Research Center (MEDTAP)
901 D Street, SW
Washington, DC 20024

(202) 479-0500
Website: www.battelle.org

(An EPC of AHCPR)
British Columbia Office of Health
Technology Assessment
Centre for Health Services & Policy Research,
University of British Columbia
429-2194 Health Sciences Mall
Vancouver, BC V6T 1Z3
Canada, (604) 822-7049
Website: www.chspr.ubc.ca

British Institute of Radiology
36 Portland Place
London, W1N 4AT
United Kingdom
(44) 171-580-4085
Website: www.bir.org.uk

Blue Cross and Blue Shield Association
Technology Evaluation Center
225 N Michigan Avenue
Chicago, IL 60601-7680
(312) 297-5530
(312) 297-6080 (publications)
Website: www.bluecares.com/new/clinical

Canadian Coordinating Office for
Health Technology Assessment
110-955 Green Valley Crescent
Ottawa ON K2C 3V4
Canada, (613) 226-2553
Website: www.ccohta.ca

Canadian Healthcare Association
17 York Street
Ottawa, ON K1N 9J6
Canada, (613) 241-8005
Website: www.canadian-healthcare.org

Catalan Agency for Health
Technology Assessment
Travessera de les Corts 131-159
Pavello Avenue
Maria, 08028 Barcelona
Spain, (34) 93-227-29-00
Website: www.aatm.es

Centre for Health Economics
University of York
York Y01 5DD
United Kingdom
(44) 01904-433718
Website: www.york.ac.uk

Center for Medical
Technology Assessment
Linköping University
5183 Linköping, Box 1026 (551-11)
Sweden, (46) 13-281-000

Center for Practice and Technology
Assessment Agency for Health
Care Policy and Research (AHCPR)
6010 Executive Boulevard, Suite 300
Rockville, MD 20852
(301) 594-4015
Website: www.ahcpr.gov

Committee for Evaluation and Diffusion of
Innovative Technologies
3 Avenue Victoria
Paris 75004, France
(33) 1-40-273-109

Conseil d'evaluation des technologies
de la sante du Quebec
201 Cremazie Boulevard East
Bur 1.01, Montreal
PQ H2M 1L2, Canada
(514) 873-2563
Website: www.msss.gouv.qc.ca

Danish Hospital Institute
Landermaerket 10
Copenhagen K
Denmark DK1119
(45) 33-11-5777

Danish Medical Research Council
Bredgade 43
1260 Copenhagen
Denmark
(45) 33-92-9700

Danish National Board of Health
Amaliegade 13, PO Box 2020
Copenhagen K, Denmark DK1012
(45) 35-26-5400

Duke Center for Clinical Health
Policy Research
Duke University Medical Center
2200 West Main Street, Suite 320

Durham, NC 27705
(919) 286-3399
Website: www.clinipol.mc.duke.edu
(An EPC of AHCPR)

ECRI
5200 Butler Pike
Plymouth Meeting, PA 19462
(610) 825-6000
(610) 834-1275 fax
Websites: www.ecri.org
www.ecriy2 k.org
www.mdsr.ecri.org

(An EPC of AHCPR)
Finnish Office for Health Care

Technology Assessment
PO Box 220
FIN-00531 Helsinki
Finland, (35) 89-3967-2296
Website: www.stakes.fi/finohta

Frost and Sullivan, Inc.
106 Fulton Street
New York, NY 10038-2786
(212) 233-1080
Website: www.frost.com

Health Council of the Netherlands
PO Box 1236
2280 CE, Rijswijk
The Netherlands
(31) 70-340-7520

Health Services Directorate
Strategies and Systems for Health
Health Promotion
Health Promotion and Programs
Branch Health Canada
1915B Tunney's Pasture
Ottawa, ON K1A 1B4
Canada, (613) 954-8629
Website: www.hc-sc.gc.ca/hppb/hpol

Health Technology Advisory Committee
121 East 7th Place, Suite 400
PO Box 64975
St. Paul, MN 55164-6358
(612) 282-6358

Hong Kong Institute of Engineers
9/F Island Centre
No. 1 Great George Street
Causeway Bay
Hong Kong

Institute for Clinical PET
7100-A Manchester Boulevard
Suite 300
Alexandria, VA 22310
(703) 924-6650
Website: www.icpet.org

Institute for Clinical
Systems Integration
8009 34th Avenue South
Minneapolis, MN 55425
(612) 883-7999
Website: www.icsi.org

Institute for Health Policy Analysis
8401 Colesville Road, Suite 500
Silver Spring, MD 20910
(301) 565-4216

Institute of Medicine (U.S.)
National Academy of Sciences

2101 Constitution Avenue, NW
Washington, DC 20418
(202) 334-2352
Website: www.nas.edu/iom

International Network of Agencies for
Health Technology Assessment
c/o SBU, Box 16158
S-103 24 Stockholm
Sweden, (46) 08-611-1913
Website: www.sbu.se/sbu-site/links/inahta

Johns Hopkins Evidence-based
Practice Center
The Johns Hopkins
Medical Institutions
2020 E Monument Street, Suite 2-600
Baltimore, MD 21205-2223
(410) 955-6953
Website: www.jhsph.edu/Departments/Epi/
(An EPC of AHCPR)

McMaster University Evidence-based
Practice Center
1200 Main Street West, Room 3H7
Hamilton, ON L8N 3Z5
Canada
(905) 525-9140 ext. 22520
Website: http://hiru.mcmaster.ca.epc/
(An EPC of AHCPR)

Medical Alley 1550 Utica Avenue, South
Suite 725
Minneapolis, MN 55416
(612) 542-3077
Website: www.medicalalley.org

Medical Devices Agency Department of Health
Room 1209
Hannibal House
Elephant and Castle
London, SE1 6TQ
United Kingdom
(44) 171-972-8143
Website: www.medical-devices.gov.uk

Medical Technology Practice
Patterns Institute
4733 Bethesda Avenue, Suite 510
Bethesda, MD 20814
(301) 652-4005
Website: www.mtppi.org

MEDTAP International
7101 Wisconsin Avenue, Suite 600
Bethesda MD 20814
(301) 654-9729
Website: www.medtap.com

MetaWorks, Inc.
470 Atlantic Avenue

Boston, MA 02210
(617) 368-3573 ext. 206
Website: www.metawork.com
(An EPC of AHCPR)

National Commission on Quality Assurance
2000 L Street NW, Suite 500
Washington, DC 20036
(202) 955-3500
Website: www.ncqa.org

National Committee of Clinical Laboratory Standards
  (NCCLS)
940 West Valley Road, Suite 1400
Wayne, PA 19087-1898
(610) 688-0100
Website: www.nccls.org

National Coordinating Center for
Health Technology Assessment
Boldrewood (Mailpoint 728)
Univ of Southampton SO16 7PX
United Kingdom, (44) 170-359-5642
Website: www.soton.ac.uk/[EQUATION]hta/address.htm

National Health and Medical Research Council
GPO Box 9848
Canberra, ACT Australia
(61) 06-289-7019

National Institute of Nursing Research, NIH
31 Center Drive
Room 5B10. MSC 2178
Bethesda, MD 20892-2178
(301) 496-0207
Website: www.nih.gov/ninr

New England Medical Center
Center for Clinical Evidence Synthesis
Division of Clinical Research
750 Washington Street, Box 63
Boston, MA 02111
(617) 636-5133
Website: www.nemc.org/medicine/ccr/cces.htm
(An EPC of AHCPR)

New York State Department of Health
Tower Building, Empire State Plaza
Albany, NY 12237
(518) 474-7354
Website: www.health.state.ny.us

NHS Centre for Reviews and Dissemination
University of York
York Y01 5DD, United Kingdom
(44) 01-904-433634
Website: www.york.ac.uk

Office of Medical Applications of Research
NIH Consensus Program Information Service

PO Box 2577, Kensington
MD 20891, (301) 231-8083
Website: odp.od.nih.gov/consensus

Ontario Ministry of Health
Hepburn Block
80 Grosvenor Street
10th Floor
Toronto, ON M7A 2C4
(416) 327-4377

Oregon Health Sciences University Division of Medical
  Informatics and Outcomes Research
3181 SW Sam Jackson Park Road
Portland, OR 97201-3098
(503) 494-4277
Website: www.ohsu.edu/epc
(An EPC of AHCPR)

Pan American Health Organization
525 23rd Street NW
Washington, DC 20037-2895
(202) 974-3222
Website: www.paho.org

Physician Payment Review Commission (PPRC)
2120 L Street NW, Suite 510
Washington, DC 20037 (202) 653-7220

Prudential Insurance Company of America Health Care
  Operations and Research Division
56 N Livingston Avenue
Roseland, NJ 07068
(201) 716-3870

Research Triangle Institute
3040 Cornwallis Road
PO Box 12194
Research Triangle Park, NC 27709-2194
(919) 541-6512
(919) 541-7480
Website: www.rti.org/epc/
(An EPC of AHCPR)

San Antonio Evidence-based Practice Center
University of Texas Health Sciences Center
Department of Medicine
7703 Floyd Curl Drive
San Antonio, TX 78284-7879
(210) 617-5190
Website: www.uthscsa.edu/
(An EPC of AHCPR)

Saskatchewan Health
Acute and Emergency
Services Branch
3475 Albert Street
Regina, SK S4S 6X6
(306) 787-3656

Scottish Health Purchasing Information Centre
Summerfield House
2 Eday Road
Aberdeen AB15 6RE
Scotland
United Kingdom
(44) 0-1224-663-456 ext. 75246
Website: www.nahat.net/shpic

Servicio de Evaluacion de
Technologias Sanitarias
Duque de Wellington 2
E01010 Vitoria-Gasteiz
Spain, (94) 518-9250
E-mail: osteba-san@ej-gv.es

Society of Critical Care Medicine
8101 E Kaiser Boulevard
Suite 300
Anaheim, CA 92808-2259
(714) 282-6000
Website: www.sccm.org

Swedish Council on Technology
Assessment in Health Care
Box 16158
S-103 24 Stockholm
Sweden
(46) 08-611-1913
Website: www.sbu.se

Southern California EPC-RAND
1700 Main Street
Santa Monica, CA 90401
(310) 393-0411 ext. 6669
Website: www.rand.org/organization/health/epc/
(An EPC of AHCPR)

Swiss Institute for Public
Health Technology Programme
Pfrundweg 14
CH-5001 Aarau
Switzerland
(41) 064-247-161

TNO Prevention and Health
PO Box 2215
2301 CE Leiden
The Netherlands
(31) 71-518-1818
Website: www.tno.n1/instit/pg/index.html

University HealthSystem Consortium
2001 Spring Road, Suite 700
Oak Brook, IL 60523
(630) 954-1700
Website: www.uhc.edu

University of Leeds
School of Public Health
30 Hyde Terrace
Leeds L52 9LN
United Kingdom
Website: www.leeds.ac.uk

USCF-Stanford University EPC
University of California
San Francisco
505 Parnassus Avenue
Room M-1490, Box 0132
San Francisco, CA 94143-0132
(415) 476-2564
Website: www.stanford.edu/group/epc/
(An EPC of AHCPR)

U.S. Office of Technology
Assessment (former address)
600 Pennsylvania Avenue SE
Washington, DC 20003
Note: OTA closed on 29 Sep, 1995.
However, documents can be accessed via the internet at
    www.wws.princeton.edu/§ota/html2/cong.html
Also a complete set of OTA publications is
available on CD-ROM; contact
the U.S. Government Printing Office
(www.gpo.gov) for more information

Veterans Administration
Technology Assessment Program
VA Medical Center (152M)
150 S Huntington Avenue
Building 4
Boston, MA 02130
(617) 278-4469
Website: www.va.gov/resdev

Voluntary Hospitals of America, Inc.
220 East Boulevard
Irving, TX 75014
(214) 830-0000

Wessex Institute of Health Research and Development
    Boldrewood Medical School
Bassett Crescent East
Highfield, Southampton SO16 7PX
United Kingdom
(44) 01-703-595-661
Website: www.soton.ac.uk/[EQUATION]wi/index.html

World Health Organization Distribution Sales, CH 1211
Geneva 27, Switzerland 2476
(41) 22-791-2111
Website: www.who.ch
Note: Publications are also available from the
WHO Publications Center, USA,
at (518) 436-9686

References

ECRI. *Healthcare Standards Official Directory*. ECRI, Plymouth Meeting, PA, 1999.

Eddy D.M. *A Manual for Assessing Health Practices & Designing Practice Policies: The Explicit Approach*. American College of Physicians, Philadelphia, PA, 1992.

Goodman C., Ed. *Medical Technology Assessment Directory*. National Academy Press, Washington, DC, 1988.

Marcaccio K.Y., ed. *Gale Directory of Databases. Volume 1: Online Databases*. Gale Research International, London, 1993.

van Nimwegen Chr., ed. *International List of Reports on Comparative Evaluations of Medical Devices*. TNO Centre for Medical Technology, Leiden, the Netherlands, 1993.

Further Information

A comprehensive listing of healthcare standards and the issuing organizations is presented in the Healthcare Standards Directory published by ECRI. The Directory is well organized by keywords, organizations and their standards, federal and state laws, legislation and regulations, and contains a complete index of names and addresses.

The International Health Technology Assessment database is produced by ECRI. A portion of the database is also available in the U.S. National Library of Medicine's new database called HealthSTAR. Internet access to HealthSTAR is through Website address http://igm.nlm.nih.gov. A description of the database may be found at http://www.nlm.nih.gov/pubs/factsheets/healthstar.html.

57

Applications of Virtual Instruments in Healthcare

Eric Rosow
Hartford Hospital

Premise Development Corporation

Joseph Adam
Premise Development Corporation

57.1 Applications of Virtual Instruments in Healthcare

Virtual Instrumentation allows organizations to effectively harness the power of the PC to access, analyze, and share information throughout the organization. With vast amount of data available from increasingly sophisticated enterprise-level data sources, potentially useful information is often left hidden due to a lack of useful tools. Virtual instruments can employ a wide array of technologies such as multidimensional analyses and Statistical Process Control (SPC) tools to detect patterns, trends, causalities, and discontinuities to derive knowledge and make informed decisions.

Today's enterprises create vast amounts of raw data and recent advances in storage technology, coupled with the desire to use these data competitively, has caused a data glut in many organizations. The healthcare industry in particular is one that generates a tremendous amount of data. Tools such as databases and spreadsheets certainly help manage and analyze these data; however databases, while ideal for extracting data are generally not suited for graphing and analysis. Spreadsheets, on the other hand, are ideal for analyzing and graphing data, but this can often be a cumbersome process when working with multiple data files. Virtual instruments empower the user to leverage the best of both worlds by creating a suite of user-defined applications which allow the end-user to convert vast amounts of data into information which is ultimately transformed into knowledge to enable better decision making.

This chapter will discuss several virtual instrument applications and tools that have been developed to meet the specific needs of healthcare organizations. Particular attention will be placed on the use of quality control and "performance indicators" which provide the ability to trend and forecast various metrics. The use of SPC within virtual instruments will also be demonstrated. Finally, a nontraditional application of virtual instrumentation will be presented in which a "peer review" application has been developed to allow members of an organization to actively participate in the Employee Performance Review process.

57.1.1 Example Application #1: The EndoTester™—A Virtual Instrument-Based Quality Control and Technology Assessment System for Surgical Video Systems

The use of endoscopic surgery is growing, in large part because it is generally safer and less expensive than conventional surgery, and patients tend to require less time in a hospital after endoscopic surgery. Industry experts conservatively estimate that about 4 million minimally invasive procedures were performed in 1996. As endoscopic surgery becomes more common, there is an increasing need to accurately evaluate the performance characteristics of endoscopes and their peripheral components.

The assessment of the optical performance of laparoscopes and video systems is often difficult in the clinical setting. The surgeon depends on a high-quality image to perform minimally invasive surgery, yet assurance of proper function of the equipment by biomedical engineering staff is not always straightforward. Many variables in both patient and equipment may result in a poor image. Equipment variables, which may degrade image quality, include problems with the endoscope, either with optics or light transmission. The light cable is another source of uncertainty as a result of optical loss from damaged fibers. Malfunctions of the charge-coupled device (CCD) video camera are yet another source of poor image quality. Cleanliness of the equipment, especially lens surfaces on the endoscope (both proximal and distal ends) are particularly common problems. Patient variables make the objective assessment of image quality more difficult. Large operative fields and bleeding at the operative site are just two examples of patient factors that may affect image quality.

The evaluation of new video endoscopic equipment is also difficult because of the lack of objective standards for performance. Purchasers of equipment are forced to make an essentially subjective decision about image quality. By employing virtual instrumentation, a collaborative team of biomedical engineers, software engineers, physicians, nurses, and technicians at Hartford Hospital (Hartford, CT) and Premise Development Corporation (Avon, CT) have developed an instrument, the EndoTester™, with integrated software to quantify the optical properties of both rigid and flexible fiberoptic endoscopes. This easy-to-use optical evaluation system allows objective measurement of endoscopic performance prior to equipment purchase and in routine clinical use as part of a program of prospective maintenance.

The EndoTester™ was designed and fabricated to perform a wide array of quantitative tests and measurements. Some of these tests include (1) Relative light loss, (2) Reflective symmetry, (3) Lighted (good) fibers, (4) Geometric distortion, and (5) Modulation transfer function (MTF). Each series of tests is associated with a specific endoscope to allow for trending and easy comparison of successive measurements.

Specific information about each endoscope (i.e., manufacturer, diameter, length, tip angle, department/unit, control number, and operator), the reason for the test (i.e., quality control, pre/post repair, etc.), and any problems associated with the scope are also documented through the electronic record. In addition, all the quantitative measurements from each test are automatically appended to the electronic record for life-cycle performance analysis.

Figures 57.1 and 57.2 illustrate how information about the fiberoptic bundle of an endoscope can be displayed and measured. This provides a record of the pattern of lighted optical fibers for the endoscope under test. The number of lighted pixels will depend on the endoscope's dimensions, the distal end geometry, and the number of failed optical fibers. New fiber damage to an endoscope will be apparent by comparison of the lighted fiber pictures (and histogram profiles) from successive tests. Statistical data are also available to calculate the percentage of working fibers in a given endoscope.

In addition to the two-dimensional profile of lighted fibers, this pattern (and all other image patterns) can also be displayed in the form of a three-dimensional contour plot. This interactive graph may be viewed from a variety of viewpoints in that the user can vary the elevation, rotation, size, and perspective controls.

Figure 57.2 illustrates how test images for a specific scope can be profiled over time (i.e., days, months, years) to identify degrading performance. This profile is also useful to validate repair procedures by comparing test images before and after the repair.

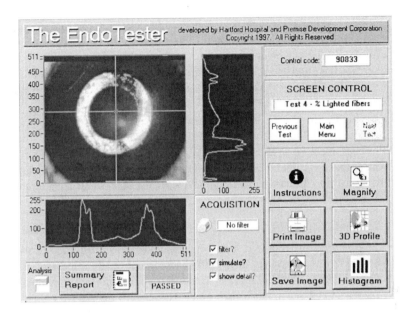

FIGURE 57.1 Endoscope tip reflection.

The EndoTester™ has many applications. In general, the most useful application is the ability to objectively measure an endoscope's performance prior to purchase, and in routine clinical use as part of a program of prospective maintenance. Measuring parameters of scope performance can facilitate equipment purchase. Vendor claims of instrument capabilities can be validated as a part of the negotiation process. Commercially available evaluation systems (for original equipment manufacturers) can cost upward of $50,000, yet by employing the benefits of virtual instrumentation and a standard PC,

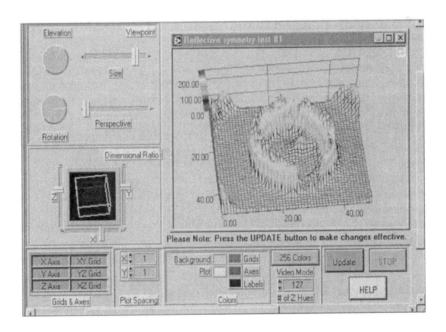

FIGURE 57.2 Endoscope profiling module.

an affordable, yet highly accurate test system for rigid and flexible fiberoptic endoscopes can now be obtained by clinical institutions.

In addition to technology assessment applications, the adoption of disposable endoscopes raises another potential use for the EndoTester™. Disposable scopes are estimated to have a life of 20–30 procedures. However, there is no easy way to determine exactly when a scope should be "thrown away." The EndoTester™ could be used to define this end-point.

The greatest potential for this system is as part of a program of preventive maintenance. Currently, in most operating rooms, endoscopes are removed from service and sent for repair when they fail in clinical use. This causes operative delay with attendant risk to the patient and an increase in cost to the institution. The problem is difficult because an endoscope may be adequate in one procedure but fail in the next which is more exacting due to clinical variables such as large patient size or bleeding. Objective assessment of endoscope function with the EndoTester™ may eliminate some of these problems.

Equally as important, an endoscope evaluation system will also allow institutions to ensure value from providers of repair services. The need for repair can be better defined and the adequacy of the repair verified when service is completed. This ability becomes especially important as the explosive growth of minimally invasive surgery has resulted in the creation of a significant market for endoscope repairs and service. Endoscope repair costs vary widely throughout the industry with costs ranging from $500 to 1500 or more per repair. Inappropriate or incomplete repairs can result in extending surgical time by requiring the surgeon to "switch scopes" (in some cases several times) during a surgical procedure.

Given these applications, we believe that the EndoTester™ can play an important role in reducing unnecessary costs, while at the same time improving the quality of the endoscopic equipment and the outcome of its utilization. It is the sincere hope of the authors that this technology will help to provide accurate, affordable and easy-to-acquire data on endoscope performance characteristics which clearly are to the benefit of the healthcare provider, the ethical service providers, manufacturers of quality products, the payers, and, of course, the patient.

57.1.2 Example Application #2: PIVIT™—Performance Indicator Virtual Instrument Toolkit

Most of the information management examples presented in this chapter are part of an application suite called PIVIT™. PIVIT is an acronym for "Performance Indicator Virtual Instrument Toolkit" and is an easy-to-use data acquisition and analysis product. PIVIT was developed specifically in response to the wide array of information and analysis needs throughout the healthcare setting.

The PIVIT applies virtual instrument technology to assess, analyze, and forecast clinical, operational, and financial performance indicators. Some examples include applications which profile institutional indicators (i.e., patient days, discharges, percent occupancy, ALOS, revenues, expenses, etc.), and departmental indicators (i.e., salary, nonsalary, total expenses, expense per equivalent discharge, DRGs, etc.). Other applications of PIVIT include 360° Peer Review, Customer Satisfaction Profiling, and Medical Equipment Risk Assessment.

The PIVIT can access data from multiple data sources. Virtually any parameter can be easily accessed and displayed from standard spreadsheet and database applications (i.e., Microsoft Access, Excel, Sybase, Oracle, etc.) using Microsoft's Open Database Connectivity (ODBC) technology. Furthermore, multiple parameters can be profiled and compared in real-time with any other parameter via interactive polar plots and three-dimensional displays. In addition to real-time profiling, other analyses such as SPC can be employed to view large data sets in a graphical format. SPC has been applied successfully for decades to help companies reduce variability in manufacturing processes. These SPC tools range from Pareto graphs to Run and Control charts. Although it will not be possible to describe all of these applications, several examples are provided below to illustrate the power of PIVIT.

57.1.3 Trending, Relationships, and Interactive Alarms

Figure 57.3 illustrates a virtual instrument that interactively accesses institutional and department specific indicators and profiles them for comparison. Data sets can be acquired directly from standard spreadsheet and database applications (i.e., Microsoft Access®, Excel®, Sybase®, Oracle®, etc.). This capability has proven to be quite valuable with respect to quickly accessing and viewing large sets of data. Typically, multiple data sets contained within a spreadsheet or database had to be selected and then a new chart of these data had to be created. Using PIVIT, the user simply selects the desired parameter from any one of the pull-down menus and this data set is instantly graphed and compared to any other data set.

Interactive "threshold cursors" dynamically highlight when a parameter is over and/or under a specific target. Displayed parameters can also be ratios of any measured value, for example, "Expense per Equivalent Discharge" or "Revenue to Expense Ratio." The indicator color will change based on how far the data value exceeds the threshold value (i.e., from green to yellow to red). If multiple thresholds are exceeded, then the entire background of the screen (normally gray) will change to red to alert the user of an extreme condition.

Finally, multimedia has been employed by PIVIT to alert designated personnel with an audio message from the personal computer or by sending an automated message via e-mail, fax, pager, or mobile phone.

The PIVIT also has the ability to profile historical trends and project future values. Forecasts can be based on user-defined history (i.e., "Months for Regression"), the type of regression (i.e., linear, exponential, or polynomial), the number of days, months, or years to forecast, and if any offset should be applied to the forecast. These features allow the user to create an unlimited number of "what if" scenarios and allow only the desired range of data to be applied to a forecast. In addition to the graphical display of data values, historical and projected tables are also provided. These embedded tables look and function very much like a standard spreadsheet.

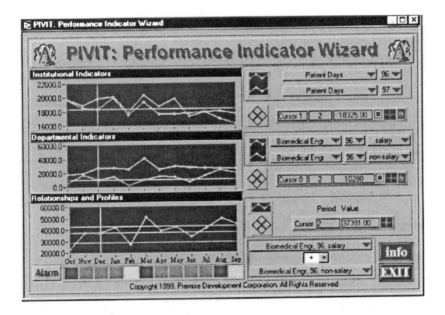

FIGURE 57.3 PIVIT™—Performance Indicator Wizard displays institutional and departmental indicators.

57.1.4 Data Modeling

Figure 57.4 illustrates another example of how virtual instrumentation can be applied to financial modeling and forecasting. This example graphically profiles the annual morbidity, mortality, and cost associated with falls within the state of Connecticut. Such an instrument has proved to be an extremely effective modeling tool due to its ability to interactively highlight relationships and assumptions, and to project the cost and/or savings of employing educational and other interventional programs.

Virtual instruments such as these are not only useful with respect to modeling and forecasting, but perhaps more importantly, they become a "knowledgebase" in which interventions and the efficacy of these interventions can be statistically proven. In addition, virtual instruments can employ standard technologies such as Dynamic Data Exchange (DDE), ActiveX, or TCP/IP to transfer data to commonly used software applications such as Microsoft Access® or Microsoft Excel®. In this way, virtual instruments can measure and graph multiple signals while at the same time send these data to another application which could reside on the network or across the Internet.

Another module of the PIVIT application is called the "Communications Center." This module can be used to simply create and print a report or it can be used to send e-mail, faxes, messages to a pager, or even leave voice-mail messages. This is a powerful feature in that information can be easily and efficiently distributed to both individuals and groups in real time.

Additionally, Microsoft Agent® technology can be used to pop-up an animated help tool to communicate a message, indicate an alarm condition, or can be used to help the user solve a problem or point out a discrepancy that may have otherwise gone unnoticed. Agents employ a "text-to-speech" algorithm to actually "speak" an analysis or alarm directly to the user or recipient of the message. In this way, on-line help and user support can also be provided in multiple languages.

In addition to real-time profiling of various parameters, more advanced analyses such as SPC can be employed to view large data sets in a graphical format. SPC has been applied successfully for decades to help companies reduce variability in manufacturing processes. It is the opinion of this author that SPC has enormous applications throughout healthcare. For example, Figure 57.5 shows how Pareto analysis can be applied to a sample trauma database of over 12,000 records. The Pareto chart may be frequency or

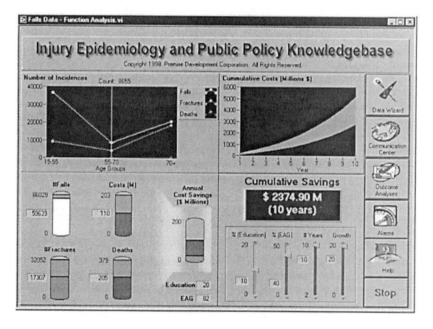

FIGURE 57.4 Injury epidemiology and public policy knowledgebase.

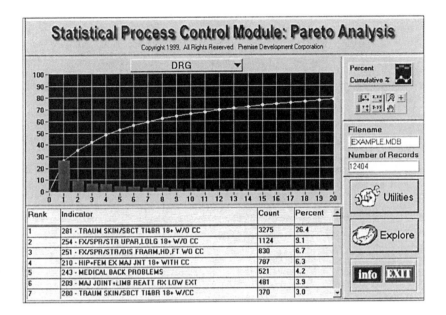

FIGURE 57.5 Statistical process control—Pareto analysis of a sample trauma registry.

percentage depending on front panel selection and the user can select from a variety of different parameters by clicking on the "pull-down" menu. This menu can be configured to automatically display each database field directly from the database. In this example, various database fields (i.e., DRG, Principal Diagnosis, Town, Payer, etc.) can be selected for Pareto analysis. Other SPC tools include run charts, control charts, and process capability distributions.

57.1.5 Medical Equipment Risk Criteria

Figure 57.6 illustrates a virtual instrument application which demonstrates how four "static" risk categories (and their corresponding values) are used to determine the inclusion of clinical equipment in the Medical Equipment Management Program at Hartford Hospital. Each risk category includes specific sub-categories that are assigned points, which when added together according to the formula listed below, yield a total score which ranges from 4 to 25.

Considering these scores, the equipment is categorized into five priority levels (High, Medium, Low, Grey List, and Non-Inclusion into the Medical Equipment Management Program). The four static risk categories are:

Equipment function (EF): Stratifies the various functional categories (i.e., therapeutic, diagnostic, analytical, and miscellaneous) of equipment. This category has "point scores" which range from 1 (miscellaneous, nonpatient-related devices) to 10 (therapeutic, life-support devices).

Physical risk (PR): Lists the "worst case scenario" of physical risk potential to either the patient or the operator of the equipment. This category has "point scores" which range from 1 (no significant identified risk) to 5 (potential for patient and/or operator death).

Environmental use classification (EC): Lists the primary equipment area in which the equipment is used and has "point scores" which range from 1 (nonpatient care areas) to 5 (anesthetizing locations).

Preventive maintenance requirements (MR): Describes the level and frequency of required maintenance and has "point scores" which range from 1 (not required) to 5 (monthly maintenance).

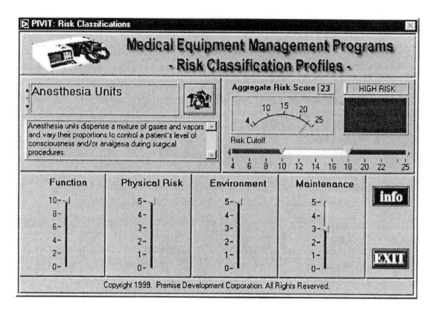

FIGURE 57.6 Medical equipment risk classification profiler.

The aggregate static risk score is calculated as follows:

$$\text{Aggregate Risk Score} = EF + PR + EC + MR \tag{57.1}$$

Using the criteria's system described above, clinical equipment is categorized according to the following priority of testing and degree of risk:

High risk: Equipment that scores between and including 18–25 points on the criteria's evaluation system. This equipment is assigned the highest risk for testing, calibration, and repair.

Medium risk: Equipment that scores between and including 15–17 points on the criteria's evaluation system.

Low risk: Equipment that scores between and including 12–14 points on the criteria's evaluation system.

Hazard surveillance (gray): Equipment that scores between and including 6 and 11 points on the criteria's evaluation system is visually inspected on an annual basis during the hospital hazard surveillance rounds.

Medical equipment management program deletion: Medical equipment and devices that pose little risk and scores less than 6 points may be deleted from the management program as well as the clinical equipment inventory.

Future versions of this application will also consider "dynamic" risk factors such as: user error, mean-time-between failure (MTBF), device failure within 30 days of a preventive maintenance or repair, and the number of years beyond the American Hospital Association's recommended useful life.

57.1.6 Peer Performance Reviews

The virtual instrument shown in Figure 57.7 has been designed to easily acquire and compile performance information with respect to institution-wide competencies. It has been created to allow every member of a team or department to participate in the evaluation of a co-worker (360° peer review). Upon

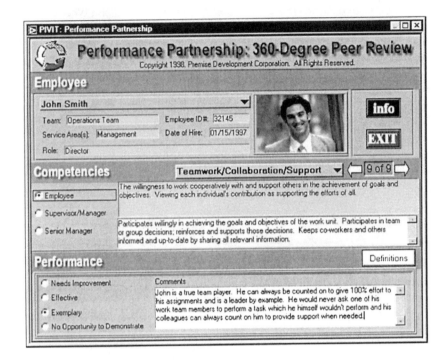

FIGURE 57.7 Performance reviews using virtual instrumentation.

running the application, the user is presented with a "Sign-In" screen where he or she enters their username and password. The application is divided into three components. The first (top section) profiles the employee and relevant service information. The second (middle section) indicates each competency as defined for employees, managers, and senior managers. The last (bottom) section allows the reviewer to evaluate performance by selecting one of four "radio buttons" and also provide specific comments related to each competency. This information is then compiled (with other reviewers) as real-time feedback.

References

1. American Society for Quality Control. *American National Standard. Definitions, Symbols, Formulas, and Tables for Control Charts*, 1987.
2. Breyfogle, F.W. *Statistical Methods for Testing, Development and Manufacturing*, John Wiley & Sons, New York, 1982.
3. Carey, R.G. and Lloyd, R.C. *Measuring Quality Improvement in Healthcare: A Guide to Statistical Process Control Applications*, 1995.
4. Fennigkow, L. and Lagerman, B. Medical Equipment Management. 1997 EC/PTSM Series/No. 1; Joint Commission on Accreditation of Hospital Organizations, 1997, pp. 47–54.
5. Frost & Sullivan Market Intelligence, file 765, The Dialog Corporation, Worldwide Headquarters, 2440 W. El Camino Real, Mountain View, CA 94040.
6. Inglis, A. *Video Engineering*, McGraw-Hill, New York, 1993.
7. Kutzner, J., Hightower, L., and Pruitt, C. Measurement and testing of CCD sensors and cameras, *SMPTE Journal*, 325–327, 1992.
8. Measurement of Resolution of Camera Systems, *IEEE Standard* 208, 1995.
9. Medical Device Register 1997, Vol. 2, Montvale NJ, Medical Economics Data Production Company, 1997.

10. Montgomery, D.C. *Introduction to Statistical Quality Control*, 2nd ed., John Wiley & Sons, New York, 1992.
11. Rosow, E. Virtual instrumentation applications with biosensors, presented at the *Biomedical Engineering Consortium for Connecticut (BEACON) Biosensor Symposium*, Trinity College, Hartford, CT, October 2, 1998.
12. Rosow, E., Adam, J., and Beatrice, F. The EndoTester': A virtual instrument endoscope evaluation system for fiberoptic endoscopes, *Biomedical Instrumentation and Technology*, 480–487, September/October 1998.
13. Surgical video systems, *Health Devices*, 24, 428–457, 1995.
14. Walker, B. *Optical Engineering Fundamentals*, McGraw-Hill, New York, 1995.
15. Wheeler, D.J. and Chambers, D.S. *Understanding Statistical Process Control*, 2nd ed., SPC Press, 1992.

Index

Living tissue electrical models (*Continued*)
   dielectric models, 10-4
   dispersions, 10-4 to 10-5
   frequency spectrum of tissue electrical model, 10-5
   impedance models, 10-4
   memristive systems and constant phase
      elements, 10-5
   Schwans multiple α, β, and γ dispersion
      model, 10-5 to 10-7
LLETZ, *see* Large loop excision of the transformation
      zone (LLETZ)
Load cell, 2-10; *see also* Pressure sensors
Load–velocity relationship, 30-10; *see also*
      Muscle strength
Local anesthetic agents, 19-3; *see also* Anesthesia
Local segment, 34-13
Lossless process, 21-6; *see also* Biomedical lasers
Low back pain (LBP), 37-2; *see also* Occupational
      medicine; Trunk
   evaluation, 37-11 to 37-13
   function-based systems, 37-5
   impairment evaluation, 37-5
   inverse and direct dynamics, 37-9 to 37-11
   isokinetic lift analysis, 37-10
   lifting strength testing, 37-8 to 37-9
   lumbar motion monitor, 37-12
   maximal and submaximal protocols, 37-5 to 37-6
   and postural sway, 37-13 to 37-16
   task and performance capacity comparison, 37-11
   trunk flexion and extension trajectories,
      37-14, 37-15
   and trunk performance, 37-5
   trunk sagittal movement profiles, 37-13
Low-frequency (LF), 10-3
Low risk, 57-8
Low vision and blindness, 41-1
   aging process, 41-5
   cataracts, 41-1, 41-3
   color blindness, 41-4
   diabetic retinopathy, 41-1, 41-2
   dyslexia, 41-4
   electronic vision systems, 41-5 to 41-6
   macular degeneration, 41-1, 41-2
   medical condition, 41-1
   retinitis pigmentosa, 41-4
   tunnel vision, 41-1, 41-3
LRMs, *see* Language representation methods (LRMs)
Lumbar motion monitor, 37-12; *see also* Low back
      pain (LBP)
LVDT, *see* Linear variable differential
      transformer (LVDT)

M

MAC, *see* Minimum alveolar concentration (MAC)
Macular degeneration, 41-1, 41-2; *see also* Low vision
      and blindness

MAE, *see* Mean absolute error (MAE)
Magnetic-based sensors, 3-1, 3-2; *see also* Magnetic
      induction-based sensors
Magnetic harmonic sensors, 3-6 to 3-7, 3-8; *see also*
      Magnetic induction-based sensors
Magnetic induction-based sensors, 3-1, 3-17; *see*
      also Inductive–capacitive resonant circuit
      sensors; Magnetoelasticity; Magnetoelastic
      resonant sensors; Radio frequency
      identification devices (RFID)
   ABICAP column, 3-5, 3-6
   BH curve, 3-7
   BH loop, 3-2
   binding of magnetic particles, 3-5
   electromotive force, 3-2
   Faraday's induction law, 3-1
   higher order harmonic fields, 3-7
   magnetically hard materials, 3-3
   magnetically soft materials, 3-2 to 3-3
   magnetic flux generation, 3-2
   magnetic harmonic sensors, 3-6 to 3-7, 3-8
   magnetic induction and magnetic materials, 3-2
      to 3-3
   magnetic markers, 3-4 to 3-6
   magnetic washing, 3-5
   VDT sensors, 3-3 to 3-4
Magnetoelasticity, 3-8, 3-17; *see also* Inductive–
      capacitive resonant circuit sensors;
      Magnetoelastic particles (MEPs)
Magnetoelastic particles (MEPs), 3-11
Magnetoelastic resonant sensors, 3-8, 3-9; *see also*
      Magnetoelasticity
   bacteria/virus and biotoxin detection, 3-11 to 3-12
   detection, 3-10 to 3-11
   magnetoelastic effect, 3-8
   magnetostriction, 3-8
   remote query, 3-9
   resonant frequency, 3-9
   response of, 3-10
   sandwich ELISA procedure, 3-12
   stress/strain sensors, 3-12 to 3-13
Magnetostriction, 3-8; *see also* Magnetoelasticity
Magnification, 46-2
Manchester encoding, 16-4
Mandatory mode, 18-3, 18-12; *see also* Mechanical
      ventilation
Mandatory standards, 55-5
Mandatory ventilation, 18-3 to 18-4; *see also*
      Mechanical ventilation
Mandatory volume-controlled inspiratory flow
      delivery, 18-8 to 18-10; *see also* Mechanical
      ventilation
MannequinPro, 38-10 to 38-11; *see also* Human
      performance engineering design and
      analysis tools
Manual muscle test (MMT), 30-11; *see also* Muscle
      strength

X

Z